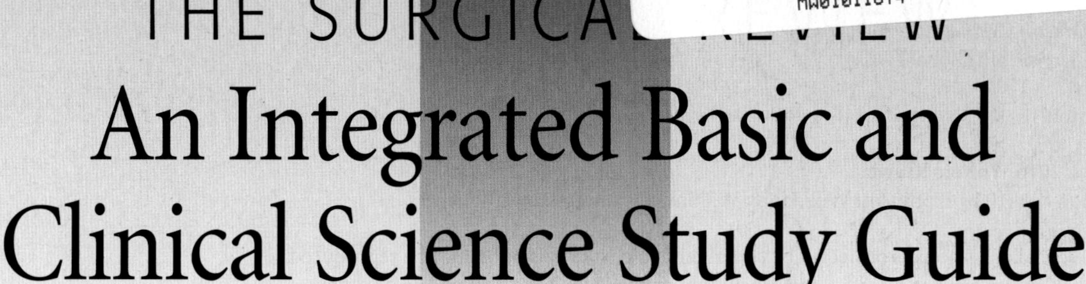

THE SURGICAL REVIEW

An Integrated Basic and Clinical Science Study Guide

FOURTH EDITION

PAIGE M. PORRETT, MD, PhD

Assistant Professor of Surgery
University of Pennsylvania
Philadelphia, Pennsylvania

PAVAN ATLURI, MD

Assistant Professor of Surgery
University of Pennsylvania
Philadelphia, Pennsylvania

GIORGOS C. KARAKOUSIS, MD

Assistant Professor of Surgery
University of Pennsylvania
Philadelphia, Pennsylvania

ROBERT E. ROSES, MD

Assistant Professor of Surgery
University of Pennsylvania
Philadelphia, Pennsylvania

Senior Editor

JEFFREY A. DREBIN, MD, PhD

Professor of Surgery
John Rhea Barton Chair of Surgery
University of Pennsylvania
Philadelphia, Pennsylvania

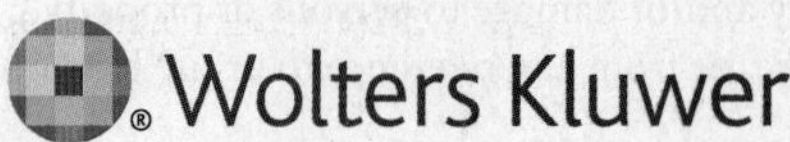

Philadelphia • Baltimore • New York • London
Buenos Aires • Hong Kong • Sydney • Tokyo

Acquisitions Editor: Keith Donnellan
Product Development Editor: Brendan Huffman
Production Project Manager: Joan Sinclair
Design Coordinator: Stephen Druding
Senior Manufacturing Coordinator: Beth Welsh
Strategic Marketing Manager: Daniel Dressler
Production Service: SPi Global

Fourth Edition

9 8 7 6 5 4 3 2 1

Printed in China

Library of Congress Cataloging-in-Publication Data
Surgical review (Kreisel)
The surgical review : an integrated basic and clinical science study guide / editors, Paige M. Porrett, Robert E. Roses, John R. Frederick, Larry R. Kasier. — Fourth edition.
p. ; cm.
Includes bibliographical references.
ISBN 978-1-4511-9332-9
I. Porrett, Paige M., editor. II. Roses, Robert E., editor. III. Frederick, John R., editor. IV. Kaiser, Larry R., editor. V. Title.
[DNLM: 1. General Surgery. 2. Surgical Procedures, Operative—methods. WO 100]
RD31
617—dc23

2015011460

This work is provided "as is," and the publisher disclaims any and all warranties, express or implied, including any warranties as to accuracy, comprehensiveness, or currency of the content of this work.

This work is no substitute for individual patient assessment based upon healthcare professionals' examination of each patient and consideration of, among other things, age, weight, gender, current or prior medical conditions, medication history, laboratory data and other factors unique to the patient. The publisher does not provide medical advice or guidance and this work is merely a reference tool. Healthcare professionals, and not the publisher, are solely responsible for the use of this work including all medical judgments and for any resulting diagnosis and treatments.

Given continuous, rapid advances in medical science and health information, independent professional verification of medical diagnoses, indications, appropriate pharmaceutical selections and dosages, and treatment options should be made and healthcare professionals should consult a variety of sources. When prescribing medication, healthcare professionals are advised to consult the product information sheet (the manufacturer's package insert) accompanying each drug to verify, among other things, conditions of use, warnings and side effects and identify any changes in dosage schedule or contradictions, particularly if the medication to be administered is new, infrequently used or has a narrow therapeutic range. To the maximum extent permitted under applicable law, no responsibility is assumed by the publisher for any injury and/or damage to persons or property, as a matter of products liability, negligence law or otherwise, or from any reference to or use by any person of this work.

LWW.com

RRS1507

CONTRIBUTORS

Cary B. Aarons, MD
Assistant Professor of Surgery at HUP and PPMC
Perelman School of Medicine
University of Pennsylvania
Philadelphia, Pennsylvania

Sean Antosh, MD
Resident in Anesthesiology and Critical Care
Department of General Anesthesia
Hospital of the University of Pennsylvania
Philadelphia, Pennsylvania

Pavan Atluri, MD
Assistant Professor of Surgery
Director, Cardiac Transplantation and Mechanical Circulatory Assist Program
Director, Minimally Invasive and Robotic Cardiac Surgery Program
Division of Cardiovascular Surgery
Department of Surgery
University of Pennsylvania
Philadelphia, Pennsylvania

David Aufhauser, MD
Resident in Surgery
Hospital of the University of Pennsylvania
Philadelphia, Pennsylvania

Edmund K. Bartlett, MD
Resident in Surgery
Hospital of the University of Pennsylvania
Philadelphia, Pennsylvania

Benjamin M. Braslow, MD
Associate Professor of Clinical Surgery
Perelman School of Medicine
University of Pennsylvania
Philadelphia, Pennsylvania

Ara A. Chalian, MD
Director, Division of Reconstructive and Facial Plastic Surgery
Professor of Head & Neck Cancer Surgery
Hospital of the University of Pennsylvania
Philadelphia, Pennsylvania

Sri Kiran Chennupati, MD
Assistant Professor of Pediatrics
Drexel University College of Medicine
Philadelphia, Pennsylvania

Christina S. Chu, MD
Associate Professor of Surgery (Surgical Oncology)
Division of Gynecologic Oncology
Fox Chase Cancer Center
Philadelphia, Pennsylvania

Jeffrey E. Cohen, MD
Resident in Surgery
Hospital of the University of Pennsylvania
Philadelphia, Pennsylvania

Brian J. Czerniecki, MD
Professor of Surgery
Perelman School of Medicine
University of Pennsylvania
Program Director PENN Breast Fellowship Program
Philadelphia, Pennsylvania

Jashodeep Datta, MD
Resident in Surgery
Hospital of the University of Pennsylvania
Philadelphia, Pennsylvania

Jeffrey A. Drebin, MD, PhD
Chairman, Department of Surgery
Hospital of the University of Pennsylvania
John Rhea Barton Professor
Perelman School of Medicine
William Maul Measey Professor of Surgical Research
Philadelphia, Pennsylvania

J. Raymond Fitzpatrick III, MD
Cardiovascular & Thoracic Surgical Associates
St. Luke's University Health Network
Bethlehem, Pennsylvania

Ian W. Folkert, MD
Resident in Surgery
Hospital of the University of Pennsylvania
Philadelphia, Pennsylvania

Douglas L. Fraker, MD
Vice Chairman for Research Department of Surgery
Jonathan E. Rhoads Professor of Surgical Science
Perelman School of Medicine
Philadelphia, Pennsylvania

Ann C. Gaffey, MD
Resident in Surgery
Hospital of the University of Pennsylvania
Philadelphia, Pennsylvania

Meera Gupta, MD
Resident in Surgery
Hospital of the University of Pennsylvania
Philadelphia, Pennsylvania

Thomas J. Guzzo, MD
Assistant Professor of Urology in Surgery at HUP
Perelman School of Medicine
University of Pennsylvania
Philadelphia, Pennsylvania

Rebecca L. Hoffman, MD
Resident in Surgery
Hospital of the University of Pennsylvania
Philadelphia, Pennsylvania

Daniel N. Holena, MD
Assistant Professor of Surgery
Perelman School of Medicine
University of Pennsylvania
Philadelphia, Pennsylvania

Matthew A. Hornick, MD
Resident in Surgery
Hospital of the University of Pennsylvania
Philadelphia, Pennsylvania

Eric D. Hudgins, MD, PhD
Instructor in Neurosurgery
The University of Pennsylvania
Philadelphia, Pennsylvania

Benjamin M. Jackson, MD
Assistant Professor of Surgery
Perelman School of Medicine
University of Pennsylvania
Philadelphia, Pennsylvania

Stephanie Jean, MD
Instructor in the Division of Gynecologic Oncology
Department of Obstetrics and Gynecology
Hospital of the University of Pennsylvania
Philadelphia, Pennsylvania

Arjun N. Jeganathan, MD
Resident in Surgery
Hospital of the University of Pennsylvania
Philadelphia, Pennsylvania

Suhail K. Kanchwala, MD
Assistant Professor of Surgery at HUP
Perelman School of Medicine
University of Pennsylvania
Philadelphia, Pennsylvania

Giorgos C. Karakousis, MD
Assistant Professor of Surgery
Perelman School of Medicine
Chair, Cancer Committee and Cancer Liaison Physician
Abramson Cancer Center Perelman School of Medicine
Philadelphia, Pennsylvania

Jane J. Keating, MD
Resident in Surgery
Hospital of the University of Pennsylvania
Philadelphia, Pennsylvania

Rachel R. Kelz, MD
Assistant Professor of Surgery
Perelman School of Medicine
Associate Program Director, General Surgery Residency Program
Department of Surgery
Perelman School of Medicine
University of Pennsylvania
Philadelphia, Pennsylvania

Patrick K. Kim, MD
Associate Professor of Surgery
Perelman School of Medicine
University of Pennsylvania
Philadelphia, Pennsylvania

John C. Kucharczuk, MD
Associate Professor of Surgery at HUP, PPMC, and PAH
Perelman School of Medicine
Chief, Division of Thoracic Surgery
University of Pennsylvania Health System
Philadelphia, Pennsylvania

Lindsay E. Kuo, MD
Resident in Surgery
Hospital of the University of Pennsylvania
Philadelphia, Pennsylvania

Meghan Lane-Fall, MD
Assistant Professor of Anesthesiology and Critical Care
Hospital of the University of Pennsylvania
Philadelphia, Pennsylvania

Kathreen P. Lee, MD
Resident in Surgery
Hospital of the University of Pennsylvania
Philadelphia, Pennsylvania

Matthew Levine, MD
Assistant Professor of Surgery
Perelman School of Medicine
University of Pennsylvania
Philadelphia, Pennsylvania

Lea Lowenfeld, MD
Resident in Surgery
Hospital of the University of Pennsylvania
Philadelphia, Pennsylvania

Niels D. Martin, MD
Co-Medical Director
Surgical Intensive Care Unit Hospital of the University of Pennsylvania
Philadelphia, Pennsylvania

Evelyn B. Marsh, MD
Instructor in Obstetrics, Gynecology and Reproductive Biology
Harvard Medical School
Boston, Massachusetts

Jeremy McGarvey, MD
Resident in Surgery
Hospital of the University of Pennsylvania
Philadelphia, Pennsylvania

Samir Mehta, MD
Assistant Professor of Orthopaedic Surgery
Chief, Division of Orthopaedic Trauma
Hospital of the University of Pennsylvania
Philadelphia, Pennsylvania

Jon B. Morris, MD
Vice Chair of Education
Department of Surgery
Associate Dean for Student Affairs
Professor of Surgery at HUP
Division of Gastrointestinal Surgery
Perelman School of Medicine
Medical Director of Admissions
Hospital of the University of Pennsylvania
Philadelphia, Pennsylvania

Douglas R. Murken, MD
Resident in Surgery
Hospital of the University of Pennsylvania
Philadelphia, Pennsylvania

Michael L. Nance, MD
Director, Pediatric Trauma Program
The Children's Hospital of Philadelphia
Philadelphia, Pennsylvania

Nikhil R. Nayak, MD
Resident in Department of Neurosurgery
Hospital of the University of Pennsylvania
Philadelphia, Pennsylvania

Elizabeth A. Nicolli, MD
Resident in Otorhinolaryngology
Head & Neck Surgery
Hospital of the University of Pennsylvania
Philadelphia, Pennsylvania

E. Carter Paulson, MD
Assistant Professor of SurgeryVeterans
Affairs Medical Center of Philadelphia
Philadelphia, Pennsylvania

Eugene J. Pietzak III, MD
Resident in Surgery
Hospital of the University of Pennsylvania
Philadelphia, Pennsylvania

Paige M. Porrett, MD, PhD
Assistant Professor of Surgery
University of Pennsylvania Medical School
Philadelphia, Pennsylvania

Steven E. Raper, MD
Associate Professor of Surgery
Perelman School of Medicine
Philadelphia, Pennsylvania

Andy S. Resnick, MD
Chief Quality Officer at Penn State
Assistant Professor of Surgery
Milton S. Hershey Medical Center
Assistant Professor of Surgery
Milton S. Hershey Medical Center
Hershey, Pennsylvania

Elijah W. Riddle, MD
Resident in Surgery
Hospital of the University of Pennsylvania
Philadelphia, Pennsylvania

Robert E. Roses, MD
Assistant Professor of Surgery at HUP
Perelman School of Medicine
University of Pennsylvania
Philadelphia, Pennsylvania

Fares Samra, MD
Resident in Surgery
Hospital of the University of Pennsylvania
Philadelphia, Pennsylvania

James M. Schuster, MD
Associate Professor of Neurosurgery
Associate Director, Neurocritical Care-Trauma
Hospital of the University of Pennsylvania
Associate Program Director
Neurosurgery Residency Program
Department of Neurosurgery
University of Pennsylvania
Philadelphia, Pennsylvania

Eric K. Shang, MD
Resident in Surgery
Hospital of the University of Pennsylvania
Philadelphia, Pennsylvania

Carrie A. Sims, MD
Associate Professor of Surgery at HUP
Perelman School of Medicine
University of Pennsylvania
Philadelphia, Pennsylvania

Sunil Singhal, MD
Assistant Professor of Surgery
Perelman School of Medicine
University of Pennsylvania School of Medicine
Assistant Professor of Medicine
Department of Medicine
Philadelphia, Pennsylvania

Andrew J. Sinnamon, MD
Resident in Surgery
Hospital of the University of Pennsylvania
Philadelphia, Pennsylvania

Danielle Spragan, MD
Resident in Surgery
Hospital of the University of Pennsylvania
Philadelphia, Pennsylvania

Matthew P. Sullivan, MD
Resident in Orthopaedic Surgery
Hospital of the University of Pennsylvania
Philadelphia, Pennsylvania

Ryan M. Taylor, MD
Resident in Orthopaedic Surgery
Hospital of the University of Pennsylvania
Philadelphia, Pennsylvania

Charles M. Vollmer Jr, MD
Associate Professor of Surgery
Perelman School of Medicine
University of Pennsylvania
Philadelphia, Pennsylvania

Jesse D. Vrecenak, MD
Resident in Surgery
Hospital of the University of Pennsylvania
Philadelphia, Pennsylvania

Heather Wachtel, MD
Resident in Surgery
Hospital of the University of Pennsylvania
Philadelphia, Pennsylvania

Grace Wang, MD
Assistant Professor of Surgery
Perelman School of Medicine
University of Pennsylvania
Philadelphia, Pennsylvania

Niamey P. Wilson, MD
UCONN Assistant Professor of Surgery
Co-Director, Breast Health Center
Saint Francis Hospital and Medical Center
Hartford, Connecticut

PREFACE

Welcome to the fourth edition of *The Surgical Review*. Once again, it has been our privilege and pleasure to bring updates in surgical practice to all practitioners of surgery. While the content and the authorship of many of the chapters has changed substantially, our primary objective has remained the same—to provide our readers with a comprehensive yet concise surgical text that can educate as well as assist in board review.

We would like to thank our partners at Wolters Kluwer for their continued support for this project as well as the many contributing authors (past and present) for their efforts in bringing this edition to life. Special thanks must also go to Ms. Tiffini Sykes and Ms. Aisha Clark for their expert assistance and administrative support. Finally, we remain deeply indebted to the original architects of *The Surgical Review*: Drs. Alexander Krupnick, Daniel Kreisel, and Larry Kaiser. We can only hope that this edition will carry on the great tradition that they started so many years ago.

Paige M. Porrett, MD, PhD
Pavan Atluri, MD
Giorgos C. Karakousis, MD
Robert E. Roses, MD

CONTENTS

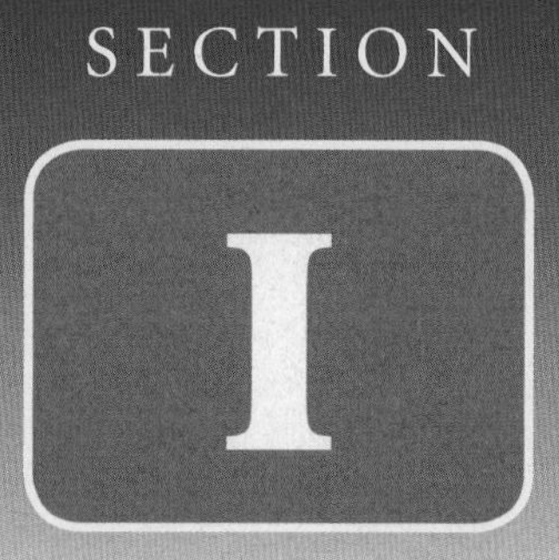

Body as a Whole

CHAPTER 1

Wound Healing

FARES SAMRA AND SUHAIL K. KANCHWALA

KEY POINTS

- Wound healing can occur by primary, secondary, or tertiary intention.
- Wound healing progresses through a well-coordinated process of three phases: inflammatory, proliferative, and maturation.
- Platelets are the first responders to a wound, causing hemostasis and secreting cytokines.
- The macrophage is the main cell of the inflammatory phase; the fibroblast is the main cell of the proliferative phase.
- The proliferative phase is composed of granulation tissue formation, neovascularization, fibroplasias, reepithelialization, and ECM production.
- Wound tensile strength reaches a peak of 80% of its uninjured counterpart by 3 months after wounding.
- A variety of systemic and local factors can contribute to the impairment of wound healing, all of which result in varying degrees of hypoxia, bacterial colonization, ischemia–reperfusion injury, altered cellular response to stress, and defects in collagen production.
- Controlling bacterial contamination, maintaining the proper amount of moisture, treating edema, and preventing further injury are the mainstays of local wound care.
- Keloids and hypertrophic scars are both examples of an exuberant fibrotic response.
- The reconstructive ladder provides a guide on how to manage progressively complicated wounds.

INTRODUCTION

Our understanding of wound healing is constantly evolving. It has long been described that the normal postnatal response to dermal injury is a well-coordinated process involving many different cell types that progress through the three phases of wound healing: inflammatory, proliferative, and maturation. With continued investigation, the underlying biology of each phase continues to be further elucidated and our understanding of additional inflammatory mediators and cellular interactions grows. Nonetheless, wound healing impairment continues to occur due to both local and systemic factors, such as diabetes mellitus, peripheral vascular disease (PVD), immunosuppression, and immobility. These conditions lead to either a defect in the wound repair mechanism or repeated wound injury and clinically manifest as chronic nonhealing wounds. Conversely, hypertrophic scars and keloid formation are examples of an exuberant fibrotic response that leads to excessive scarring. This chapter will review the biology for a thorough understanding of the wound healing process, as well as outline some of the local and systemic factors that impair wound healing. Noninvasive therapies and wound healing adjuncts are discussed, as well as plastic surgical techniques employed to prevent wound breakdown or manage the chronic wound.

BASICS OF WOUND HEALING

Categories

Wound closure has classically been divided into three basic categories: primary intention, secondary intention, and tertiary intention. Healing by primary intention is achieved when wound edges are reapproximated within hours of initial injury. For primary intention to be successful, a wound should be relatively acute and clean. Wounds that are contaminated or have been open for a prolonged period of time should not be closed primarily due to increased risk of infection. These wounds are often managed by secondary intention, which occurs when a wound is left open and allowed to close by granulation tissue formation, wound contracture, and reepithelialization. The final category of wound healing is tertiary intention, which is also known as delayed primary closure. Tertiary intention occurs when a wound is left open and treated with local wound care as a temporizing measure. Then, when it appears clean, absent of infection, and suitable for closure, the wound is closed surgically. This can accelerate healing and reduce scar formation when performed in a minimally contaminated wound. The different categories of wound healing, along with clinical examples of each, are outlined in Figure 1.1.

Phases

Normal wound healing progresses through three distinct phases (Fig. 1.2). The *inflammatory phase* begins early with platelet aggregation and hemostasis. It continues with the production of cytokines and growth factors and the recruitment of inflammatory cells, such as neutrophils, macrophages, and lymphocytes, to the wound. As the inflammation subsides, the *proliferative phase*, which consists of granulation tissue formation, neovascularization, fibroplasia, reepithelialization, and extracellular matrix (ECM) production, becomes prominent. The major cell type in the proliferative phase is the fibroblast. The *maturation phase* is characterized by wound contraction and remodeling of the ECM, including collagen cross-linking.

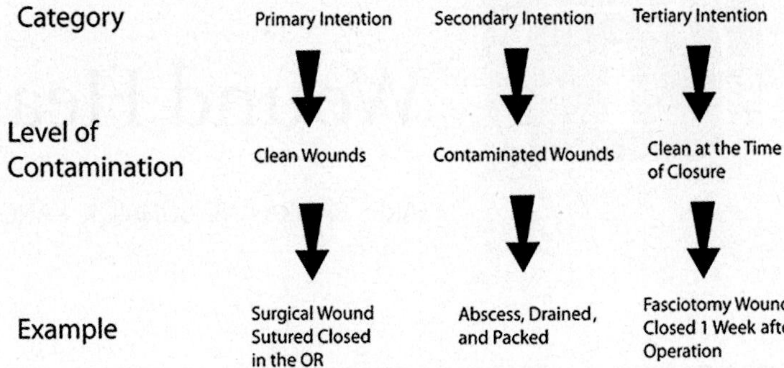

FIGURE 1.1 Categories of wound healing. Wound healing can progress through primary, secondary, or tertiary intention. The most important factor in determining whether to close a wound is the level of contamination.

Inflammation

The inflammatory phase begins immediately after creation of a wound. The first step in this phase is hemostasis. Circulating platelets, which are derived from megakaryocytes in the bone marrow, are activated by subendothelial collagen and basement membrane proteins. The von Willebrand factor (vWF) mediates initial platelet adherence by binding both platelet cell surface receptors and subendothelial collagen. Platelets are also bound by molecules such as glycoprotein IIb/IIIa, which is responsible for binding fibrinogen and mediating aggregation of platelets at the wound site. Platelet cross-linking by fibrin forms the platelet plug that results in hemostasis and creates the provisional matrix for the ensuing cellular response. Of note, another potent stimulator of platelet aggregation is thromboxane A2, the eicosanoid inhibited by aspirin therapy.

Activated platelets at the site of a fresh wound also secrete biologically active molecules that affect wound healing. Platelets have two kinds of granules, known as alpha granules and dense granules, which are synthesized and packaged by the megakaryocyte. Alpha granules contain growth factors, cytokines, ECM proteins, and clotting factors. These include platelet-derived growth factor (PDGF), transforming growth factor-β (TGF-β), platelet factor-4, thrombospondin, fibronectin, fibrinogen, and vWF. Dense granules contain vasoactive substances, such as epinephrine, serotonin, adenosine diphosphate, calcium, and histamine. Initially, release of the dense granules leads to vasoconstriction, which helps to control hemorrhage. Later, these granules promote vasodilation and increase capillary permeability, thus promoting the recruitment of inflammatory cells to the wound. Release of PDGF and TGF-β from alpha granules is an important first step in initiating the cellular response.

Once hemostasis is achieved, vasodilation and increased capillary permeability cause infiltration of inflammatory cells to the wound site. Neutrophils, monocytes, fibroblasts, and endothelial cells deposit on the fibrin scaffold formed by platelet activation. Once in the wound, neutrophils are responsible for phagocytosis of microbes and debris. After 48 hours, the wound is relatively decontaminated and the number of neutrophils in the wound declines. If the wound is not successfully decontaminated, chemotaxis of neutrophils to the wound will continue, resulting in persistent inflammation and delayed healing. It is important to note that although they are the first to arrive and play a significant role in the wound healing process, neutrophils are not the most important cells in the healing process. In fact, the absence of neutrophils was not shown to affect wound healing in uninfected wounds. Moreover, as stated above, the persistence of neutrophils may be responsible for the release of free oxygen radicals and other cytokines that contribute to chronic wounds. Macrophages, on the other hand, are vital to wound healing. Along with neutrophils, macrophages are responsible for decontaminating the wound of microbes and devitalized tissue via phagocytosis. They also degrade ECM components and

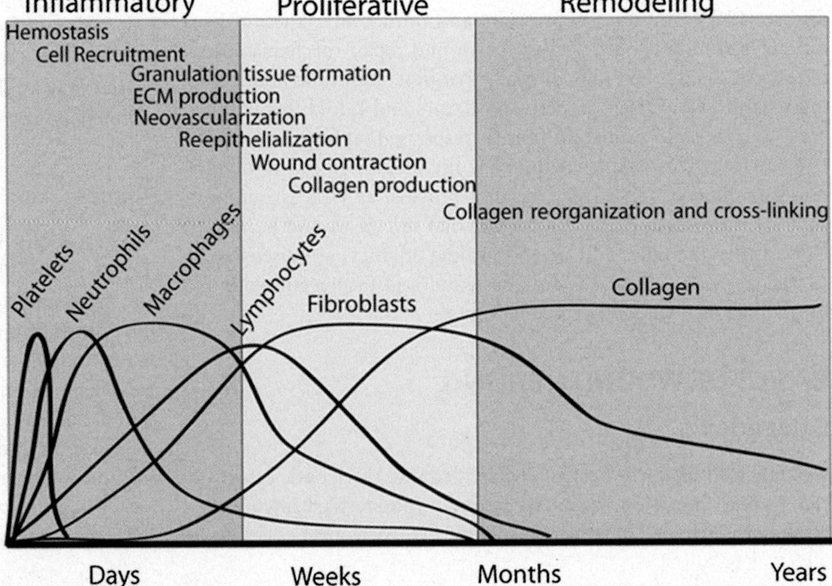

FIGURE 1.2 Phases of wound healing. Wound healing progresses through inflammatory, proliferative, and remodeling phases. Cells are recruited to the wound and proliferate in an organized sequence that results in hemostasis, granulation tissue formation, ECM production, neovascularization, reepithelialization, wound contraction, collagen production, and collagen reorganization and cross-linking. The end result is scar formation and wound closure. ECM, extracellular matrix.

secrete cytokines and growth factors that coordinate the cellular response, driving recruitment of additional cells to the wound, apoptosis of neutrophils, and stimulation of fibroblast proliferation. In fact, macrophages are known to be the source of more than 30 different growth factors and cytokines important to the wound healing process. Lymphocytes also play a small but poorly understood role in the inflammatory phase. They appear in small numbers and secrete cytokines that have effects on other cells in the wound, including macrophages and fibroblasts. It is thought that they likely play a role in mediating the inflammatory response in chronic wounds.

Proliferation

As the inflammatory phase comes to a close, wound healing shifts toward the proliferative phase and the processes of granulation tissue formation, neovascularization, reepithelialization, and ECM production. Fibroblast migration, in response to cytokines produced by platelets and macrophages during the inflammatory phase, ushers in this next chapter of the wound healing process. PDGF and TGF-β are two of the most important cytokines driving fibroblast chemotaxis and activation, but there are several other cytokines that play an important role in the inflammation phase as well, and these are outlined in Table 1.1.

The initiation of neovascularization can be divided into the separate processes of angiogenesis and vasculogenesis. Angiogenesis results in the formation of new blood vessels from existing blood vessels, while vasculogenesis is the *de novo* formation of new blood vessels from bone marrow–derived progenitor cells known as endothelial progenitor cells (EPCs). Angiogenesis occurs in response to a number of cytokines and growth factors, including PDGF, fibroblast growth factor (FGF), epidermal growth factor (EGF), Insulin-like growth factor I (IGF-I), and vascular endothelial growth factor (VEGF). The process proceeds with endothelial cells in the wound releasing several proteases including matrix metalloproteinases (MMP), resulting in degradation of the surrounding ECM. This allows for endothelial cells to migrate and form immature blood vessels that later mature into functional capillaries. Vasculogenesis first requires the homing of EPCs to the site of the wound. Stromal-derived factor-1α (SDF-1α) and other chemokines control the recruitment of EPCs to the wound. EPCs are multipotent and have the ability to differentiate into the various cell types that combine to form blood vessels. Once in the wound, EPCs secrete cytokines and growth factors affecting other cells in a paracrine fashion. EPC differentiation is likely mediated by many of the same cytokines that control angiogenesis; however, the exact mechanism is still under investigation. Neovascularization and ECM production results in the formation of granulation tissue in the wound bed. Clinically, granulation tissue can be identified as a clean, highly vascular, beefy red wound base.

The epithelium is an important part of the body's barrier defense system, and wounding creates a defect in this defense. The process of reepithelialization is initiated very early in the wound healing process. Clot provides a temporary barrier between the wound bed and the outside environment while keratinocytes migrate across the epithelial gap and proliferate in response to cytokines and interactions with the ECM. The granulation tissue provides a tissue scaffold for the migrating keratinocytes to follow; however, reepithelialization can occur without significant granulation tissue formation. Keratinocyte differentiation follows the migrating edge until the wound is covered with a layer of normal epithelium. Generally, a larger wound will take longer to reepithelialize than a

TABLE 1.1 Summary of notable inflammatory cytokines

Cytokine	Cells of origin	Role in inflammatory response	Clinical application
EGF	Platelets, macrophages, fibroblasts	Angiogenesis, re-epithelialization	Decreased in chronic wounds
FGF	Macrophages, mast cells, T lymphocytes	Fibroblast recruitment	Decreased in chronic wounds
IFNα	Monocytes, macrophages	Decreases collagen production	Used to treat hypertrophic keloid scars
PDGF	Platelets, macrophages, fibroblasts	Fibroblast recruitment, myofibroblast stimulation	Recombinant form used to treat diabetic ulcers
TNFα	Macrophages, T lymphocytes, keratinocytes	Leukocyte chemoattraction	Elevated levels linked to deficient healing
TGFβ	Platelets, fibroblasts, macrophages	Reepithelialization, wound fibroplasia	Elevated in hypertrophic and keloid scars
IL-I	Keratinocutes, neutrophils, macrophages	Leukocyte chemoattraction, wound fibroplasis	Increased in chronic wounds
IL-8	Macrophages, endothelial cells	Reepithelialization, angiogensis	Increased levels in delayed-healing wounds
IL-10	Monocytes, Lymphocytes	Down-regulation of other cytokines, limits fibroblast proliferation	Necessary for scarless fetal wound healing

EGF, epidermal growth factor; FGF, fibroblast growth factor; IFNα, interferon alpha; PDGF, platelet-derived growth factor; TNFα, tumor necrosis factor-alpha; TGFβ; transforming growth factor-beta; IL, interleukin.

Derived from Henry G, Garner W. Inflammatory mediators in wound healing. *Surg Clin North Am.* 2003;83:483–507; and Barrientos S, Stojadinivic O, Golinko MS, et al. Growth factors and cytokines in wound healing. *Wound Repair Regen.* 2008;16:585–601.

From Janis JE, Harrison B. Wound healing: part I. Basic science. *Plast Reconstr Surg.* 2014;133:2, with permission.

smaller wound. Incisional wounds closed primarily will reepithelialize within 24 hours.

While granulation tissue formation, neovascularization, and reepithelialization are all important components of wound healing, it is the production of collagen that gives the wound its strength. As these other processes are occurring, fibroblasts are being activated and proliferating within the granulation tissue. The ECM is degraded at the same time as collagen production is occurring, so there is an increase in the wound strength over time. Once the collagen fibers are deposited, the wound begins to mature with remodeling and cross-linking, processes that continue to improve the wound strength.

Collagen is the most abundant structural protein in the human body, comprising a major portion of skin, tendon, cartilage, bone, blood vessels, and cornea. There are many types of collagen, but the most common in humans are types I, II, III, IV, and V. Type I collagen is the major type in adult skin with type III comprising a smaller fraction of the total collagen. Collagen is made primarily by fibroblasts and composed of three polypeptide chains wound together to form a triple helix. Hydroxylation of proline and lysine amino acids by prolyl hydrolase and lysyl hydrolase leads to intermolecular hydrogen bonds, which give collagen its strength and stability. These hydroxylation reactions require vitamin C and oxygen to proceed. This explains one mechanism by which vitamin C deficiency and hypoxia cause impaired wound healing. A triple-helix collagen molecule is secreted as procollagen by the fibroblast into the ECM, where it is cleaved by proteases to form tropocollagen. Tropocollagen is cross-linked with other tropocollagen molecules to form fibrils, and then fibrils assemble to form fibers.

As the processes of fibroplasia, neovascularization, reepithelialization, and ECM production are occurring, the wound also begins to contract. Wound contraction is primarily driven by myofibroblasts and fibroblasts. Activated fibroblasts can differentiate into myofibroblasts, which express α-smooth muscle actin and have similarities with smooth muscle cells. Wound contraction occurs as a result of interactions between the cells and the ECM in and around the wound. It not only lessens the time to wound closure but also reduces the final size of the scar.

Maturation and Remodeling

Once closed, the wound begins the remodeling process to achieve maximum strength as it matures. Wound strength increases quickly over the first 6 to 8 weeks and then continues to slowly gain strength and can change in appearance over the next year. This is a result of the reorganization of the collagen within the wound and an increase in cross-linking. The early collagen formed during the wound healing process is very disorganized. MMPs break down the disorganized collagen, and new collagen is produced and oriented in line with the tensile forces present. The net amount of collagen in the wound stays roughly even, but the turnover leads to greater organization, which improves the biomechanical properties of the scar as the wound matures. Of note, breaking strength of the wound is only 3% at 1 week, but this increases to 20% after 3 weeks and reaches its peak of 80% of its uninjured counterpart by 3 months after wounding.

As described, normal wound healing progresses through a defined series of events that include an inflammatory phase, a proliferative phase, and a remodeling phase. When one of these phases is prolonged or altered, wound healing can be either impaired or exuberant. Both of these are pathologic conditions.

IMPAIRED WOUND HEALING

There are many different factors that can alter the course of normal wound healing. Many systemic conditions, such as diabetes mellitus, PVD, smoking, malnutrition, immunosuppression, and age, affect the wound healing process as a part of their greater effect on the patient. Other local factors, such as pressure-induced ischemia, infection, and radiation, can also potentiate chronic wounds. Ultimately, hypoxia, bacterial colonization, ischemia–reperfusion injury, altered cellular response to stress, and defects in collagen production are the primary mechanisms of wound healing impairment present to varying degrees in all of these conditions. The aim of treatment is to correct these defects and thus restore the wound healing process to normal.

Systemic Factors

Diabetes mellitus is a chronic condition affecting greater than 20 million Americans. The impairment in wound healing seen with diabetes is multifactorial in nature. Hyperglycemia causes a modification of many of the proteins and enzymes involved in healing, resulting in their dysfunction. Diabetic wounds have also been shown to be deficient in growth factor production, including PDGF, KGF, TGF-β, HGF, and VEGF. Furthermore, these wounds have an abnormal cellular response to growth factors, including decreased cell recruitment, angiogenesis, reepithelialization, ECM production, and wound contracture. The effects of hyperglycemia are also seen at the level of the basement membrane, resulting in dysfunctional permeability of cells as well as accessibility of nutrients to the wound bed. There is therefore an altered inflammatory response, impaired leukocyte function, and greater susceptibility to soft tissue infection—an additional cause of inhibited wound repair. As diabetes results in microvascular and macrovascular disease, these wounds are subject to both limited blood flow and insufficient oxygen delivery. The tissue hypoxia in diabetes also prevents normal reduction–oxidation reactions in wound healing as well as appropriate hydroxylation of collagen, resulting in diminished tensile strength of the wound. Although large vessel ischemia can often be treated with endovascular or open procedures, small vessel disease and tissue hypoxia often still remain. In addition to the systemic ischemic impairment of the wound healing processes, diabetic neuropathy increases the likelihood of repeated pressure-induced ischemic injury of wounds. Repeated injury not only increases the wound size due to mechanical disruption but it can also cause repeated ischemia–reperfusion injury and inflammation. Since diabetic wound healing impairment is multifactorial in nature, the treatment of diabetic wounds requires therapies to correct multiple defects in the wound healing process.

PVD, secondary to the ischemia and hypoxia it causes, is another systemic illness that causes chronic wounds. Hyperlipidemia, hypertension, diabetes, smoking, male sex, old age, and family history are all risk factors for PVD. When the partial pressure of oxygen in tissues drops below 30 mm Hg, healing is impaired. Hypoxia impairs the normal cellular function of neutrophils and fibroblasts, resulting in an increased risk of infection and inhibited intermolecular cross-linking of collagen molecules. Ischemic wounds occur most commonly on the distal portion of the lower extremities, and therefore chronic wounds of the lower extremities should include assessment of pulses, ankle–brachial index, and segmental pressures to assess for the presence and degree of PVD.

Smoking is especially harmful to wound healing as it not only is a risk factor for PVD but also causes hypoxia through increased carbon monoxide levels in the blood, reduction of blood flow velocity through vasoconstriction, increased platelet adhesiveness causing thrombosis, and inhibition of erythrocyte, macrophage, and fibroblast proliferation. Cessation of smoking is beneficial to wound healing but can be difficult to achieve due to the highly addictive nature of cigarettes. Although there is no consensus on duration of abstinence, it has been recommended to have patients attempt to at least abstain from smoking for 4 weeks prior to and following surgery. Nicotine replacement has often been used to help patients with cravings during these periods of abstinence, but the effect of nicotine supplementation on wound healing has not been clearly established. In addition to smoking cessation, treatment of ischemic wounds should follow basic wound care principles of limiting bacterial contamination, preventing prolonged pressure on the wound, and avoiding repeated injury. If a chronic wound will not heal in the face of adequate wound care, revascularization may help to improve local tissue oxygenation and allow for wound healing.

Chronic venous disease, another form of PVD, can also lead to persistent nonhealing wounds. Venous hypertension can result from incompetent venous valves in the lower extremities, chronic deep venous thrombosis, or vascular trauma. It causes extremity edema, vascular congestion, and local tissue hypoxia. Chronic lower extremity edema is accompanied by extravasation of fluid and protein, including fibrinogen, into the ECM. Increased ECM fluid and the formation of fibrin sleeves around capillaries prevent the normal diffusion of oxygen and nutrients between the ECM and the capillaries and disrupt the normal mechanisms of wound healing. Treatment of chronic wounds in the face of venous disease requires compression therapy, which aims to promote healing by limiting the edema. Pressure therapy in conjunction with aggressive local wound care is the standard treatment of these wounds.

Patient nutrition, typically measured by albumin and prealbumin, is of paramount importance in wound healing. Surgery and trauma are both known to increase metabolic demand, and underlying nutritional deficiencies can play a significant inhibitory role in the healing process. Protein malnutrition is particularly important to assess and correct in the wounded patient, as it has been associated with increased wound dehiscence and compromised wound healing. In addition, specific vitamin or elemental deficiencies can also lead to wound healing impairment. Scurvy is the condition caused by vitamin C deficiency. Posttranslational hydroxylation of proline and lysine residues, which gives collagen its tensile strength, is dependent on vitamin C as a cosubstrate. Scurvy manifests as fragile vessels, bleeding mucous membranes, loss of teeth, and nonhealing wounds. Minerals such as zinc and magnesium are important in enzymatic reactions that take place during wound healing. Zinc plays a role in RNA and DNA polymerase, and its deficiency diminishes wound strength and epithelialization. It is often used in the treatment of venous stasis ulcers as a part of Unna boots. Magnesium also acts as a cofactor in protein and collagen synthesis and is found in some topical wound healing applications. The treatment of nutritional deficiencies attempts to replace the deficient component. Nutritional supplementation above and beyond the required amount, however, will not further improve wound healing in a well-nourished patient.

It is well established that immunosuppression has a negative impact on wound healing. In particular, immunosuppressive drugs have a deleterious effect on the inflammatory phase. Steroids interfere with prostaglandin synthesis, leukocyte migration, cytokine production, fibroblast proliferation, and collagen synthesis. Vitamin A has also been shown to play a role in wound repair and is often used for supplementation in patients on steroids. Although it does not reverse the effects of steroids, it does promote epithelialization and collagen synthesis. Vitamin A is given orally in doses of 25,000 IU/day preoperatively and for 4 days postoperatively.

Advanced age is another factor that affects normal wound healing. The elderly heal more slowly and with less scarring. Age has been shown to decrease collagen synthesis, growth factor production, angiogenesis, and reepithelialization. Laboratory studies have also demonstrated a decreased proliferative potential for aged fibroblasts and epithelial cells. Although this can lead to finer scars and an improved cosmetic result, it also implicates a delay in restoration of tensile strength. Furthermore, older patients are more likely to have comorbidities leading to wound healing impairment, such as diabetes, malnutrition, or PVD. As such, it is paramount to medically optimize elder patients as well as allow a greater amount of time for restoration of tensile strength while managing their wounds.

Local Factors

Patients with partial or complete immobility often suffer with chronic pressure-induced wounds. Paralysis, stroke, dementia, advanced age, and chronic illness are just a few of the conditions that can lead to patients being confined to a bed or wheelchair and place them at risk for pressure ulcer development. Pressure sore pathophysiology involves cyclical prolonged pressure over a bony prominence followed by destructive tissue reperfusion injury. The most frequent locations for pressure-induced wounds include the sacrum, trochanter, and ischium, although it is not uncommon to develop pressure wounds over the heel, ankle, knee, or posterior scalp. Once a pressure ulcer has formed, relieving pressure on the wound with specially designed mattresses and frequent repositioning is essential for healing. Surgical flap closure of pressure ulcers is often contraindicated because the same factors that lead to pressure ulcer development will prevent healing of a surgical flap. Contained infection or necrotic tissue in the wound should be treated aggressively with drainage or debridement. Finally, it is important to maximize nutrition to facilitate healing in patients who have developed pressure ulcers since these patients often are malnourished.

Chronic infection can be seen in many different clinical situations and can prevent normal healing irrespective of etiology. Bacterial contamination can trap a wound in the inflammatory phase and prevent healing. All open wounds become colonized with bacteria; however, bacterial counts greater than 10^5 bacteria/mm^3 can stimulate the patient's immune response. Increased inflammatory cell recruitment to the wound will change the cytokine milieu, augment the release of proteases, and affect the cellular response of other cells in the wound such as fibroblasts. Wounds with uncontrolled infection require measures to decrease the bacterial burden. Sharp debridement of necrotic tissue, drainage of purulence, antibiotics, and frequent dressing changes can all help rid the wound of infection and promote normal healing when used appropriately.

Ionizing radiation plays a well-established role in the management of various malignancies, including breast, prostate, skin, rectal, brain, and some lung cancers. Radiation has subsequently become a common cause of wound healing morbidity in surgical patients. Radiation damages DNA and creates free radicals that damage proteins and cell membranes causing microvascular damage, fibrosis, and atrophy. Furthermore, fibroblast migration, proliferation, and contraction are all impaired in the radiated wound. The sum of these effects results in a wound with slower epithelialization, decreased tensile strength, and higher infection and dehiscence rates. The most effective treatment is prevention, by limiting the extent of radiation damage in the first place.

HYPERTROPHIC SCARS AND KELOIDS

Hypertrophic scarring and keloid formation both result from an exuberant wound healing response leading to excessive ECM production and disfiguring scar formation. Hypertrophic scars remain within the boundary of the original injury, regress spontaneously, and rarely recur after surgical excision. Keloids, in contrast, extend beyond the boundaries of the original injury, continue to grow over time, commonly recur after excision, and are present for a minimum of 1 year. Histologically, keloids can be distinguished from hypertrophic scars by the presence of large collagen bundles. Keloids also tend to occur in periods of physiologic growth, and most commonly form in patients between the ages of 10 and 30 years. Both hypertrophic scars and keloids can occur in people of all races; however, they are more commonly found in dark-skinned patients. Keloids in particular affect 15 times as many patients with darkly pigmented skin as compared to those with lighter skin. Keloids are also known to have a familial predisposition.

The pathophysiology of keloid formation involves ongoing inflammation and excessive accumulation of ECM. This is primarily driven by dysfunctional fibroblasts, which produce high levels of collagen, elastin, fibronectin, and proteoglycan and show abnormal responses to cell signaling. The dysfunctional signaling pathways is demonstrated by an increased production of multiple cytokines, including TGF-β, IGF-1, PDGF, interleukins, and VEGF. In contrast, hypertrophic scar fibroblasts have an increased rate of collagen production, but they respond appropriately to growth factors.

The best treatment for keloids is prevention, that is, avoidance of incisions in patients known to form keloids whenever possible. Multiple treatments have been tried, including silicone sheeting, pressure therapy, radiotherapy, steroid injections, verapamil injections, and 5-fluorouracil injections. The absence of a single therapy speaks to the difficulty of treating keloids.

WOUND MANAGEMENT

The majority of wounds can be treated by diligently utilizing basic wound care methods aimed at controlling bacterial contamination, maintaining the proper amount of moisture in the wound, treating edema, and preventing further injury. Furthermore, it is essential to assess the most appropriate surgical approach for each wound. Janis' 2011 work on the new reconstructive ladder provides a good guide on how to surgically manage progressively complicated wounds (Fig. 1.3). Several of these principles are outlined in this chapter. Providers should have a low threshold for involving plastic surgeons in the management of more complex wounds requiring greater levels of sophistication for appropriate treatment and closure.

Bacterial contamination can usually be controlled by debridement of any necrotic or grossly infected tissue, drainage of purulence, and frequent dressing changes. If untreated, the presence of infection keeps the wound in a state of inflammation and prevents progression into the later stages of wound healing. Debridement effectively removes inflamed tissue and converts the wound from a chronic one to an acute one. All wounds produce fluid and exudates to some degree. Frequent dressing changes help to control the wound exudate, which can act as a culture medium for bacterial growth. Classic wet-to-dry gauze dressing changes also cause some mild debridement of dead tissue when the packing is removed. This type of dressing contrasts with a wet-to-wet dressing, which promotes wound healing instead of debridement. Sometimes wounds produce a large amount of fibrinous exudate that collects on the wound surface. This should be debrided either mechanically or enzymatically, as it can act as a biofilm harboring bacteria. There are several commercially available products that enzymatically remove exudates that collect in the wound bed. Finally, there is also the option of using antibiotics either topically or systemically to control infection. If the wound is associated with surrounding cellulitis, treatment with systemic antibiotics should be instituted. Antibiotics should be used selectively, as inappropriate use can lead to resistant organisms and complications such as pseudomembranous colitis.

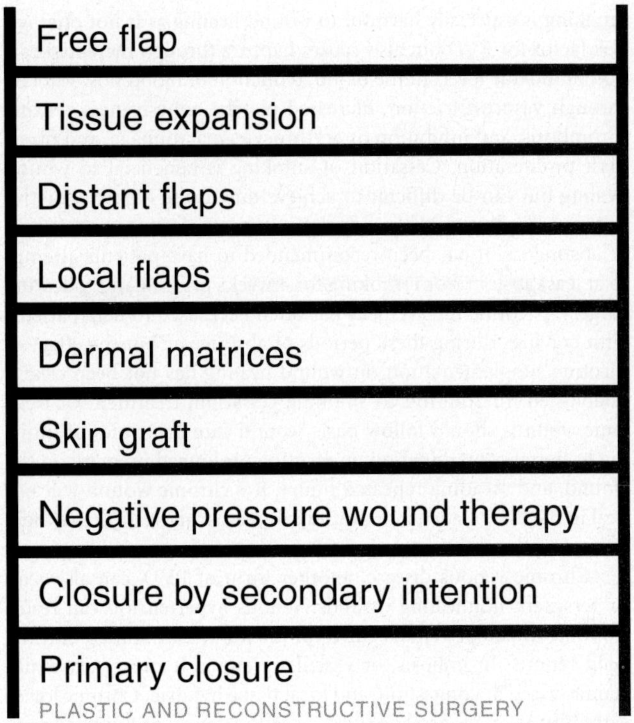

Controlling the level of moisture in the wound is important not only to limit bacterial growth but also to promote healing and prevent skin breakdown. Studies have demonstrated that wound moisture promotes reepithelialization. Therefore, if a wound has a clean base, a dressing that retains moisture is the best choice to promote wound healing. However, in cases of infected wounds, or those that produce a large amount of exudate, an absorptive dressing is needed to prevent further excess moisture from leading to maceration of the skin at the wound edges.

FIGURE 1.3 New reconstructive ladder demonstrating progressive sophistication required for surgical closure. From Janis JE, Kwon RK, Attinger CE. The new reconstructive ladder: modifications to the traditional model. *Plast Reconstr Surg.* 2011;127:1S, with permission.

Negative pressure wound therapy has gained great popularity in the treatment of chronic wounds. It has many potential benefits, including controlling exudates, promoting granulation tissue formation, improving blood supply to the wound, decreasing bacterial burden, maintaining moisture, lessening edema, and protecting the wound from trauma. Suspected mechanisms include exertion of tensile forces on the local tissue environment, resulting in cellular deformation, which causes increased mitotic activity and cellular proliferation. Exudate removal also promotes an appropriately moist environment while removing excess fluid, which could otherwise provide a platform for bacterial growth or a reservoir of inflammatory cytokines and MMP. Negative pressure wound therapy is not recommended in the setting of exposed vessels, malignancy, necrotic tissue, untreated osteomyelitis, or nonenteric and unexplored fistulas. These dressings should also be used with caution on abdominal wounds with defects in the fascia, as bowel fistula formation is a theoretical complication. Similarly, caution should be exercised in patients who are anticoagulated or those with active bleeding or grossly infected wounds.

Hyperbaric oxygen therapy has gained popularity in an effort to combat the problem of hypoxia in chronic wounds. By increasing the atmospheric pressure and delivering 100% inspired oxygen, the partial pressure of oxygen in the wound can be increased. This can promote angiogenesis, fibroblast proliferation, leukocyte oxidative killing, and toxin inhibition. Clinically it has shown to be of benefit in the treatment of chronic wounds, especially those associated with diabetes. It does not replace traditional wound care but rather is an adjunctive therapy that may provide benefit in the treatment of impaired wounds.

There are several relatively new wound care options that have been taken from the bench to the bedside and shown significant promise. Currently, PDGF (i.e., becaplermin topical gel [Regranex]) is the lone FDA-approved topical growth factor used in the treatment of chronic wounds when applied once daily to the wound. While it has shown some efficacy, good basic wound care is still required. Furthermore, topical growth factor therapy does have its limitations. There are many growth factors involved in normal wound healing, all of which require the proper concentration delivered to the right place at the right time. While topically delivered single growth factor therapy can replace deficient growth factors, it does not address the issues of timing, concentration, or the complex milieu of biologically active molecules in the wound healing process. Gene therapy is an active area of research aimed at delivering deficient growth factors to wounds. The half-life of topically applied growth factors is likely short, and gene therapy offers the opportunity to have constant production at the desired site. The safety of gene therapy has not been fully evaluated and is still in experimental stages.

CONCLUSIONS

Wound healing requires a complex coordinated series of events involving multiple cell types for the progression from an acute wound to a well-healed scar. The normal healing process advances through inflammatory, proliferative, and remodeling phases. Failure to progress through this sequence normally leads to a pathologic spectrum ranging from chronic nonhealing wounds to deforming keloids. Identifying the reason why a wound fails to progress through the normal phases of healing may allow for correction of the specific pathology. In cases of wound healing impairment, hypoxia, bacterial colonization, ischemia–reperfusion injury, altered cellular response to stress, and defects in collagen production are the primary mechanisms present to varying degrees. Local wound care, providing adequate oxygenation and perfusion of tissues, treatment of nutritional deficiencies, and minimization of pressure on chronic wounds are all examples of modifying treatment to fit the specific etiology of wound healing impairment. Conversely, keloid management is focused on prevention in susceptible patients, as other treatment modalities have failed to prove highly successful. New therapies such as growth factor therapy, hyperbaric oxygen, and negative pressure wound therapy have helped in the treatment of chronic wounds, and emerging therapies such as gene therapy are actively being developed. The complex biology behind chronic wounds and the comorbidities inherent in patients with these wounds will continue to make chronic wounds a significant health care problem for many patients. Diligence in utilizing established methods and continued research to develop new treatment strategies provide hope to minimize the effects of this problem.

ACKNOWLEDGMENTS

The authors would like to acknowledge the contributions of Benjamin J. Herdrich and Kenneth W. Liechty to previous editions of this chapter.

Suggested Readings

Broughton G II, Janis JE, Attinger CE. Wound healing: an overview. *Plast Reconstr Surg.* 2006;117:7S.

Galiano RD, Mustoe TA. Wound healing. In: Mullholland MW, Lillemoe KD, Doherty GM, et al., eds. *Greenfield's Surgery: Scientific Principles and Practice.* 5th ed. Philadelphia: Lippincott Williams & Wilkins; 2011.

Janis JE, Harrison B. Wound healing: part I. Basic science. *Plast Reconstr Surg.* 2014;133:2.

Janis JE, Harrison B. Wound healing: part II. Clinical applications. *Plast Reconstr Surg.* 2014;133:3.

Janis JE, Kwon RK, Attinger CE. The new reconstructive ladder: modifications to the traditional model. *Plast Reconstr Surg.* 2011;127:1S.

CHAPTER

2 Hemostasis and Coagulation

JEREMY MCGARVEY AND GRACE WANG

KEY POINTS

- Hemostasis is characterized by vasospasm, platelet plug formation, and appropriate initiation of the clotting cascade.
- Normal platelet function requires adhesion, activation, aggregation, and cross-linking. Platelet disorders are characterized by a deficiency in these steps.
- Secondary hemostasis *in vivo* involves activation of serial clotting factors via three cell-based steps: initiation, amplification, and propagation.
- *In vitro* coagulation function involves activation of either intrinsic (aPTT) or extrinsic (PT/INR) coagulation cascades.
- Hereditary and acquired conditions may affect platelet function and coagulation. Treatment of these disease processes relies on knowledge of the underlying pathology and directed correction of these deficiencies.
- Novel oral anticoagulants offer directed inhibition of either factor Xa or thrombin and do not require routine therapeutic monitoring. Specific antidotes do not exist and may complicate surgical patient management.

INTRODUCTION

Understanding hemostasis, thrombosis, and coagulation is fundamental to the perioperative management of any surgical patient. Because bleeding is inherent to most surgical procedures, the surgeon should be aware of the biologic processes underlying the body's intrinsic mechanisms to limit blood loss, as well as appreciate factors that may potentiate or antagonize these pathways.

In this chapter, we discuss the normal hemostatic and coagulation mechanisms in addition to inherited and acquired pathologic conditions that may affect them. This chapter also discusses commonly used pharmacologic agents in the treatment of thrombotic or coagulation disorders, as well as monitoring tests available to assess therapeutic efficacy. Lastly, we briefly discuss the use and risks of donated blood transfusion products in the management of bleeding and coagulopathy.

HEMOSTASIS

Primary Hemostasis

Endothelium and Vessel Injury

Endothelial cells function as a highly active barrier between the vessel lumen and the subendothelial wall components. In the normal uninjured environment, the endothelium is critical in the preservation of nonthrombotic interface. Anticoagulant effects of the endothelium are in large part maintained through sustained production of prostacyclin (PGI_2), nitric oxide (NO), thrombomodulin, tissue plasminogen activator (tPA), tissue factor pathway inhibitor (TFPI), and heparin and dermatan sulfate. PGI_2 and NO secretion results in vasodilation and platelet inhibition, which in turn prevents intravascular platelet aggregation. Thrombomodulin production results in activation of protein C and subsequent inhibition of factors Va and VIIIa, while local TFPI release reversibly inhibits factor Xa. Endogenous heparin and dermatan sulfate expression results in antithrombin III (ATIII) binding—thus inactivating thrombin and preventing propagation of clot.

The blood vessel is shifted from a nonthrombotic state toward a procoagulant microenvironment during injury and endothelial disturbance. Vasoconstriction is an early mediator of primary hemostasis as a result of neuromyogenic reflexes within the vascular smooth muscle. Vascular contraction is further augmented shortly thereafter by paracrine signaling via ADP, thromboxane A_2, and serotonin from nearby adherent platelets. Concurrently, exposure of subendothelial tissue factor (TF) and collagen provides a nidus for platelet and leukocyte adhesion. Increased endothelial cell production of von Willebrand factor (vWF), expression of cellular TF and platelet-activating factor (PAF), and reduced thrombomodulin availability improves coagulation protein and platelet binding. Additionally, surface expression of cell adhesion molecules (e.g., E- and P-selectin) initiates the leukocyte adhesion cascade, which—in turn—potentiates the inflammatory and procoagulant response by release of interleukin-1 (IL-1) and tumor necrosis factor-alpha (TNFα).

Platelets

Platelet adhesion, activation, and the formation of the platelet plug are all critical components of early hemostasis and propagation of the coagulation cascade (Fig. 2.1). Platelets are derived from bone marrow megakaryocytes and have a typical lifespan of 9 to 12 days. Approximately one third of the body's platelet pool is stored in the spleen. Mature, inactivated platelets are spherical, anucleated, and contain cytoplasmic exosomes (alpha-, lambda-, and dense granules) that potentiate thrombosis and coagulation.

Exposed extracellular matrix results in prompt adherence of circulating platelets by collagen-specific binding with surface glycoprotein Ia/IIa. Platelet adhesion is further strengthened by the presence of vWF, which mediates the binding of collagen with glycoprotein Ib/IX. Collagen interaction with glycoprotein VI

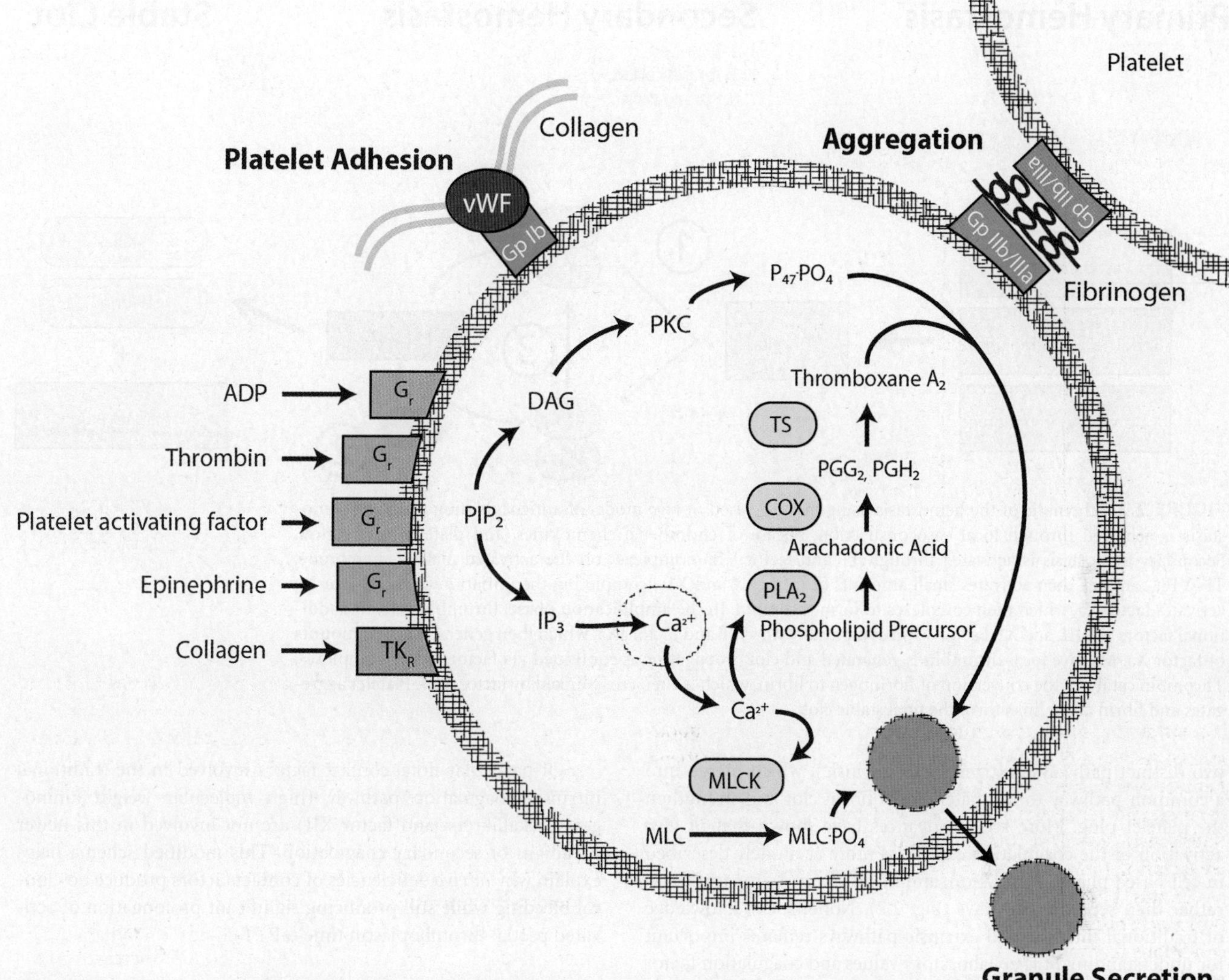

FIGURE 2.1 The normal platelet response to endothelial injury and receptor-mediated activation leading to platelet adherence, aggregation, and granule release. COX, cyclooxygenase; DAG, diacylglycerol; Gp, glycoprotein; G_R, G-protein–linked receptor; TK_R, tyrosine kinase–linked receptor; IP_3, inositol triphosphate; MLC, myosin light chain; MLCK, myosin light chain kinase; PIP_2, phosphatidylinositol bisphosphate; PGG_2, prostaglandin G_2; PGH_2, prostaglandin H_2; PKC, protein kinase C; PLA_2, phospholipase A_2; PLC, phospholipase C; PO_4, phosphate; TS, thromboxane synthase; vWF, von Willebrand factor.

initiates a signaling cascade that activates the platelet, promotes tight adhesion to the extracellular matrix via surface integrins, stimulates the activation of nearby platelets, and propagates platelet–platelet binding. Activation of the platelet is accompanied by a shape change from spherical to stellate with many pseudopods. Release of alpha (platelet factor 4 [PF4], β-thromboglobulin, thrombospondin, platelet-derived growth factor, fibrinogen, vWF) and dense (ADP, serotonin) granule contents results in autocrine and paracrine signaling that improves vascular vasoconstriction and additional platelet activation. Thromboxane A_2 production by activated platelets results in improved affinity for fibrinogen by the glycoprotein IIb/IIIa membrane receptor—promoting platelet cross-linking and the formation of a platelet plug within 1 to 3 minutes of endothelial injury. Clot stabilization occurs within 10 minutes of injury and is aided in part by negative feedback from endothelial cell PGI_2 release.

Following platelet plug formation, procoagulant protein complexes (i.e., prothrombinase, tenase) form on platelet phospholipid surfaces and augment the production of thrombin via the coagulation cascade. In all, this process allows localized and rapid hemostatic control and limits on going blood loss.

Secondary Hemostasis

Secondary hemostasis is a process by which circulating inactive serine protease zymogens (i.e., coagulation factors) sequentially activate and interact with one another. The liver is responsible for the production of all coagulation factors with the exception of factor VIII and vWF, which are produced by endothelial cells. Factors II, VII, IX, and X are formed through vitamin K–dependent reactions and of particular importance for pharmacologic anticoagulation. Historically, the coagulation cascade was thought to involve

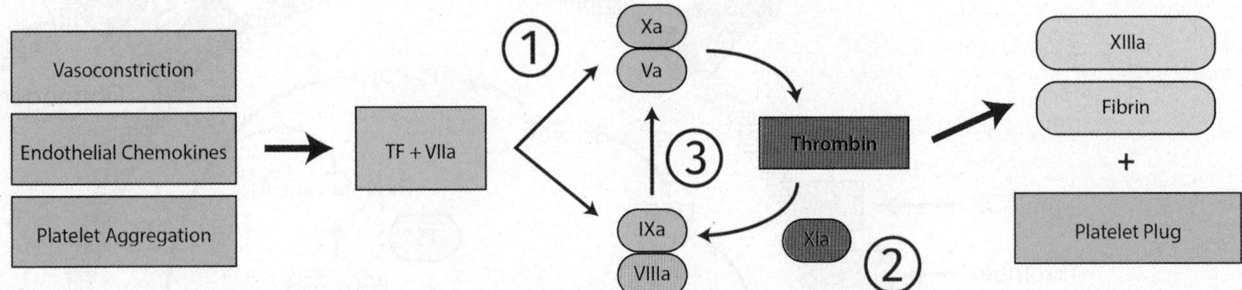

FIGURE 2.2 Schematic of the hemostasis using the cell-based *in vivo* model of anticoagulation. Primary hemostasis is achieved through local vasoconstriction, release of endothelial chemokines, and platelet aggregation. Secondary hemostasis is activated through TF and factor VIIa complexes on the activated platelet membrane. TF–VIIa complex then activates small amounts of factors X and XI—completing the initiation phase. Factor Xa activates factor Va, which then complexes to form thrombin. In the amplification phase, thrombin activates additional factors V, VIII, and XI. Factor VIIIa complexes with vWF and factor IXa, which then generates large amounts of factor Xa. Massive local thrombin is generated and clot propagation is continued via factor Xa–Va complexes. Thrombin catalyzes the conversion of fibrinogen to fibrin, which is then cross-linked by factor XIII. Platelet aggregates and fibrin cross-links form the final stable clot.

two distinct pathways (extrinsic and intrinsic), which merge into a common pathway to ultimately form fibrin clot and strengthen the platelet plug. More recent advances have shown that *in vivo* activation of the coagulation cascade is more accurately described in cell-based phases—initiation, amplification, and propagation—rather than separate pathways (Fig. 2.2). Nonetheless, knowledge of traditional intrinsic and extrinsic pathways remains important for understanding *in vitro* laboratory values and coagulation factor deficiencies (Fig. 2.3).

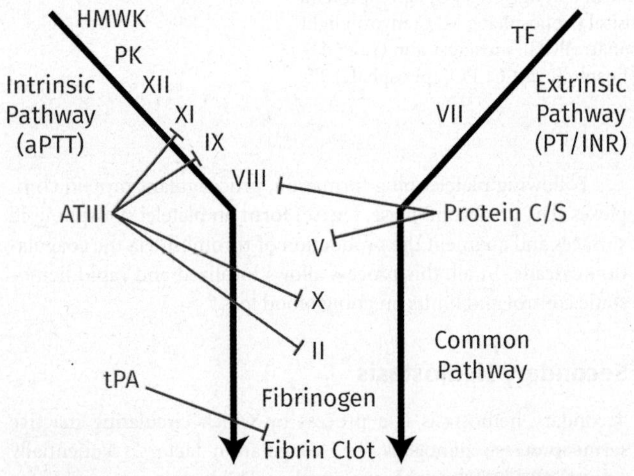

FIGURE 2.3 Schematic of the traditional *in vitro* clotting cascade with extrinsic, intrinsic, and common pathways. Factors are represented by roman numerals; ATIII, antithrombin III; aPTT, activated partial thromboplastin time; HMWK, high molecular weight kininogen; INR, international normalized ratio; PK, prekallikrein; PT, prothrombin time; tPA, tissue plasminogen activator; TF, tissue factor.

Of particular note, contact factors involved in the traditional intrinsic coagulation pathway (high molecular weight kininogen, prekallikrein, and factor XII) are not involved in this newer paradigm of secondary coagulation. This modified schema helps explain why *in vivo* deficiencies of contact factors produce no clinical bleeding while still producing significant prolongation of activated partial thromboplastin time (aPTT).

Initiation and Amplification

TF released by the injured vascular endothelium is bound to factor VII to form TF–VIIa complexes. This complex then activates factors X and IX to form Xa and IXa, respectively. Factor Xa interacts with factor Va to form the factor Xa–Va complex (prothrombinase complex), which resides on the activated platelet membrane. The prothrombinase complex converts small amounts of factor II (prothrombin) to factor IIa (thrombin)—*initiation*. The thrombin produced from this initial reaction serves to activate additional factor V, factor VIII, factor XI, and platelets via a positive feedback loop (*amplification*).

Propagation

Factor IXa (created from both the original TF–VIIa complex and factor XIa) is able to interact with factor VIIIa to form factor IXa–VIIIa complex (tenase complex), which also resides on the activated platelet membrane. Tenase complex converts additional factor X to factor Xa, which then forms more prothrombinase complexes. Large amounts of thrombin are generated, leading to the formation of fibrin from fibrinogen. Fibrin monomers are covalently cross-linked by factor XIIIa, which was activated by thrombin. Cross-linked fibrin weaves throughout the platelet plug to form a stable fibrin clot.

Negative Feedback and Fibrinolysis

Regulation of clot formation/expansion and fibrinolysis are important negative feedback mechanisms to limit pathologic intravascular thrombosis. In addition to the endogenous anticoagulants produced by the endothelium previously described, ATIII, protein C, and protein S are important natural anticoagulants.

ATIII is a 70-kD glycoprotein in the serine protease inhibitor family. This protein directly inhibits factors IIa (thrombin), IXa, Xa, and XIa. Heparin sulfate produces a conformational change in the molecule that accelerates the inhibitory reactions up to 40,000-fold.

Protein C is a vitamin K–dependent natural anticoagulant, which is activated by thrombin–thrombomodulin complexes on the endothelial cell surface following the formation of clot. Activated protein C (APC) competitively binds factors Va and VIIIa, which accordingly limits thrombin production. Protein S is a vitamin K–dependent cofactor in the formation of APC.

Fibrinolysis describes the process by which fibrin clot is degraded into soluble fragments. Plasminogen, tPA, and α_2-antiplasmin are important regulatory and precursor proteins necessary for fibrin degradation. These proteins are incorporated into the polymerized fibrin clot as it forms. Further, thrombin formation positively up-regulates the release of tPA release from nearby endothelial cells. tPA acts to convert plasminogen to plasmin, which in turn binds fibrin and degrades the polymer into soluble split products (fragment E and D-dimer). α_2-Antiplasmin serves as a negative regulator of plasmin and binds and inactivates circulating excess plasmin. Accordingly, continuously secreted plasmin is actively bound by α_2-antiplasmin until a critical threshold is reached—thus allowing early clot formation during vascular injury without immediate degradation.

MONITORING

Platelet Count and Bleeding Time

The platelet count is a normal component of the complete blood count (CBC) and is used to assess quantitative deficiencies. The normal platelet count is 150,000 to 400,000/μL of blood. Patients with counts below 50,000/μL are subject to easy bruising and bleeding, but spontaneous bleeding does not typically occur unless counts are below 20,000/μL (Table 2.1).

Bleeding time is a measure of qualitative platelet dysfunction and is performed using a standardized small superficial incision on a patient's forearm (Ivy method) or pinprick on the fingertip (Duke method). With the Ivy method, a blood pressure cuff is inflated proximally on the arm to 40 mm Hg. In both methods, blood is wiped away every 30 seconds, and time is recorded from initiation of cut until no additional bleeding is noted. Bleeding times between 2 and 10 minutes are considered normal. Times between 10 and 15 minutes are considered abnormal and associated with low-to-moderate risk for bleeding, while greater than 15 minutes is serious risk for spontaneous bleeding and severe platelet dysfunction or thrombocytopenia.

Prothrombin Time and International Normalized Ratio

Prothrombin time (PT) is a measure of the function of the extrinsic and common pathways of the *ex vivo* coagulation cascade. Accordingly, PT measures the function of factors VII, V, X, II, and I (fibrinogen). Because the PT can vary from laboratory to laboratory due to variations in reagents and detectors, the international normalized ratio (INR) was developed to standardized values across institutions independent of methods. A normal INR is 1.0. Prolongation in PT/INR usually occurs when factor levels fall below 30% to 50% normal range. Warfarin therapy typically prolongs PT/INR due to depletion of vitamin K–dependent factors II, VII, IX, and X—with a more marked reduction of factor VII due to a short half-life.

Partial Thromboplastin Time and Activated Clotting Time

The aPTT is a measure of the *ex vivo* intrinsic coagulation cascade compromising high molecular weight kininogen, prekallikrein, and factors XI, IX, VIII, V, X, II, and I. Factor levels less than 30% of

TABLE 2.1 Summary of platelet and coagulation monitoring values in hemostatic disorders

Condition	Platelet Count	Bleeding Time	PT/INR	aPTT
Warfarin	Unaffected	Unaffected	Increased	Normal or mildly increased
Heparin	Unaffected	Unaffected	Normal or mildly increased	Increased
Aspirin	Unaffected	Increased	Unaffected	Unaffected
DIC	Decreased	Increased	Increased	Increased
von Willebrand disease	Unaffected	Increased	Unaffected	Normal or mildly increased
Glanzmann's thrombasthenia	Unaffected	Increased	Unaffected	Unaffected
Hemophilia	Unaffected	Unaffected	Unaffected	Increased
Thrombocytopenia	Decreased	Increased	Unaffected	Unaffected
Liver failure, early	Unaffected	Unaffected	Increased	Unaffected
Liver failure, end stage	Decreased	Increased	Increased	Increased
Uremia	Unaffected	Increased	Unaffected	Unaffected

normal are usually required to affect aPTT. Heparin results primarily in prolonged aPTT due to depletion of intrinsic pathway factors as a result of ATIII-mediated inactivation.

Activated clotting time (ACT) is a test similar to aPTT but used in clinical situations requiring high-dose heparin administration (cardiopulmonary bypass, endovascular interventions, ECMO). ACT measures the time required for whole blood to clot in the presence of an activator and—as such—is also influenced by platelet count and function in addition coagulation factors.

Thromboelastography

Rotational thromboelastography (TEG) is a viscoelastic hemostatic assay that measures whole-blood coagulation kinetics and biomechanical properties. Unlike bleeding time, PT, and aPTT, TEG provides a quantitative measure of all aspects of hemostasis, including platelet aggregation, clot strengthening, fibrin cross-linking, and fibrinolysis. Metrics available from TEG include latency time, time to achieve a certain clot strength, fibrin cross-linking speed, maximum clot strength, and clot lysis time. Advantages of TEG analysis lie in its quantification of thrombodynamics, its ability to differentiate between platelet and plasma coagulative disorders, and the rapidity of its results (approximately 10 minutes and performed at bedside); however, interpretation of results can be complex, and its widespread clinical use remains limited.

DISORDERS OF PLATELETS

Inherited Platelet Disorders

von Willebrand's Disease

von Willebrand's disease (vWD) is the most common congenital bleeding disorder—affecting as much as 1% of the population. Because of its role in platelet aggregation and as a carrier protein for factor VIII, clinical manifestations often include epistaxis, menorrhagia, and petechiae. Laboratory findings include prolonged bleeding time, mildly prolonged aPTT, and abnormal platelet binding as measured by a depressed ristocetin cofactor assay. Many subtypes of vWD have been identified; however, there are three major groups and inheritance patterns. Type I vWD, which is inherited in an autosomal dominant pattern, is characterized by quantitative reduction in vWF levels with normal protein structure and function. Type II vWD is inherited variably and characterized by abnormal qualitative protein function. Type III vWD is inherited in an autosomal recessive pattern and associated with severe bleeding with absent vWF production.

Treatment of vWD is dependent on the underlying pathology. For type I and II diseases, D-deoxydesmopressin arginine vasopressin (DDAVP) is typically a first-line therapy and stimulates release of vWF from endothelial cells. For type III disease surgical prophylaxis or bleeding, transfusion with cryoprecipitate or factor VIII:vWF concentrate is necessary due to absent endogenous production.

Glanzmann's Thrombasthenia

Glanzmann's thrombasthenia is a rare congenital platelet disorder that is a result of defective or decreased synthesis of glycoprotein IIb/IIIa. As a result, platelets are unable to bind fibrinogen and lack the ability to form platelet aggregates. Clinically, patients with this disorder present with epistaxis, menorrhagia, easy bruising, and mucosal bleeding. In laboratory tests, this manifests as increased bleeding time. Treatment is often focused on reducing symptoms (i.e., oral contraceptives and dental hygiene); however, in severe bleeding, platelet transfusion may be necessary to provide phenotypically normal platelets.

Acquired Platelet Disorders

Renal Failure and Uremia

Platelet dysfunction in renal disease is a result of numerous changes to protein function and intraluminal fluid dynamics. Uremic patients are associated with dysfunctional vWF, decreased levels of thromboxane A_2, and altered platelet granules—all of which are necessary for platelet plug formation. Additionally, anemia associated with renal failure results in decreased red blood cell laminar flow within the vessel. As a result, platelets are not naturally forced to the vessel wall as they are in normal conditions—thus decreasing platelet adhesion and aggregation. Treatment of uremic platelet dysfunction depends on severity of symptoms/bleeding risk and relies on correction of the uremia with dialysis, as well as adjunctive therapies including: erythropoietin to improve anemia and DDAVP/cryoprecipitate to increase vWF levels.

Extracorporeal Oxygenation

Extracorporeal bypass circuitry (i.e., cardiopulmonary bypass, ECMO) gives rise to abnormal platelet activation in part due to fibrinogen accumulation within the oxygenation membrane. As a result, platelets form aggregates, change shape, and release granule contents. Adherent platelets to the oxygenation membrane can also break away or fragment. Consequently, consumption and loss of platelets from the circulating pool result in thrombocytopenia as well as qualitative dysfunction.

Continuous thrombin generation resulting from blood contact with the nonendothelial cell surfaces also quickly overwhelms the body's natural anticoagulant capabilities. As such, extracorporeal oxygenation is not possible without aggressive anticoagulation—typically in the form of systemic unfractionated heparin given intravenously and intermittently into the extracorporeal circuit to maintain therapeutic anticoagulation levels. Venoarterial bypass (VA ECMO) is associated with higher thrombotic complications and increased morbidity than venovenous bypass (VV ECMO) due to outflow into the systemic circulation. Thrombin reduction strategies have also been employed, including use of heparin-coated circuitry and separating salvaged red blood cells with the use of CellSaver devices.

Heparin-Induced Thrombocytopenia

Heparin-induced thrombocytopenia (HIT) is a serious adverse drug reaction to exogenous heparin administration. HIT may develop in two forms: type 1 and type 2. Type I HIT is associated with transient mild thrombocytopenia and is a result of nonimmunologic platelet sequestration from direct heparin interactions. Type 1 HIT may occur in as many as 10% of patients receiving unfractionated heparin and typically resolves spontaneously within 96 hours of heparin cessation. Type 2 HIT is an unusual immunologic complication affecting 1% to 3% of patients following administration of unfractionated heparin and approximately 0.2% following administration of low molecular weight heparin (LMWH). Following administration, heparin binds with PF4, which is released from platelet alpha granules. In cases of HIT, IgG antibodies form against the heparin–PF4 complex within 5 to 10 days following exposure that, in turn, strongly activates platelet adhesion and aggregation. Activation via the FcγRIIa receptor also stimulates additional granule release—resulting in increased PG4 and a self-perpetuating cascade.

Clinical concern for HIT should be raised when platelet counts decrease by greater than 50% from preheparin levels. Platelet counts typically fall within 5 to 15 days of initial heparin exposure; however, onset may also be rapid (prior heparin exposure) or delayed in rare cases. Bleeding complications from HIT are rare, while thrombotic events are common. Massive platelet activation and platelet plug formation (white clot) predisposes the patient to venous thrombosis, thromboembolism, limb ischemia, stroke, and myocardial infarction.

Confirmation of HIT and heparin–PF4 antibodies can be accomplished by serotonin release assay (SRA), heparin-induced platelet aggregation (HIPA) assay, or immunoassay (ELISA). SRA is a functional assay that utilizes control platelets tagged with radiolabeled serotonin and patient serum. Heparin is titrated into the mixture, and C^{14}-serotonin release is detected as an indicator of antibody-mediated platelet activation. SRA has a sensitivity and specificity of greater than 95%; however, its application is limited by technical complexity. The HIPA assay is a functional assay that also employs test platelets in the presence of a patient's platelet-poor plasma. Platelet aggregation is then measured in the presence of low and high heparin concentrations. HIPA is associated with excellent specificity (>90%), however, lacks sensitivity (approximately 80%). Lastly, ELISA immunoassays for heparin–PF4 antibodies more directly measures antibody binding *in vitro* via enzyme-linked secondary antibodies to the antibody–heparin–PF4 complex. This test is associated with excellent sensitivity (>97%)—making ELISA one of the more common screening tests in clinical use; however, low specificity leads to false positives that may necessitate a confirmatory functional test (SRA).

With suspicion for HIT or positive laboratory findings, treatment involves immediate cessation of all heparin therapies (including heparin-coated catheters, LMWH, and heparin flushes) as well as prevention of thromboembolic complications. Non–heparin-based anticoagulation strategies (i.e., argatroban, bivalirudin, warfarin) are encouraged unless there is a clinical contraindication. Avoidance of platelet transfusion is appropriate to help propagation of white clot. Duration of treatment following HIT diagnosis has not yet been clearly defined. Antibodies typically disappear within 2 to 3 months; however, lifelong avoidance should be recommended unless clinically necessary (e.g., cardiac or vascular procedures with a single heparin administration).

Idiopathic Thrombocytopenic Purpura

Idiopathic thrombocytopenic purpura (ITP) is an acquired disorder arising from pathologic destruction of platelets due to autoantibody formation. While the precipitating event is not often clear, ITP commonly occurs at times of infection (often viral) or altered immune homeostasis (malignancy, lymphoproliferative disorders, concurrent autoimmune disease). B-cell IgG production against platelet glycoprotein IIb/IIIa receptors is thought to drive antibody-mediated destruction and impaired production of platelets; however, autoantibodies are not always detectable in patients with ITP. Accordingly, routine testing for platelet autoantibodies in patients with suspected ITP is not recommended. Diagnosis is clinical and one of exclusion after ruling out other potential etiologies of thrombocytopenia through history, physical, and laboratory testing. Initial therapies for ITP patients with platelet count less than 30,000/μL are focused toward prevention of bleeding and include glucocorticoids and intravenous immune globulin (IVIG). Nonresponders to first-line therapies may require splenectomy. If surgery is contraindicated or ineffective, rituximab has also been shown to improve thrombocytopenia, although with lower response rates when compared to splenectomy.

DISORDERS OF COAGULATION

Inherited Coagulopathies

Hemophilia A/B

Factor VIII and IX deficiency underlies hemophilia A and B, respectively. Both hemophilias are passed through an X-linked receive inheritance pattern and affect 1 in 5,000 (hemophilia A) to 30,000 (hemophilia B) males in the United States. Deficiency in these factors results in impaired formation of the tenase (VIIIa–IXa) complex—impacting the amplification phase of coagulation and leading to decreased factor Xa and thrombin creation. Clinically, hemophilia is often diagnosed in early childhood due to a known family history of the disease; however, a minority of hemophiliacs are diagnosed later in life due to spontaneous or exaggerated bleeding. Symptoms may include mucosal bleeding, excessive bleeding during circumcision, hemarthrosis, and—most severely—intracranial hemorrhage. Laboratory testing confirms diagnosis, with elevated aPTT and decreased factor VIII or IX levels.

Management of hemophilia is focused toward improving deficient circulating factor levels. Acute bleeds are often managed with either recombinant factor replacement or transfusion. For hemophilia A, management of acute bleeding or for surgical prophylaxis involves administration of recombinant factor VIII, cryoprecipitate transfusion, and/or desmopressin (increases circulating vWF–VIII complexes). For hemophilia B, acute blood loss control and surgical prophylaxis are achieved with use of recombinant factor IX and fresh frozen plasma (FFP) or cryoprecipitate transfusion. Desmopressin is not effective in the management of hemophilia B, as release of endothelial vWF has no effect on circulating factor IX levels. Recombinant factor prophylaxis is now the standard of care for both hemophilia A and B long-term management in order to reduce spontaneous bleeding and its chronic complications (joint damage).

Acquired Coagulopathies

Disseminated Intravascular Coagulation

Disseminated intravascular coagulation (DIC) is clinical syndrome resulting from unchecked activation of the normal coagulation response with loss of localization. Sepsis is the most common cause of DIC; however, burns, trauma, malignancy, and obstetrical complications are also associated. The pathogenesis of DIC stems from systemic microvascular activation of platelets, diffuse activation of clotting factors, deposition of fibrin with microangiopathic thrombosis, and subsequent fibrinolytic pathway activation. In sepsis, this cascade is typically initiated via widespread synthesis of proinflammatory cytokines, which leads to up-regulation of TF on monocytes. Although the biology underlying DIC is primarily procoagulant, thrombotic complications alone actually represent only 5% to 10% of cases. Paradoxically, massive consumption of platelets and coagulation factors typically leads to severe thrombocytopenia and hemorrhage.

Clinical diagnosis of DIC is based on exclusion of other etiologies of bleeding and thrombocytopenia (i.e., liver failure, hypothermia, HIT, etc.), the presence of a known underlying disorder associated with DIC, and scored using the following metrics: platelet count, fibrinogen level, presence of fibrin degradation products, and prothrombin time. Additionally, peripheral blood smear will show evidence of schistocytes, which are fragmented red blood cells that have been split by fibrin strands within microvasculature.

Successful management of DIC remains treatment of the inciting pathology. Additionally, supportive care with replacement coagulation factors and platelets to maintain an INR less than 1.5 and platelet count greater than 50,000/mm^3 is recommended. Heparin use in patients with thrombotic complications from DIC has been described; however, its use remains controversial and without consensus recommendation. Similarly, antifibrinolytic agents to control severe hemorrhage have been described; however, their use is not generally recommended due to unabated fibrin deposition and thrombotic complications.

Liver Failure and Vitamin K Deficiency

The liver is responsible for the production of thrombopoietin and all major coagulation factors with the exception of factor VIII and vWF. Consequently, hepatic failure as a result of cirrhosis, intoxications, shock, and trauma has the potential to impact platelet production and the normal coagulation response. In addition, biliary pathology with reduced bile salt secretion impairs ileal absorption of lipid-soluble vitamin K, further impairing activity of factors II, VII, IX, and X. Treatment of bleeding secondary to hepatic failure is centered on correction of factor and platelet deficiencies with blood component management. Patients with vitamin K deficiency or synthetic impairment should also be treated routinely with vitamin K supplementation.

Hypothermia

Hypothermia is a commonly seen cause of altered coagulation in the surgical population as a result of trauma, massive resuscitation, extended exposure to open body cavities during procedures, or iatrogenic hypothermia for cerebral or myocardial protection. Procoagulant proteolytic enzyme kinetics show reduced activity in moderate-to-severe hypothermia (<34°C), resulting in a functional coagulopathy. Additionally, hypothermia is associated with impaired platelet function and decreased collagen-induced platelet aggregation.

Treatment of hypothermia is determinate on the cause and severity. Prompt treatment of the underlying cause and limiting evaporative heat loss (e.g., closure of the incision, removal of wet garments) is recommended if possible. Mild hypothermia (>34°C) can often be treated with passive rewarming techniques (warm blankets, increased room temperature) alone. Moderate hypothermia (30°C to 34°C) should be treated with active rewarming, including forced warm air blankets and warmed intravenous fluids. Severe hypothermia (<30°C) is associated with profound cardiovascular instability and coagulopathy. In addition to external passive and active rewarming methods, internal rewarming techniques should be considered—including warm esophageal lavage, warm bladder irrigation, peritoneal lavage, and extracorporeal circulation.

Massive Transfusion

Massive transfusion is defined as replacement of a patient's blood volume with packed red blood cells (pRBCs) in a 24-hour period or acute transfusion of over half the patient's blood volume per hour. Banked pRBCs are typically refrigerated at 4°C, while FFP is stored at −30°C. Consequently, large-volume blood product resuscitation can result in severe hypothermia leading to coagulopathy. Furthermore, only trace levels of procoagulant proteins and platelets are present in pRBCs, and large transfusions with only pRBCs can result in a significant dilutional coagulopathy and thrombocytopenia. Data from trauma literature have recently supported the implementation of a standardized massive transfusion protocol utilizing a 1:1:1 ratio of pRBC, FFP, and platelet administration. Careful monitoring of temperature, calcium, and potassium levels is critical during large transfusions and is discussed in greater detail later.

Inherited Thrombophilias

Factor V Leiden

Factor V Leiden is the most common hereditary procoagulant disorders—affecting approximately 5% of the Caucasian North American population. The disorder is caused by a single nucleotide polymorphism in the factor V gene and is inherited in an autosomal dominant pattern. Mutation of the factor V protein prevents APC-mediated inactivation, thereby increasing risk for uncontrolled clot formation. Heterozygotes exhibit a 5- to 7-fold risk in thromboembolic events, while homozygous carriers of the factor V Leiden mutation have up to 50-fold increased risk for thromboembolism. Smoking, cancer, pregnancy, oral contraceptive use, and surgery increase risk further. Clinical presentation typically involves venous thromboembolism with deep venous thrombosis (DVT) or pulmonary embolism (PE)—with 30% of carriers having an event by 60 years of age. Definitive demonstration of factor V Leiden and APC resistance is made by performing aPTT with and without APC. Confirmatory testing using PCR of the factor V gene can also be performed. Thromboembolic events in the setting of a factor V Leiden mutation are typically treated with short-term anticoagulation; however, lifelong anticoagulation is not typically necessary unless additional risk factors are present (e.g., recurrent thromboembolic events, homozygous state, multiple thrombophilic defects).

Antithrombin III Deficiency

ATIII, as previously discussed, is a natural anticoagulant that inactivates thrombin and factors Xa, IXa, and XIa. This process is accelerated 4,000-fold in the presence of heparin binding to ATIII. Functional or quantitative deficiency of ATIII is inherited in an autosomal dominant pattern and the result of more than 120 described mutations in the protein that affect synthesis or ligand binding. Deficiency is rare—affecting only 0.05% of the population. Carriers are at an eightfold risk for having a thrombotic event.

Iliofemoral DVT is the most common site of thrombosis, while arterial events are rare. Forty percent of individuals will present with spontaneous thromboembolism, while the remainder while develop in the setting of another risk factor (i.e., trauma, pregnancy, surgery). ATIII-deficient individuals will develop recurrent thromboembolic episodes in approximately 60% of cases. Because of its function as a cofactor in heparin-based anticoagulation, ATIII-deficient patients may also be identified due to therapeutic heparin resistance. Diagnosis may be confirmed using an ATIII–heparin cofactor assay, which looks at inactivation of thrombin or factor Xa. During attempted heparin anticoagulation, known or suspected deficiency is treated with FFP transfusion or ATIII concentrate. ATIII-deficient individuals with a spontaneous thromboembolic event are often treated with long-term/indefinite oral anticoagulation due to the high lifetime risk for recurrence.

Protein C/S Deficiency

Protein C and S are both vitamin K–dependent natural anticoagulants involved in the neutralization of factors Va and VIIIa. Protein C and S deficiencies are inherited in an autosomal dominant pattern and affect approximately 0.2% of the population. Affected individuals are at 7- to 8.5-fold lifetime risk of developing thrombosis. Serum protein C and S levels below normal limits confirm the diagnosis. Venous thromboembolism is the most common clinical manifestation of these deficiencies; however, rare reports of arterial thrombosis with both protein C and S deficiencies have been described. Thromboembolic events are typically treated with short-term anticoagulation. Indefinite anticoagulation is not typically necessary unless additional risk factors are present or in cases of recurrent events. Because the half-life of both protein C and S is shorter than that of the procoagulant factors, warfarin-induced skin necrosis is a known risk factor for patients with decreased protein C and S levels due to a transient procoagulant state during initiation of the drug. As such, warfarin-based anticoagulation should be initiated slowly and with caution. Systemic heparinization is recommended, and protein C or S concentrates or FFP may be used to increase serum levels prior to warfarin administration.

Acquired Thrombophilias

Within the surgical population, a number of conditions may predispose patients to thromboembolic events, including but not limited to immobility/stasis, malignancy, obesity, smoking, prior thrombotic events, trauma, inflammatory bowel disease, recent surgery, pregnancy, myeloproliferative disorders, mechanical valves, and central venous catheters. In the absence of contraindications, perioperative thromboprophylaxis with intermittent pneumatic compression devices and/or pharmacologic agents (heparin, LMWH) is recommended by current CHEST society guidelines. In high-risk cancer patients undergoing abdominopelvic surgery, extended-duration prophylaxis for up to 4 weeks is recommended. Thromboembolic event management is often focused on treatment of the underlying process and anticoagulation. Duration of anticoagulation therapy is dependent on the type of event, its magnitude, predisposing factors, and the risks of anticoagulation.

Patients who are previously receiving anticoagulant or antiplatelet therapy for acquired thromboembolic diseases during the perioperative period also require consideration. In general, moderate- to high-risk patients on aspirin therapy for secondary prevention of cardiovascular events should be continued on aspirin throughout the perioperative period unless contraindicated due to bleeding complications. For noncardiac surgery patients with recent cardiovascular stenting, postponement of surgery beyond 6 weeks for bare metal stenting and 6 months for drug-eluting stenting is recommended if possible. For procedures performed within this period, dual antiplatelet therapy (i.e., aspirin and clopidogrel) should be continued. For procedures outside of this window, patients should be continued on aspirin therapy; however, additional antiplatelet agents can be temporarily held. Patients being treated for atrial fibrillation, mechanical valves, or venous thromboembolic disease with vitamin K antagonists (warfarin), LMWH, or novel oral anticoagulants should be triaged based on the likelihood of thromboembolic disease and bleeding risk within the perioperative period.

COAGULATION PHARMACOLOGY

Antiplatelet Agents

Aspirin (acetylsalicylic acid, ASA) is a nonsteroidal anti-inflammatory drug (NSAID) that irreversibly inhibits cyclooxygenase isoforms (COX-1 and COX-2). COX-1 is an enzyme found in most of tissues and mediates synthesis of prostaglandins and thromboxane A_2. COX-2 is preferentially expressed in inflammatory tissues following exposure to proinflammatory cytokines. At low doses (81 mg/day), aspirin primarily inhibits COX-1–mediated thromboxane A_2 synthesis, thereby limiting local vasoconstriction and preventing platelet aggregation due to impaired cross-linking and decreased glycoprotein IIb/IIIa affinity for fibrinogen. At higher doses, aspirin also irreversibly inhibits COX-2 activity—resulting in an anti-inflammatory affect. Because COX activity is irreversibly inhibited due to acetylation from aspirin, platelets are unable to synthesize new protein, and the drug maintains its effects for the life span of the platelet (7 to 9 days). Accordingly, significant aspirin-mediated bleeding is treated with platelet transfusion (Table 2.2).

Ticlopidine (Ticlid), **prasugrel** (Effient), and **clopidogrel** (Plavix) are drugs within the thienopyridine family of antiplatelet agents. These agents irreversibly inhibit activity of the ADP-$P2Y_{12}$ receptor on the platelet membrane, which in turn impairs glycoprotein IIb/IIIa–mediated platelet cross-linking and aggregation. Clopidogrel is currently labeled for use in the United States in patients with acute coronary syndromes, recent myocardial infarction or stroke, and established peripheral arterial disease. Off-label usage is common, including intolerance of aspirin therapy, prevention of coronary artery bypass graft closure, stable coronary artery disease, peripheral or coronary artery stenting, and symptomatic carotid artery stenosis. Prasugrel is a new agent within the thienopyridine family that is labeled for use in acute coronary syndromes during percutaneous coronary intervention. Prasugrel has also found use clinically in a significant subset of patients (16% to 50%) whom have resistance to clopidogrel therapy and continue to have high platelet reactivity. Clopidogrel resistance is thought to be due to a polymorphism in the hepatic cytochrome pathway (CYP2C19*2), which impairs the formation of clopidogrel's active metabolite. Pharmacodynamic studies have also found prasugrel to inhibit platelet aggregation more rapidly and consistently compared to clopidogrel. Like aspirin therapy, the most common side effect of thienopyridine usage is bleeding, and this risk may be

TABLE 2.2 Summary of antiplatelet and anticoagulant agents

Drug	Class	Mechanism of Action	Monitoring	Reversal Agent
Aspirin	Antiplatelet	COX inhibition → decreased platelet aggregation	Bleeding time	Irreversible; platelet transfusion
Ticlopidine, Clopidogrel, Prasugrel	Antiplatelet	ADP receptor antagonism → decreased platelet aggregation/activation	Bleeding time	Irreversible; platelet transfusion
Cilostazol	Antiplatelet	Phosphodiesterase III inhibition → vasodilation and decreased platelet activation	N/A	No specific antidote
Abciximab, Eptifibatide, Tirofiban	Antiplatelet	Glycoprotein IIb/IIIa inhibition → decreased platelet activation		No specific antidote
Unfractionated Heparin	Antithrombin III agonist	Potentiates ATIII inhibition of factors IIa, IXa, Xa, XIa	aPTT	Protamine
LMWH	Antithrombin III agonist	Potentiates ATIII inhibition of factor Xa	Anti–Factor Xa level	Protamine
Warfarin	Vitamin K antagonist	Inhibits vitamin K–dependent synthesis of factors II, VII, IX, X	PT, INR	Vitamin K
Bivalirudin, Argatroban	Direct thrombin inhibitor (parenteral)	Binds active site of thrombin → inhibits clot formation	PT, INR, aPTT	No specific antidote
Dabigatran	Direct thrombin inhibitor (oral)	Binds active site of thrombin → inhibits clot formation	No routine monitoring	No specific antidote In emergencies: prothrombin complex, factor VIIa, dialysis
Rivaroxaban, Apixaban, Edoxaban	Direct factor Xa inhibitors (oral)	Factor Xa inhibition → inhibits clot formation	No routine monitoring	No specific antidote In emergencies: prothrombin complex, factor VIIa
Recombinant Tissue Plasminogen Activator	Fibrinolytic	Activates plasminogen-mediated clot breakdown	No routine monitoring. fibrinogen level to assess bleeding risk	No specific antidote

increased with dual antiplatelet therapy. In one study comparing clopidogrel with prasugrel in patients with acute coronary syndromes, the latter was associated with decreased thrombotic events but with an increased risk of bleeding and a similar mortality rate. Because of its irreversible effects on platelet aggregation, antiplatelet effects can be demonstrated for the lifespan of the platelet. As previously discussed, discontinuation of COX and ADP inhibitors prior to surgery due to bleeding risk should be weighed against the risk of thromboembolic events.

Cilostazol (Pletal) is a member of the phosphodiesterase inhibitor family, which is approved clinically for intermittent peripheral arterial claudication. Inhibition of phosphodiesterase III results in increased intracellular cyclic AMP, which results in activation of protein kinase A (PKA) and inhibition of platelet aggregation. Additionally, increased PKA activity also prevents myosin light chain kinase activation in vascular smooth muscle—preventing vasoconstriction and smooth muscle proliferation. Onset of action is typically slow and may require up to 12 months before symptomatic relief is noticeable. Use of cilostazol in patients with a known diagnosis of heart failure is contraindicated due to decreased survival with phosphodiesterase inhibition.

Glycoprotein IIb/IIIa inhibitors are a family of antiplatelet agents that directly inhibit platelet aggregation by blocking integrin binding with fibrinogen. These agents include **abciximab** (ReoPro), **eptifibatide** (Integrilin), and **tirofiban** (Aggrastat) and are commonly adjuncts to heparin and aspirin therapy. Usage of these drugs is typically limited to prevention of cardiac ischemic events before, during, and after percutaneous coronary intervention and stenting. Abciximab is a chimeric human/mouse monoclonal antibody against the glycoprotein IIb/IIIa receptor. The half-life of abciximab is short at 10 minutes; however, a functional effect on platelets can be detected for up to 7 days after administration. Eptifibatide is a peptide-based drug derived from pygmy rattlesnake venom and reversibly binds glycoprotein IIb/IIIa. Onset of action with eptifibatide is approximately 1 hour, with return of normal platelet function within 4 hours of discontinuation. Tirofiban is a synthetic, non–peptide-based reversible inhibitor of glycoprotein IIb/IIIa. Onset of action is approximately 10 minutes with return of normal platelet function to baseline within 4 to 8 hours. As expected, bleeding is the major drug-related complication associated with all drugs in the glycoprotein IIb/IIIa inhibitor family.

Anticoagulants

Antithrombin III Agonists

Unfractionated **heparin** and **LMWH** (e.g., **enoxaparin, dalteparin**) constitute members of the ATIII agonist family of anticoagulants. As previously discussed, ATIII is a potent endogenous inhibitor of anticoagulation by inactivating factors IIa, IXa, Xa, and XIa. Heparin and LMWH interact with and produce a conformational change in ATIII that increases its activity up to 40,000-fold. Unfractionated heparin primarily affects components of the intrinsic and common pathways of the *in vitro* coagulation cascade, and, accordingly, aPTT is typically used to measure therapeutic efficacy—with a target aPTT range of approximately 1.5 to 2.5 times the baseline aPTT value. LMWH differs from unfractionated heparin due to its size (<8 kDa) and its preferential activity against factor Xa. Dosing of LWMH is typically via subcutaneous injection and weight based. Because LMWHs strongly inhibit factor Xa only and the anticoagulant effects are more predictable than unfractionated heparin, routine therapeutic monitoring is not performed with LMWH but can be assessed if necessary using an anti–factor Xa assay. Bleeding and thrombocytopenia are the most common side effects of both unfractionated heparin and LMWH, although LMWH is associated with a lower incidence of HIT and clinically significant thrombocytopenia.

Vitamin K Antagonists

Warfarin (Coumadin) is a commonly used anticoagulant in clinical practice that prevents vitamin K–dependent γ-carboxylation of factors II, VII, IX, and X. Inhibited carboxylation of glutamic acid residues on these factors impairs their ability to bind their respective substrates—making them inactive. Additionally, warfarin competitively inhibits vitamin K reactivation through the vitamin K epoxide reductase complex (VKORC), which in turn results in depletion of functional vitamin K stores and reduced vitamin K–dependent factor synthesis. Paradoxically, initiation of warfarin therapy is associated with a transient procoagulant state due to inhibition of proteins C and S, which are also vitamin K dependent and have shorter half-lives than the procoagulant factors. This phenomenon can lead to warfarin-induced skin necrosis and is particularly noteworthy in patients known to have protein C or S deficiency or those who have received large loading doses of warfarin. Therapeutic anticoagulation onset typically takes at least 24 to 72 hours, during which time previously carboxylated vitamin K–dependent anticoagulant factors are degraded and new factors are synthesized. Since warfarin principally affects members of the extrinsic and common pathways of *in vitro* coagulation, anticoagulation effect is measured using the PT and INR. Warfarin is degraded via the hepatic cytochrome P-450 system and, accordingly, numerous coadministered drugs and food products can either inhibit or induce its degradation.

Direct Thrombin Inhibitors

Direct thrombin inhibitors (DTIs) compromise a class of anticoagulants that function by inactivating circulating and clot-bound thrombin, which in turn prevents clot amplification and propagation. Parentally administered DTIs include **argatroban** and **bivalirudin**. Argatroban is a small molecule DTI that blocks the active site of thrombin and is currently approved for use in patients with a contraindication to heparin administration due to anti–heparin–PF4 antibodies (HIT). Therapeutic monitoring of argatroban is performed using aPTT measurements, although dose-dependent increases in PT may also be seen and falsely elevate INR during warfarin conversion. Argatroban is metabolized by the liver and should not be used in patients with diminished liver function. Bivalirudin functions by binding the active site and exosite I of thrombin and is currently approved for use in patients with acute coronary syndromes undergoing percutaneous coronary revascularization—particularly those with a contraindication to heparin. Bivalirudin is metabolized renally. **Dabigatran** (Pradaxa) is a novel oral DTI that is currently labeled for use in the treatment/prevention of DVT, PE, and non–valvular atrial fibrillation–associated stroke. Dabigatran reaches peak plasma levels within 2 hours of administration and has a renally excreted half-life of 12 to 17 hours. There is currently no widespread or standardized monitoring technique for dabigatran, and, accordingly, routine blood test monitoring is not performed. Assessment of dabigatran anticoagulant activity in emergency situations and overdose may be assessed with a DTI assay or ecarin clotting time; however, this is rarely done. Additionally, dabigatran has no specific antidote or reversal agent. In emergent situations, recombinant prothrombin complex concentrate, recombinant factor VIIa, cryoprecipitate, or even dialysis may be necessary to quickly reduce anticoagulant effects. Antibody-mediated reversal of dabigatran with the humanized antibody fragment idarucizumab is currently undergoing phase III clinical trials.

Factor Xa Inhibitors

In addition to novel oral DTI agents, oral direct factor Xa inhibitors have recently become commercially available, including **rivaroxaban** (Xarelto), **apixaban** (Eliquis), and **edoxaban** (Lixiana). Like dabigatran, these medications are approved for use in prevention and treatment of venous thromboembolism and nonvalvular atrial fibrillation. Peak onset of the direct factor Xa inhibitors are approximately 2 to 4 hours after administration. Their half-lives are typically shorter than that of dabigatran at 7 to 14 hours and excreted through both feces and urine. The pharmacokinetics of these drugs are very predictable and dose dependent, obviating the need for routine therapeutic monitoring. Circulating concentrations of these drugs do not correlate well with standard laboratory testing (aPTT, PT, thrombin time), requiring anticoagulant effect to be measured by anti–factor Xa activity when necessary. A specific antidote is not available for this class of drug, and, because the majority of circulating drug is protein bound, oral factor Xa inhibitors are not easily dialyzable. Animal studies and small cohort studies have shown prothrombin complex concentrates to be effective against rivaroxaban-associated bleeding. Directed antidotes against factor Xa inhibitors are currently in development. For patients with normal renal function, current recommendations suggest discontinuing novel oral anticoagulants (including dabigatran and factor Xa inhibitors) 1 to 2 days prior to elective low-risk and high-risk surgery, respectively, with no need for bridging anticoagulation. For patients with impaired renal function, up to 4 days of therapy cessation may be necessary.

Thrombolytics

Recombinant tissue plasminogen activator (r-tPA, alteplase, reteplase, tenecteplase) is manufactured in exogenous tPA that catalyzes plasminogen to plasmin, thereby initiating fibrinolysis. r-tPA is currently approved for use in acute ST-segment elevation myocardial infarction, acute ischemic stroke, and acute massive PE. Thrombolysis with r-tPA is also commonly utilized for acute peripheral artery occlusion, parapneumonic effusions, and central venous catheter thrombosis. Hemorrhagic stroke or other major bleeding risks are contraindications for r-tPA use. r-tPA is rapidly cleared from the circulation—with 80% metabolized within 10 minutes of therapy cessation. Therapeutic monitoring is not routinely performed; however, bleeding risk while undergoing r-tPA administration can be indirectly measured with serum fibrinogen level (bleeding risk increased when serum fibrinogen is <150 mg/dL).

Procoagulants

Topical Hemostatic Agents

Topical hemostatic agents are commonly employed intraoperatively as an adjunct to control minor bleeding not amenable to electrocautery or standard surgical technique. Physical agents promote coagulation by providing a scaffold that stimulates coagulation and supports thrombus formation. Oxidized regenerated cellulose (**Surgicel Nu-Knit, Surgicel Fibrillar**) products are frequently used as topical mesh placed on sites of bleeding to promote coagulation. Because of their low pH, oxidized regenerated cellulose materials have also been shown to have bactericidal properties *in vitro*. Gelatin matrix (**Gelfoam, Surgifoam**) products are hydrocolloid gelatin created from hydrolyzed porcine collagen. These materials can absorb blood up to 40 times their weight and serve as the foundation of a hemostatic plug. Biologically active topical products, unlike physical agents, augment normal coagulation by providing exogenous procoagulants directly to the site of bleeding. Topical thrombin (**FloSeal, Surgiflo**) and fibrin sealants (**Tisseel, Cryoseal**) are commonly used bioactive topicals that augment hemostasis via directed factor II (thrombin) or fibrinogen application, respectively. Biologically active agents are often used in practice combined with a physical agent (i.e., thrombin-soaked gelatin sponges or granules).

Antifibrinolytics

Aminocaproic acid (Amicar) and **tranexamic acid** (Cyklokapron) are commercially available procoagulants that interfere with normal plasmin-mediated fibrin clot degradation. Aminocaproic acid interferes with fibrinolysis by competitively blocking the fibrin-binding site on plasminogen, thereby preventing conversion to plasmin. Accordingly, Amicar is currently labeled for use in the prevention of fibrinolytic bleeding due to cardiac surgery, congenital hematologic disease, cirrhosis, and malignancy. Similarly, tranexamic acid displaces fibrin from the plasminogen-binding site as well as directly inhibiting plasmin-based fibrinolysis. Tranexamic acid is currently labeled for use in hemophiliac patients undergoing dental procedures as well as in treatment of menorrhagia. Clinically, tranexamic acid is also used in the prevention of cardiac and orthopedic surgical bleeding and has been shown to increase survival following early administration in patients with massive traumatic bleeding (CRASH-2 trial).

Desmopressin

Desmopressin (DDAVP, 1-desamino-8-D-arginine vasopressin) is a synthetic analog to endogenous vasopressin that is used clinically for treatment of diabetes insipidus, nocturia, management of bleeding secondary to hemophilia A, type 1 and 2 vWD, and prevention of surgical bleeding in uremic patients. vWF release is stimulated by DDAVP binding to the V2 receptor on endothelial cells—resulting in increased plasma vWF and vWF:VIIIa complexes. Accordingly, platelet aggregation and secondary hemostasis are improved. Administration can be via intravenous or intramuscular injection, oral administration, or intranasal spray. For perioperative vWD and hemophilia A patients, dosing is recommended approximately 30 minutes (IV) or 2 hours (intranasal) prior to the procedure with repeat dosing based on clinical condition, aPTT, or bleeding time. Uremic patients with surgical bleeding may be treated with 0.3 mg/kg DDAVP intravenously and monitored with improvement in bleeding time. Repeat dosing of DDAVP in bleeding uremic patients is typically of limited utility due to tachyphylaxis related to depletion of intracellular vWF stores.

Anticoagulant Reversal Agents and Antidotes

Protamine sulfate reverses the effects of heparin and LMWHs by binding circulating drug and forming a salt complex with no anticoagulant activity. The ion complex formed from heparin–protamine binding is then cleared from circulation. In general, 1 mg of protamine should be administered to neutralize approximately 100 units of heparin. Serious adverse side effects of protamine include hypotension, hypersensitivity reactions/anaphylaxis, and pulmonary hypertension. Appropriate heparin reversal following protamine administration can be measured with either aPTT or ACT.

Phytonadione (**vitamin K**) antagonizes the effects of warfarin by increasing hepatic synthesis and carboxylation of vitamin K–dependent coagulation factors II, VII, IX, and X. Vitamin K is typically given in either oral or intravenous forms, although intravenous administration is associated with severe hypersensitivity reactions and should be limited to emergency reversal if possible. Onset of action with oral forms is approximately 6 to 10 hours versus 1 to 2 hours with intravenous therapy. For minor bleeding in setting of warfarin use, current guidelines recommend 2.5 to 5 mg oral vitamin K with INR monitoring to ensure efficacy. With more severe bleeding, 5 to 10 mg IV vitamin K should be administered and—if emergent—coadministered with recombinant prothrombin complex concentrate.

TRANSFUSION MEDICINE

Blood component therapy remains a critical component in the management of the surgical and critically ill population. Whole blood donation from normal healthy volunteers is typically separated into two or more components, including red blood cells, plasma, cryoprecipitate, and platelets. Fresh whole blood is rarely transfused in clinical practice due to the availability of component therapies; however, studies in austere combat environments suggest a continuing role for whole blood transfusion in the resuscitation of massive hemorrhage—particularly when component therapy is not readily available. For the scope of this discussion, however, we will focus on individual component therapies and their respective uses and risk. Additionally, manufactured recombinant factor replacement has become increasingly prevalent clinically—allowing precise treatment of specific factor deficiencies or abnormalities.

Packed Red Blood Cells

Red cell concentrates are derived from whole-blood donation and used in the treatment of blood loss and anemia. Each unit of pRBCs contains approximately 200 mL of red blood cell concentrate and an additional 100 mL of preservation solution. The hematocrit of pRBC concentrate is approximately 65% to 85% using a citrate-based solution—which allows storage for up to 42 days at 4°C—and is expected to raise the recipient hematocrit approximately 3% to 4% in the abscess of continued blood loss. Because citrate binds free calcium, plasma ionized calcium levels can fall during transfusion and should be monitored during significant pRBC transfusions. Additionally, oxygen release by stored blood is impaired by loss of 2,3-BPG concentrations during storage, which shifts the oxyhemoglobin dissociation curve leftward. Additional treatment techniques (i.e., leukoreduction, irradiation, or washing) of stored red blood cells may be performed for recipients at risk for complications due to donor leukocyte or plasma interactions. Although storage capacity has improved with the advent of new preservation solutions, recent studies have shown increased complication rates and mortality associated with increased storage time.

Plasma

FFP and frozen plasma (FP-24) is derived from donor whole blood that has been separated and frozen (between −18°C and −30°C) within 8 and 24 hours, respectively. Once thawed, plasma contains near-normal levels of the majority of plasma proteins, including natural pro- and anticoagulant factors. FFP and FP-24 are indicated in the treatment of multiple coagulation factor deficiencies, massive transfusion protocols, and when specific factor concentrates are not available. Current guidelines recommend a dose between 10 and 20 mL/kg to restore factor levels required for hemostasis. Despite increasing clinical use of FFP over the past decade, indications for its use have narrowed due to the expansion of commercially available factor concentrates that, in general, are more efficacious and have a favorable safety profile.

Cryoprecipitate

Cryoprecipitate is generated from controlled thawing of frozen plasma at 1°C to 6°C—precipitating high molecular weight proteins. These precipitatable proteins include high concentrations of fibrinogen, factor VIII, factor XIII, and vWF. Typically transfused in pools of 4 to 6 individual units (10 to 15 mL each), cryoprecipitate is indicated in the use of massive transfusion protocols, hypofibrinogenemia, factor VIII deficiencies (hemophilia A) when factor concentrates are not available, and bleeding associated with vWD when factor concentrates or DDAVP are not available. Like FFP, indications for cryoprecipitate use have declined with the advent of numerous recombinant factor concentrates.

Platelets

Platelets are typically collected from single donors using plateletpheresis techniques and are stored from no more that 5 days at room temperature. Platelet concentrates contain approximately 7×10^{10} platelets per 50 mL, and each unit should increase platelet levels by at least 5,000/μL. Typical indications for platelet concentrate transfusions include massive transfusion, hereditary platelet dysfunction (Glanzmann's thrombasthenia), drug-induced platelet dysfunction, cardiopulmonary bypass surgery–related platelet destruction, and platelet underproduction (liver dysfunction, malignancies, myelosuppression). In preparation for surgical procedures, platelet counts are typically recommended to be above 50,000/μL. Spontaneous bleeding risk is significantly increased with platelet counts less than 5,000/μL, although unprovoked bleeding can even occur in thrombocytopenic patients with platelet counts above 50,000/μL.

Recombinant Coagulation Factors and Factor Concentrates

Individual factor isolation techniques and the manufacture of DNA recombinant coagulation factors have led to focused management of bleeding diatheses and other isolated deficiencies. Isolated and recombinant factors currently available include **fibrinogen concentrate** (RiaSTAP) for use in hypofibrinogenemia, **recombinant thrombin** for topical application, **recombinant factors VIII and IX** for use in the treatment of hemophilia, **vWF concentrate** for treatment of vWD, and **antithrombin concentrate** for hereditary antithrombin deficiency. Of particular note in surgical populations are **prothrombin complex concentrates** (**PCCs**) and **recombinant factor VIIa** (**NovoSeven**). PCC consists of an isolated concentrate containing all vitamin K–dependent clotting factors (II, VII, IX, II, protein C, and protein S). This concentrate is currently labeled for use in emergency reversal of vitamin K antagonist therapy due to major bleeding or urgent surgery. Dosage is based on pretreatment INR, and onset of action is rapid—showing INR decline within 10 minutes of administration and lasting for 6 to 8 hours. Recombinant factor VIIa concentrate is currently labeled for use in hemophiliacs with bleeding or undergoing surgery who have developed inhibitors to isolated factor replacement, congenital factor VII deficiency, acquired hemophilias with uncontrollable hemorrhage, and refractory bleeding after cardiac surgery. Because factor VII is TF dependent, NovoSeven administration activates the coagulation cascade at sites of endothelial injury or increased TF expression—thereby limiting widespread thrombosis (although this is a known potential complication of recombinant VIIa administration). Perioperative dosing in adults with acquired hemophilia is typically 70 to 90 μg/kg, with repeat dosing every 2 to 3 hours until hemostasis is achieved.

Transfusion-Related Complications

Transfusion reactions are rare but can potentially lead to life-threatening complications. Reactions can be broadly categorized into early or late events. Early reactions may be related to product storage conditions (i.e., hypocalcemia, hypothermia, hyperkalemia, dilutional coagulopathy), hemolytic reactions due to ABO incompatibility, nonhemolytic fevers due to donor leukocyte interactions, allergic reactions, bacterial transmissions, and transfusion-associated lung injury (TRALI). Nonhemolytic fevers are the most common adverse event associated with transfusion and can be treated with antipyretics and reduction in rate or discontinuation of transfusion. Rarely, nonhemolytic fevers may progress to cardiovascular collapse. Evidence of a hemolytic process (brown urine output, indirect hyperbilirubinemia, myoglobinuria) should result in prompt cessation of transfusion, repeat crossmatching, and aggressive fluid resuscitation. Onset of dyspnea or acute respiratory distress syndrome (ARDS) within 6 hours of transfusion should raise suspicion for TRALI—occurring with a frequency of approximately 1 in 5,000 transfusions and carrying a mortality of 6% to 9%. The mechanism of lung injury is a result of donor antibodies against recipient neutrophils, which activate an acute-phase response and accumulate in lung microvasculature. Pulmonary endothelial damage from the host immune response causes capillary leakage and fluid accumulation within alveolar spaces. Treatment is mainly supportive and may require advanced mechanical ventilation for ARDS.

Delayed transfusion reactions are typically limited to recipient immune response to donor antigens (immune sensitization) and transmission of infections. Immune sensitization to donor blood is of particular importance in organ transplant populations. Limiting foreign HLA exposure using leukoreduced transfusions can reduce allosensitization risk. With improvements in donor screening, viral transmission related to transfusion has decreased significantly. The estimated current risk for hepatitis B transmission is approximately 1 in 100,000. The estimated current risk for hepatitis C and HIV transmission is less than 1 in 1,000,000 and 4,000,000, respectively.

Suggested Readings

Fawole A, Daw HA, Crowther MA. Practical management of bleeding due to the anticoagulants dabigatran, rivaroxaban, and apixaban. *Cleve Clin J Med.* 2013;80(7):443–451.

Franchini M. Heparin-induced thrombocytopenia. *Thromb J.* 2005;3:14.

Guyatt GH, Akl EA, Crowther M, et al. *Executive Summary: Antithrombotic Therapy and Prevention of Thrombosis.* 9th ed. American College of Chest Physicians Evidence-Based Clinical Practice Guidelines. *Chest.* 2012;14:7S–47S.

Hunt BJ. Bleeding and coagulopathies in critical care. *N Engl J Med.* 2014;370(9):847–859.

Khan S, Dickerman JD. Hereditary thrombophilia. *Thromb J.* 2006;4:15.

Konkle BA. Acquired disorders of platelet function. *Hematology.* 2011;2011:391–396.

Kumar R, Carcao M. Inherited abnormalities of coagulation. *Pediatr Clin N Am.* 2013;60:1419–1441.

Makaryus JN, Halperin JL, Lau JF. Oral anticoagulants in the management of venous thromboembolism. *Nat Rev Cardiol.* 2013;10:397–408.

Maxwell MJ, Wilson MJA. Complications of blood transfusion. *Cont Educ Anaesth Crit Care Pain.* 2006;6(6):225–229.

McGillicuddy EA, Maxfield MW, Salameh B, et al. Bleeding diatheses and preoperative screening. *J Surg Educ.* 2013;70(3):423–431.

Stanworth SJ. The evidence-based use of FFP and cryoprecipitate for abnormalities of coagulation tests and clinical coagulopathy. *Hematology.* 2007:179–186.

CHAPTER 3

Surgical Infectious Disease

REBECCA L. HOFFMAN AND DANIEL N. HOLENA

KEY POINTS

- The toxic properties of gram-negative bacterial endotoxin rest in the lipid A moiety of the LPS molecule. The endotoxin stimulates the hypothalamus to produce fever and stimulates macrophages to release TNF-α, which can result in septic shock.
- Bacterial inoculation of the peritoneal cavity results in (a) *phagocytosis* of the bacteria by macrophages, (b) *clearance* of the bacteria via translymphatic absorption, and (c) *sequestration* of the remaining intraperitoneal bacteria by inflammatory exudates.
- The most common cause of a surgical site infection in a clean case is a break in sterile technique.
- Prophylactic antibiotics should be administered 30 to 60 minutes prior to incision and should be selected based upon the anticipated case classification.
- A guiding principle in the management of surgical infections is source control.

Antibiotic	Action	Mechanisms of Resistance
β-Lactams	Inhibit cell wall synthesis	Bacterial β-lactamase Reduced penetration
Vancomycin	Inhibits cell wall synthesis	Reduced penetration
Tetracyclines Aminoglycosides Macrolides Chloramphenicol	Bind to ribosomes and inhibit RNA transcription	Down-regulation of transport mechanisms
Fluoroquinolones	Inhibit DNA helicase	Alteration of target binding sites

INTRODUCTION

Joseph Lister dramatically changed the practice of surgery with his 1867 landmark document *On the Antiseptic Principle in the Practice of Surgery*. The incorporation of antiseptic techniques had an immediate impact on morbidity and mortality, reducing postoperative infections from 90% to 10%. Surgical infectious diseases include infections that require surgical intervention and infections that result from surgical intervention. An understanding of host defenses, microbiology, antimicrobial therapies, and proper antiseptic technique is required of all practicing surgeons.

HOST DEFENSE MECHANISMS

Barriers

The body has many natural barriers that serve important roles in preventing infection. These include the skin, respiratory epithelium, and gastrointestinal (GI) and genitourinary (GU) adaptations. The *skin* is the first line of defense against infectious disease. It functions as a mechanical barrier against microbial invasion and provides an unfavorable environment for microbial growth with its acidic pH (5 to 6) and relative lack of water. Its constant epithelial cell proliferation allows daily cell turnover and sloughing of both dead cells and resident flora.

Throughout the epithelial surface of the respiratory tract lies a mucous blanket that contains immunoglobulin A. The *mucociliary mechanism* captures inhaled particulates within the superficial mucous blanket resting on the ciliated respiratory epithelium from the larynx to the terminal bronchioles. The mucus is steadily rolled toward the mouth by the motion of the cilia. The regularly beating cilia convey particles and alveolar macrophages embedded in the mucous blanket from the distal airways toward the pharynx where they are expelled by coughing. This process efficiently clears particles by the mucociliary mechanism every 14 minutes. Secretory immunoglobulin A (S-IgA), produced by the lymphoid tissue throughout the respiratory tract, offers additional protection to the host by preventing bacterial adherence to the respiratory epithelium.

The *acidic pH* of gastric secretions prevents the growth of most bacteria in the stomach, keeping it essentially sterile. However, the introduction of antacids compromises this natural barrier, and the stomach becomes vulnerable to bacterial and/or fungal colonization. Aspiration in the setting of gastric pH neutralization may pose an increased risk of developing pneumonia.

The small and large intestines are colonized with abundant bacterial flora, and there is an increasing gradient in the concentration of bacteria proceeding from the small to the large bowel. *Peristalsis* and *a normal motility pattern* keep the bacterial population of the small bowel constant. Bacterial content increases significantly in the colon.

The urinary tract is normally sterile except at the urethral orifice. Urine also contains IgA, which prevents bacterial adherence to the urothelium. The most important natural defense of the bladder in males is the long urethra, which is quite distant and thus protected from the anus. The incidence of urinary tract infections (UTIs) is increased in women because the urethra is short and in close proximity to the fecal stream.

Microbial Flora

Microbes themselves contribute to host defense, particularly in the GI tract. The gut, which is sterile *in utero*, is initially exposed to microbes during birth and during the initial feedings. Thereafter, the GI tract becomes colonized, and the composition of the resident flora continues to changes as the host diet changes. The normal microflora of the GI tract adds to host defense by occupying potential epithelial binding sites, which limits pathologic microbial penetration. This is known as *colonization resistance* or *tropism*. The resident microflora also functions as a physical mycobacterial barrier, which is constantly maintained by rapid cell turnover, the shedding of enterocytes, mucous production, and bacterial growth. The presence of microflora in the GI tract also promotes the development of gut-associated lymphoid tissue.

The distal small intestine and colon harbor the largest concentrations of microorganisms in the GI tract. Bacterial anaerobes (*Bacteroides fragilis*, *Fusobacterium*, *Peptostreptococcus*) outnumber aerobes (*Escherichia coli*, *Enterococcus faecalis*) in the colon by a ratio of 300:1. The total concentration of bacteria in stool is 10^{12} CFU/g, which represents approximately 30% of the dry weight of feces.

Immunology

Phagocytic leukocytes, in concert with the cellular adaptive and humoral immune systems, constitute the host's most formidable defense mechanism against infection. Macrophages, monocytes, and granulocytes initiate the eradication of bacteria and fungi by ingesting these pathogens in a process known as *phagocytosis*. This is the single most important process in the control of infection. Phagocytes in the circulating blood are monocytes and granulocytes (neutrophils, eosinophils, and basophils). Macrophages are differentiated monocytes that reside in all living tissues of the body but are heavily concentrated in the lungs, liver, and spleen. These noncirculating cells are referred to as the reticuloendothelial system. While phagocytes can eliminate microbes independently, they also play an important role in the host's immune response by serving as antigen-presenting cells to T lymphocytes. Circulating phagocytes migrate to areas of inflammation by following a gradient of chemoattractant molecules in a highly efficient process known as *chemotaxis*. At the site of inflammation, opsonization facilitates phagocytic recognition of the pathogenic species. *Opsonization* is the process by which opsonins (immunoglobulins and complement) bound to the surface of microbes, interact with receptors on the phagocyte, and promote ingestion. Disorders in opsonization result in a failure to clear the offending microbe and place the host at a high risk of bacterial infection, especially from encapsulated bacteria. Opsonization and subsequent phagocytosis are the host's primary method of eliminating extracellular pathogens.

Microbes that live inside cells (primarily viruses) are cleared by the host's cellular immune system. Cellular immunity consists of an afferent limb that is responsible for recognizing foreign antigen and an efferent limb that destroys the infected cell. Upon induction of an immune response, macrophages, as well as other professional antigen-presenting cells such as B cells and dendritic cells, process and then present antigen on their cell surface in conjunction with major histocompatibility complex (MHC) molecules. MHC molecules are transmembrane proteins, subdivided into class I and class II, which are critical in stimulating T-cell responses (see Chapter 5). The antigen–MHC class II complex binds to T lymphocytes that express the CD4 molecule and are known as *helper T cells*. Helper T cells interact with the antigen-presenting macrophages and proliferate into a subpopulation of T-cell clones that recognize the specific antigen(s) and amplify the immune response. These cells produce specific lymphokines that promote B-cell differentiation into antibody-generating plasma cells and coordinate the effector arm of the immune response. *Effector cells* consist of monocytes, macrophages, granulocytes, and cytotoxic T cells that express the CD8 molecule. Cytotoxic CD8 T cells can kill virally infected cells by direct contact. Although the contributions of the cytotoxic T cells are significant, the majority of antigen elimination is handled by the monocytes, macrophages, and granulocytes. In this manner, a small number of sensitized T lymphocytes can respond to a microbial invasion, stimulate a large immune response, and eliminate infection from the host.

Humoral responses to infection are dependent on immunoglobulins and complement. *Immunoglobulins* are primarily directed against extracellular pathogens. They protect the host from infection by (a) neutralizing viruses and bacterial toxins, (b) inhibiting microbial attachment to host cells, (c) opsonizing pathogens for elimination by phagocytes, and (d) activating the complement cascade. Five classes of immunoglobulins are produced by B-cell–derived plasma cells: IgG, IgA, IgM, IgD, and IgE. IgM, IgG, and IgA are most directly involved in microbial defense. IgM is the first immunoglobulin produced in the initial response to antigen and is a potent activator of complement. IgG is transported across the placenta from the mother to the fetus and protects the newborn until the 4th month of life and is also the predominant immunoglobulin produced and circulating during anamnestic responses. IgA is a monomer in the circulating blood and combines with a secretory component and an amino acid chain (J chain) to form the polymeric S-IgA. S-IgA acts as a first line of defense against pathogens by preventing bacterial adherence to the mucosal epithelium of the respiratory, GI, and GU tracts. IgA deficiency is the most common immunoglobulin deficiency. Patients with IgA deficiency can present with recurrent mucosal infections resulting in bronchitis, allergies, or GI malabsorption.

The *complement* system is a nonspecific defense system that allows for an immediate response to invading organisms. It is an efficient and self-regulated cascade that requires the binding of only a few molecules of antibody to activate large amounts of complement. The proteins that constitute the complement system are inactivated by themselves, but interaction with antigen–antibody complexes or microbial cell surfaces activates these substances and initiates a cascade of reactions, which ultimately results in cell lysis. The complement cascade can be activated through two separate pathways, which converge into a common final pathway (Fig. 3.1).

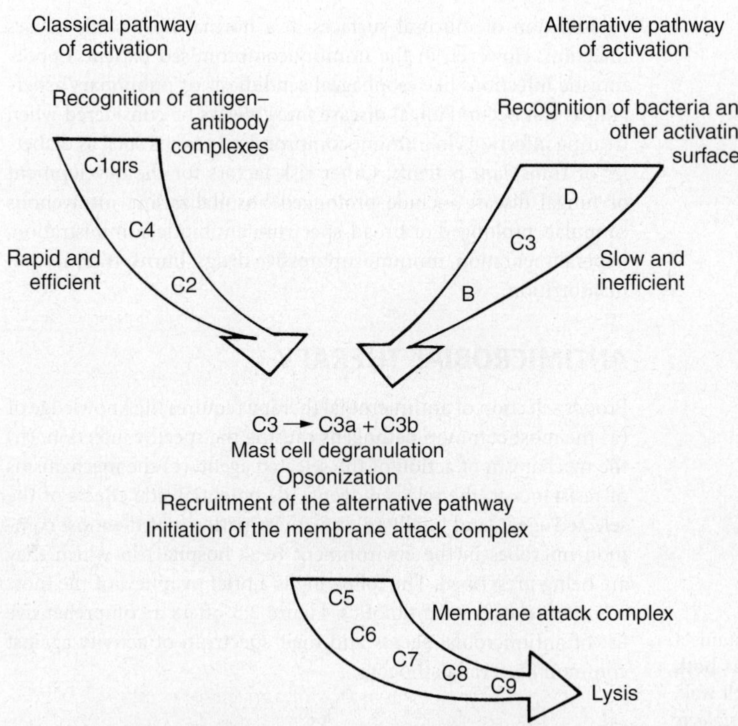

FIGURE 3.1 Pathways of complement activation. (From O'Leary JP, ed. *The Physiologic Basis of Surgery*. 3rd ed. Philadelphia: Lippincott Williams & Wilkins; 2002:179, with permission.)

The majority of microbial elimination is carried out by the phagocytic leukocytes. These effector cells are attracted to the area of inflammation by chemokines released during mast cell degranulation and engulf the opsonized pathogens. Patients with recurrent infections should be screened for complement deficiencies. The most serious is C3 deficiency, which results in recurrent infections with gram-negative and encapsulated organisms.

SURGICAL MICROBIOLOGY AND PATHOGENICITY

Viruses

Viruses are obligate intracellular pathogens composed of a central core of genetic material (DNA or RNA) surrounded by a protein coat (the capsid), which protects the nucleic acid and serves as a vehicle of transmission from one cell to another. Some viruses have an outer membrane (the envelope) that comprises lipids acquired from the host's nuclear membrane. Viruses do not contain any cell machinery and therefore depend entirely upon the host cell to provide the energy and the biosynthetic organelles for viral replication. As the virus replicates, the process continues until the host cell lyses or the virus buds off to infect another cell. Viruses cause disease by cell lysis or by interfering with normal cell machinery to cause cellular dysfunction. One concern during viral infection is the associated risk of bacterial superinfection. This may occur in part due to the impaired phagocytic capacity of virally infected macrophages or polymorphonuclear leukocytes (PMNs) rendering the host more vulnerable to bacterial infection. Viral infections can cause congenital malformations (TORCH viruses; toxoplasmosis, other, rubella, cytomegalovirus, herpes simplex), chromosomal damage (herpes), altered immune function (human immunodeficiency virus [HIV]), and increased cellular proliferation and oncogenesis (HTLV-I). Viruses have been implicated in surgical diseases such as appendicitis (enterovirus), ulcerative colitis (cytomegalovirus [CMV]), and intussusception (adenovirus). Viral illnesses rarely require surgical intervention. One exception is hepatitis B or C infection causing cirrhosis, hepatocellular carcinoma, and end-stage liver disease that may require liver transplantation (see Chapter 13).

Bacteria

Bacteria generate their own energy and contain all the biosynthetic machinery necessary for self-replication. Their structure includes a single circular molecule of DNA, ribosomes, a cytoplasmic membrane, and a cell wall. Some bacteria carry plasmids, which are autonomously replicating strands of DNA that may carry genes conferring resistance to antibiotics. Bacteria are prokaryotes and have no nuclear membrane. They have three general shapes: rods, spheres, and spirals. Differences in cell wall structure determine whether bacteria stain gram positive or gram negative (Fig. 3.2).

The initial step in bacterial pathogenicity is adherence to an epithelial surface. Once attached to the host, bacteria cause disease by invading tissues, producing toxins, or inciting pathologic immune responses. *Streptococcus pneumoniae* is an example of a bacterial species that invades tissue. Other bacteria produce toxins that can be subdivided into two classes: *exotoxins* and *endotoxins*. Protein exotoxins cause hemolysis of red blood cells, white blood cell death, necrosis of tissues, degradation of intercellular substances, and clotting of plasma. Important surgical diseases resulting from bacterial exotoxins include necrotizing fasciitis caused by *Clostridium perfringens*, *Streptococcus pyogenes* (group A Strep), and *Staphylococcus aureus* and toxic megacolon caused by *Clostridium difficile*. Endotoxins are macromolecular complexes of phospholipids, polysaccharide, and protein, which form the outer layer of the cell wall of gram-negative bacteria. *Lipopolysaccharide*

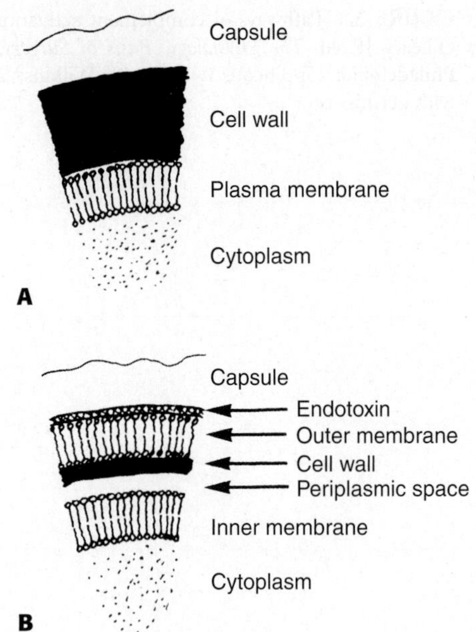

FIGURE 3.2 The wall of the gram-positive organism **(A)** contains a much larger cell wall, while the gram-negative bacteria **(B)** has both an inner and an outer membrane around the relatively thin cell wall. (From Fry DE. Surgical infections. In: O'Leary JP, ed. *The Physiologic Basis of Surgery*. 2nd ed. Philadelphia: Lippincott Williams & Wilkins; 1996:185, with permission.)

(LPS or endotoxin) is composed of a "core" polysaccharide region and a unique "O antigen" polysaccharide region, which are covalently bound to the "lipid A" region. The toxic properties of LPS largely rest with the lipid A moiety of the molecule. LPS induces fever by direct action on the hypothalamus and by stimulating the release of pyrogens like IL-1, IL-6, and tumor necrosis factor (TNF). It can cause septic shock by activating the complement system, causing the release of vasoactive substances, prostaglandins, collagenases, and serotonin, and inducing disseminated intravascular coagulation, platelet aggregation, and thrombocytopenia.

Fungi

Fungi are primitive eukaryotes, which contain DNA in their nucleus and organelles capable of biosynthesis and energy generation in their cytoplasm. External to their plasma membrane lies a rigid cell wall that protects the cell from osmotic rupture. Most medically important fungi are molds. *Molds* are multicellular fungi that form long filaments called hyphae and reproduce by forming spores. *Yeasts* are unicellular fungi that reproduce by budding. Many fungi are dimorphic and grow as either form depending on their environment. An immunocompetent host rarely develops invasive fungal infections. However, there are three main mechanisms by which fungi can gain access to human tissues and cause disease: (a) inhalation, (b) inoculation of the subcutaneous tissues, and (c) colonization of mucosal surfaces. Histoplasmosis, blastomycosis, and coccidioidomycosis are examples of fungal diseases caused by inhalation of spores into the lung. Inoculation of the subcutaneous tissues by spores occurs in sporotrichosis. In this uncommon occupational disease, gardeners who injure their skin with contaminated thorns or branches present with nodules and ulcers on their hands and feet that may require surgical drainage. Fungal colonization of mucosal surfaces in a normal host rarely causes infection. However, in the immunocompromised patient, opportunistic infections like esophageal candidiasis or pulmonary aspergillosis can occur. Fungal disease must always be considered when treating infections in immunocompromised groups such as diabetics or transplant patients. Other risk factors for the development of fungal disease include prolonged hospitalization, intravenous cannulae, prolonged or broad-spectrum antibiotic administration, hyperalimentation, immunosuppressive drugs, burns, trauma, and malnutrition.

ANTIMICROBIAL THERAPY

Proper selection of antimicrobial therapy requires the knowledge of (a) the most common pathogens causing the specific infection, (b) the mechanism of action of the selected agent, (c) the mechanisms of resistance to the selected agent, (d) potential side effects of the selected agent, and finally (e) sensitivity patterns of the most common microbes in the environment (e.g., hospital) in which they are being prescribed. The following is a brief overview of the most common classes of antibiotics. Figure 3.3 offers a comprehensive list of antimicrobial agents and their spectrum of activity against common bacterial pathogens.

Inhibitors of Cell Wall Synthesis

The majority of antimicrobial agents that inhibit cell wall synthesis share a common structural element, a β-lactam ring. The *β-lactam ring* binds to division plate proteins on the bacteria and inhibits cell wall peptidoglycan synthesis, thus inducing autolytic bacteriolysis. Side chains of the β-lactam ring distinguish the agents of this class from one another and are responsible for the variance in their activity. The major mechanism of resistance against this class of antibiotics is bacterial production of the enzyme *β-lactamase*, which disrupts the β-lactam ring.

Penicillin G, the prototypical β-lactam, has excellent bactericidal activity against most gram-positive and anaerobic organisms. The broad-spectrum penicillins (e.g., ampicillin, piperacillin) add coverage against gram-negative organisms. β-Lactamase activity can be overcome by the addition of enzymatic inhibitors, such as sulbactam or tazobactam, to the parent antibiotic. The most common adverse effect of the penicillins is the development of an allergic reaction that can range from a benign rash to, on rare occasions, anaphylactic shock.

The cephalosporins are also broad-spectrum β-lactams, which are classified by generations on the basis of their antimicrobial activity. First-generation cephalosporins have strong gram-positive, modest gram-negative, and poor anaerobic coverage. Second-generation cephalosporins have increased gram-negative and anaerobic activity but weaker gram-positive activity. Third-generation cephalosporins target gram-negative enteric organisms, and fourth-generation cephalosporins have extended activity against *Pseudomonas* species. Fifth-generation cephalosporins retain all the activity of the prior generations but are also active against methicillin-resistant *Staphylococcus aureus* (MRSA). Despite their broad spectrum of activity, all cephalosporins are ineffective against enterococcal infections. There is a 1% incidence of cross-allergic reaction between cephalosporins and penicillins, with the majority of reactions occurring with early-generation cephalosporins (e.g., cefazolin).

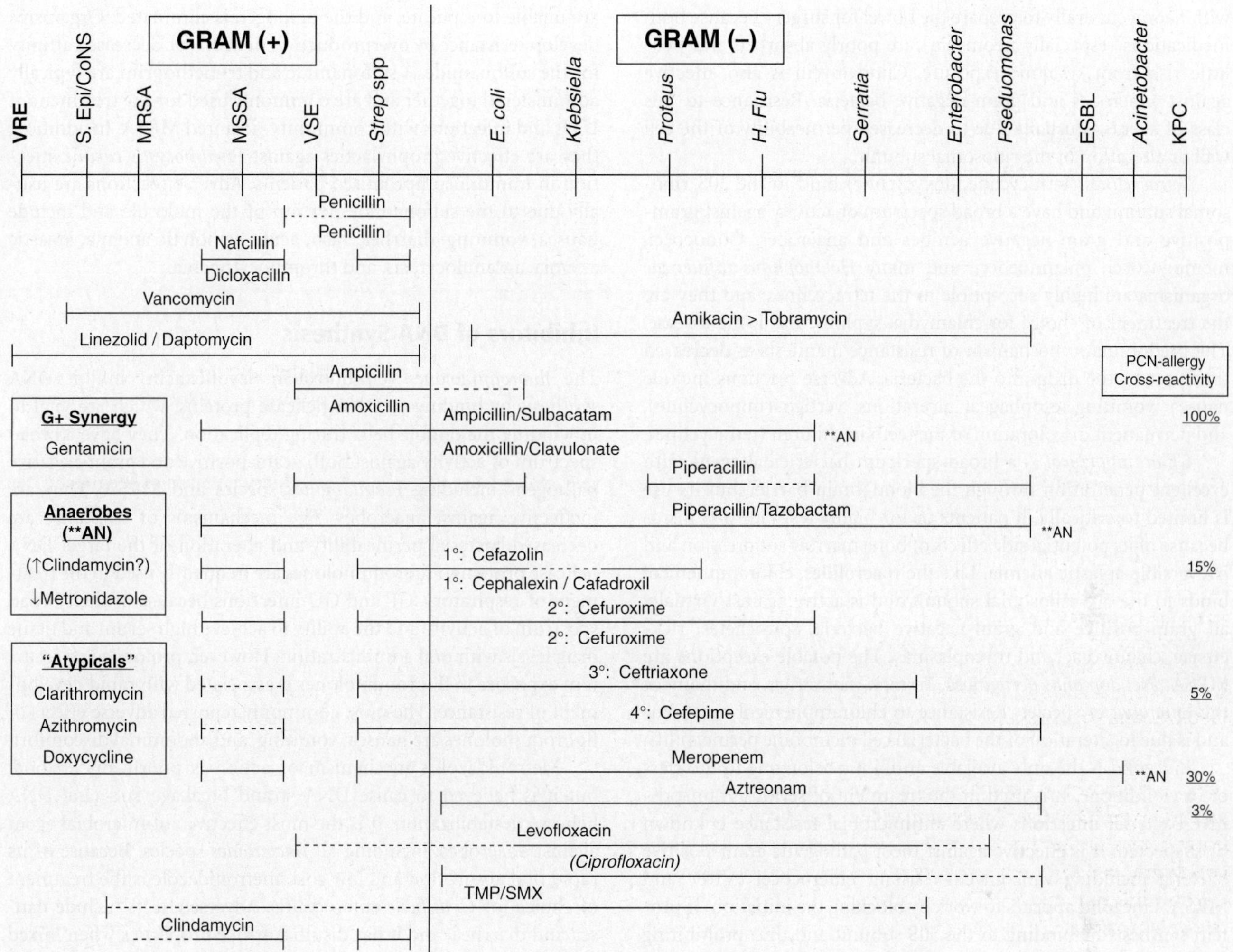

FIGURE 3.3 Spectrum of activity of commonly used antimicrobial agents. VRE, vancomycin-resistant enterococcus; MRSA, methicillin-resistant *Staphylococcus aureus*; CoNS, coagulase-negative staphylococci; VSE, vancomycin-sensitive enterococcus; ESBL, extended-spectrum beta-lactamase; CRE, carbapenem-resistant enterobacteriaceae. **Percentages of MRSA coverage are specific to each individual institution. Numbers presented here represent coverage rates at the Hospital of the University of Pennsylvania only. (Figure courtesy of the Division of Infectious Diseases, Hospital of the University of Pennsylvania.)

Other synthetic β-lactams include imipenem and meropenem, which offer the broadest range of activity (gram positive, gram negative, *Pseudomonas*, and anaerobes) of all antibiotics. Aztreonam provides good gram-negative and pseudomonal coverage and is unique in that it does not pose a danger in patients with an allergy to either penicillin or cephalosporins. Vancomycin does not contain a β-lactam ring in its structure, but it inhibits cell wall synthesis by preventing glycopeptide polymerization. It is effective against the majority of gram-positive organisms and is the treatment of choice for MRSA and *Staphylococcus epidermidis* infections. However, it has poor tissue penetration and may not be an optimal antibiotic for severe pneumonia or soft tissue infection.

Inhibitors of Ribosomal Protein Synthesis

Aminoglycosides, *macrolides*, *tetracyclines*, *glycylcyclines*, and *chloramphenicol* inhibit bacterial protein synthesis by interfering with ribosomal activity. All of these agents are considered *bacteriostatic* except for the aminoglycosides, which are *bactericidal*. The *aminoglycosides* (amikacin, streptomycin, gentamicin) bind irreversibly to the 30S subunit of bacterial ribosomes and are especially active against aerobic gram-negative bacilli, *Pseudomonas* sp., and *S. aureus*. They are ineffective against anaerobes. The most common mechanism of resistance is plasmid-induced modification of the aminoglycoside, which decreases its ability to penetrate the bacteria and reduces its binding affinity for the ribosome. Other less common mechanisms include modified bacterial enzymes that reduce aminoglycoside transport into the bacteria and the evolution of bacteria deficient in aminoglycoside binding sites. The two most common adverse effects of the aminoglycosides are nephrotoxicity and ototoxicity, although these effects are seen mostly with prolonged exposure to high trough levels of the medication.

The *macrolides* (erythromycin, clindamycin) bind to the 50S ribosomal subunit to prevent protein synthesis. This class of agents has a broad spectrum of activity against gram-positive bacteria and cover *Mycoplasma* well. Erythromycin is commonly combined with neomycin orally to prepare the bowel for surgery because both medications (especially neomycin) are poorly absorbed and pose little risk from systemic exposure. Clindamycin is also effective against anaerobes and gram-negative bacteria. Resistance to this class of agents is usually due to decreased permeability of the cell wall or alteration of the ribosomal subunit.

Tetracyclines (tetracycline, doxycycline) bind to the 30S ribosomal subunit and have a broad spectrum of activity against gram-positive and gram-negative aerobes and anaerobes. Gonococci, meningococci, pneumococci, and many *Haemophilus influenzae* organisms are highly susceptible to the tetracyclines, and they are the treatment of choice for chlamydia, syphilis, and Lyme disease. The predominant mechanism of resistance manifests as decreased transport of the drug into the bacteria. Adverse reactions include nausea, vomiting, esophageal ulcerations, vertigo (minocycline), and permanent discoloration of the teeth in children (tetracycline).

Chloramphenicol is a broad-spectrum bactericidal agent with excellent penetration through the blood–brain barrier, but its use is limited to critically ill patients or for highly resistant organisms because of its potential side effects of bone marrow suppression and irreversible aplastic anemia. Like the macrolides, chloramphenicol binds to the 50S ribosomal subunit and is active against virtually all gram-positive and gram-negative bacteria, spirochetes, rickettsiae, chlamydiae, and mycoplasmas. The notable exceptions are MRSA, *Pseudomonas aeruginosa*, *Serratia marcescens*, and many of the *Enterobacter* species. Resistance to chloramphenicol can occur and is due to alteration of the bacterial cell membrane permeability.

Linezolid is the only available antibiotic belonging to the class of oxazolidinone. It is used in the treatment of serious gram-positive bacterial infections where antimicrobial resistance is known or suspected. It is effective against most pathogenic gram-positive bacteria including vancomycin-resistant enterococci (VRE) and MRSA. Linezolid appears to work by blocking the initiation of protein synthesis by binding to the 50S subunit and thus prohibiting the binding of tRNA. While relatively safe over short periods of use, serious long-term adverse effects may include bone marrow suppression, thrombocytopenia, and peripheral neuropathy.

Tigecycline is the first available antibiotic of the glycylcyclines, which are structurally similar to tetracyclines. Tigecycline is a bacteriostatic antibiotic that inhibits protein synthesis by binding to the 30S ribosomal subunit and preventing docking of tRNA. It has broad-spectrum activity against both gram-positive and gram-negative bacteria, including resistant strains of *Acinetobacter baumannii* and MRSA. The adverse event profile is similar to tetracycline and includes nausea and vomiting as well as permanent discoloration of the teeth in children.

Inhibitors of Folic Acid Synthesis

Sulfonamides and *trimethoprim* are bacteriostatic antimicrobial agents, which inhibit bacterial DNA replication by interfering with the folic acid synthetic pathway. *Sulfonamides* are structurally similar to *para*-aminobenzoic acid (PABA) and are readily incorporated into the folic acid biosynthetic pathway. *Trimethoprim* inhibits dihydrofolate reductase, a vital enzyme in the pathway. These agents work synergistically to inhibit the production of folic acid. Without folic acid, bacteria are unable to synthesize the purine bases which, along with the pyrimidines, are necessary to form the backbone of DNA strands (humans get folic acid through their diet, and therefore, host purine synthesis is unaffected). Bacteria are unable to replicate, and the pathogen is eliminated. Organisms develop resistance by overproduction of PABA or decreased affinity for the sulfonamide. A sulfonamide and trimethoprim are typically administered together and are commonly used for the treatment of UTIs and infections with community-acquired MRSA. In addition, they are effective prophylactics against *Pneumocystis carinii* infection in immunocompromised patients. Adverse reactions are usually due to the sulfonamide portion of the molecule and include nausea, vomiting, diarrhea, rash, acute hemolytic anemia, aplastic anemia, agranulocytosis, and thrombocytopenia.

Inhibitors of DNA Synthesis

The *fluoroquinolones* (ciprofloxacin, levofloxacin) inhibit DNA synthesis by binding to DNA helicase proteins, which are vital to unwinding the double helix during replication. They have a broad spectrum of activity against both gram-positive and gram-negative pathogens including *Pseudomonas* species and MRSA. They are ineffective against anaerobes. The mechanisms of resistance are decreased bacterial permeability and alteration of the target DNA helicase proteins. Fluoroquinolones are frequently used in the treatment of respiratory, GI, and GU infections because of their broad spectrum of activity and the ability to achieve high serum and tissue drug levels with oral administration. However, prolonged or recurrent exposure to fluoroquinolones is associated with rapid development of resistance. The most commonly reported adverse effects of fluoroquinolones are nausea, vomiting, and abdominal discomfort.

Metronidazole's mechanism of action is poorly understood, but it is believed to cause DNA strand breakage and fatal DNA helicase destabilization. It is the most effective antimicrobial agent against anaerobes, including all *Bacteroides* species. Because of its rapid oral absorption and low cost, metronidazole is the treatment of choice for *C. difficile* enterocolitis. Adverse effects include nausea and diarrhea, and it has disulfiram-like properties when mixed with alcohol, resulting in severe abdominal cramping, flushing, and vomiting. Despite its frequent use, resistance to metronidazole by anaerobes is extremely rare.

Antifungal Therapy

Amphotericin B, fluconazole, and caspofungin are the most commonly prescribed antifungal agents in surgical patients. Amphotericin B has a broad spectrum of activity against fungi and can be used for the majority of fungal infections. It is a polyene macrolide that binds to fungal membrane sterols to cause cell lysis and is considered the definitive treatment for all systemic fungal infections. It is a potent drug, but it is also toxic, and its side effects can limit its use. Frequent adverse effects at the onset of therapy include fever, chills, nausea, vomiting, and hypotension. Nephrotoxicity is the most common serious side effect associated with amphotericin B and develops in up to 80% of patients. Amphotericin B can also cause anaphylaxis, reversible normocytic anemia, thrombocytopenia, leukopenia, severe electrolyte disturbances, and thrombophlebitis at the injection site. It is also available in a liposomal form (AmBisome), which is associated with a lower toxicity profile but is more expensive. Resistance to amphotericin B is very rare.

Fluconazole is a safer alternative to amphotericin B in the treatment of many fungal diseases. Its mechanism of action is the disruption of fungal membrane sterol synthesis. It is most commonly used for infections caused by the *Candida* species except *Candida*

TABLE 3.1 General spectrum of activity of commonly used antifungal agents

Organism	Amphotericin	Fluconazole	Caspofungin	Voriconazole
Candida albicans	Excellent	Moderate	Excellent	Excellent
Candida glabrata	Moderate	Poor	Excellent	Poor
Candida tropicalis	Excellent	Excellent	Excellent	Excellent
Candida krusei	Moderate	Poor	Excellent	Poor
Cryptococcus neoformans	Excellent	Excellent	None	Excellent
Aspergillus spp.	Moderate	Poor	Moderate	Excellent
Histoplasma	Excellent	Poor	None	Moderate
Coccidioides	Excellent	Excellent	None	Moderate

glabrata (*Torulopsis*). Increasingly, *Candida albicans* is also becoming resistant to this agent. It is highly effective in the treatment of mucosal candidiasis and candiduria and is administered as lifelong maintenance therapy (after induction therapy with amphotericin B) for HIV-infected patients with cryptococcal meningitis. Life-threatening infection by any of these fungi usually requires amphotericin B or caspofungin treatment. Nausea, vomiting, and diarrhea are the most commonly reported side effects of fluconazole.

Caspofungin, an echinocandin, is also a safer alternative to amphotericin B and differs from fluconazole in that it has broader antifungal activity. As with the other antifungal agents, its mechanism of action involves disruption of fungal cell wall synthesis. Because of its broad spectrum and low toxicity, caspofungin is the preferred agent for empiric fungal coverage in patients with severe sepsis or septic shock. The spectra of coverage for the commonly used antifungal agents are listed in Table 3.1.

SURGICAL PROPHYLAXIS

Surgical site infections (SSIs) are the most common nosocomial infections among surgical patients. Up to 5% of all patients undergoing an operation develop infections that result in prolonged hospitalizations, increased costs, and significant morbidity. The majority of SSIs can be attributed to endogenous contamination from the host's resident microflora (e.g., skin and GI tract) or exogenous contamination from a break in sterile technique. Careful maintenance of sterile technique is sometimes overlooked during prolonged or emergent operations. Endogenous contamination of the surgical site is a persistent threat starting from the time of incision until the sterile incision reepithelializes, at approximately 48 hours. There are also patient-related factors that contribute to the development of SSIs, which include extremes of age, nutritional status, obesity, diabetes, and tobacco use. SSIs are classified into three types: superficial incisional, deep incisional, and organ/space, and by definition, must occur within 30 days from the procedure (or up to 1 year after the implantation of a prosthetic device). A superficial incisional SSI involves the skin and/or subcutaneous tissue, a deep incisional SSI involves the deep soft tissue layers such as muscle or fascia, and an organ/space SSI can involve any part of the body (other than the skin and soft tissue) that was opened or manipulated during the procedure.

In 2004, hospitals began collecting data on their rates of SSIs as part of the Surgical Care Improvement Project (SCIP), which defines a set of core measures used to quantify the quality of health care delivery in hospitals across the country (Fig. 3.4). As a result, factors such as the timing, selection and dosing of preoperative antimicrobials, and skin preparation, which have been shown to decrease the rate of SSIs, are now incorporated into the complete preparation of a patient for surgery.

While it is perhaps intuitive that patients undergoing clean-contaminated or contaminated (see Table 3.2) surgical procedures should be treated with antimicrobial prophylaxis, data suggest that the relative risk reduction in SSI is the same in a clean case as the higher-risk procedures. Therefore, the use of prophylaxis in clean cases is justified, but the decision should be based on both cost and the risk and benefits of the therapy. The optimal time of antibiotic administration is 30 to 60 minutes prior to skin incision so that therapeutic blood levels are achieved by that time. Prolonged operations or operations associated with a large amount of blood loss require an additional dose; however, postoperative dosing does not significantly alter the rate of infection and may lead to the development of resistant organisms and an increased risk of adverse reactions.

Specific antimicrobial recommendations follow from the most common pathogens causing an SSI for a particular procedure (Table 3.3). For clean cases, gram-positive organisms such as *S. aureus* and *S. epidermidis* are most commonly responsible, and therefore, cefazolin, a first-generation broad-spectrum cephalosporin, is commonly used as the prophylactic agent for the majority of surgical procedures. If gram-negative bacteria and anaerobes are anticipated in the operative site (e.g., clean-contaminated or contaminated cases such as bowel surgery), the second-generation cephalosporins cefotetan or cefoxitin may be superior. For patients allergic to β-lactams, clindamycin and vancomycin are good alternatives, but they lack gram-negative and anaerobic activity so must be supplemented (Table 3.3). Certain operative sites have higher risks of infections and require additional prophylaxis. Historically, patients undergoing colorectal surgery have benefited from mechanical cleansing of the bowel and oral administration of erythromycin and neomycin to reduce the bacterial concentration within the colon. Recently, there are new data suggesting that mechanical bowel preparation may not significantly alter wound infection rate but may increase morbidity by causing the patient to be dehydrated prior to surgery, although this remains controversial.

Immunotherapy is rarely used to prevent surgical infections, but it is very successful in preventing tetanus. The tetanus toxin

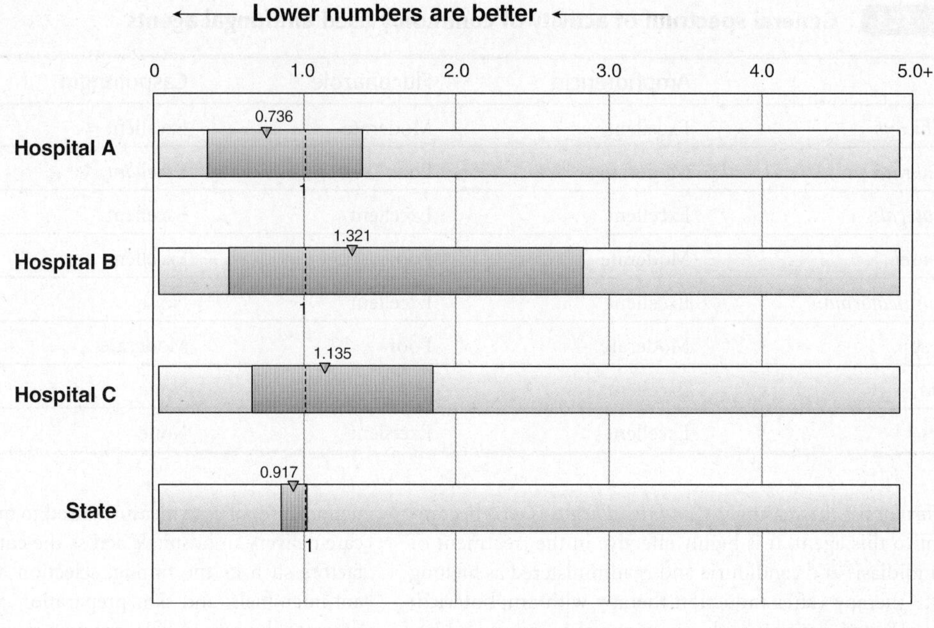

FIGURE 3.4 The rate of SSIs following colon surgery for three hospitals in the United States compared to each other and the state average. Available from http://www.medicare.gov/hospitalcompare (last Accessed January 15, 2015).

is produced by the organism *Clostridium tetani* and inhibits neurotransmitter release, leading to spastic paralysis. After a full course of active immunization (full childhood series or three doses in adults), passive immunization with a booster injection of the toxoid protects adults for as long as 10 years. Patients with dirty wounds should receive a booster injection of the toxoid if their last booster was more than 5 years prior to the current event. It is imperative to ask all patients with wounds about their tetanus immunization history. Patients with unclear or incomplete immunization histories and those who have never received immunization should receive the tetanus immunoglobulin and toxoid booster at the same time in different injection sites.

While there is no evidence that removing hair from skin prior to surgery reduces rates of SSIs, if hair removal is otherwise indicated, clippers rather than a razor should be used. The use of razors is associated with significantly more SSIs (RR 2.09, 95% CI, 1.15 to 3.80). Prior to the application of a sterilizing solution, the operative site should be cleansed with a germicidal detergent to ensure that there is no evidence of gross contamination (dirt, debris).

After ensuring a clean operative field, there are several options for the application of an antimicrobial solution. Most modern antimicrobial preparations contain either iodophores or chlorhexidine gluconate, both of which are bactericidal. Furthermore, antimicrobial agents are available in either aqueous or alcohol-based

TABLE 3.2 Classification of operative wounds and the corresponding risk of SSI

Classification	Criteria	Risk (%)
Clean	Elective, not emergency, nontraumatic, primarily closed; no acute inflammation; no break in technique; respiratory, GI, biliary, and GU tracts not entered	<2
Clean contaminated	Urgent or emergency case that is otherwise clean; elective opening of respiratory, GI, biliary, or GU tract with minimal spillage (e.g., appendectomy) not encountering infected urine or bile; minor technique break	<10
Contaminated	Nonpurulent inflammation; gross spillage from GI tract; entry into biliary or GU tract in the presence of infected bile or urine; major break in technique; penetrating trauma <4-hour old; chronic open wounds to be grafted or covered	~20
Dirty	Purulent inflammation (e.g., abscess); preoperative perforation of respiratory, GI, biliary, or GU tract; penetrating trauma >4-hour old	~40

Adapted from Bratzler DW, Dellinger EP, Olsen KM, et al. Clinical practice guidelines for antimicrobial prophylaxis in surgery. *Am J Health-Syst Pharm.* 2013;70:195–283.

TABLE 3.3 Current recommendations for antimicrobial prophylaxis in selected general surgery procedu

Type of Procedure	Recommended Antimicrobial	Recommended Adult Dose
Cardiac	Cefazolin	2 g[a]
	Cefuroxime	1.5 g
Thoracic	Cefazolin	2 g[a]
	Ampicillin–sulbactam	3 g
Gastrointestinal		
Gastroduodenal with and without lumen entry	Cefazolin	2 g[a]
Open biliary tract	Cefazolin	2 g[a]
	Cefoxitin	2 g
	Cefotetan	2 g
	Ampicillin–sulbactam	3 g
Laparoscopic procedure, low risk	None	
Laparoscopic procedure, high risk	Cefazolin	2 g[a]
	Cefoxitin	2 g
	Cefotetan	2 g
	Ceftriaxone	2 g
	Ampicillin–sulbactam	3 g
Appendectomy, uncomplicated appendicitis	Cefazolin + metronidazole	2 g[a] + 500 mg
	Cefoxitin	2 g
	Cefotetan	2 g
Small intestine, nonobstructed	Cefazolin	2 g[a]
Small intestine, obstructed	Cefazolin + metronidazole	2 g[a] + 500 mg
	Cefoxitin	2 g
	Cefotetan	2 g
Hernia repair	Cefazolin	2 g[a]
Colorectal	Cefazolin + metronidazole	2 g + 500 mg
	Cefoxitin	2 g
	Ampicillin–sulbactam	3 g
	Ceftriaxone + metronidazole	2 g + 500 mg
	Ertapenem	1 g
Transplant		
Liver	Piperacillin–tazobactam	3.375 g
	Cefotaxime + ampicillin	1 g + 2 g
Pancreas, pancreas–kidney	Cefazolin	2 g
	Fluconazole (if high risk)	400 mg
Heart, lung	Cefazolin	2 g
Vascular	Cefazolin	2 g

Those patients with a beta-lactam allergy undergoing cardiac, thoracic, or vascular procedures, and hernia repairs should be treated with clindamycin or vancomycin. Those undergoing procedures involving the GI tract (including liver, pancreas, and kidney transplantation) should be treated with clindamycin or vancomycin + aminoglycoside or aztreonam or a fluoroquinolone.

[a]Dosing should be 3 g if the patient's weight is >120 kg.

Adapted from Bratzler DW, Dellinger EP, Olsen KM, et al. Clinical practice guidelines for antimicrobial prophylaxis in surgery. *Am J Health-Syst Pharm.* 2013;70:195–283.

solutions. Aqueous, iodophore-containing solutions, such as povidone–iodine, have traditionally been the most commonly used skin preparation because of its efficacy and safety on nearly all skin surfaces, including mucosa. The antimicrobial activity of povidone–iodine is limited, however, to the time that the agent is in contact with the skin. On the other hand, aqueous-based chlorhexidine solutions provide a longer period of bactericidal activity after their application. Whereas the application of both of these agents is at least a two-step process, the application of alcohol-based solutions that contain iodine or chlorhexidine is much faster, and their duration of action is much longer (up to 48 hours of bactericidal activity after surgery). Care must be taken to apply alcohol-based solutions only on hair-free areas and to allow the solution to completely dry before applying drapes, as they are flammable. In addition, these solutions should not be used on mucosal surfaces. Despite these limitations, alcohol-based, iodine-containing solutions have been shown to reduce the rate of incisional SSIs threefold when compared to iodine alone and are therefore the preferred agent when appropriate and available.

There are additional precautions that surgeons can take to reduce the risk of SSIs. For instance, if the respiratory, GI, or GU tracts are entered during the procedure, a separate set of instruments should be used and then removed from the field. Everyone involved in the operation should change their gloves after the "dirty" portion of the procedure is complete. Technical aspects of surgery that are known to decrease the incidence of wound infection include obliteration of dead space, removal of devitalized tissue, wound closure without tension, and hemostasis without compromise of the vascular supply to the wound. The presence of hematoma, seroma, and dead tissue supplies sufficient growth media for bacteria to thrive. Although drains were originally designed to evacuate hematoma and reduce the risk of infection, open drains (e.g., Penrose) have been shown to increase infection rates by serving as an entry portal for bacteria. Closed suction drains (e.g., Jackson–Pratt bulb suction) enable the drain tip to remain sterile and have proven effective in reducing infection rates in certain settings. Generally, the presence of any foreign body, including drains, increases the risk of infection, and therefore, drains should only be used when the accumulation of blood or fluid is anticipated.

Not all infections related to surgery are located at the surgical site, yet they are still the responsibility of the surgical team to prevent and address. Catheter-associated urinary tract infections (UTIs) are the most common hospital-acquired infection, accounting for than 1 million cases a year in the United States. Where there was once liberal insertion of the urinary catheter during surgical procedures, the modern trend is toward a minimalist approach to their use. Indications for urinary catheter placement in the operating room include anticipating a long procedure, performing urologic or low pelvic surgery, and the need to monitor fluid balance. The necessity of a urinary catheter should warrant careful consideration, and in most cases, the catheter should be removed at the conclusion of the procedure. If a catheter is needed, it should be placed prior to prepping the surgical site. The easily applied principles of antibiotic administration, proper skin preparation, surgical technique, and urinary catheter placement can have a dramatic impact on reducing the incidence of infections in surgical patients.

SPECIFIC INFECTIONS

The types of infections that are most important to surgeons include those that occur as a result of a surgical procedure itself and those that require surgical intervention. Surgical infections differ from medical infections in that they are usually the result of impaired host defenses, such as injury to an epithelial barrier, or a depressed immunologic response, such as in trauma, cancer, or diabetic patients. In addition, whereas medical infections are commonly caused by a single type of organism, surgical infections are typically polymicrobial and characterized by organisms that are part of the host's native flora. The guiding principle in the management of all surgical infections is source control. Source control refers to the identification and management of the offending cause. This often amounts to the surgical removal or control of the source, such as abscess drainage, debridement of devitalized or infected tissue, and exploration with washout and correction of the underlying problem.

Intra-abdominal Infections

The mortality rate from a serious intra-abdominal infection is between 5% and 50%, so recognition and early intervention is of utmost importance. The risk of death and complications in the setting of an intra-abdominal infection increases with patient age, the presence of a serious underlying comorbidity and poor nutritional status. Intra-abdominal infections can occur following surgical procedures, called organ space infections (see "Surgical Prophylaxis"), or spontaneously. Organ space infections are typically the result of visceral perforations at sites of ischemic or devitalized tissue, anastomotic leakage, or persistent contamination from the primary process. A similar pathophysiology occurs in the case of spontaneously occurring infections in nonhospitalized patients. Common examples of these infections include inflammation and perforation of the appendix (appendicitis) and colon (diverticulitis). Peritonitis, or inflammation of the peritoneum and peritoneal cavity, as a result of these processes, is termed *secondary peritonitis*. Secondary peritonitis should be distinguished from primary peritonitis, or inflammation in the absence of perforation, in that it is first and foremost a surgically treated disease.

Clinical signs and symptoms of intra-abdominal infection include fever, hypotension, tachycardia, severe abdominal pain, and nausea and/or vomiting. Physical examination may demonstrate signs of peritonitis, or inflammation of the peritoneum and peritoneal cavity, such as rebound tenderness, involuntary guarding, or boardlike rigidity of the abdominal wall. In hospitalized patients in particular, the first sign of an infection may manifest as new-onset signs of end-organ dysfunction (such as acute kidney injury). In patients who have altered mental status or are immunosuppressed, physical examination findings may be blunted or absent, and thus, a high index of clinical suspicion is required to diagnose an intra-abdominal infection.

The host response to microbial invasion of the peritoneal cavity occurs by three different mechanisms: phagocytosis, clearance, and sequestration. Following a bacterial inoculation of the peritoneal cavity, bacteria undergo *phagocytosis* by resident macrophages. These activated macrophages release cytokines, which attract additional phagocytic leukocytes (e.g., PMNs) to assist them in engulfing the invading organisms and eliminating them from the peritoneal cavity. The resident macrophages represent the host's first line of defense. *Clearance* occurs via translymphatic absorption of bacteria, fluid, and other particles through specialized structures in the peritoneal mesothelium on the underside of the diaphragm. The bacteria transit through stomata located between mesothelial cells into lymph vessels, which drain into the thoracic duct. The bacteria gain access to the bloodstream when the thoracic duct empties into the left subclavian vein. Clearance of the peritoneal cavity is a highly efficient process that results in bacteremia within minutes of bacterial invasion into the peritoneal cavity. Pathogens that escape phagocytosis and clearance undergo *sequestration*. It is hypothesized that once the mesothelial cells of the peritoneal cavity recognize infection or injury, they produce an inflammatory exudate rich in opsonins and fibrinogen. This exudative fluid forms fibrin polymers that, along with the omentum and other mobile viscera, wall off contaminated enteric contents, seal perforations, and prevent further bacterial seeding of the peritoneal cavity. If the inflammatory fluid and fibrin deposition completely isolate bacteria from the host's phagocytic cells, a cavity is created that promotes bacterial proliferation and results in the formation of an *abscess* (which may manifest as localized peritonitis). In the event that the infection is not contained within an abscess, generalized contamination of the peritoneal cavity ensues, resulting in generalized secondary peritonitis and often, hemodynamic compromise.

An average of four to five isolates usually occur in patients with secondary intra-abdominal infections, and 80% to 90% of specimens contain both aerobic and anaerobic bacteria. Commonly encountered aerobic isolates seen with secondary peritonitis include gram-negative bacilli (*E. coli*, *Enterobacter* sp., *Klebsiella* sp.), gram-positive cocci (streptococci, staphylococci, and enterococci species), and the *Bacteroides* species (especially *B. fragilis*). *Clostridium* and the anaerobic cocci are the other common anaerobes isolated.

The principles of treatment of most serious intra-abdominal infections include either percutaneous abscess drainage or open surgical intervention for source control, hemodynamic support, and the early administration of antimicrobial therapy. The decision to pursue percutaneous drainage versus open drainage should be based upon the patient's clinical state and the presence or absence of an easily accessible abscess cavity. Often, if there is a clearly defined abscess, percutaneous image-guided drain placement results in both source control and identification of the offending bacteria. If the abscess is not easily accessible, or the patient has generalized contamination, open surgical exploration with culture of the peritoneal fluid is often warranted.

Antibiotic therapy should be initiated as soon as the diagnosis of peritonitis is established and should cover a wide spectrum of microorganisms. If the likelihood of resistant gram-negative rod infection is small, then ampicillin/sulbactam, piperacillin/tazobactam, or a second-generation cephalosporin is a good initial option. If the suspected perforated viscus is in the lower rather than upper GI tract, anaerobic coverage should be included. Antibiotics should be tailored on the basis of the results of intraoperative cultures and should be continued postoperatively. General guidelines for the discontinuation of antibiotics include (a) when the patient is hemodynamically stable, well appearing, and afebrile for 48 hours; (b) when the leukocyte count has normalized for 48 hours; and (c) when the band count is less than 3%.

Clostridium difficile Colitis

Clostridium difficile is a gram-positive, spore-forming bacteria that causes inflammation of the colon via toxin-mediated damage to the mucosa. In 2% to 5% of adults, the presence of this bacteria is a normal, albeit minor, component of the host flora. However, alterations in the microbial balance of the host environment, such as that caused by treatment with antibiotics, allow this bacteria to become pathogenic. Even just one dose of an antibiotic may be enough to incite disease. The other primary risk factor for the development of *C. difficile*–associated colitis is hospitalization. Therefore, given the nature of surgical practice, which often includes the preoperative antibiotic prophylaxis, hospitalization, and concomitant management with antibiotics, *C. difficile* colitis is becoming an increasingly important disease to the surgeon. In fact, surgical patients make up 45% to 55% of all patients presenting with *C. difficile* colitis. Surgical consultation to aid in the management of severe *C. difficile* colitis in medical patients is also increasing in regularity.

C. difficile is a particularly virile pathogen for several reasons. First, the spores that it produces are heat resistant and can survive on inanimate objects, often persisting in the environment for months to years. In addition, the bacteria produces an enterotoxin (toxin A), which causes cell rounding and mucosal damage and inflammation, and a cytotoxin (toxin B), which also causes cell rounding. Both toxins A and B are potent stimulators of the inflammatory response. The transmission of the bacteria occurs via the fecal–oral route.

The spectrum of disease caused by *C. difficile* varies from an asymptomatic, carrier state to toxic megacolon resulting in death. The overall mortality rate in patients with a *C. difficile* infection is 23% at 30 days. Watery, foul-smelling diarrhea, which may or may not be hemocult positive, is the most common presenting symptom of infection. In mild-to-moderate disease, other systemic signs of disease are generally absent. In more severe disease, such as that which forms pseudomembranous colitis, the diarrhea may be accompanied by abdominal cramping and tenderness, anorexia, dehydration, tachycardia, and a leukocytosis. This manifestation develops in up to 40% of patients who are symptomatic. Fulminant colitis, manifested by worsening clinical symptoms and systemic toxicity, develops in 2% to 5% of patients despite antibiotic therapy. It should be noted that diarrhea may be absent in some of these patients. Toxic megacolon is the most feared complication of infection with *C. difficile* and is characterized by obstipation, a dilated colon, and severe systemic hemodynamic compromise. Recurrent disease occurs in 25% to 35% of patients.

The most commonly utilized test for the diagnosis of *C. difficile* infection is an enzyme-linked immunosorbent assay (ELISA) for both toxins and the glutamate dehydrogenase antigen (GDH) in a stool sample. Performed together, these tests are inexpensive, have a rapid turn-around time, and have very high sensitivities and specificities (both greater than 90%). The gold standard for the diagnosis of this pathogen is the cytotoxin neutralization assay, which tests for toxin activity. This test, however, is labor intensive and takes 24 to 48 hours to perform and, therefore, has largely fallen out of favor. Diagnosis can also be made or confirmed using endoscopy, which in mild disease shows patchy erythema and muscosa, or in more severe disease, the presence of pseudomembranes. Computed tomography (CT) scanning is most useful in the case of toxic megacolon, where a substantially dilated, edematous, and thick-walled colon is diagnostic.

The effective treatment of *C. difficile* infection requires prompt removal of offending agents (i.e., discontinuation of antibiotics, if possible), initiation of appropriate antibiotic therapy, and in more concerning cases, prompt surgical involvement and potential intervention. Metronidazole, given orally or intravenously, is the first-line antimicrobial therapy in mild-to-moderate disease. Vancomycin is, given *orally* or in enema form, also effective and is used more frequently in more severe cases or in the case of recurrent disease. Typically, these medications are administered for a 2-week course, but a clinical response should be expected in 3 to 4 days. A newly FDA-approved macrolide antibiotic, fidaxomicin, has been shown to be superior to metronidazole and vancomycin in terms of eradicating infection and preventing recurrence. This drug, however, has yet to gain widespread use due to its high associated cost. Antimotility agents should be avoided. Surgical intervention is warranted in cases of colonic perforation or toxic megacolon, failure of medical therapy, or in the presence of severe systemic toxicity, and definitive surgical therapy consists of a total abdominal colectomy with creation of an end ileostomy. An alternative surgical approach involves the creation of a loop ileostomy, intraoperative colonic irrigation with a warmed polyethylene glycol 3350/electrolyte solution via the ileostomy, and postoperative colonic antegrade lavage with vancomycin flushes. This approach shows promise in terms of treating the infection while preserving the colon and reducing the mortality associated with severe disease and a large operation, but level I data are lacking. More recently, the concept of fecal microbiota transplant for the treatment of recurrent or refractory *C. difficile* infection has been popularized. The treatment modality is based upon the understanding that the most basic pathophysiologic principle of this disease process is a disruption in the normal colonic microflora. By reintroducing donor feces, there is near-immediate restoration of appropriate bacterial diversity, and residual *C. difficile* spores are eradicated. Transplant has been shown to be effective in greater than 90% of patients with this disease.

Cutaneous Abscesses

The term "cutaneous abscess" refers to an infectious process within the dermis and superficial soft tissues that is characterized by a semiliquid, necrotic center (pus) and a highly vascularized shell of inflammatory tissue. The pus is composed of debris from local tissue, dead and dying monocytes, components of blood and plasma, and of course, bacteria. An abscess is categorized as a surgical infection because without drainage, the process would not resolve with antimicrobial therapy alone. For this reason, it is important to distinguish an abscess from cellulitis, which is a superficial soft tissue infection with an intact blood supply and viable tissue, and therefore no pus. Cellulitis is treated with antibiotics only. Subcutaneous abscesses may form anywhere, but common locations producing surgical consultation include perirectal abscesses and breast abscesses. A pilonidal cyst is a special type of abscess that commonly occurs at the natal cleft of the buttocks, near the coccyx, and is an abscess that contains hair, skin, and other debris. Hidradenitis suppurativa is a chronic condition characterized by clusters of abscesses and sebaceous and epidermoid cysts in areas bearing apocrine sweat glands (such as the underarms, under the breasts, inner thighs, groin, and buttocks).

The diagnosis of an abscess is typically made with physical examination alone, although ultrasound can be used to confirm the diagnosis and provide additional anatomic information. Physical examination findings consistent with the diagnosis include pain, swelling, erythema, and fluctuance at the site. These lesions are commonly polymicrobial, with the predominant species dependent on location. Abscesses on the trunk, head, and neck are most commonly caused by *S. aureus* combined with streptococcus species, whereas abscesses in the axilla have a greater gram-negative component, and abscesses below the waist often contain mixed aerobic and anaerobic gram-negative flora. Abscesses causes by *S. aureus* alone constitute about 25% of lesions overall.

Treatment of an abscess involves incision of the lesion, evacuation of the pus, and probing of the cavity to break up any loculations. The cavity should be allowed to close by secondary intention from the inside out, as to prevent recurrent infection in the same cavity should the epidermis close first. Gram stain, culture, and systemic antibiotics are rarely necessary in the case of an uncomplicated abscess. When there are multiple lesions, impaired host defenses, severe surrounding cellulitis, or systemic signs of infection (such as fever), treatment with an antibiotic tailored to the offending microbe are warranted.

Necrotizing Soft Tissue Infections

Necrotizing soft tissue infections (*NSTIs*) are the most serious of all soft tissue infections and are associated with a mortality rate of 40% or higher. They typically develop in the deep subcutaneous tissue, superficial or deep fascia, muscle, or any combination of those. Immunosuppression caused by diseases such as diabetes mellitus, malignancy, and HIV/AIDS, as well as exposure to certain medications causing immunosuppression (steroids, monoclonal antibodies), intravenous drug use, and trauma, can all predispose patients to the development of an NSTI. Diagnosing these infections can be challenging, and a high index of suspicion is critical because the classic signs of infection are often absent. The infection is introduced through a break in the skin (e.g., incision, perineal decubitus ulcer, enterostomy), although the inciting event is not identified in up to 50% of cases. Signs of an NSTI may include skin discoloration or necrosis, subcutaneous crepitus, blebs, or a thin, grayish foul-smelling drainage. Often, the overlying skin may have a relatively normal appearance, masking significant infection of the underlying tissues. The presence of gas on x-ray or CT scans of the involved soft tissue may aid in the diagnosis; however, the absence of gas does not rule out the diagnosis. A failure to respond to conventional nonoperative therapy, rapid progression of any clinical signs of soft tissue infection, or a significant change in the patient's hemodynamic status may be the earliest signs of an NSTI necessitating urgent operative intervention.

Surgical intervention is the mainstay of treatment and includes radical debridement of all infected and necrotic tissue back to margins that are grossly normal, as evidenced by the appearance of bleeding, healthy tissue. Patients require an average of three surgical debridements, spaced 12 to 36 hours apart, to obtain control of the infection. Very rarely, amputation of extremities may be required to gain control of this infection. Wounds are left open and packed loosely with a gauze that is changed frequently. These infections tend to be polymicrobial and synergistic in nature, and both aerobic and anaerobic organisms are usually present. Empiric broad-spectrum antibiotic therapy, which includes an antibiotic or antibiotic combination that treats aerobic, anaerobic, gram-positive cocci and gram-negative rods, should be initiated immediately. Often, high doses of penicillin G are included in the regimen to treat *Clostridium* sp. Because of the recent marked increase in the prevalence of MRSA, however, vancomycin should also be given. Gram stain and culture data sent from intraoperative specimens can aid in subsequent direction of the postoperative antibiotic regimen.

Hyperbaric oxygen has been as an adjunctive therapy in the management of some NSTI, but the benefit of this intervention remains unclear. It should be emphasized that the mainstay of therapy for NSTI is early radical debridement with adjunctive antibiotics; delays in operative management for the provision of hyperbaric oxygen are unwarranted and potentially lethal.

Sepsis and Early Goal-Directed Therapy

Patients often come to surgical attention because they are manifesting severe systemic signs of infection, or sepsis, as a result of either a surgical infectious process or an infectious process that has resulted in such severe hypoperfusion that surgical intervention is warranted. The systemic inflammatory response syndrome (SIRS) is the most basic physiologic derangement of the spectrum of diseases that characterize a systemic inflammatory response and includes any two of the following criteria: body temperature less than 36°C (96.8°F) or greater than 38°C (100.4°F), heart rate greater than 90 beats per minute, tachypnea greater than 20 breaths per minute or an arterial partial pressure of carbon dioxide less than 32 mm Hg, and a white blood cell count greater than 4,000 cells/mm^3 or greater than 12,000 cells/mm^3 or the presence of greater than 10% bands. The pathophysiology of SIRS begins with the activation of a cytokine cascade and the elaboration of a host of secondary inflammatory mediators, such as arachidonic acid metabolites (prostaglandins and leukotrienes), nitric oxide (causing vasodilation), oxygen free radicals (causing cell damage), and platelet-activating factor (causing increased platelet deposition, vasodilation, increased capillary permeability, and coagulation pathway activation, which leads to end-organ dysfunction via the formation of microthrombi). The degree of physiologic derangement then defines the more severe levels of disease, such that SIRS+ a documented infection is known as sepsis, SIRS+systolic blood pressure less than 90 mm Hg is septic shock, and an altered function of two or more organ systems is called multiple organ dysfunction syndrome (MODS). Fever, decreased systemic vascular resistance (hypotension), increased cardiac output, and elevated lactate are clinical features of this spectrum of diseases. Of particular interest to the general surgeon is the effect of hypoperfusion on the bowel, as the gut is particularly sensitive to decreases in blood flow. Bowel hypoxia and subsequent ischemia contribute to the overall inflammatory process via bacterial translocation across dead or dying tissue.

Mortality increases with the evolution of this spectrum of diseases, such that sepsis carries a rate of 15%, septic shock a rate of 50%, and MODS a rate of 90%. Factors that predispose patients to this disease include old age, disability, malnutrition, immunosuppression, prior or concurrent antimicrobial administration, renal insufficiency, diabetes mellitus, congestive heart failure, malignancy, the presence of a central line, and respiratory or urinary tract intubation.

While many different organisms can cause this devastating septic cascade, gram-negative bacterial sepsis is most commonly caused by *E. coli*. Blood cultures confirm the diagnosis, but gram-negative sepsis is usually suspected when septic physiology is recognized, especially in the setting of a known source of infection. The tenets of treatment for sepsis are aimed at correction of the main pathophysiologic mechanisms: infection, inadequate tissue perfusion, and a persistent inflammatory state. Treatment targeted specifically to these components is called "early goal-directed therapy." In patients with suspected SIRS, the initiation of broad-spectrum antibiotics should not be delayed. The choice of antibiotics should be based on the suspected etiology, whether the process is community acquired versus hospital acquired and local resistance patterns. It has been shown that when appropriate antimicrobials are considered early in patient's disease course, mortality is significantly reduced. Prompt support and correction of inadequate tissue perfusion is accomplished with the aggressive administration of crystalloid resuscitative fluids (at least 30 mL/kg) to achieve a target mean arterial pressure greater than or equal to 65 mm Hg, a urine output greater than or equal to 0.5 mL/kg/h, or a central venous pressure of 8 to 12 mm Hg. Vasopressor medications are indicated if fluid resuscitation fails to achieve these goals. Of course, source control is the definitive management of sepsis, and a comprehensive effort should be made to identify and treat the process. Correction of the underlying disease process will have the biggest effect on controlling the infection and removing the stimulus that contributes to the inflammatory state.

Nonsurgical Infections in Surgical Patients

Urinary Tract Infections

UTIs are the most common cause of gram-negative bacterial sepsis in hospitalized patients. The presence of 10^5 CFU/mL of urine in a patient is diagnostic of a UTI. Many antimicrobial agents concentrate in the urine facilitating efficient therapies. Culture and sensitivity reports should be obtained, and follow-up specimens should be sent to the laboratory to confirm eradication. Over 80% of UTIs are due to *E. coli*; other common pathogens include *Klebsiella*, *Proteus*, *Pseudomonas*, and *Enterobacter* species.

Catheter and Prosthetic Device Infections

Many patients require long-term indwelling intravenous catheters for chemotherapy or parenteral hyperalimentation. Infection is a major problem with such devices. The most common pathogenic organisms involved are *S. aureus* and *S. epidermidis*, which produce a biofilm that facilitates adherence to the catheters and prevents antimicrobial penetration. Fungal and gram-negative organisms also infect indwelling catheters, especially in immunocompromised patients who have been receiving long-term antibiotic therapy. Optimal treatment of these types of infections consists of device removal and initiation of an appropriate antimicrobial agent. In patients receiving long-term hyperalimentation without alternative intravenous access sites, the catheter may be left in place and treated with a prolonged course of antibiotic therapy. However, sepsis, bacteremia, or fungemia necessitates catheter removal regardless of the circumstances.

Postoperative Pneumonia

Postoperative pneumonia is the most common infection in surgical intensive care units (ICUs). Pneumonia is the leading cause of ICU mortality and is the result of compromised host defenses. Postoperative pneumonia can be classified into three categories: ventilator-associated pneumonia (VAP), non–ventilator-associated pneumonia, and aspiration-associated pneumonia. VAP is defined as the development of a pulmonary infection after the initiation of mechanical ventilation and is classified as early (within 4 days of the initiation of mechanical ventilation) or late (after 4 days of mechanical ventilation). Endotracheal intubation allows the microflora of the oropharynx direct access to the tracheobronchial tree, eliminates the host's natural defense mechanism of coughing, and disrupts the competency of the glottis. The mortality rate of VAP is 40% to 70%. Early VAP tend to be caused by community-acquired microbes (methicillin-sensitive *S. aureus*, *Haemophilus* sp., *Streptococcus* sp.), whereas late VAP is frequently due to nosocomial infection (*Pseudomonas, Acinetobacter*, MRSA).

Non–ventilator-associated pneumonia begins with the development of atelectasis from reduced tidal volumes. Decreased tidal volumes in the postoperative patient are secondary to the lingering effects of general anesthesia, postoperative pain and splinting, and reduced respiratory drive from narcotics. The collapse of airways in atelectatic lung segments impairs the mucociliary mechanism and prevents clearance of bacteria. This leads to local bacterial proliferation in an enclosed space, which can progress into a lobar pneumonia.

The development of aspiration-associated pneumonia may or may not be preceded by an obvious aspiration event. Gross aspiration, commonly due to an altered sensorium and a distended stomach, causes a chemical pneumonitis that places the lung at a high risk of bacterial infection. Microaspiration causes pneumonia in a more subtle manner.

In healthy patients, microaspiration of normal oropharyngeal flora is typically a benign event that stimulates the cough reflex and results in expectoration of the aspirated microbes. Postoperative patients have an impaired cough reflex, and the composition of their oropharyngeal flora may be altered by gastric acid–reducing medications. These medications alkalinize the normally acidic milieu of the stomach, which results in gastric proliferation of intestinal bacteria and retrograde colonization of the oropharynx. In this circumstance, microaspiration may pose an increased risk of pneumonia, as each occult event exposes the tracheobronchial tree to more virulent gram-negative enteric pathogens.

Restoration of the normal host defenses is the key to preventing postoperative pneumonia. This includes early extubation, ambulation, coughing, deep breathing, and postural chest physiotherapy. Aggressive suctioning of the airways helps manage secretions and prevents mucous plugging in both ventilated and nonventilated patients. Aspiration precautions include gastric decompression and an upright position during oral intake. Treatment of postoperative pneumonia consists of the maintenance of the pulmonary toilet by the methods described earlier and broad-spectrum or culture-directed antibiotics.

HIV in the Surgical Patient

The *HIV* epidemic over the past 25 years has created new infectious disease challenges for the surgeon. This blood-borne virus is transmitted by exposure to infected blood or body fluids. The virus infects CD4 lymphocytes and releases RNA and the enzyme *reverse transcriptase*. This enzyme, using the host cell machinery, produces multiple copies of viral DNA (cDNA) from the template RNA. This cDNA incorporates itself into the host's chromosomes, and new virions are produced. Viral synthesis continues until the capacity of the cell has been exceeded and the T lymphocyte ruptures, releasing multiple copies of the virus into the blood to infect other host CD4 lymphocytes. This ultimately results in depletion of host CD4 cells and immunosuppression. When the CD4 count drops below 200 cells/μL or the patient manifests an indicator condition/infection (e.g., *P. carinii pneumonia*, toxoplasmosis, cryptosporidiosis), the patient is considered to have *acquired immunodeficiency syndrome (AIDS)*.

Patients with AIDS often present with abdominal pain requiring the attention of a surgeon. Because of their immunocompromised state, these patients are susceptible to a variety of opportunistic infections and often have uncommon presentations of *common* diseases. In fact, only about 10% of HIV-positive patients have an opportunistic infection as the cause of their abdominal pain. The most common surgical causes of abdominal pain in patients with HIV are bowel perforation, bowel obstruction, appendicitis, and cholecystitis (see Table 3.4).

The most common nonsurgical causes of abdominal pain in the HIV/AIDS patient population are pancreatitis, infectious enteritis/gastritis, and NHL. A less common cause is splenomegaly. The high incidence of pancreatitis is related to the use of protease inhibitors. Enteritis/gastritis is frequently due to opportunistic infection with CMV, fungi, or mycobacterial species. Treatment is based on restoring immune competence and antibiotic therapy. Splenomegaly can develop most commonly as a result of CMV, *Salmonella*, or mycobacterial infection and is present in up to 70% of patients with AIDS but is usually asymptomatic. Splenectomy is indicated in cases complicated by refractory thrombocytopenia (which is not due to bone marrow failure), splenic abscess, splenic infarct with abdominal pain, or hemorrhage due to rupture.

Infectious Diseases and the Surgeon

The operating theater presents the most significant risk for needlestick injuries among all health care workers. In particular, medical students and surgical residents are at the greatest risk given the amount of time spent in the operating room and the relative unfamiliarity with the technical aspects of the procedure and/or the equipment. In 2005, it was estimated that 20% to 38% of surgical procedures in an urban academic hospital involved exposure to HIV, hepatitis B virus (HBV), or hepatitis C virus (HCV). The average risk of infection following an injury is 0.3% for HIV, 6% to 30% for HBV, and 1.8% for HCV, although ultimately these risks depend on the viral load of the patient, and in the case of HBV, the vaccination status of the exposed individual.

In general, the Centers for Disease Control and Prevention (CDC) has identified four factors associated with increased risk of

TABLE 3.4 Common offending agents in the etiology of surgical infectious diseases in the HIV patient

Appendicitis	Obstruction	Enteritis/Gastritis	Splenomegaly
Cytomegalovirus	Cytomegalovirus	Cytomegalovirus	Cytomegalovirus
Kaposi Sarcoma (KS)	Kaposi Sarcoma (KS) Non-Hodgkin's Lymphoma (NHL) Mycobacteria	Mycobacteria	Mycobacteria

Note: Cytomegalovirus may also be responsible for cholangitis.

infection. These include a deep injury, visible blood on the transmission tool, injury with a needle that has been placed directly in the patient's artery or vein, or injury occurring with a patient who has a high viral load or an untreated patient with a terminal HIV-related illness.

The prevention of needlestick injuries begins with following universal precautions, which means treating all bodily fluids as if they were infected with a blood-borne pathogen. Masks, gowns, and gloves should be worn in any situation where exposure may be anticipated. Wearing two sets of gloves in the operating room has been shown to decrease the risk of blood contamination by a factor of 7 to 8. Additional preventative measures include the use of blunt-tip suture needles when closing fascia or muscle, the avoidance of needle recapping, and prompt disposal of sharps into an appropriate container.

In the event of an injury, the CDC recommends washing the area immediately and thoroughly with soap and water and seeking immediate evaluation by health care professionals qualified in the management of occupational exposures. Despite the prevalence of these blood-borne pathogens in the surgical patient population, the increased propensity for trainees to sustain a needlestick injury, and the well-documented policies and processes for handling such events, these incidents are grossly underreported. A 2007 study of surgical residents found that while 99% had sustained at least one injury by their final year of training, only 49% were reported to an employee health service. Yet reporting the injury allows the injured to gain access to appropriate counseling regarding the risk of the exposure, the prevention of secondary transmission (which has implications for significant others and other patients), and may help to alleviate anxiety, as well as to provide the appropriate follow-up testing, postexposure prophylaxis with antiretroviral therapy, and vaccinations, if warranted. A culture of occupational safety is imperative for the protection of both employees and patients, and one should never feel embarrassed or too rushed to take the appropriate steps in the event of an exposure.

Suggested Readings

Bloodborne Infectious Diseases: HIV/AIDS, Hepatitis B, and Hepatitis C in Workplace Safety and Health Topics. Centers for Disease Control and Prevention. Accessed June 22, 2014 at www.cdc.gov/niosh/topics/bbp.

Bratzler DW, Dellinger EP, Olsen KM, et al. Clinical practice guidelines for antimicrobial prophylaxis in surgery. *Am J Health-Syst Pharm.* 2013;70:195–283.

Dellinger EP. Surgical infections and choice of antibiotics. In: Townsend CM Jr, Beauchamp RD, Evers BM, et al., eds. *Sabiston Textbook of Surgery.* 18th ed. Philadelphia: WB Saunders; 2008:299–327; Chapter 14.

Dunn DL, Rotstein OD. Diagnosis, prevention, and treatment of infection in surgical patients. In: Greenfield LJ, Mulholland MW, Oldham KT, et al., eds. *Surgery: Scientific Principles and Practice.* 3rd ed. Philadelphia: Lippincott Williams & Wilkins; 2001:178–202.

Makary MM, Al-Attar A, Holzmueller CG, et al. Needlestick injuries among surgeons in training. *N Eng J Med.* 2007;356:2693–2699.

Pacheco SM, Johnson S. Important clinical advances in the understanding of *Clostridium difficile* infection. *Curr Opin Gastroenterol.* 2013;29:42–48.

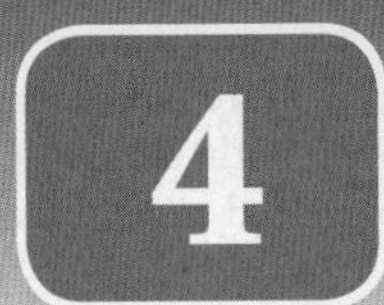

CHAPTER 4

Nutrition, Digestion, Absorption

MATTHEW A. HORNICK AND NIELS D. MARTIN

KEY POINTS

- After 24 hours of starvation or major stress, glycogen stores are depleted and the body utilizes fat as its primary energy source.
- The response to starvation in times of stress or injury is maladaptive and is characterized by hypermetabolism, negative nitrogen balance, glucose intolerance, and lipolysis.
- Given that albumin has a half-life of 18 days, prealbumin (half-life 1.3 days) and transferrin (half-life 8.5 days) are more sensitive indicators of acute protein loss.
- Respiratory quotient (RQ—ratio of carbon dioxide produced to oxygen consumed) reflects substrate utilization at any single point in time: RQ less than 0.7 suggests fat metabolism (underfeeding), whereas RQ greater than 1.0 suggests carbohydrate metabolism (overfeeding).
- Enteral feeding is preferred over parenteral nutrition because enteral feeding preserves gut immune function and avoids central venous catheter–associated complications.

DIGESTION AND ABSORPTION

Mouth and Pharynx

Mechanical digestion begins in the mouth through gross breakdown of food by the teeth and tongue. Chemical digestion of food also begins in the mouth as food mixes with saliva containing α-amylase, RNase, DNase, lysozyme, peroxidase, and lingual lipase.

Saliva begins as an isotonic solution secreted by the acinar cells and is chemically altered along its course through the salivary ducts. The ductal cells absorb sodium and chloride and, to a lesser extent, secrete potassium and bicarbonate, with the degree of ion exchange determined by the transit time of the saliva within the ducts. Slower rates increase exchange, producing hypotonic saliva rich in potassium and bicarbonate. Regulation of salivary production and flow is controlled by the autonomic nervous system with norepinephrine and acetylcholine as the two main agonists (Fig. 4.1).

The mouth and pharynx initiate the act of swallowing. During the oral or voluntary phase of swallowing, the tongue propels the food bolus toward the hypopharynx. Tactile receptors coordinate the transition to the pharyngeal phase as the bolus moves into the esophagus, with respiration reflexively inhibited. The soft palate moves upward to prevent entry into the nasopharynx, and the epiglottis covers the opening of the larynx to prevent aspiration into the trachea. Contraction of the superior pharyngeal muscles propels the bolus past the upper esophageal sphincter (UES) as it relaxes. Failure of UES relaxation elevates intrapharyngeal pressure and can lead to the formation of a *Zenker diverticulum*. During the esophageal phase of swallowing, the bolus passes beyond the UES into the esophagus and is propelled toward the stomach by peristaltic waves (Fig. 4.2).

Esophagus

The esophagus is a muscular conduit that connects the oropharynx to the stomach, functioning primarily to transport the food bolus. Measuring approximately 25 to 30 cm in length, the esophagus begins at the level of the cricoid cartilage and ends at the level of the 11th thoracic vertebra. The esophageal lumen is lined predominantly by

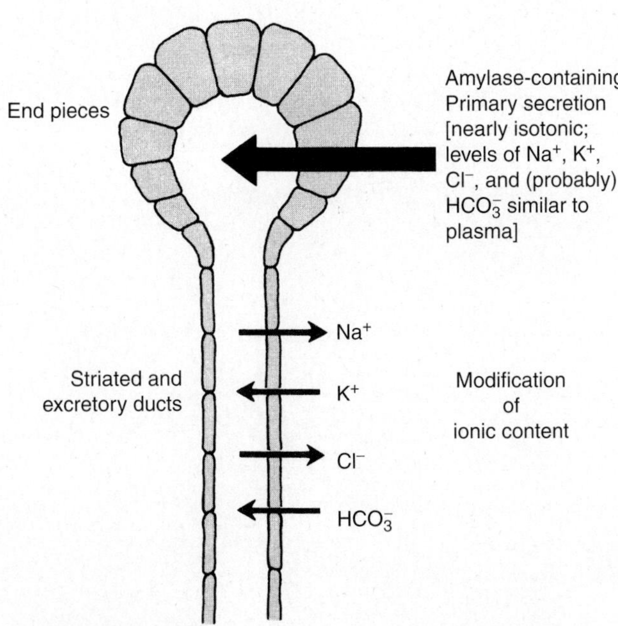

FIGURE 4.1 Salivary secretion. (From Berne RM, Levy MN, eds. *Physiology*. 2nd ed. St. Louis: Mosby; 1988, with permission.)

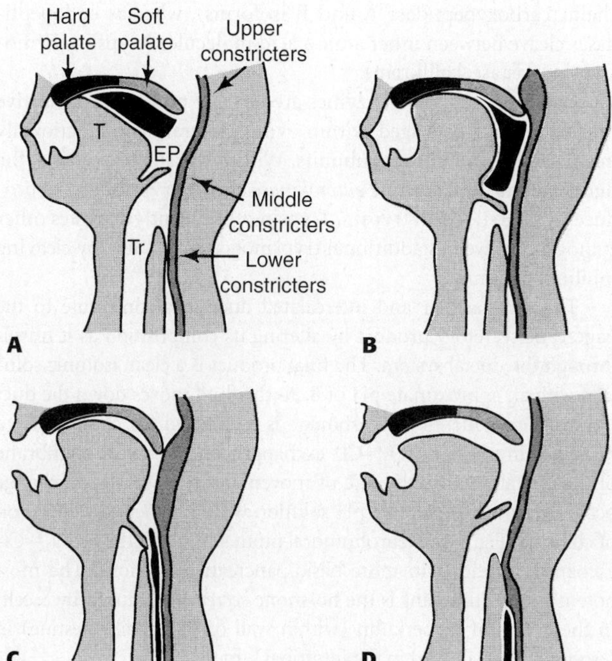

FIGURE 4.2 The oral and pharyngeal phases of swallowing involve the (**A**) separation of the bolus of food between the tongue and the soft and hard palate and (**B**) advancement of the bolus into the oropharynx. As respiration is inhibited, the bolus of food is propelled through the (**C**) pharynx by the sequential peristalsis of the superior, middle, and inferior constrictor muscles and advanced into the (**D**) upper esophagus, initiating the esophageal phase of swallowing. (From Johnson LR. Motility. In: Johnson LR, ed. *Essential Medical Physiology*. Philadelphia: Lippincott–Raven Publishers; 1999:432, with permission.)

squamous epithelium, except for the most distal aspect, which is lined by junctional columnar cells. The muscular layer is heterogeneous along its length—the proximal third consists of voluntary striated muscle, whereas the distal two thirds consists of involuntary smooth muscle. Unique to the esophagus is the absence of an outer serosal layer.

During the act of swallowing, the UES relaxes to allow passage of the food bolus, and a primary peristaltic wave propels the bolus toward the stomach. Smooth muscle cells are stimulated by local distention and will continue to initiate waves until the food bolus passes through the lower esophageal sphincter (LES) and into the stomach. The LES is a high-pressure zone situated between the positive-pressure intra-abdominal cavity and the negative-pressure intra-thoracic cavity, serving as a functional sphincter and barrier against regurgitation of gastric contents. Tonic contraction is regulated by vagal cholinergic innervation. Several substances have been shown to decrease local LES tone, including atropine, caffeine, isoproterenol, secretin, calcium channel blockers, tobacco, ethanol, and prostaglandin E_2. Decreased LES tone may manifest as gastroesophageal reflux disease, whereas increased tone may play a role in the development of achalasia.

Stomach

The stomach is a reservoir where mechanical digestion continues to completion in preparation for delivery to the small intestine. Anatomically, the stomach can be divided into three main sections. The cardia is located just distal to the gastroesophageal junction and contains no acid-secreting parietal cells. The corpus, or body, is responsible for the storage of chyme, and its proximal portion is called the fundus. The antrum is the distal portion of the stomach, responsible for proper emptying of chyme into the intestine. The cardia and fundus are covered by columnar epithelium and gastric pits, which are lined by a variety of cell types. Mucous cells in the neck of the pits produce a protective coat of mucus that shields the gastric epithelium from the acidic intraluminal environment. *Parietal cells* and *chief cells* deeper within the pits secrete acid and pepsinogen, respectively. Additionally, parietal cells secrete intrinsic factor, a protein required for vitamin B_{12} absorption in the distal ileum. The antral epithelium is dominated by mucus cells and gastrin-secreting G cells (Fig. 4.3).

Gastric relaxation is triggered by the act of swallowing via a vagally mediated parasympathetic feedback loop called the *vasovagal reflex*. When receiving the food bolus, relaxation of the proximal stomach and LES allows for an increase in gastric volume without a proportional increase in pressure. The enteric nervous system (ENS) contributes by stimulating active dilation of the fundus in response to gastric distention, termed "gastric accommodation." Once the bolus enters the stomach, it is churned vigorously into chyme. Ingested nutrients are dissolved and solubilized to facilitate enzymatic digestion.

Although the majority of enzymatic digestion occurs in the small bowel, protein breakdown is initiated in the stomach by *pepsinogens*, a group of aspartic proteinases secreted by chief cells as zymogens. Pepsinogen secretion is stimulated primarily by (1) acetylcholine, released as a vagal reflex in response to declining pH,

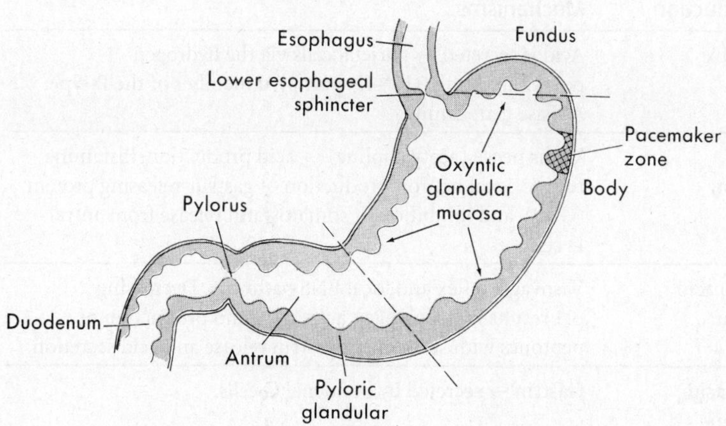

FIGURE 4.3 The stomach. (From Berne RM, Levy MN, eds. *Physiology*. 2nd ed. St. Louis: Mosby; 1988:633, with permission.)

and (2) gastrin, secreted by antral G cells in response to the presence of amino acids. Secretin and cholecystokinin (CCK), produced by duodenal S cells and I cells, respectively, also stimulate pepsinogen release. Activation of pepsinogens occurs by spontaneous cleavage of the *N*-terminus fragment when gastric pH is between 1.8 and 3.5.

The stomach provides a uniquely acidic environment (Table 4.1) that serves as a barrier to pathogens and regulates digestion by activating enzymes and signaling the production of hormones. Acid is secreted by parietal cells via the hydrogen–potassium pump (H^+–K^+ pump), a member of the P-type ATPase gene family. The three acid secretagogues are acetylcholine, gastrin, and histamine, which bind to their respective receptors on the parietal cell membrane and function synergistically through a G protein–coupled pathway. Acetylcholine and gastrin also act indirectly via histamine release from enterochromaffin-like (ECL) cells in the lamina propria.

Inhibition of acid secretion is accomplished by a negative feedback loop. The delivery of acid, lipids, and hyperosmolar solution to the duodenum results in production of somatostatin by D cells, which inhibits release of antral gastrin and down-regulates parietal cell H^+–K^+ pump activity. Duodenal enteroendocrine cells release CCK and gastrin inhibitory protein (GIP), both of which inhibit acid secretion directly.

Pancreas

The pancreas is a retroperitoneal endocrine gland embraced by a C-shaped loop of the duodenum. It weighs on average between 75 and 125 g and manufactures a vast majority of digestive enzymes, delivered to the duodenum through a branched ductal system. The functional unit of the exocrine pancreas is the acinus, which consists of 15 to 100 acinar cells surrounding the proximal end of a small intercalated duct. The ducts secrete a bicarbonate-rich solution that neutralizes the acidic chyme. The ductal system eventually coalesces into the main pancreatic duct (Wirsung) and the accessory duct (Santorini).

The pancreas generates over 1.5 L of enzyme-rich fluid each day (Table 4.2), containing approximately 20 different zymogens. These enzymes are classified by their substrates and include proteases, amylases, lipases, and nucleases. Proteases are further classified by their location of cleavage within the substrate protein molecule: exopeptidases cleave protein molecules at the end of the amino acid chain (carboxypeptidase A and B isoforms), whereas endopeptidases cleave between inner amino acid molecules (trypsin, chymotrypsin, elastase, kallikrein).

Pancreatic digestive enzymes are initially produced as inactive precursors and packaged within zymogen granules, functionally inactivated by inhibitory subunits. Within the small intestine, the duodenal mucosal enzyme *enterokinase* cleaves trypsinogen to produce its catalytic form trypsin. Trypsin subsequently activates other zymogens, as well as additional trypsinogen molecules, by cleaving inhibitory subunits.

The centroacinar and intercalated duct cells contribute to the pancreatic secretory product by altering its composition as it travels through the ductal system. The final product is a clear, isotonic solution with an approximate pH of 8. As the fluid moves down the duct toward the duodenum, bicarbonate is exchanged for chloride via a protein pump, the HCO_3^-–Cl^- exchanger, on the apical membrane of the ductal cells. As the rate of movement increases, less exchange occurs, resulting in a lower pH solution with a higher concentration of chloride (Fig. 4.4). Neurohumoral input stimulates the HCO_3^-–Cl^- exchanger, resulting in more basic pancreatic secretions. The most potent pump stimulant is the hormone *secretin*, produced by S cells in the crypts of Lieberkühn (within wall of the small intestine) in response to bile or acid in the intestinal lumen.

Biliary System

Enzymatic digestion and intestinal absorption are dependent on solubilization and dissolution of ingested nutrients into a hydrophilic solution. Bile is a mixture of phospholipids, salts, cholesterol, and pigments, which functions to dissolve fat through organization into micelles, making them vulnerable to lipases. As bile passes through the canaliculi and bile ducts of the liver, it is altered by the addition of bicarbonate, a process augmented by exposure to secretin.

After entering the gallbladder, bile is further concentrated 10- to 20-fold. This process affects the solubility of calcium and cholesterol, sometimes inducing precipitation and stone formation. The gallbladder epithelium secretes mucus glycoproteins that form a protective barrier against the detergent effects of bile salt. Hydrogen ions are also secreted to acidify the solution and increase calcium solubility. While fasting, the gallbladder is filled by tonic contraction of the ampullary sphincter with periods of relaxation

TABLE 4.1 Four phases of gastric acid secretion

Secretory Phase	Stimulus	Acid production	Mechanisms
Basal	Interdigestive	Constitutive	Acid is secreted by parietal cells via the hydrogen–potassium pump (H^+–K^+ pump), a member of the P-type ATPase gene family.
Cephalic	Senses (i.e., taste, smell), swallowing	30% acid production	Vagus nerve (acetylcholine) → acid production, histamine release, local neuron production of gastrin-releasing protein (GRP), and inhibition of somatostatin release from antral D cells.
Gastric	Gastric distention/ peptones	50%–60% acid production	Vasovagal reflex and local ENS pathways. Decreasing pH results in pepsinogen activation and production of peptones with subsequent gastrin release and acid secretion.
Intestinal	Duodenal peptones/ amino acids	5%–10% acid production	Gastrin → secreted by duodenal G cells.

TABLE 4.2 **Pancreatic secretory phases**

Secretory phase	Stimulus	Mechanism
Cephalic	Senses (i.e., taste, smell)	Modest increase in fluid and electrolyte production, but largely enhances enzyme secretion.
Gastric	Gastric distention	Enzymatic secretion modulated by release of hormones, neural mediation, altered pH, and the delivery of nutrients to the proximal intestine (peptide-induced gastrin release and the vasovagal reflex initiated by gastric distention).
Intestinal	Chyme within duodenum	Secretin, CCK, vasovagal enteropancreatic reflex. "Liquid meal" elicits about 60% of the maximum secretory potential; solid meal → results in a prolonged pancreatic response. Long-chain fatty acids elicit the strongest response.

CCK, cholecystokinin.

and partial emptying. During digestion, *cholecystokinin (CCK)* is released from the duodenal mucosa and stimulates the gallbladder to contract while simultaneously relaxing the sphincter of Oddi. Within 30 to 40 minutes, 50% to 70% of the gallbladder's contents pass into the duodenum. Ninety-five percent of secreted bile is ultimately actively absorbed by the terminal ileum. It is carried through the portal blood by albumin and lipoprotein to the liver where it is extracted and reused. Bile that enters the colon is deconjugated

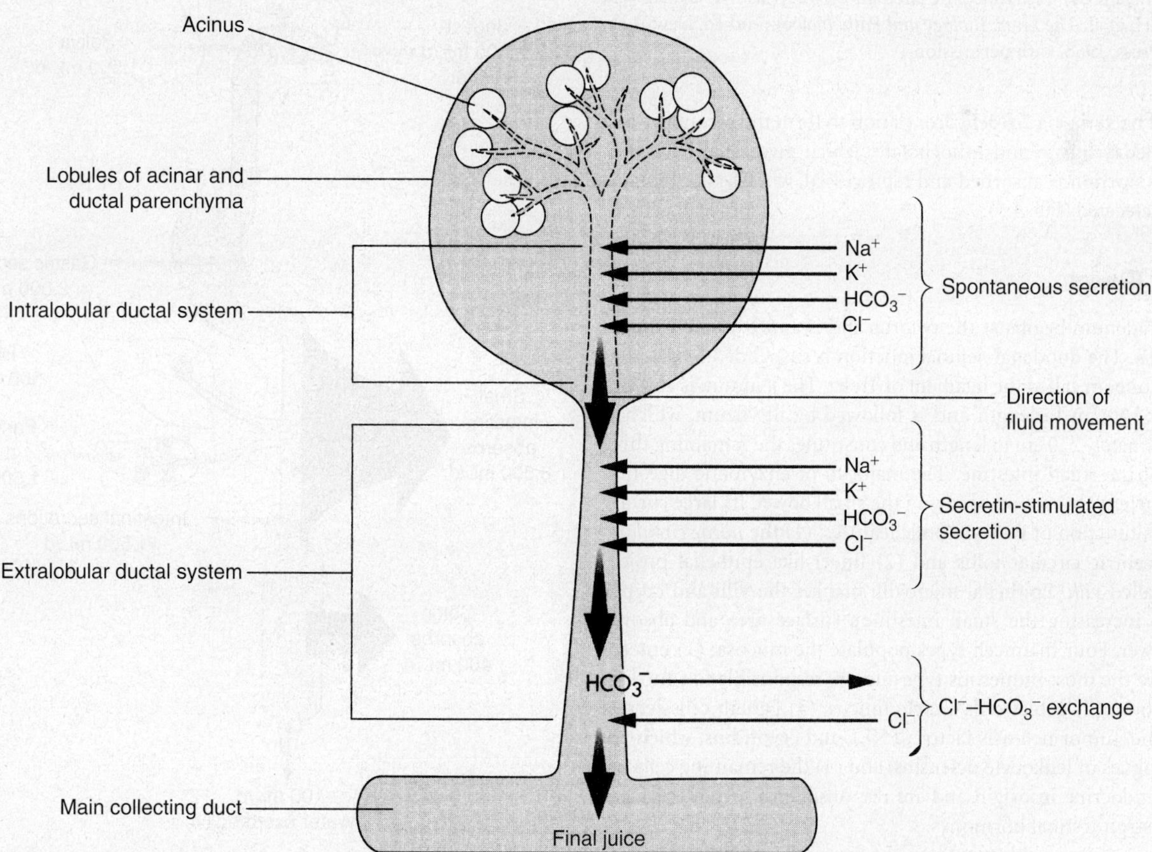

FIGURE 4.4 Pancreatic secretion. (From Savage E, Fishman S, Miller L. *Essentials of Basic Science in Surgery.* Philadelphia: J.B. Lippincott; 1993:189, with permission.)

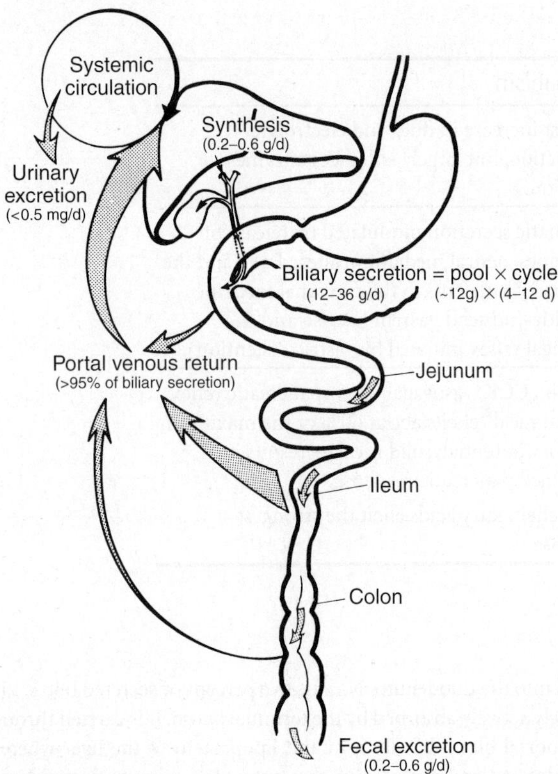

FIGURE 4.5 Enterohepatic circulation of bile acids. (From Carey MC, Cahalane MJ. Enterohepatic circulation. In: Arias IM, Jakoby WB, Popper H, et al. *The Liver: Biology and Pathobiology.* 2nd ed. New York: Raven Press; 1988, with permission.)

by local bacteria via 7α-dehydroxylation to form the secondary bile acids, deoxycholate and lithocholate, which give stool its brown color. A portion is absorbed and reprocessed, whereas the remainder is defecated (Fig. 4.5).

Small Bowel

The duodenum begins at the pylorus and is approximately 20 cm in length. The duodenal–jejunal junction is suspended by a strand of peritoneum called the ligament of Treitz. The jejunum is approximately 150 cm in length and is followed by the ileum, which is approximately 250 cm in length and constitutes the remaining three fifths of the small intestine. The majority of enzymatic digestion and nutrient absorption occurs in the small bowel. Its large surface area is a function of two anatomic features: (1) the *plicae circulares* or concentric circular folds and (2) finger-like epithelial projections called *villi.* Epithelial microvilli blanket the villi and crypts, further increasing the small intestine's surface area and absorptive power. Four main cell types populate the mucosa: (1) enterocytes are the most numerous type and are responsible for nutrient absorption; (2) goblet cells secrete mucus; (3) Paneth cells secrete lysozyme, tumor necrosis factor (TNF), and cryptidins, which are homologues of leukocyte defensins; and (4) the remaining cells are enteroendocrine in origin and are responsible for producing specific gastrointestinal hormones.

The semipermeable membrane of the small intestine is ideal for both secretion and absorption of simple molecules such as water, carbohydrates, lipids, proteins, minerals, and vitamins. Approximately 9 L of fluid pass through the small intestine each day (approximately 7 L of which is endogenously secreted), with only 500 to 1,000 mL reaching the cecum (Fig. 4.6). Water absorption is generally coupled to the movement of solutes and nutrients, which occurs via passive diffusion, solvent drag, and active transport. Passive diffusion is the energy-free movement of electrolytes down an electrochemical gradient (through a membrane channel or between cells) and occurs mostly in the jejunum. Solvent drag is the coupling of solute absorption to the movement of water across the membrane. Active transport is an energy-dependent mechanism that moves simple molecules against an electrochemical gradient created by the sodium–potassium ATPase pump. In an ATP-dependent process, this pump exchanges sodium and potassium across the basolateral membrane (against their respective concentration gradients), creating an electrochemical gradient that enables sodium and chloride to move intracellularly (with water following) in exchange for potassium and bicarbonate.

Colon

The colon, measuring approximately 1.5 m in length, is responsible for water and electrolyte absorption, as well as the storage and elimination of nonabsorbable fecal material. Approximately 1,000 mL of chyme reaches the cecum each day, of which only about 100 to 200 mL is defecated. As in the small intestine, the

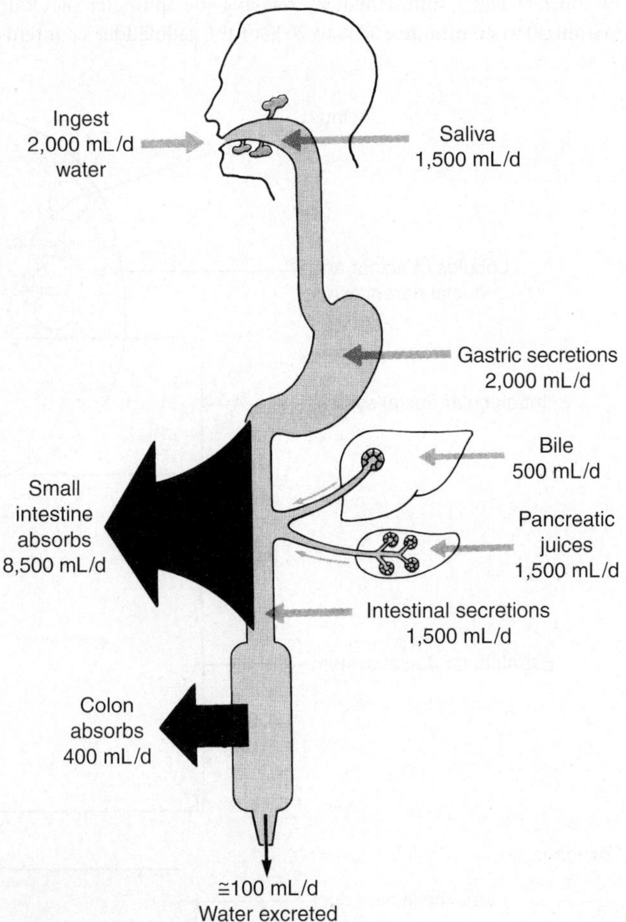

FIGURE 4.6 Fluid balance in the gastrointestinal tract. (From Berne RM, Levy MN, eds. *Physiology.* 2nd ed. St. Louis: Mosby; 1988:633, with permission.)

sodium–potassium ATPase pump plays a critical role in water and electrolyte absorption.

NUTRITION AND METABOLISM

Protein

Nonessential amino acids are synthesized endogenously, whereas *essential amino acids* must be obtained exogenously from the diet because they cannot be synthesized. Amino acids are utilized in both protein synthesis and energy-producing catabolic reactions. It is important to note that protein is an inefficient energy source, in that the degradation of protein yields only 25% of the energy required for its synthesis.

The protein requirement for an average healthy adult is approximately 0.8 g/kg/d, with each gram of protein yielding 4 kcal of energy (Table 4.3). In an acutely ill patient, the requirement may be substantially higher because of protein wasting. *Nitrogen balance* is calculated by subtracting nitrogen output, or the sum of all nitrogen found in excretions and secretions (urine, feces, or fistula drainage), from nitrogen intake, or the sum of all nitrogen entering the body via enteral and parenteral means. Nitrogen output can be estimated by measuring urea nitrogen excreted in a 24-hour period, with the addition of a correction factor (4 g per 24 hours) to approximate insensible nonurea urinary nitrogen and fecal losses. Additional correction factors can be used to estimate nitrogen output from other sources such as fistulas. One gram of nitrogen is equivalent to 6.25 g of protein.

$$\textit{Nitrogen balance} = (\text{protein intake in grams} / 6.25) - (\text{urinary urea nitrogen} + 4\text{ g})$$

In general, a positive nitrogen balance suggests an anabolic state, whereas a negative nitrogen balance suggests catabolism or protein wasting. Most healthy individuals have a nitrogen balance in relative equilibrium. Avoiding negative nitrogen balance is a central tenet of many perioperative nutrition paradigms.

Carbohydrates

Glucose fuels the vast majority of metabolic processes. Red blood cells (RBCs) and white blood cells require glucose because of their limited cellular machinery, and the brain prefers glucose as its energy source (but can adapt to other fuel sources over time). Glucose oxidation yields approximately 3.4 kcal of energy per gram of substrate (Table 4.3). After absorption by the intestine, glucose can be immediately oxidized, stored as glycogen in muscle and liver cells, or converted into fat if glycogen stores are replete. Once glucose enters the cell, it is phosphorylated to glucose-6-phosphate (G6P) and thereby confined to the cytosol. In conditions of excess, G6P is polymerized into glycogen via glycogen synthetase in muscle and liver cells. In conditions of need, only glycogen stored in the liver can be utilized systemically, because hepatocytes alone are able to dephosphorylate G6P to form glucose, which can readily leave the cell.

Lipids

Lipids are essential nutrients that constitute the most efficient energy reserve, with the oxidation of 1 g of fat yielding 9 kcal of energy (Table 4.3). Heart, liver, and skeletal muscle rely on fatty acids as a major fuel source. Lipids are also processed into important structures such as cell membranes and myelin sheaths around axons.

The storage of energy as fat begins with fatty acid synthesis in the cell cytosol. Lipids are stored in adipose cells as triglyceride molecules consisting of a glycerol backbone with three covalently bound fatty acids. When glycogen stores are depleted, triglycerides are broken down via lipolysis, and fatty acid molecules are oxidized for energy. Fatty acids are combined with coenzyme A (CoA) and adenosine triphosphate (ATP) to yield fatty acyl-CoA, which undergoes beta-oxidation to generate a two-carbon acetyl-CoA molecule that enters the TCA cycle (Fig. 4.7). During starvation conditions, acetyl-CoA is shunted away from the TCA cycle and toward the formation of ketones, which provides vital energy for the brain, heart, and skeletal muscle.

Vitamins

Vitamins serve as crucial cofactors for many biochemical pathways and are necessary for growth, maintenance, and reproduction. There are four fat-soluble and nine water-soluble vitamins (Table 4.4).

The *fat-soluble vitamins* include A, D, E, and K. In addition to its role in wound healing, vitamin A plays a role in wound healing and is important for maintaining sight because it limits keratinization of epithelium in the eye. Vitamin D is essential for the intestinal absorption of calcium and phosphorus. Vitamin E is a family of tocopherols with seven members that participate in many biochemical processes. Vitamin K is a critical cofactor in the hepatic synthesis of several clotting factors, specifically factors II, VII, IX,

TABLE 4.3 Summary of nutrient caloric yield and metabolism

	Yield (kcal/g)	Storage	Synthesis	Degradation
Protein	4.0	None	*Essential*: ingested *Nonessential*: protein synthesis using amino acid substrate	Proteolysis: pyruvate → gluconeogenesis Urea → urea cycle
Carbohydrate	3.4	Glycogen	Gluconeogenesis using amino acid substrate during starvation	Glycolysis: CO_2, H_2O, and ATP
Fat	9.0	Triglycerides	Lipogenesis using acetyl-CoA	Lipolysis: pyruvate → gluconeogenesis Acetyl-CoA → CO_2, H_2O, and ATP

ATP, adenosine triphosphate.

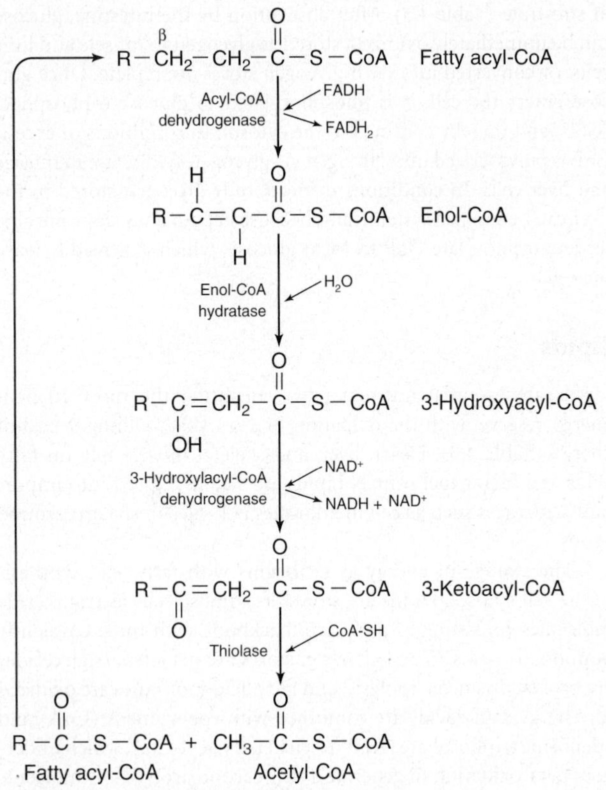

$R{-}\overset{\beta}{C}H_2{-}CH_2{-}C(=O){-}S{-}CoA$ Fatty acyl-CoA

Acyl-CoA dehydrogenase (FADH → $FADH_2$)

$R{-}CH{=}CH{-}C(=O){-}S{-}CoA$ Enol-CoA

Enol-CoA hydratase (H_2O)

$R{-}C(OH){=}CH_2{-}C(=O){-}S{-}CoA$ 3-Hydroxyacyl-CoA

3-Hydroxylacyl-CoA dehydrogenase (NAD^+ → $NADH + NAD^+$)

$R{-}C(=O){=}CH_2{-}C(=O){-}S{-}CoA$ 3-Ketoacyl-CoA

Thiolase (CoA-SH)

$R{-}C(=O){-}S{-}CoA + CH_3{-}C(=O){-}S{-}CoA$

Fatty acyl-CoA Acetyl-CoA

FIGURE 4.7 Fatty acid β-oxidation.

and X. Vitamin K levels are sensitive to intestinal bacterial overgrowth because a significant amount of vitamin K is produced and absorbed by the colon. All fat-soluble vitamins depend on the presence of bile for absorption.

Water-soluble vitamins include B complex vitamins and ascorbic acid (vitamin C). Vitamin B_{12} is important for DNA synthesis, and its deficiency may manifest as macrocytic anemia and neuropathy. Because vitamin B_{12} is the only water-soluble vitamin that can be stored in the liver and recycled for a substantial length of time, its deficiency is rare except in patients with certain disease states, such as pernicious anemia or after intestinal bypass surgery. Folate is the most common water-soluble vitamin and also plays a role in DNA synthesis. Folate deficiency may manifest as leukopenia, megaloblastic anemia, steatorrhea, sprue, and glossitis. Vitamin C is required for the hydroxylation of proline residues in collagen synthesis, and hence, its deficiency manifests as impaired wound healing and bleeding tendencies due to fragile capillaries.

Trace Elements

The trace elements include iron, iodine, cobalt, zinc, copper, selenium, manganese, and chromium. They comprise less than 0.1% of the diet but have important roles in metabolism, immune function, and wound healing. Zinc is stored predominantly in muscle, and during proteolysis zinc is mobilized and excreted in the urine. Patients who are acutely ill are susceptible to zinc deficiency, often presenting as diarrhea, CNS disturbances, eczematoid dermatitis, and alopecia. Zinc also contributes to wound healing. Chromium is a cofactor for insulin, and its deficiency causes glucose intolerance and peripheral sensory neuropathy. Selenium is a component of the RBC enzyme glutathione peroxidase, which plays an important role in protecting RBCs from lipid peroxidation (Table 4.5).

Fluid and Electrolytes

Water comprises approximately 60% of total body weight in men and 50% of total body weight in women. Two thirds of total body water (TBW; 40% of total body weight) is intracellular, and one third (20% of total body weight) is contained either within the vasculature as plasma (5%) or within the interstitium as lymphatic fluid (15%). *Serum osmolality* can be calculated from serum glucose, sodium, and urea levels:

$$\textit{Serum osmolality} = \left(2\text{Na}^+ + \text{urea}/2.8\right) + \left(\text{glucose}/18\right)$$

TABLE 4.4 Vitamin functions and deficiency states

Vitamin	Function	Deficiency state
Fat soluble		
A (retinol)	Rhodopsin synthesis	Xerophthalmia, keratomalacia
D (cholecalciferol)	Intestinal calcium absorption, bone remodeling	Rickets (children), osteomalacia (adults)
E (α-tocopherol)	Antioxidant	Hemolytic anemia, neurologic damage
K (naphthoquinone)	τ-Carboxylation of glutamate in clotting factors	Coagulopathy (deficiency in factors II, VII, IX, and X)
Water soluble		
B_1 (thiamine)	Decarboxylation and aldehyde transfer reactions	Beriberi, neuropathy, fatigue, heart failure
B_2 (riboflavin)	Oxidation–reduction reactions	Dermatitis, glossitis
B_5 (niacin)	Oxidation–reduction reactions	Pellagra (dermatitis, diarrhea, dementia, death)
B_6 (pyridoxal phosphate)	Transamination and decarboxylation reactions	Neuropathy, glossitis, anemia
B_7 (biotin)	Carboxylation reactions	Dermatitis, alopecia
B_9 (folate)	DNA synthesis	Megaloblastic anemia, glossitis
B_{12} (cyanocobalamin)	DNA synthesis, myelination	Megaloblastic anemia, neuropathy
C (ascorbic acid)	Hydroxylation of hormones, hydroxylation of proline in collagen synthesis, antioxidant	Scurvy

TABLE 4.5 Trace elements

Trace Element	Function	Deficiency
Chromium	Promotes normal glucose utilization in combination with insulin	Glucose intolerance, peripheral neuropathy
Copper	Component of enzymes	Hypochromic microcytic anemia, neutropenia, bone demineralization, diarrhea
Fluorine	Essential for normal structure of bones and teeth	Caries
Iodine	Thyroid hormone production	Endemic goiter, hypothyroidism, myxedema, cretinism
Iron	Hemoglobin synthesis	Hypochromic microcytic anemia, glossitis, stomatitis
Manganese	Component of enzymes, essential for normal bone structure	Dermatitis, weight loss, nausea, vomiting, coagulopathy
Molybdenum	Component of enzymes	Neurologic abnormalities, night blindness
Selenium	Component of enzymes, antioxidant	Cardiomyopathy
Zinc	Component of enzymes involved in metabolism of lipids, proteins, carbohydrates, nucleic acids	Alopecia, hypogonadism, olfactory and gustatory dysfunction, impaired wound healing, acrodermatitis enteropathica, growth arrest

Sodium

Hyponatremia is defined as a serum sodium level less than 130 mEq/L. Declining levels should be monitored cautiously if severe fluid shifts are expected, such as with shock, high-output enteric fistulas, or aggressive diuresis. When serum sodium values fall below 120 mEq/L, patients are at high risk for neuropsychiatric symptoms, including lethargy, anorexia, vomiting, and decreased consciousness. When values fall below 110 mEq/L, life-threatening seizures may ensue. Serum sodium less than 130 mEq/L necessitates assessment and correction. The most common cause of hyponatremia is fluid overload, although it can also occur in volume-deficient or euvolemic states. Pseudohyponatremia is a falsely low serum sodium laboratory value as a result of hyperglycemia or hyperlipidemia.

Urine sodium levels are valuable in the assessment of hypovolemic hyponatremia. If the circulating volume is low and the urine sodium level is greater than 20 mEq/L, hyponatremia is typically due to renal wasting caused by diuretic use or renal dysfunction. A urine sodium concentration less than 20 mEq/L suggests an extrarenal source of sodium loss, such as diarrhea, nasogastric suction, or enteric fistula. Euvolemic hyponatremia is most commonly associated with syndrome of inappropriate antidiuretic hormone (SIADH), in which excessive ADH stimulates renal sodium reabsorption. To correct hyponatremia, hypovolemic patients should be resuscitated with isotonic saline or lactated Ringers, whereas patients with volume overload or SIADH should be treated with fluid restriction. Excessively rapid correction of hyponatremia may result in *central pontine myelinolysis*, and levels should be monitored carefully. The suspected duration of hyponatremia helps guide the appropriate rate of correction. In patients who are acutely symptomatic (<48 hours), the goal is to increase serum sodium by 1 to 2 mEq/L/h for 3 to 4 hours, until neurologic symptoms resolve or until serum sodium is greater than 120 mEq/L. In patients with chronic hyponatremia, the rate of correction should not exceed 0.5 to 1.0 mEq/L/h, with total sodium correction limited to 8 to 12 mEq/L/d.

Hypernatremia typically occurs when a net negative water balance is sustained, resulting in serum sodium concentration greater than 145 mEq/L. Symptoms include lethargy, weakness, and irritability. Major GI losses or massive burns are frequent causes of hypovolemic hypernatremia. Hypervolemic hypernatremia is most commonly seen after sodium bicarbonate infusion or excessive exogenous sodium administration. Euvolemic hypernatremia may occur when hypotonic losses are replaced with isotonic solutions, such as total parenteral nutrition (TPN). It may also occur with fever or head injury causing central diabetes insipidus, characterized by deficient vasopressin production and excessively dilute urine output.

Free water deficit (measured in liters) can be calculated with the following equation:

$$\text{Total body weight (TBW) deficit} = 0.6W - \left(0.6W \times \left[140 / P_{Na}\right]\right)$$

where W is weight in kilograms, 0.6 or 60% is the percentage of free body water in men (0.5 should be used for women), and P_{Na} is the serum sodium concentration. Rapid correction of hypernatremia may result in cerebral edema; it is recommended that the free water deficit be replaced over 48 to 72 hours. Central diabetes insipidus is treated with intranasal or parenteral desmopressin or desmopressin acetate (DDAVP).

Potassium

Potassium is the dominant intracellular cation, with only 2% of total body potassium in the extracellular space. The Na^+/K^+ pump maintains the intracellular sequestration of potassium while extruding sodium into the extracellular compartment. The movement of potassium across cell membranes contributes to a vast number of physiologic reactions, including axon depolarization. Although potassium balance is under predominantly renal control, small amounts are also excreted by the GI tract. Increased renal excretion is stimulated by high plasma potassium concentrations, alkalosis, ADH, aldosterone, and elevated sodium delivery to the distal renal tubules.

Hypokalemia is defined as serum potassium concentration below 3.3 mEq/L. Renal potassium losses often occur in the setting of aggressive diuretic administration. Extrarenal losses from the GI tract (vomiting or diarrhea), decreased oral intake, and certain medications may also contribute to low serum concentrations. Mild hypokalemia is generally asymptomatic, but when the concentration falls below 3.0 mEq/L, muscle weakness, ileus, and cardiac conduction abnormalities may result. ECG manifestations include T-wave depression, prominent U waves, and prolongation of the QT interval. Oral formulations can be used to correct mild hypokalemia, unless oral repletion is contraindicated. Parenteral formulations can be administered safely at a rate of 10 to 20 mEq/L/h and should be used if severe or symptomatic hypokalemia is present. Magnesium may need to be repleted prior to correcting potassium.

Hyperkalemia is defined as serum potassium concentration greater than 5.5 mEq/L. Renal dysfunction is the most common etiology, but other common causes include crush injuries, cell lysis (such as in rhabdomyolysis), reperfusion injury, adrenal insufficiency, and certain drugs including succinylcholine, β-receptor agonists, and digitalis. The most feared complication of hyperkalemia is cardiac arrhythmia, which may occur when potassium levels approach or exceed 6.5 mEq/L. Possible ECG changes include peaked T waves, prolonged QRS interval, and deepening of the S wave into a sinusoidal pattern, all of which may forebode a life-threatening arrhythmia. While mild hyperkalemia can be treated with oral intake restriction and loop diuretics, severe hyperkalemia must be addressed urgently, particularly in the setting of ECG changes. In these circumstances, calcium chloride is frequently infused to stabilize the myocardial membrane. Sodium bicarbonate and insulin administration lowers serum potassium levels immediately by causing potassium to shift intracellularly but do not permanently eliminate potassium; the administration of oral or rectal potassium-binding resins is necessary for excretion. The most rapid and definitive treatment for hyperkalemia is hemodialysis, which may be initiated if hyperkalemia is life threatening or in patients with renal failure.

Calcium

Calcium is a divalent cation with important roles in muscle contraction, coagulation, cell division, and neural function. Calcium is especially critical in cell signaling mechanisms, often serving as a second messenger. About 99% of calcium resides within bone, and serum calcium levels are controlled by parathyroid hormone (PTH) and calcitonin. Forty-five percent of serum calcium exists in its biologically active ionized form, with the remainder bound to albumin and other plasma proteins. When assessing serum calcium levels, it is important to note that most laboratories sum the ionized and plasma-bound fractions. Since a large fraction of serum calcium is bound to albumin, the assay is sensitive to albumin depletion. The ionized fraction is physiologically significant and is unchanged by fluctuations in the albumin concentration.

PTH is the main modulator of calcium homeostasis and is released from the parathyroid gland when serum calcium concentrations decline. PTH increases serum calcium by three separate mechanisms involving bone resorption, renal reabsorption, and intestinal absorption. Vitamin D contributes to osteoclast activation and renal calcium reabsorption and is the chief stimulus of enteric calcium absorption (Fig. 4.8).

Hypocalcemia is commonly seen following parathyroid and thyroid operations. It may occur due to manipulation, ischemia, or unintentional excision of parathyroid glands during thyroid surgery, or limited PTH production from the atrophic glands remaining after resection of a parathyroid adenoma. Hypocalcemia can also occur as a result of vitamin D deficiency secondary to malnutrition or malabsorption. Typical clinical manifestations of hypocalcemia include hyperactive muscle contraction and reflexes, with muscle cramps and perioral tingling as early warning signs. Chvostek's sign is a facial muscle spasm that occurs with tapping the facial nerve, and Trousseau sign is carpal–pedal spasm after application of a blood pressure cuff on the limb. If hypocalcemia is severe, ECG may show a prolonged QT interval and prolonged ST segment, and tetany and/or ventricular arrhythmias may ensue. Immediate treatment with intravenous calcium gluconate is appropriate in these situations.

The most common etiology of *hypercalcemia* is primary hyperparathyroidism, occurring secondary to parathyroid adenoma, parathyroid hyperplasia, and rarely parathyroid carcinoma. Another frequent cause of hypercalcemia, particularly in the hospital setting, is malignancy with associated metastatic disease or PTH-like activity, with certain tumors of the lung, breast, thyroid, and kidney most often implicated. Hypercalcemia may also result from thiazide diuretics, multiple myeloma, Paget disease, hyperthyroidism, prolonged immobilization, and sarcoidosis. When serum levels approach or exceed 12 mg/dL, hypercalcemia can be associated with renal stones; polyuria; GI symptoms including nausea, vomiting, ileus, and pancreatitis; cardiovascular manifestations including hypotension and shortened QT intervals on ECG; and neurologic symptoms including confusion and coma. Metastatic calcification refers to the deposition of calcium salts in otherwise normal tissue, principally affecting interstitial tissues of blood vessels, lungs, and kidneys but also potentially leading to cutaneous manifestations (as in calciphylaxis). Severe hypercalcemia deserves immediate attention, and treatment should aim to maximize renal excretion via normal saline infusion and loop diuretics. Calcitonin, a thyroid-derived hormone that inhibits calcium resorption, has been effectively used to treat hypercalcemia associated with malignancy. Mithramycin may also be used on a long-term basis to inhibit bone resorption in patients with metastatic disease. The mainstay of treatment for hypercalcemia in primary hyperparathyroidism is resection of the hyperfunctioning parathyroid gland(s).

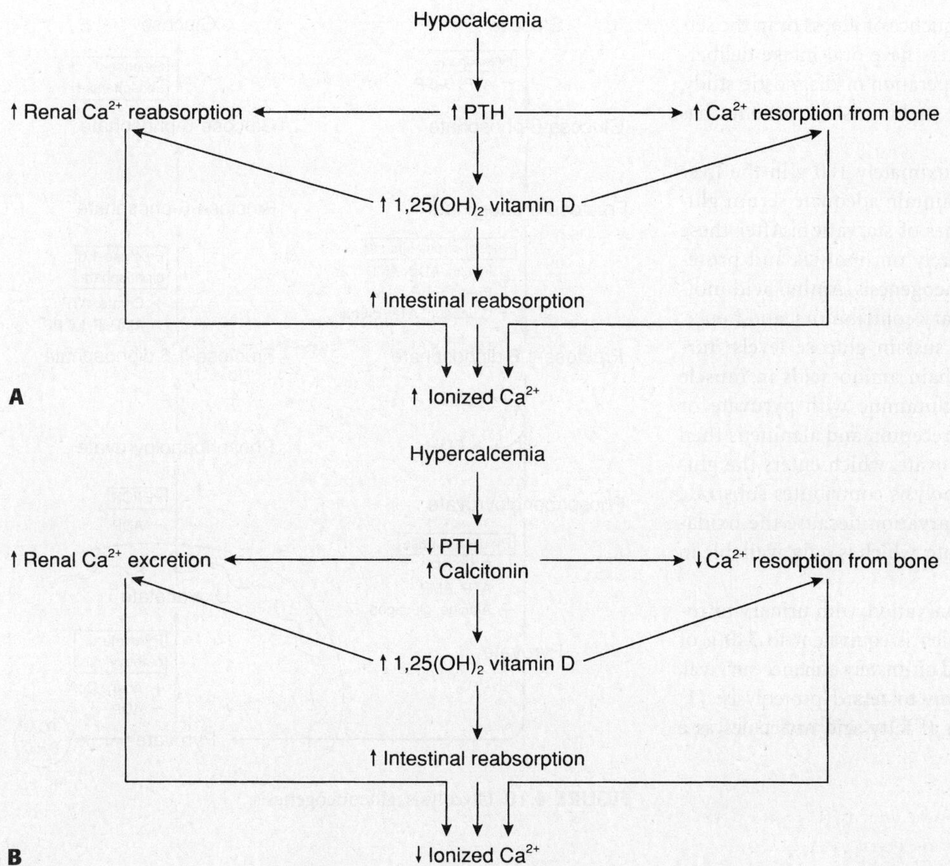

FIGURE 4.8 Physiologic compensatory effects of **(A)** hypocalcemia and **(B)** hypercalcemia. (From Wait RB, Kahng KU, Dresner LS. Fluids and electrolytes and acid–base balance. In: Greenfield LJ, Mulholand MW, Oldham KT, et al., eds. *Surgery: Scientific Principles and Practice.* 2nd ed. Philadelphia: Lippincott–Raven Publishers; 1997:258, with permission.)

Magnesium

Magnesium is second only to potassium as the most abundant intracellular cation. It often serves as a cofactor in enzymatic reactions and plays an important role in the activity of electrically excitable cells. In addition, magnesium facilitates the movement of calcium into muscle and is critical for muscle contraction. Magnesium is absorbed in the small intestine, and 50% is stored in bone reserves. It is excreted via the kidneys and is not under any known hormonal control.

Hypomagnesemia is caused by excessive renal losses (diuretic therapy, primary hyperaldosteronism, renal dysfunction) or GI losses (malabsorptive states, nutrition deficiency). Clinical signs of hypomagnesemia are similar to hypocalcemia, typically manifesting as muscle weakness, spasm, and hyperreflexia. Widening of the QRS and prolongation of the QT interval may be evident on ECG. Mild deficiencies can be treated with oral supplementation, but levels below 1 mEq/L should be repleted with intravenous magnesium sulfate at a rate no greater than 1 to 2 g/h.

The primary etiology of *hypermagnesemia* is renal failure. Other rare causes include severe crush injury, rhabdomyolysis, severe dehydration, and metabolic acidosis. Clinical signs include depression of deep tendon reflexes and neuromuscular activity, potentially progressing to paralysis, coma, and cardiac arrhythmia. Sinus bradycardia and prolongation of the PR, QRS, and QT intervals may be seen on ECG. As with hypercalcemia, initial treatment of severe hypermagnesemia consists of infusing normal saline in combination with a loop diuretic. Hemodialysis may be necessary to rapidly lower the serum magnesium concentration. The infusion of calcium gluconate may play a role in cell membrane stabilization.

Phosphorus

The organic form of phosphorus contributes significantly many important metabolic intermediates, including the energy molecule ATP. Its inorganic form, representing 85% of its stores, resides in the bone, contributing strength and structure. *Hypophosphatemia* can be the result of GI loss, excessive renal excretion, or intracellular electrolyte shifts. While usually clinically silent, hypophosphatemia has the potential to cause skeletal and cardiac muscle weakness, resulting in weak respiratory effort and decreased cardiac output. If the deficiency is mild, oral replacement is sufficient. Intravenous replacement is reserved for severe deficiencies, especially if the patient develops weakness or if oral replacement is contraindicated. *Hyperphosphatemia* is exceedingly rare outside of renal failure but can result from large-scale cell lysis in the setting of tumor or rhabdomyolysis. If mild, sucralfate or aluminum-containing antacids can be used as binders. If severe, or in the case of renal failure, hemodialysis may be necessary.

Metabolism in Starvation

The physiology of starvation evolved to enhance survival in times of famine. Starvation conditions are often encountered in surgical patients, both pre- and postoperatively. Many patients have limited oral tolerance, either as a direct consequence of illness or in the setting of specific treatments, while others have oral intake deliberately withheld in anticipation of an operation or diagnostic study. Perioperative nutritional support in malnourished patients has become a priority.

Systemic glycogen reserve (approximately 100 g in the liver and 250 g in skeletal muscle) can maintain adequate serum glucose levels for about 24 hours in times of starvation. After these stores are depleted, the body must rely on lipolysis and proteolysis to provide substrate for gluconeogenesis. Amino acid molecules from proteolysis are the primary contributors, and hence, protein breakdown is necessary to sustain glucose levels during times of starvation. Branched-chain amino acids in muscle are transaminated to alanine and glutamine with pyruvate or α-ketoglutamate as the usual amine receptor, and alanine is then deaminated by the liver to form pyruvate, which enters the gluconeogenesis pathway (Fig. 4.9). Lipolysis contributes substrate to a lesser extent during times of starvation because the oxidation of fatty acids requires oxaloacetate, which is only available in limited supply (Fig. 4.10).

Proteolysis is dominant in early starvation, with urinary nitrogen losses between 8 and 12 g/d, which is equivalent to 340 g of tissue per day. To conserve protein and ultimately enhance survival, the body employs several mechanisms to retard proteolysis: (1) peripheral tissues increase utilization of fatty acid molecules as a fuel source and (2) the brain increases utilization of ketone bodies (fat derived), which reduces dependence on gluconeogenesis and its required proteolytic substrates.

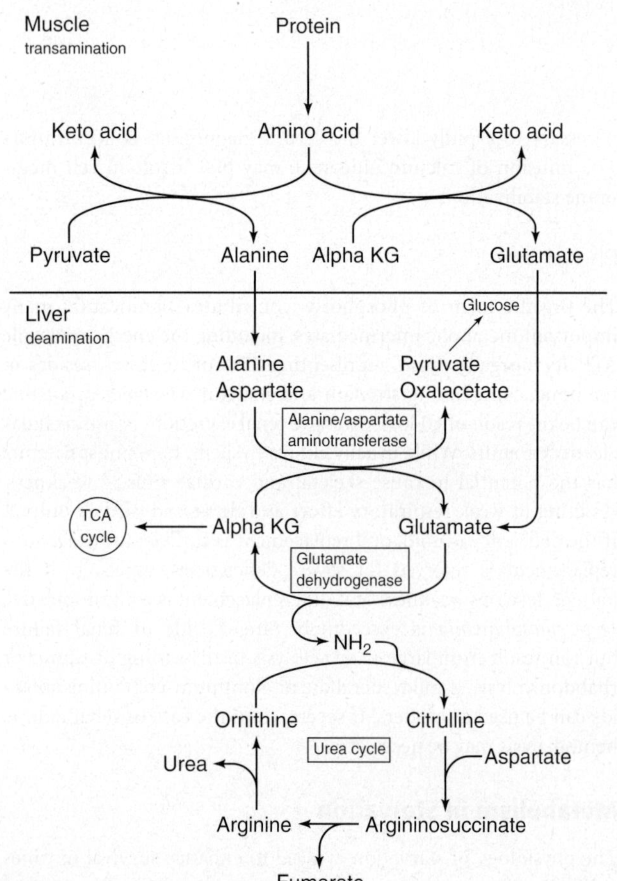

FIGURE 4.9 Protein metabolism.

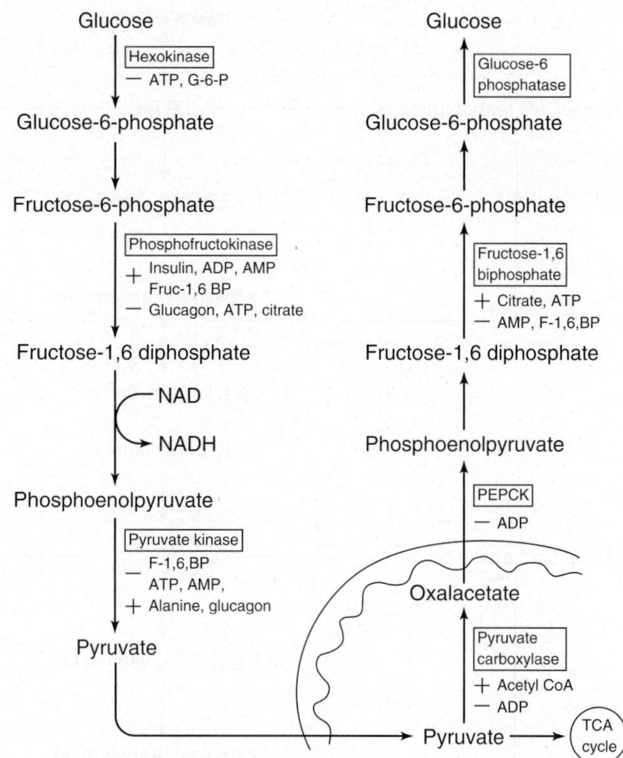

FIGURE 4.10 Glycolysis, gluconeogenesis.

Metabolism in Stress/Injury/Sepsis

The physiologic response to starvation in times of stress or injury, as in the days immediately following a major abdominal operation, is maladaptive. Even during starvation, stress or injury results in increased basal metabolic rate in an attempt to mount an inflammatory response and optimize wound healing. This hypermetabolic response is catecholamine induced and mediated by the sympathetic nervous system. Rising levels of adrenocorticotropic hormone, cortisol, catecholamines, glucagon, and growth hormone all contribute to a hyperglycemic state, with peripheral glucose intolerance despite elevated serum insulin. Glucagon is chiefly responsible for driving hepatic gluconeogenesis, while peripheral glucose intolerance is mediated by cortisol and catecholamines. The brain and peripheral tissues fail to "ketoadapt" and continue their preference for glucose. Therefore, demand for glucose remains high, and the only supply is through breakdown of valuable protein molecules.

The derangement in glucose metabolism is not the only force behind increasing proteolysis and its corresponding nitrogen loss. Amino acids are required by the liver for synthesis of inflammatory molecules and acute-phase reactants involved in coagulation and opsonization. The bone marrow also requires amino acid substrate for production of hematopoietic cells needed for the immune response and wound healing. In total, exogenous protein requirements may increase by up to threefold.

Fat metabolism is accelerated by the sympathetic nervous system in times of stress or injury. Despite accelerated lipolysis, plasma lipid levels typically remain normal because lipid consumption increases in peripheral tissues. Unlike in simple starvation, ketone production declines in stress/injury, most likely due to elevated levels of several ketogenesis inhibitors including insulin, glucagons, glucose, alanine, and lactate.

Caloric Requirements

To ensure adequate caloric and nutritional intake during times of stress/injury, it becomes necessary to obtain or estimate energy and protein requirements. One method for approximating caloric need is *indirect calorimetry*, in which the patient breathes into a spirometer or *metabolic cart* that measures oxygen consumption (VO_2) and carbon dioxide production (VCO_2). These values are then used to calculate the metabolic rate.

$$\begin{aligned}\textit{Metabolic rate}\left(\text{kcal}/\text{m}^2/\text{h}\right) = &\left(3.9\times \text{VO}_2[\text{L}/\text{min}]\right)\\ &+1.1\times \text{VCO}_2(\text{L}/\text{min})\\ &\times 60(\text{min}/\text{h})/\text{body surface area}\left(\text{m}^2\right)\end{aligned}$$

Metabolic cart values can also be used to derive the *respiratory quotient* (*RQ*), which is the ratio of expired carbon dioxide to consumed oxygen. Because RQ reflects a single time point, frequent reassessment is required, especially in the acutely ill patient with rapidly changing metabolism. The RQ provides information about substrate utilization—an RQ of 1.0 is indicative of carbohydrate metabolism, 0.8 is indicative of protein metabolism, and 0.7 is indicative of fat metabolism. An RQ greater than 1.0 suggests overfeeding, since excess carbohydrates are converted to carbon dioxide. Overfeeding may manifest as increased respiratory rate (to expire excess carbon dioxide) and ultimately may lead to difficulty weaning from the ventilator. Conversely, an RQ less than 0.7 is seen in starvation, since fat metabolism does not increase carbon dioxide production but oxygen consumption increases. Unfortunately, indirect calorimetry is not available at many institutions because the metabolic cart is labor intensive and expensive.

While less accurate than indirect calorimetry, a variety of other methods can be used to predict energy requirements. The *Harris–Benedict equation* estimates basal energy expenditure (BEE) on the basis of weight, height, age, and gender and can be adjusted to estimate total energy expenditure (TEE) by accounting for an individual's activity level.

$$\text{BEE}(\text{women}) = 655 + (9.6W) + (1.8H) - (4.7A)$$
$$\text{BEE}(\text{men}) = 66 + (13.7W) + (5H) - (6.8A)$$

where W is weight in kilograms, H is height in centimeters, and A is age in years. TEE can be estimated by multiplying BEE by an activity factor of 1.3 for hospitalized patients and 1.5 for outpatients.

NUTRITIONAL ASSESSMENT AND SUPPORT

Nutritional Assessment

In the 1930s, the relationship between disease-related malnutrition and postoperative morbidity and mortality was first recognized. There remains considerable debate regarding optimal strategies for assessing perioperative nutritional status.

A comprehensive assessment should begin with a thorough history and physical examination. The history and review of systems should expose impediments to appropriate oral intake or efficient intestinal absorption. These obstacles may include the inability to chew or swallow, severe alcoholism, malabsorptive disorders such as Crohn's disease, a history of surgical procedures or trauma, and any other chronic medical problems. During the examination, peripheral edema, ascites, and signs of vitamin and mineral deficiency should be noted. Severe caloric deficiency, or *marasmus*, may manifest as decreased subcutaneous fat and a cachectic appearance with muscle wasting. *Kwashiorkor*, an isolated protein deficiency seen infrequently, can be difficult to diagnose in the obese and postsurgical populations, but typical signs include peripheral edema and a protuberant abdomen secondary to ascites and hepatomegaly.

Multiple nutritional screening tools have been devised, but all objective parameters and subjective scoring systems have limitations, and no consensus exists. Weight and BMI alone are thought to be relatively unreliable measures of nutritional risk, because these parameters poorly reflect lean body mass and do not account for confounding variables such as age, gender, and underlying disease process. Levels of serum transport proteins such as *albumin*, *prealbumin*, and *transferrin* are useful indicators of visceral protein mass. Albumin has a half-life in the serum of 18.2 days and therefore is limited in its ability to detect acute changes in the critically ill patient. Because of their shorter half-lives, prealbumin (1.3 days) and transferrin (8.5 days) have increased sensitivity in the detection of acute protein loss.

Utilizing a combination of measures to assess nutritional status is currently the most accurate and reliable method in identifying malnourished patients. *Subjective global assessment* (*SGA*) is a comprehensive assessment tool, accounting for factors such as recent weight loss, dietary intake, lean body mass, functional capacity, and GI symptoms that might suggest poor absorptive capacity (Fig. 4.11). *NRS 2002* (*Nutritional Risk Screening*) grades degree of nutritional impairment and indications for nutritional support on the basis of both objective weight loss parameters and severity of metabolic stress associated with underlying procedure or disease state, with major abdominal surgery considered a moderately severe stressor (Fig. 4.12). Patients deemed severely malnourished on the NRS 2002 scale (score >5) have been shown to derive the most benefit from perioperative nutritional support.

In recent years, several large interdisciplinary organizations have published broad guidelines for nutritional assessment and support in critical care and perioperative settings. The European Society of Parenteral and Enteral Nutrition (ESPEN) recommends use of NRS 2002, SGA, and serum albumin to determine nutritional risk and need for supplementation. Under ESPEN parameters, patients with at least one of the following criteria should receive 7 to 10 days of preoperative TPN: weight loss greater than 10% to 15% within 6 months, BMI less than 18 kg/m^2, SGA grade C, and serum albumin less than 30 g/L. The Society of Critical Care Medicine and the American Society of Parenteral and Enteral Nutrition (SCCM/ASPEN) recommend evaluating weight loss and nutrient intake prior to admission/operation, disease severity, comorbid conditions, and GI function in assessing need for perioperative nutritional support.

Enteral Access

Nutritional support may be administered via enteral or parenteral routes or a combination of both. Short-term enteral feeds can be

Features of subjective global assessment (SGA)

(Select appropriate category with a checkmark, or enter numberical value where indicated by "#.")

A. History

1. Weight change
   Overall loss in past 6 months: amount = # ________ kg; % loss = # ________
   Change in past 2 weeks: ________ increase,
   ________ no change,
   ________ decrease.
2. Dietary intake change (relative to normal)
   ________ No change,
   ________ Change, ________ duration = # ________ weeks.
   ________ type: ________ suboptimal solid diet, ________ full liquid diet
   ________ hypocaloric liquids, ________ starvation.
3. Gastrointestinal symptoms (that persisted for >2 weeks)
   ________ none, ________ nausea, ________ vomiting, ________ diarrhea, ________ anorexia.
4. Functional capacity
   ________ No dysfunction (e.g., full capacity),
   ________ Dysfunction ________ duration = # ________ weeks.
   ________ type: ________ working suboptimally
   ________ ambulatory,
   ________ bedridden.
5. Disease and its relation to nutritional requirements
   Primary diagnosis (specify) ________
   Metabolic demand (stress): ________ no stress, ________ low stress,
   ________ moderate stress, ________ high stress,

B. Physical (for each trait specify: 0 = normal, 1+ = mild, 2+ = moderate, 3+ = severe).

________ loss of subcutaneous fat (triceps, chest)
________ muscle wasting (quadriceps, deltoids)
________ ankle edema
________ sacral edema
________ ascites

C. SGA rating (select one)

________ A = Well nourished
________ B = Moderately (or suspected of being) malnourished
________ C = Severely malnourished

FIGURE 4.11 Subjective global assessment. (From Detsky AS, McLaughlin JR, Baker JP, et al. What is subjective global assessment of nutritional status? *J Parenter Enteral Nutr.* 1987;11(1):8–13. Reprinted by Permission of SAGE Publications.)

given via nasogastric tube or postpyloric nasoenteric tube. Surgical gastrostomy or jejunostomy tubes are an option when long-term enteral supplementation is anticipated. Gastrostomy tubes can be placed percutaneously (percutaneous endoscopic gastrostomy) or via laparotomy. PEG cannot be performed if upper endoscopy is contraindicated or if the gastric lumen cannot be safely accessed percutaneously due to patient anatomy or prior abdominal operations. Jejunostomy tubes may be inserted in an open or laparoscopic fashion, approximately 30 cm distal to the ligament of Treitz. In patients susceptible to aspiration, postpyloric access is preferred for enteral feeding, but otherwise, there are no data to suggest that gastric or postpyloric feeds are physiologically superior. Gastric feeds may be administered continuously or bolused intermittently. While continuous gastric feeding may be associated with lower gastric residual volumes, bolus gastric feeding allows for periods of gastric acidosis between feeds (when acid production is not suppressed), which ultimately limits bacterial overgrowth in the lower GI tract.

Enteral Nutrition

Enteral nutrition, whenever feasible, is generally preferred over parenteral nutrition in postoperative and critical care settings. Several studies stress the immunologic benefits of enteral feeding and its association with improved clinical outcomes. In postoperative patients, enteral nutrition has been shown to be associated with lower incidence of infections and complications (including anastomotic leak and superficial/deep fascial surgical site infections), improved wound healing, and shorter hospital stay. Enteral nutrition is thought to prevent gastrointestinal villous atrophy, thereby maintaining immune function (IgA secretion) and limiting bacterial translocation. Recently, an evidence-based initiative to "enhance recovery after surgery" (ERAS) has challenged traditional dogmas regarding the timing of postoperative enteral feeding, suggesting that very early enteral feeding enhances outcomes with no detrimental effects on anastomotic integrity. Under ERAS protocols, postoperative patients are encouraged to resume enteral nutrition (either oral or supplemental) as soon as tolerated, as early as 4 hours after colorectal surgery and within 24 hours after upper GI surgery.

While both enteral and parenteral routes carry risks, the complication profile associated with enteral feeding is thought to be far less morbid. Enteral access tubes are often responsible for skin breakdown and superficial site infections. More serious, albeit very rare, mechanical complications of enteral access include intestinal perforation (during insertion or after tube dislodgement) or bowel obstruction at the site of tube entry (particularly jejunostomy tubes). Depending on the specific route of administration, enteral feeding may also cause vomiting and increase risk for aspiration. Despite these issues, enteral nutrition is perceived to be safer than TPN because it obviates the risk of catheter-related complications.

Table 1 Initial screening			
		Yes	No
1	Is BMI <20.5?		
2	Has the patient lost weight within the last 3 months?		
3	Has the patient had a reduced dietary intake in the last week?		
4	Is the patient severely ill? (e.g. in intensive therapy)		
Yes: If the answer is 'Yes' to any question, the screening in Table 2 is performed. **No:** If the answer is 'No' to all questions, the patient is re-screened at weekly intervals. If the patient e.g. is scheduled for a major operation, a preventive nutritional care plan is considered to avoid the associated risk status.			

Table 2 Final Screening			
Impaired nutritional status		**Severity of disease (≈ increase in requirements)**	
Absent **Score 0**	Normal nutritional status	Absent **Score 0**	Normal nutritional requirements
Mild **Score 1**	Wt loss >5% in 3 mths of Food intake below 50–75% of normal requirement in preceding week	Mild **Score 1**	Hip fracture* Chronic patients, in particular with acute complications: cirrhosis*, COPD*. *Chronic hemodialysis, diabetes, oncology*
Moderate **Score 2**	Wt loss >5% in 2 mths or BMI 18.5 – 20.5 + impaired general codition or Food intake 25–60% of normal requirement in preceding week	Moderate **Score 2**	Major abdominal surgery* Stroke* *Severe pneumonia, hematologic malignancy*
Severe **Score 3**	Wt loss >5% in 1 mths (> 15% in 3 mths) or BMI < 18.5 + impaired general condition of Food intake 0–25% of normal requirement in preceding week in preceding week.	Severe **Score 3**	Head injury* Bone marrow transplantation* *Intensive care patients (APACHE > 10).*
Score:	+	**Score:**	**= Total Score:**
Age	if ≥ 70 years: add 1 to total score above	**= age-adjusted total score**	
Score ≥ 3: the patient is nutritionally at-risk and a nutritional care plan is initiated **Score ≥ 3:** weekly rescreening of the patient. If the patient e.g. is scheduled for a major operation, a preventive nutritional care plan is considered to avoid the associated risk status.			

FIGURE 4.12 Nutritional risk screening (NRS) 2002. (From Kondrup J, Allison SP, Elia M. ESPEN guidelines for nutrition screening 2002. *Clin Nutr.* 2003;22:415–421, with permission from Elsevier.)

Parenteral Nutrition

Parenteral nutrition is indicated when enteral feeding is contraindicated or poorly tolerated, or enteral access is not feasible. Contraindications to enteral feeding include intestinal obstruction, anastomotic leak, high-output fistulas, intestinal ischemia, and shock with impaired splanchnic perfusion (vasopressor requirement serves as a proxy). Following abdominal surgery, short-term intestinal dysfunction may limit patients' tolerance of enteral nutrition, but ileus typically resolves within a short time. Parenteral nutrition is typically reserved for patients unable to tolerate enteral feeds or unable to meet goal energy requirements on enteral feeds for greater than approximately 7 days and in whom duration of parenteral supplementation is anticipated to be 7 days or longer. Parenteral supplementation provided for less than 5 to 7 days has not been shown to have a beneficial effect on clinical outcome and thus should be avoided given risks inherent to central venous access. In patients on long-term TPN, efforts should be made to reinstitute enteral nutrition, but TPN should not be discontinued until the patient is receiving greater than 60% of energy requirements via enteral route. Recent evidence suggests that combined parenteral and enteral regimens may reduce nosocomial infections and improve outcomes in ICU patients who fail to meet nutritional requirements after 5 days of enteral feeding alone.

Parenteral nutrition formulas are hyperosmolar solutions (primarily dextrose-containing, see Table 4.6) that tend to cause venous sclerosis in peripheral veins and hence must be administered through a central venous catheter. PICC lines are often used for short-term parenteral access, whereas Broviac or Hickman lines are preferred for longer-term central venous access. Line infection and venous thrombosis are relatively common in patients receiving TPN, particularly those requiring chronic central access. Long-term TPN may also contribute to the development of liver injury, including steatosis and cirrhosis. Other drawbacks of parenteral nutrition include the risk of overfeeding and its higher cost relative to enteral feeding regimens.

TABLE 4.6 Calculating total parenteral nutrition

1	Estimate daily caloric (25–35 kcal/kg) and protein (1–2 g/kg) requirements.
2	Calculate the volume required to deliver the protein requirement with a 5% amino acid solution (50 g/L).[a] This volume is initially infused over 24 h.
3	Determine the amount of calories (kcal) provided by the dextrose in the above volume.
4	The remainder of the caloric requirement, not met by the dextrose solution, is provided by lipids as a 10% lipid emulsion (1 kcal/mL). This can be infused separately or as a mixture with the $A_{10}D_{50}$.[b]
5	Add standard electrolytes, multivitamins, and trace elements.[c]

[a]Solution of 10% amino acids mixed in equal parts with 50% dextrose ($A_{10}D_{50}$), whose final concentration is 5% amino acids and 25% dextrose.
[b]Some multivitamin preparations are not compatible with lipid emulsions.
[c]The amount of various electrolytes added to the TPN solution should be adjusted daily on the basis of patient disease and serum chemistries.
TPN, total parenteral nutrition.

Refeeding Syndrome

Refeeding syndrome describes a constellation of metabolic and electrolyte disturbances seen in malnourished patients after reinitiating enteral or parenteral supplementation and can be fatal if not recognized. When nutrition is reinitiated, carbohydrate delivery raises insulin levels considerably, leading to massive influx of glucose, potassium, magnesium, and phosphorus into cells. As the body shifts from catabolic to anabolic processes, the high demand for phosphorus in the intracellular synthesis of phosphorylated compounds causes a precipitous decline in serum phosphorus levels. Severe hypophosphatemia, in turn, can result in several life-threatening complications, including cardiac failure, respiratory failure, seizures, and arrhythmias. Patients deemed high risk for refeeding syndrome should have serum electrolyte levels carefully monitored while feeds are advanced to goal.

Preoperative Supplementation

Preoperative nutritional supplementation is often indicated in patients anticipating major surgery. In patients with gastrointestinal disease, limited oral tolerance, and/or intake secondary to underlying disease state may severely impair nutrition status prior to operation. As mentioned, several studies have observed lower complication rates and shorter hospital stays in severely malnourished patients receiving perioperative nutritional support. At least 7 to 10 days of preoperative supplemental nutrition is generally recommended (can often be administered at home) and should be continued in the initial postoperative period until enteral feeds are tolerated. As with postoperative patients, preoperative enteral feeding is the preferred route of administration, but TPN is indicated if patient disease restricts enteral access or enteral tolerance.

Carbohydrate Loading

Surgery predisposes to hyperglycemia by causing a transient reduction in insulin sensitivity postoperatively, which may be compounded by preoperative fasting (fasting increases glucagon and depletes insulin levels). Poor glycemic control, particularly in critically ill patients and following major surgery, has been shown to be associated with increased infectious complications, longer hospital stays, and increased mortality. Recent research suggests that preoperative carbohydrate loading (with a "CHO drink") may help preserve insulin sensitivity by stimulating levels of insulin release analogous to levels observed after a mixed meal. Larger randomized controlled trials are necessary to better clarify the clinical benefits of preoperative carbohydrate supplementation.

Immunonutrition

Several studies have demonstrated improved outcomes after preoperative oral supplementation with immune-modulating formulas. Currently, glutamine, arginine, and omega-3 fatty acids are the most common supplements in immunonutrition regimens and have been shown to enhance postoperative small bowel function and preserve T-lymphocyte responsiveness following major surgery. In a recent meta-analysis of multiple randomized controlled trials, immunonutrition reduced postoperative infection rates and decreased length of hospital stay. Preoperative treatment for 5 to 7 days optimized cost-effective benefits of immune-modulating regimens.

Considerations in Obesity

Assessment of nutritional status and provision of supplementation can be particularly challenging in obese patient populations. Because malnutrition can occur in obese patients with low muscle mass, fat-free mass index is thought to be a better predictor for risk of adverse events. ASPEN recommends the Penn State University 2010 predictive equation to assess energy requirements in critically ill or hospitalized obese patients:

$$\textit{Resting energy expenditure}\ (\text{kcal/day}) = \text{MSJ}(0.96) + \left[T_{\max}(167) \times V_E(31)\right] - 6{,}212$$

$$\text{MSJ (Mifflin-St. Jeor equation)} = 5 + 10\ (\text{weight in kg}) + 6.25 + \text{height (cm)} - 5\ (\text{age in years})$$

$$V_E = \text{minute ventilation (L/min)}$$

$$T_{\max} = \text{maximum body temperature over previous 24 hours (Celsius)}$$

To avoid overfeeding, low-calorie regimens are typically administered to obese patients. Complications of overfeeding include insulin resistance, glucose intolerance, hyperlipidemia, nonalcoholic fatty liver disease, and hypoventilation syndrome. Obese patients are predisposed to many of these conditions at baseline and thus more susceptible to adverse events in the setting of overfeeding. Permissive underfeeding (typically at 60% to 70% of goal energy requirements) allows for proportionately deficient calories and protein, while hypocaloric/high-protein regimens provide deficient calories while ensuring adequate protein. Smaller studies have shown some benefit with respect to hypocaloric/high-protein feeding (reduced duration of ventilator dependence, ICU stay, antibiotic course), but one larger randomized controlled trial showed no difference in outcomes between hypocaloric and eucaloric regimens in obese populations. Adequate protein intake does appear to confer a survival advantage, so high-protein regimens are generally preferred over permissive underfeeding regimens in which protein may be deficient.

Suggested Readings

Arnold M, Barbul A. Reconstructive nutrition and wound healing. *Plast Reconstr Surg.* 2006;117(suppl):42s.

Boron WF, Boulpaep EL, eds. *Medical Physiology: A Cellular and Molecular Approach.* 1st ed. Philadelphia: WB Saunders; 2003.

Burke DJ, Alverdy JC, Aoys E, et al. Glutamine-supplemented total parenteral nutrition improves gut function. *Arch Surg.* 1989; 124:1396–1399.

Carney DE, Meguid MM. Current concepts in nutritional assessment. *Arch Surg.* 2002;137:42–45.

Cerantola Y, Hubner M, Grass F, et al. Immunonutrition in gastrointestinal surgery. *Br J Surg.* 2011;98(1):37–48.

Choban P, Dickerson R, Malone A, et al. A.S.P.E.N. clinical guidelines: nutritional support of hospitalized adult patients with obesity. *J Parenter Enteral Nutr.* 2013;37(6):714–744.

DeWitt RC, Wu Y, Renegar KB, et al. Bombesin recovers gut-associated lymphoid tissue (GALT) and preserves immunity to bacterial pneumonia in TPN-fed mice. *Ann Surg.* 2000; 231:1–8.

Gustafsson UO, Ljungqvist O. Perioperative nutritional management in digestive tract surgery. *Curr Opin Clin Nutr Metab Care.* 2011;14:504–509.

Heidigger CP, Berger MM, Graf S, et al. Optimization of energy provision with supplemental parenteral nutrition in critically ill patients: a randomized controlled clinical trial. *Lancet.* 2013;381(9864): 385–393.

Jie B, Jiang ZM, Nolan MT, et al. Impact of preoperative nutritional support on clinical outcome in abdominal surgical patients at nutritional risk. *Nutrition.* 2012;28:1022–1027.

Kondrup J, Allison SP, Elia M. ESPEN guidelines for nutrition screening 2002. *Clin Nutr.* 2003;22:415–421.

Li J, Kudsk KA, Janu P, et al. Effect of glutamine-enriched TPN on small intestine gut associated lymphoid tissue (GALT) and upper respiratory tract immunity. *Surgery.* 1997;121:542–549.

Li L, Wang Z, Ying X, et al. Preoperative carbohydrate loading for elective surgery: a systematic review and meta-analysis. *Surg Today.* 2012;42(7):613–624.

Marino PL. *The ICU Book.* 2nd ed. Philadelphia: Lippincott Williams & Wilkins; 2007.

McClave SA, Martindale RG, Vanek VW, et al. Guidelines for the provision and assessment of nutrition support therapy in the adult critically ill patient: Society of Critical Care Medicine (SCCM) and American Society for Parenteral and Enteral Nutrition (A.S.P.E.N.). *J Parenter Enteral Nutr.* 2009;33(3): 277–316.

Stroud M, Duncan H, Nightingale J. Guidelines for enteral feeding in adult hospital patients. *Gut.* 2009;52(7):vvi1–vvi12.

Townsend CM, Beauchamp DR, Evers MB, et al., eds. *Sabiston Textbook of Surgery: The Biological Basis of Modern Surgical Practice.* 16th ed. Philadelphia: WB Saunders; 2001.

Varadhan KK, Neal KR, Dejong CH, et al. The enhanced recovery after surgery (ERAS) pathway for patients undergoing major elective open colorectal surgery: a meta-analysis of randomized trials. *Clin Nutr.* 2010;29:434–440.

CHAPTER 5

Immunology and Transplantation

DAVID AUFHAUSER AND MATTHEW LEVINE

KEY POINTS

- T lymphocytes orchestrate allograft rejection and recruit B lymphocytes and other inflammatory cells into the process.
- When a recipient and a donor are crossmatched, the reactivity of recipient serum antibodies with donor lymphocytes is quantified and used to predict the probability of rejection. In particular, a positive crossmatch is predictive of hyperacute/accelerated rejection mediated by antibodies produced by presensitized B lymphocytes.
- Acute cellular rejection is a major cause of early allograft dysfunction across all type of solid organ transplants. It is typically treated with steroids and antilymphocyte antibodies.
- Chronic rejection is a major cause of late graft failure and loss and is challenging to treat. Induction of long-lasting transplantation tolerance may require prevention of the chronic immune responses to organ transplants.
- Calcineurin inhibitors are the foundation of modern maintenance immunosuppression for solid organ transplantation. However, their nephrotoxicity has made renal insufficiency and failure a major late complication of organ transplantation.
- The first line of treatment for PTLD is reduction of immunosuppression. PTLD is primarily caused by an EBV-infected B-lymphocyte compartment.

INTRODUCTION

The evolution of solid organ transplantation into a standard of care for the treatment of end-stage organ failure was a remarkable achievement of 20th-century surgery. This success hinged on the development and refinement of novel operative techniques and pharmacologically effective means of inhibiting immunologic rejection. Despite these innovations and the implementation of chronic immunosuppressive therapies, the alloimmune response continues to pose a major challenge to the long-term success of organ transplants. Therefore, the major basic scientific objective of transplantation surgery remains the development of practical immunotherapeutic strategies for the induction of immunologic tolerance.

Allograft rejection is the end result of a coordinated immunologic assault on the transplanted organ (i.e., *alloimmunity*). On the basis of the kinetics of its onset and diagnosis, allograft rejection is described as *hyperacute* (minutes to hours), *acute* (days to weeks), or *chronic* (months to years). These clinical rejection categories correlate with distinct but overlapping pathologic processes. Understanding the mechanistic basis of immunologic rejection of organ allografts is an important requirement for both intelligent clinical practice and the development of novel immunotherapeutic strategies.

All organisms, from simple unicellular protozoa to complex multicellular mammals, have evolved mechanisms to detect and eliminate invasive foreign pathogens. The *innate immune system* comprises cellular and molecular elements whose function is to detect and eliminate foreign pathogens on the basis of a broad range of molecular/cellular markers. Prominent examples of these cellular, molecular, and soluble agents of *innate immunity* include (a) the *natural killer (NK)* cells, which recognize infected or malignant cells on the basis of an MHC class I deficiency; (b) the family of *Toll-like receptors* (TLRs), which recognize pathogen-associated molecular patterns (PAMPs) (e.g., lipopolysaccharide, staphylococcal enterotoxin) and deliver activation signals to a broad range of cells, including lymphocytes; and (c) the *complement cascade* of soluble proteins, which serves to opsonize and neutralize pathogens and foreign antigenic epitopes. These innate immune mechanisms in transplantation mediate much of the allograft damage from ischemia–reperfusion injury incurred during organ donation and implantation and initiate and regulate many aspects of the adaptive immune response.

The *adaptive immune system* is a relatively recent product of immunologic evolution with the capacity to generate highly specific immune responses to a wide spectrum of distinct pathogens based on more subtle antigenic disparities. The functional characteristics of the adaptive immune system are oriented along four distinct axes: (a) *specificity*, the ability to generate a highly specific and tailored response to an enormously diverse array of offending microorganisms; (b) *inducibility*, the capacity to recognize and activate the cellular immunologic machinery upon recognition of an offending microorganism; (c) *memory*, the development of a kinetically and quantitatively greater response, termed a "recall" or "presensitized" response, following repeated exposure to the same pathogen; and (d) *tolerance to self*, the ability of the immune system to distinguish between "self" versus "non–self-"antigens. Basic scientific research in transplantation immunology has established the critical role of the adaptive immune system in the rejection of organ allografts. As such, a basic knowledge of the core principles underlying the function of the adaptive immune system is of key importance.

Specificity

A process of *pseudorandom combinatorial rearrangement* of antigen receptor gene segments (i.e., immunoglobulins and T-cell receptors [TCRs]) is the molecular mechanism underlying the generation of antigen receptor diversity. This process is a unique example of a somatic cell (i.e., the T or B lymphocyte) acquiring a specialized ability for clonal expression of a unique antigen receptor by rearranging its genomic DNA. In the case of B lymphocytes, these receptors are expressed on the cell surface and are referred to as *membrane Ig* (*mIg*) or the *B-cell receptor* (*BCR*). When secreted by B lymphocytes, these antigen receptors are known as *antibodies*. In the case of T lymphocytes, the *TCR* is expressed on the cell surface and permits recognition of a diverse array of foreign antigenic peptides presented in the context of *major histocompatibility complex* (*MHC*) proteins (see the following text).

Inducibility

Following the engagement of their cell surface antigen receptors, both B and T cells are stimulated to enter the cell cycle and produce an array of effector inflammatory cytokines and chemokines, which regulate the inflammatory response to the foreign agent. Typically, the productive activation of both T and B cells requires the delivery of signals through the cell membrane antigen receptors (i.e., "signal 1") in addition to the delivery of costimulatory signals (i.e., "signal 2") via the cell surface (e.g., B7-CD28, CD40-CD40L) or soluble mediators (e.g., IL-2, IL-4). Costimulatory signals provide the context within which the antigen is recognized, helping to determine the type and magnitude of response. In the case of T cells, IL-2, interferon-γ, tumor necrosis factor (TNF), and IL-4 are among prominent soluble effectors induced following activation. Additionally, cytotoxic T cells rely on *perforin* molecules to mechanically lyse infected or foreign cells. In the case of B cells, antigen-specific IgM or IgG antibodies are the primary effector mediators. Soluble antibodies, through their capacity to activate the *classical complement pathway* of the innate immune system, lead to the formation of the *membrane attack complex* (*MAC*) on the surface of foreign or infected cells.

Memory

A key characteristic of the adaptive immune system is its capacity to quickly recall previously encountered antigen. This trait is known as the *memory response* and is mediated by both memory T and B lymphocytes. The differentiation of naive T and B cells into memory cells occurs following the primary immune response; results in the generation of phenotypically distinct, long-lived memory cells; and leads to the organism's capacity to mount a faster immune response upon antigen reencounter. Immunologic memory is the basis for the impressive efficacy of modern-day vaccines in preventing infectious disease epidemics. However, this memory response also imposes an extremely difficult challenge on the acceptance of organ transplants in *presensitized* recipients.

Tolerance to Self

The random generation of antigen receptors by developing B and T cells gives the adaptive immune system the ability to recognize a diverse and endless array of existing and emerging foreign antigenic epitopes. This ability provides a formidable challenge to the acceptance of organ transplants from genetically disparate individuals. The random generation of receptor diversity also leads to the generation of T and B cells with high affinity for *self*-antigens (i.e., *autoantigens*), the so-called *autoreactive* T- and B-cell clones. The fact that the majority of mammalian organisms do not suffer from autoimmune diseases attests to the efficacy and existence of regulatory mechanisms to keep autoreactive T and B lymphocytes in check. *Negative selection* of autoreactive lymphocytes occurs early in the course of lymphocyte development. Following encounter with their cognate autoantigen, immature autoreactive T cells undergo death in the thymus, whereas autoreactive B cells undergo death in the bone marrow (BM). Unlike their mature counterparts, immature T and B lymphocytes undergo *programmed cell death* (i.e., *apoptosis*) upon encounter with their antigen. In this fashion, the mature T- and B-cell repertoires are purged of clones with specificity for self. In addition to negative selection, another well-described mechanism that ensures tolerance to self is *anergy*. Anergic T and B cells are unable to become activated following antigen encounter. Finally, *immunologic ignorance* is thought to be an important tolerance mechanism and is the result of either (a) an immunologically privileged anatomic site (i.e., the anterior chamber of the eye, testes, etc.) or (b) the presence of antigen-specific anergic $CD4^+$ regulatory cells (i.e., T*reg*) capable of inhibiting T-cell–mediated immune responses. Failure of either of these three tolerance mechanisms can lead to an autoimmune disease. In the realm of transplantation immunology, major research efforts are directed at harnessing these immunologic tolerance mechanisms to induce a state of donor-specific tolerance to transplanted tissues.

The Major Histocompatibility Complex

MHC proteins are a group of cell surface molecules that play a critical role in adaptive immunity. In humans, there are six principal MHC genes that map to a region of chromosome 6. These molecules are also known as *human leukocyte antigens* (*HLA*) and are divided into two classes. A child inherits one set of HLA molecules linked together on a single chromosome (or *haplotype*) from each biologic parent. Siblings have a 50% chance of sharing one haplotype with one another, a 25% chance of being HLA haplotype identical, and a 25% chance of being completely haplotype disparate.

MHC class I is expressed by all nucleated cells and is typically loaded with intracellular peptides, both self and viral proteins. Conceptually, one can consider MHC class I to be presenting antigens from within the cell. Humans express three MHC class I loci, HLA-A, B, and C. These genes are expressed codominantly, and most individuals are heterozygous at each locus. Therefore, most patients express six different class I molecules. The α chain of class I molecules, also known as the heavy chain, is a 45-kDa transmembrane protein, containing a peptide-binding groove. It binds noncovalently to the $\beta 2$ microglobulin protein, also known as the light chain. $\beta 2$-Microglobulin is a 12-kDa soluble protein and binds to the extracellular domain of the α chain and stabilizes it. NK cells, part of the innate immune system, are inhibited by MHC class I. Malignant transformation can result in down-regulation of MHC class I, and transformed cells are thus targets for destruction by NK cells.

MHC class II is expressed constitutively on the thymic epithelium and *antigen-presenting cells* (*APCs*). MHC class II molecules are loaded with phagocytosed proteins that are processed into peptides with the APC. Thus, the MHC class II typically presents antigens present in the extracellular space. In humans, there are three MHC class II loci: HLA-DP, DQ, and DR, all of which are expressed codominantly. MHC class II comprises an α and a β chain, which together form a peptide-binding groove.

Antigen-Presenting Cells

APCs are a diverse but functionally related group of cells that express the MHC class II antigen-presenting molecule. These cells are capable of providing both "signal 1" (i.e., MHC–peptide ligands for the TCR) and "signal 2" (i.e., membrane-bound and soluble costimulatory molecules), thereby activating CD4$^+$ cells (see following text) and initiating a productive immune response. *Dendritic cells* (*DCs*), *tissue macrophages*, and B cells are members of this class of cells.

T Lymphocytes

T lymphocytes develop in the thymus from BM-derived progenitors. Key to the development of T cells is the fact that TCR molecules have evolved to recognize foreign antigenic epitopes presented to them in the context of MHC molecules. During their development, individual T cells undergo TCR gene complex recombination to generate an antigen receptor. Depending on whether its TCR has affinity for class I or class II MHC molecules, the immature T cell differentiates into a CD8$^+$ or CD4$^+$ lineage cell, respectively. T lymphocytes with too high an affinity for self-MHC molecules are negatively selected in the thymus. Upon egress from the thymus, mature CD4$^+$ and CD8$^+$ T cells hone to primary lymphoid organs (i.e., lymph nodes and spleen) and continuously recirculate throughout the body, thereby maximizing their potential to detect and respond to foreign antigens. Upon TCR recognition of foreign antigens presented in the context of MHC molecules along with appropriate costimulation, T cells are induced to differentiate into effector cells capable of orchestrating a coordinated immune response (i.e., CD4$^+$ helper T cells) or destroying infected cells and tissues (i.e., CD8$^+$ cytotoxic T cells). CD4$^+$ T cells are activated via MHC class II–TCR interactions, whereas CD8$^+$ T cells are activated via MHC class I–TCR interactions.

CD4$^+$ helper T cells act as modulators of the immune response and are divided into several subsets by their gene expression, biochemical mediators, and target cells. TH1 cells promote the cellular immune response through the activation of macrophages via production of the cytokines interferon-γ and TNF-β. TH2 cells enhance the humoral immune response through the production of IL-4, IL-5, and IL-13, which target B cells, basophils, and eosinophils. TH17 cells increase neutrophil activity through the secretion of IL17-A, IL17-F, L-21, and IL-22 and are thought to play a role in autoimmune diseases and immune responses against extracellular bacteria and fungi. *Regulatory T cells* (*Treg*) maintain immune tolerance and suppress the immune response through IL-10 and TGF-β. Treg cells play an antagonistic role against the proinflammatory actions of the other CD4$^+$ subsets.

The T-cell response against transplanted organs is primed via two complementary pathways of antigen presentation. In the *direct* pathway, donor MHC molecules expressed by APCs originating from the allograft directly activate alloreactive host T cells. In the *indirect* pathway, donor-derived antigens are processed and presented by recipient APCs. In experimental models of transplantation, organ allografts are not rejected in the absence of T lymphocytes. As such, T-cell–directed immunosuppression is currently the mainstay of antirejection immunotherapy at the time of transplantation.

B Lymphocytes

Like the T lymphocytes, B cells undergo BCR gene complex recombination to generate an antigen receptor in the BM. This BCR is then expressed in the form of IgM and IgD immunoglobulin molecules on the surface of immature BM B cells. At this early developmental stage, immature B cells are susceptible to *negative selection* via *apoptosis* upon BCR binding to a cognate autoantigen. Following the immature developmental checkpoint, the mature B lymphocyte enters the primary B-cell compartment as a *follicular* (*FO*) B cell in the spleen and lymph nodes. Alloreactive FO B cells are able to participate in generating a *germinal center* (*GC*) reaction through cognate interaction with alloreactive CD4$^+$ T cells following transplantation. This cognate T- and B-cell interaction occurs via MHC class II molecules expressed by B lymphocytes. The end result of this GC reaction is the generation of high-affinity alloreactive IgG-producing *plasma cells* and *memory B cells*. An equivalent process can occur from presentation of foreign MHC after blood transfusion or pregnancy leading to *alloantibody* formation in the absence of prior transplantation.

Alloantibodies pose a major challenge to the survival of organ allografts. These alloantibodies are detected via crossmatch assays in clinical HLA laboratories at transplant centers. Prior to transplantation, the presence of specific alloantibodies to the donor portends a poor prognosis for allograft survival and, in many cases, prevents the patient from receiving an organ transplant. Different transplanted organs may have different susceptibility to antibody-mediated damage, with the liver typically considered to be more resistant to this type of injury. Furthermore, appearance of alloantibodies following transplantation is tightly correlated with *chronic rejection* and *acute humoral rejection*. Despite this, the mainstay of immunosuppressive therapy for organ transplantation does not typically include agents that specifically target the B lymphocyte. An important focus of transplantation research is the development of novel immunotherapeutic approaches to curtail the alloantibody response and promote donor-specific B-lymphocyte tolerance.

Rejection

Hyperacute rejection occurs within minutes of graft revascularization and is the result of preformed antibodies directed against donor alloantigens. These alloantibodies are typically present as a result of blood transfusions, pregnancy, or previous organ transplantation. Following recognition of the allograft by the preformed alloantibody, the complement cascade injures the graft's endothelium, and hemorrhagic necrosis of the graft ensues, thanks in part to fibrin and platelet deposition, vasoconstriction, and neutrophil adhesion. As opposed to acute and chronic rejection, hyperacute rejection is a rare phenomenon since it can be prevented by screening recipients for alloantibodies in two ways. In the *panel reactive antibody* (*PRA*) assay, serum IgG and IgM antibodies contained in the recipients' serum are tested for binding to a panel of cells expressing a range of different HLA haplotypes. The PRA assay gives a "percent positive" readout, which directly indicates the proportion of cells (representing possible donors) with which the recipient serum is reactive. The traditional PRA assay has been largely replaced with a calculated PRA, which screens recipient serum against single antigen beads covering the spectrum of HLA molecules. This calculated PRA helps predict alloreactivity against a specific donor organ with a known HLA haplotype prior to transplantation. Further confirmation of alloreactivity can be seen with *crossmatching*, where a recipient's serum IgG and IgM antibodies are specifically tested for binding to donor-derived lymphocytes using flow cytometry or complement cytotoxicity assays. A positive crossmatch between the recipient and potential donor portends a poor prognosis for transplantation.

Prospective crossmatches are performed routinely for kidney and pancreas transplants as these grafts are most susceptible to hyperacute rejection and can tolerate the extra ischemia time required to perform the crossmatch assay.

A unique circumstance where a crossmatch for a kidney transplant is not always required is when the kidney is transplanted together with a liver from the same donor. Liver transplants are relatively resistant to humoral rejection. Indeed, even in the case of a multiply transplanted recipient, a prospective crossmatch for liver transplants is often not performed. This resistance of liver allografts to hyperacute rejection is presumably due to the liver's ability to absorb the alloantibodies from the recipient circulation. The tissue regenerative capacity of the liver may also play a role. This process is efficient enough that by the time the kidney is transplanted and perfused, there are no longer sufficient titers of circulating alloantibodies to trigger hyperacute kidney rejection.

Acute rejection is the most frequent form of rejection seen clinically and is thought to be the result of alloreactive T-cell activation via the direct and indirect pathways of antigen presentation. It typically occurs within a few weeks of transplantation but can occur episodically at any time during the transplant course, particularly in the face of suboptimal immunosuppression. In experimental models of transplantation, $CD4^+$ T cells are required for acute rejection to occur. This fact is consistent with the important role of $CD4^+$ T cells as central regulators of the adaptive immune response. Once activated, $CD8^+$ cytotoxic T cells recognize donor MHC class I antigen on transplant tissue parenchyma and kill the allograft cells. Additionally, the cytokines produced by both $CD4^+$ and $CD8^+$ T cells promote the nonspecific activation of macrophages, neutrophils, mast cells, and NK cells, which also contribute to graft injury. In cases of severe acute rejection, IgG antibodies may also result from $CD4^+$ T-cell interactions with B lymphocytes.

Chronic rejection remains the major cause of late graft failure. Pathologic examples of chronic rejection include obliterative bronchiolitis, cardiac allograft vasculopathy (CAV), and glomerulosclerosis. In the case of liver transplants, "ductopenic" chronic rejection is a well-described entity. Chronic rejection occurs over months to years after transplantation. Although chronic rejection is thought to have a T-cell–mediated component, alloantibodies produced by B lymphocytes also appear to have a key role. Nonimmune mechanisms such as ischemia–reperfusion injury, infections, and donor–recipient size mismatching may play a role in late graft failure as well.

ORGAN DONATION

The majority of transplanted organs are procured from brain dead patients, although the percentage of live donor kidney transplants has increased to greater than 33%. Brain death is determined by two in-hospital examinations 12 hours apart, usually performed by a neurologist or neurosurgeon, confirming (a) loss of cerebral function (no response to painful stimuli and no movement except for spinal reflexes) and (b) loss of brain stem function (fixed pupils; absence of corneal, oculovestibular, oculocephalic, and gag reflexes; and no respiratory effort after 3 minutes at a $p\text{CO}_2 \geq 60$ mm Hg). Declaration of brain death may be made 6 hours earlier with a brain scan documenting lack of cerebral blood flow. Because of the potential for conflict of interest, the surgical transplant team is never involved with the care of the donor or in the determination of brain death.

Some patients have irreversible neurologic injury but do not fulfill the criteria of true brain death. If families decide to withdraw life support, these patients can qualify as *non–heart-beating donors* (*NHBDs*) and their organs can be used after cessation of circulatory and respiratory function (*donation after cardiac death* [*DCD*]). These donors have an intrinsic variable phase of hypotension followed by cardiac arrest before organ recovery can begin. Initially, only the kidneys were used from NHDBs, but there has been increased utilization of other grafts including the liver, pancreas, lung, and even heart from such donors. Recipients of the kidneys from NHBDs have a higher risk of *delayed graft function* (DGF), where the transplanted kidney may not provide sufficient renal function to avoid dialysis early after the transplant but generally have equivalent long-term function likely to selection of high-quality donors. Livers from NHBDs have higher rates of biliary complications due to longer warm ischemic times.

The two main exclusion criteria for organ donation are malignancy and infection. Active donor malignancies typically preclude transplantation due to risk of transmission to the recipient, although exceptions are made for nonmelanoma skin cancers and central nervous system tumors. Treated donor malignancies are evaluated on an individual basis by tumor type, extent of disease, and disease-free interval to assess the risk of transmission. Although HIV infection historically excluded donation, recent legislation will allow HIV+ organs to be used for HIV+ recipients. Donor hepatitis, cytomegalovirus (CMV), and syphilis serologies are always determined, but positive serologies do not preclude organ donation. Organs from donors with positive hepatitis serologies are generally allocated only to recipients who are also positive or immune to hepatitis B and/or C. CMV and syphilis, should they occur in the recipient following transplantation, can be treated. A history of tuberculosis, active hepatitis B (sAg+), active herpes simplex virus (HSV) encephalitis, and seropositivity for human lymphotropic virus-1 (HTLV-1) or HTLV-2 in the donor may preclude donation.

DONOR OPERATION

A midline incision extending from the suprasternal notch to the pubis is made to enter the abdomen and thorax. A sternotomy is performed and the pericardium opened. The chest and abdomen are carefully explored to exclude any neoplasia or infection. In the thorax, the superior vena cava and aorta are dissected to allow later occlusion of the inflow and outflow tracts. In the abdomen, a right medial visceral rotation is performed, exposing the aorta, inferior vena cava (IVC), and inferior mesenteric vein (IMV). The left triangular ligament of the liver and the gastrohepatic ligament are divided, and the supraceliac aorta is prepared for cross-clamping. Heparin is given systemically. Cannulae are inserted into the distal abdominal aorta, IMV, and ascending aorta. After aortic cross-clamping, the heart is cooled with a potassium-rich cardioplegia solution through the ascending aortic cannula, and cold preservative solution is infused through the distal aortic and IMV cannulae. Ice is packed around the abdominal organs, and blood is vented through the IVC into the chest.

Blanching of the heart occurs within a few seconds, and the heart is removed first. After inflation of the lungs, the endotracheal tube is removed, and the trachea is stapled in preparation for removal of the lungs. The liver is removed with a diaphragmatic patch around the suprahepatic IVC, and the infrahepatic IVC is divided just above the renal veins. The gastroduodenal artery is divided, the portal vein is divided near the junction of the SMV and splenic veins, and the common bile duct (CBD) is divided near the duodenum. The hepatic artery is traced back to the origin of the celiac axis, where it is removed with a cuff of aorta. The pancreas is removed with the duodenum and a short segment of proximal jejunum, the spleen, and the origin of the superior mesenteric artery. The intestines can be kept in continuity with the liver if they are being used in a composite liver–intestine graft. The ureters are divided at the pelvic brim with their surrounding periureteral tissue. The kidneys can then be removed *en bloc* with the aorta and IVC kept in continuity or separated. The iliac arteries and veins are taken in the event vascular reconstruction of either the pancreatic or the liver; vasculature is required for successful implantation.

ORGAN PRESERVATION

To slow metabolic activity, hypothermia is induced by flushing the organs with 4°C preservation solution and storing them on ice. Nevertheless, metabolism continues, and the buildup of lactate, free fatty acids, and nucleotide breakdown products is accompanied by the depletion of glycogen, glutathione, and other reducing agents, making the organ sensitive to reperfusion injury. University of Wisconsin preservation fluid ("UW solution") was the original preservation solution developed to counteract these effects, and a number of different formulations now exist. The cationic composition of these solutions (high K+, low Na+) resembles the intracellular composition to minimize diffusion down electrochemical gradients. Lactobionate is impermeable and acts as an osmotic agent to suppress hypothermia-induced cell swelling. Calcium chelators suppress the activity of calcium-dependent enzymes such as phospholipases and proteases that would otherwise autodigest the cell. By chelating iron, they also may help suppress oxidative damage during reperfusion. Phosphate buffers are included to counteract the accumulated acids and, together with adenosine and dextrose, represent an effort to provide an energy source for the cells. Each organ can tolerate a different duration of cold ischemia (Table 5.1).

TABLE 5.1 Cold storage time (hours) for solid organs

Organs	Maximum Ischemic Time	Clinical Practice
Kidney	72	24–30
Kidney on pump	120–168	30
Liver	48	12–20
Pancreas	72	10–20
Small bowel	10	10
Heart	4	4
Lung	8	8
Lung with EVLP	12	10

RENAL TRANSPLANTATION

The majority of kidney transplants are performed in patients with insulin-dependent diabetes mellitus, glomerulonephritis, and hypertensive nephrosclerosis. Other causes of renal failure leading to transplant include polycystic kidney disease, systemic lupus erythematosus, Alport disease, IgA nephropathy, obstructive nephropathy, recurrent pyelonephritis, nephrosclerosis, and interstitial nephritis. Complications of prior transplants, including failure of an initial renal allograft and calcineurin inhibitor toxicity following transplantation of other organs, are growing indications for additional transplants. The potential kidney transplant recipient should be screened for occult infections at hemodialysis and peritoneal dialysis sites as well as underlying malignancies or infectious processes that are likely to complicate transplantation. Furthermore, a full cardiac, peripheral vascular, and neurologic exam is warranted given the association of end-stage renal disease (ESRD) with chronic cardiovascular disorders.

The usual exclusion criteria of active infection and malignancy apply to cadaveric kidney donors. *Expanded criteria donors* (*ECDs*) are those greater than 60 years of age or those over 50 years old with two of the following: a history of hypertension, terminal creatinine over 1.5, or death from a stroke. ECD kidneys are commonly used in appropriate patients. The ECD classification is being replaced by a *kidney donor profile index* (*KDPI*) that accounts for a number of donor risk factors and which will become a factor in renal allocation.

Living donors are generally young and without comorbidities, but donors of increasing age, body mass index, and treated hypertension can be approved to donate if otherwise healthy. The presence of two normal kidneys is confirmed by measuring serum chemistries and creatinine clearance, performing a urinalysis, and by imaging the kidney using a combined MRI/MRA or CT angiography.

Transplant outcomes in the case of renal allografts from living donors are substantially better than those from deceased donors. This difference is due to several factors including the fact that living donor kidneys are in better condition, the time of transplant from a living donor may be optimized for the recipient, and the recipient and donor may be better matched for HLA haplotype. Moreover, living donor kidneys are less likely to suffer from DGF or acute tubular necrosis (ATN) because cold ischemia time is kept to a minimum. In addition, deceased donor kidneys may have suffered multiple physiologic insults while still in the donor because of the physiologic derangements that occur during brain death. In terms of timing of transplant for the recipient, waiting times for a deceased donor kidney depend on blood type and region of the country and vary from 2 to 7 years or longer. Longer waiting time translates into an increased risk of death, even after transplantation. It is often possible to avoid dialysis altogether with a living donor transplant or early listing for deceased donor kidneys. This strategy is known as preemptive transplantation. Although patients are fully evaluated and medically optimized for surgery at the time of evaluation, it is difficult to maintain this status during the long waiting time. Finally, the potential for improved HLA matching contributes to the longer half-life of living donor kidneys and may lower the risk of sensitizing the recipient for subsequent transplants.

Most living donor operations are performed laparoscopically both on the left and the right side. The procedure can be performed with a hand port, with total laparoscopic technique, or with single port technology. In any of these approaches, an incision must be made to remove the kidney in transplantable condition. A longer renal vein and easier access to the renal artery make the left kidney the graft of choice. Exceptions to this strategy are donors who have multiple left renal arteries demonstrated by preoperative imaging. Gonadal and adrenal veins are typically ligated. The ureter is divided first proximal to the bladder, and the distal stump is ligated. The renal artery is divided as close to its origin from the aorta as possible. Subsequently, the renal vein is divided near its junction with the vena cava. The kidney is removed, and blood is flushed from the kidney by instilling cold heparinized preservative solution into the artery, and the kidney is immersed in an icy slush during the interval before transplantation. Living donor nephrectomies can also be performed as an open surgery with an oblique flank incision. Although operating room costs are greater for laparoscopic donor nephrectomies, this is compensated for by quicker return to work and daily living, shorter hospital stays, and an improved quality of life.

The kidney recipient operation is typically performed through an extraperitoneal approach via an oblique incision in the left or right lower quadrant, although a midline incision and intraperitoneal approach may be employed in pediatric recipients or when surgically indicated (Fig. 5.1). The lymphatics overlying the iliac vessels should be ligated to avoid lymphocele formation following transplantation. Typically, the donor renal artery is anastomosed in an end-to-side fashion to the external iliac artery. The renal vein is anastomosed end-to-side to the external iliac vein. The donor ureter is usually attached to the recipient bladder (ureteroneocystostomy), but urinary tract continuity can also be established by anastomosing the recipient ureter to the donor renal pelvis (ureteropyelostomy) or donor ureter (ureteroureterostomy) if there are problems with either the donor's ureter or the recipient's bladder. Before unclamping the vessels at the end of the operation, most surgeons administer mannitol and furosemide to promote diuresis.

DGF occurs in up to 30% of deceased donor transplants. This is typically due to ATN stemming from ischemic insult and resulting reperfusion injury. As expected, these pathologies occur much more rarely in living donor transplants. This condition is generally self-limited, but it is important to distinguish it from other causes of low urine output such as rejection or technical complications requiring intervention. Technical complications with the vascular anastomoses can be ruled out with transplant ultrasound or a radioisotope nuclear perfusion scan. If ultrasound shows a correctable cause of poor renal function such as anastomotic problems, thrombosis, or hematoma, urgent reexploration is required. If the kidney does not recover despite vascular patency, a biopsy should be performed to exclude rejection. Urine leaks can present as fluid collections or a persistently elevated creatinine due to urine reabsorption. The cause of such leaks may be technical in nature, but typically, they develop as a result of ischemia of the distal ureter. Such leaks are usually treated with stenting and percutaneous drainage of the collection, although reoperation and surgical revision is performed if the leak is large. Mild ischemia can lead to late strictures in the ureter and may require surgical reconstruction if dilation and stenting fail. *Renal transplant artery stenosis* (*RTAS*) generally presents with hypertension and decreased renal function and can be due to either technical or immunologic causes. It occurs 3 months to 2 years after transplantation. Percutaneous transluminal angioplasty with occasional stenting can be successful at treating RTAS.

Rejection of the graft remains the most frequent cause of early graft failure. Hyperacute rejection is rare because of prospective crossmatching. In this condition, alloreactive antibodies fix and activate complement, thereby rendering the endothelium prothrombotic. Deposition of fibrin thrombi and platelet aggregates causes rapid compromise of renal allograft perfusion, leading to a bluish discoloration of the graft and cessation of graft function. This devastating complication necessitates immediate removal of the graft. Acute cellular rejection is the most common form of rejection and typically occurs within months of transplantation. Patients may present with fever, graft tenderness, malaise, oliguria, or elevation in serum creatinine. A renal biopsy, usually obtained percutaneously, is the gold standard for the diagnosis of acute graft rejection. When acute rejection is diagnosed, prompt rescue therapy with intravenous high-dose steroids and/or antilymphocyte antibodies is initiated. Chronic rejection causes a gradual decline of renal function over years and is an important contributor to late graft loss. Clinical signs include proteinuria and microscopic hematuria, which are usually accompanied by a progressive rise

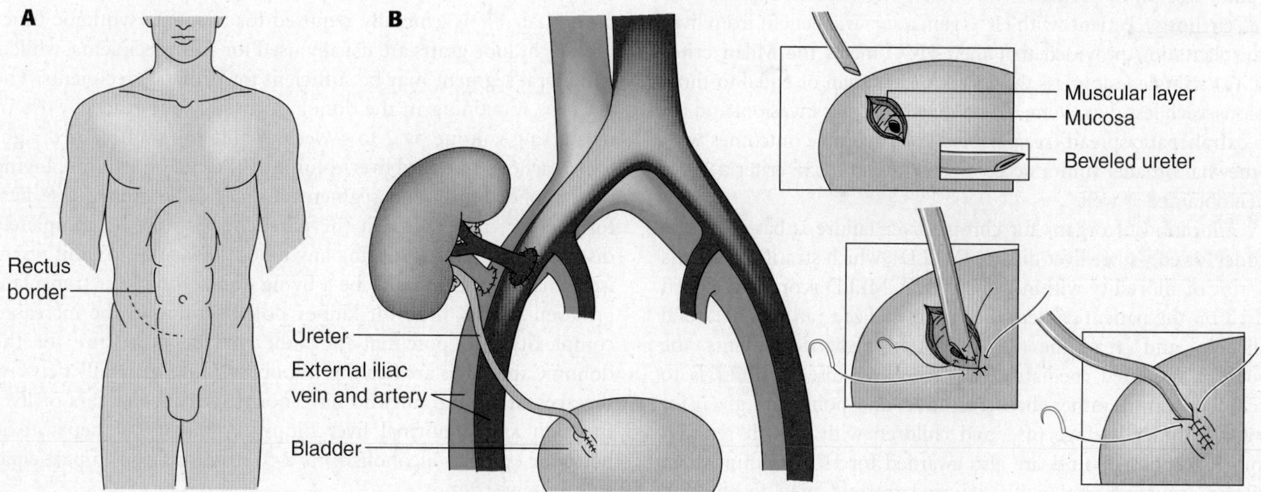

FIGURE 5.1 Renal transplantation incision **(A)** and completed implantation **(B)**. (From Mulholland MW. *Greenfield's Surgery: Scientific Principles and Practice*. 5th ed. Philadelphia: Lippincott Williams & Wilkins; 2011.)

in serum creatinine. The diagnosis of chronic rejection is made by renal biopsy, which shows thickening of the glomerular basement membranes, interstitial fibrosis, and proliferation of arterial smooth muscle cells. It is generally accepted that the emergence of alloantibodies is a main factor contributing to the pathogenesis of chronic rejection. There is no consensus treatment for chronic rejection, with different centers attempting rescue therapy using a variety of approaches.

One-year graft survival for HLA identical living-related kidney transplants exceeds 95%, 5-year graft survival is over 90%, and 10-year graft survival is over 65%. One-year graft survival of one-haplotype–matched living-related kidneys is over 90%. For deceased donor renal transplants, 1-year graft survival rates are over 88% and 5-year graft survival is over 66%. Among deceased donor renal grafts, six-antigen–matched grafts have a superior 1-year (93%) and 5-year (77%) graft survival. Organ quality has a significant independent impact on expected graft survival. National sharing of six-antigen–matched organs has been limited to highly sensitized recipients.

LIVER TRANSPLANTATION

Indications for liver transplantation include (a) decompensated hepatic cirrhosis, (b) intractable portal hypertension, (c) nonresectable tumors isolated to the liver (predominately *hepatocellular carcinoma* [*HCC*]), and (d) recurrent cholangitis not amenable to conventional surgical treatment. Causes of cirrhosis and portal hypertension include alcoholic liver disease, chronic hepatitis B or C, nonalcoholic steatotic hepatitis (NASH), primary sclerosing cholangitis (PSC), primary biliary cirrhosis (PBC), Wilson's disease, hemochromatosis, rare forms of α1-antitrypsin deficiency, amyloidosis, Budd–Chiari syndrome, and congenital hepatic fibrosis. Fulminant liver failure can be due to viral hepatitis (Hep A > Hep B > Hep C), autoimmune hepatitis, drug toxicity (especially acetaminophen), or ingestion of various *Amanita* mushrooms. Liver transplantation following acute liver failure is associated with a significantly higher acute mortality than following chronic liver disease. However, the long-term prognosis of patients receiving liver transplants following acute liver failure is superior. Often resection of HCC cannot be undertaken because of insufficient hepatic reserve in patients with underlying chronic liver disease (i.e., cirrhosis). Patients with HCC gain a survival benefit from liver transplantation provided that their HCC meets the Milan criteria: (a) a single lesion less than 5 cm or less than or equal to three lesions, each less than 3 cm; (b) no macrovascular invasion; and (c) no extrahepatic spread (see Chapter 13). Favorable outcomes with somewhat broader tumor acceptance criteria (UCSF criteria) have been obtained as well.

Allocation of organs for chronic liver failure is based on the model for end-stage liver disease (MELD), which stratifies patients by risk of mortality within 3 months. A MELD score is assigned based on the patient's international normalized ratio (INR), total bilirubin, and creatinine (Table 5.2). In pediatric patients, the model is modified (pediatric end-stage liver disease [PELD]) to include albumin, rather than creatinine, and points are given for children under the age of 1 and children with growth retardation. "Exception" points are also awarded for HCC within Milan criteria, recurrent cholangitis, inborn errors of metabolism, and hepatopulmonary syndrome. Status 1 designation pertains only to patients with fulminant hepatic failure and to those with primary graft failure or early hepatic artery thrombosis following transplant.

TABLE 5.2 MELD and PELD calculations

MELD = 9.57 × log e (creatinine) + 3.78 × log e × (bilirubin) + 11.2 × log e (INR) + 6.43
PELD = 4.8 × log e (bilirubin) + 18.57 × log e (INR)−6.87 × log e (albumin) + 4.36 (if patients are <1 y of age) + 6.67 (if the patient has height or weight ≤2 standard deviations below average for age)
Calculated score is rounded to the nearest whole number.

MELD, model for end-stage liver disease; PELD, pediatric end-stage liver disease; INR, international normalized ratio.

As discussed earlier, though donor–recipient pairs are usually chosen with ABO blood group compatibility in mind, HLA matching and prospective crossmatching are not performed in the case of liver transplantation.

Uncontrolled infections or cardiovascular instability are the most frequent reasons that exclude patients from receiving liver transplants. Hepatorenal syndrome is not an absolute contraindication to liver transplantation, as patients receiving up to 6 weeks of dialysis see recovery of their renal function with liver transplant alone in most cases. Simultaneous kidney transplants can be performed if indicated. Evidence of severe brain edema in fulminant hepatic failure suggests irreversible brain damage and is considered a contraindication to transplantation.

The shortage of donor organs, particularly in the pediatric population, has led to the development of alternatives to the standard orthotopic liver transplant procedure. Specifically, lobar or segmental transplantation of part of a donor liver (either deceased or living) is possible due to the liver's regenerative capacity as well as its segmental internal architecture (see Chapter 13). Thus, two recipients can benefit from one donor, and the reduced size livers can fit into the abdominal cavity of a child.

Another approach to increase the donor pool is *living-donor liver transplantation*. Potential advantages of living-related liver transplantation are similar to those of living-related renal transplantation: shortened waiting times, shorter cold ischemia time, improved histocompatibility, and use of an organ from a physiologically normal donor. Because a graft-to-body weight ratio of more than 1% is generally required for adequate synthetic function, right lobe grafts are usually used for adult recipients, while a left lateral segment may be sufficient for pediatric recipients. The left lobe remaining in the donor of a right lobe reaches 90% of its starting volume by 2 to 4 weeks, while the transplanted right lobe reaches a standard liver volume by the end of 1 month. Living donor lobectomies and segmentectomies differ from those performed for cancer in that the parenchyma must be completely dissected before interrupting any blood flow so as to limit warm ischemia time. Criteria to be a living donor for a liver transplant are even stricter than for kidney donation due to the increased complexity and potential morbidity of the procedure for the donor. Candidates are healthy, nonobese adults generally between the ages of 21 and 50 who have normal serum markers of liver function and a normal liver biopsy. A history of hepatotoxic behavior (such as alcoholism) is a contraindication to participation as a liver donor.

The liver transplant recipient operation (Fig. 5.2) is performed through a bilateral subcostal incision with midline extension. Portal hypertension and coagulopathy may contribute to blood loss.

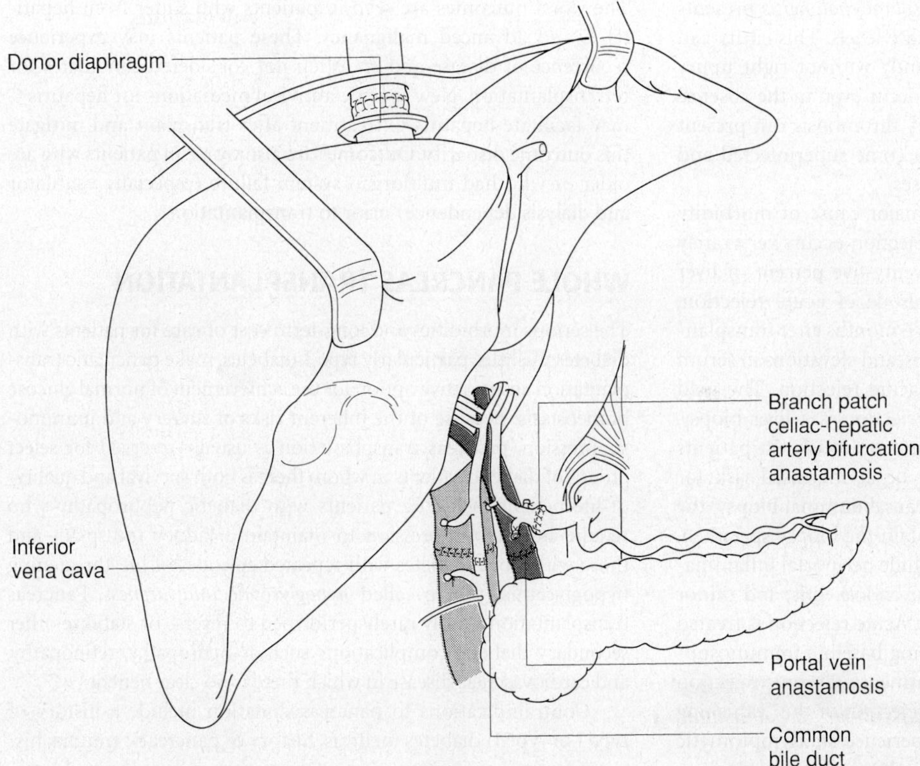

FIGURE 5.2 Completed liver transplantation. (From Greenfield LJ. *Surgery: Scientific Principles and Practice.* 1st ed. Philadelphia: J.B. Lippincott; 1993:534, with permission.)

The right and left branches of the hepatic artery, the CBD, and the cystic duct are divided at the hilum. Clamps are placed on the portal vein and suprahepatic vena cava/hepatic veins. Because caval and portal blood flow interruption is poorly tolerated for significant periods, this clamping is done just prior to removing the native liver. In some cases, "piggyback" technique (see below) or venovenous bypass are used to mitigate hemodynamic changes. The suprahepatic IVC anastomosis can be performed end-to-end followed by an end-to-end anastomosis at the infrahepatic IVC. Alternatively, recipient hepatectomy can be performed leaving the IVC in place, and an end-to-side anastomosis is done to the combined orifices of the recipient's hepatic veins ("piggyback") followed by ligation of the donor infrahepatic IVC. This technique does not require caval occlusion. The preservative fluid is flushed out of the liver by infusing lactated Ringer's solution through the portal vein. Subsequently, the portal vein is anastomosed end to end, and then, the liver is reperfused. The hepatic artery may be anastomosed to a branch patch of the recipient hepatic artery system before or after portal reperfusion.

On reperfusion, hypotension, arrhythmias, and, occasionally, cardiac arrest may occur because of the bolus of cold, hyperkalemic, and acidotic blood–solution mixture traveling from the donor liver to the heart. Biliary reconstruction can be performed as an end-to-end anastomosis of donor and recipient CBD or as a Roux-en-Y choledochojejunostomy between donor CBD and a defunctionalized limb of recipient jejunum.

Technical complications include intra-abdominal bleeding, hepatic artery thrombosis, and bile leak. Postoperative bleeding is occasionally due to surgical bleeding from varices or one of the vascular anastomoses, although it is also relatively common not to find a site of bleeding upon reexploration of the patient. Postoperative coagulopathy and thrombocytopenia result in diffuse oozing from extensive dissection planes. Intra-abdominal clot and blood then promotes fibrinolysis, causing persistent oozing even when the INR and platelet count are corrected. Patients with a persistent blood transfusion requirement may benefit from reoperation for evacuation of hematoma to interrupt the fibrinolytic cycle even if there is no surgical bleeding to repair. *Hepatic artery thrombosis* is a particular problem in pediatric patients because of the small size of the vessels involved. Because the vascular supply of the bile duct, particularly the donor CBD, arises from the hepatic artery, these patients may present with a biliary leak or even necrosis and complete dehiscence of the CBD accompanied by deteriorating liver function. This complication often requires retransplantation. *Biliary leaks* resulting from aggressive skeletonization of the donor duct, or technical errors in the placement of stitches, sometimes respond to conservative management when adequately drained. These patients are at increased risk of developing late strictures because of scar tissue around the duct.

Nontechnical reasons for graft dysfunction or failure include *primary nonfunction* (*PNF*), *early allograft dysfunction* (*EAD*), and early rejection. PNF occurs in 2% to 5% of liver transplants and is attributable to ischemia–reperfusion injury, steatosis, poor nutritional status of the donor, and an incompletely characterized humoral immune response. Clinically, the patient develops fulminant hepatic failure early after liver transplantation. Retransplantation is generally required within a few days. If retransplantation can be accomplished within the first week, the results are equivalent to those of a primary transplant. EAD occurs in around 23% of liver transplants and is characterized by persistent hyperbilirubinemia, persistent transaminitis, or failure to correct coagulopathy at 1 week following liver transplant. Risk factors for the development of EAD include older donor age and higher recipient MELD score preceding transplant. Although many allografts that develop EAD eventually recover biochemical function, EAD is associated with higher mortality and higher rates of graft loss.

In addition to the infections common to all transplant patients, clinicians should understand that certain infections are unique to the liver transplant population. *Posttransplant cholangitis* presents as rising bilirubin and alkaline phosphatase levels. This entity can arise with or without fevers and frequently without right upper quadrant (RUQ) pain. Moreover, it can occur even in the absence of biliary obstruction. Late hepatic artery thrombosis can present with areas of necrosis in the liver that become superinfected and present with fevers caused by liver abscesses.

Liver allograft rejection remains a major cause of morbidity after liver transplantation. Hyperacute rejection occurs very rarely in hepatic transplantation. Fifteen to twenty-five percent of liver transplants recipients experience an episode of acute rejection, most commonly during the first 7 days to 6 months after transplantation. Fever, graft tenderness, leukocytosis, and elevations in serum bilirubin and hepatic enzymes suggest acute rejection. The gold standard for diagnosing acute hepatic rejection is a liver biopsy. These biopsies are typically obtained percutaneously. In patients with ascites or coagulopathy who may be at increased risk for complications following percutaneous transabdominal biopsy, the internal jugular vein is cannulated to obtain the biopsy specimen. Histologic findings of acute rejection include periportal inflammatory infiltrates, destructive cholangitis or endothelitis, and minor inflammatory changes in hepatic lobules. Acute rejection is treated with a rescue course of steroids, increasing baseline immunosuppression, or antithymocyte antibody treatments. Chronic rejection has also been referred to as ductopenic rejection or the "vanishing bile duct syndrome." Patients usually experience an asymptomatic rise in alkaline phosphatase and gamma-glutamyl transpeptidase. These patients eventually develop jaundice and pruritus. Severe cases of chronic rejection are treated with retransplantation.

Currently, the 1-year patient survival rate after liver transplantation is greater than 85% at most institutions. The 10-year patient survival rate is over 60%. Survival rates are dependent on the indication for the procedure. The best results are obtained in patients who undergo hepatic transplantation for cholestatic liver disease. The worst outcomes are seen in patients who suffer from hepatitis C and advanced malignancy. These patients may experience recurrence of disease and are often not considered candidates for retransplantation. New specific antiviral mediations for hepatitis C may facilitate hepatitis C treatment after transplant and mitigate this outcome disparity. Outcomes are also worse in patients who are older or who had multiorgan system failure (especially ventilator and dialysis dependence) prior to transplantation.

WHOLE PANCREAS TRANSPLANTATION

The serious morbidities and long-term cost of care for patients with diabetes mellitus, particularly type 1 diabetes, make pancreatic transplantation an attractive option for the achievement of normal glucose homeostasis. Because of the inherent risks of surgery and immunosuppression, pancreas transplantation is usually reserved for select groups of diabetic patients in whom there is both survival and quality-of-life benefit including patients with diabetic nephropathy who require immunosuppression to maintain a kidney transplant and those with labile diabetes with repeated episodes of life-threatening hypoglycemia, the so-called *hypoglycemic unawareness*. Pancreas transplantation is only rarely performed to reverse or stabilize other secondary diabetic complications such as neuropathy, retinopathy, and cardiovascular disease in which there is no clear benefit.

Contraindications to pancreas donation include a history of type I or type II diabetes mellitus, history of pancreatic trauma, history of prior pancreatic surgery, pancreatitis, severe atherosclerosis, and significant intra-abdominal contamination. Although segmental pancreatic grafts have been reported, most centers transplant whole pancreaticoduodenal allografts.

The pancreas is transplanted ectopically into the iliac fossa with the arterial blood supply coming from the recipient iliac artery (Fig. 5.3). Venous drainage is established by anastomosing the donor portal vein to the recipient iliac vein (i.e., systemic drainage)

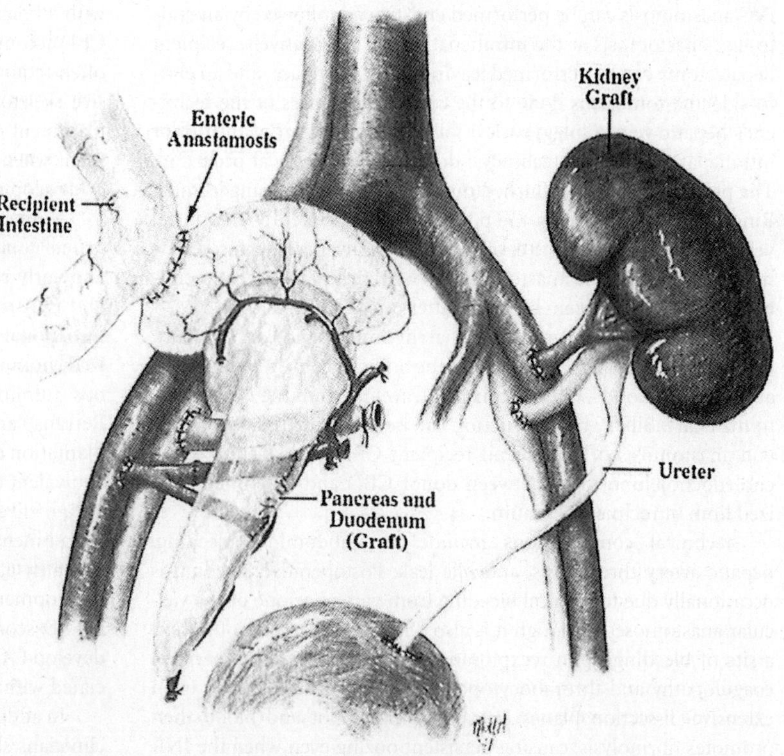

FIGURE 5.3 Enterically drained simultaneous pancreas and kidney transplant with systemic venous drainage. (From LeRoith D, Olefsky JM, Taylor SI. *Diabetes Mellitus: A Fundamental and Clinical Text.* 3rd ed. Philadelphia: Lippincott Williams & Wilkins; 2004:735, with permission.)

or to the superior mesenteric vein (i.e., portal drainage). Exocrine drainage is generally managed through enteric or bladder drainage via the duodenal segment with enteric drainage now the more common technique. Advantages of bladder drainage include the ability to diagnose rejection by urinary amylase levels, cystoscopic access for transduodenal needle biopsies, lower rates of infection, and relative technical ease. The main disadvantages are hematuria and cystitis/urethritis secondary to biochemical irritation from the pancreatic exocrine drainage. Metabolic acidosis resulting from loss of bicarbonate in the urine is also a frequently encountered entity. Conversion to enteric drainage can be performed operatively if these complications of bladder drainage occur.

Glucose levels are followed closely postoperatively, and patients may be initially maintained on insulin infusions to keep serum glucose levels below 200 mg/dL. Particular attention needs to be paid to fluid balance as well as bicarbonate and electrolyte losses in the initial postoperative period. Serum amylase and lipase are frequently elevated initially as a result of ischemia–reperfusion pancreatitis. These typically are rapidly diminished shortly after transplantation.

One-year patient survival in the case of pancreatic transplants exceeds 90%. One-year pancreas graft survival, as defined by complete insulin independence, is greater than 70%. One-year pancreas survival for simultaneous pancreas–kidney transplants is higher at greater than 80%. Despite the relatively good outcomes associated with pancreas transplantation, clinical vigilance must be maintained to detect and treat potential posttransplant complications. Because rejection is the major etiology for pancreatic allograft loss, early diagnosis and treatment is critical to the outcome of pancreas transplantation. Rejection of the exocrine gland typically precedes rejection of the endocrine pancreas. Therefore, hyperglycemia indicates advanced rejection and potentially irreversible damage to the graft. Pancreatic graft rejection can be suggested by changes in exocrine and endocrine parameters in the serum (and urine for the bladder-drained pancreas allograft). Such episodes of rejection are sometimes treated empirically with antilymphocyte antibody therapy if there is high clinical suspicion. In combined kidney–pancreas transplants, elevation of serum creatinine, combined with renal graft biopsy, is a convenient way to guide therapy. Another cause of graft failure is *donor splenic vein thrombosis*, which can progress into the SMV/portal confluence and prevent venous outflow from the graft. This entity generally presents with pain and an elevated serum amylase, lipase, and glucose and is best diagnosed by magnetic resonance venography (MRV) or ultrasound. Anticoagulation is sometimes sufficient for nonocclusive thrombi, but percutaneous or surgical thrombectomy can also be used as a treatment modality.

INTESTINAL TRANSPLANTATION

Intestinal transplantation is indicated in patients with irreversible intestinal failure resulting in permanent parental nutrition dependence and with complications of parenteral nutrition use including cholestatic liver disease, thrombosis of at least two central veins, recurrent or severe catheter-associated bloodstream infections, and persistent fluid and electrolyte disturbance. Intestinal failure is most commonly the result of massive surgical resection of the small bowel leading to *short-bowel syndrome* (*SBS*). In adults, the underlying causes of such operations include mesenteric ischemia, Crohn's disease, traumatic injury, and radiation injury. In children, SBS is seen following necrotizing enterocolitis, gastroschisis, and congenital intestinal anomalies. Indications outside of the setting of SBS include malabsorptive disorders, motility disorders, and rarely tumors.

Intestinal transplantation is subdivided into three distinct procedures: (a) isolated intestinal transplantation of the jejunoileum, (b) liver–intestinal transplantation of the liver and jejunoileal axis, and (c) multivisceral transplantation of the stomach, duodenum, liver, pancreas, jejunum, and ileum. The choice of procedure is dictated principally by the presence of concurrent liver failure related to parenteral nutrition and comorbid disease of the pancreas, stomach, or colon. Isolated intestinal transplantation is conducted through a midline laparotomy incision with unilateral or bilateral extension. Typically, an extensive lysis of adhesions is required prior to recipient enterectomy given the extensive surgical history that usually precedes SBS. The donor intestine must be carefully matched to the size of the recipient's abdominal cavity due to a high rate of abdominal wall complications associated with this procedure (see the following text). Arterial blood supply is established by anastomosing the donor SMA with an aortic patch to the recipient infrarenal aorta. Venous drainage typically consists of an anastomosis of the donor SMV to the recipient's portal vein, SMV, or splenic vein, although caval drainage can be used if the portal system is inaccessible due to thrombosis or prior surgery. Enteric inflow is achieved with an end-to-end jejunojejunostomy, and enteric outflow usually consists of an end-to-side ileocolostomy. A temporary loop ileostomy is raised at the skin surface to facilitate endoscopic surveillance of the allograft. A jejunostomy tube is fashioned in the proximal jejunum to provide access for postoperative enteral nutrition. The surgical technique for combined liver–intestinal transplantation and multivisceral transplantation are more complicated and are beyond the scope of this chapter.

Technical complications of intestinal transplantation include bleeding, thrombosis, anastomotic leak, and abdominal compartment syndrome. Because most intestinal transplant recipients have complicated prior abdominal surgical history, abdominal wall closure is often challenging. Many patients develop loss of domain of the abdominal cavity and require techniques such as pretransplant abdominal tissue expanders, temporary mesh closure, abdominal myocutaneous flaps, or abdominal wall transplant to restore domain.

Acute cellular rejection can be particularly devastating in intestinal transplantation and has a high incidence (60%) compared to other solid organ transplants. It usual presents in the first month following transplantation and initially presents with fever, abdominal pain, nausea, vomiting, and increased ostomy output. It can progress to bacteremia or fungemia and septic shock as bacteria and fungi translocate across the injured mucosa. Severe acute cellular rejection is associated with high rates of graft loss. Because of the severity of acute cellular rejection, the patient typically undergo routine endoscopy with biopsy or zoom endoscopy without biopsy twice weekly via ileostomy for the first month after transplantation. Acute cellular rejection is treated with increased calcineurin inhibition, corticosteroids, or antilymphocyte antibodies. Chronic rejection presents later with anorexia, intestinal stricture or obstruction, gastrointestinal (GI) bleeding, or chronic diarrhea and often requires graft excision. Further complicating the immunologic management of intestinal transplant recipients, intestinal transplant recipients exhibit a higher rate of *graft versus host disease* (*GVHD*) than seen in other solid organ transplants. GVHD occurs when immune cells from the transplanted allograft recognize the recipient as "foreign" and mount an immune response against the recipient. GVHD can affect a number of different systems with cutaneous, GI, ocular, hematopoietic, and renal manifestation seen most frequently. GVHD is seen in around 7% of intestinal transplant recipients; this contrasts with an incidence of less than 0.5% in recipients of other solid organ transplants.

Despite these challenges, 1-year patient survival after intestinal transplantation is now greater than 75% with higher survival reported at individual centers. Five-year patient survival is greater than 55%. Combined liver–intestinal transplants typically fare better than isolated intestinal allograft, probably because the liver affords the intestine some protection from the alloimmune response.

HEART TRANSPLANTATION

Heart transplantation is performed for end-stage heart disease that is refractory to medical management. One-year survival rates are above 80%, and 5-year survival rates are well above 70%. Improvements in medical management, revascularization techniques, and mechanical ventricular assist devices have decreased the rate of death while on the waiting list. The most common etiologies of heart failure requiring transplantation are idiopathic dilated cardiomyopathy and ischemic heart disease. More unusual etiologies include ventricular dysfunction secondary to valvular or congenital disease and malignant ventricular arrhythmia. Congenital heart disease is the primary indication for heart transplantation in children. Contraindications to cardiac transplantation include cancer, recent pulmonary emboli, active infection, and fixed pulmonary resistance greater than 6 Wood units that does not respond to vasodilators.

Donors and recipients must be ABO and size (within 20% total body weight) compatible. HLA matching is done only if recipients have a high PRA on workup; sensitization in this population can occur because many have had blood transfusions associated with previous cardiac surgery, including previous transplant. Therefore, an extremely conservative approach to blood transfusions, particularly in younger patients undergoing routine cardiac surgery, may afford a great survival advantage should these patients subsequently require a cardiac allograft. Contraindications to heart donation include infection, extracranial malignancy, ventricular dysrhythmias (which may occur primarily as a result of the physiologic changes of brain death), and death from carbon monoxide poisoning with a blood carboxyhemoglobin level greater than 20%. Donor management frequently requires a Swan–Ganz catheter to guide hemodynamic monitoring, and donors above 40 to 45 years of age may get a cardiac catheterization to exclude coronary atherosclerosis. An echocardiogram must show normal valvular anatomy and ventricular function.

Most hearts are transplanted orthotopically. The biatrial technique involves four anastomoses: the left and right atria, the pulmonary artery, and the aorta (Fig. 5.4). The bicaval heart transplant begins with complete excision of the recipient heart except for a cuff of left atrial tissue around the ostia of the paired pulmonary veins and small cavoatrial cuffs requiring five anastomoses. Total orthotopic implantation utilizes pulmonary venous cuffs, necessitating six anastomoses. Proponents of the latter two methods argue that they are associated with improved atrial function, a reduction of atrial arrhythmias, as well as improved tricuspid and mitral valve function. However, many surgeons feel that these advantages are marginal and are outweighed by the longer ischemic times and higher risk for anastomotic complications.

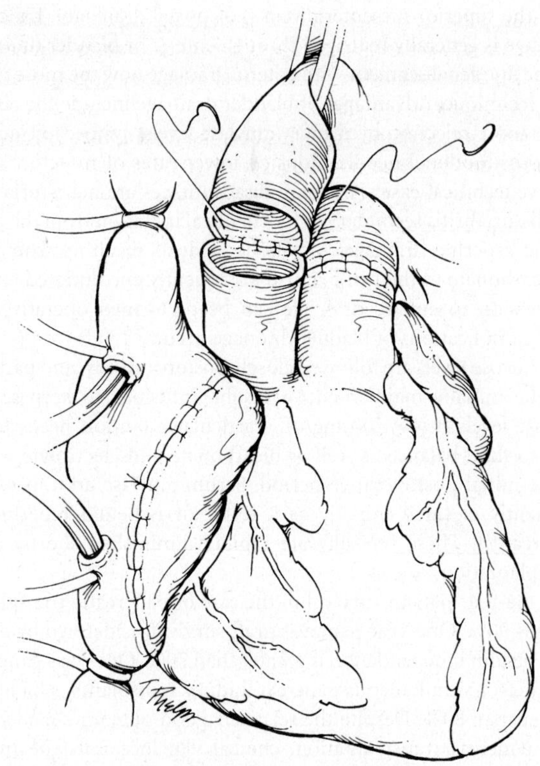

FIGURE 5.4 Aortic anastomosis at completion of orthotopic cardiac transplantation. (From Kaiser LR, Kron IL, Spray TL. *Mastery of Cardiothoracic Surgery*. 1st ed. Philadelphia: Lippincott Williams & Wilkins; 1998:506, with permission.)

Right ventricular dysfunction occurs commonly in the early posttransplant period, usually as a result of ischemic injury and elevated pulmonary vascular resistance. Inotropic support and pulmonary vasodilators are frequently used during the first 2 to 3 days posttransplantation. Loss of vagal innervation to the transplanted heart results in a resting heart rate of approximately 100 beats/minute. In addition, the transplanted heart is unresponsive to digoxin and atropine. Early postoperative bradyarrhythmias are usually the result of donor sinoatrial and atrioventricular dysfunction caused by surgical trauma, ischemic injury, and long bypass time. Most of these bradyarrhythmias respond well to pharmacologic agents such as isoproterenol or to temporary epicardial pacing. However, permanent pacemakers will occasionally be required.

Acute rejection is common during the first few months after transplantation but accounts for fewer than 10% of early deaths after cardiac transplantation. The most frequent symptom of rejection is fatigue, and one of the early signs of rejection is tachyarrhythmia. Endomyocardial biopsy is the gold standard for diagnosis of acute cardiac allograft rejection. Surveillance biopsies are frequently done during the first year after transplantation. Acute allograft rejection typically responds quite well to steroid rescue therapy. Cytolytic agents are reserved for episodes of severe rejection associated with hemodynamic compromise or episodes resistant to steroids. The major cause of morbidity and mortality after the first year following transplant is CAV. This pathologic process is thought to be mediated by alloantibodies and results in diffuse narrowing of the epicardial coronary arteries, intramyocardial arterioles, and venous structures. Because reinnervation is incomplete, most cardiac

CAV: Cardiac allograft vasculopathy.

transplant patients do not experience chest pain. Cardiac ischemia in heart transplant recipients typically presents not as angina but as heart failure or sudden death. Either coronary angiography or intravascular coronary ultrasound is necessary to diagnose CAV. Acute rejection ischemia–reperfusion injury, drug toxicity, hyperlipidemia, and hypertension may contribute to the development of CAV. The only definitive treatment for CAV is retransplantation. Infections are responsible for 10% of early deaths and 30% of late deaths. Heart transplant recipients are particularly susceptible to infections with the herpes viruses, namely CMV, Epstein–Barr virus (EBV), varicella zoster virus, and several HSV subtypes.

LUNG TRANSPLANTATION

The most common indications for lung transplantation are chronic obstructive pulmonary disease (30%), idiopathic pulmonary fibrosis (29%), and cystic fibrosis (16%). Other causes of end-stage lung disease treated with transplantation include α1-antitrypsin deficiency, idiopathic pulmonary arterial hypertension, and retransplantation. Septic diseases such as cystic fibrosis are treated with double-lung replacement to remove septic foci and avoid contamination of the donor allograft by the native lung. Lung and combined heart–lung transplants are performed for end-stage pulmonary parenchymal and vascular disorders and for patients with congenital heart disease complication by refractory pulmonary hypertension. Each disease process has specific guidelines (e.g., values for forced expiratory volume in 1 second [FEV_1], vital capacity, or pulmonary artery pressure) for the timing of referral for transplant, but the general indications for transplantation include failure of other therapies, high risk of death within 2 years, and functional disability without loss of the ability to ambulate. Active cigarette smokers are not considered candidates for lung transplant. High-dose steroid therapy and ventilator dependence are relative contraindications to transplant. One-year patient survival after lung transplantation is 83%, 2-year patient survival is 73%, and 5-year patient survival is 54%, the lowest of all solid organ transplants.

The donor and recipient must be ABO and size compatible. HLA matching is not performed. When accepting the donor lungs, it is important to rule out infectious processes and malignancy. In addition, the PO_2 at 100% oxygen and 5 cm H_2O of positive end-expiratory pressure (PEEP) ideally should exceed 350 mm Hg. Bronchoscopy is routinely performed. Because the lung graft can maintain a low level of aerobic metabolism by utilizing oxygen that diffuses from the alveoli to endothelial and parenchymal cells, the lungs are removed from the donor by clamping the trachea after a full volume of ventilation, maintaining them in an inflated state.

The lung is generally the most fragile organ in cadaveric donors and is the least likely organ to be suitable for transplantation. Normothermic *ex vivo lung perfusion* (EVLP) has also emerged as a technique to expand the donor pool. Marginal quality donor lungs are perfused and ventilated in an extracorporeal circuit to allow them time to heal from the injuries sustained with brain death, resuscitation, and the recovery operation. Following a period of EVLP, potential lung grafts are reassessed for suitability in transplantation. EVLP may help predict posttransplant performances of high-risk donor lungs, particularly those allografts from DCD, and thereby expand the use of previously discarded organs.

Single-lung transplants have traditionally been performed through a posterolateral thoracotomy, although there is an increasing trend toward the use of muscle-sparing thoracotomies, anterior thoracotomies, and sternotomies to minimize postoperative discomfort. In the case of single-lung transplants, the lung receiving less blood as determined by nuclear perfusion scan is typically the one replaced. Double-lung transplants have traditionally been performed through a clamshell incision (bilateral thoracosternotomy) with division of both internal mammary arteries, although some centers use a median sternotomy. Cardiopulmonary bypass (CPB) is used routinely for patients whose native lung function is sufficiently poor that they do not tolerate single-lung ventilation. Most single-lung transplant procedures are performed without CPB.

Complications in the early postoperative period usually involve the bronchial anastomosis, generally as a result of ischemia of the donor segment of bronchus. Superficial patches of necrosis usually heal without clinical sequelae, but necrosis at the suture line may lead to disruption of the airway. This may manifest as an air leak, sepsis associated with mediastinal infection, or a bronchopulmonary fistula. Complete dehiscence or bronchopulmonary fistulas both require immediate surgical correction or retransplantation. However, partial dehiscence can be treated with gentle mechanical debridement, pleural drainage, and reduction in corticosteroid dosing to facilitate anastomotic healing. Long-term bronchial ischemia can lead to airway stenosis. This complication is often managed by repeated dilation and placement of an endobronchial stent. During the first 72 hours posttransplantation, pulmonary edema can develop, ranging from mild, transient hypoxemia to acute severe respiratory distress requiring prolonged mechanical ventilation, inhaled nitric oxide, or prostacyclin. This phenomenon is pathologically similar to *acute respiratory distress syndrome* (ARDS), and its most severe form is termed primary graft failure. It is associated with mortality rates as high as 60%, and emergency retransplantation does not result in an improvement in survival.

Since the lung is directly exposed to airborne pathogens, it is particularly susceptible to various bacterial, viral, and fungal infections. Lung transplant recipients have a rate of infection several times higher than that of other organ recipients. *Pseudomonas aeruginosa* and other gram-negative organisms as well as *Staphylococcus aureus* are most often isolated. CMV pneumonitis is also of particular concern in lung transplant patients. Both infections and acute rejection present with fever, leukocytosis, dyspnea, increased secretions, and infiltrates/pleural effusions on chest radiographs. Bronchoscopy with transbronchial biopsies and bronchoalveolar lavage for microbiologic cultures are essential to differentiate these processes. Acute rejection episodes usually respond well to pulse treatment with steroids. Failure to respond to steroids may lead to the use of antithymocyte globulin.

The primary cause of late mortality and morbidity after lung transplantation is *bronchiolitis obliterans* (BOS). More than a third of all lung transplant recipients develop this fibroproliferative process of the small airways, leading to luminal obstruction and airflow limitation. Alloantibodies are detected in only a minority of patients with BOS, although donor-specific antibodies do significantly increase the risk of developing BOS. Clinically, a third of patients present with a steady decline over many years, a third demonstrate a drop and plateau pattern, and the final third have an accelerated decline that is not reversible. Acute rejection, respiratory virus, CMV infection, and gastroesophageal reflux disease are significant risk factor in the development of BOS.

VASCULARIZED COMPOSITE ALLOTRANSPLANTATION

Vascularized composite allotransplantation (VCA), consisting mainly of face and upper extremity limb transplantation, has recently emerged as a new therapy for disfiguring facial injuries and limb loss. Currently performed only on experimental basis, VCA may offer significant functional and cosmetic benefits over conventional reconstruction options. VCA recipients, like solid organ transplant recipients, require lifelong immunosuppression to prevent rejection, although optimal immunosuppression approaches are evolving as greater clinical data and experience accrues.

IMMUNOSUPPRESSION

A thorough understanding of transplant immunology is necessary for the optimal care of the postoperative transplant patient, specifically when it comes to the management of immunosuppression. This is true even if the surgeon is not primarily responsible for managing the immunosuppression. There are several different classes of agents employed to protect the transplant allograft from rejection.

Steroids

Corticosteroids suppress the immune system via inhibition of DNA and RNA synthesis. By binding to their intracellular receptors, they inhibit transcription of cytokines such as IL-1, IL-2, IL-6, IFN-γ, and TNF-α. In addition, they act in an anti-inflammatory fashion by inhibiting lymphocyte transmigration across endothelium, decreasing chemotaxis, and impairing macrophage and granulocyte function. Long-term administration of corticosteroids is associated with side effects including hypertension, hyperlipidemia, hyperglycemia, cataract formation, osteoporosis, psychosis, pancreatitis, GI tract bleeding, ulceration and perforation, poor wound healing, and growth retardation.

Calcineurin Inhibitors

Calcineurin is a Ca^{+}-dependent serine/threonine phosphatase and dephosphorylates a number of DNA transcription factors, including NFAT. Following dephosphorylation, NFAT localizes to the nucleus and binds to the promoter region of the *IL-2* gene, resulting in up-regulation of IL-2 expression. Cyclosporine is a cyclic peptide drug derived from a fungus and binds to cyclophilin-A, a peptidyl-prolyl isomerase that normally facilitates cellular protein folding. The complex of cyclosporine and cyclophilin binds and inhibits the phosphatase activity of calcineurin, resulting in the inhibition of IL-2 production. One of the most serious long-term side effects of cyclosporine use is *nephrotoxicity*, which is pathologically manifested as vasoconstriction and interstitial nephritis. Other side effects include gingival hyperplasia, hypertension, and hyperkalemia. Cyclosporine is metabolized by the cytochrome P-450 system in the liver. As such, its dosing must be tightly guided by serum trough levels especially when given with other drugs that interact with the P-450 system.

Tacrolimus (FK506/Prograf) is functionally related to cyclosporine. It was first isolated from *Streptomyces* and binds to a cellular protein named FK506-binding protein (FKBP). The complex of tacrolimus and FKBP inhibits calcineurin activity thereby inhibiting IL-2 expression, similarly to cyclosporine. Tacrolimus also inhibits production of IL-3, IL-4, IFN-γ, and IL-2 receptor expression. Like cyclosporine, tacrolimus causes significant nephrotoxicity, hypertension, and hyperkalemia. Hypomagnesemia is another electrolyte abnormality associated with tacrolimus. Tacrolimus-induced central nervous system (CNS) toxicity is a well-described entity and presents as headaches, tremors, mental status changes, or even seizures. Another serious side effect of tacrolimus is diabetes mellitus, which seems to be related to inhibition of insulin gene transcription as well as some degree of islet β-cell toxicity rather than insulin resistance. Tacrolimus-associated diabetes is potentially reversible after withdrawal of the drug. Overall, the high incidence of nephrotoxicity associated with the use of calcineurin inhibitor agents needs to be balanced with their efficacy at preventing T-cell–mediated acute rejection. Development of novel immunotherapeutic drugs capable of preventing rejection without reliance on this class of immunosuppressive agents is an important goal of transplantation research in large part due to concern over nephrotoxicity.

Cell Cycle Inhibitors

Sirolimus (rapamycin/Rapamune) also binds to FKBP. However, it does not exert its immunosuppressive activity via the calcineurin pathway. Rather, the complex of sirolimus and FKBP binds to and inhibits a kinase named FRAP (FKBP–rapamycin/sirolimus-associated protein), also known as "mammalian target of rapamycin" (mTOR). FRAP/TOR kinase activity is required to activate cyclin-dependent kinases and is necessary for T cells to progress from G1 to S phase during the proliferative response to IL-2 and IL-6. Sirolimus causes less nephrotoxicity than calcineurin inhibitors. However, it does cause hyperlipidemia, hypertension, pneumonitis, acne, rashes, and interferes with wound healing to such a degree that it is not typically used immediately after transplant surgery. There is a FDA black box warning for the use of sirolimus in liver transplantation due to early increased risk of hepatic artery thrombosis in one study, although this finding remains a point of controversy. *Everolimus* (*Zortress*) is a derivative of sirolimus that also inhibits mTOR. It has been approved for use as an immunosuppressant in renal and liver transplantation and as an antineoplastic agent against some malignancies. Everolimus is used as a component of calcineurin inhibitor–sparing immunosuppression regimens and may offer additional benefit in preventing fibrosis progression in HCV-positive liver transplant recipients and as antineoplastic agent in transplant recipients with malignancies (such as recurrent HCC). Everolimus carries a FDA black box warning for increased risk of arterial and venous thromboses in kidney transplantation and for increased mortality when used in the first 3 months following heart transplantation.

Antimetabolites

Mycophenolate mofetil (MMF/CellCept/Myfortic) is hydrolyzed *in vivo* to mycophenolic acid (MPA), which is its active form. MPA inhibits the activity of inosine monophosphate dehydrogenase (IMPDH), an enzyme active in the *de novo* guanine synthesis pathway. B and T cells are dependent on *de novo* guanine synthesis for proliferations because they lack the salvage pathway upon which other rapidly dividing cells frequently depend. MPA inhibits lymphocyte proliferation, without the skin, hair, and GI side effects that other antimetabolites cause. It also blocks glycosylation of adhesion molecules, inhibiting leukocyte recruitment and adhesion to endothelial cells. MMF has no renal toxicity, but it does cause BM suppression and GI symptoms such as nausea, diarrhea, and vague abdominal pain. It is contraindicated in pregnancy.

Currently, *azathioprine* (Imuran) is used primarily in patients intolerant of MMF. It contains an imidazole linked to 6-mercaptopurine, which is converted to its active form, 6-thioguanine, in the liver by hypoxanthine–guanine phosphoribosyltransferase (HGPRT). The substituted purine sufficiently resembles the unsubstituted purine in that it is incorporated into DNA but does not allow for DNA replication and RNA transcription. Adverse effects include increased risk of malignancy, hepatitis, myelosuppression (especially leukopenia), cholestasis, alopecia, and pancreatitis. Azathioprine is contraindicated in pregnancy. It is contraindicated in patients on angiotensin-converting enzyme (ACE) inhibitors as the combination can result in severe anemia and pancytopenia.

Methotrexate is rarely used, with pediatric heart transplant recipients being an exception. Methotrexate inhibits DNA and RNA synthesis by blocking folic acid metabolism. It also inhibits macrophage chemotaxis. Adverse effects include myelosuppression, GI toxicity, hepatic dysfunction, nephrotoxicity, and dermatitis.

Anti–T-Lymphocyte Antibodies

The development of monoclonal antibodies for use in the clinical setting represented a major advance for clinical transplantation. Currently, polyclonal and monoclonal antibodies directed toward cell surface proteins on T lymphocytes are used as part of immunosuppressive induction therapies or for the treatment of steroid-resistant acute rejection.

Thymoglobulin is a polyclonal preparation purified from the serum of rabbits immunized with human thymocytes. *ATGAM* is similar to Thymoglobulin, except that it prepared from the serum of immunized horses. Once T cells are bound by antibody, they are depleted from the circulation through opsonization and complement-mediated, antibody-dependent cell-mediated cytotoxicity. Damaged T cells are cleared by the lymphoreticular system.

Basiliximab (Simulect) is a humanized IgG1 mouse anti-human IL-2 receptor alpha chain (a.k.a., CD25). CD25 is expressed on activated T lymphocytes and permits high-affinity binding to IL-2. Simulect binds but does not activate the IL-2 receptor and functions as a competitive inhibitor for endogenous IL-2. *Daclizumab* (Zenapax) is another humanized monoclonal antibody and is specific for a different epitope of CD25. Both are primarily utilized as induction agents for renal transplantation and have been used with impressive success in the setting of clinical islet transplantation in patients with type 1 diabetes.

Alemtuzumab (Campath) is a recombinant IgG1 monoclonal antibody that binds CD52, a surface protein expressed on mature T- and B-cell lymphocytes and that depletes both classes of leukocytes. It was initially approved as a treatment for B-cell chronic lymphocytic leukemia, but its use has expanded to include the treatment of multiple sclerosis and GVHD after hematopoietic stem cell transplantation. In solid organ transplantation, it is utilized in primarily as an induction agent in kidney, pancreas, and lung allografts.

Belatacept (Nulojix) is a fusion protein composed of the Fc domain of human IgG1 and the extracellular domain of CTLA-4 that acts as costimulation blocker to inhibit T-cell activation. It is employed as an alternative to calcineurin inhibitors in maintenance immunosuppression and may improve graft survival compared to calcineurin inhibitors because of less nephrotoxicity and fewer metabolic side effects. Belatacept application is limited to EPV-seronegative patients due to an increased risk of *posttransplant lymphoproliferative disease* (*PTLD*; see below under "Malignancy") in EPV seropositive patients.

Anti–B-Lymphocyte Antibodies

Rituximab (Rituxan) is another humanized monoclonal antibody specific for the B-lymphocyte marker CD20. Rituxan effectively depletes peripheral B cells. It is frequently used to treat non-Hodgkin B-cell lymphoma. However, it has also been extensively utilized in clinical transplantation for treatment of steroid-resistant antibody-mediated rejection or rejection with evidence of vasculitis, especially in cases exhibiting peritubular C4d-positive immunohistochemical staining as a marker for humoral rejection. Unfortunately, plasma cells do not express high levels of CD20, thereby rendering Rituxan inefficient for the depletion of alloantibodies in the presensitized recipient. Therefore, the development of novel B-cell–directed agents capable of eliminating plasma and memory B cells is an important goal of transplantation immunology researchers.

POSTTRANSPLANT COMPLICATIONS

Infections

As a consequence of pharmacologic immunosuppression, transplant recipients are at increased risk for the development of multiple infections. The potential development of any particular infection is influenced by the time interval posttransplant. During the first month posttransplantation, patients are at increased risk for bacterial infections in the wound, urine, and lung. Perioperative antibiotics help limit the incidence of wound infection. Every effort should be made to remove the urinary catheter as soon as possible. Low-grade fevers and elevated white blood cell counts, even in the absence of symptoms, require a full culture workup. In the first 6 months following transplantation, patients are at increased risk for opportunistic infections and viral infections, including *Pneumocystis carinii*, *Candida*, and *CMV* infection in particular. CMV infections in immunosuppressed individuals can plague a range of organ systems. Posttransplantation, CMV infection presents as esophagitis, GI bleeding and ulceration, colitis, hepatitis, leukopenia, pneumonia, renal insufficiency, or CNS changes evolving into coma. CMV infection of the GI tract is not always associated with positive serum CMV titers and is diagnosed by endoluminal biopsy. Patients are frequently placed on Bactrim, nystatin, and acyclovir, ganciclovir, or valganciclovir as prophylaxis against these infections following transplant. Bactrim also helps to prevent urinary tract infections.

Malignancy

The increased risk of neoplasia in transplant patients has been attributed to (a) suppression of immunologic surveillance mechanisms that would normally destroy malignant cells expressing mutant proteins (especially in cancers that are associated with viral pathogenesis) and (b) the direct carcinogenic effect of immunosuppressive drugs. The risk of developing malignancy in transplant patients is several times greater when compared to normal age-matched populations. Most common among transplant patients are cervical cancer (associated with the human papillomavirus [HPV]), carcinoma of the vulva and perineum (HSV), squamous cell carcinomas of the skin and lip (HPV), Kaposi sarcoma (EBV), and lymphomas (EBV and HTLV-1). Renal cancers, hepatobiliary carcinomas, and various sarcomas are also somewhat more prevalent in transplant patients.

PTLD is generally an EBV-driven proliferative disorder of B cells, the manifestation of which can range from polyclonal B-cell hyperplasia to monoclonal B-cell lymphoma. All levels of clonality and histology can be found at different sites in the same patient. The incidence of PTLD (1% to 2% in renal transplants, 2% to 5% in liver and heart, 10% in heart–lung recipients) is related to the degree of immunosuppression used with each organ more than the type of organ transplanted. Antilymphocyte antibody therapy in particular is associated with increased risk for development of PTLD. PTLD can present in a variety of manners including (a) unexplained fevers without other symptoms, (b) a mononucleosis-like syndrome or hepatitis, (c) bleeding mesenteric masses or intestinal obstruction, or (d) with CNS symptoms including seizures, altered mental status, or focal neurologic dysfunction as a consequence of neurologic tumor burden. The absence of adenopathy on radiographic imaging does not rule out PTLD; the disease can be entirely extranodal. Definitive diagnosis is made using tissue biopsy.

The mainstay of treatment for PTLD is to decrease the level of immunosuppression. Up to 86% of patients have regression of PTLD with reduction of immunosuppression. However, this is not effective if PTLD has progressed to a true monoclonal B-cell lymphoma. CHOP chemotherapy used in the case of non-Hodgkin's lymphoma has been used for the treatment of PTLD. Additionally, there have been promising results with the anti–B-cell monoclonal antibody Rituxan.

Suggested Readings

Busuttil RW, Kilntmalm GB. *Transplantation of the Liver*. 2nd ed. Philadelphia: Elsevier Publishing; 2005.

Kirk A, Knechtle SJ, Larsen CP, et al. *Textbook of Organ Transplantation*. Chicester: John Wiley & Sons; 2014.

Kirklin JK, Young JB, McGiffin DC. *Heart Transplantation*. New York: Elsevier Publishing; 2002.

Morris P, Knechtle SJ. *Kidney Transplantation*. 7th ed. Philadelphia: Saunders Publishing; 2013.

Murphy K. *Janeway's Immunobiology*. 8th ed. New York: Garland Publishing; 2011.

Wilkes DS, Burlingham WJ. *Immunobiology of Organ Transplantation*. New York: Springer Publishing; 2004.

CHAPTER

6 Statistics and Epidemiology

MEERA GUPTA, E. CARTER PAULSON, AND RACHEL R. KELZ

KEY POINTS

- The *median* of a distribution is the value that equals the 50th percentile.
  The *mean* is the arithmetic average of the distribution.
  The *mode* is the value of the distribution that occurs most frequently.
- *The mean and standard deviation* should be used to describe data that are normally distributed.
  The median and percentiles should be used to describe data that are not normally distributed.
- A confidence interval for an odds ratio or risk ratio that includes "1" indicates that the result is not statistically significant and the corresponding *p* value will be greater than 0.05.
- *t Tests and ANOVA* are used to analyze data sets that contain noncategorical, *normally distributed*, variables.
  t tests compare the means between two groups.
  ANOVA compares the means of more than two groups.
- The *chi-square* test is used to analyze categorical data or compare proportions.
- *Sensitivity* = TP/(TP + FN) = the percentage of patients with disease who have a positive test result.
- *Specificity* = TN/(FP + TN) = the percentage of patients who do not have disease and who have a negative test result.
- *Positive predictive value* (PPV) = TP/(TP + FP) = probability that a patient with a positive test result actually has the disease.
- *Negative predictive value* (NPV) = TN/(TN + FN) = probability that a patient with a negative test result actually is disease free.
- *Multipredictor regression modeling* allows study of the effect of a single variable on an outcome while adjusting for other covariates associated with the outcome. Examples of these regression models include *linear, logistic, Poisson, Cox proportional hazards (survival), repeated measures, and generalized linear models.*

FUNDAMENTALS OF STUDY DESIGN

Epidemiology is defined as the study of the distribution of health and disease in groups of people as well as the study of factors influencing this distribution. There are two basic categories of epidemiologic studies: descriptive and analytic. *Descriptive studies* observe and describe the health and factors influencing it in selected groups of people. Information from descriptive studies serves as a context for developing hypotheses and designing further *analytic studies.* Analytic studies allow inferences about causality using formal hypothesis testing. *Biostatistics* is the science of describing, analyzing, and interpreting biologic or health data collected in these studies using statistical methods. An understanding of study design and analysis is essential both for conducting clinical research and for interpreting the medical literature and applying it to clinical practice. This chapter covers study design and basic descriptive and analytic statistics and reviews the fundamentals of interpreting diagnostic tests.

Descriptive Studies

Descriptive studies include case reports, case series, and correlational studies. The *case report* is a detailed clinical description of a single patient, often used to document a rare or uncommon presentation of a disease and its management. For example, a case report could present the use of single-incision laparoscopy to perform a living donor nephrectomy for transplantation. No statistical analyses can be performed on the sample of one, and observations are not generalizable to other subjects. Case reports may suggest hypotheses for further study.

The individual case report can be expanded to a *case series*, which is a clinical description of a group of patients with a specific disease or condition. It usually provides descriptions of diagnoses as well as of the interventions and outcomes. An example of a case series is the description of the use of single-incision laparoscopy to perform living donor nephrectomy in a group of similar patients. Similar to case reports, lacking a comparison or control group, statistical analyses beyond descriptive statistics or subgroup comparisons within the series are not possible. Case series cannot prove causation but can be used for hypothesis generation. For example, the hypothesis that laparoscopy is a safe and effective method for performing colon resections for cancer could arise from a case series. Such hypotheses then must undergo more rigorous testing using one of the analytic approaches discussed later in the chapter.

A third type of descriptive study, the *correlational study*, evaluates the relationship between two or more variables for a given set of subjects. Of note, it does not examine the effect of one variable on the other. A well-known example of such a study correlated breast cancer mortality rates in 28 countries in the 1960s to the countries' average per capita pork intake. There was a strong correlation between higher breast cancer rates in countries with high per capita pork intake (1). Correlational studies have many limitations. For example, it is impossible to determine if the women getting breast cancer were the same as those eating pork. In addition, it is possible that pork intake was simply a marker for other behaviors, such as smoking or eating high-fat diets, which were actually responsible for high cancer rates. As with the case report and case series, correlational studies cannot reveal causality and are useful mainly to generate hypotheses for future analytic testing.

		Null Hypothesis	
		True	False
Hypothesis Test	Non-Significant: Accept Null	No Error	Type II Error Beta set to prevent
	Significant: Reject Null	Type I Error – Alpha set to prevent	No Error

FIGURE 6.1 Relationship between the null hypothesis and the results of the hypothesis test.

Analytic Studies

Unlike descriptive studies, analytic studies allow quantitative analysis of relationships between risk factors and health outcomes. Analytic study designs fall into two broad categories: observational and interventional (experimental). Both designs are used to test specific, defined hypotheses regarding the association between potential causative factors and health outcomes. Of note, while factors evaluated in individual observational studies can be significantly associated with health outcomes, one cannot state that they are actually causal.

Hypothesis Testing

When conducting analytic studies, the null and alternative hypotheses must be defined prior to data collection and analysis. The null hypothesis (H_0), which is assumed true prior to the study, states that there is no difference between the two study groups or that there is no relationship between the factor under investigation and the outcome of interest. For example, if one were comparing a new drug for the treatment of peptic ulcer disease (PUD) to an old drug, the null hypothesis states that there is no difference in outcome between the two drugs. The alternative hypothesis (H_a) would state that there is a significant difference between the study groups or that there is a significant association between a causative factor and an outcome. For example, in the clinical trial of a new peptic ulcer drug, the alternative hypothesis might be that the new drug has a different effect, on average, compared with that of the current drug. In general, the goal of hypothesis testing is to use experimental data to determine whether the null or the alternative hypothesis is more likely to represent reality.

All hypothesis tests have unavoidable, but quantifiable, risks of reaching the wrong conclusion (Fig. 6.1). A type I error occurs when an investigator rejects the null hypothesis, when, in fact, it is true. Using the above example, the investigator would, on the basis of the results of the clinical trial, conclude that the new ulcer drug is more effective than the old one, when, in reality, there is no difference. Prior to data collection, an alpha level (α) for the study should be stated. The alpha level is the probability of making a type I error and is most often set at 0.05. This means that an investigator is willing to accept a 5% possibility that differences deemed significant are due to chance rather than true differences.

A type II error occurs when an investigator does not reject the null hypothesis, when, in fact, the alternative hypothesis is true (Fig. 6.1). On the basis of the above example, a type II error occurs if the investigator concluded that the two ulcer drugs had the same effectiveness, when, in reality, the new drug was better (or worse). Similar to the alpha level, researchers should specify a beta level for their study prior to commencement of data collection. Beta level (β) is defined as the probability of making a type II error and is most often set at 0.2, which means that the investigator is willing to accept a 20% chance that no difference will be found on the basis of the study, when a difference truly exists.

Frequently, beta is used to calculate a study power, defined as 1-beta. The power of a study, which is usually 0.8, is the ability of a study to detect prespecified differences between groups assuming those differences are real. The power of a study is determined by the sample size, the magnitude of the difference an investigator hopes to detect, the variability in the sample, and the selected alpha level. Small sample sizes, small differences between study groups, large variability within groups, and a small alpha limit a study's power. Meanwhile large samples, large differences, little variability, and larger alpha values increase power.

Ideally, an investigator should define alpha and beta levels as well as the magnitude of the difference they want to detect and use these values to determine a sample size prior to beginning the study. Often, however, funding or logistics create a finite sample size for the study. Using this sample size, an investigator can determine the power his or her study has to detect differences of various magnitudes between the study groups. Generally, if a sample size is small, a study has adequate power to detect true differences only if their magnitude is large. Studies with large sample sizes have the power to detect smaller differences (Fig. 6.2).

Choosing appropriate alpha and beta levels and performing appropriate sample size and power calculations prior to the start of data collections minimize the risk of both type I and type II errors. This is true for both observational and interventional analytic studies.

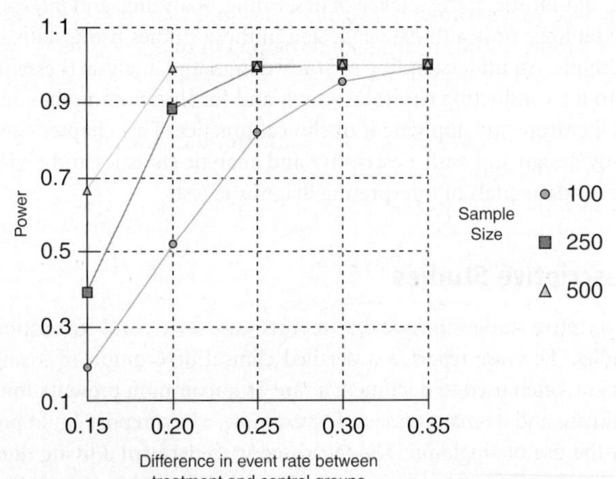

FIGURE 6.2 Relationship between power, sample size, and the magnitude of difference between treatment and control groups.

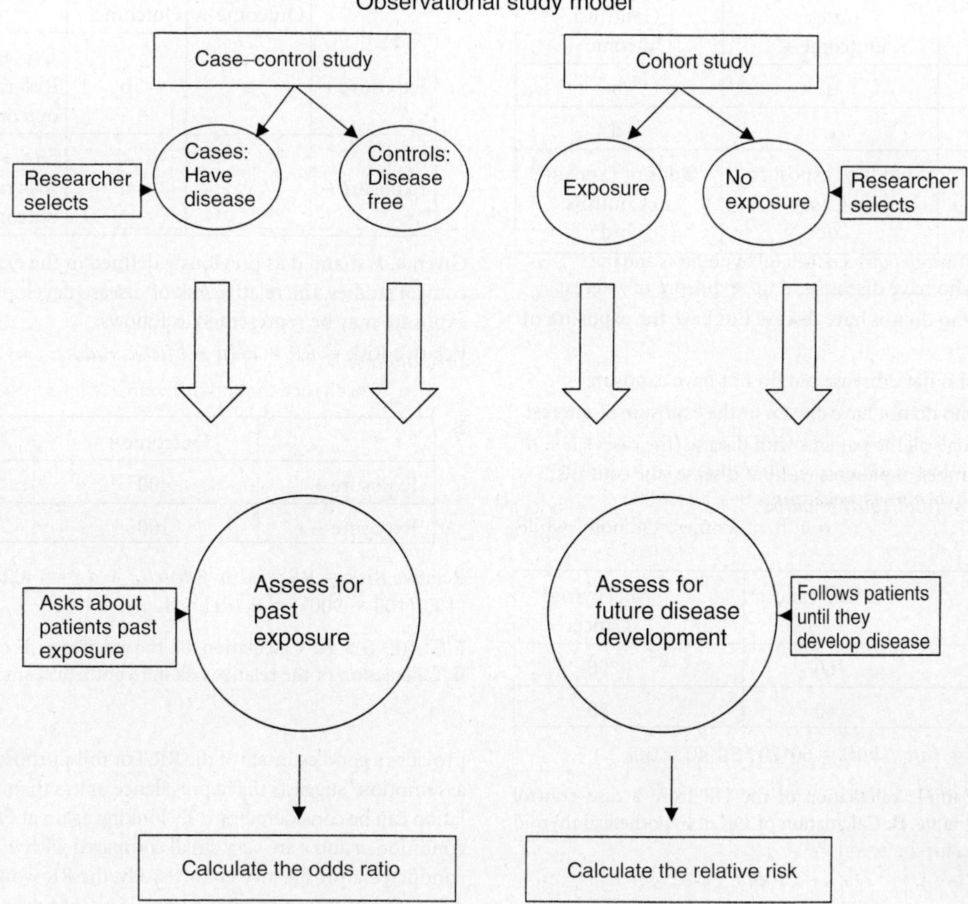

FIGURE 6.3 Schematic representation of the difference between a case–control and a cohort study.

Observational Studies

Observational studies include case–control and cohort studies. In a *case–control study*, the study group is identified on the basis of the presence of a condition or outcome of interest (cases) and is compared with a control group where the condition is absent (Fig. 6.3). Participants are interviewed or their medical records are reviewed to identify exposures to possible risk factors and statistical tests used to determine if a significant association exists between a prior exposure and subsequent development of a disease. The proportion of case patients with a history of exposure is compared to the proportion of control patients without the exposure to evaluate the association between the exposure and outcome. This may be expressed as a risk ratio (RR), the proportion of subjects with (or without) the exposure who develop the outcome with (or without) exposure, or as an odds ratio (OR).

In case–control studies, the association between exposure and disease is most often reported as an OR, defined as the odds of developing disease given exposure to a risk factor relative to the odds of developing disease given no exposure. Examining a 2 × 2 contingency table shows that the odds of exposure for those with disease would be *a*/*c* and the odds of exposure for those without disease would be *b*/*d* (Fig. 6.4A). The OR would then be *a*/*c* ÷ *b*/*d*, or *ad*/*bc*.

An example of a simple case–control design is a study in which the last 100 cases of thyroid cancer seen at one institution are matched with 100 normal controls. Prior radiation exposures would be determined for all subjects to see whether patients with thyroid cancer were exposed to more radiation than controls. In the example shown (Fig. 6.4B), 60 of the thyroid cancer patients had a history of radiation exposure, whereas only 30 of the noncancer patients had exposure to radiation. The OR for radiation exposure and the development of cancer is 3.5; that is, the odds of developing thyroid cancer in a patient exposed to radiation is 3.5 times that for an unexposed patient.

The case–control design is simple and is particularly well suited to investigations of rare diseases or diseases that take a long time to develop. Otherwise, many subjects would need to be followed for a very long time to generate a sufficient number of diseased individuals to produce accurate results. For instance, identifying children exposed to radiation and following them until they develop thyroid cancer as adults would be expensive, time consuming, and logistically difficult. In addition, the case–control design allows evaluation of multiple exposures that might be associated with a specific disease process using a single data set.

Case–control studies often require relatively small sample sizes and may be completed quickly and economically. Their simplicity, however, can be deceiving, as these studies require meticulous case and control selection and thorough and accurate exposure history to avoid biased and inaccurate results. If exposure is ascertained through subject interview, subjects may selectively recall past events introducing *recall bias*. Patients with lung cancer may, for example, more accurately recall their smoking history, whereas a patient

A

	Cases: Outcome +	Controls: Outcome −
Exposure +	a	b
Exposure −	c	d
	Odds of exposure in Cases: a/c	Odds of exposure in Controls: b/d

a = the subjects who have disease and the exposure of interest
b = the subjects who do not have disease but have the exposure of interest
c = the subjects who have disease but do not have exposure
d = the subjects who do not have disease or the exposure of interest.
Note that $a + c$ equals all the patients with disease (the cases); $b + d$ equals the total number of patients without disease (the controls).
Odds ratio = $OR = (a/c)/(b/d) = ad/bc$

B

	Thyroid cancer	No Thyroid Cancer
Radiation +	60	30
Radiation −	40	70

Odds ratio = $OR = (a/c)/(b/d)$ = 60*70 / 30*40 = 3.5

FIGURE 6.4 A. Sample calculation of the OR from a case–control study using a 2 × 2 table. **B.** Calculation of OR in hypothetical thyroid cancer scenario.

A

	Outcome +	Outcome −	
Exposure +	a	b	a/(a + b) Risk rate of developing outcome in exposed
Exposure −	c	d	c/(c + d) Risk rate of developing outcome in unexposed

Given *a, b, c,* and d as previously defined in the example for case-control studies, the relative risk of disease development given exposure may be represented as follows:
Relative Risk = $RR = a/(a + b)/c/(c + d)$.

B

	Outcome +	Outcome −
Exposure +	400	600
Exposure −	100	900

Relative Risk = $RR = a/(a + b)/c/(c + d)$ = (400/(400 + 600)) / (100/(100 + 900)) = 0.4/0.1 = 4

FIGURE 6.5 A. Calculation of the relative risk of a cohort study. **B.** Calculation of the relative risk in hypothetical smoking scenario.

without lung cancer may underreport their true history. *Interviewer bias* occurs when an interviewer more thoroughly interviews case subjects than control subjects in an effort to elucidate an exposure he or she believes to be associated with the outcome being studied. *Selection bias* occurs when the exposure status differentially affects selection of diseased and nondiseased subjects for study inclusion.

In a cohort study, subjects are identified on the basis of presence or absence of an exposure and then followed to document the development of one or many outcomes (Fig. 6.3). A simple example of a cohort study is following a group of smokers and a group of nonsmokers to assess the development of outcomes, including lung cancer, heart disease, emphysema, or other selected diseases.

The association between the risk factor (exposure) and disease in a cohort study is reported as the *relative risk*, or RR, which is calculated using the 2 × 2 contingency table as $a/(a + b) \div c/(c + d)$ (Fig. 6.5A). The RR is the risk of disease in the exposed population divided by the risk of disease in the unexposed population. If the relative risk is above 1, the exposure of interest increases risk of the outcome; if less than 1, it reduces risk. In the hypothetical smoking example described earlier, 1,000 smokers and 1,000 nonsmokers are followed. Four hundred smokers and one hundred nonsmokers eventually develop lung cancer. The relative risk of smoking and lung cancer is 4.0 (Fig. 6.5B); that is, smokers have four times the risk of developing lung cancer compared with nonsmokers.

In case–control studies, because subjects are selected on the basis of disease status, it is not possible to determine the rate of development of disease; therefore, a relative risk cannot be determined. However, if the disease in a case–control study is rare, the OR provides a good estimate of the RR. For this purpose, the "rare disease assumption" suggests that a prevalence of less than 10% of the population can be considered rare. By looking again at Figure 6.5, in a rare condition, *a* and *c* are very small compared with *b* and *d*. If one then conducted a prospective cohort study, the RR would be $a/(a + b) \div c/(c + d)$, but as *a* and *c* are very small $(a + b) \approx b$ and $(c + d) \approx d$. The equation then becomes $a/b \div c/d$, which equals the OR ad/bc.

One advantage of cohort studies is that they allow the study of multiple outcomes such as the development of lung cancer, stroke, and cardiac disease in a cohort of smokers. These studies are well suited to investigating the risks of rare exposures, including rare occupational exposures such as occur to those working in a vinyl chloride factory. Cohort studies also provide information on the temporal relationship between exposure and disease important in proving causality. Some of the disadvantages of cohort studies are the expenses involved, the long interval needed for follow-up, and the potential for patient withdrawal and loss to follow-up.

A *nested study* is considered a combination of a case–control and cohort study in which subjects are selected from a population whose characteristics are known because its members are already the subjects of an existing larger cohort. In a *case–cohort study*, all cases in the cohort are compared to a random sample of participants who do not develop the outcome. In a *nested case–control study*, cases are compared to only a predetermined selection of controls from the cohort based off of a case's matched risk set in a ratio of, that is 1:2 or 1:4, depending on the minimal sample size requirement to detect a significant association between the exposure and outcome. This makes the analysis more efficient by controlling factors such as age and ethnicity, but limits its generalizability.

Intervention Studies

Intervention studies can be thought of as a type of prospective cohort study where subjects are identified on the basis of exposure status and followed to determine outcome. The defining feature of an intervention study is that the investigator determines the exposure status of each participant. Ideally, the subjects are randomly allocated to a treatment (exposure) group on the basis of some chance mechanism, a design also known as a *randomized controlled trial* (RCT). This maximizes the likelihood that unrecognized risk factors, or confounders, are allocated equally between the two groups, thereby minimizing bias. Blinding is an important aspect of RCTs that may further reduce bias. In *open trials*, both the patient and physician know the full details of treatment. This design has the potential for placebo and treatment bias but is sometimes unavoidable, particularly in studies of surgical techniques, where it may not be possible or ethical to hide from the patient or investigator the patient's group membership (which treatment they receive). In *single-blind trials*, the patient, but not the investigator, is unaware of group membership. This limits placebo effect but does not address the possibility of treatment bias, for example, an investigator treating a patient differently knowing he or she is receiving the new drug versus the placebo. In a *double-blind RCT*, neither the investigator nor the patient knows group membership, further minimizing potential bias. Generally, RCTs, particularly double-blind RCTs, are considered the most sophisticated form of epidemiologic research providing the most scientifically rigorous and unbiased results (i.e., level 1 evidence). These studies, however, can be expensive and may be subject to large subject attrition over the potentially lengthy follow-up period. Ethical and logistic considerations also may limit the use of this study design.

DESCRIPTIVE STATISTICS

After completing data collection, the investigator must organize and report the data in a concise, comprehensible form. An important part of this process is collapsing the data into summary statistics, which are then used to evaluate relationships between study groups. This section reviews basic methods used for presenting and summarizing data.

Levels of Measurement

It is critically important to understand the level of measurement for each study variable, since knowing it helps one decide how to interpret that variable and what statistical analyses are appropriate. In general, there are four levels of measurement: nominal, ordinal, interval, and ratio. At the *nominal* level of measurement, numbers or other symbols are assigned to a set of categories for the purpose of classifying the observations. Gender and race are examples of nominal-level variables. There is no intrinsic ordering to nominal variables; one variable is not "better or worse" or "higher or lower" than another.

An *ordinal* variable is similar to a nominal variable except that there is a clear ordering of the categories. Common examples are pain scales recorded as no pain, moderate pain, and severe pain or social class represented as low, middle, and high, which exhibit an underlying order. Although ordinal variables can be rank ordered, it is important to recognize that the distances between variables do not have any meaning. For example, on a pain scale, severe pain is worse than moderate pain, but it is impossible to determine how much worse or whether that amount of worsening is equal to that between moderate and mild pain. Nominal and ordinal variables together often are referred to as *categorical variables*. In *interval* measurement, variables have intrinsic order, and the distance between the values does have meaning. Common examples include body temperature, dates, and IQ scores.

With all these variables, we can compare values not only in terms of which is larger or smaller but also in terms of how much larger or smaller one is compared with another. For example, something that is 80°F is 10°F warmer than something that is 70°F, which is the same difference between two things that are 40°F and 30°F. A special type of interval measurement is a *ratio* measurement. The special feature of ratio variables is that there is a meaningful absolute zero, which makes it possible to calculate meaningful ratios. Weight is an example of a ratio variable. It is meaningful to report that someone who weighs 100 kg is twice as heavy as someone weighing 50 kg. In comparison, by using interval variables, it is not meaningful to report that something that is 80°F is twice as hot as an object that is 40°F.

A variable may additionally be categorized as *discrete* or *continuous*. Discrete data only take on certain values within a given range with no intermediate levels. An example is the number of patients operated on in 1 month; you cannot operate on 10.2 patients, only on 10 or 11. Continuous variables have no such limitation and can assume all possible values along a continuum within a specified range. Most clinical parameters are continuous, including, for example, blood pressure, temperature, height, weight, and cholesterol level. All nominal and ordinal variables are discrete; interval and ratio measurements may be either discrete or continuous.

Once one has examined the data and understands the levels of measurement for each variable, it is important to understand how to describe the data and what analytic tests to use. Often this is based on the distinction between *categorical* and *noncategorical* data. In general, nominal and ordinal data are considered *categorical*, while interval and ratio data are *noncategorical*. Occasionally, if an ordinal variable has many categories, such as a 10-level pain scale, it may be treated as an interval variable.

Describing the Data

There are three properties commonly present in the description and evaluation of noncategorical data: (i) distribution, (ii) measure of central tendency, and (iii) variability.

Distribution

One of the first steps in analyzing noncategorical data is to determine the distribution of the data, as distribution plays an important role in the selection of descriptive statistics and analytic methods. The most well-known distribution is the normal distribution. The shape of a normal distribution resembles that of a bell and is referred to as the "bell curve" distribution (Fig. 6.6A). The properties of a normal distribution are symmetry around the mean and unimodality. The normal distribution can be completely specified by two parameters: the mean and the standard deviation (SD) (see below).

The empirical rule states that for a normal distribution, 68% of the data fall within 1 SD of the mean and 95% fall within 2 SDs of the mean. Almost all (99.7%) data fall within 3 SDs of the mean. There are statistical tests that allow determination of normality for noncategorical data. However, plotting the data as a histogram (described below) is simpler and often allows visual confirmation of the distribution. Many of the descriptive and analytic statistical methods described below are contingent on the data being normally distributed. There are numerous other distributions that are beyond the scope of this text. It is important to recognize nonnormally distributed data so that correct statistical analyses, outlined in the following sections, are performed.

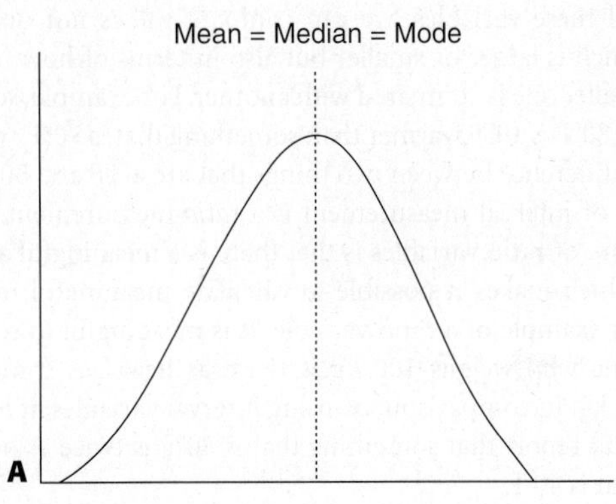

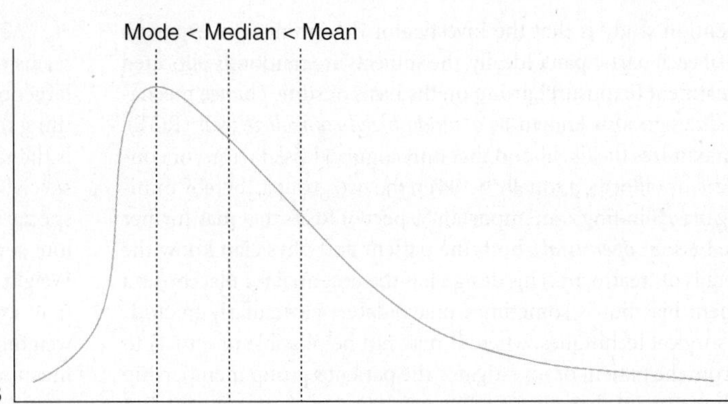

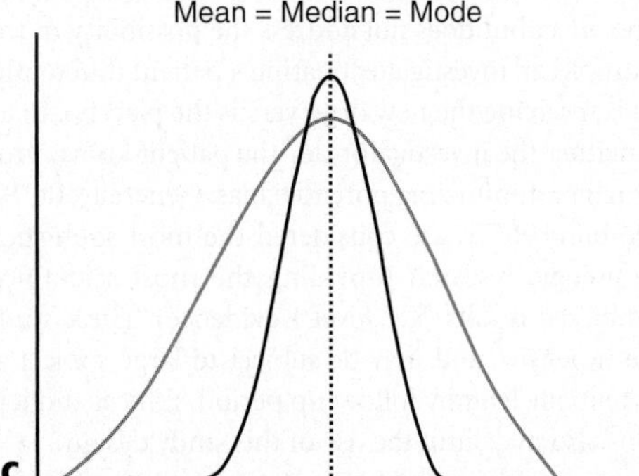

FIGURE 6.6 A. Representation of a normal distribution. Note, the mean, median, and mode of a normal distribution are equivalent. **B.** Example of a right-skewed distribution. **C.** Example of two normal distributions in which the mode, median, and mean are similar but the variances differ.

Measure of Central Tendency

The three most commonly used measures of the center of the data are the mean, median, and mode. The mean, also known as the average, is defined as the sum of the values of the observations divided by the number of observations. Although the most commonly reported of the three measures, it can be significantly affected by a few exceptionally large or small values. In general, the mean should only be reported for data that are normally distributed. The median is the midpoint of the observations when arranged in order. If there are odd number of observations, the median is the middle observation. If there is an even number of observations, the median is the sum of the middle two values divided by 2. In practice, half of the observations in a data set lie below the median and half lie above. Unlike the mean, the median is not greatly affected by large or small outlying data points. Generally, the median should be reported for data that are not normally distributed. The mode is the value occurring most frequently in a set of observations. Some distributions may be bimodal and have two values that occur with equal frequency. The mode is reported rarely for noncategorical data as it may be far from the center of the data.

For normally distributed data the mean, median, and mode are all the same (Fig. 6.6A). If the data are skewed, however, or nonnormally distributed, these values may differ from each other. A skewed distribution is one in which more observations fall on one side of the mean than on the other side. For example, in a right-skewed distribution (Fig. 6.6B), there is a longer tail in the higher values, resulting in mean > median > mode. Right-skewed distributions are common in clinical studies because many clinical and biologic variables have a natural lower boundary but no definitive upper boundary. For example, hospital length of stay can be no shorter than 1 day but might be as long as several hundred days.

It generally does not make sense to calculate means or medians for categorical data. For example, one cannot calculate the mean race of a study group or the median gender. Instead, categorical data are described using percentages or other ratios. In a study looking at the association between hair color (brown, blond, black, and red) and colon cancer, for instance, the number of patients in each hair color category in the colon cancer group might be presented as four percentages, which total 100%. Similarly, the percentage of patients with each hair color in the noncancer group would be presented. The mode can also be used to describe categorical data. Again, it may not make sense to describe the mean or median hair color of cancer patients, but it does make sense to speak about the most frequent (modal) hair color.

Variability

Two data sets can have the same mean and median but have significantly different variability (Fig. 6.6C). Therefore, an adequate summary of the data requires both a measure of center and also a measure of variability. Measures of variability include the SD and percentiles, which are reported in conjunction with the mean and median of the data, respectively, and the range. The range is calculated by simply subtracting the lowest from the highest value in the data, but it is rarely reported. The most common measures of variability are the variance and its related function, the SD. Both of these parameters describe the spread of individual observations around the center of a normally distributed data set when the center is expressed as a mean. The variance is computed by calculating the difference between each observation and the mean. These differences are squared, and the resulting values are summed. This total sum is divided by the number of observations minus one, or $n-1$.

$$\sqrt{\left[\frac{\Sigma(\text{obs}-\text{mean})^2}{\text{no.of obs}-1}\right]}$$

The term "$n-1$" is used in the denominator to adjust for the fact that in studies we are typically looking at samples rather than the entire population. The mean of the sample estimates the mean of the underlying population. If data represent the entire population, then n may be used rather than $n-1$. The SD is the square root of the variance and can be thought of as the average distance of observations from the mean. Like the mean, the SD is greatly affected by large outliers.

When the median is used to describe the center, the variability is described using percentiles. The xth percentile is the value that x% of the data are below and the remainder are above. The median is the 50th percentile. Frequently, the 25th and 75th percentiles are reported and are known as the lower and upper quartiles of the data. Similar to the median, percentiles are not dramatically affected by the presence of outliers.

Graphical Display

It is often easier to understand and more efficient to interpret data presented graphically as opposed to descriptively or in tabular form since a graphic display often provides a quick, overall impression. Covered below are some of the more common graphic methods for conveying information about data.

Line Graphs

Line graphs show the behavior of one variable in relation to another. Often a variable is plotted in relation to time on the horizontal axis. Generally, line graphs are used for noncategorical data and can be used to compare several variables or categories at the same time. In the example, the rate of recurrence of thyroid cancer is plotted on the y-axis versus time on the x-axis (Fig. 6.7). Multiple line graphs are plotted simultaneously to show differences in recurrence rate over time on the basis of size of the initial tumor.

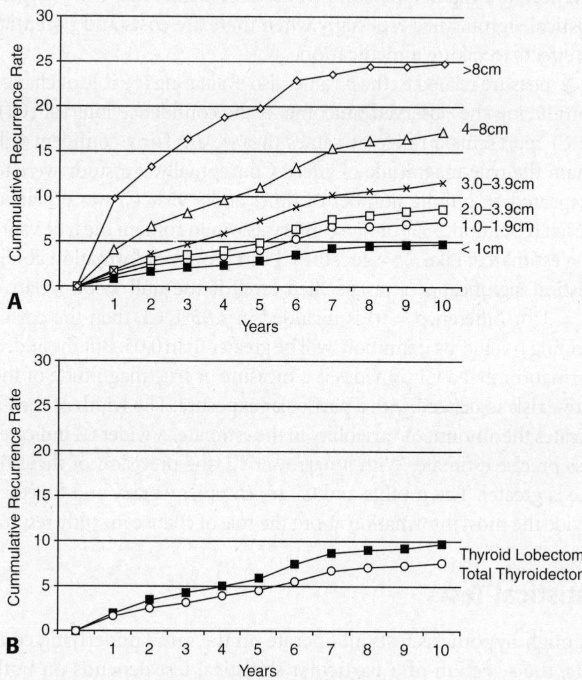

FIGURE 6.7 Use of a line graph to show recurrence rates based on size of initial thyroid tumors over time. (From Bilimoria K, Bentrem DJ, Ko CY, et al. Extent of surgery affects survival for papillary thyroid cancer. *Ann Surg.* 2007;246(3):375–381, with permission.)

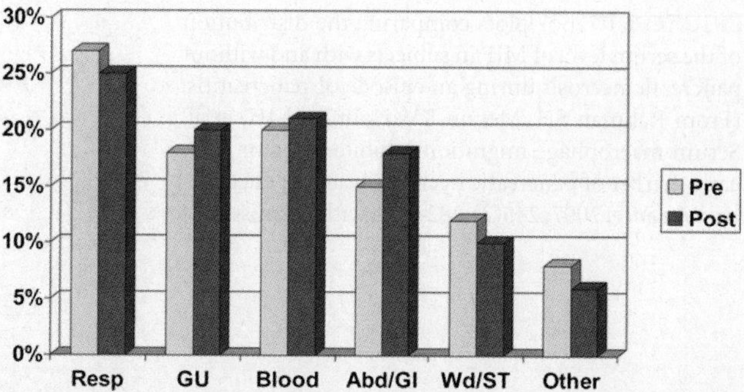

FIGURE 6.8 Use of a bar graph to compare infection rates among surgical site and study group. (From Scalea T, Bochicchio GV, Bochicchio KM, et al. Tight glycemic control in critically injured trauma patients. *Ann Surg.* 2007;246(4):605–610, with permission.)

Bar Graphs

Bar graphs are used to compare categorical variables and are preferable when groups are characterized by nonnumeric attributes such as nonsmoker/light smoker/heavy smoker. Here, there are no formal x-axis units, as each bar across the x-axis represents a different category or variable. In the example given, the rate of infection (y-axis) is compared by surgical site category (x-axis) and by study group (Fig. 6.8).

Histograms

Histograms look similar to bar graphs, but they serve a different purpose. Rather than displaying occurrence in some number of categories, a histogram represents the sampling distribution of one variable. The sampling distribution demonstrates how often a variable assumes each possible value across the possible set of values. The y-axis represents frequency, and most statistical programs mark the x-axis in equally spaced units of the variable values. Histograms visually display data distribution that provides information regarding range, normalcy, and skewness. The histogram shown depicts the number of hospitals that perform different numbers of gastrectomies per year and demonstrates a right-skewed distribution (Fig. 6.9).

Box Plots

Box plots also show the distribution of the data and are especially useful for comparing the distributions of two or more variables graphically. They are created from five numbers describing the data: the median, the 25th percentile, the 75th percentile, the minimum

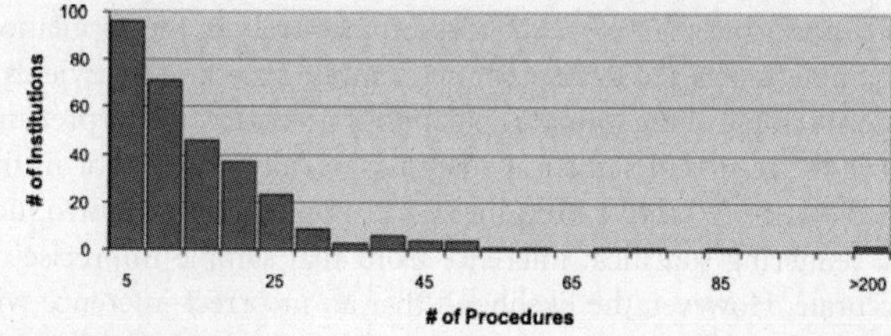

FIGURE 6.9 Histogram showing the distribution of the number of hospitals performing varying numbers of gastrectomies per year. It is an example of a right-skewed distribution. (From Enzinger P, Benedetti JK, Meyerhardt JA, et al. Impact of hospital volume on recurrence and survival after surgery for gastric cancer. *Ann Surg.* 2007;245(3):426–434, with permission.)

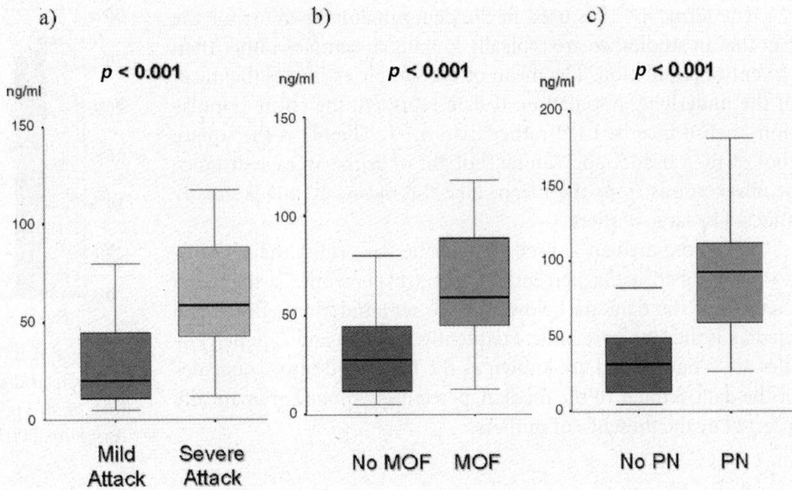

FIGURE 6.10 Box plots comparing the distribution of the serum level of MIF in subjects with and without pancreatic necrosis during an episode of pancreatitis. (From Rahman SH, Menon KV, Holmfield JH, et al. Serum macrophage migration inhibitory factor is an early marker of pancreatic necrosis in acute pancreatitis. *Ann Surg.* 2007; 245(2):282–289, with permission.)

data value, and the maximum data value. The ends of the box represent the 25th and 75th percentiles, and the line in the middle of the box is drawn at the median. The interval between the 25th and 75th percentiles is known as the *interquartile range*. The two points connected to the box by a line may represent either the 95th and 5th percentile or the maximum and minimum values of the data. This plot allows visualization of the range and variability of the data and permits comparison between multiple groups. In the example, the distribution of the serum migration inhibitory factor (MIF) level is shown grouped by presence or absence of pancreatic necrosis during an episode of pancreatitis (Fig. 6.10). It is clear that patients without pancreatic necrosis not only have a lower median serum level but also experience less variation in the serum level.

ANALYTIC METHODS

An important goal of statistics is making inferences about differences and relationships across groups at the population level using data from relatively limited samples. Biostatistics is the branch of statistics that applies statistical methods to medical and biologic questions. Analysis of epidemiologic studies involves determining if associations between exposure and disease observed in a sample result from true associations in the underlying population or because of chance, that is, the probability that observations of associations or differences seen in samples represent real relationships at the population level or chance occurrences.

Understanding the role of chance as an alternative explanation is important in determining associations. It is also particularly important in understanding the process and goals of statistical inference. *Inference* is using a sample to make assumptions about the population the sample is believed to represent. A sampling method that yields a random sample of the source population is necessary to interpret and believe the results of statistical analysis. Poor design or error in the methods used to sample from the source population may introduce bias, rendering statistical inference from that sample imprecise or inaccurate. However, the likelihood that an incorrect inference will be made about the true characteristics of the population on the basis of representative sample decreases as the size of the sample increases.

Once data are collected, a variety of statistical tests may be employed. Each statistical test results in a probability statement, or *p* value. The *p* value is the likelihood of obtaining a result at least as extreme as that observed in the study sample by chance alone. Thus, a *p* value of 0.10 indicates that there is a 10% chance that the results obtained were due to chance, whereas a *p* value of 0.001 means that there is only a 1 in a 1,000 probability that the results were due to chance. In general, the accepted cutoff for the predetermined alpha level is most often 0.05. This ensures that there is no more than a 5% risk that the observed differences in the study are due to chance rather than a real association at the population level when the *p* value reaches alpha or less. Results with a *p* value less than the predetermined alpha are said to be "statistically significant."

Although a result may be statistically significant, it is important to remember that statistical significance does not necessarily mean clinical significance. For example, a new drug may be tested and found to lower a person's cholesterol by 1 mg, a result that turns out to be statistically significant. However, from a clinical standpoint, a reduction of 1 mg in a person's cholesterol means very little despite statistical significance especially when there are costs and potential side effects to taking a medication.

A measure related to the *p* value, also evaluating the role of chance in producing the observed outcome, is the confidence interval (CI). The CI represents a range of values that we are fairly confident will contain the true magnitude of effect. Conceptually, if a study were to be repeated an infinite number of times and a 95% CI was obtained for each repetition, 95% of those intervals would contain the true value being estimated. Like a *p* value, the CI can provide information about statistical significance at a specified level. If the null value (relative risk = 1 or difference = 0) is included in a 95% CI, then the corresponding *p* value, by definition, will be greater than 0.05. But the added information that a CI provides is a measure of true magnitude of the relative risk associated with a particular exposure. The width of the CI indicates the amount of variability in the estimate. A wider CI indicates a less precise estimate. With a narrower CI, the precision of the estimate is greater. The *p* value and CI are complementary and together provide the most information about the role of chance in study results.

Statistical Tests

Although hypothesis tests all operate on the same underlying concepts, the selection of a particular statistical test depends on both the data characteristics and the specific hypothesis being evaluated. To go into great detail about the different tests is beyond the scope of this chapter; however, there are certain tests that appear frequently in the literature.

t Test

A *t test* evaluates the observed difference between calculated mean values of two study groups to determine statistical significance. If the variance of the underlying population is known, or if the sample size is large enough, the standard normal distribution is used to determine the test statistic. It usually is the case, however, that the variance of a population is not known and a *t* distribution is used. Once a *t* test is performed, a *t* statistic is obtained and converted into a *p* value with the use of a *t table* (available online and in most books on statistics) or, more often, directly by statistical software. *t* Tests are used with noncategorical, normally distributed or parametric data, including clinical measurements such as height, blood pressure, or cholesterol level.

A *paired t test* is a version of a *t* test used in studies that look at pre- and posttreatment effects, with patients serving as their own controls, or in studies where patients in the two treatment groups are closely matched. An example would be the effects of an antihypertensive drug where the mean value of a patient's blood pressure level is compared before and after the new therapy. A *t* statistic would be calculated with accompanying *p* value to determine if the difference in observed effect was statistically significant.

Analysis of variance (ANOVA) is used to compare means among three or more normally distributed groups. It provides an overall test of equality of several means but does not specify which individual group mean or means are different. If one were to test the effect of three different diets on cholesterol levels, a significant ANOVA result would only indicate that the means of the three groups were not the same, but one would need to perform additional tests, known as post hoc tests, to determine which diet group(s) had different mean levels in cholesterol.

When data do not follow a normal distribution or cannot be defined by certain parameters, such as the mean and SD, nonparametric statistical tests are appropriate. Examples of nonparametric tests are the *signed rank*, *Wilcoxon rank-sum*, and *Kruskal–Wallis* tests. These tests are used when data are nonnormally distributed or when the data are ordinal but not interval scaled, so that the spacing between adjacent values cannot be assumed constant. Nonparametric tests have less power than parametric alternatives because they make no assumption about the shape or distribution of the data, and some of the information is ignored. For example, the precise distance between two data points is ignored and instead only the relative order is used when the data are ranked. Because parametric tests do not ignore aspects of the data, they are more powerful and should be used whenever possible.

Chi-Square Test

For categorical data, the chi-square test is a simple and common method to determine whether differences in proportions between study groups are statistically significant. The chi-square test is analogous to the *t* test for comparing means between two study groups, but it compares proportions rather than means. This test compares the expected proportion of individuals with a certain outcome against the proportion that is observed in the sample being analyzed. Expected values are determined on the basis of the assumption that the null hypothesis is true. There is no difference in the proportions between the two groups.

Usually, a 2 × 2 contingency table is used to present the observed data. One can also use an *r* × *c* contingency table that contains counts of observations in *r* rows and *c* columns representing the various levels of disease and exposure. An example of an *r* × *c* table would have disease status represented as a binary outcome (yes/no) in columns and exposure status as categories in rows. Examples of categorical exposure status are age categories (ages 20 to 29, 30 to 39, etc.) or smoking level (never, light smoker [<1 pack per day], heavy smoker [>1 pack per day]). Statistical programs compute the expected values from the observed values and compute the chi-square statistic. As with other test statistics, the larger the chi-square value, the smaller the *p* value, or the less likely the differences in proportions between categories are due to chance. When the categorical data being evaluated are paired, as happens in a matched case–control study, a variant of the chi-square test called *McNemar test* is appropriate. Another chi-square variant is the *Fisher exact test*, used when sample sizes are small. The Fisher exact test must be used when any one of the expected frequencies (or one "bin") in the *r*× *c* table is less than 5 subjects, a situation that can be seen in a study if there are very few "events" or cases of disease.

DIAGNOSTIC TESTS

In clinical practice, diagnostic test results often guide patient management. A patient with a constellation of signs and symptoms is the basis of any diagnostic process. Diagnostic tests are most often used to classify patients according to a binary outcome variable such as disease status (yes/no). Diagnostic tests can also classify patients according to categorical outcome variables such as low, intermediate, and high probability in cases of suspected pulmonary emboli. Physicians are required to interpret the results of these tests and make treatment decisions on the basis of their interpretation. Understanding and interpreting results of diagnostic tests are important applications of biostatistical methods.

A 2 × 2 contingency table provides the simplest structure for analyzing the results and characteristics of a diagnostic test. The 2 × 2 method, however, requires that two assumptions be met. The diagnostic test of interest is compared to a "gold standard" diagnostic method that gives truly accurate disease status results. In reality, most gold standards are not 100% accurate. In addition, the diagnostic test must yield a binary result that can be considered positive or negative. Again, this assumption is not always true. Many tests have either multiple levels (e.g., VQ scan) or continuous results (e.g., white blood cell [WBC] count). More complicated diagnostic test analysis, however, is beyond the scope of this text. The following sections focuses on using the 2 × 2 contingency table method to determine a diagnostics test's sensitivity, specificity, positive predictive value (PPV), and negative predictive value (NPV).

Constructing the 2 × 2 table is the first step in performing calculations for diagnostic tests. By convention, the test results are on the left side of the table in rows, and the true disease status is across the top of the table in the columns (Fig. 6.11). There are four possible combinations in the table: test positive:disease positive, test positive:disease negative, test negative:disease negative, and test negative:disease positive. These combinations are referred to as the test result being a true positive (TP), false positive (FP), true negative (TN), and false negative (FN), respectively. For the following discussion, consider this clinical example. There is a new test for PUD administered to 1,000 subjects. The subjects also undergo endoscopy as the gold standard for ulcer diagnosis. Endoscopy is able to identify ulcer disease in 250 of the 1,000 subjects. Of those 250 patients, where endoscopy identified ulcer disease, the new

	Disease +	Disease –
Test +	True Positive (TP)	False Positive (FP)
Test –	False Negative (FN)	True Negative (TN)

Sensitivity = *TP*/(*TP* + *FN*) = the percentage of patients with a positive test result who truly have disease = true positive rate
Specificity = *TN*/(*FP* + *TN*)= the percentage of patients with a negative test result who do not have disease = true negative rate
Prevalence = (*TP* + *FN*) / (*TP* + *FP* + *FN* + *TN*)
Positive predictive value (PPV) = *TP*/(*TP* + *FP*) = the percentage of patients with a positive test who truly have disease
Negative predictive value (NPV) = *TN*/(*FN* + *TN*) = the percentage of patients with a negative test who are truly disease free

FIGURE 6.11 Representative 2 × 2 table used in the calculation of the test-operating characteristics of a diagnostic test.

test is able to identify the ulcer disease in only 150. The new test also is positive for ulcer disease in 150 of the subjects who have no ulcer disease based on endoscopy. These results are presented in Figure 6.12A.

When describing a new diagnostic test, the first parameters usually defined are the test sensitivity and specificity. The *sensitivity* of a test is the ability of a test to detect disease when it is present, or the probability of having a positive test, given that the patient has disease. Sensitivity is often referred to as the *true-positive rate.* It is calculated by dividing the number of TP patients by all the patients with disease in the study population. In the example given, the sensitivity of the test is 0.60. The *specificity* of a test is the ability of a test to identify patients without disease, or the probability of having a negative test, given that the patient does not have disease. Specificity is often referred to as the *true-negative rate.* It is calculated by dividing the number of TN patients by all the patients without disease in the study population. The specificity of the hypothetical ulcer test, therefore, is 0.80. Of note, sensitivity and specificity are characteristics of the test and remain constant regardless of the underlying prevalence of the disease of interest.

Although they are important test characteristics, sensitivity and specificity are not useful for clinical decision making. Most patients do not present with a gold standard diagnosis. Rather most clinicians and patients want to know the probability of having disease when a patient has a positive or negative test result. That information is provided by the PPVs and NPVs of a diagnostic test. The PPV is the probability that a subject who has given a positive test result has disease and is calculated by dividing the number of TP subjects by all subjects with positive test results. Conversely, the NPV is the probability that a subject with a negative test result is in fact disease free. NPV is calculated by dividing the number of TN subjects by all subjects with negative test results. Unlike sensitivity and specificity, which remain constant for a given test, the PPV and NPV change as the prevalence of disease in the underlying population changes. *Prevalence* is the proportion of individuals in a population who have the disease at a specific instant. For example, in Figure 6.12A, the prevalence of disease is 25%. *Incidence* is the proportion of individuals in the population who develop the disease within a certain time (i.e., 1 year). The PPV of a positive test is 0.50, which means that a subject with a positive test result has a 50% probability of having disease. The NPV in this example is 0.86. Assume, however, that the prevalence of disease in the population was twice as high, that is, 50% (Fig. 6.12B). The sensitivity and specificity remain the same. Now, however, the PPV of the test is 0.75 and the NPV is 0.67. A subject with a positive test in this population, where disease prevalence is higher, is much more likely to have the disease, whereas a patient with a negative test is less likely to truly be disease negative.

Often a physician's decision to perform a given medical intervention is based on the determination that the benefit of the intervention outweighs the risk of providing the therapy. The decision-making process can be represented schematically (Fig. 6.13). The *treatment threshold* X represents the probability of disease at which a physician could choose either to treat or to observe. Below this threshold, the probability of disease is low enough for a physician to decide not to provide intervention. Beyond the treatment threshold, the probability of disease is high enough that intervention is warranted. The prevalence of disease is also known as the *pretest* (or prior) *probability*, and it is the chance that a patient has disease, given no other information. Thus, if this probability were higher than the treatment threshold, no test would be necessary and treatment would be given. Often, the pretest probability is lower than the treatment threshold, so diagnostic tests

	Ulcer	No Ulcer
Test +	150	150
Test –	100	600
	250	750

Sensitivity = TP/(TP + FN) = 150/(150 + 100) = 0.60
Specificity = TN/(TN + FP) = 600/(600 + 150) = 0.80,
Prevalence = (TP + FN)/(TP + FN + TN + FP)
= (150 + 100)/(150 + 100 + 600 +150) = 0.25
PPV = TP/(TP + FP) = 150/(150 + 150) = 0.50
NPV = TN/(TN + FN) = 600/(600 + 100) = 0.86

	Disease +	Disease –
Test +	300	100
Test –	200	400
	500	500

Sensitivity = TP/(TP + FN) = 300/(300 + 200) = 0.60
Specificity = TN/(TN + FP) = 400/(400 + 100) = 0.80,
Prevalence = (TP + FN)/(TP + FN + TN + FP)
= (300 + 200)/(300 + 200 + 400 +100) = 0.50
PPV = TP/(TP + FP) = 300/(300 + 100) = 0.75
NPV = TN/(TN + FN) = 400/(400 + 200) = 0.67

FIGURE 6.12 A. Example of diagnostic test for PUD in sample population with 25% prevalence of ulcers. **B.** Example of diagnostic test for PUD in sample population with 50% prevalence of ulcers.

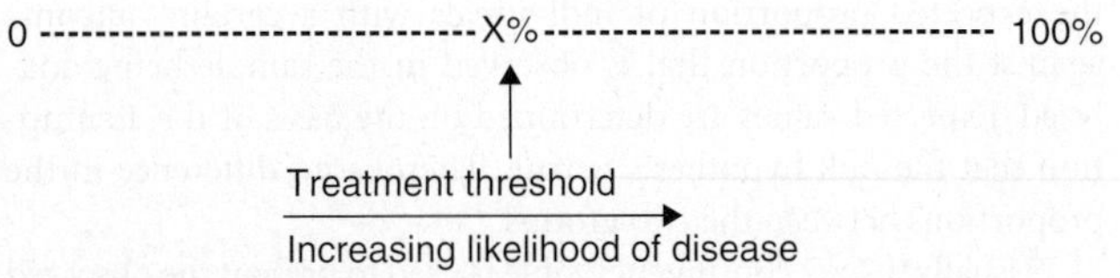

FIGURE 6.13 Decision to treat based on the results of a test.

are used to increase, or decrease, the estimated disease probability (known as *posttest probability*), so that there is less ambiguity in the decision-making process. Depending on the test characteristics (sensitivity and specificity) and the prevalence of disease in the population being studied, the posttest probability of disease will vary. Treatment should depend on whether the posttest probability is higher or lower than the predefined treatment threshold. The treatment threshold is physician dependent and varies with factors such as physician experience, availability of diagnostic testing, and disease severity. In the example mentioned earlier, when the prevalence of PUD was 50%, a clinician might not be certain about whether to start treatment for PUD; with a positive test, however, the patient now has a posttest probability of 75%, which might lend more weight toward treatment.

MULTIPREDICTOR REGRESSION MODELING

Multipredictor regression modeling is a branch of statistics that is used when there are multiple factors (also known as predictors, covariates, or independent variables) that are related to a single outcome or dependent variable. These statistical techniques allow the investigator to study the association between one or more factors of interest and an outcome while adjusting for other clinically or statistically relevant factors. To describe in great detail about different regression models and how to compute them requires the expertise of a statistician and the use of a statistical program; this is beyond the scope of this chapter. However, given the growing emphasis on higher-level statistics in clinical and translational research, a basic understanding of each model is useful for clinicians.

Univariable regression describes the relationship between the primary independent variable of interest and a dependent variable. Each covariate selected for generating a multivariable regression model is selected based on whether they meet nominal significance in the univariable regression analysis. Nominal significance is set by the investigational team prior to running the analyses. It is often determined by the p values. A p value less than 0.10 or p value less than 0.20 is often set as the threshold. Covariates may be included even if they do not demonstrate nominal significance when they are considered clinically meaningful. *Multivariable regression* models are used to measure the relationship between a primary independent factor and an outcome while adjusting for other covariates also known to be associated with the primary factor and the outcome. The additional covariates are known as potential confounders because their significant association with both the factor of interest and the outcome in the univariate analysis indicates that the potential confounder may influence the relationship between the factor and the outcome. Other covariates related to the factor of interest and the outcome may function as effect modifiers. Models can be built in a variety of ways including the forward stepwise or backward elimination methodology. A covariate is identified as a *confounder* on the primary independent variable, when the covariate correlates with both the primary independent variable and the dependent variable of interest. *Effect modification*, or interaction, occurs when there is a combined nonadditive influence of two independent variables on the third dependent variable. To control for effect modification, an interaction variable must be added to the model.

Commonly used regression models include *linear, logistic, Poisson, Cox proportional hazards (survival), repeated measures, and generalized linear models.*

Linear regression is a model used for assessing the relationship of a single (simple) or the joint relationships of multiple (multiple) independent factors ($x_1, x_2, \ldots, x_k$) with a continuous outcome variable y. For a *simple linear regression model*, the regression line is defined as $y = \beta_0 + \beta_1 * x$, or the mean value of the outcome y given a single predictor value x. For example, we can measure the volume of a child's pulmonary dead space (mL) [y] as a function of height (cm) [x] where the mean pulmonary dead space is 66.93 mL and average height is 144.6 cm. Therefore, $y = 66.93 + \beta_1 * (x, - 144.6)$. If we were given $\beta_1 = + 1.03$ mL, one would state that for every 1 cm increase in height, the pulmonary dead space would change by 1.03 mL. Of note, when you have a single dichotomous variable (x), simple linear regression gives the same result as a t-test. For *multiple linear regression model*, the regression line is defined as $y = \beta_0 + \beta_1 * x_1 + \beta_1 * x_2 + \beta_1 * x_k$, where each independent covariate x contributes a coefficient β to the relationship with the outcome y. The independent factors (x's) may be continuous or categorical in a linear regression model.

We have discussed identifying associations involving binary outcomes using contingency tables. These tables, however, are limited when considering multiple independent variables, continuous and multilevel categorical variables. *Logistic regression* is used to identify multiple possible predictors for increased or decreased odds of a particular categorical outcome. Logistic regression can be binomial (dependent variable is binary, i.e., "case" vs. "noncase"; "dead" vs. "alive") or multinomial (dependent variable has three or more possible outcomes, i.e., disease "A," "B," or "C"). The odds are defined as the probability that a particular outcome is a case divided by the probability that it is a noncase. While the basic structure of the logistic model mirrors that of the other regression models, the univariable and multivariable functions are described: $\text{OR} = e^{\beta 0 + \beta 1 * x1} = y$ and $\text{OR} = e^{\beta 0 + \beta 1 * x1 + \beta 1 * x2 + \beta 1 * xk} = y$, respectively.

Poisson regression is often used for modeling count data of events and person time. This type of analysis utilizes a log-linear model that permits the investigator to model rates, or an *incidence rate ratio* (IRR). Number of events $(y) = e^{\beta 0 + \beta 1 * x1} + e^{(\text{offset})}$ and $y = e^{\beta 0 + \beta 1 * x1 + \beta 1 * x2 + \beta 1 * xk} + e^{(\text{offset})}$, where the *offset* is the person-time such as person-years, follow-up time, or number of office visits. These functions represent the univariable and multivariable Poisson functions, respectively. A hypothetical scenario for Poisson regression: the number of chronic conditions is associated with number of hospitalizations using the number of hospitalizations and number of office visits (offset) to find that the isolated crude IRR of hospitalizations ($e^{\beta 0}$). If there are 4.4 hospitalizations per 100 office visits for the sample population and if the IRR for every additional chronic condition x_n (ordinal variable) increases the odds of hospitalization by 1.13 (CI, 1.09 to 1.18; $p < 0.001$), then the Poisson regression is written as: $\ln(y/\text{offset}) = e^{4.4 + 1.13 * \text{number of chronic conditions}}$ or $y/\text{offset} = 4.4 + 1.13 *$ number of chronic conditions.

Survival analysis is used for studying time to event or multiple events (i.e., time to death/disease recurrence/treatment failure or response). Study time starts at time zero (t_0) when the patient enters the study and contributes time until the event is reached or until the patient is censored. A *censored observation* is defined as an observation with incomplete information. There are four different types of censoring possible: right truncation, left truncation, right censoring, and left censoring. Right censoring includes only the time during which a patient enrolled at t_0 exits the study (stops contributing time) but does not experience the event of interest (i.e., is lost to follow-up, dies without the occurrence of event, or meets the end of the study period).

Disease-free survival, recurrence-free survival, and overall survival are frequently used terms for these studies. Kaplan–Meier curves for a categorical variable of interest are used to estimate instantaneous risk of the event occurring on a continuous time plot, using the log-rank test to compare the survival distribution of groups each time an event occurs.

A *Cox proportional hazards model* is used to determine the association between a variable or multiple variables of interest and survival while controlling for covariates. The main assumption of this analysis is that the hazards are proportional over time. For an instantaneous time (t), the hazard rate is the probability that an individual will experience an event at time t while that individual is at risk for having an event. The cumulative hazards function provides an estimate of the average hazard or risk of the event given the independent variable compared to a set reference group or absence of the independent variable. As an example, 50 nursing home subjects are enrolled in a study to either use or not use a protective barrier ("protect": yes = 1, no = 0) to protect them from developing a sacral pressure ulcer (event) and are followed for a period of 40 months. A Kaplan–Meier survival graph (Fig. 6.14) is generated to determine if there is an association between use of the barrier and risk of pressure ulcer known as the unadjusted hazard ratio (HR) for time to pressure ulcer; HR = 0.19 (CI, 0.08 to 0.42) reveals that those who used the protective barrier had a significantly lower risk (HR < 1.0) of pressure ulcer in the study. Similar to other regression models, a multivariable regression model can be developed using variables found to be significant on univariate analysis (nominal significance set at $p < 0.20$) such as patient age and nutritional status. Controlling for covariates, confounders, and effect modifiers in this model, we can determine that the adjusted relative HR of developing a pressure ulcer in the setting of the protective barrier is 0.17 times that of those who did not use the barrier (HR = 0.17; CI, 0.07 to 0.38).

Repeated measures (longitudinal) regression involve the use of the same subjects in a study more than once over time. In repeated measures designs, each subject is observed before and one or more times after an intervention. A common example is a pre- and post-test of the competency of participants attending a course of lectures. A *crossover study* is a type of longitudinal study in which subjects receive a sequence of different treatments (or exposures) as well as placebo, thereby having the subject serve as his or her own control. The observations made on a subject during the duration of the study form a correlated cluster of responses, where each response relates the response prior to it or one taken at a later date both on an individual and population level. Therefore, outcomes are correlated across observations, and predictor variables can be associated with different levels of hierarchy.

Simple repeated measures studies can be analyzed using ANOVA/ANCOVA (analysis of covariance), while more correlation structures such as clustered, hierarchical, longitudinal, and multilevel repeated measures data may require analysis of difference scores, generalized estimating equations, random effects, and mixed models. Repeated measures designs have the obvious advantage of eliminating the difference in responses between individuals. But there are also some problems that one should be aware of: the carryover effect, learning effect, and latent effect. *Carryover effects* occur when a new or additional exposure occurs before the effects of the previous exposure have worn off. *Learning effects* are observed when the response (outcome) improves each time subjects take a test; for example, previous test's questions and answers are remembered by the subject when he or she takes the test again. Finally, *latent effects* occur when one exposure can instigate the dormant effects of a prior exposure.

Predictive models can be reduced to numerical estimates of probabilities that determine the overall likelihood of an event such as disease recurrence, graft failure, or death. This can be graphically displayed as a *nomogram*, or analogs (i.e., scales) of predictors that when depicted properly will generate a single line representing the cumulative overall probability or risk score for the outcome.

In summary, basic statistical tools can be used to evaluate important clinical relationships. However, as surgery is a complex field, more sophisticated statistical tools are often required to properly examine the relationship between factors and outcomes. While commercially available statistical packages facilitate the use of these tools without the need for much advanced training, consultation with a statistician is generally advisable prior to employing complex

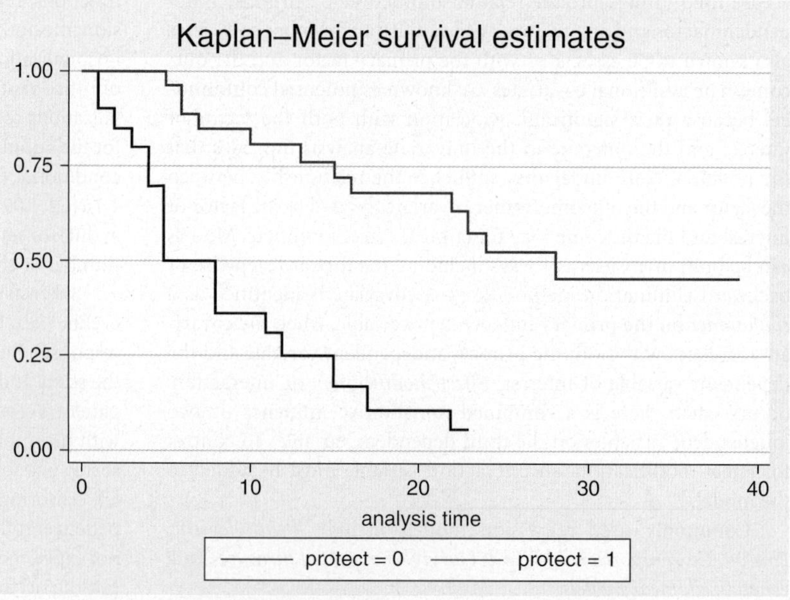

FIGURE 6.14 Kaplan–Meier Curve Time to Sacral Ulcer by Utilization of a Protective Barrier. Variable protect: 1 = sample population using protective barrier; 0 = Sample population not using the protective barrier.

statistical tools independently. However, these more sophisticated methods are frequently used more and more to generate much of the publicly reported information used by consumers and insurers to determine the quality of care provided by individual surgeons and organizations. Therefore, it is increasingly important for surgeons to have an at least basic familiarity with statistical modeling.

ACKNOWLEDGMENTS

The authors of this chapter would like to thank Dr. Seema Sonnad for her contributions to the prior editions of this chapter.

References

Collett D. *Modelling Survival Data in Medical Research.* 2nd ed. Boca Raton: Chapman & Hall/CRC; 2003.

Hosmer DW, Lemeshow S, May S. *Applied Survival Analysis: Regression Modeling of Time-to-Event Data.* New York: John Wiley & Sons, Inc.; 2008.

Juul S, Frydenberg M. *An Introduction to Stata for Health Researchers.* 3rd ed. College Station: StataCorp LP; 2010.

Research Methods II. *Chapter 10. Analysis of Longitudinal Studies: Repeated Measures Analysis.* 99–112; http://www.oxfordjournals.org/our_journals/tropej/online/ma_chap10.pdf (Last accessed 5/18/2014)

Suggested Readings

Detsky AS, Naglie IG. A clinician's guide to cost-effectiveness analysis. *Ann Intern Med.* 1990;113(2):147–154.

Glick HA, Doshi JA, Sonnad SS, et al. *Economic Evaluation in Clinical Trials.* New York: Oxford University Press; 2007.

Hennekens CH, Buring JE. In: Mayrent SL, ed. *Epidemiology in Medicine.* Philadelphia: Lippincott Williams & Wilkins; 1987.

Rosner B. *Fundamentals of Biostatistics.* 7th ed. Boston, MA: Brooks/Cole, Cengage Learning; 2011.

Vittinghof E, Glidden DV, Shiboski SC, et al. *Regression Methods in Biostatistics: Linear, Logistic, Survival, and Repeated Measures Models.* New York: Springer Science & Business Media; 2005.

Anesthesia

SEAN ANTOSH AND MEGHAN LANE-FALL

KEY POINTS

- The preoperative assessment is geared at defining and decreasing the patient's risk for adverse perioperative outcomes. The history (including functional status) and physical examination are as important as laboratory studies in preoperative assessment. Different preoperative tests (e.g., ECG and complete blood count) will be indicated depending on the patient's age, comorbidities, and the nature of surgery.
- All inhaled anesthetics cause a dose-dependent decrease in systemic and venous resistance, decrease in cardiac contractility, decrease in ventilatory drive, decrease in cerebral metabolic drive, and increase in ICP and cerebral blood flow.
- Nitrous oxide will expand closed air spaces and should be avoided in cases where a bowel obstruction or a pneumothorax is present as well as for cases involving middle ear surgery.
- Severe hyperkalemia may be seen after the administration of succinylcholine to patients with muscular dystrophy, paralysis, extensive burns, and crush injury. The risk of hyperkalemia may occur as soon as 24 to 48 hours after initial injury and may last for months.
- Local anesthetics work by preventing ion flow through neural sodium channels. Speed of onset, potency, and duration of action are dependent on chemical properties such as lipophilicity and pKa. Epinephrine prolongs the duration of local anesthetic action.
- A multimodal approach to pain management, using various medications with different pharmacologic properties, is optimal for treating pain in the perioperative period.
- Early signs of malignant hyperthermia include an increase in carbon dioxide production, tachycardia, hypertension, and a metabolic acidosis.

INTRODUCTION

Anesthesia, which is a temporary state of unconsciousness, loss of memory, lack of pain, and muscle relaxation (see Table 7.1), has its roots in the United States. On October 16, 1846, William T.G. Morton, who was actually a dentist, gave the first public demonstration of general anesthesia at the Massachusetts General Hospital. On that day, after the patient had been anesthetized; a tumor was removed from his neck. From this initial display, the discipline of anesthesiology was born. Given the need for anesthesia to facilitate most surgical interventions, it is imperative that the surgeon be familiar with the basic concepts of anesthesia and the role of the perioperative anesthesiologist. To function most effectively in the operating room, the surgeon and the anesthesiologist must work together as a team. For example, it is important that the surgeon relay to the anesthesiologist information pertaining to sudden or large amounts of blood loss, adequacy of relaxation, and clamping or unclamping of major vessels, which may affect the management of the patient's hemodynamics. The anesthesiologist, in turn, has a responsibility to inform the surgeon of important physiologic information, such as hemodynamic instability and changes in respiratory status.

TABLE 7.1 The "A" components of operative anesthesia

Amnesia	Inability to form memories
Anesthesia	Lack of sensation
Analgesia	Relief/lack of perception of pain
Akinesia	Lack of movement in response to surgical stimulus
Areflexia	Blunting of autonomic reflexes—attenuation of reflexic hemodynamic responses to surgical stimulus
Anxiolysis	Decrease in procedure-related anxiety

PREOPERATIVE ASSESSMENT

An anesthetic begins with the preoperative assessment, which includes a detailed history, a physical examination, and a review of pertinent data and studies. The goal of the preoperative assessment is to summarize the patient's health status to formulate an anesthetic plan. The evaluation may take place on the day of surgery, in the patient's hospital room the night before surgery, or in a physician's office or preoperative evaluation center days to weeks prior to an elective procedure. The obvious advantage of an evaluation one or more days before surgery is that it allows further studies to be performed, if indicated, and interventions to take place so that the patient may be "optimized" (i.e., the patient's risk of perioperative complications is minimized). In today's medical environment focused on efficiency and cost savings, the first time the anesthesiologist meets the patient is often on the day of surgery. To maximize time and resources, the surgeon should know what information to acquire preoperatively, so that the anesthesiologist's assessment can be made easily and expediently.

Clinical History

Assessment of each organ system is necessary, with special attention paid to cardiac and pulmonary function, as many perioperative complications are cardiopulmonary in nature. The preanesthetic assessment of the cardiovascular, respiratory, and gastrointestinal (GI) systems is reviewed in further detail in the following text.

Cardiovascular System

A thorough interrogation of a patient's cardiac status is necessary prior to surgery. This evaluation may be as simple as asking focused questions or may involve additional (and sometimes invasive) testing such as echocardiography or cardiac catheterization. The anesthesiologist will ask questions regarding hypertension, coronary disease, arrhythmias, valvular problems, as well as overall functional status. Active cardiac conditions such as decompensated heart failure, severe valvular disease, significant arrhythmias, or unstable coronary syndromes (including myocardial infarction within 7 days) must be evaluated and treated before noncardiac surgery. In patients *without* active cardiac disease, the assessment of cardiac risk has been aided by the American College of Cardiology (ACC) and American Heart Association (AHA), which jointly publish, and regularly update, a series of guidelines regarding perioperative care. They classify surgical procedures as elevated or low risk, depending on the association with perioperative cardiac complications (Table 7.2). Elevated-risk procedures include aortic, other major vascular, or peripheral vascular surgery. Five clinical predictors of cardiac risk, which are independent of the surgical procedure, include (1) ischemic heart disease, (2) history of heart failure, (3) cerebrovascular disease, (4) diabetes mellitus, and (5) renal insufficiency.

As part of the cardiac evaluation, a level of functional status should be elicited, which can be expressed in metabolic equivalents (METs). Perioperative cardiac morbidity is increased in those unable to achieve four METs. Examples of four MET activities include climbing stairs, walking up a hill, or running a short distance (Table 7.3).

TABLE 7.2 Cardiac risk[a] stratification for noncardiac surgical procedures

Risk level	Procedure
Elevated[b] (reported cardiac risk ≥1%)	• Aortic and other major vascular • Peripheral vascular • Anticipated prolonged surgical procedures associated with large fluid shifts and/or blood loss • Carotid endarterectomy • Head and neck • Intraperitoneal and intrathoracic • Orthopedic • Prostate
Low[c] (reported cardiac risk generally <1%)	• Cataract • Plastic surgery

[a]Combined incidence of cardiac death and nonfatal myocardial infarction.

[b]These two categories were previously divided into three categories: low, intermediate, and high risk

[c]Do not generally require further preoperative cardiac testing.

From Fleisher LA, Fleischmann KE, Auerbach AD, et al. 2014 ACC/AHA guideline on perioperative cardiovascular evaluation and management of patients undergoing noncardiac surgery: executive summary: a report of the American College of Cardiology/American Heart Association Task Force on Practice Guidelines. *Circulation.* 2014;130. doi: 10.1161/CIR.0000000000000105, with permission.

TABLE 7.3 Estimated energy requirements for various activities

1–2 METs	• Sitting quietly; riding in a vehicle • Playing a musical instrument
4–5 METs	• Playing golf without a cart • Gardening without lifting; mowing lawn with power mower; raking lawn • Swimming slowly
>10 METs	• Playing squash • Jogging (10-min mile) • Jumping rope

MET, metabolic equivalent.

From Fletcher GF, Balady GJ, Amsterdam EA, et al. Exercise standards for testing and training: a statement for healthcare professionals from the American Heart Association. *Circulation.* 2001;104:1694–1740, with permission.

Respiratory System

The evaluation of the pulmonary system includes an inquiry about reactive airway disease, chronic obstructive pulmonary disease (COPD), tobacco use, oxygen requirement, obstructive sleep apnea (OSA) symptoms, and recent upper respiratory tract infections. The value of preoperative pulmonary function tests (PFTs) remains controversial, except in the case of lung resection. Clinical findings and patient exercise capability are more predictive of perioperative outcomes than spirometry. However, PFTs may be useful to determine if recent interventions have optimized a patient's lung function, and a patient with an FEV1 less than 70% of predicted may be at an increased risk of pulmonary complications. Regardless of pulmonary status, patients should be strongly encouraged to refrain from tobacco use before surgery. Just 24 hours of smoking abstinence will reduce carboxyhemoglobin levels, and mucociliary transport can be improved after several weeks of smoking cessation. Some concern has been raised that smoking cessation immediately before surgery may increase cough and sputum production, but this has not been borne out by evidence.

Gastrointestinal System

The anesthesiologist must determine the patient's risk for gastric aspiration during induction as well as emergence of anesthesia. Aspiration occurs in these settings because of a decreased level of consciousness and loss of airway reflexes. If the airway is not protected intraoperatively with an endotracheal tube (ETT), the patient may be at risk for aspiration during maintenance of anesthesia. Situations that increase the risk of aspiration are shown in Table 7.4. If a patient is at increased risk for aspiration, a rapid sequence induction is often necessary, and heavy sedation should not be administered without an ETT to protect the airway.

Medications

The patient's current medications need to be reviewed during the preoperative assessment. In general, most cardiovascular drugs should be

TABLE 7.4 Risk factors for aspiration during surgery and anesthesia

- Recent ingestion of food (<8 h for heavy meals, <6 h for light solid food, <2 h for clear liquids)
- Trauma
- GI dysfunction (e.g., bowel obstruction and gastroparesis)
- Increased intra-abdominal pressure (e.g., pregnancy and laparoscopy)
- Use of opioids

continued up to the day of surgery, although certain classes of medications can predispose to physiologic derangements (Table 7.5).

Much attention is focused on the use of β-blockade during the perioperative time. ACC/AHA guidelines recommend the continuation of β-blocker therapy in any patient taking the drugs for hypertension, angina, or symptomatic arrhythmia (class I recommendation). The guidelines also advocate the use of β-blockers in patients undergoing vascular surgery who were found to have ischemia on preoperative testing. The use of β-blockers in other populations is more controversial. β-Blocker therapy is likely to be of benefit in patients with multiple cardiac risk factors, as described earlier, but this effect has not been definitively demonstrated. Regardless of clinical scenario, β-blockers should probably be started days to weeks before surgery if perioperative β-blockade is desired, in order to minimize the risk of hypotension during β-blocker titration.

Physical Examination

A targeted physical examination with special emphasis on the vital signs, airway, heart, lungs, and central nervous system (CNS) should be performed prior to anesthetic induction. Height and weight are necessary for accurate dosing of drugs. The anesthesiologist places particular emphasis on the airway evaluation to predict the degree of difficulty with mask ventilation and intubation. The airway examination, which can be remembered with the acronym "LEMON" (see Table 7.6), includes visual examinations of the external face and neck structures as well as visual inspection of the open mouth. Predictors of difficulty with ventilation include obesity, presence of a beard, edentulousness, presence of OSA symptoms, and advanced age.

TABLE 7.5 Medication classes and effects on anesthetic course during surgery

Medication class	Possible effects
Diuretics	Hypovolemia and hypotension Electrolyte abnormalities and ECG changes
ACE inhibitors, certain antiarrhythmics	Refractory vasodilation and hypotension
Antiplatelet agents, anticoagulants	Possible increased blood loss Increased risk of epidural hematoma formation on epidural catheter placement or removal
Insulin, oral hypoglycemics	Hypoglycemia, altered level of consciousness
MAO inhibitors	Life-threatening hypertension or hyperthermia when used with sympathomimetics or meperidine

ECG, electrocardiogram; ACE, angiotensin-converting enzyme; MAO, monoamine oxidase.

Diagnostic Testing

Laboratory data and diagnostic studies should be ordered on the basis of findings on history and physical examination, keeping in mind the planned procedure. The uniform ordering of a "standard" battery of laboratory tests is expensive and rarely of any utility. A general guideline for ordering laboratory studies is provided in Table 7.7.

TABLE 7.6 Airway examination and predictors of more difficult intubation

Physical signs	Less difficult intubation	More difficult intubation
Look externally	• Normal face/neck • No known pathology	• Known face or neck pathology • Abnormal face shape • Sunken cheeks • Receding mandible • Narrow mouth
Evaluate the 3-3-2 rule	• Mouth opening >3 F • Hyoid–chin distance >3 F • Thyroid cartilage–mouth floor distance >2 F	• Mouth opening <3 F • Hyoid–chin distance <3 F • Thyroid cartilage–mouth floor distance <2 F
Mallampati[a]	• Classes I and II	• Classes III and IV
Obstruction	• None	• Pathology within and/or around the upper airways (epiglottis, abscess, etc.)
Neck mobility	• Can extend and flex neck normally	• Limited range of motion

[a]The Mallampati score is a 4-point system for describing the visualization of airway structures on visual exam of the open mouth. Lower scores (I and II as compared to III or IV) indicate more visible airway structures.

TABLE 7.7 Recommended laboratory testing system utilized at the Johns Hopkins Hospital

Diagnostic test	Clinical indicators for testing
Electrocardiogram	Age 50 or older Significant cardiocirculatory disease, current or past Diabetes mellitus (age 40 or older) Renal disease Other major metabolic disease Procedure level 5[a]
Chest x-ray	Asthma or COPD that is debilitating or with change of symptoms or acute episode within past 6 mo Cardiothoracic procedure Procedure level 5[a]
Serum chemistries	Renal disease Adrenal or thyroid disorders Diuretic therapy Chemotherapy Procedure level 5[a]
Urinalysis	Diabetes mellitus Renal disease Genitourologic procedure Recent genitourinary infection Metabolic disorder involving renal function Procedure level 5[a]
Complete blood count	Hematologic disorder Vascular procedure Chemotherapy Procedure level 4[a]
Coagulation studies	Anticoagulation therapy Vascular procedure Procedure level 5[a]
Pregnancy test	Patients for whom pregnancy might complicate the surgery Patients of uncertain status by history

[a]Five surgical categories are defined, with a higher category denoting increasing invasiveness. Blood loss and estimated risk are also taken into account in this system. Procedure level 4, defined as highly invasive procedures with blood loss >1,500 mL and major risk to patients independent of anesthesia, includes major orthopedic surgery, reconstruction of the GI tract, and vascular repair without an ICU stay. Procedure level 5 is similar to level 4 but includes a usual postoperative ICU stay with invasive monitoring.

COPD, chronic obstructive pulmonary disease; GI, gastrointestinal; ICU, intensive care unit.

From Pasternak LR. Screening patients: strategies and studies. In: McGoldrick K, ed. *Ambulatory Anesthesiology: A Problem-Oriented Approach*. Baltimore: Williams & Wilkins; 1995, with permission.

The decision to obtain preoperative cardiac evaluation studies is aided by the ACC/AHA guidelines and depends on the urgency of the surgery, the patient's clinical risk predictors, the risk of the surgery itself, the patient's functional status, and results of previous cardiac evaluations or interventions (Fig. 7.1). It is important to keep in mind that these are only guidelines and every patient should be considered individually. The role of a consultant (e.g., internist, cardiologist) in the perioperative assessment is important but is often misunderstood. The consultant's role is not to provide "medical clearance" for surgery. The consultant should define the patient's medical conditions in terms of severity and interpret the results of previous studies as they pertain to their field of expertise. In addition, recommendations on the necessity of further evaluations should be made. Finally, the consultant should make recommendations on how to optimize the patient's medical status preoperatively. The decision to proceed with surgery should be made by the surgeon and the anesthesiologist, with assistance from the consultant.

On the basis of the patient's state of health, a physical status (PS) is assigned (Table 7.8). PS is a means of classifying patients on the basis of their overall condition and does not take the planned procedure into account. The PS is typically used to help anesthesiologists communicate with each other to quickly summarize a patient's overall health status. An elevated PS has been shown to correlate with increased perioperative mortality.

MONITORING

Standard Monitors

Certain tools have become standard intraoperative monitors for virtually all anesthetics in modern operating rooms. They include the pulse oximeter, noninvasive blood pressure monitor, electrocardiogram (ECG), temperature monitor, and a means of assessing adequacy of ventilation, usually with an end-tidal carbon dioxide ($EtCO_2$) monitor (see Table 7.9).

All operating rooms employ end-tidal capnometry to measure the level of CO_2 in the breathing circuit. The presence of sustained CO_2 in exhaled gas is the gold standard for successful endotracheal intubation, although the presence of $EtCO_2$ cannot rule out an endobronchial (i.e., mainstem) intubation. Capnometry serves as a noninvasive measure of systemic partial pressure of CO_2, albeit an indirect one. However, the difference between $EtCO_2$ and P_aCO_2 does indicate the extent of dead space ventilation. With normal lungs, $EtCO_2$ is approximately 5 to 6 mm Hg below arterial CO_2, which is due to anatomic dead space ventilation and normal intrapulmonary right to left shunting. An increase in the gap suggests that an increase in dead space ventilation has occurred, usually because perfusion to part of the lung has become compromised (i.e., physiologic dead space has increased). An extreme example of this occurs during cardiac arrest or a pulmonary embolism, as the $EtCO_2$ concentration acutely and profoundly decreases (see Table 7.10). An obstruction to expiration such as bronchospasm can be detected by a delayed upstroke of the $EtCO_2$ tracing.

There are various ventilator monitors and alarms built into most modern anesthesia machines. Mass spectrometry can be used to measure the exhaled concentration of oxygen, nitrogen, nitrous oxide, and inhalational anesthetics, permitting a real-time correlation between exhaled concentration of gases and anesthetic levels. Although some form of end-tidal anesthetic gas monitoring is typical, oxygen monitoring is mandatory, and low–oxygen

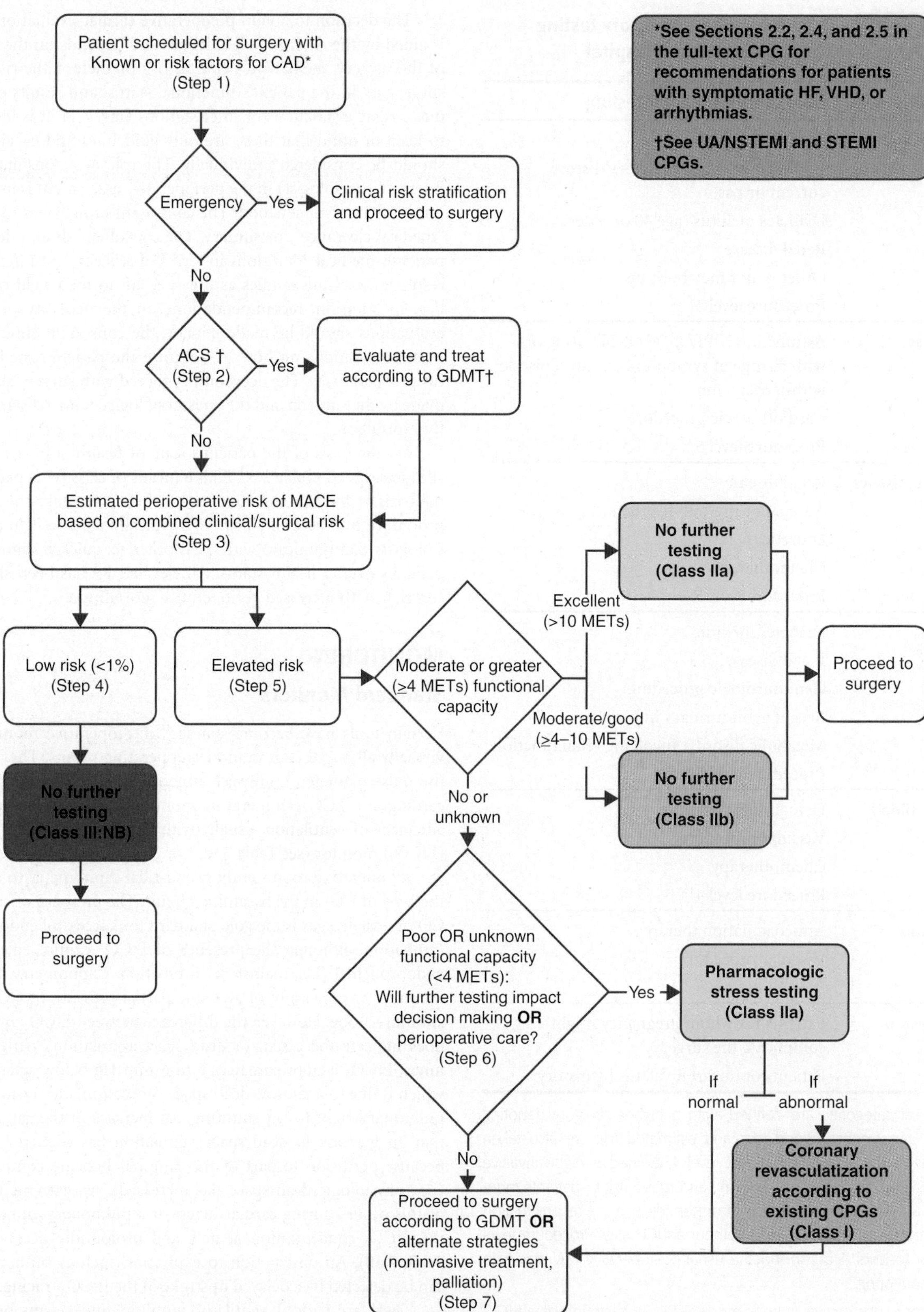

FIGURE 7.1 Stepwise Approach to Preoperative Cardiac Assessment.
Steps are discussed in text. Subsequent care may include cancellation or delay of surgery, coronary revascularization followed by noncardiac surgery, or intensified care. CHF, congestive heart failure; ECG, electrocardiogram; MET, metabolic equivalent; MI, myocardial infarction. (From Fleisher LA, Fleischmann KE, Auerbach AD, et al. 2014 ACC/AHA guideline on perioperative cardiovascular evaluation and management of patients undergoing noncardiac surgery: executive summary: a report of the American College of Cardiology/American Heart Association Task Force on Practice Guidelines. *Circulation.* 2014;130. DOI: 10.1161/CIR.0000000000000105, with permission.)

TABLE 7.8 The physical status classification of the american society of anesthesiologists

Physical status	Degree of systemic disease
1	No systemic disease
2	Mild systemic disease
3	Severe systemic disease
4	Severe systemic disease that is a constant threat to life
5	A moribund patient who is not expected to survive without the operation
6	Brain death present, organ donor

[a]NOTE: The letter "E" is added to the PS designation in emergency cases, as in "4E."

From ASA Physical Classification System. Available at: http://www.asahq.org/clinical/physicalstatus.htm. Accessed October 18, 2014, with permission.

TABLE 7.10 Factors that may change $EtCO_2$ during anesthesia

Increases in $EtCO_2$	Decreases in $EtCO_2$
Elements that change CO_2 production	
Increases in metabolic rate	**Decreases in metabolic rate**
Hyperthermia	Hypothermia
Sepsis	Hypothyroidism
Malignant hyperthermia	
Shivering	
Hyperthyroidism	
Elements that change CO_2 elimination	
Hypoventilation	Hyperventilation
Rebreathing	Hypoperfusion
	Pulmonary embolism

From Greenberg SB, Murphy GS, Vender JS. Standard monitoring techniques. In: Barash PG, Cullen BF, Stoelting RK, eds. *Clinical Anesthesia*. 7th ed. Philadelphia: Lippincott Williams & Wilkins; 2013, with permission.

concentration alarms are universal. A low-pressure alarm will signal decreased airway pressure and allow the detection of a circuit disconnection. A kink in the circuit, main stem bronchus intubation, patient respiratory effort, and bronchospasm will often set off the high-pressure alarm. Spirometry allows the measurement of minute ventilation and tidal volumes.

Cutaneous application of a peripheral nerve stimulator allows an objective assessment of the level of neuromuscular blockade when paralytic agents are used. A sequence of four electrical stimuli (i.e., "train of four") of 50 to 60 mA is applied at a frequency of 2 Hz over a peripheral nerve, which is meant to simulate nerve conduction. Typically, the ulnar nerve, which innervates the adductor pollicis muscle, is stimulated, and thumb opposition is monitored for effect. When nondepolarizing neuromuscular blocking (NMB) drugs (e.g., pancuronium and cisatracurium) are used, the train of four demonstrates "fade," with the last twitch amplitude smaller than the first. This is analogous to the "fatigue" seen with myasthenic patients. This allows the anesthesiologist the ability to assess muscle relaxation and guide when the patient needs more paralysis.

TABLE 7.9 Anesthetic monitors

Standard monitors
- Noninvasive blood pressure measurement
- ECG
- Pulse oximetry
- Temperature probes (e.g., skin, esophageal, nasopharyngeal, and bladder)
- Oxygen analyzer
- Capnometer and volatile agent concentration detector
- Peripheral nerve stimulator ("twitch monitor")

Additional anesthetic monitors (use depends on clinical scenario)
- Arterial blood pressure monitoring
- CVP measurement
- Pulmonary artery catheterization
- EEG, SSEPs
- Processed EEG (e.g., BIS monitor)
- TEE

EEG, electroencephalogram; SSEP, somatosensory-evoked potential.

Advanced Monitors

Additional specialized or invasive monitors may be employed depending on the patient's past medical history and the planned surgical procedure. An intra-arterial catheter (arterial line) may be inserted for "beat-to-beat" blood pressure monitoring or frequent blood gas and electrolyte monitoring. Cannulation of a central vein may be performed to provide large bore venous access for administration of vasoactive or caustic medications or central venous pressure (CVP) monitoring. The CVP may be used as a surrogate of left ventricular end-diastolic pressures (LVEDPs) to monitor intravascular volume. However, the absolute CVP value is often difficult to interpret, especially in the setting of positive-pressure ventilation, although the overall trend may give valuable information.

Traditionally, pulmonary artery catheters (PACs) are placed in situations where the CVP is not a reliable indicator of LVEDP. Conditions in which the pulmonary artery occlusion pressure (PAOP) is a more accurate measure of LVEDP and ultimately left ventricular end-diastolic volume (LVEDV) include abnormalities of the tricuspid valve, the right ventricle, the pulmonary vasculature, or the pericardium. The use of PAOP as an indicator of LVEDV relies on the assumption that there is a predictable relationship between the PAOP, the left atrial pressure (LAP), LVEDP, and the LVEDV. Mitral valve disease, aortic insufficiency, positive-pressure ventilation, positive end-expiratory pressure, catheter position in the lung, and alterations in left ventricular compliance can all confound the relationship between PAOP and LVEDV. Many studies have shown a poor relationship between PAOP and echocardiographic measurements of LVEDV.

The PAC can provide other important information. Pulmonary artery pressures can be measured as well as cardiac output. Newer catheters have the ability to measure mixed venous saturations (SVO_2) and provide continuous cardiac output measurements.

Fluid therapy can be titrated to cardiac output and stroke volume. Systemic vascular resistance can be calculated using CVP and cardiac output. Although most studies have failed to show any improvement in perioperative morbidity or mortality with the use of PACs, it must be kept in mind that many of them have been retrospective, non-blinded, or underpowered, and most have been designed to evaluate the use of PACs in intensive care rather than perioperative settings. In addition, the PAC is a monitor, not an intervention. Thus, its value depends on what the physician does with the information obtained from it, making its utility difficult to prove in a study.

Transesophageal echocardiography (TEE) is currently employed primarily in the cardiac surgical suites and may be used instead of, or in concert with, the PAC. TEE permits real-time evaluation of left ventricular wall motion, end-diastolic volume, and valvular function. It is used to detect air embolism, aortic dissection, valve malfunction, endocarditis, and myocardial ischemia. Anesthesiologists usually undergo additional specific training in the use and interpretation of TEE.

For neurologic monitoring, a number of specialized monitors may be employed during procedures where the integrity of the CNS may be compromised. Electroencephalographic (EEG) monitoring is used for carotid endarterectomies and during some cardiac surgical procedures. Somatosensory-evoked potentials (SSEPs) are useful for monitoring the spinal cord and its vascular supply, such as in thoracic aneurysm repair or scoliosis repair. Monitoring may be done by the anesthesiologist or more typically by a dedicated neurophysiology technician. These advanced neurologic monitors require different anesthetic choices in order to avoid degradation of their signals.

The BIS (bispectral index) monitor has been developed to assess the depth of anesthesia. It integrates analyses of EEG with more traditional spectral and burst suppression analyses to monitor the effects of many, although not all, hypnotic intravenous (IV) and inhalational agents on the EEG. The BIS index decreases as consciousness decreases and has been shown to correlate well with the loss of consciousness caused by these agents. Use of the BIS index has the potential to reduce the incidence of intraoperative recall, but it has many limitations. For example, it is a poor predictor of the likelihood of movement under anesthesia. It also correlates poorly with loss of consciousness induced by ketamine, nitrous oxide, and high-dose opioids.

ANESTHETIC TECHNIQUES

On the basis of proposed surgery, the patient's condition and preference, the surgeon's needs, and the anesthesiologist's judgment, an anesthetic technique is chosen. General anesthesia, regional anesthesia, and monitored anesthesia care (MAC) represent the various options (Table 7.11). In general, there are three phases of anesthetic care: induction, maintenance, and emergence. Each phase has its own unique challenges and considerations.

INDUCTION AND MAINTENANCE OF ANESTHESIA

Induction of anesthesia is the first phase of any anesthetic. For most situations employing general anesthesia, the goal of induction is loss of consciousness with maintenance of ventilation using an ETT or laryngeal mask airway (LMA). This goal is usually accomplished with a combination of IV and inhalational agents, which are detailed below. During this period of time, the patient is usually preoxygenated, or denitrogenated, with 100% oxygen delivered from a face mask with as tight of a seal as possible. The ultimate goal of this is to bring the end-tidal concentration of oxygen greater than 80% with an SaO_2 of 100% to allow for the most apnea time possible for intubation without desaturation.

Intravenous Agents

These are a group of unrelated medications that are administered intravenously (IV) to provide hypnosis. Most of these agents work by facilitating γ-aminobutyric acid (GABA) pathways in the brain.

TABLE 7.11 Types of anesthesia and their characteristics

Anesthetic type	Characteristics
General anesthesia	• Loss of consciousness (see Table 7.1 for the "As" of general anesthesia) • Maintenance of anesthesia with inhaled and/or intravenous agents • Support of ventilation (usually) with endotracheal tube, LMA, or face mask
Regional anesthesia	
Neuraxial	• Injection of local anesthetic into the epidural or intrathecal space to prevent nerve transmission of surgical stimuli or to treat postoperative pain • Often supplemented with sedation or general anesthesia
Peripheral nerve block	• Infiltration of nerve(s) with local anesthetic to anesthetize a specific sensory distribution for surgery or postoperative pain control • Often supplemented with sedation
MAC	• Administration of sedation and analgesics for patient comfort • Monitoring of physiologic parameters (blood pressure, pulse oximetry, ECG) • Typically used for minor procedures

LMA, laryngeal mask airway; MAC, monitored anesthesia care; ECG, electrocardiogram.

IV induction agents include barbiturates, propofol, etomidate, ketamine (*N*-methyl-D-aspartic acid [NMDA] antagonist), and benzodiazepines. Traditionally, these medications have been used for the induction of anesthesia because of their fast onset. This property derives from their high lipid solubility, which allows them to traverse cell membranes, specifically the blood–brain barrier, rapidly. The high lipid solubility also leads to fast offset because of extensive redistribution out of the brain into the blood and then into peripheral tissues. During prolonged infusions, the drugs begin to accumulate in peripheral tissues, such as muscle and fat, which prolong awakening once the infusion is discontinued. In these situations, the offset of the drug is dependent more on metabolism (largely hepatic) and clearance (largely renal) than on redistribution.

Propofol

Propofol is the most common induction agent currently used in the United States, mainly due to its rapid onset and short duration because of redistribution. Propofol causes large decreases in vascular tone and cardiac contractility, therefore must be used with caution in patients with low cardiac reserve. Propofol decreases cerebral metabolic rate for oxygen ($CMRO_2$), cerebral blood flow (CBF), and intracranial pressure (ICP). An additional benefit of propofol is its antiemetic properties. Continuous infusions of propofol can be used in combination with other agents, such as opioids, for maintenance of anesthesia, termed total intravenous anesthesia (TIVA).

Etomidate

Etomidate is an imidazole-containing compound well suited for the induction of anesthesia in patients with compromised hemodynamics, as it causes minimal cardiorespiratory depression. Subcortical inhibition may lead to occasional myoclonic activity during induction. It can suppress adrenal hormone synthesis even after a single dose for up to 5 to 6 hours. The significance of this suppression in the short term is unknown. However, the use of long-term infusions in critically ill patients has been associated with increased mortality, presumably from adrenal suppression.

Benzodiazepines

Benzodiazepines are primarily used as anxiolytics. However, they may also be used for anesthetic induction, usually in combination with other agents. Benzodiazepines have no analgesic properties and are therefore often combined with opioids and should not be used as a single anesthetic agent for a surgical procedure. Midazolam, because of its short duration of action, is the predominant benzodiazepine encountered in anesthetic practice. Midazolam has profound amnestic properties. Overdose with benzodiazepines can be treated with flumazenil, a specific benzodiazepine antagonist. Bolus administration of flumazenil may cause seizure activity in patients on chronic benzodiazepine therapy.

Ketamine

Ketamine is a phencyclidine derivative that induces a dissociative state of anesthesia by inhibition of thalamocortical pathways and activation of the limbic system. Ketamine's CNS effects are mediated via inhibition of NMDA receptors, which stimulate the sympathetic nervous system (SNS), resulting in an increased heart rate, blood pressure, and cardiac output. Ketamine has negligible effects on ventilatory drive and induces bronchodilatation. It may therefore be desirable for induction of anesthesia in patients who must maintain spontaneous breathing (e.g., awake/sedated endotracheal intubation) or in patients with reactive airway disease. Ketamine also possesses potent analgesic properties and may be used as an adjunct in patients with chronic pain to decrease overall intraoperative opioid usage. CBF and oxygen consumption are increased with the administration of ketamine. Therefore, it is undesirable in patients with head injury and/or elevations in ICP. Its stimulation of the SNS makes ketamine relatively contraindicated in the presence of coronary artery disease or uncontrolled hypertension. Emergence dysphoria and hallucinations are common following ketamine-based anesthesia. Benzodiazepines can be used to decrease these complications.

Opioids

Opioids are not sedative–hypnotics and have minimal amnestic properties. They interact with opioid receptors in the CNS and mediate effects on pain, mood, respiration, circulation, and bowel and bladder function. In general, opioids are not associated with a decrease in cardiac contractility, therefore may be ideal as anesthetic adjuncts for patients with compromised cardiac function undergoing cardiac surgery. However, blood pressure may fall as a result of vagally mediated bradycardia and blunting of the SNS, so opioids must be dosed with caution in this setting.

Some opioids tend to be used only in the operating theater. Fentanyl has minimal cardiovascular effects, no active metabolites, and a short half-life. Remifentanil has an ultrashort half-life, as it is metabolized by plasma pseudocholinesterase (which also metabolizes the muscle relaxant succinylcholine), and it is commonly administered via infusion as part of TIVA. Longer-acting opioids, such as morphine, hydromorphone, and meperidine, may be used during surgery as anesthetic adjuncts and after surgery for postoperative analgesia.

Opioids have important side effects. They cause a direct dose-dependent depression of ventilation. Opioids have a prominent effect on the GI tract, as peristalsis is slowed and gastric emptying is delayed. Nausea and vomiting, as well as constipation and urinary retention, are common side effects of opioids. Morphine and meperidine have been associated with histamine release, causing flushing and sometimes hypotension. Both these drugs have active metabolites that are renally excreted, and meperidine's metabolites can lower the seizure threshold.

Barbiturates

Sodium thiopental was the most commonly used barbiturate but is no longer commercially available in the United States. It is included here for historical reasons and because it may still be in use in other countries.

When administered in bolus fashion, thiopental causes profound respiratory depression, peripheral vasodilation, and myocardial depression. The dose should be decreased in the presence of decreased protein-binding states (chronic renal failure and cirrhosis) and in those with decreased central blood volume (elderly and hypovolemia), as the free-drug concentration in plasma will be higher in these situations. A beneficial effect of barbiturates is a reduction of cerebral metabolism and oxygen consumption. They may provide cerebral protection in the face of focal ischemia but not in the event of global ischemic episodes like cardiac arrest. A contraindication to barbiturate administration is acute intermittent porphyria, as an attack may be precipitated.

Inhalational Agents

The CNS is the primary effector site of anesthetic gases, with the lungs providing a conduit for delivery of gas to it. The standard measure of potency for inhaled anesthetics is defined as the *minimum alveolar concentration* (MAC) of a given gas at 1 atmosphere that produces immobility in 50% of subjects exposed to a noxious stimulus.

The inhalational agents in common use today include the volatile anesthetics isoflurane (MAC = 1.2%), sevoflurane (MAC = 2%), and desflurane (MAC = 6.6%) as well as the gas nitrous oxide (MAC = 104%). The more soluble the agent is in the blood, the slower is its rise in partial pressure in the brain, and the slower the onset of anesthesia. Increased solubility of inhaled anesthetics in tissues leads to an increased uptake in the muscle and fat, which prolongs awakening once administration of the agent has been discontinued. All volatile anesthetics cause dose-dependent cardiac depression; decreases in systemic, pulmonary, and venous vascular resistance; respiratory depression; bronchodilation; decreases in $CMRO_2$; and increases in ICP. When choosing an inhaled anesthetic, the anesthesiologist considers an agent's side effect profile, its potential for airway irritation, and its degree of metabolism in the body.

Desflurane is the most insoluble agent in the blood, thereby allowing a very quick onset and offset of anesthesia. However, desflurane is both pungent odor and has a propensity to induce airway irritation, as well as laryngospasm, which make it relatively unsuitable for mask inductions. Additionally, catecholamine surges may occur from rapid increases in inspired concentrations, which may result in significant tachycardia. *Sevoflurane* is a nonpungent agent, which makes it ideal for mask inductions, especially in pediatrics or in patients without IV access. Its blood solubility falls between that of isoflurane and desflurane. Sevoflurane is metabolized in the liver with the production of fluoride ions, which are excreted via the kidneys and has not been shown clinically to impair renal function. *Isoflurane* is the oldest and least expensive of the three inhaled anesthetics discussed here. It is more pungent than sevoflurane and undergoes minimal metabolism. Isoflurane's comparatively high solubility and consequent tissue accumulation lead to longer emergence times than those observed with sevoflurane or desflurane, especially during procedures of short to medium duration.

Nitrous oxide is a colorless, odorless gas, which has a very low solubility in blood and has the lowest tissue solubility of the volatile anesthetic agents. It has a very low potency, which results in its use only as an adjuvant anesthetic at relatively high inspired concentrations. Its major shortcoming is a tendency to diffuse into closed air-containing spaces; therefore, it is contraindicated in the presence of a pneumothorax, small bowel obstruction, air embolism, and middle ear surgery. Nitrous oxide will activate the SNS and increase $CMRO_2$. The use of nitrous oxide has been associated with an increased incidence of postoperative nausea.

MUSCLE RELAXANTS

NMB agents are used to facilitate intubation as well as to enhance surgical exposure, to ensure immobility, and to enable a patient to be anesthetized with lower concentrations of inhalational agents. The degree of paralysis can be objectively assessed with a peripheral nerve stimulator.

The two major classes of NMB agents include depolarizing and nondepolarizing agents (Table 7.12). The only depolarizing agent used in the United States today is *succinylcholine*. Succinylcholine binds to nicotinic acetylcholine (ACh) receptors at the neuromuscular junction (NMJ), causing an initial depolarization that leads to a diffused noncoordinated muscle contraction referred to as a fasciculation. A stylized picture of the NMJ is found in Figure 7.2. Succinylcholine remains bound to the ACh receptor, and flaccid paralysis follows. It eventually dissociates from the receptor and diffuses into the bloodstream, where it is metabolized by plasma pseudocholinesterase. The major advantage of succinylcholine is its rapid onset, provision of reliable intubating conditions in 60 seconds, and an ultrashort duration of action of 3 to 5 minutes.

Succinylcholine, however, is associated with various adverse side effects (Table 7.13). Succinylcholine can cause the release of potassium from muscle, with a rise of 0.5 to 1 mEq/L, because of its depolarizing effects at the ACh receptor. In susceptible patients, life-threatening hyperkalemia may ensue. The patients at risk include patients with extensive burns, massive tissue injuries, neurologic injuries (spinal cord injuries or hemiparesis), and neuromuscular disorders (muscular dystrophy or amyotrophic lateral

TABLE 7.12 Commonly used muscle relaxants

Agent	Intubating dose (mg/kg)	Duration (min)	Clearance	Autonomic effects	Notes
Depolarizing					
succinylcholine	1.5–2.0	3–5	Enzymatic	Vagotonic	↑ K^+, arrhythmias
Nondepolarizing					
Pancuronium	0.08–0.1	90	Renal	Vagolytic	Tachycardia
Cisatracurium	0.2	60	Enzymatic		
Vecuronium	0.1	30	Renal, hepatic		No CV effects
Rocuronium	0.6–1.0	30–60	Hepatic		Rapid intubating conditions

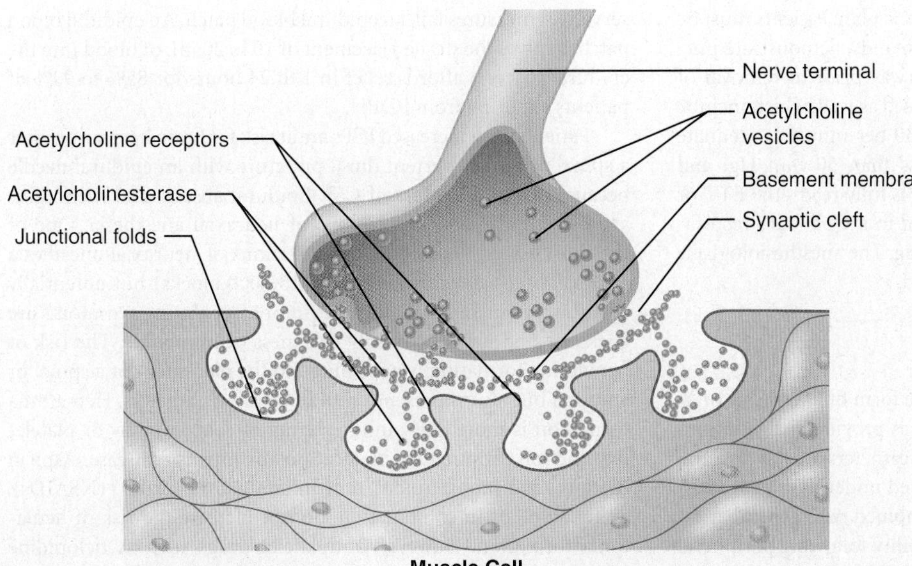

FIGURE 7.2 The neuromuscular junction. (From Neuromuscular blocking agents. In: Barash PG, Cullen BF, Stoelting RK, eds. *Clinical Anesthesia*. 7th ed. Philadelphia: Lippincott Williams & Wilkins; 2013, with permission.)

sclerosis [ALS]). The common pathway appears to be either the loss of neurologic innervation of the NMJ or defective muscle membranes. Regardless, there is a subsequent diffusion of nicotinic receptors from the NMJ to the rest of the muscle membrane and increased risk of hyperkalemia with succinylcholine administration. Patients may be at risk for severe hyperkalemia with succinylcholine as soon as 24 to 48 hours after the acute injury and stay at risk for months to years later. Relative contraindications to succinylcholine include its use in patients with intracranial hypertension or open orbital injuries due to a sudden but brief increase in ICP or intraocular pressure. Succinylcholine use is relatively contraindicated in children, given the prevalence of subclinical or undiagnosed myopathies. Succinylcholine can also precipitate the life-threatening disorder malignant hyperthermia (MH) (discussed later in the chapter).

Nondepolarizing NMB agents do not activate the ACh receptor; they competitively inhibit ACh binding at the NMJ. The elimination of most nondepolarizing NMBs is via hepatic and renal mechanisms. The choice of a particular agent usually depends on the desired length of paralysis and the presence of any hepatic or renal disease (Table 7.12).

TABLE 7.13 **Adverse effects of succinylcholine**

- May trigger malignant hyperthermia
- Has prolonged duration of action in patients with abnormal plasma cholinesterase or severe liver disease
- Can increase intragastric, intraocular, and intracranial pressures
- Vagotonic effects can cause cardiac arrhythmias such as bradycardia, junctional rhythms, or ventricular dysrhythmias
- Associated with transient hyperkalemia that can be life threatening in patients with severe burns, paralysis, or major trauma
- Usually contraindicated in pediatric patients because of hyperkalemia risk in patients with undiagnosed muscular dystrophies

MAINTENANCE OF PHYSIOLOGIC STABILITY

During surgery, the anesthesiologist is responsible for maintaining optimal operating conditions for the surgeon while maintaining the hemodynamics and physiologic conditions of the patient. The surgical stress response, combined with the anesthetic-induced decrease in sympathetic tone, as well as the cardiorespiratory depressant effects of the anesthetic drugs, can often make this challenging. Superimposed on these challenges is the presence of any intrinsic disease state. Hypovolemia is common due to fluid deficits from either preoperative fasting or bowel preparation. Isotonic crystalloids are typically used for maintenance fluids, administered at approximately 2 mL/kg/h. Blood loss is replaced with either crystalloid or colloids until transfusion becomes necessary. Often large fluid volumes are administered to replenish the intravascular volume due to fluid sequestration in the interstitial spaces from capillary leaks. "Third space losses" from large abdominal procedures can require up to 10 mL/kg/h of crystalloid for replacement.

EMERGENCE FROM ANESTHESIA

When an operation is over, the paralysis induced by nondepolarizing NMB agents should be reversed with acetylcholinesterase inhibitors (e.g., neostigmine), which is assessed by the magnitude of neuromuscular blockade via twitch monitor. The greater the number of twitches obtained reflects a greater degree of spontaneous recovery; however, if no twitches are obtained, the blockade is too intense for reversal. Even with four out of four twitches obtained, a patient may still have up to 70% of NMJ receptors blocked. Acetylcholinesterase inhibitors mechanism of action is via inhibition of ACh breakdown at the NMJ, leading to a rise in intrasynaptic levels of ACh. Reversal will increase ACh levels at muscarinic receptors as well, resulting in a diffuse vagal response resulting in severe bradycardia and possibly asystole. To counteract this, anticholinergics such as glycopyrrolate or atropine are administered with the acetylcholinesterase inhibitors.

Once the patient has been reversed from his or her neuromuscular blockade and all anesthetic agents have been discontinued, extubation is the next phase in the anesthetic plan. Patients must be able to breathe on their own, follow commands, demonstrate purposeful movements, and protect their airway prior to removal of the ETT. Some objective criteria may be used as well, which include a reasonable respiratory rate (>8 and <30 per minute), adequate tidal volumes (>5 mL/kg), a $PaCO_2$ less than 50 mm Hg, and hemodynamic stability. When the patient is fully ready, the ETT or LMA is removed with close attention paid to the patient's respiratory mechanics and comfort with breathing. The anesthesiologist is always prepared for reintubation if needed.

REGIONAL ANESTHESIA

Regional blockade may be used as the sole form of anesthesia or as an adjunct to general anesthesia, as well as provide analgesia into the postoperative period, especially when catheters are left in place. Studies have shown that surgery performed under neuraxial anesthesia, or when neuraxial blockade is combined with general anesthesia, results in higher rates of graft viability following peripheral revascularization, decreased intraoperative blood loss, and lower rates of deep venous thrombosis for hip surgery.

Epidural anesthesia is achieved by the administration of local anesthetics (discussed later) into the epidural space. A needle is used to traverse the skin, subcutaneous tissue, supraspinous ligament, interspinous ligament, and ligamentum flavum, after which the epidural space is reached. Typically, a catheter is threaded into the epidural space to allow redosing during the procedure or the administration of epidural analgesics in the postoperative period. Placement of a spinal needle is similar to that of an epidural; however, the epidural space is traversed and the subarachnoid space entered, which is heralded by return of cerebrospinal fluid (CSF). A much finer needle is typically employed for spinal anesthesia, and it is less common to place an indwelling catheter. As the spinal cord terminates at the L1–L2 level in adults, at least one interspace below this is chosen for spinal anesthesia.

The systemic implications of neuraxial anesthesia may be significant. In addition to their sensory and motor effects, local anesthetics create a chemical sympathectomy in the affected body region that results in vasodilation. When the block is proximal to the high thoracic cardiac accelerator fibers, bradycardia can also ensue. The combination of bradycardia and peripheral pooling of blood can cause profound hypotension. Mental status changes from impaired CBF may occur. Treatment of hypotension includes fluid administration, vasoconstrictors, and inotropic agents. Occasionally, anticholinergics are required for severe bradycardia.

Other than hypotension, there are several other important complications of neuraxial anesthesia. A "total spinal" implies a regional block that spreads throughout the entire spinal cord. The block may inhibit the muscles of respiration, requiring temporary positive-pressure ventilation. However, apnea often resolves with the restoration of a normal blood pressure. A postdural puncture headache (PDPH) may occur following spinal anesthesia or after inadvertent dural puncture with attempted epidural placement. The pathophysiology of a PDPH is the result of CSF leakage, which leads to sagging of the brain in the cranial vault causing traction on the pain-sensitive dural fibers. These headaches, which are usually occipital or frontal in location, are exacerbated by the erect position and ameliorated by assumption of a supine position. Visual and auditory disturbances can occasionally occur. Treatment of PDPH includes bed rest, IV hydration, caffeine, and if these "conservative" measures fail, an epidural blood patch. An epidural blood patch involves the sterile placement of 10 to 20 mL of blood into the epidural space. It affords relief in 1 to 24 hours for 85% to 90% of patients suffering from PDPH.

Patients with increased ICPs are at risk for brain herniation after a spinal or an inadvertent dural puncture with an epidural needle because of a sudden loss of CSF. Epidural abscess and meningitis are two infectious complications of neuraxial anesthesia. One of the most feared neurologic complications of neuraxial anesthesia is an *epidural hematoma*, a rare (1:150,000 blocks) but potentially devastating outcome. The most common presenting symptoms are backache and lower extremity weakness or numbness. The risk of hematoma formation is not limited to the placement of a spinal or epidural but also is present upon removal of catheters. Hematoma formation is more likely in the setting of coagulopathy or platelet dysfunction, from either medications or intrinsic disease. Aspirin therapy and nonsteroidal anti-inflammatory drugs (NSAIDs), either alone or in combination, do not increase the risk of hematoma formation. However, antiplatelet drugs such as ticlopidine and clopidogrel do increase the risk. The current American Society of Regional Anesthesia guidelines recommend discontinuing ticlopidine for 14 days and clopidogrel for 7 days prior to performing neuraxial anesthesia. If a hematoma is suspected, an emergent MRI is indicated, followed by surgical decompression. The chance for recovery is significantly decreased if surgery occurs greater than 8 hours after the event.

Commonly used peripheral nerve blocks include those of the brachial plexus, the sciatic and femoral nerves, the intercostal nerves, the ilioinguinal nerve, and the nerves of the ankle. Advantages of peripheral nerve blocks over neuraxial blockade include greater hemodynamic stability and less risk of serious neurologic injury. Complications of peripheral nerve block include hematoma, block failure, intravascular injection, and rarely, infection or nerve damage. Intercostal, interscalene, supra-, or infraclavicular nerve blocks may cause pneumothorax, which may result in respiratory decompensation. An interscalene block can also cause phrenic nerve paralysis. Additional relative contraindications to regional nerve blocks include sepsis, skin infection in the area of proposed needle placement, and preexistent neurologic deficit/neuropathy.

LOCAL ANESTHETICS

Local anesthetics act on the sodium channels of nerve membranes. They bind to specific receptors within the inner portion of sodium channel and stabilize the channel in the inactivated state, thus terminating the initiation and conduction of action potentials. Local anesthetics can be classified as either amides (e.g., *lidocaine* and *bupivacaine*) or esters (e.g., *procaine*) on the basis of their intermediate linkage structure. Plasma cholinesterase is responsible for the metabolism of the ester family of agents, while local anesthetics with an amide linkage undergo hepatic metabolism. Esters have a higher incidence of "true" allergic reactions based on a cross-sensitivity to para-aminobenzoic acid, which is a product of ester metabolism.

Local anesthetics may be used topically, subcutaneously, and in a wide variety of perineural locations for major nerve blocks. The choice of agent is based on the location to be blocked, desired duration of action, and toxicity. The addition of epinephrine, which causes vasoconstriction in that region, will prolong an agent's duration of action, limit systemic absorption and toxicity, and may serve as a marker for intravascular injection by inducing tachycardia.

Local anesthetics are weak bases; therefore, alkalinization of a local anesthetic solution with bicarbonate will speed onset, as it increases the percentage of local anesthetic present in the nonionized form. It is the nonionized form of these weak bases that penetrates nerve cell membranes.

The major concern regarding the use of local anesthetics is their cardiovascular and CNS toxicity. CNS symptoms tend to precede cardiovascular symptoms. The first signs of neurologic toxicity may be a metallic taste in the mouth, circumoral tingling, or tinnitus. CNS depression may be followed by excitation in the form of tonic–clonic seizures. Local anesthetic–induced seizures may be terminated with barbiturates or benzodiazepines. Larger doses of local anesthetics are needed to produce cardiovascular toxicity than are needed to produce convulsions. Lidocaine toxicity typically produces bradycardia and vasodilation. Bupivacaine can cause significantly more cardiac toxicity than the other local anesthetics. Although it suppresses cardiac contractility to the same degree as lidocaine, it can have profound effects on cardiac conduction. Bupivacaine binds avidly to cardiac sodium channels and dissociates very slowly. The first sign of bupivacaine toxicity may be a ventricular arrhythmia or cardiovascular collapse. Treatment often involves lipid emulsion therapy, cardiopulmonary resuscitation (CPR), and may require temporary cardiopulmonary bypass.

Toxicity is frequently said to occur at a given dose for a given weight. However, toxicity is primarily related to the plasma concentration. The accidental injection of a small amount of lidocaine into the vertebral artery may cause a seizure, while subcutaneous infiltration of large amounts of lidocaine has minimal side effects. Systemic blood levels vary as a function of the rate of absorption from a particular injection site. Drugs injected for intercostal nerve blocks are absorbed much more rapidly than drugs infiltrated subcutaneously. Therefore, the intercostal nerve block will result in a higher peak plasma concentration and a higher risk for toxicity.

Lidocaine is perhaps the most commonly used local anesthetic, having a wide margin of safety and a moderate duration of action. The maximum dose of lidocaine for infiltration is 5 mg/kg, and 7 mg/kg if epinephrine is added. Bupivacaine is an amide agent that provides excellent sensory and motor blockade and lasts approximately twice as long as lidocaine. The maximum dose for infiltration is 3 mg/kg. Ropivacaine is a newer amide agent. It shares a similar pharmacokinetic profile with bupivacaine. The major advantage of ropivacaine over bupivacaine is decreased cardiac toxicity.

POSTOPERATIVE PAIN MANAGEMENT

A multimodal approach to pain management is ideal when treating pain in the perioperative period. A multimodal approach uses various medications that all have different pharmacologic properties to achieve the goal of a comfortable recovery for the patient. Examples of such agents include NSAIDs, opioids, and adjunctive medications.

NSAIDS inhibit the activity of cyclooxygenase-1 (COX-1) and cyclooxygenase-2 (COX-2), which decrease the synthesis of prostaglandins and thromboxanes. With the addition of NSAIDs to postoperative pain management, patients report an overall decrease in pain intensity, as well as a reduction in opioid consumption by as much as 30%. However, there is an increased risk of GI and postoperative bleeding, which may make a surgeon reluctant to prescribe such medications. Additionally, COX-2 inhibitors, such as celecoxib or valdecoxib, have increased cardiovascular risk when used during the preoperative period.

TABLE 7.14 Opioid equianalgesic table

Drug	PO/PR (mg)	SQ/IV (mg)
Morphine	30	10
Hydromorphone	7.5	1.5
Oxycodone/ hydrocodone	20	Na
Methadone	10	5

Opioids are the most common medication used to control postoperative pain. Opioids bind to specific receptors throughout the nervous system and exert their effects mostly on mu, kappa, and delta receptors. Parenteral opioids are usually prescribed postoperatively until the patient can be safely transitioned to oral analgesics. A commonly employed approach to parenteral opioid administration is patient-controlled analgesia (PCA), which allows the patient to determine when they need additional medication. With a PCA, a patient's pain is usually better controlled, leading to higher satisfaction.

The conversion from parenteral to oral opioid analgesics may be challenging due to prior chronic opioid use or high requirements. When making the transition, the provider should utilize a conversion chart to determine the needed dosing, while allowing for cross tolerance (see Tables 7.14 and 7.15).

MALIGNANT HYPERTHERMIA

MH is an extremely rare but potentially lethal complication of anesthesia, with known triggers of MH includes all volatile agents as well as succinylcholine. It has an incidence of 1 in 12,000 anesthetics in children and 1 in 40,000 anesthetics in adults. Susceptible patients have a genetic predisposition. The pathophysiology of MH is the inability of the sarcoplasmic reticulum to reaccumulate calcium in skeletal muscle, which causes sustained muscle contractions. A laboratory test to detect susceptibility to MH is available.

MH is a clinical diagnosis. The first sign is frequently an elevation in the $EtCO_2$ level. Other findings include tachycardia, dysrhythmias, skeletal muscle rigidity, and eventually, an elevated body temperature. Laboratory abnormalities include a combined

TABLE 7.15 Fentanyl patch conversion table

Fentanyl transdermal	Morphine mg/24 h PO	Hydromorphone mg/24 h PO
25 μg/h	45 (30–75)	10
50 μg/h	90 (76–117)	20
75 μg/h	135 (118–150)	30
100 μg/h	180 (151–196)	40

50 μg/h Fentanyl = 1 mg/h IV morphine.

metabolic and respiratory acidosis, hyperkalemia, and extremely high levels of creatine kinase.

Therapy includes immediate discontinuation of volatile anesthetics, hyperventilation with 100% oxygen, conclusion of surgery as quickly as possible, maintenance of urine output to protect the kidneys from myoglobin, and active cooling measures. *Dantrolene* is the drug of choice for treatment of MH. It acts by interfering with the release of calcium from the sarcoplasmic reticulum.

CONCLUSION

Surgical practice is facilitated by the safe practice of anesthesia, which requires open and frequent communication between the surgery and anesthesia teams before, during, and after a surgical intervention. Surgeons' familiarity with anesthetic techniques and physiologic concerns enables efficient use of perioperative resources and promotes optimal patient outcomes.

Suggested Readings

Barash PG, Cullen BF, Stoelting RK, eds. *Clinical Anesthesia*. 7th ed. Philadelphia: Lippincott Williams & Wilkins; 2013.

Butterworth J, Mackey D, Wasnick J. *Morgan & Mikhail's Clinical Anesthesiology*. 5th ed. New York: McGraw-Hill; 2013.

Fleisher LA, Fleischmann KE, Auerbach AD, et al. 2014 ACC/AHA guideline on perioperative cardiovascular evaluation and management of patients undergoing noncardiac surgery: executive summary: a report of the American College of Cardiology/American Heart Association Task Force on Practice Guidelines. *Circulation.* 2014;130. doi: 10.1161/CIR.0000000000000105

Horlocker TT, Wedel DJ, Benzon H, et al. Regional anesthesia in the anticoagulated patient: defining the risks (The Second ASRA Consensus Conference on Neuraxial Anesthesia and Anticoagulation). *Reg Anesth Pain Med.* 2003;28(3):172–197.

Miller RD, ed. *Miller's Anesthesia*. 7th ed. Philadelphia: Churchill Livingstone; 2009.

SECTION

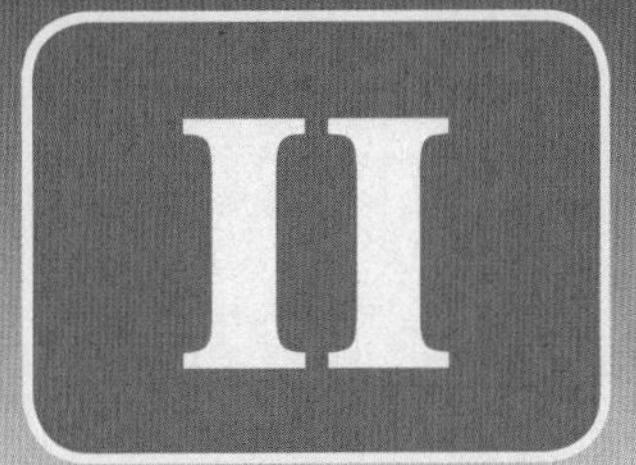

Abdomen and Gastrointestinal Tract

CHAPTER

8 Hernias

LEA LOWENFELD, JON B. MORRIS, AND ANDY S. RESNICK

KEY POINTS

- A hernia is a defect in the abdominal wall that allows protrusion of the abdominal contents beyond their inherent domain.
- A reducible hernia can be returned to its usual anatomic location. An incarcerated hernia cannot be reduced. A strangulated hernia has compromise of the vascular supply resulting in ischemia.
- Borders of the inguinal canal include the aponeurosis of the external oblique anteriorly, the transversalis fascia posteriorly, the aponeurosis of the internal oblique superiorly, and the inguinal ligament inferiorly.
- A direct inguinal hernia herniates through the floor of Hesselbach's triangle, medial to the epigastric vessels. An indirect hernia herniates through the internal ring toward the external ring and scrotum, lateral to the epigastric vessels.
- Borders of a femoral hernia include the femoral vessels laterally, inguinal ligament superiorly, lacunar ligament medially, and Cooper's ligament inferiorly.
- Femoral hernias should all be repaired due to a higher incidence of incarceration and strangulation.
- Open inguinal hernia repair techniques include the Bassini repair, the Shouldice repair, the McVay repair, the tension-free mesh Lichtenstein repair, and the Rutkow plug and patch repair.
- Laparoscopic inguinal hernia repair techniques include transabdominal preperitoneal (TAPP) repair, total extraperitoneal (TEP) repair, and intraperitoneal onlay mesh (IPOM) repair.
- Complications of inguinal hernia repair include recurrence, bleeding, infection, testicular atrophy/ischemia, and neuralgia.

INTRODUCTION

A hernia, coming from the Latin word for "rupture," is a defect in the abdominal wall allowing for protrusion of its contents beyond their inherent domain. A large part of any general surgical practice is devoted to the diagnosis and treatment of hernias and their complications. As such, it is important to understand the types of hernias that can occur, the pertinent regional anatomy, their natural history, and the treatment options available.

DEFINITIONS AND TERMS

Hernias may develop in any of the structures surrounding or supporting the abdominal cavity. Congenital maldevelopment of an abdominal support structure and acquired physical stresses each play a significant role. Factors that weaken the integrity of fascial tissue and collagen strength (e.g., overexpression of matrix metalloproteinases involved in extracellular matrix synthesis and degradation, Marfan's syndrome, and steroid use) and factors that increase intra-abdominal pressure (e.g., morbid obesity, pregnancy, chronic pulmonary disease, constipation, and urinary obstruction) can increase the risk of developing hernias.

Several terms are used to describe hernias and their contents. A *reducible* hernia is one in which the herniated contents can return to their anatomic position spontaneously or can be returned to their anatomic position with manual manipulation. An *incarcerated* hernia is one in which the herniated contents cannot be returned to their anatomic position in a nonsurgical manner, and may be acute or chronic. An incarcerated hernia containing bowel can cause a bowel obstruction. An incarcerated hernia with vascular compromise is referred to as a *strangulated* hernia. A strangulated hernia containing bowel can result in ischemia and perforation. When a portion of the hernia sac is composed of the herniating organ (e.g., bladder, cecum, sigmoid), this is a *sliding* hernia. When less than the full circumference of the bowel wall is trapped in the hernia, this is a *Richter's* hernia. A Richter's hernia can present with incarceration, ischemia, and bowel perforation without obstruction. A *Littre's* hernia refers specifically to a *Richter's* hernia containing a Meckel's diverticulum.

GROIN HERNIAS

Groin hernias are by far the most common type of abdominal hernias, representing approximately 90% of cases. Two thirds of inguinal hernias are *indirect*, passing lateral to the epigastric vessels, through the internal inguinal ring toward the external inguinal ring and into the scrotum. Indirect inguinal hernias occur in men due to a persistent processus vaginalis, the peritoneal continuation between the abdominal cavity and the scrotum. In females, the canal of Nuck is the analogous embryologic remnant related to the migration of the gubernaculum of the round ligament to the labium majus. The remaining inguinal hernias are *direct*, passing medially to the epigastric vessels and the internal inguinal ring directly through the floor of the inguinal canal (Fig. 8.1). A *pantaloon* hernia has both indirect and direct components. Despite the anatomic distinction, repair of these types of hernias are the same.

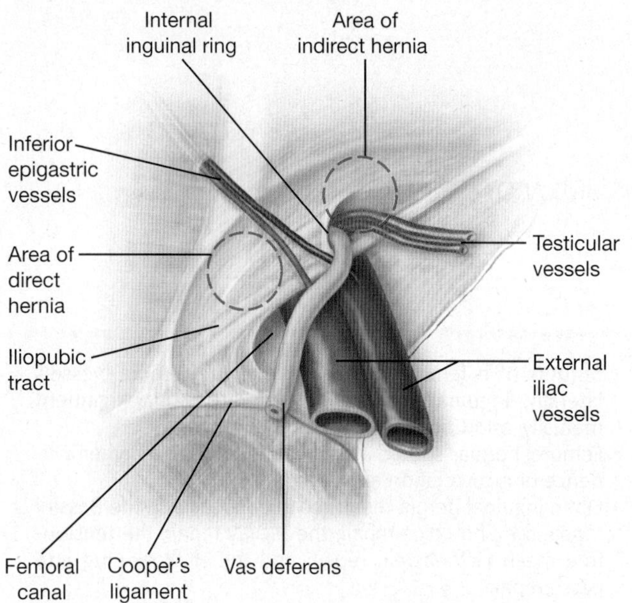

FIGURE 8.1 Direct and indirect inguinal hernias. (From Jones D, ed. *Master Techniques in Surgery: Hernia.* Philadelphia: Wolters Kluwer Health; 2013.)

Anatomy of the Lower Abdominal Wall

The lower abdominal wall is made up of three musculoaponeurotic layers (external oblique, internal oblique, and transverses abdominis) covered by subcutaneous fat and skin (Figs. 8.2 and 8.3; Table 8.1). The *external oblique muscle* arises from the lower eight ribs interdigitating with the serratus anterior and the latissimus dorsi laterally with its fibers running in an inferomedial direction.

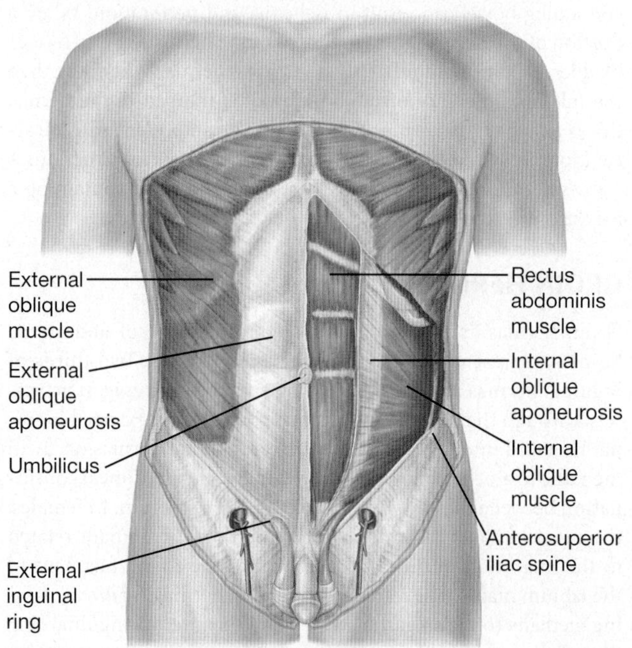

FIGURE 8.2 Muscles of the anterior abdominal wall. (From Jones D, ed. *Master Techniques in Surgery: Hernia.* Philadelphia: Wolters Kluwer Health; 2013.)

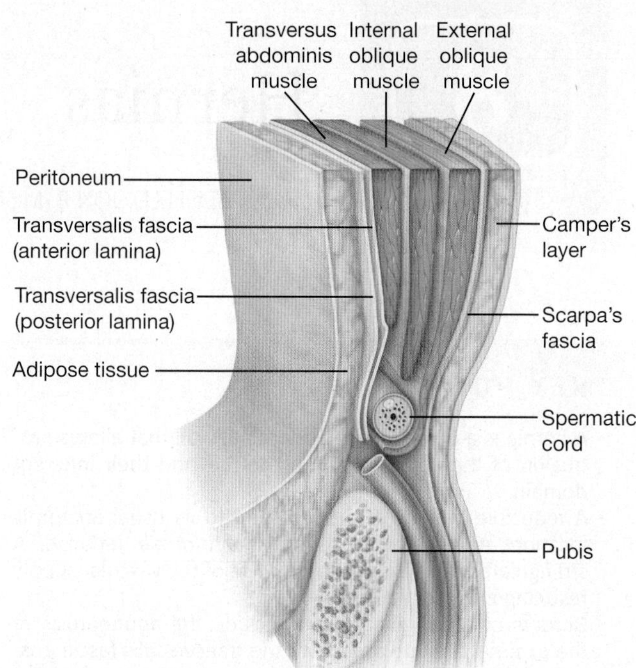

FIGURE 8.3 Layers of the anterior abdominal wall: Skin, Camper's fascia, Scarpa's fascia, external oblique aponeurosis and muscle, internal oblique aponeurosis and muscle, transversus abdominis aponeurosis and muscle, transversalis fascia, preperitoneal fat, and peritoneum. (From Jones D, ed. *Master Techniques in Surgery: Hernia.* Philadelphia: Lippincott Williams & Wilkins; 2013.)

The aponeurosis contributes to the anterior rectus sheath before inserting into the linea alba in the midline. The portion of the external oblique aponeurosis that stretches between the anterior superior iliac spine and the pubic tubercle is somewhat thickened and folds back onto itself, forming the *inguinal* (Poupart) *ligament*. Medially, the inguinal ligament reflects back onto the pectin pubis as the *lacunar ligament*. The *internal oblique muscle* is the middle layer of the abdominal wall musculature. Its fibers course in a superomedial direction. Above the arcuate line, the aponeurosis of the internal oblique splits and contributes to both the anterior and posterior rectus sheaths; below the arcuate line, it solely contributes to the anterior rectus sheath. The *transversus abdominis* forms the

TABLE 8.1 Layers of the anterior abdominal wall

Skin
Subcutaneous fat
Camper's fascia Scarpa fascia
External oblique muscle
Internal oblique muscle
Transversus abdominis muscle
Transversalis (endoabdominal) fascia
Properitoneal fat
Peritoneum

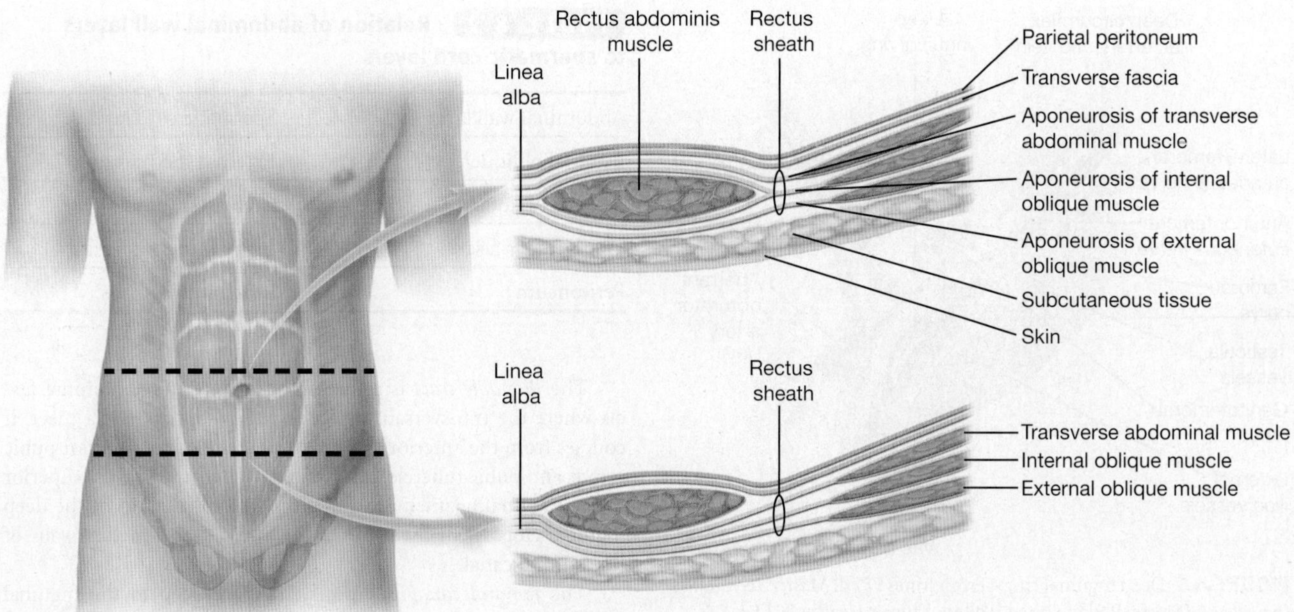

FIGURE 8.4 Rectus sheath. (From Jones D, ed. *Master Techniques in Surgery: Hernia*. Philadelphia: Wolters Kluwer Health; 2013.)

innermost muscular layer of the abdominal wall. The transversus abdominis courses transversely. Above the arcuate line, the aponeurosis contributes to the posterior rectus sheath along with the internal oblique; below the arcuate line, it joins the internal and external oblique to form the anterior rectus sheath (Fig. 8.4).

The *inguinal canal* courses from the *deep inguinal ring* to the *superficial inguinal ring* (Fig. 8.5). The *deep inguinal ring* is a natural defect in the transversalis fascia approximately halfway between the anterior superior iliac spine and the pubic tubercle through which the spermatic cord in men or the round ligament in women exits the abdominal cavity and enters the inguinal canal (Fig. 8.6). The *superficial inguinal ring* is a triangular opening in the aponeurosis of the external oblique muscle just superior to the medial part of the inguinal ligament (Fig. 8.7). The external oblique fascia forms the anterior border of the inguinal canal. The arching fibers of the internal oblique and transversus abdominis muscles (*falx inguinalis*) form the superior border. The inguinal and lacunar ligaments form the inferior border. The transversalis fascia forms the posterior border or floor.

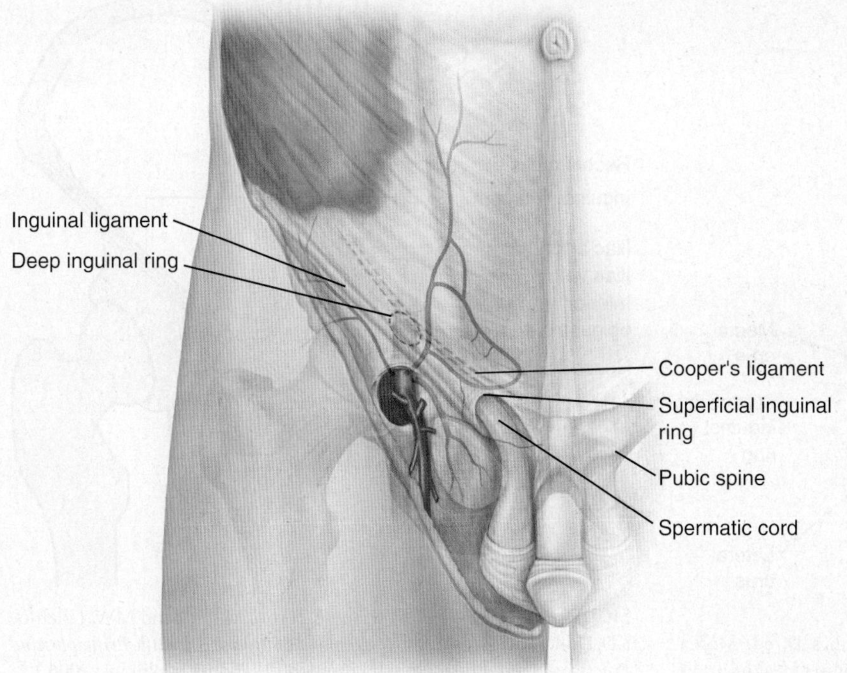

FIGURE 8.5 The inguinal canal. (From Jones D, ed. *Master Techniques in Surgery: Hernia*. Philadelphia: Wolters Kluwer Health; 2013.)

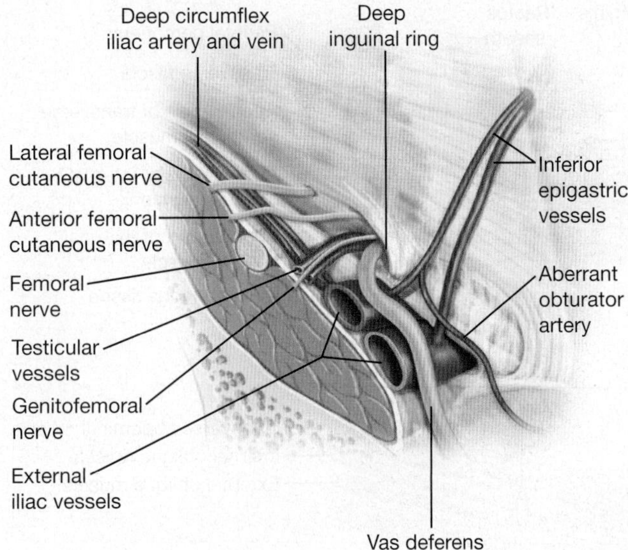

FIGURE 8.6 Deep inguinal ring. (From Jones D, ed. *Master Techniques in Surgery: Hernia*. Philadelphia: Wolters Kluwer Health; 2013.)

The *spermatic cord* passes through the deep inguinal ring and consists of the vas deferens, testicular artery, pampiniform venous plexus, and the usually obliterated processus vaginalis. The transversalis fascia extends onto the cord forming the internal spermatic fascia as the cord passes through the deep inguinal ring. The internal oblique muscle extends fibers onto the cord as the cremaster muscle. The external oblique muscle fascia adds the external spermatic fascia at the superficial inguinal ring (Table 8.2).

Hesselbach's triangle defines a region of the abdominal wall through which a *direct* inguinal hernia protrudes. The triangle is bounded by the inferior epigastric artery laterally, the inguinal ligament inferiorly, and the rectus sheath medially. An *indirect* inguinal hernia protrudes lateral to the inferior epigastric artery and anteromedial to the spermatic cord (Fig. 8.8).

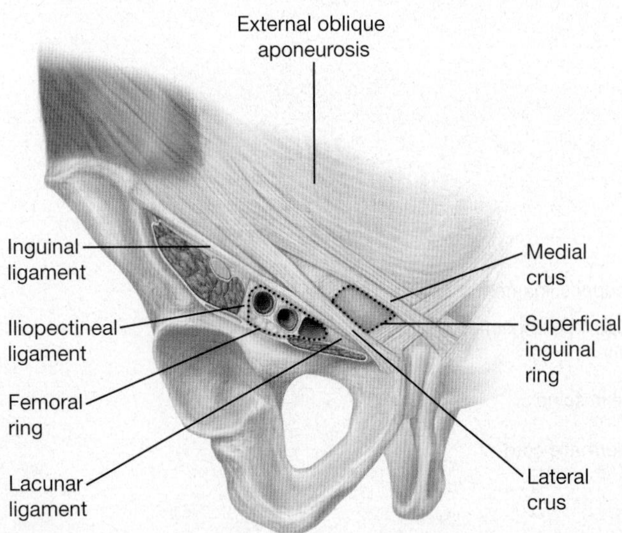

FIGURE 8.7 Superficial inguinal ring. (From Jones D, ed. *Master Techniques in Surgery: Hernia*. Philadelphia: Wolters Kluwer Health; 2013.)

TABLE 8.2 Relation of abdominal wall layers to spermatic cord layers

Abdominal wall layer	Spermatic cord layer
External oblique	External spermatic fascia
Internal oblique	Cremaster muscle
Transversalis fascia	Internal spermatic fascia
Peritoneum	Processus vaginalis

The *iliopubic tract* is a thickening of the endoabdominal fascia where the transversalis fascia and the iliopsoas fascia meet. It courses from the anterior superior iliac spine to the superior pubic ramus and pubic tubercle. It is located deep to and slightly superior to the inguinal ligament, forming the inferior margin of the deep inguinal ring. Medially, it forms the anterior and medial walls of the femoral canal.

The *femoral canal* is a potential space deep to the inguinal ligament. It is bounded laterally by the common femoral vein, superoanteriorly by the inguinal ligament, posteriorly by Cooper's ligament, and medially by the lacunar ligament. A femoral hernia represents a peritoneal outpouching through the femoral canal (Fig. 8.9).

There are three nerves that are encountered during inguinal hernia repair. The *ilioinguinal nerve* arises from the L-1 nerve root and runs superior to the spermatic cord through the superficial inguinal ring to innervate the scrotum or labium majus. The *iliohypogastric nerve* arises with the ilioinguinal nerve from the L-1 nerve root and courses between the internal oblique and transverses abdominis where it braches into an anterior branch, which innervates the hypogastric region, and a lateral branch, which innervates the gluteal region. The genital branch of the *genitofemoral nerve*

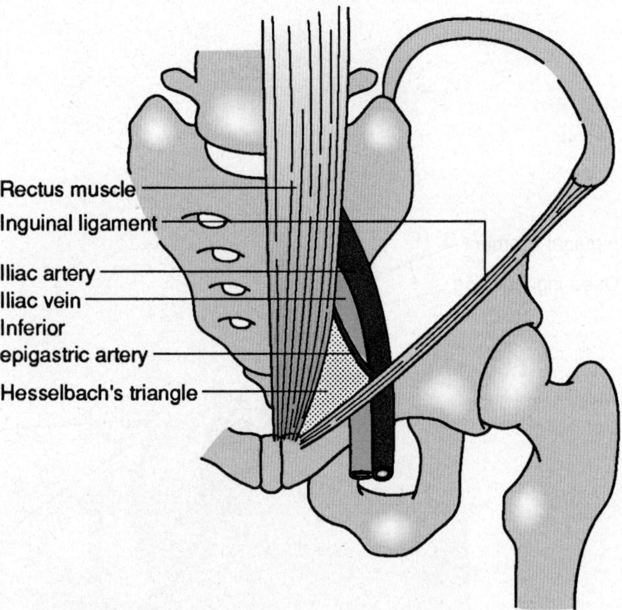

FIGURE 8.8 Hasselbalch's triangle. (From Mulholland MW, Lillemoe KD, Doherty GM, et al., eds. *Greenfield's Surgery: Scientific Principles and Practice*. 4th ed. Philadelphia: Lippincott Williams & Wilkins; 2006.)

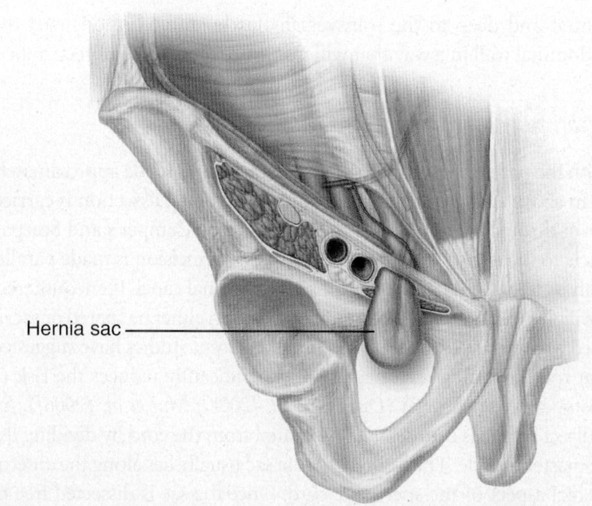

FIGURE 8.9 The femoral canal. (From Jones D, ed. *Master Techniques in Surgery: Hernia*. Philadelphia: Wolters Kluwer Health; 2013.)

arises from the L-1 and L-2 nerve roots and enters the inguinal canal inferior to the deep inguinal ring. It provides motor innervation for the cremaster muscle and sensory innervation to the scrotum and medial thigh (Fig. 8.10).

Clinical Presentation and Assessment of Groin Hernias

The diagnosis of a groin hernia is primarily made by history and physical examination.

History

Most commonly, the patient will present with complaints of pain and/or swelling in the groin. The pain may radiate into the scrotum, may be intermittent or continuous, may get worse after extended periods of standing, and may improve with rest. It is important to ask about symptoms of bowel obstruction—nausea, vomiting, abdominal distension, abdominal pain, and constipation, which would suggest that a loop of bowel has become entrapped in the hernia sac.

Physical Exam

The inguinal region should be visually and manually examined with the patients standing and in the supone position with and without the patient performing a Valsalva maneuver (e.g., bearing down, coughing). Erythema of the skin overlying the hernia is concerning for strangulation and ischemia of the hernia contents. In men, the examination finger is invaginated into the scrotum and directed up toward the superficial inguinal ring. While palpating the superficial inguinal ring, the examiner may ask the patient to perform a Valsalva maneuver,

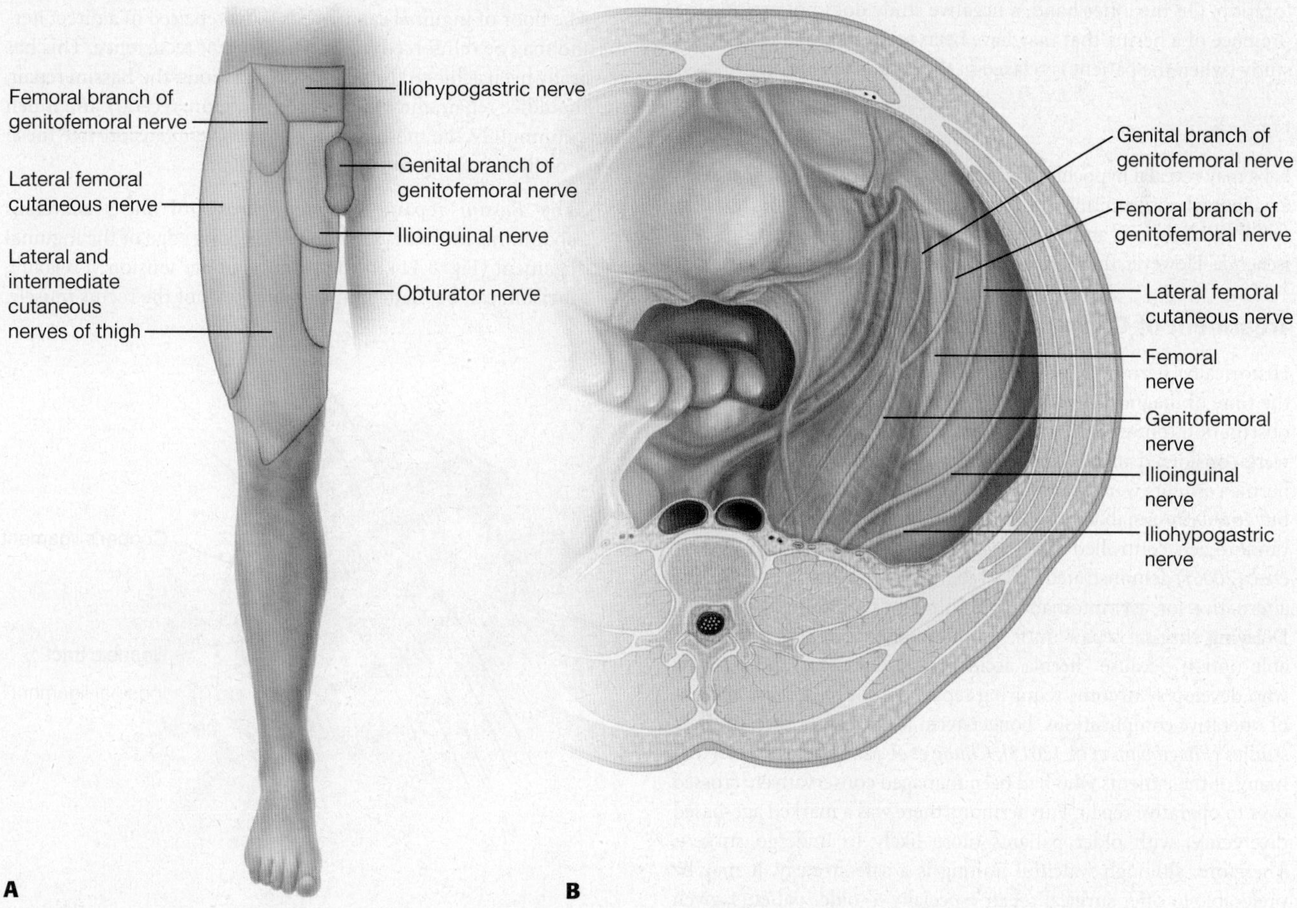

FIGURE 8.10 Inguinal nerves and their cutaneous innervations. (From Jones D, ed. *Master Techniques in Surgery: Hernia*. Philadelphia: Wolters Kluwer Health; 2013.)

which in turn may elicit a "tap" against the finger, suggesting an indirect inguinal hernia. With the examination finger in this position, the integrity of the floor of the inguinal canal can also be assessed for evidence of a direct inguinal hernia. Clinical assessment of inguinal hernias can be more challenging in women. The small external ring does not easily admit the examining finger; however, the round ligament may be thickened and palpable as it courses toward the labia. Women who report a history of a palpable or reducible mass in the appropriate location should be considered for surgical exploration and hernia repair even if physical exam is negative. A complete physical exam should also include an abdominal exam. Abdominal distension may suggest a bowel obstruction due to an incarcerated hernia. Peritonitis may suggest a bowel perforation due a strangulated hernia. Even without diffuse peritonitis, bowel perforation may occur in an incarcerated and strangulated hernia that is isolated from the abdominal cavity.

Imaging

A strong clinical history supported by physical exam findings of a hernia is sufficient indication for inguinal exploration, and additional imaging studies are often unnecessary. Ultrasound or a CT scan may be used to confirm the diagnosis in cases with atypical symptoms or inconclusive physical findings. Alternate diagnoses include inguinal adenopathy, undescended testis, spermatocele, varicocele, hydrocele, lipoma, or testicular cancer. Imaging can also be useful in identifying the hernia contents and can show evidence of a small bowel obstruction, bowel wall ischemia, or intestinal perforation. On the other hand, a negative study does not exclude the presence of a hernia that may have been reduced at the time of the study (when the patient is relaxed in the supine position).

Labs

Labs may reveal a hypochloremic, hypokalemic metabolic alkalosis in a patient who is vomiting due to a small bowel obstruction. Labs may reveal a leukocytosis and an elevated lactate in a patient with intestinal ischemia. However, there are no labs that are diagnostic of a hernia.

Treatment of Groin Hernias

Historically, herniorrhaphy was recommended for all hernias at the time of diagnosis in order to avoid a "hernia accident"—bowel obstruction, bowel ischemia, or bowel perforation. Small hernias were considered more dangerous than larger hernias because the hernia contents were more likely to get trapped in the small hernia but could presumably move freely in and out of a larger defect. Two randomized controlled trials (*Fitzgibbons et al. [2006]; O'Dwyer et al. [2006]*) demonstrated that "watchful waiting" was an acceptable alternative for asymptomatic or minimally symptomatic patients. Delaying surgical repair until symptoms increased was an acceptable option because "hernia accidents" rarely occur and patients who develop symptoms requiring repair do not have a greater risk of operative complications. Longer-term follow-up of each of these studies (*Fitzgibbons et al. [2013]; Chung et al. [2011]*) has shown that many of the patients who had been managed conservatively crossed over to operative repair. Furthermore, there was a marked age-based divergence, with older patients more likely to undergo surgery. Therefore, although watchful waiting is a safe strategy, it may be preferable to offer surgical repair especially to older patients, given that eventually these patients will require surgery.

The goal of both open and laparoscopic groin hernia repair is to restore the herniated structures to their previous anatomic position behind and deep to the transversalis fascia, and to reconstruct the abdominal wall in a way that will minimize the chance of recurrence.

Open Repair

With the patient positioned supine, an incision is made approximately 2 cm above and parallel to the inguinal ligament. Dissection is carried down through the skin, subcutaneous fat, and Camper's and Scarpa's fascia to the external oblique aponeurosis. An incision is made parallel with its fibers and spread to expose the inguinal canal. If encountered, the iliohypogastric and ilioinguinal nerves can either be spared or sacrificed to prevent postoperative neuralgia. Recent studies have suggested that routine ilioinguinal neurectomy significantly reduces the risk of postoperative neuralgia (*Dittrick et al. [2004]; Mui et al. [2006]*). An indirect hernia is exposed and separated from the cord by dividing the cremaster muscle. The indirect hernia sac usually lies along the anteromedial aspect of the spermatic cord. Once the sac is dissected free of the cord, the hernia contents can be replaced into the peritoneal cavity, and the hernia sac can either be replaced into the peritoneal cavity as well or it can be divided and ligated at its base, near the internal ring. A direct hernia appears as a bulge in the posterior wall of the inguinal canal. Without opening or excising the sac, the hernia is reduced and the posterior wall of the inguinal canal is repaired. If the sac extends into the scrotum, no attempt should be made to retrieve the sac distal to the pubic tubercle. Instead, the sac should be divided at the pubic tubercle, and the distal end can be left open or marsupialized to prevent a hydrocele from forming and to minimize trauma to the cord.

The floor of inguinal canal needs to be repaired in a direct hernia and may be reinforced in order to prevent recurrence. This has classically been achieved by one of four methods: the Bassini repair, the Shouldice repair, the McVay repair, or, more recently and much more commonly, the mesh repair—Lichtenstein tension-free mesh repair or Rutkow plug and patch mesh repair.

1. The *Bassini* repair: The aponeurosis of the transversus abdominis muscle is sewn to the shelving edge of the inguinal ligament (Fig. 8.11). If the repair is under tension, a relaxing incision can be made in the aponeurosis of the rectus muscle.

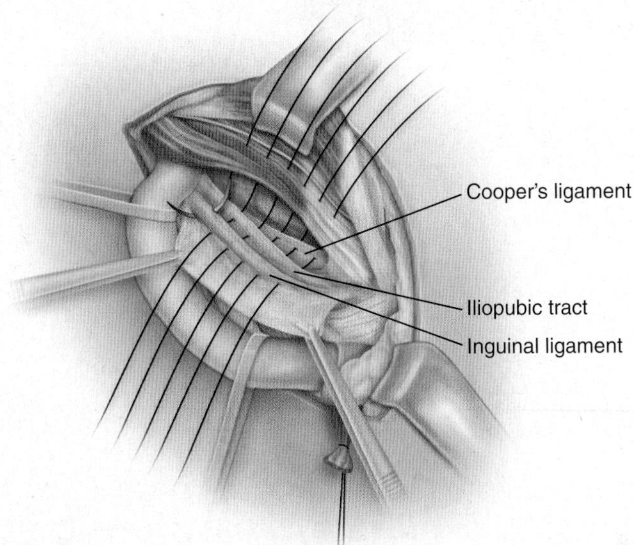

FIGURE 8.11 The Bassini inguinal hernia repair. (From Jones D, ed. *Master Techniques in Surgery: Hernia*. Philadelphia: Wolters Kluwer Health; 2013.)

Recurrence rates vary from 5% to 20% depending on the size of the initial hernia.

2. The *Shouldice* repair: The transversalis fascia is divided from the internal ring to the pubic tubercle. The fascia is then imbricated onto itself and sewn to the inguinal ligament with two suture lines (Fig. 8.12). As with the Bassini repair, relaxing incisions may be necessary. Recurrence rates, at least as reported by the Shouldice Clinic, are much lower, at 0.6%.
3. The *McVay* or *Cooper's ligament* repair: The floor of the inguinal canal is excised and reconstructed by sewing the conjoined tendon (the fused aponeuroses of the internal oblique and the transversus abdominis) to the femoral sheath and inguinal ligament laterally and Cooper's ligament medially from the pubic tubercle to the femoral vein (Fig. 8.13). Relaxing incisions are often necessary in this procedure. This repair closes off the femoral canal and, therefore, is the procedure of choice for femoral hernia repairs.

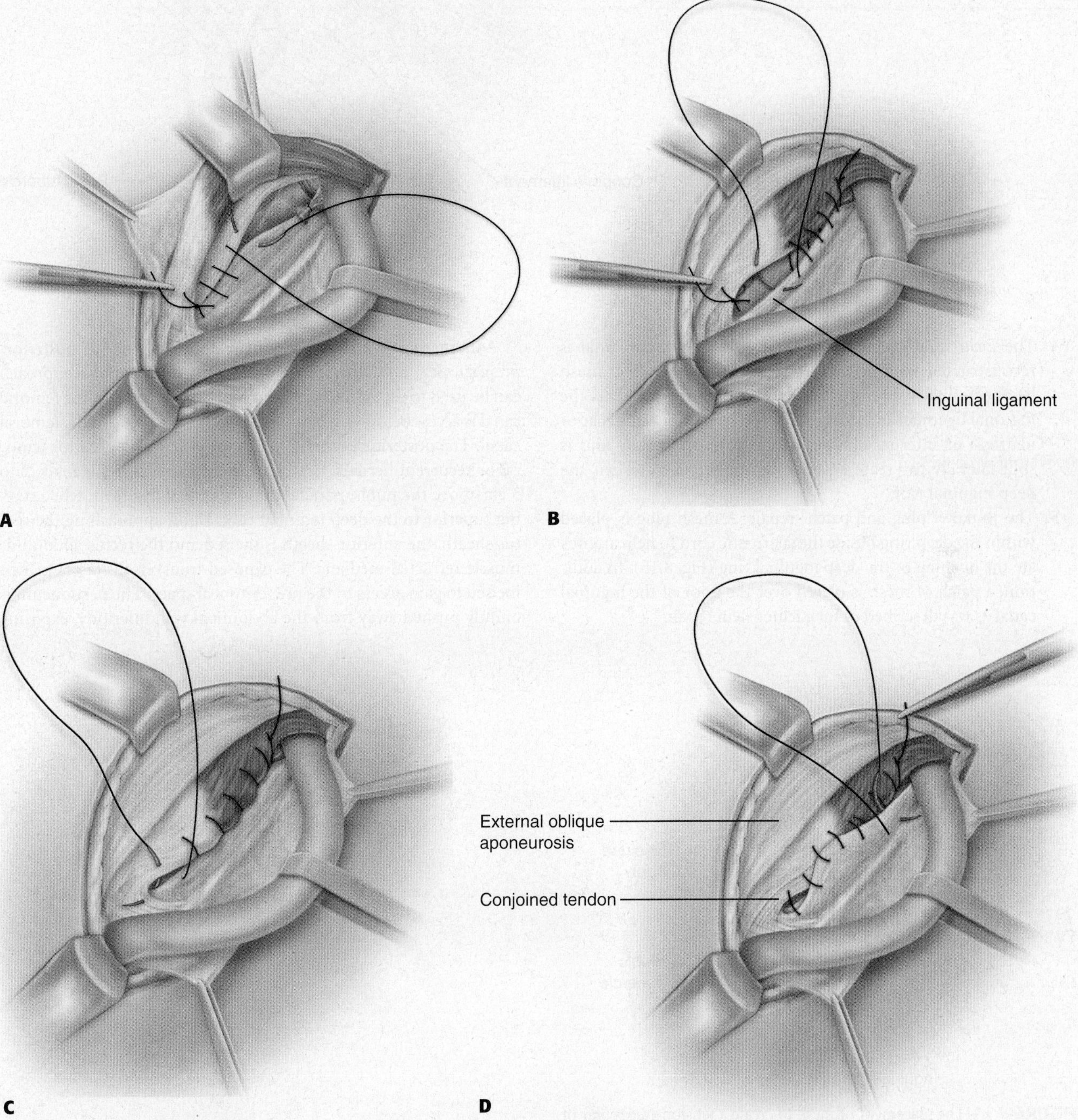

FIGURE 8.12 The Shouldice inguinal hernia repair. The first line of suture proceeds from the superficial inguinal ring toward the deep inguinal ring and then reverses direction back toward the superficial inguinal ring. The second line of suture starts at the deep inguinal ring and proceeds toward the superficial inguinal ring before reversing its course and ending at the deep inguinal ring. (From Jones D, ed. *Master Techniques in Surgery: Hernia.* Philadelphia: Wolters Kluwer Health; 2013.)

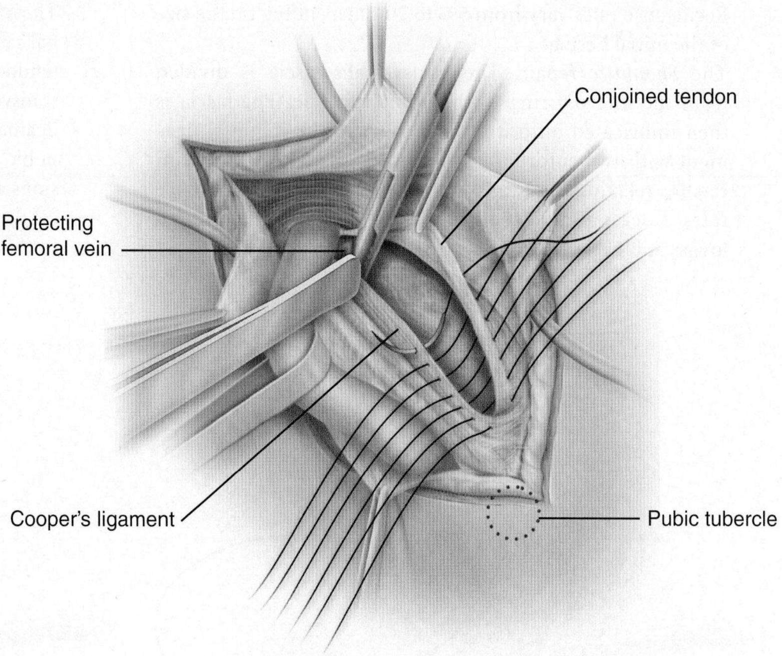

FIGURE 8.13 The McVay or Cooper's ligament repair. (From Jones D, ed. *Master Techniques in Surgery: Hernia*. Philadelphia: Wolters Kluwer Health; 2013.)

4. The *Lichtenstein* repair: The floor of the inguinal canal is reconstructed with prosthetic mesh (Fig. 8.14). The mesh lies posterior to the spermatic cord and is sutured to the inguinal ligament inferiorly and transversus abdominis aponeurosis or internal oblique aponeurosis superiorly and is split laterally to create an opening for the cord to exit the deep inguinal ring.
5. The Rutkow "plug and patch" repair: A mesh plug is placed within the deep ring beside the spermatic cord to help attenuate the opening of the deep inguinal ring (Fig. 8.15). In addition, a patch of mesh is placed over the floor of the inguinal canal as was described in the Lichtenstein repair.

Alternatively, an infrainguinal approach or a posterior/preperitoneal approach can be used. An infrainguinal approach can be used to repair femoral hernias. In this approach, the femoral canal is access below the inguinal ligament and a plug in the femoral canal. The posterior/preperitoneal approach is also used for femoral or recurrent hernias. In this approach, an incision is made 2 to 3 cm above the pubis, parallel to the inguinal ligament, while staying superior to the deep inguinal ring. Upon approaching the rectus sheath, the anterior sheath is incised and the rectus abdominis muscle retracted medially. The exposed transversalis fascia is then incised to gain access to the preperitoneal space. The peritoneum is bluntly pushed away from the abdominal wall inferiorly, exposing

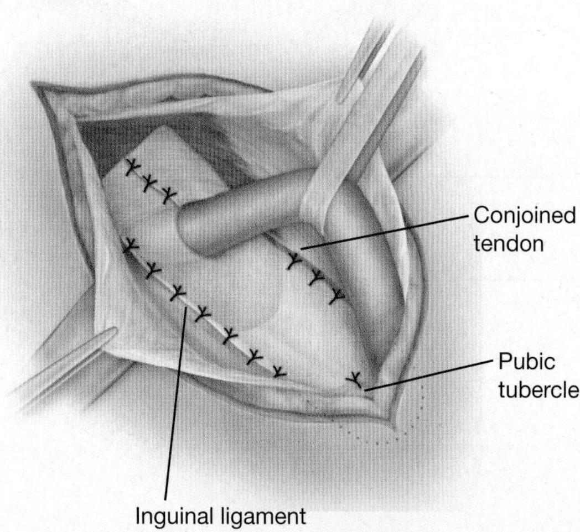

FIGURE 8.14 The placement of mesh to create a tension-free repair of an inguinal hernia was initially popularized by Lichtenstein. The mesh is sewn medially to the pubic tubercle, caudally to the inguinal ligament, and cephalad to the conjoined tendon. (From Jones D, ed. *Master Techniques in Surgery: Hernia*. Philadelphia: Wolters Kluwer Health; 2013.)

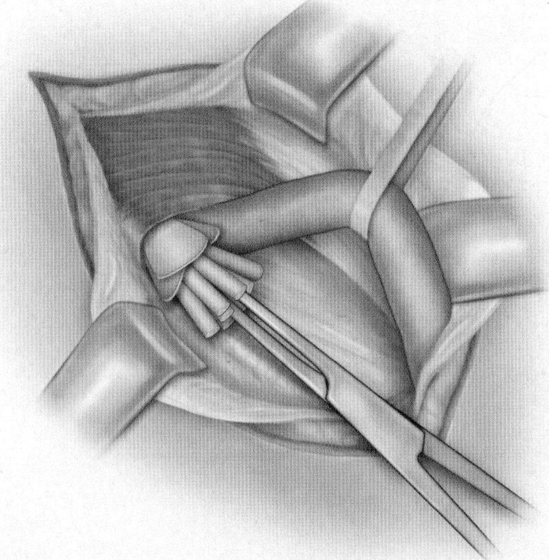

FIGURE 8.15 The placement of a mesh plug used in a "plug and patch" repair to help minimize the aperture of the deep inguinal ring. (From Jones D, ed. *Master Techniques in Surgery: Hernia*. Philadelphia: Wolters Kluwer Health; 2013.)

the internal surface of the inguinal region. After reducing the hernia by gentle traction, the sac is amputated, and the hernia defect is repaired either by approximating the transversus abdominis aponeurosis to Cooper's ligament medially and the iliopubic tract laterally or by suturing or tacking a piece of prosthetic mesh to the posterior aspect of the abdominal wall.

Groin hernias that are strangulated with a high suspicion for ischemic bowel or bowel perforation should be approached via a lower midline incision to facilitate examination of the bowel for viability and resection of the diseased segment. In this approach, the hernia is pulled into the peritoneal cavity rather than pushed in from the inguinal canal. Sometimes both a midline incision and an inguinal incision are required to reduce the hernia from both directions.

Laparoscopic Repair

Laparoscopic inguinal hernia repair has traditionally been advocated for bilateral and recurrent inguinal hernia repair because the approach can access both sides and uses planes that have not been violated; however, many more minimally invasive surgeons now recommend laparoscopic repair for the majority of their patients because it is associated with less postoperative pain, fewer postoperative restrictions on activity, and earlier return to work. There are three different methods of laparoscopic repair: the transabdominal preperitoneal (TAPP) repair, the total extraperitoneal (TEP) repair, and the intraperitoneal onlay mesh (IPOM) repair. All three procedures involve placement of a mesh patch over the deep inguinal ring and the floor of the inguinal canal.

1. TAPP repair: The peritoneal cavity is entered in the standard fashion with a periumbilical camera port followed by placement of 5-mm ports lateral to the rectus sheath, also at the level of the umbilicus. The peritoneum on the posterior surface of the anterior abdominal wall is incised transversely well above the level of the hernia and then reflected inferiorly. This flap exposes the preperitoneal space, allowing identification of the hernia defect, epigastric vessels, the pubic tubercle, Cooper's ligament, and the iliopubic tract (Fig. 8.16). Indirect hernias are mobilized and dissected away from the cord structures if possible, although a large sac may need to be divided. Direct hernias are isolated from the transversalis fascia. Following this, a mesh patch is placed to reinforce the pelvic floor and fixed to Cooper's ligament, the pubic tubercle, the posterior rectus, and the transverses abdominis with tacks. When performing a TAPP repair, it is critical to resecure the peritoneal flap to the abdominal wall after placement of the mesh. This not only protects the mesh from the intra-abdominal contents but also prevents potential bowel migration into the flap and subsequent bowel obstruction.
2. TEP repair: A periumbilical incision is used, and the anterior rectus sheath is incised on the side opposite the hernia (or opposite the larger hernia, if bilateral). Reflecting the rectus muscle laterally, a dissecting balloon is placed into the preperitoneal space, between the muscle and the posterior sheath (Fig. 8.17). Insufflation of the balloon opens and defines the preperitoneal space for the camera, and 5-mm working trocars are placed either in the midline, inferior to the camera port, or laterally. The remainder of the TEP repair proceeds exactly as described above in the TAPP repair, but peritoneal closure is not necessary.

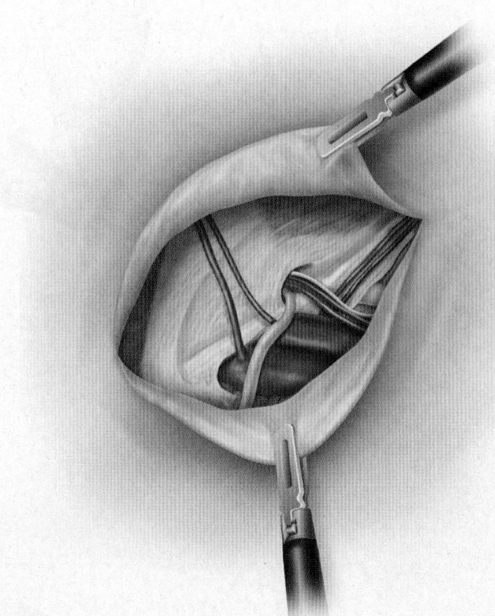

FIGURE 8.16 Access to the preperitoneal space for the TAPP repair—creation of the peritoneal flap. (From Jones D, ed. *Master Techniques in Surgery: Hernia*. Philadelphia: Wolters Kluwer Health; 2013.)

3. IPOM repair: Laparoscopic entry into the peritoneal cavity is achieved in a similar fashion to the TAPP repair. In the simplified IPOM repair, however, there is no peritoneal flap raised. Instead, the mesh is fixed directly to the peritoneum. Due to the inability to tack mesh posterior to the iliopubic tract and no peritoneal flap to cover the mesh in this area, there is a risk of bowel herniation under the mesh; therefore, the IPOM repair has largely been abandoned in inguinal hernia repair.

Complications of Groin Hernia Repair

As with any operation, there is a risk of bleeding and infection. If the hernia contains ischemic bowel requiring bowel resection, the risk of infection is increased. Infection in the setting of mesh repair may require removal of the mesh. Therefore, a hernia repair in the setting of a bowel resection should be done primarily or with biologic mesh that carries a lower risk of infection.

Additional complications unique to groin hernia repair include testicular atrophy, neuralgia, and recurrence. Testicular atrophy occurs as a consequence of ischemic orchitis, which may occur secondary to thrombosis of the delicate veins of the pampiniform plexus due to traumatic handling of the spermatic cord during dissection or may occur secondary to venous outflow obstruction due to creation of a tight internal ring. Primary arterial ischemia to the testicle is much more rare because of the rich blood supply to the testicle (the testicular artery from the aorta, the artery of the ductus deferens from the superior vesical artery, and the cremasteric artery from the inferior epigastric artery). Clinical manifestations often become apparent 2 to 5 days following the repair and most commonly present as marked testicular swelling associated with scrotal and testicular pain rather than incisional pain. The process lasts 6 to 12 weeks, resulting in either complete resolution or testicular atrophy. Doppler flow studies or a nuclear medicine flow scan can be used to establish a diagnosis. Care is supportive pain management.

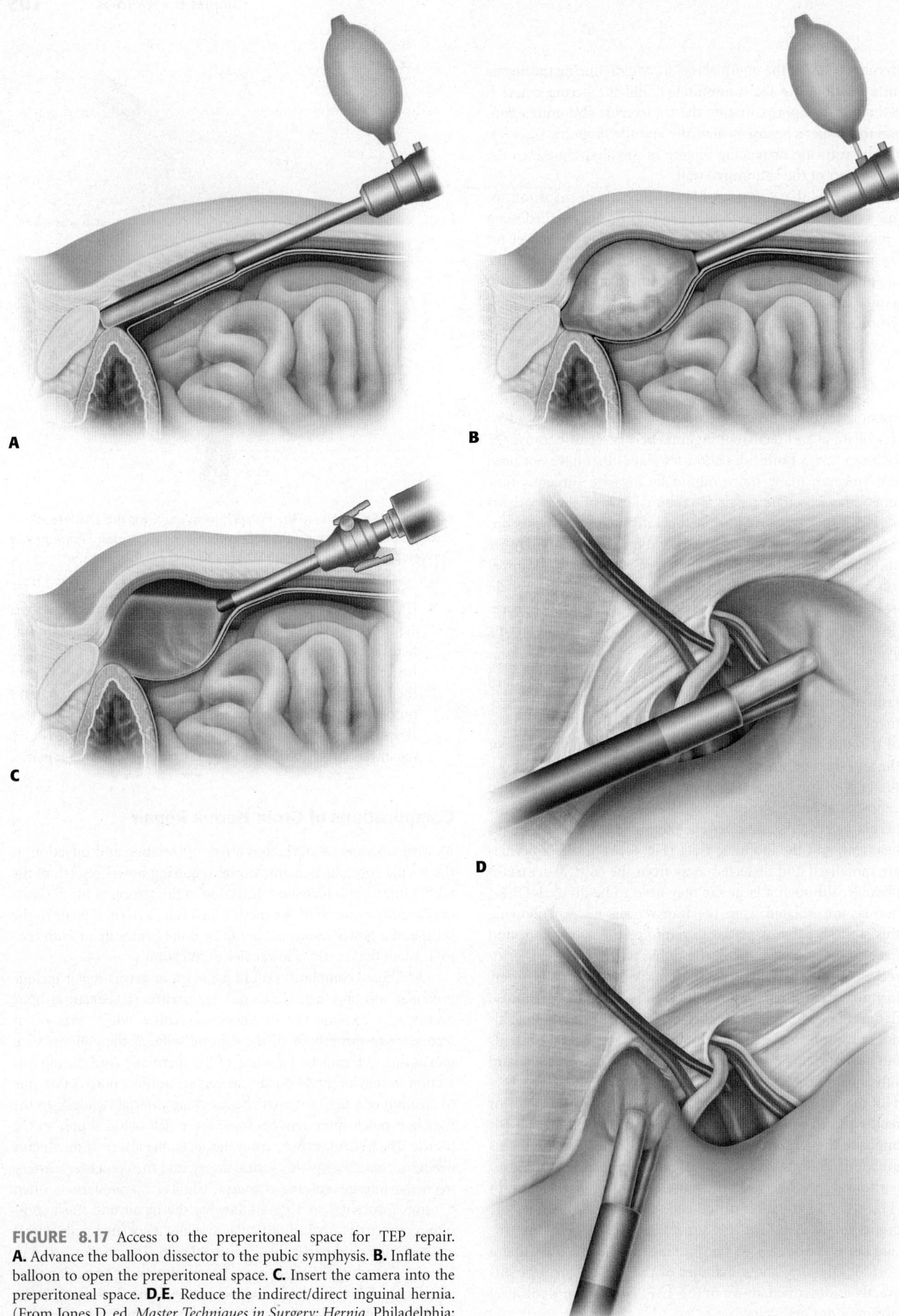

FIGURE 8.17 Access to the preperitoneal space for TEP repair. **A.** Advance the balloon dissector to the pubic symphysis. **B.** Inflate the balloon to open the preperitoneal space. **C.** Insert the camera into the preperitoneal space. **D,E.** Reduce the indirect/direct inguinal hernia. (From Jones D, ed. *Master Techniques in Surgery: Hernia*. Philadelphia: Wolters Kluwer Health; 2013.)

Orchiectomy is indicated only for intractable pain or lack of blood flow to the testicle. Rarely, antibodies may develop in the atrophic testicle, which may be associated with an increased risk of infertility and is another indication for orchiectomy.

Neuralgia may result from surgical trauma to the sensory nerves in the groin or secondary to nearby inflammatory and fibrotic responses. Neuroma is a special case of residual neuralgia, which results from a proliferation of nerve fibers outside the neurilemma of a partially or completely divided nerve. Pain associated with a neuroma is variable and may present as a burning pain at the incision with intermittent shooting pain that radiates into the scrotum with or without skin hypersensitivity. Management of postherniorrhaphy neuralgia is difficult and may involve analgesics, antidepressants, anxiolytics, transcutaneous electrical stimulation, and steroid injections. Ilioinguinal and iliohypogastric nerve blocks, or in the case of the genitofemoral nerve, a paravertebral block at L-1 and L-2 can be both therapeutic and diagnostic. Surgical treatment is reserved for those cases that cannot be managed with oral pain medications and have been shown to get relief with local anesthetic blocks. Surgery traditionally involved excision of the mesh and triple neurectomy. However, recently a less invasive approach of selective/directed neurectomy, which only excises the ilioinguinal nerve or the nerve that has been identified with a dyed nerve block, has been shown to be equally effective.

Laparoscopic groin hernia repair shares the same risks associated with all laparoscopic procedures including injury to surrounding structures during port placement (i.e., major and minor blood vessels, bowel, and bladder), port site hernia, gas embolism, and bowel obstruction secondary to adhesions in the TAPP and IPOM repairs that enter the peritoneum. Recurrent hernias with previously placed preperitoneal mesh or previous pelvic or preperitoneal surgery can make preperitoneal dissection in the scarred plane difficult. Additionally, laparoscopic inguinal hernia repair requires general anesthesia, so patients at high risk for general anesthesia should undergo an open repair that can be performed under local anesthesia. Finally, although certain nerve injuries (e.g., ilioinguinal) are much less common with laparoscopic repair, inadvertent tacks placed posterior to the iliopubic tract, lateral to the cord, in the triangle of pain (Fig. 8.18), can lead to nerve injuries, rarely, if ever seen, following open repair (e.g., lateral femoral cutaneous and genitofemoral nerves). Similarly, while injuries to the femoral vessels are less common in laparoscopic repair, injuries to the iliac vessels can occur when dissection or tack placement occurs in the triangle of doom (Fig. 8.18).

ANTERIOR ABDOMINAL WALL HERNIAS

Umbilical hernias are commonly congenital in origin but may be acquired in adults. The umbilicus is a site of potential weakness where the round ligament, urachus, and obliterated umbilical arteries converge. In the pediatric population, they rarely

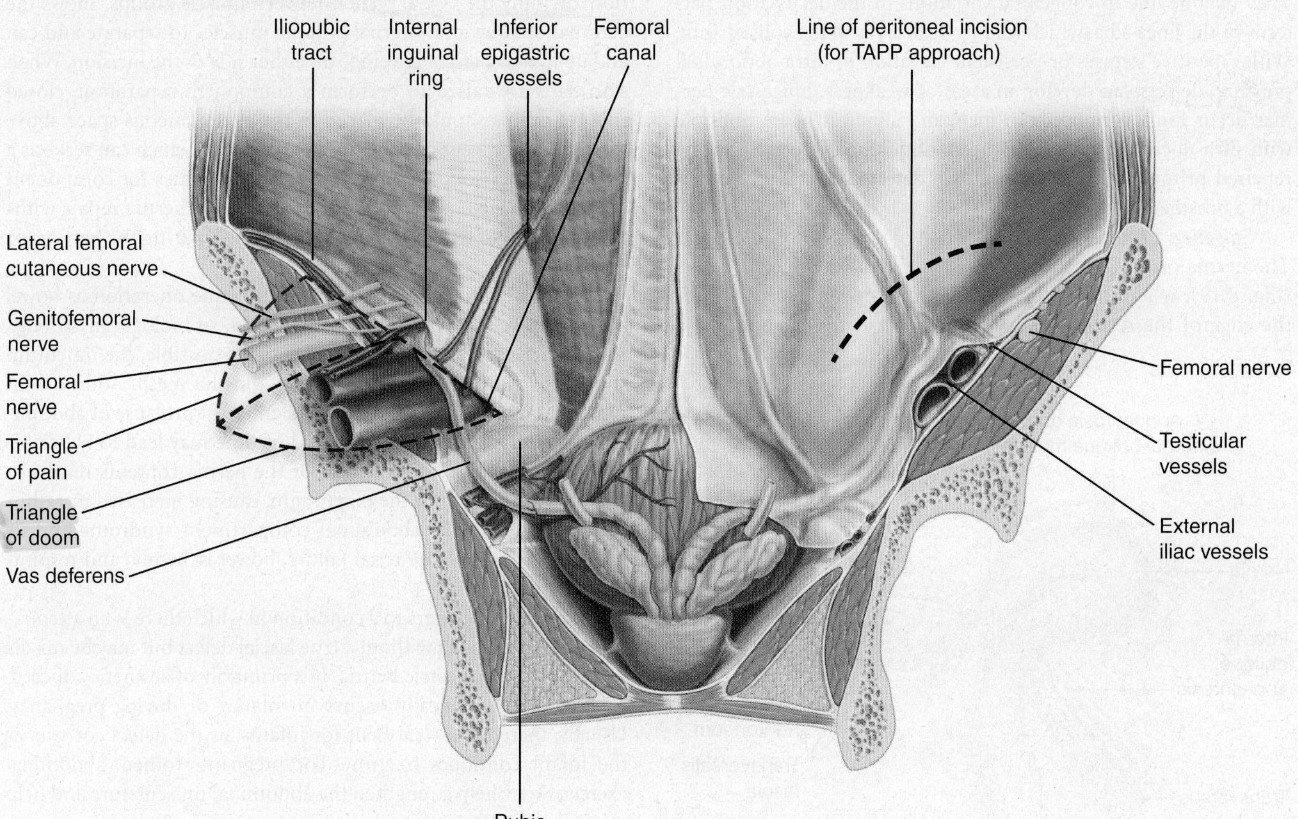

FIGURE 8.18 The triangle of doom, containing the iliac vessels, is bounded superiorly by the internal ring, medially by the vas deferens, and laterally by the spermatic vessels. The triangle of pain, containing the lateral femoral cutaneous and genitofemoral nerves, is bordered by the iliopubic tract superiorly and the spermatic vessels medially. (Jones D, ed. *Master Techniques in Surgery: Hernia*. Philadelphia: Wolters Kluwer Health; 2013.)

present with incarceration or strangulation and most spontaneously close within the first 2 to 3 years of life. Therefore, surgical repair is deferred until at least the age of 2 (some advocate waiting until age 4 to 5) unless there is abdominal pain referable to the hernia, incarceration, skin maceration, or a very large hernia. Pediatric hernias that necessitate surgical repair can be closed primarily. In adults, umbilical hernias occur secondary to conditions leading to increased intra-abdominal pressure and straining and do not spontaneously regress. The repair is performed by making a periumbilical curvilinear incision and identifying the hernia sac, the fascial defect, and the intact surrounding fascia. The hernia and its contents are reduced or excised, and the fascial edges are reapproximated primarily for small defects (<1 cm) or brought together using a piece of mesh to reinforce the repair and relieve tension on the fascia. The mesh can be placed as an underlay with the fascia closed over the top, as an overlay with the fascia closed beneath, or as a bridging piece if the defect is large and the fascia will not come together without tension. Cirrhotic patients with ascites are a population that is particularly at risk for developing hernias and are at higher risk for incarceration and strangulation as well as a higher risk of perioperative morbidity and mortality. If the hernia is filled with ascites alone, repair can be performed electively. However, if the hernia is not reducible and shows evidence of strangulation, repair needs to be done emergently.

Epigastric hernias occur in the linea alba above the umbilicus. They may be due to congenital variations in the decussation patterns of the linea alba, which lead to weak areas in the epigastrium. With repetitive stresses or persistent elevation in intra-abdominal pressure, defects can develop in areas of weakness. Epigastric hernias occur more commonly in men, and about 20% are multiple with 80% located slightly off the midline. Small defects can be repaired primarily. Larger or multiple defects may require repair with a prosthetic mesh.

Spigelian hernias are hernias of the lateral abdominal wall. The hernia protrudes through a weakness in the spigelian fascia (Fig. 8.19), where the transversus abdominis aponeurosis joins the edge of the rectus sheath forming the semilunar line. Most

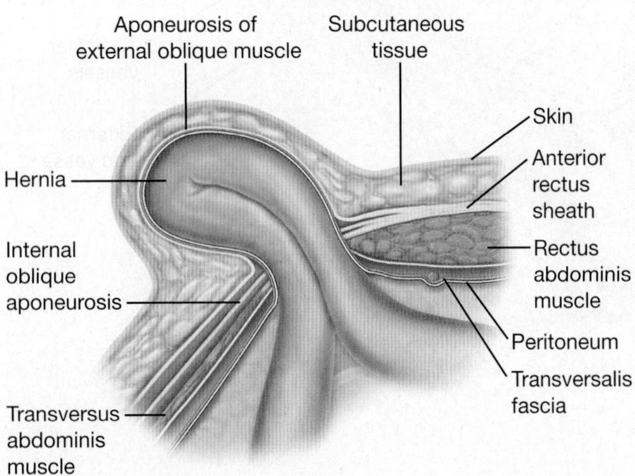

FIGURE 8.19 A spigelian hernia protrudes through the linea semilunaris. (From Jones D, ed. *Master Techniques in Surgery: Hernia.* Philadelphia: Wolters Kluwer Health; 2013.)

of these occur where the spigelian fascia crosses the arcuate line in the lower abdomen. Depending on body habitus and size of hernia, these hernias can be difficult to diagnose by physical examination alone. Given the high likelihood of incarceration or strangulation of a spigelian hernia, repair is indicated when identified.

Incisional hernias develop at the site of a previous surgical incision in the abdominal wall. These most commonly involve vertical midline incisions of the anterior abdominal wall but may also occur from incisions in the lumbar and perineal regions. Incidence varies from 0.5% to 13.9% of patients undergoing abdominal surgery. Factors contributing to the development of incisional hernias include poor technique, poor postoperative wound healing, wound infection, use of steroids, obesity, increased intra-abdominal pressure, and nutritional depletion.

Smaller hernias can be closed primarily, while larger hernias may require relaxing incisions along the lateral aspects of the anterior rectus sheath to enable approximation of the medial edges of the anterior rectus sheath and/or require prosthetic polypropylene or polytetrafluoroethylene (PTFE) mesh repair. The mesh should be secured using nonabsorbable monofilament sutures and have significant overlap with the fascia (4 to 8 cm). The recurrence rate for incisional hernias is 30% to 50%. With mesh repair, the recurrence rate is as low as 10%.

Very large defects that cannot be brought together without tension may require component separation. Component separation, dividing the fascial planes between muscle groups, allows the external oblique and internal oblique muscles to separate and can add up to 3 to 4 cm of coverage on either side of the incision. When skin flaps are raised to perform a component separation, closed suction drains should be placed in the subcutaneous space above the mesh to prevent postoperative collections, which can serve as a nidus for infection. Newer endoscopic techniques for component separation have been described to allow open hernia repair without the need for extensive lateral dissection, sparing the perforator vessels.

When a hernia repair is done at the same operation as bowel surgery, there is a higher risk of infection, so biologic mesh (e.g., AlloDerm) should be used, and, whenever possible, the omentum should be placed between the bowel and the mesh. Additionally, repair of larger hernias that exhibit significant prolapse of abdominal contents for an extended period of time may lead to (1) respiratory compromise as reduction of the hernia contents results in superior dislocation of the diaphragm, causing increased intrathoracic pressure or (2) abdominal compartment syndrome and its manifestations as acute renal failure, bowel ischemia, and respiratory failure.

Diastasis recti refers to a condition in which there is an attenuation of the linea alba without a true fascial defect but may be misdiagnosed as an epigastric hernia. It is primarily of aesthetic concern. This condition typically occurs in infancy or during pregnancy. Usually, there is no treatment for infants, as the defect corrects as the infant continues to grow. For pregnant women, abdominal exercises may help strengthen the abdominal musculature and help minimize the attenuation.

Laparoscopic Repair

All types of ventral hernias can be considered for laparoscopic repair. Entrance into the abdomen can be achieved via open or

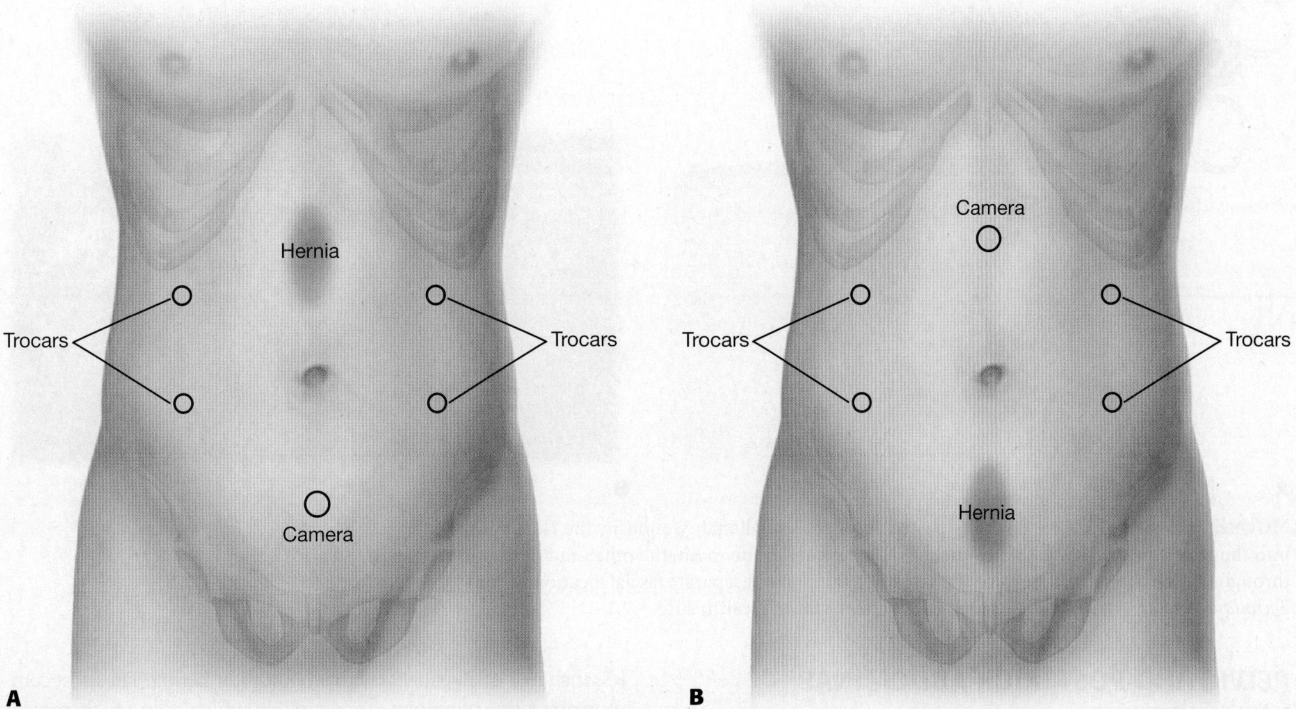

FIGURE 8.20 Trocar placement for laparoscopic ventral hernia repair. (From Jones D, ed. *Master Techniques in Surgery: Hernia*. Philadelphia: Wolters Kluwer Health; 2013.)

closed technique, depending on the surgical history and experience of the surgeon. Port placement varies depending on hernia location and presence of adhesions. Several 5- and 10-mm working trocars are placed under direct vision on either side of the abdomen (Fig. 8.20). Adhesions and the hernia sac are carefully dissected away from the abdominal wall. On completion of the adhesiolysis, the fascial defect can usually be easily and safely visualized (Fig. 8.21). A piece of mesh is chosen and cut down to a size that will cover the defect with significant overlap onto the abdominal wall fascia. The coated side of the mesh, which will face the intra-abdominal contents, can be composed of PTFE, collagen,

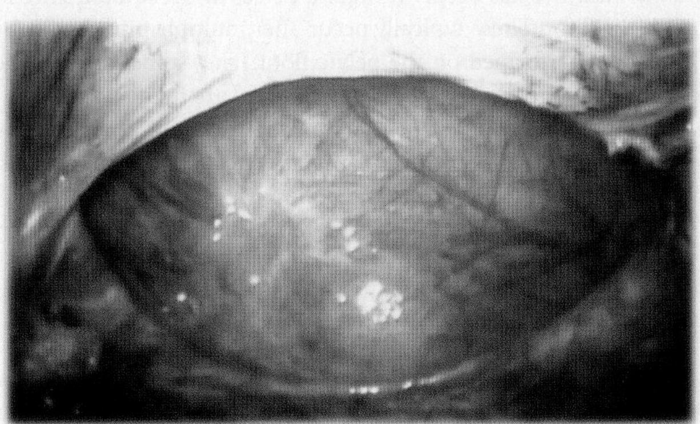

FIGURE 8.21 Laparoscopic view of large fascial defect. (From Jones D, ed. *Master Techniques in Surgery: Hernia*. Philadelphia: Wolters Kluwer Health; 2013.)

cellulose, or some form of biologic or composite material. A combination of stay sutures (at 3, 6, 9, and 12 o'clock) and tacks (spaced in between) are used to secure the mesh at 1-cm intervals circumferentially, with 3 to 5 cm overlap with healthy fascia surrounding the defect (Fig. 8.22).

Advantages

Laparoscopic ventral hernia repair does not require any extensive flap dissection, and thus there is a lower incidence of postoperative soft tissue infections. Additionally, laparoscopy also allows visualization of the entire abdominal wall and the discovery of additional previously unrecognized fascial defects, which can then be covered with mesh. Finally, as with other laparoscopic procedures, recovery time is shorter, with studies showing decreased lengths of hospital stay and shorter duration of time out of work.

Disadvantages

As with any laparoscopic procedure, there is a risk of enterotomy during port placement and adhesiolysis, especially in patients who have had extensive previous abdominal surgeries. Unrecognized enterotomy can be catastrophic. Additionally, both tacks and transfascial sutures can cause chronic pain symptoms. Finally, laparoscopic ventral hernia repairs are also commonly associated with seroma formation, which may require percutaneous drainage or excision of the mesh if it becomes infected.

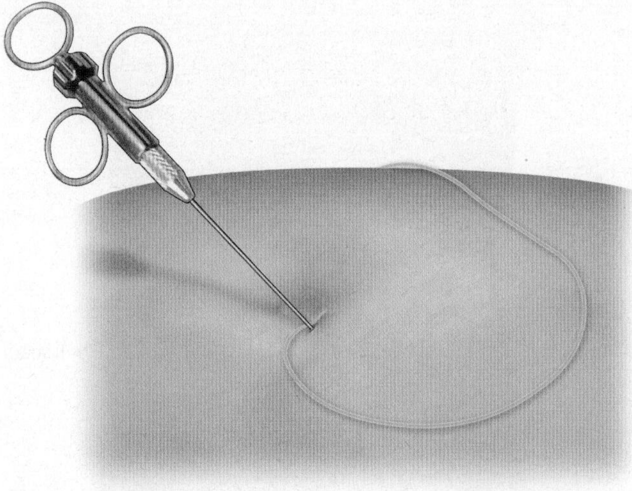

A

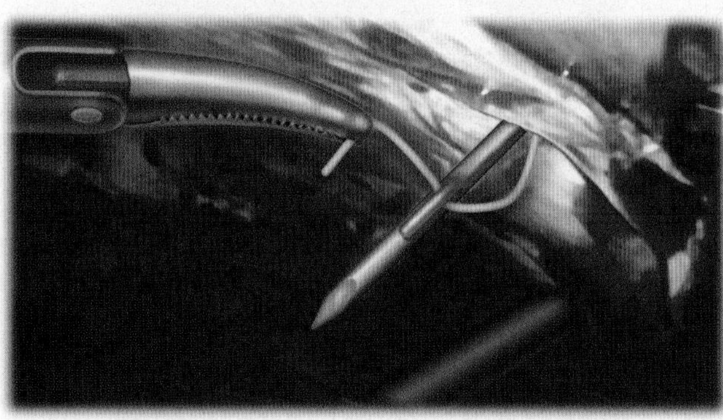

B

FIGURE 8.22 (*A*) A suture passer is passed through a small stab wound in the skin, through the fascia, and into the abdominal cavity. (*B*) After anchoring the suture to the mesh, the other end of the suture is passed back through the abdominal wall through the same skin incision but separate fascial location. (From Jones D, ed. *Master Techniques in Surgery: Hernia*. Philadelphia: Wolters Kluwer Health; 2013.)

PELVIC AND POSTERIOR ABDOMINAL WALL HERNIAS

Pelvic hernias comprise a rare group that occurs as protrusions through muscles that make up the pelvic floor, including *obturator* hernias, *sciatic* hernias, and *perineal* hernias.

Obturator hernias are defects that occur through the obturator canal, which course along the tract taken by the obturator neurovascular bundle as it exits the pelvis (Fig. 8.23). These present primarily in elderly women and are associated with radicular pain extending down the medial thigh with abduction or internal rotation of the thigh. This is known as the classic *Howship–Romberg* sign, though it is present in less than half of all patients with an obturator hernia. The most common presenting symptoms are crampy abdominal pain and those associated with small bowel obstruction. On physical examination, a mass may be felt on vaginal or rectal examination. Given the high mortality associated with an obturator hernia, accurate diagnosis and prompt treatment is critical. Obturator hernias are repaired via a transabdominal approach. Any nonviable bowel is resected, and the hernia sac is excised. An attempt is made to close the fascial defect primarily, but a prosthetic patch may be used if primary closure is under tension or felt to be inadequate. Recurrences are rare following an appropriate repair.

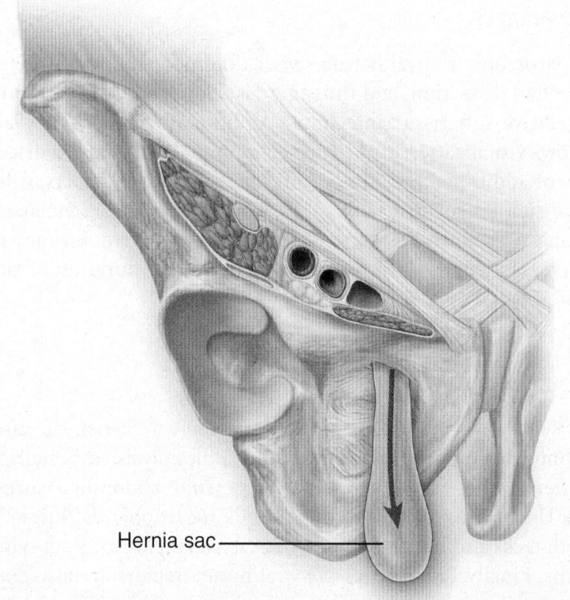

FIGURE 8.23 An obturator hernia protrudes through the obturator canal. (From Jones D, ed. *Master Techniques in Surgery: Hernia*. Philadelphia: Wolters Kluwer Health; 2013.)

Sciatic hernias are defects that occur through the greater or lesser sciatic foramina. Patients present with a gradually enlarging mass in the infragluteal region. Sciatic nerve compression may result along with symptoms of bowel obstruction and ischemia. A CT scan or an ultrasound may be necessary to definitively establish the diagnosis. Sciatic hernias can be repaired through either the transabdominal or transgluteal approach, with the transabdominal approach preferred when signs of bowel obstruction or strangulation are present. As with obturator hernias, a prosthetic mesh patch may be needed to facilitate the repair.

Perineal hernias occur through a defect in the levator sling in the pelvic floor. These typically occur after multiple pregnancies or operations performed on the pelvic floor. They appear as a bulge just lateral to the midline perineal raphe and are frequently asymptomatic and reducible. Depending on their location, they may be associated with pain on sitting or a variety of urinary complaints, most commonly dysuria. Strangulation or incarceration is rare. Diagnosis can be confirmed by a detailed history and a thorough physical examination, paying particular attention to the vaginal and rectal examinations. These hernias may be repaired via a transabdominal approach with or without prosthetic material.

LUMBAR HERNIAS

Lumbar hernias arise through the posterior abdominal wall either spontaneously or from previous surgical incisions (eg: nephrectomy). Spontaneous lumbar hernias usually occur at one of two sites. The superior lumbar triangle, also called Grynfeltt triangle, is the most

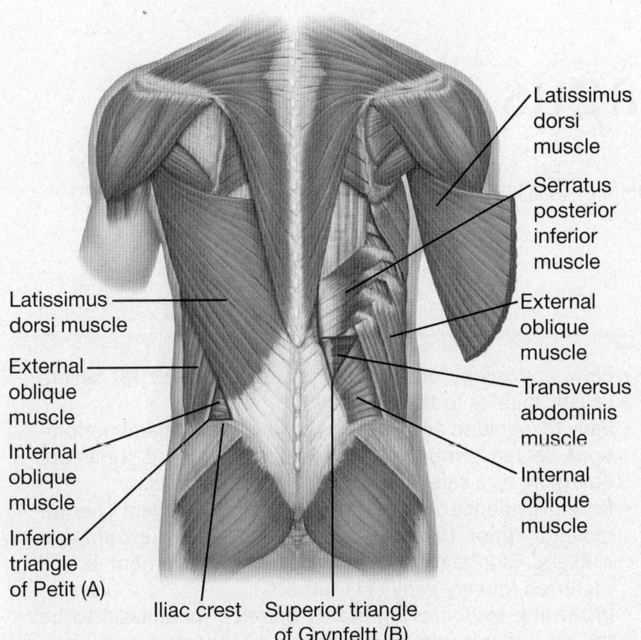

FIGURE 8.24 A hernia in the lumbar region can occur through the (*A*) inferior lumbar triangle or the (*B*) superior lumbar triangle. (From Jones D, ed. *Master Techniques in Surgery: Hernia*. Philadelphia: Wolters Kluwer Health; 2013.)

common. The inferior lumbar triangle, also called Petit triangle, is less commonly involved (Fig. 8.24). These hernias present most commonly as a mass in the flank that may or may not be associated with pain. Lumbar hernias progress in size over time and have a 10% incidence of incarceration and strangulation. They may be repaired primarily or with mesh but are associated with a high incidence of recurrence. When a lumbar hernia occurs as a result of trauma, mostly surgical, a true fascial defect should be confirmed rather than a diastasis from denervation and weakness of the lateral abdominal wall.

Suggested Readings

Cameron JL, Cameron AM. *Curr Surg Ther*. 11th ed. Philadelphia: Saunders; 2014.

Chung L, Norrie J, O'Dwyer PJ. Long-term follow-up of patients with a painless inguinal hernia from a randomized clinical trial. *Br J Surg*. 2011;98:596–599.

Dittrick GW, Ridl K, Kuhn JA, et al. Routine ilioinguinal nerve excision in inguinal hernia repair. *Am J Surg*. 2004;188:736–740.

Fischer JE, Jones DB, Pomposelli FB, et al., eds. *Fischer's Mastery of Surgery 6E*. Philadelphia: Lippincott Williams & Wilkins; 2011.

Fitzgibbons RJ Jr, Giobbie-Hurder A, Gibbs JO, et al. Watchful waiting vs repair of inguinal hernia in minimally symptomatic men: a randomized clinical trial. *JAMA* 2006;295:285–292.

Fitzgibbons RJ, Greenburg AG, eds. *Nyhus and Condon's Hernia*. Philadelphia: Lippincott Williams & Wilkins; 2002.

Fitzgibbons RJ, Ramanan B, Arya S, et al. Long-term results of a randomized controlled trial of a nonoperative strategy (watchful waiting) for men with minimally symptomatic inguinal hernias. *Ann Surg*. 2013;258(3):508.

Jacob, BP, Ramshaw B. *The SAGES Manual of Hernia Repair*. New York: Springer; 2013.

Jones D. *Master Techniques in Surgery: Hernia*. Philadelphia: Lippincott Williams & Wilkins; 2012.

Mui WL, Ng CS, Fung TM, et al. Prophylactic ilioinguinal neurectomy in open inguinal hernia repair: a double-blind randomized controlled trial. *Ann Surg*. 2006;244:27–33.

Mulholland MW, Lillemoe KD, Doherty GM, et al., eds. *Greenfield's Surgery: Scientific Principles and Practice*. 5th ed. Philadelphia: Lippincott Williams & Wilkins; 2011.

O'Dwyer PJ, Norrie J, Alani A, et al. Observation or operation for patients with an asymptomatic inguinal hernia: a randomized clinical trial. *Ann Surg* 2006;244:167–117.

Scientific American Surgery. New York: Decker Intellectual Properties, Inc. 2014. Available at: http://www.ACSSurgery.com

Townsend CM, Beauchamp RD, Evers BM, et al., eds. *Sabiston Textbook of Surgery*. 19th ed. Philadelphia: WB Saunders; 2012.

CHAPTER

9

The Esophagus

ANDREW J. SINNAMON AND JOHN C. KUCHARCZUK

KEY POINTS

- An extensive submucosal lymphatic network and the absence of a serosa contribute to early and distant lymph node metastasis in esophageal cancer.
- Laparoscopic Heller esophagocardiomyotomy with partial fundoplication is the procedure of choice for achalasia.
- Many esophageal motility disorders present with chest pain; a synchronous cardiac cause must always be excluded.
- Surgical treatment for a pulsion diverticulum of the esophagus must consist of esophagomyotomy to address the concomitant dysmotility causing elevated intraluminal pressure.
- Early endoscopy and antibiotics are indicated for severe caustic injuries to the esophagus.
- Early recognition and primary repair of esophageal perforations decrease mortality. Endoscopically placed stents are emerging as a safe alternative in select patients.
- Recent evidence supports the use of neoadjuvant chemoradiation prior to esophagectomy for many esophageal cancers. Esophagectomy as primary management is still preferred for very early (T1) tumors.
- Increasing evidence implicates Barrett's metaplasia to be the precursor lesion to esophageal adenocarcinoma.
- The sole blood supply for the gastric conduit following esophagectomy is the right gastroepiploic artery.

ANATOMY

The esophagus develops from the embryonic foregut between the 4th and 5th weeks of gestation. Similar to other segments of the gastrointestinal tract, the esophagus is a tube composed of mucosa, muscularis mucosa, submucosa, and an inner circular and outer longitudinal muscularis layer. However, in contradistinction to the rest of the alimentary tract, the esophagus lacks a true serosal layer, which is a contributing factor for direct extension of esophageal carcinoma to nearby structures.

The esophagus can be divided into three anatomic regions—cervical, intrathoracic, and intra-abdominal—and the surgical incisions to approach each region are generally selected on this basis. The cervical esophagus begins in the distal oropharynx at the level of the cricopharyngeus, which is the first constriction seen on endoscopy approximately 15 cm from the incisors. The cervical esophagus continues for about 5 cm to the thoracic inlet at the level of T1. The striated muscles of the proximal esophagus are located just inferior to the cricopharyngeus muscle, which is a continuation of the inferior pharyngeal constrictor. This region has clinical significance, because the junction of the cricopharyngeus and thyropharyngeus fibers in the inferior oropharynx is an area of potential weakness known as Killian triangle. This is the area in which Zenker diverticulum occurs, and it is also the most common site of iatrogenic perforation during esophageal instrumentation. The cervical esophagus lies slightly to the left of the midline, allowing for adequate access via a left cervical incision, but it may also be approached from the right neck as the situation indicates.

The thoracic esophagus begins at the thoracic inlet, just to the right of midline, in proximity to the brachiocephalic vessels. The membranous trachea abuts the upper thoracic esophagus, and, as a result, esophageal tumors can compress, invade, or fistulize to the trachea. The thoracic esophagus beyond the tracheal bifurcation (about 25 cm endoscopically) has a trajectory anterior and to the left of the descending thoracic aorta. In general, a right thoracotomy provides the ideal exposure for surgery of the thoracic esophagus. The distal esophagus (beyond 35 cm endoscopically) and gastroesophageal (GE) junction can be approached through a left thoracotomy or thoracoabdominal incision. (Figure 9.1 outlines the pertinent topography of the esophagus.) The thoracic duct

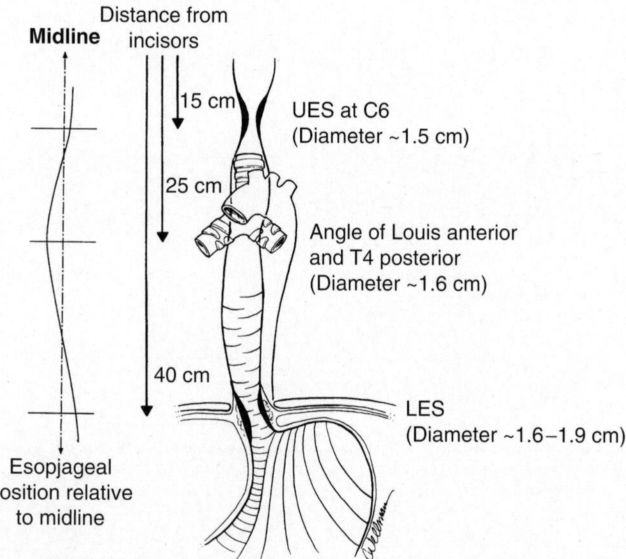

FIGURE 9.1 Topography of the esophagus with pertinent clinical endoscopic measurements in adults. (From Baker RJ, Fischer JE, eds. *Mastery of Surgery*. 4th ed. Philadelphia: Lippincott Williams & Wilkins; 2001:742, with permission.)

enters the chest to the right of the distal esophagus, crosses the midline at the level of T5 as it passes posterior to the aorta, and terminates near the junction of the internal jugular and left subclavian vein. This close relationship renders the thoracic duct vulnerable to injury during esophageal surgery.

The vascular supply of the esophagus is segmental. The cervical esophagus is supplied mainly by the inferior thyroid artery, a branch of the thyrocervical trunk. The thoracic portion of the esophagus receives its blood supply from the bronchial arteries and from arterial branches arising directly from the descending thoracic aorta. The remaining intra-abdominal portion of the esophagus receives its blood supply from the left gastric and inferior phrenic arteries. Venous drainage follows a similar segmental pattern. Importantly, the left gastric vein drains into the portal venous system, accounting for the formation of esophageal varices in patients with portal hypertension. (Figure 9.2 details the segmental arterial blood supply.)

Lymphatic drainage also occurs in a segmental fashion. The cervical esophagus drains into the internal jugular, paratracheal, and deep cervical lymph nodes. The midthoracic esophagus drains into the subcarinal and pulmonary ligament nodes. The lower one third of the esophagus drains into the periesophageal and celiac nodes. Because of the rich network of submucosal lymphatics in the esophagus, malignant tumors that penetrate into the submucosa tend to spread within the submucosa and to distant (>4 cm away) lymph nodes (key point: lymph node metastasis in esophageal cancer).

Esophageal motility is coordinated by both sympathetic and parasympathetic innervations. The left and right vagus nerves course along the esophagus, with the left vagus coursing anteriorly and the right vagus coursing posteriorly as they enter the abdomen. The vagus nerve and its recurrent laryngeal branches provide sympathetic innervation to the striated portion of the esophagus and the upper esophageal sphincter (UES) to coordinate the initiation

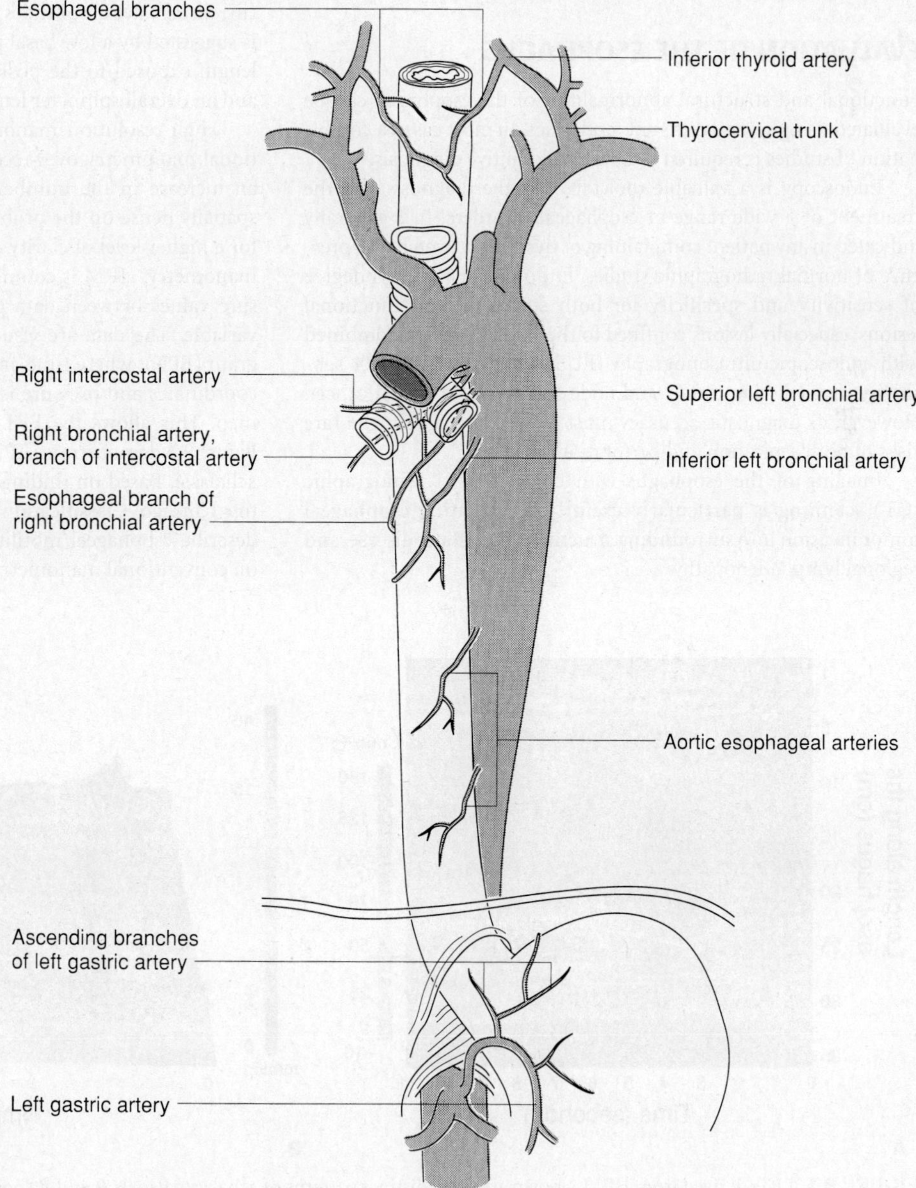

FIGURE 9.2 Arterial blood supply of the esophagus. (From Baker RJ, Fischer JE, eds. *Mastery of Surgery*. 4th ed. Philadelphia: Lippincott Williams & Wilkins; 2001:744, with permission.)

of esophageal peristalsis. These nerves are particularly vulnerable during mobilization of the cervical esophagus, and this can contribute to postoperative difficulties manifested mainly by aspiration. The remainder of the esophagus receives parasympathetic innervation from the vagus nerve and an intrinsic autonomic nerve plexus located in the submucosa of the esophageal wall.

ESOPHAGEAL PHYSIOLOGY

During the swallowing phase, as food enters the esophagus, the cricopharyngeus muscle (or UES) reaches twice its normal resting pressure of 30 mm Hg and initiates a primary peristaltic wave in the upper esophagus. Smooth muscle activation continues the peristaltic wave through the remainder of the esophagus, allowing food to overcome the pressure gradient of approximately 10 mm Hg from the chest into the abdomen. Further relaxation of the lower esophageal sphincter (LES) allows food to easily enter the stomach. Secondary peristaltic waves continue to clear the esophagus of food and refluxed gastric contents.

EVALUATION OF THE ESOPHAGUS

Functional and structural abnormalities of the esophagus can be evaluated using several different modalities. In most cases, a combination of studies is required to obtain a definitive diagnosis.

Endoscopy is a valuable tool for both the diagnosis and the treatment of a wide range of esophageal disorders. It is generally indicated in any patient complaining of dysphagia, even in the presence of normal radiographic studies. Endoscopy has a high degree of sensitivity and specificity for both structural and functional lesions, especially lesions confined to the mucosa. When combined with endoscopic ultrasonography (EUS), endoscopy has 90% sensitivity in predicting tumor and node status in esophageal cancer. However, its diagnostic accuracy must be weighed against the rare risks of both aspiration and perforation.

Imaging of the esophagus with computerized tomographic (CT) scanning is particularly useful for evaluating esophageal tumor invasion into surrounding structures, metastatic disease, and regional lymphadenopathy.

A barium swallow provides both structural and functional information. Aspiration can be documented by residual contrast in the larynx after swallowing. Esophageal peristalsis is seen with a stripping wave after a swallowed bolus of contrast. The addition of motion-recording techniques greatly facilitates the evaluation of function.

Esophageal manometry allows precise measurement of the contractility and resting pressures of various portions of the esophagus. The test is indicated in any patient with a suspected motor abnormality when barium swallow or endoscopy does not show a clear structural defect. A conventional manometric study consists of four parts: the assessment of the LES, measurement of LES relaxation, esophageal body manometry, and assessment of the UES. Manometry is most widely used in conjunction with pH monitoring in the diagnosis of GE reflux disease. A normal manometric test would include (i) a resting basal LES pressure of 10 to 45 mm Hg with complete relaxation during the average of 10 wet swallows (swallows performed with the administration of a small water bolus), (ii) peristaltic wave progression at a rate of 2 to 8 cm/s, and (iii) distal wave amplitudes of 30 to 180 mm Hg. An abnormal LES is suggested by a low basal pressure less than 6 mm Hg, an average length exposed to the positive-pressure abdomen less than 1 cm, and an overall sphincter length of less than 2 cm.

High-resolution manometry (HRM) has risen from conventional manometry over recent years, with the key difference being an increase in the number of pressure sensors. These are more spatially dense on the probe, in 1-cm intervals or less. This allows for a higher level of clarity and is more accurate than conventional manometry. HRM is commonly interpreted by interpolating pressure values between data points to create a continuous pressure variable. The data are visualized as an esophageal pressure topogram (EPT), where time and anatomic location are given X and Y coordinates and pressure is represented by color, such as in a heat map. This allows the EPT to provide three dimensions of data. Figure 9.3 demonstrates EPTs for patients with different subtypes of achalasia. Based on findings in normal and symptomatic patients, the Chicago Classification criteria have been defined to better describe esophageal motility disorders not previously identifiable on conventional manometry.

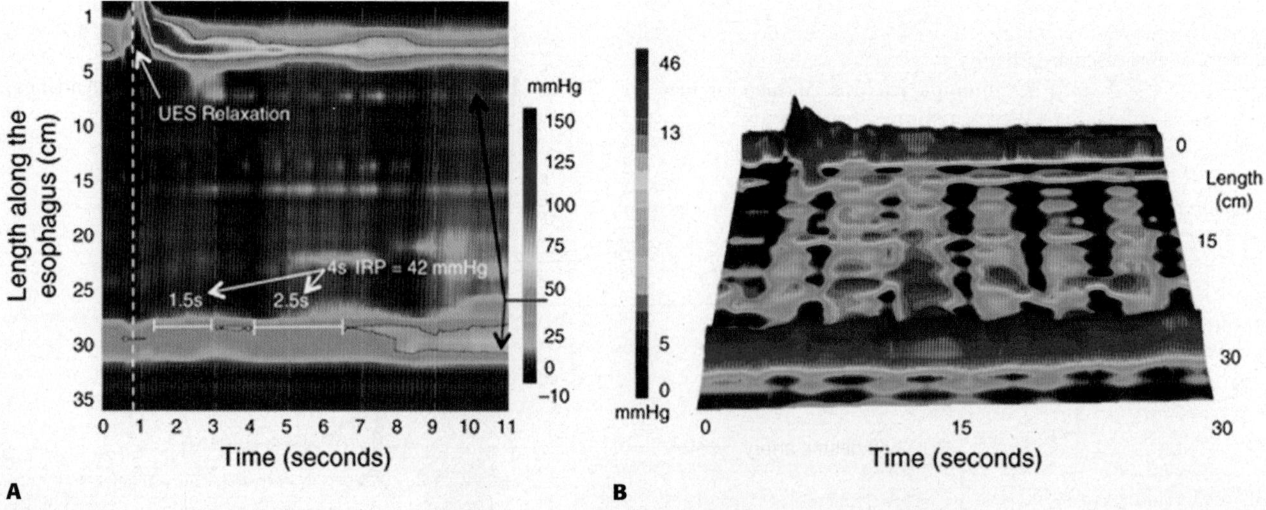

FIGURE 9.3 EPTs derived from HRM. Shown are three distinct patterns of achalasia. Panels **A** and **B** show classic achalasia;

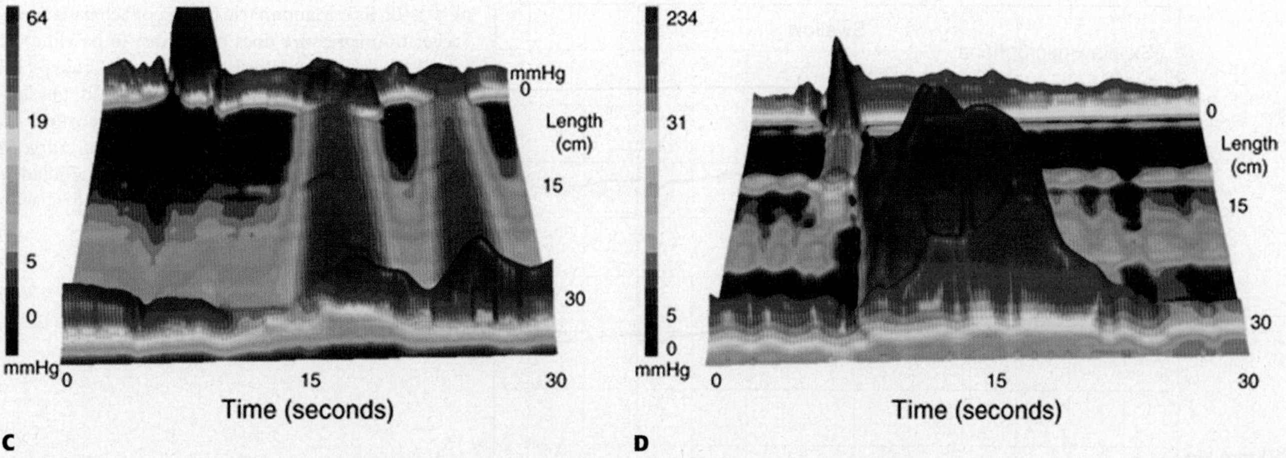

FIGURE 9.3 (*Continued*) panels **C** and **D** show achalasia subtypes with contraction of the esophageal body. (From Kahrilas PJ. *Esophageal motor disorders in terms of high-resolution esophageal pressure topography: what has changed? Am J Gastroenterol.* 2010;105:981–987, with permission.)

Twenty-four–hour pH monitoring is performed by placement of a pH probe 5 cm superior to the LES (as determined by manometry). Monitoring of pH is not a test for reflux but rather a measure of the severity and duration of esophageal acid exposure. It is also used to correlate the patient's symptoms with documented acid exposure, as the patient is instructed to keep a diary while the probe is in place. The test is indicated in patients with reflux-like symptoms, who have failed to respond to a 12-week course of acid suppression therapy, and in the preoperative evaluation in patients being considered for an antireflux procedure.

MOTILITY DISORDERS

An esophageal dysmotility evaluation is indicated in patients presenting with either dysphagia or chest pain when other primary cardiac or esophageal disorders (i.e., stricture, malignancy) are absent. There are four basic categories of primary motor disorders of the esophagus: inadequate relaxation of the LES (achalasia), uncoordinated contractions (diffuse esophageal spasm [DES]), hypercontraction (nutcracker esophagus and hypertensive LES), and hypocontraction (ineffective esophageal motility). Regardless of the type of disorder, the etiology of most primary motility disorders remains unknown. However, neuromuscular impairment resulting from cerebrovascular ischemia, myasthenia gravis, Parkinson's disease, motor neuron disease, multiple sclerosis, collagen vascular diseases, and polymyositis often complicates the clinical picture.

Achalasia is a rare disorder (1 per 100,000) and refers to the final stages of esophageal aperistalsis accompanied by failed relaxation of the LES. This results in a functional obstruction in the distal esophagus rendering the patient unable to eat normally. Loss of nitric oxide–producing inhibitory ganglion cells in the esophageal body and LES appears to be the mechanism behind achalasia, but the etiology of the disease is unknown and likely multifactorial. The diagnosis is typically made late in the course because of the gradual onset of symptoms and the ability of most patients to compensate for the impaired function of the LES. Patients eventually present with progressive dysphagia, chest pain, weight loss, and occasionally regurgitation. If regurgitation occurs, it is usually associated with meals and may be accompanied by respiratory symptoms resulting from aspiration. In addition, these patients can also suffer from pneumonitis, bronchiectasis, hemoptysis, or esophagitis. End-stage achalasia causes dilation of the esophagus resulting in an air–fluid level and a characteristic *bird's beak* appearance on barium esophagogram as shown in Figure 9.4. Manometric findings include incomplete relaxation of the LES to less than 8 mm Hg and

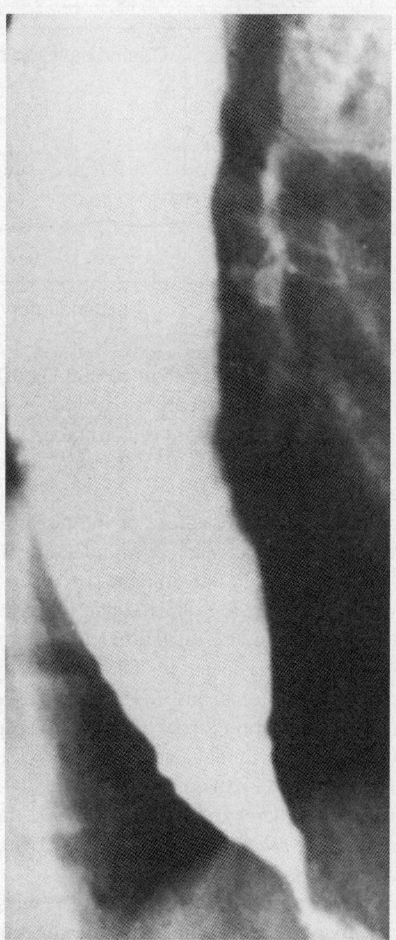

FIGURE 9.4 Barium esophagogram in a patient with achalasia demonstrating a persistent "bird's beak" taper at the GE junction. (From Bell RH, Rikkers LF, Mulholland MW. *Digestive Tract Surgery: A Text and Atlas.* Philadelphia: Lippincott–Raven Publishers; 1996:34, with permission.)

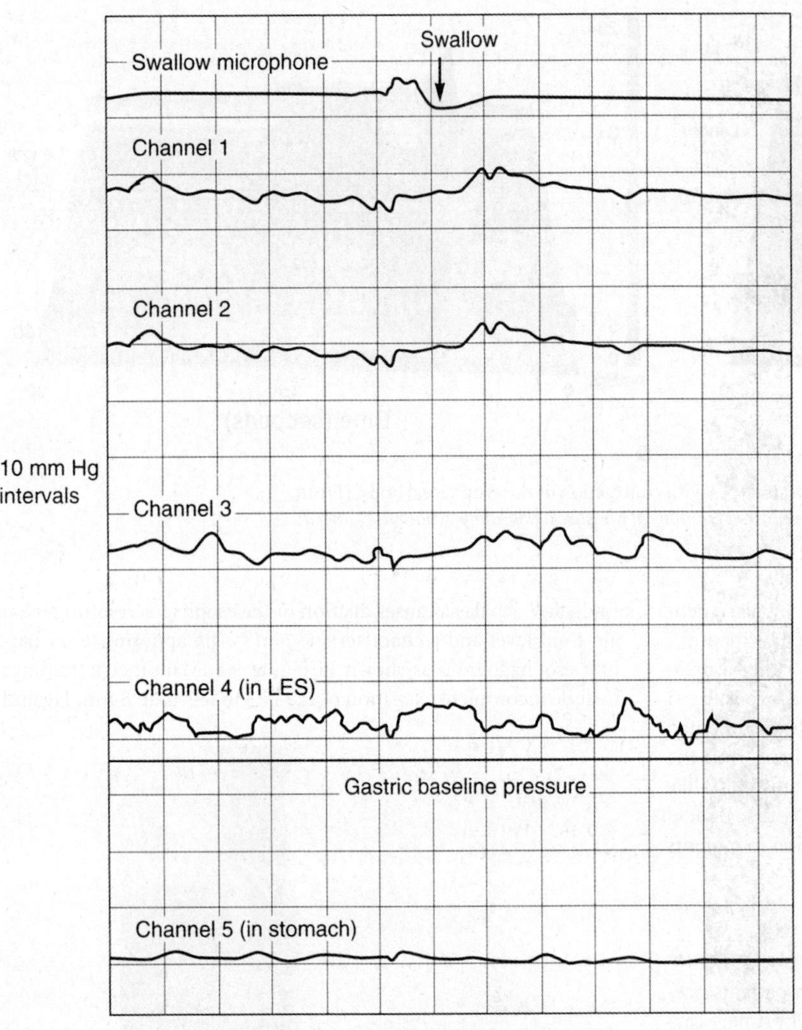

FIGURE 9.5 Manometric tracing of achalasia; nonrelaxation (pressure does not return to baseline) of the LES and absent peristalsis. (From Crookes PF, Demeester TR. Esophageal anatomy and physiology, and gastroesophageal reflux. In: Greenfield LJ, Mulholland M, Oldham KT, et al., eds. *Surgery: Scientific Principles and Practice*. 2nd ed. Philadelphia: Lippincott–Raven Publishers; 1997:676, with permission.)

low-amplitude contractions of less than 40 mm Hg of the esophageal body after swallowing or aperistalsis with so-called *mirror imaging* (Fig. 9.5). This condition is considered premalignant, with squamous cell carcinoma (SCC) occurring in 1% to 10% of patients over 15 to 25 years.

Because of the progressive nature of the disease and lack of effective medical therapies, all patients with documented achalasia should be evaluated for surgical treatment. Two major nonsurgical therapies are used in poor surgical candidates or when the diagnosis is in question—pneumatic dilatation and injection of botulinum toxin. With pneumatic dilatation, the vast majority of patients experience relief of symptoms, but it is frequently short lived. In addition, pneumatic dilatation carries a 5% risk of esophageal perforation. Botulinum toxin inhibits acetylcholine release from the excitatory neurons in the LES and can be injected endoscopically directly into the LES, thereby reducing its resting pressure. This results in symptomatic relief in the majority of patients, but again, this is temporary.

The most effective and durable method to reduce resting LES pressure in patients with achalasia and relieve the functional obstruction is surgical esophagomyotomy (Heller). The myotomy involves division of both the longitudinal and the circular muscle layers from 5 cm proximal and 2 cm distal to the GE junction without injury to the underlying mucosa. In most cases, myotomy can be performed using a laparoscopic approach. In the presence of a proximal motility disorders or progressive disease despite a laparoscopic myotomy, a right thoracoscopy or thoracotomy can be performed for a complete esophagocardiomyotomy (see Fig. 9.6). Alleviation of dysphagia, regurgitation, and chest pain can be expected in 80% to 90% of patients at 5 years. Since the Heller myotomy results in the obliteration of the majority of the antireflux mechanism of the LES, most surgeons combine the myotomy with a partial fundoplication.

Uncoordinated esophageal contraction is best characterized by DES. DES is primarily a disorder of the esophageal body, demonstrated by manometry with frequent simultaneous esophageal contractions of high amplitude (>30 mm Hg), with normal relaxation of the LES. The etiology of DES is unknown. Patients often present with angina-like chest pain or dysphagia and must always undergo cardiac evaluation prior to considering an esophageal cause. DES often resembles a "corkscrew" esophagus on barium esophagogram as shown in Figure 9.7. Treatment is usually conservative with the use of calcium channel blockers and long-acting nitrates to help attenuate the esophageal contractions. Surgery, usually a long esophagomyotomy, is recommended only for the most severe cases, when symptoms become refractory to conservative management (see Fig. 9.8).

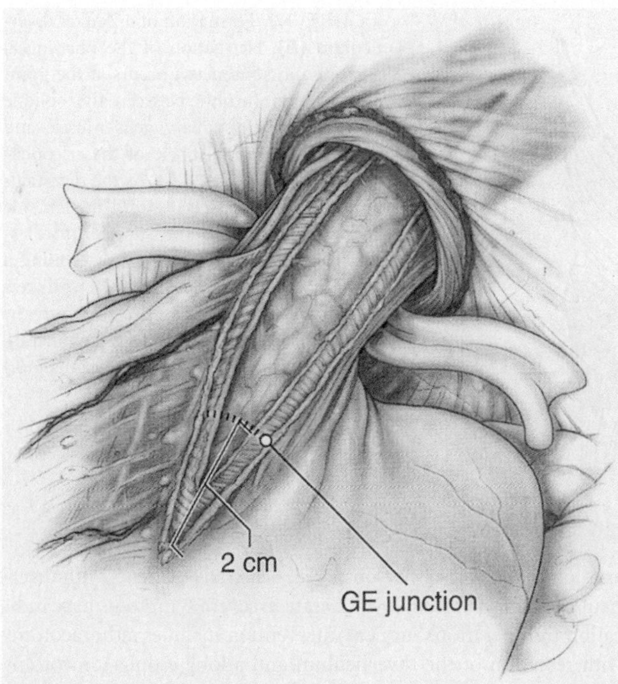

FIGURE 9.6 Heller esophagocardiomyotomy, revealing intact esophageal and gastric mucosa. (From Baker RJ, Fischer JE, eds. *Mastery of Surgery*. 4th ed. Philadelphia: Lippincott Williams & Wilkins; 2001:808, with permission.)

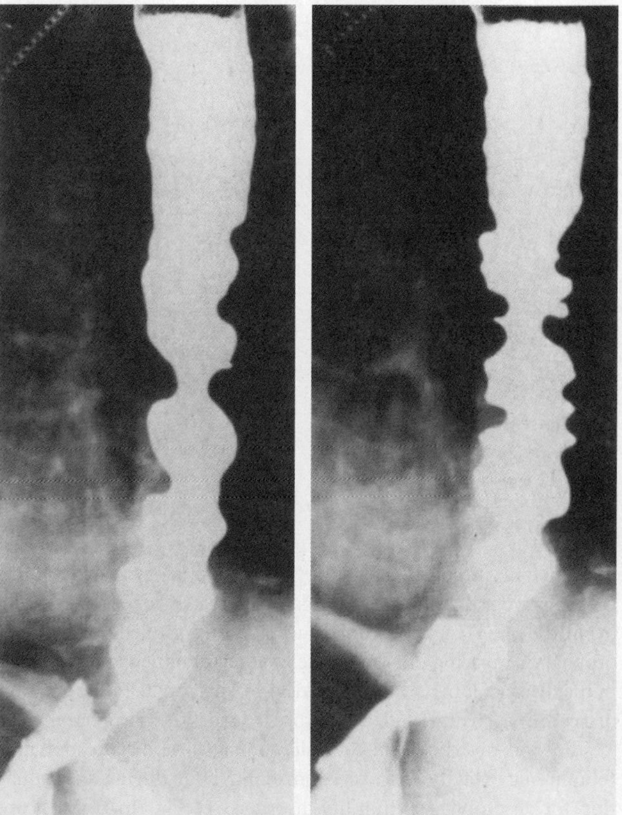

FIGURE 9.7 Barium esophagogram demonstrating tertiary contractions of the circular muscle "corkscrew" characteristic of DES. (From Bell RH, Rikkers LF, Mulholland MW. *Digestive Tract Surgery: A Text and Atlas*. Philadelphia: Lippincott–Raven Publishers; 1996:38, with permission.)

Esophageal hypercontraction or "nutcracker esophagus" is the most common motility disorder observed in patients with noncardiac chest pain. Manometric amplitudes of the esophageal body two standard deviations greater than normal (peaks >180 mm Hg) characterize this disorder. These peaks occur within the context of peristalsis, and this feature distinguishes nutcracker esophagus from DES. For this reason, dysphagia is uncommon. Similar to patients with DES, patients with esophageal hypercontraction often present with crushing chest pain occurring frequently at rest. Again, the mainstay of treatment is the conservative management with the use of calcium channel blockers and nitrates.

ESOPHAGEAL DIVERTICULA

Esophageal diverticula are mucosa-lined pouches that protrude outward from the esophageal lumen. *Pulsion diverticula* arise from elevated intraluminal pressures that force mucosa and submucosa through the muscular layer and are most commonly associated with dysmotility. *Traction diverticula* result from an adjacent inflammatory process (usually mediastinal granulomatous disease such as histoplasmosis or tuberculosis). Esophageal diverticula are often asymptomatic. A proximal diverticulum may produce dysphagia, halitosis, or aspiration. All esophageal diverticula can be associated with regurgitation of undigested food or recurrent aspiration, and depending on the severity, these may be indications for operation. Dependent diverticula may be associated with an increased risk of malignancy because of stasis and inflammation of the pouch, though this is not well defined. In patients with a diverticula associated with a motility disorder, the motility disorder is more likely to produce symptoms than the diverticula.

A *pharyngoesophageal (Zenker) diverticulum* is an uncommon entity; a false diverticulum arising from the area of weakness inferior to the oblique fibers of the thyropharyngeus and the horizontal fibers of the cricopharyngeus or UES, as illustrated in Figure 9.9. Dysfunction of the cricopharyngeus, usually a discoordination that results in a delay in opening the cricopharyngeus in response to the presence of a food bolus, causes increased intraluminal pressure that ultimately results in the formation of a false diverticulum consisting of protruding mucosa. Surgical treatment includes cervical esophagomyotomy with resection of the diverticulum (small diverticula

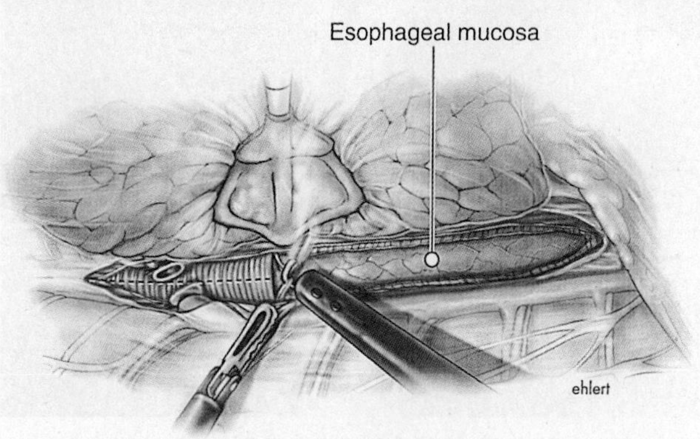

FIGURE 9.8 Long esophagomyotomy. (From Fischer JE, ed. *Mastery of Surgery*. 5th ed. Philadelphia: Lippincott Williams & Wilkins; 2007:750, with permission.)

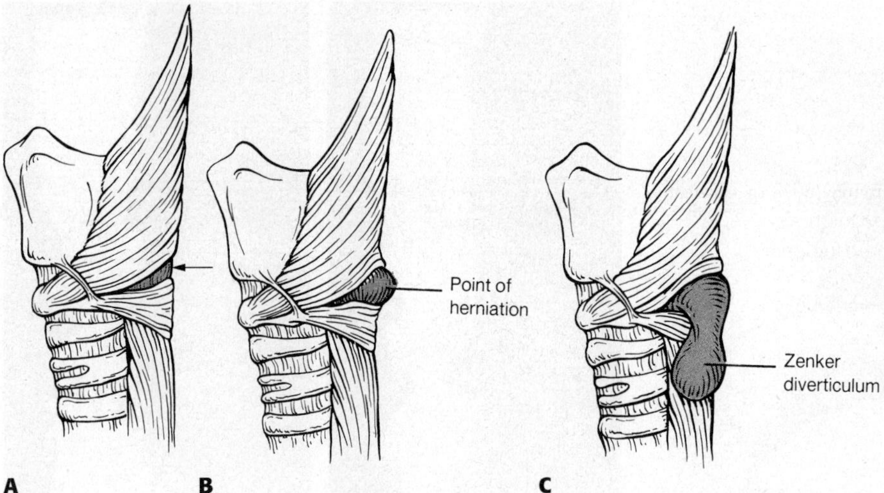

FIGURE 9.9 Formation of a Zenker diverticulum **(A)**. Herniation of the pharyngeal mucosa and submucosa occurs at the point of transition (*arrow*) between the oblique fibers of the thyropharyngeus muscle and the more horizontal fibers of the cricopharyngeus muscle **(B** and **C)**. As the diverticulum enlarges, it dissects toward the left side and downward into the superior mediastinum in the prevertebral space, forming a false diverticulum. (From Bell RH, Rikkers LF, Mulholland MW. *Digestive Tract Surgery: A Text and Atlas*. Philadelphia: Lippincott–Raven Publishers; 1996:33, with permission.)

can be left in situ) or diverticulopexy with cricopharyngeal myotomy. Cricopharyngeal myotomy can also be performed endoscopically by introducing an endoscopic linear cutting stapler through the oropharynx, placing one jaw in the esophageal lumen and the other in the diverticulum and firing the device. This results in the creation of a common channel and in the process divides the cricopharyngeus.

Pulsion diverticula in the midesophagus or distal esophagus (epiphrenic) may be discovered incidentally or during an evaluation for an esophageal motility disorder (see Fig. 9.10). Most are asymptomatic and can be observed. Generally, patients with diverticula greater than 3 cm or moderate to severe symptoms have indication for operation. Surgical intervention includes a thoracotomy with resection of the diverticulum and a long esophagomyotomy on the side of the esophagus opposite to the diverticulum. A partial fundoplication can be added in patients with poor esophageal motility to reduce the incidence of GE reflux following a distal esophagomyotomy.

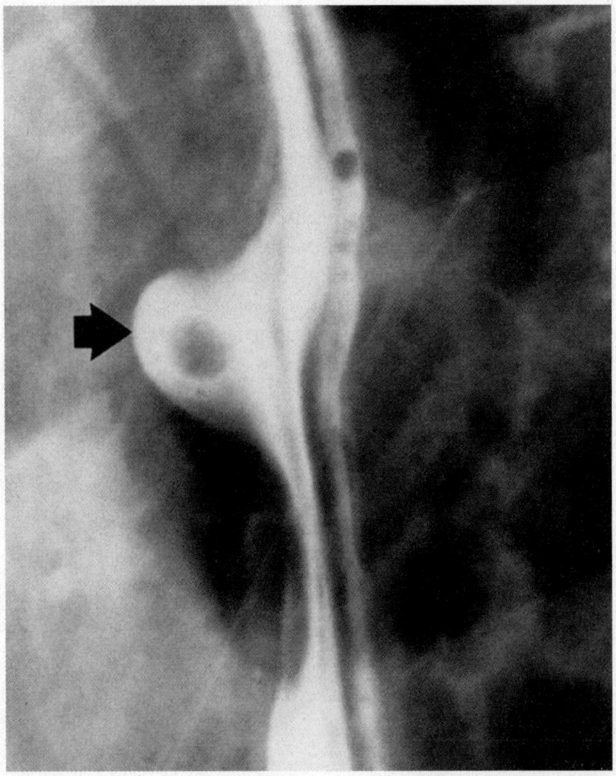

FIGURE 9.10 Esophagogram of a patient with a large epiphrenic pulsion diverticulum, indicated by *Arrow*. (From Brant WE, Helms C, eds. *Fundamentals of Diagnostic Radiology*. 4th ed. Philadelphia: Wolters Kluwer Health; 2012.)

ESOPHAGEAL PERFORATION

The absence of a serosa investment predisposes the esophagus to rupture at lower pressures than other parts of the alimentary tract. Clinical and radiographic manifestations reflect the size and location of the tear. Cervical perforations typically present with dysphagia, cervical pain, subcutaneous emphysema, or fever. Lower esophageal rupture usually drains into the left thoracic cavity or abdomen, whereas rupture of the midesophagus may drain into either the left or the right thoracic cavity. Clinical presentation in these scenarios may include a pleural effusion, pneumothorax, pneumomediastinum, subcutaneous emphysema, chest or back pain, tachycardia, tachypnea, and fever. Perforation of the intra-abdominal esophagus results in abdominal pain and peritonitis. Esophageal perforation is caused by spontaneous rupture in approximately 15% of cases, traumatic rupture in 20%, and iatrogenic rupture in 60%. If any of the above signs or symptoms is present following esophageal instrumentation, a diagnostic evaluation is mandatory, as delay in diagnosis may be lethal.

Iatrogenic perforation is most commonly caused by esophagoscopy; a higher risk is associated with endoscopic intervention. Most iatrogenic injuries occur at the level of the cricopharyngeus. Other less frequent causes include operative injury, foreign body ingestion, trauma, and esophageal or tracheal intubation.

Spontaneous rupture can occur from increased pressure against a closed glottis, where the perforation typically localizes to the left lateral wall, just superior to the diaphragm. This is known as *Boerhaave syndrome* and classically presents with the *Mackler's triad*: vomiting, lower thoracic pain, and subcutaneous emphysema.

Early diagnosis of esophageal perforation can dramatically reduce the morbidity and mortality associated with this problem. Physical examination may reveal crepitus in the neck or anterior chest, a finding that indicates subcutaneous emphysema caused by swallowed air leaking out of the esophageal disruption. An upright chest radiograph may identify pneumomediastinum or pneumothorax, which can be present in up to 40% of patients with perforation. Often a pleural effusion is present. The diagnostic modality of choice is a water-soluble contrast esophagogram followed by a dilute barium esophagogram. This modality will accurately image approximately 60% of cervical perforations and up to 90% of mediastinal perforations. Serial barium esophagograms may be required if the initial esophagogram is negative, and the clinical suspicion remains high as long as the clinical situation of the patient is stable and does not worsen. A high index of suspicion should prompt a trip to the operating room and endoscopy for definitive diagnosis. A rent in the esophagus is easily visualized at the time of esophagoscopy, but no attempt should be made to place the endoscope through the perforation. Esophagoscopy has high sensitivity for perforations caused by external trauma. CT scans may suggest perforation with the presence of extraluminal air, esophageal thickening, or fluid collections. Pleural fluid collected by thoracentesis is suggestive of perforation with a pH less than 6.0, the presence of food particles, or elevated salivary amylase.

Treatment options include both operative and nonoperative management, depending on the time from injury to diagnosis and the degree of injury, the extent of the injury, the clinical status of the patient, and the location of the injury. Operative management has traditionally been the treatment of choice for patients presenting with any signs or symptoms of systemic toxicity such as tachycardia, hypotension, or end-organ failure; this includes most patients with esophageal perforation. Other signs of significant contamination, such as pneumomediastinum, pneumothorax, or extensive subcutaneous emphysema, are associated with a higher incidence of sepsis and are definitive indications, in most cases, for operation. Several operative options exist, but the goals are debridement of devitalized tissue, primary repair, and adequate drainage. The surgeon must always consider appropriate treatment of the perforation as well as any underlying esophageal pathology that may have predisposed to the perforation or the instrumentation. For example, an intra-abdominal perforation in the context of pneumatic dilatation for achalasia mandates an esophagomyotomy in addition to primary repair of the perforation and a partial fundoplication for reinforcement and reflux control. In cases of severe necrosis or an underlying esophageal carcinoma, an esophagectomy should be performed if the clinical situation permits this, as attempts at repair will most often fail. Well-contained cervical perforations are treated with cervical incision and drainage alone. Several options exist for the management of intrathoracic perforations including primary repair with or without local flap reinforcement, in addition to extensive debridement and exposure of the mediastinum to allow drainage (Fig. 9.11). Delayed presentation or a patient in extremis necessitates expeditious surgery, often drainage, debridement, and proximal diversion and distal ligation or T tube placement. Regardless of type of primary repair or time to presentation, the lowest mortality rates are achieved in patients managed operatively, ranging from 0% to 31% and averaging 12%.

General criteria for nonoperative management include minimal symptoms, absence of systemic signs of infection, effluent draining back into the esophagus without contamination of body cavities, and an absence of associated pathology (malignancy, stricture, motility disorder). Patients should be fluid resuscitated, placed on broad-spectrum antibiotics, and given nothing by mouth for 7 to 10 days, at which point another contrast study is undertaken.

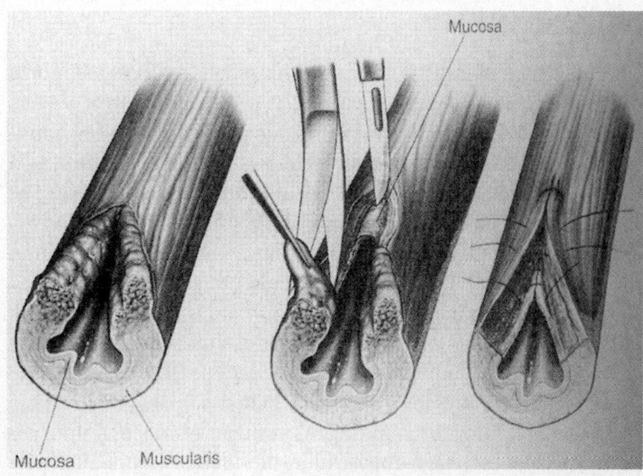

FIGURE 9.11 Closure of the perforated esophagus requires debridement of necrotic tissue and closure of mucosal and muscular laceration. (From Baker RJ, Fischer JE, eds. *Mastery of Surgery*. 4th ed. Philadelphia: Lippincott Williams & Wilkins; 2001:846, with permission.)

Clinical deterioration indicates treatment failure and mandates an operation. Nonoperative management is most successful in patients with perforations recognized early following instrumentation and in patients who present later when the clinical consequences of the perforation have already declared themselves. The mortality rate in select groups is reported to be low, averaging 18%.

Unfortunately, operative morbidity and mortality associated with surgical repair can be high. Repair is technically difficult due to the absence of esophageal serosa. For this reason, the use of endoscopically placed esophageal stents is emerging as a potential alternative to open surgery. Initially explored in perforations associated with esophageal malignancy, stents have now been used to manage iatrogenic and spontaneous perforations, fistulae, and anastomotic leaks after esophagectomy. They afford the rapid control of leakage of esophageal contents, potential for early oral nutrition, and the avoidance of well-established operative morbidity. As demonstrated by Freeman and colleagues, stent placement may be safely considered in patients who would otherwise be managed surgically, with low rates of mortality and failure in their series (<3% and 8%, respectively). Factors associated with failure include a leak of the proximal cervical esophagus, a leak traversing the GE junction, an injury longer than 6 cm, or a leak site other than esophagogastrostomy after esophagectomy. Potential complications include stent migration requiring adjustment and failure to control a leak requiring traditional surgical repair. Stents can, and should be, removed once the leak has healed, as esophagoaortic fistulae have been described, presumably resulting from radial force exerted by stents over an extended period of time.

Morbidity and mortality from esophageal perforation remain high. The etiology clearly determines outcome, with spontaneous perforations associated with a mortality of 36%, iatrogenic perforations of 19%, and traumatic perforations of 7%. In addition, cervical perforations are associated with the lowest mortality of 6%, whereas thoracic and abdominal perforations are associated with mortality rates of 27% and 21%, respectively. The most critical determinant remains the time from injury to definitive treatment. Patients treated less than 24 hours after the perforation have a mortality rate of approximately 10% to 15%, while those diagnosed later have rates upward of 50%.

CAUSTIC INJURY

The incidence of caustic injury to the esophagus has a bimodal distribution, with its peak occurring at ages younger than 5 years followed by a secondary peak later in adolescence and young adulthood. The latter group usually swallows greater quantities as a result of suicide attempts, resulting in more extensive injury. The most common ingested chemicals include alkali (65%), acid (16%), and bleach. Alkali, an odorless and tasteless liquid, usually causes the most damage via liquefaction necrosis to surrounding tissues. Acid injury results in coagulation necrosis and is less severe, though upper airway injury can complicate the clinical sequelae. Bleaches are esophageal irritants and do not cause serious esophageal injury.

Patients may present with oral and chest pain, hypersalivation, dysphagia, bleeding, or vomiting. Assessment of mucosal injury is performed by esophagoscopy within the first 24 hours after presentation. Because of the risk of perforation, the endoscope should not be passed beyond the proximal lesion. Treatment consists of fluid resuscitation and broad-spectrum antibiotics. Attention must be paid to maintenance of a safe airway, which can require urgent tracheostomy if the caustic injury is accompanied by an associated laryngeal burn. Corticosteroids have been shown to decrease the severity and persistence of esophageal strictures following second- and third-degree injuries in several small studies, but routine use is controversial. Emetics are contraindicated. Early surgical intervention is reserved for patients with perforation, extensive hemorrhage, or extensive necrosis. If gastric necrosis is present, a transhiatal esophagogastrectomy with end-cervical esophagostomy, mediastinal drainage, and feeding jejunostomy are required. Gastrointestinal continuity is restored at a later date with colonic interposition.

After the acute phase of injury is past, surgical management is directed toward the prevention of strictures. Strictures will develop in 20% of patients and occur within the first 2 months. The highest risk exists in those patients with deep circumferential injury or transmural necrosis. Satisfactory treatment is usually achieved with early, repeated bougie dilatation. Surgical intervention is needed in less than 10% of patients with stricture and is reserved for refractory or complete stenosis. Esophageal resection with gastric, colonic, or jejunal interposition is the procedure of choice unless severe periesophagitis precludes safe dissection of the esophagus in which case a substernal bypass with esophageal exclusion may be performed.

FOREIGN BODIES

Foreign body ingestion occurs frequently in the pediatric population. Generally, ingested foreign bodies lodge in the regions of anatomic narrowing. Foreign bodies are usually easily diagnosed with chest x-ray, dilute barium esophagogram, or flexible endoscopy. Objects can usually be removed with flexible endoscopy. Sharp foreign bodies should always be removed because of a 15% to 30% risk of perforation at the ileocecal valve. Surgical removal is indicated for objects that cannot be removed endoscopically, a situation that occurs rarely.

BENIGN ESOPHAGEAL LESIONS

Benign neoplasms of the esophagus are extremely rare and account for 0.5% of all esophageal masses. Approximately 80% of these lesions occur in the distal two thirds of the esophagus and are multiple in 10% of patients.

Leiomyomas are slow-growing tumors, and patients with these lesions present with a long history of generalized upper gastrointestinal symptoms of regurgitation, belching, dysphagia, and pain. Diagnosis is usually made by barium esophagogram, which shows a smooth concave defect with sharp borders. Endoscopy with EUS also reveals a lesion with normal overlying mucosa and a freely movable mass with narrowing but not complete obstruction of the lumen. Biopsy is contraindicated, since mucosal interruption will complicate subsequent surgical excision.

The majority of small lesions can be followed with expectant management and surveillance, utilizing routine radiography and endoscopy. Indications for surgical excision include unremitting symptoms, tumor size greater than 3 cm in diameter, progressive increase in tumor size, mucosal ulceration, and confirmation of a histopathologic diagnosis. The procedure is performed via thoracotomy or thoracoscopy with a longitudinal esophageal myotomy, enucleation of the mass, and reapproximation of the muscularis. Outcomes are excellent, and recurrence is rare. Esophageal resection is usually required with lesions greater than 8 cm or with lesions that involve the entire circumference of the esophagus.

Esophageal duplication cysts are part of the spectrum of bronchopulmonary foregut abnormalities and can present as a mass lesion. They are lined with various types of epithelium and can occur anywhere along the length of the thoracic esophagus. Enteric and bronchogenic cysts are the most common and are of foregut origin. Only rarely is there a communication with the esophageal lumen. They usually present in childhood, are located on the right side in 60% of cases, and are associated with vertebral and spinal cord abnormalities. Because of the risk of ulceration, bleeding, or superinfection, surgical excision is recommended.

A *Schatzki ring* is a ring of mucosa and submucosa encircling the esophagus at the squamocolumnar junction that is associated with GE reflux disease. Etiology is unknown. Symptoms of dysphagia generally arise during the ingestion of food. The treatment of choice is endoscopic dilatation, but intervention is reserved for symptomatic patients. Recurrence is common after dilation but may be prevented by maintenance acid-suppressive therapy.

MALIGNANT ESOPHAGEAL NEOPLASMS

The prevalence of esophageal carcinoma varies worldwide, primarily because of the influence of local dietary and environmental factors. In high-risk areas such as China and Iran, the prevalence can be as high as 180 per 100,000 men. Approximately 18,000 new cases are diagnosed and 15,000 deaths occur per year in the United States. These numbers represent a 15% to 20% increase over the last two decades, but there is some evidence that this sharp rise in incidence may currently be at a plateau.

Histologically, SCC or adenocarcinoma accounts for 90% of esophageal cancers. Melanomas, leiomyosarcomas, carcinoids, and lymphomas comprise the other 10%. Approximately three fourths of adenocarcinomas arise in the distal two thirds of the esophagus, whereas SCC arises more commonly in the middle and upper third of the esophagus. Risk factors for both types of cancer include cigarette smoking (both quantity and duration of smoking), exposure to carcinogens including *N*-nitrosamines, and a prior history of radiotherapy to the mediastinum. Unlike adenocarcinoma, SCC is associated with chronic irritation associated with alcohol, achalasia, chronic esophagitis, diverticula, caustic injury, and possibly human papillomavirus (HPV).

The incidence of adenocarcinoma has increased considerably in Western countries for unclear reasons, particularly among white men. Patients with reflux symptoms have an eightfold increased risk of adenocarcinoma of the esophagus. The most important reason is likely linked to GE reflux and the development of Barrett's columnar cell. Increasing evidence supports the hypothesis that Barrett's metaplasia may be the precursor lesion to esophageal adenocarcinoma. Patients with Barrett's esophagus are at a high risk for adenocarcinoma, although the absolute risk of malignant transformation to adenocarcinoma is 0.12% per year according to current evidence. This can be much higher if dysplasia is present. Obesity is also a risk factor for adenocarcinoma.

Patients with esophageal cancer usually present with dysphagia (first to solids), anorexia, and weight loss. Cervical lymphadenopathy (Virchow node), hepatomegaly, or pleural effusions are highly suggestive of metastatic disease. Screening has not been advocated in the United States, except in high-risk patients such as those with Barrett esophagus, because of the high cost and low prevalence of the disease. In these patients, endoscopy is recommended every 3 to 5 years and more frequently in the presence of low-grade dysplasia. Treatment with proton pump inhibitors may be associated with reversal of metaplasia to normal squamous mucosa, but their benefit in this regard has not been proven, and whether this reduces the overall risk of cancer remains unknown. High-grade dysplasia is an indication for esophagectomy. Without treatment, up to one half of patients with high-grade dysplasia will develop adenocarcinoma within 3 years, and a significant number of patients who undergo esophagectomy for high-grade dysplasia are found to have an invasive lesion. Alternative strategies for management of high-grade dysplastic Barrett esophagus include endoscopic ablation and endoscopic mucosal resection. While these techniques avoid the potential morbidity and mortality of esophagectomy, they carry the risk of failure to eradicate all dysplastic or possibly neoplastic tissue.

Tumors are classified according to the 2010 American Joint Committee on Cancer (AJCC) Tumor Node Metastasis (TNM) system. Recent data show that prognosis is dependent on T stage, histology, grade, and tumor location in lymph node–negative tumors, which is reflected in the current staging system. SCCs and adenocarcinomas are therefore staged separately, with tumor location taken into account for SCCs (Tables 9.1–9.3). Number of lymph nodes involved with tumor defines N stage rather than location of regional nodes. For SCC, overall 5-year survival rates are approximately 70% for stage IA, 60% for stage IB, 55% for stage IIA, 40% for stage IIB, 25% for stage IIIA, and 15% for stages IIIB and IIIC. For adenocarcinoma, overall 5-year survival rates are approximately 75% for stage IA, 65% for stage IB, 50% for stage IIA, 40% for stage IIB, 25% for stage IIIA, and 15% for stages IIIB and IIIC.

Prior to initiation of therapy, definitive diagnosis and accurate staging are critical to pursuing the most appropriate treatment course. Esophagoscopy with biopsy is the preferred diagnostic modality.

TABLE 9.1 TNM classification for esophageal SCC and esophageal adenocarcinoma

Primary tumor (T)	
Tx	Primary tumor cannot be assessed
T0	No evidence of primary tumor
Tis	High-grade dysplasia
T1	Tumor invades lamina propria, muscularis mucosa, or submucosa
T1a	Tumor invades lamina propria or muscularis mucosa
T1b	Tumor invades submucosa
T2	Tumor invades muscularis propria
T3	Tumor invades adventitia
T4	Tumor invades adjacent structures
T4a	Resectable tumor invading pleura, pericardium, or diaphragm
T4b	Unresectable tumor invading other adjacent structures, such as aorta, vertebral body, trachea, etc.
Regional lymph nodes (N)	
Nx	Regional lymph node(s) cannot be assessed
N0	No regional lymph node metastasis
N1	Metastasis in 1–2 regional lymph nodes
N2	Metastasis in 3–6 regional lymph nodes
N3	Metastasis in 7 or more regional lymph nodes
Distant metastasis (M)	
M0	No distant metastasis
M1	Distant metastasis
Histologic grade (G)	
Gx	Grade cannot be assessed—stage grouping as G1
G1	Well differentiated
G2	Moderately differentiated
G3	Poorly differentiated
G4	Undifferentiated—stage grouping as G3 squamous

TABLE 9.2 TNM staging for esophageal SCC

Stage	T	N	M	Grade	Tumor location[a]
0	Tis	N0	M0	1, X	Any
IA	T1	N0	M0	1, X	Any
IB	T1	N0	M0	2–3	Any
	T2–3	N0	M0	1, X	Lower, X
IIA	T2–3	N0	M0	1, X	Upper, middle
	T2–3	N0	M0	2, 3	Lower, X
IIB	T2–3	N0	M0	2–3	Upper, middle
	T1–2	N1	M0	Any	Any
IIIA	T1-2	N2	M0	Any	Any
	T3	N1	M0	Any	Any
	T4a	N0	M0	Any	Any
IIIB	T3	N2	M0	Any	Any
IIIC	T4a	N1-2	M0	Any	Any
	T4b	Any	M0	Any	Any
	Any	N3	M0	Any	Any
IV	Any	Any	M1	Any	Any

[a]Tumor location defined by the position of the upper (proximal) edge of the tumor.

EUS has emerged as the best way to stage local invasion (T classification). In addition, EUS is sensitive in detection of regional lymph node metastases, and guided fine needle aspiration can be performed for diagnostic purposes. EUS has 90% accuracy in determining T stage in 80% to 90% of patients. Nodal involvement (N stage) is best evaluated by a combination of EUS and chest CT with intravenous contrast. A good-quality CT scan of the chest and upper abdomen is critical to evaluate the liver, lungs, and lymph nodes for changes suspicious for metastatic disease (M stage) that preclude surgical resection. Local invasion into adjacent structures (trachea, heart, great vessels) can also be detected on CT. Combined PET-CT scanning is effective at detecting (PET) and localizing (CT) potentially metastatic disease.

TABLE 9.3 TNM staging for esophageal adenocarcinoma

Stage	T	N	M	Grade
0	Tis	N0	M0	1, X
IA	T1	N0	M0	1–2, X
IB	T1	N0	M0	3
	T2	N0	M0	1–2, X
IIA	T2	N0	M0	3
IIB	T3	N0	M0	Any
	T1–2	N1	M0	Any
IIIA	T1–2	N2	M0	Any
	T3	N1	M0	Any
	T4a	N0	M0	Any
IIIB	T3	N2	M0	Any
IIIC	T4a	N1-2	M0	Any
	T4b	Any	M0	Any
	Any	N3	M0	Any
IV	Any	Any	M1	Any

Source: From Edge S, Byrd DR, Compton CC, et al., eds. *American Joint Commission on Cancer Staging Manual*. 7th ed. New York: Springer; 2010, with permission.

While esophagectomy has traditionally been the primary treatment for early esophageal cancer, recent experience supports multimodal therapy including neoadjuvant chemotherapy and radiation to improve survival. Early-stage esophageal cancer (stage I T1N0M0 and possibly T2N0M0) is best treated by esophagectomy prior to consideration of chemotherapy or radiotherapy. Evidence from several trials suggests that more advanced disease (stage I T2–T3, stage II, and stage III) may be better treated by neoadjuvant chemoradiation prior to surgical resection. Because of decreased oral intake and tumor cachexia, consideration should be given to pretreatment alimentation with a jejunal tube or esophageal stent. This is particularly true in patients who have lost more than 10% body weight, though preoperative alimentation has not been shown to be associated with decreased postoperative morbidity. Jejunal tube placement may be valuable for patients who are planning to undergo preoperative chemoradiation to maintain their nutritional status with a future operation in mind.

Multiple surgical approaches are available. Tumor location and surgeon preference are the most important factors for selection of the approach. All approaches involve resection of the esophagus with anastomosis most commonly to the gastric remnant placed in the posterior mediastinum or in the neck. Reconstruction with a gastric conduit involves division of the short gastric vessel, the left gastric, left gastroepiploic, and right gastric arteries, with the sole blood supply via the right gastroepiploic artery. Lymph nodes should be removed from perigastric as well as periesophageal locations. Placement of a feeding jejunostomy tube should be considered at time of surgery.

The *Ivor–Lewis* operation involves a right thoracotomy combined with an upper midline laparotomy to create an intrathoracic anastomosis. Laparotomy is performed first for mobilization of the stomach and creation of a gastric tube as described above, followed by mobilization of the GE junction and distal esophagus. The laparotomy incision is then closed, the patient repositioned in left lateral decubitus, and a right thoracotomy performed. The intrathoracic esophagus is then mobilized and the proximal esophagus divided. The gastric remnant is delivered into the chest and an esophagogastric anastomosis performed at the level of the azygos vein. A cervical incision can be added to remove more of the proximal esophagus (Fig. 9.12), with the anastomosis placed in the neck (the *McKeown's procedure*). A right thoracotomy allows for a more thorough mediastinal lymph node dissection, as well as better visualization and control for midthoracic tumors that abut the aorta or trachea. The advantage of a cervical anastomosis, in addition to resulting in a total esophagectomy with a better functional result, is that a leak in this location has a lower mortality rate when compared to an intrathoracic leak. Disadvantages of the Ivor–Lewis and McKeown's procedures include increased rates of postoperative pulmonary complications due to thoracotomy and risk of life-threatening mediastinitis if anastomotic leak occurs.

Transhiatal esophagectomy is another popular approach, particularly for tumors of the lower third of the esophagus. This involves gastric mobilization and lower mediastinal dissection through a laparotomy incision combined with a cervical incision for upper mediastinal dissection and anastomosis (see Figs. 9.13 and 9.14). Lower

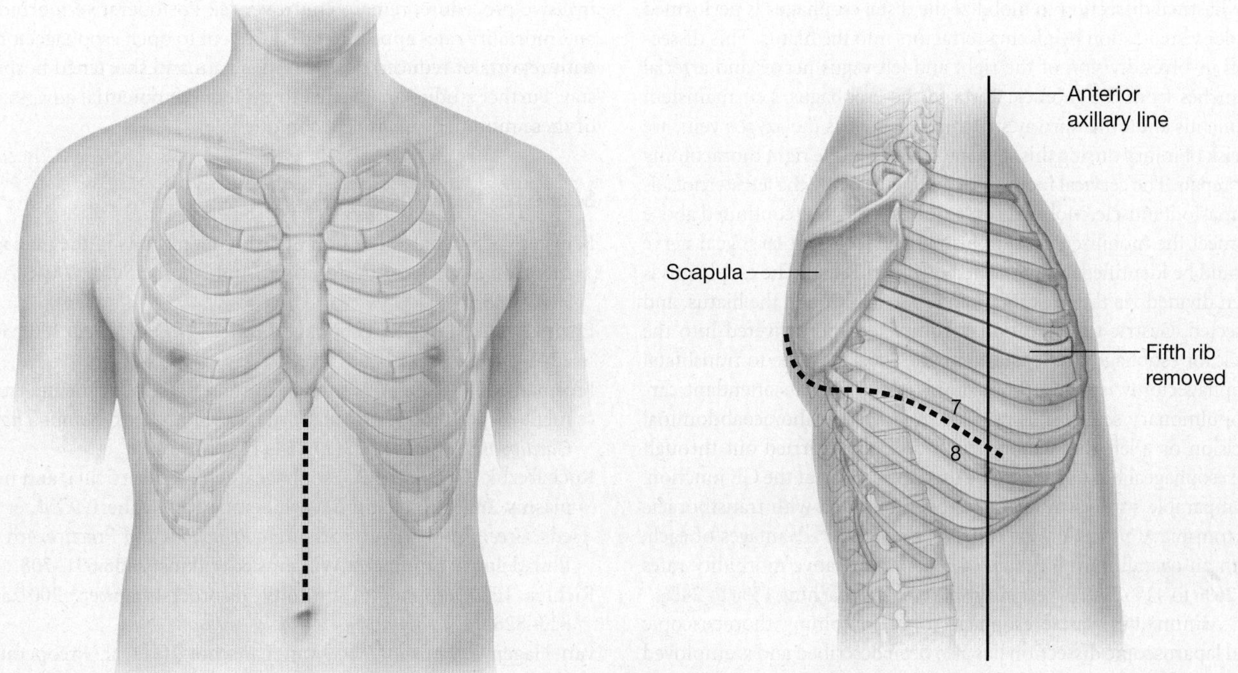

FIGURE 9.12 Incisions for Ivor Lewis Esophagectomy. A neck incision can be added for additional resection and cervical anastomosis. (From Luketich JD, ed. *Master Techniques in Surgery: Esophageal Surgery*. Philadelphia: Wolters Kluwer Health; 2014.)

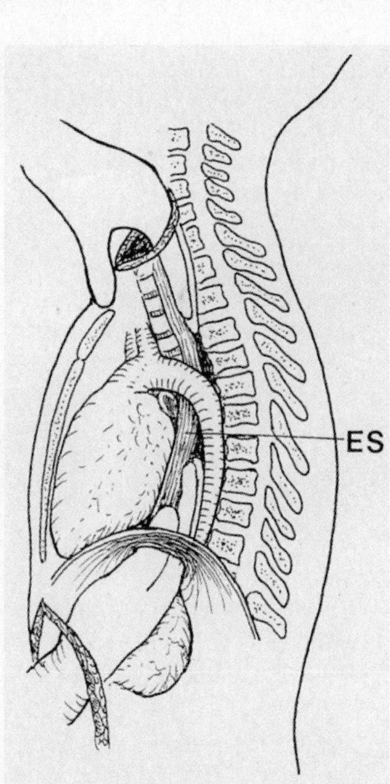

FIGURE 9.13 Transhiatal mobilization of the esophagus (ES) from the neck and abdomen. (From Baker RJ, Fischer JE, eds. *Mastery of Surgery*. 4th ed. Philadelphia: Lippincott Williams & Wilkins; 2001:829, with permission.)

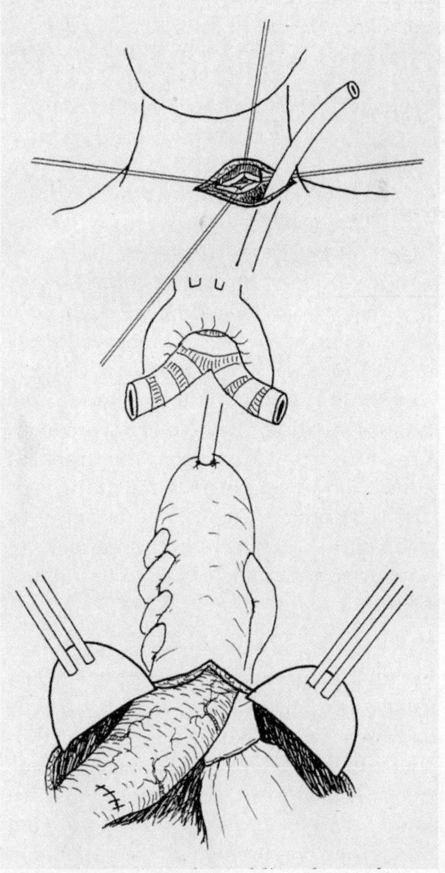

FIGURE 9.14 After esophageal resection, the gastric conduit is delivered through the posterior mediastinum to the neck. (From Baker RJ, Fischer JE, eds. *Mastery of Surgery*. 4th ed. Philadelphia: Lippincott Williams & Wilkins; 2001:831, with permission.)

mediastinal dissection to mobilize the distal esophagus is performed under visualization by placing retractors into the hiatus. This dissection involves division of the right and left vagus nerves and arterial branches from the thoracic aorta to the esophagus. Left mainstem bronchus and other airway structures, as well as the azygos vein, are at risk of injury during this step and would require right thoracotomy for repair. The cervical incision is then made along the left sternocleidomastoid muscle. Mobilization of the esophagus is continued above to meet the mobilized portion below. The recurrent laryngeal nerve should be identified and protected during this step. The esophagus is then divided via the neck incision, retracted through the hiatus, and resected. Gastric tube creation is completed and delivered into the neck for esophagogastric anastomosis. The advantage to transhiatal esophagectomy is that a thoracotomy, along with its attendant cardiopulmonary sequelae, is avoided. A single left thoracoabdominal incision or a left thoracotomy with dissection carried out through the esophageal hiatus can also be used for tumors at the GE junction. Comparable survival results have been reported with transthoracic or transhiatal procedures despite the theoretical advantages of each, with an overall mortality rate of 5%, perioperative morbidity rates of 26% to 41%, and 5-year survival rates approaching 15% to 24%.

Minimally invasive esophagectomy combining thoracoscopic and laparoscopic dissection has also been described and is employed by a number of surgeons with comparable results to the classic open procedures. The advantages, if any, conferred by this minimally invasive procedure, remain controversial. Postoperative morbidity and mortality rates appear to be equivalent to open esophagectomy, with reports of reduced postoperative pain and shortened hospital stay. Further studies are needed to explore the potential advantages of these minimally invasive techniques.

Suggested Readings

Brinster CJ, Singhal S, Lee L, et al. Evolving options in the management of esophageal perforation. *Ann Thorac Surg.* 2004;77(4): 1475–1483.

Enzinger PC, Mayer RJ. Esophageal cancer. *N Engl J Med.* 2003;349: 2241–2252.

Freeman RK, Ascioti AJ. Esophageal stent placement for the treatment of perforation, fistula, or anastomotic leak. *Semin Thorac Cardiovasc Surg.* 2011;23(2):154–148.

Kucharczuk JC, Kaiser LR. Esophageal injury, diverticula, and neoplasms. In: Mulholland MW, Lillemoe KD, Doherty GM, et al., eds. *Greenfield's Surgery: Scientific Principles and Practice.* 4th ed. Philadelphia: Lippincott Williams & Wilkins; 2006:691–708.

Richter JE. Oesophageal motility disorders. *Lancet.* 2001;358: 823–828.

van Hagen P, Hulshof MC, van Lanschot JJ, et al. Preoperative chemoradiotherapy for esophageal or junctional cancer. *N Engl J Med.* 2012;336(22):2074–2084.

CHAPTER 10

The Stomach

DOUGLAS R. MURKEN AND ROBERT E. ROSES

KEY POINTS

- Bleeding peptic ulcers refractory to endoscopic intervention should be controlled with the *three-suture technique*, and truncal or selective vagotomy should be considered. When performed, vagotomy should be coupled with pyloroplasty to facilitate gastric emptying.
- The indications for antireflux surgery include persistent symptoms despite optimal medical management for 4 weeks or more, complications, manometric evidence of a defective LES, and 24-hour pH test demonstrating GERD.
- Candidates for bariatric surgery include patients with severe obesity (BMI > 35 kg/m^2) who have an obesity-related complication, and patients with morbid obesity (BMI > 40 kg/m^2).
- The majority of gastric cancer patients have micrometastasis at the time of presentation.
- Multimodality therapy including perioperative chemotherapy or postoperative chemoradiotherapy is appropriate for the majority of patients with resectable gastric cancer.

ANATOMY

The stomach and duodenum develop from the caudal portion of the embryonic foregut during the 5th week of gestation. The primitive stomach is invested within the ventral and dorsal mesenteries. In postnatal life, the ventral mesentery is represented by the lesser omentum, consisting of the falciform, gastrohepatic, and hepatoduodenal ligaments. The greater omentum (former dorsal mesentery) forms the gastrosplenic and gastrophrenic ligaments. Rotation of the gut leads to the anterior position of the left vagal trunk and the posterior location of the right trunk at the level of the gastroesophageal (GE) junction. The stomach rests between the 10th thoracic and the 3rd lumbar vertebral segments, fixed at these points by the GE junction proximally and retroperitoneal attachments of the duodenum distally.

The stomach can be divided into four functional parts, serving as guidelines in planning surgical resection (Fig. 10.1). The *cardia* is located immediately distal to the GE junction, while the *fundus* extends above the GE junction. The *body* (corpus) is the central portion of the stomach, marked distally by the *angularis incisura*, a crease on the lesser curvature, just proximal to the terminal nerves of Latarjet (terminal posterior branches of the vagus to the antrum). The distal thickened segment of the stomach is the *pylorus*. The *antrum* is the inferior portion of the stomach just proximal to the pyloric sphincter.

An abundant network of extramural and intramural vascular collaterals exists in the stomach. The blood supply of the stomach is primarily derived from branches of the celiac trunk. The *left gastric artery*, the first branch of the celiac trunk, and the *right gastric artery*, a branch of the hepatic artery, supply the lesser curvature. The *vasa brevia*, also known as the *short gastric arteries*, and the *left gastroepiploic artery*, both of which arise from the *splenic artery*, form a collateral network with the *right gastroepiploic artery*, a branch of the gastroduodenal artery, to supply the greater curvature. The venous drainage parallels the arterial supply (Fig. 10.2). The left gastric vein is more commonly known as the coronary vein.

Lymphatic drainage from the proximal lesser curve of the stomach traverses the superior gastric lymph nodes surrounding the left gastric artery, while that from the distal lesser curve traverses the suprapyloric lymph nodes. Pancreaticosplenic nodes and subpyloric and omental nodes drain the proximal and the antral portions of the greater curve, respectively. Ultimately, all the perigastric lymphatics converge at the celiac axis. Metastatic disease can bypass the primary nodes owing to extensive intramural and extramural communications.

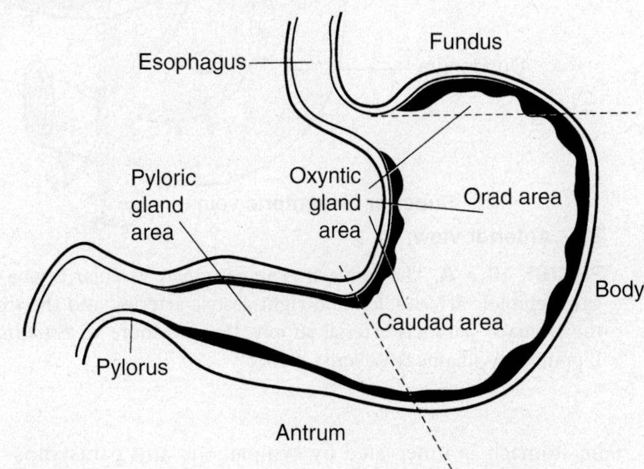

FIGURE 10.1 The stomach is anatomically divided into four parts with different anatomic functions.(From Johnson LR. Secretion. In: Johnson LR, ed. *Essential Medical Physiology*. New York: J.B. Lippincott; 1992:482, with permission.)

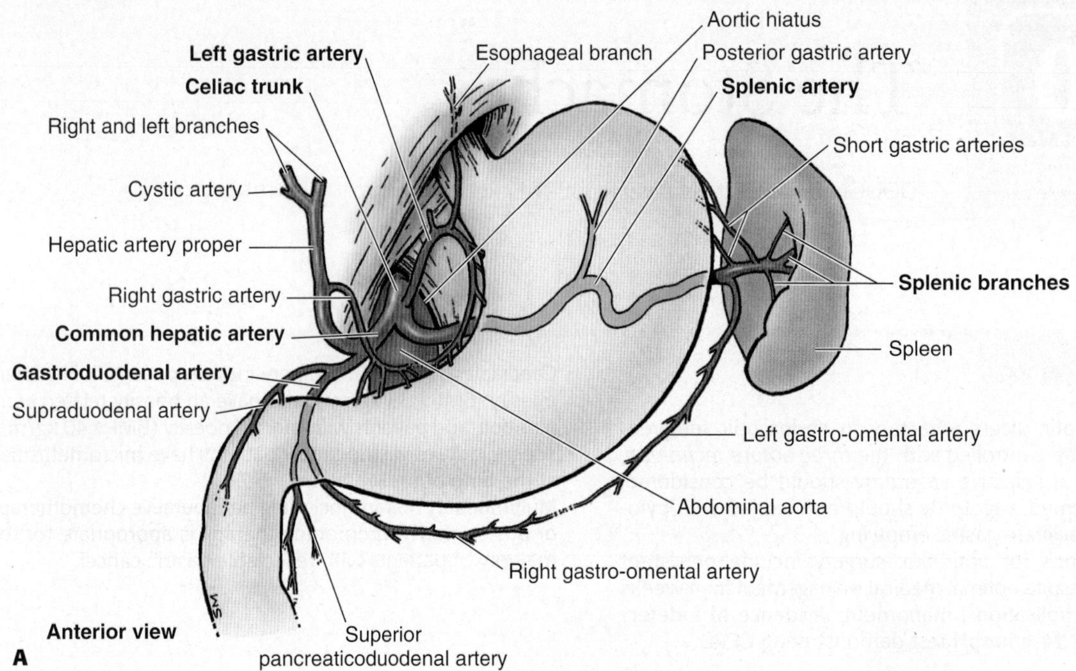

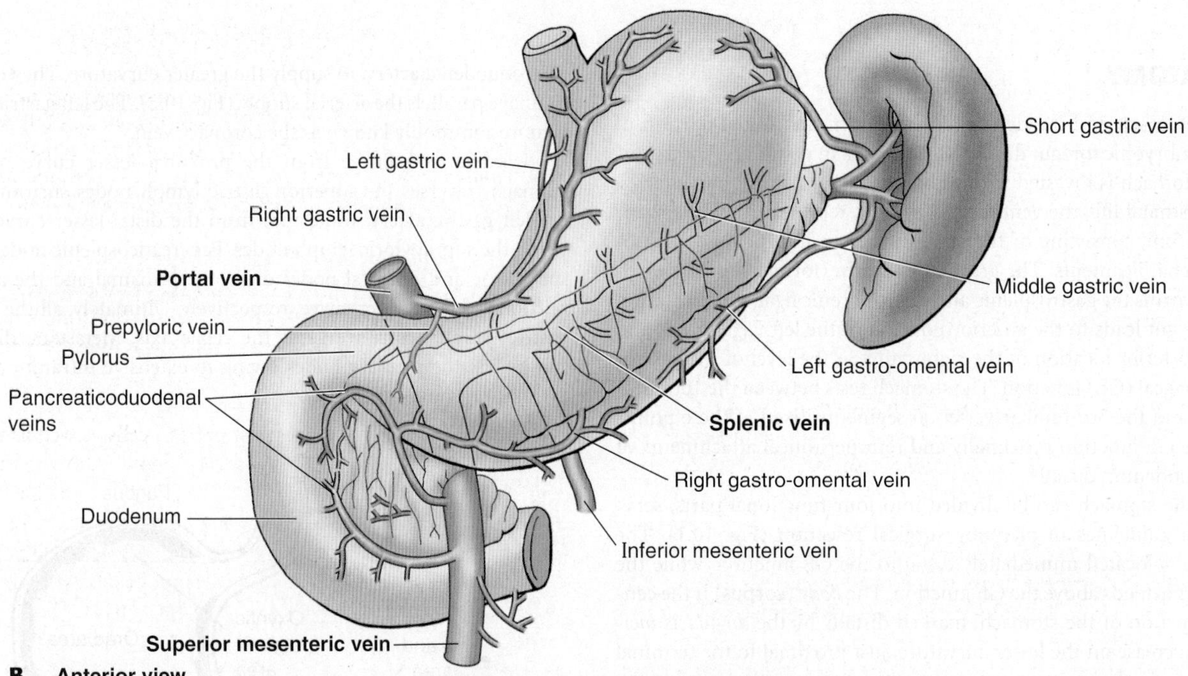

FIGURE 10.2 A. The stomach is an extremely vascular organ with blood supply from the left and right gastroepiploic arteries, left and right gastric arteries, and the short splenic vessels. **B.** Venous drainage of the stomach parallels arterial supply. (From Moore K. *Essential Clinical Anatomy*. 6th ed. Philadelphia: Lippincott Williams & Wilkins; 2010.)

The stomach is innervated by sympathetic and parasympathetic fibers. Thoracic sympathetic nerves transmit pain via the greater splanchnic nerve and celiac plexus. Parasympathetic fibers convey largely afferent signals along two discrete vagal trunks emerging through the esophageal hiatus of the diaphragm. The left trunk, which runs along the anterior surface of the esophagus, gives off a hepatic branch and then courses along the lesser curvature (Fig. 10.3). The right trunk, in its posterior position between the esophagus and the aorta, branches into the celiac division and the posterior division, which supplies the posterior gastric wall. A high branch known as the *criminal nerve of Grassi* should be identified during truncal vagotomy.

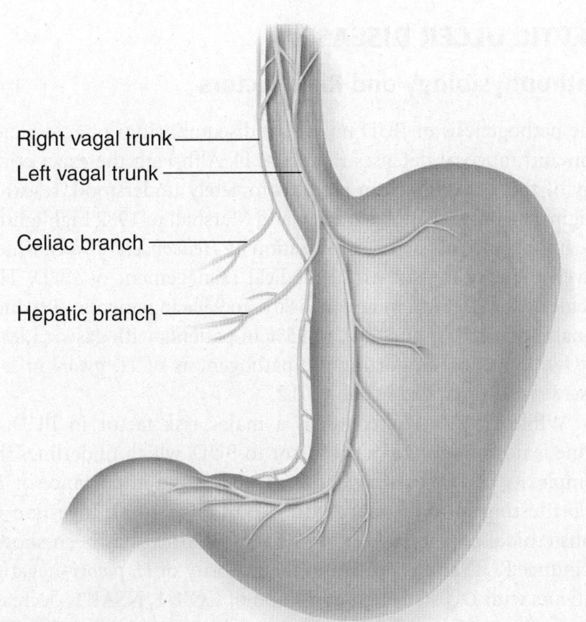

FIGURE 10.3 The vagus nerve forms two vagal trunks on the anterior and posterior surfaces of the stomach. The anterior vagal trunk gives off the hepatic vagal branch. (From Sawers JL. Selective vagotomy and pyloroplasty. In: Nyhus LM, Baker RJ, eds. *Mastery of Surgery*. 2nd ed. Philadelphia: Little, Brown and Company; 1992:674, with permission.)

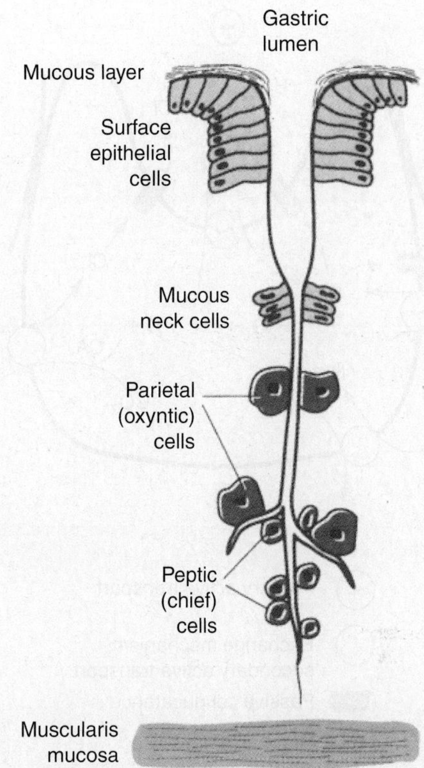

FIGURE 10.4 The oxyntic gland is divided into three regions: (i) the surface, containing mucosal cells; (ii) the neck, containing mainly parietal cells and a few mucosal cells; and (iii) the base, containing mainly chief cells. (From Johnson LR. Secretion. In: Johnson LR, ed. *Essential Medical Physiology*. New York: J.B. Lippincott; 1992:482, with permission.)

HISTOLOGY

The gastric mucosa is largely composed of simple columnar cells. Interspersed within the mucosa are three types of specialized glands—cardiac, oxyntic, and antral—each with a distinct function and distribution within the stomach. Cardiac glands occupy the narrow transition zone between squamous epithelium of the esophagus and simple columnar cells of the stomach. The cardiac glands secrete mucus. The fundus and body of the stomach contain tubular oxyntic glands, in which acid-secreting parietal cells are prominent (Fig. 10.4). Oxyntic glands also contain chief cells that synthesize pepsinogen. Each oxyntic gland can be divided into three regions: (i) isthmus, containing surface mucosal cells and a few parietal cells; (ii) neck, containing a high concentration of parietal cells and few mucosal cells; and (iii) base, containing chief cells, a few parietal cells, scattered mucosal cells, and undifferentiated cells. Endocrine cells are found in all three regions of oxyntic glands. Antral glands are located in the distal stomach, or antrum, as well as in the pyloric channel. Gastrin-secreting cells are a distinctive feature of these glands and can be identified morphologically by numerous dense granules containing this hormone. On stimulation, gastrin diffuses through the basal membrane and into the bloodstream.

PHYSIOLOGY

The complex physiologic function of the stomach is discussed elsewhere in this text. Several elements of gastric physiology most pertinent to the disease processes that are subsequently discussed in this chapter bear emphasis.

Gastric acid is a known contributor to the pathogenesis of peptic ulcer disease (PUD). Under normal circumstances, the stimulation of acid secretion occurs in three phases: cephalic, gastric, and intestinal. Basal acid secretion is 2 to 5 mEq/h in a fasting state and is modulated by histamine secretion and vagal tone. The *cephalic phase* of acid secretion begins with the thought, sight, and smell of food, which increase vagal tone, resulting in cholinergic stimulation of gastrin-secreting cells and parietal cells as well as relaxation of gastric smooth muscle tone to accommodate a food bolus. Loss of this "receptive relaxation" is associated with the postprandial nausea and vomiting seen in postvagotomy patients. Entry of food into the stomach initiates the *gastric phase*; partially hydrolyzed food and gastric distention stimulate the release of gastrin. Gastrin binds to receptors on the basolateral parietal cell membrane, resulting in acid secretion via the apical membrane-bound parietal cell proton pump (Fig. 10.5). The *intestinal phase* begins as gastric contents empty into the duodenum. The hormones enterooxyntin, secretin, somatostatin, peptide YY, gastric inhibitory peptide, and neurotensin all play a role during this phase of gastric acid secretion.

After every meal, the stomach secretes approximately 1,000 mL of gastric juice composed mainly of mucus, HCO_3 ions, pepsinogen, and intrinsic factor. To achieve such an acidic environment within the gastric lumen, parietal cells create a significant transmembrane hydrogen ion gradient via "proton pump" H^+/K^+ ATPase channels located in their apical membranes. Three major signaling molecules—histamine, acetylcholine, and gastrin—bind to their respective receptors along the basolateral membrane of the parietal

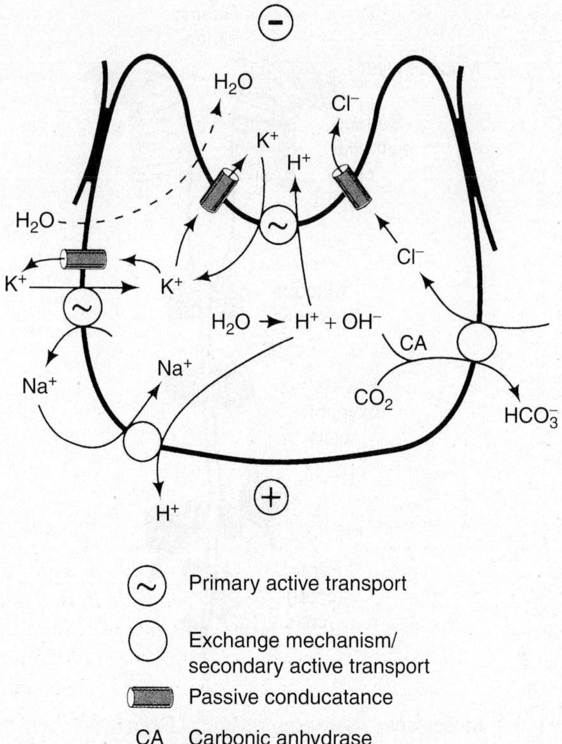

FIGURE 10.5 The gastric parietal cell produces hydrochloric acid and creates an acidic intraluminal gastric environment. (From Johnson LR. Secretion. In: Johnson LR, ed. *Essential Medical Physiology*. New York: J.B. Lippincott; 1992:485, with permission.)

cell, stimulating this acid secretion. Of these three, histamine has a dominant effect, which helps explain the efficacy of H2-blockers in gastric acid reduction. Mucus, produced by the oxyntic glands, is 95% water combined with high molecular weight glycoproteins. This mucoid gel forms a protective layer on the gastric mucosal surface known as the *unstirred layer*. HCO_3 ions formed as a by-product of acid secretion are trapped in this layer and maintain neutrality over the gastric mucosa, despite the low luminal pH. The combination of HCO_3 ions and the unstirred layer of mucoid gel acts as a mechanical barrier to the effects of acid. *Pepsinogen* is synthesized by chief cells and is stored as a zymogen, which is activated by a falling pH level, resulting in cleavage of a polypeptide fragment to the active enzyme pepsin. Pepsin catalyzes hydrolysis of peptide bonds containing phenylalanine, tyrosine, and leucine. The most important pathway for pepsin secretion is stimulation of muscarinic receptors of the M1-type (cholinergic). The major function of pepsin is to initiate protein digestion, and pepsin functions optimally at a pH of 2.0 and is irreversibly denatured at a pH of 7.0 or greater. Finally, a mucoprotein, *intrinsic factor*, is secreted by parietal cells of the gastric mucosa. This factor is necessary for the absorption of cobalamin (vitamin B_{12}) from the terminal ileum. Histamine, acetylcholine, and gastrin stimulate intrinsic factor secretion. Atrophy of the parietal cells results in a deficiency of intrinsic factor and pernicious anemia. This deficiency can be corrected by parenteral administration of vitamin B_{12}. Total gastrectomy results in the permanent dependency of parenteral vitamin B_{12} administration.

PEPTIC ULCER DISEASE

Pathophysiology and Risk Factors

The pathogenesis of PUD involves a disequilibrium of acid secretion and mucosal defenses (Table 10.1). Although the exact etiology of this disequilibrium is not completely understood, research originating from work by Warren and Marshall in 1982 highlighted the importance of gastric colonization by *Helicobacter pylori*, which paved the way for successful medical management of PUD. The incidence of *H. pylori* infection is 80% to 95% in patients with duodenal ulcers (DUs) and 60% to 95% in patients with gastric ulcers (GUs). Evidence supporting the pathogenesis of *H. pylori* in DU disease is summarized in Table 10.2.

While *H. pylori* infection is a major risk factor in PUD, it alone is not *sufficient* as a precursor to PUD, which underlines the complexity of PUD pathogenesis as well as the importance of *H. pylori* testing in all patients with PUD (Table 10.3). Ingestion of nonsteroidal anti-inflammatory drugs (NSAIDs) has been shown to induce PUD and is present in the majority of *H. pylori*–negative patients with DU. Through inhibition of COX-1, NSAIDs decrease the cytoprotective and antisecretory effects of prostaglandins. The U.S. Food and Drug Administration (FDA) estimates the rate of NSAID-induced ulcers to be 2% to 4% per patient-year. The effects of *H. pylori* and NSAID exposure are synergistic, and empiric *H. pylori* testing on individuals committed to long-term NSAID therapy has been advocated. Other risk factors for PUD include smoking, hyperacidity (as an independent risk factor in DU and prepyloric GU), physiologic stress states (including trauma, burns, and sepsis), steroids, and polygenetic inheritance, as evident by a possible association with blood group O. A relationship between PUD and alcohol abuse is less clear, and there is no evidence that diet influences risk.

Clinical Features and Treatment

Many patients present with epigastric pain; often worse in the morning and relieved by eating or taking antacids. Pain referred to the back may signal perforation or penetration into the head of the pancreas. Physical examination is typically nonspecific in uncomplicated cases. The differential diagnosis includes dyspepsia, gastric and duodenal neoplasia, cholelithiasis, pancreatitis, and pancreatic neoplasia. Upper endoscopy is diagnostic and has replaced contrast radiography as the gold standard. Acid secretory studies are no longer routinely used.

TABLE 10.1 Factors modulating gastric mucosal protection

Stimulation	Inhibition
cAMP	NSAIDs
Prostaglandins	α-Adrenergic agonists
Cholinomimetics	Bile acids
CCK	Acetazolamide
Glucagon	Ethanol

cAMP, cyclic adenosine monophosphate; CCK, cholecystokinin; NSAIDs, nonsteroidal anti-inflammatory drugs.

TABLE 10.2 Support for the role of *helicobacter pylori* in ulcer disease

1. *H. pylori*–positive patients almost always demonstrate antral gastritis, characterized by nonerosive mucosal inflammation.
2. *H. pylori* binds only to gastric epithelium.
3. Eradication of *H. pylori* results in resolution of gastritis with antimicrobials, and recurrence is associated with reinfection.
4. Intragastric administration of isolated organism in animal models and in two humans resulted in lesions of chronic superficial gastritis.

From Mulholland MW. Duodenal ulcer. *Surgery: Scientific Principles and Practice*. 2nd ed. Philadelphia: Lippincott–Raven Publishers; 1997:768, with permission.

Of all dyspeptic patients referred for endoscopy, 13% have DUs, 10% have GUs, 2% have gastric cancer, and up to 15% have esophagitis. Benign ulcers have a typical appearance with sharp edges and a clean smooth base. Recent hemorrhage is characterized by an eschar or exudate. Histopathologic evaluation demonstrates nonspecific inflammation. Malignant ulcerations of gastric cancer, on the other hand, typically have thick, irregular margins and protrude into the gastric lumen. Even if a GU appears benign on endoscopy, the strong association between gastric cancer and ulceration mandate biopsy; at least four biopsies should be obtained by the endoscopist. Despite the predilection for higher acid secretion in patients with DUs, circulating serum gastrin levels are typically normal (50 to 100 pg/mL), and measuring gastrin levels is only helpful if *Zollinger–Ellison syndrome* (ZES) is suspected.

Diagnosis and eradication of *H. pylori* infection are paramount to successful therapy. For patients with an ulcer at endoscopy, biopsy of the tissue for urease testing (e.g., CLO or Campylobacter-like organism test) is highly accurate and allows rapid diagnosis. In the setting of acute bleeding, however, its sensitivity is decreased.

TABLE 10.3 Postulated pathogenetic factors in patients with DUs

Acid secretion
Increased acid secretory capacity
Increased basal secretion
Increased pentagastrin-stimulated output
Increased meal response
Abnormal gastric emptying
Environment
Cigarette smoking
NSAIDs
Helicobacter infection
Mucosal defense
Decreased duodenal HCO_3 ion production
Decreased gastric mucosal prostaglandin production

From Mulholland MW. Duodenal ulcer. In: Greenfield LJ, Mulholland MW, Oldham KT, et al., eds. *Surgery: Scientific Principles and Practice*. 2nd ed. Philadelphia: Lippincott–Raven Publishers; 1997:759, with permission.

Culture of *H. pylori* from a biopsied specimen, preferably from the antrum, is an alternative. *H. pylori* infection can also be achieved reliably with the urea breath test. Labeled urea is converted into ammonia and labeled carbon dioxide by the *H. pylori* urease in the stomach. The carbon dioxide diffuses into the rich bloody supply within the stomach wall and can be detected upon expiration. The sensitivity of urea breath testing is unaffected by active bleeding but decreases with antisecretory therapy. Other nonendoscopic means of diagnosis include stool antigen testing and serologic testing.

Medical therapy is directed toward both the reduction of acid secretion and eradication of *H. pylori*, if present. Successful treatment of *H. pylori* infection has dramatically reduced recurrent ulceration, which usually signifies reinfection (10% of cases). Various therapeutic combinations exist, and treatment with bismuth subsalicylate, metronidazole, tetracycline, and omeprazole has the highest cure rate (94% to 98%), but compliance is difficult to achieve. Antisecretory drugs include histamine receptor (H2) antagonists and proton pump inhibitors (PPIs). As mentioned previously, the parietal cell secretes acid into the stomach in response to three major stimuli: acetylcholine released by vagal postsynaptic neurons, histamine released in a paracrine fashion, and gastrin released by antral G cells. Histamine is the dominant of these three pathways, as the other two serve to enhance this interaction. As such, H2 antagonists effectively reduce parietal cell acid secretion. However, subsequent identification of the hydrogen–potassium ATPase "proton pump" as the final common pathway in acid secretion led to the development of PPIs. Subsequent meta-analyses demonstrated the superiority of PPIs over H2-blockers in healing gastroduodenal ulcers. Current recommendations for duration of PPI therapy for acute, uncomplicated GU and DU are 8 and 4 weeks, respectively. Current recommendations for complicated PUD (bleeding, perforation) include maintenance therapy with a PPI, although the long-term effects of sustained hypergastrinemia are not known. Another attractive option is *sucralfate*, an aluminum salt of sulfated sucrose. This polymer acts by providing a protective coat over the gastric and duodenal mucosa, which binds bile acids and inhibits pepsin while stimulating mucus, prostaglandin, and HCO_3 ion secretion. Side effects are minimal, and systemic absorption is virtually negligible. It is also the drug of choice for ulcer therapy during pregnancy. When administered at a dose of 1 g four times a day, eradication is achieved within 4 weeks in 80% of patients. *Misoprostol*, a prostaglandin analog, counters the prostaglandin-depleting effects of NSAIDs and is a useful adjunct for patients committed to long-term NSAID therapy. *Antacids* should be used as supplements to the antisecretory drugs mentioned earlier.

Surgical treatment for PUD is indicated for complications of PUD: hemorrhage, perforation, obstruction, or failure of medical management. Widely used procedures include (i) *truncal vagotomy and antrectomy*, (ii) *truncal vagotomy with drainage*, and (iii) *highly selective vagotomy*. Complete acid reduction is achieved by truncal vagotomy combined with resection of the gastric antrum. This entails a 50% resection of the distal stomach with a gastroduodenal (Billroth I resection) or gastrojejunal (Billroth II resection) anastomosis (Fig. 10.6). Truncal vagotomy must be combined with a drainage procedure, as denervation will result in impaired pyloric coordination and delayed gastric emptying of solids as first described by Dragstedt. The use of *pyloroplasty* offers the advantage of preserving continuity of the duodenal loop (hence the integrity of the hormonal milieu) and avoids the morbidity associated with

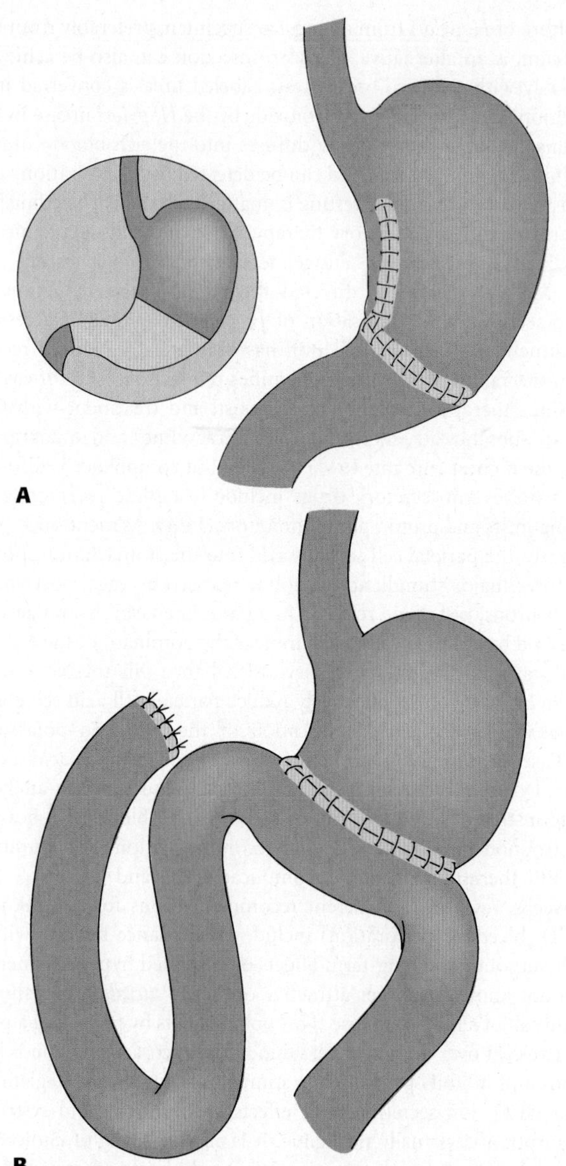

FIGURE 10.6 The anatomic differences between an antrectomy with **(A)** a Billroth I reconstruction and **(B)** a Billroth II resection. (From Mulholland MW, Lillemoe KD et al., eds. *Surgery: Scientific Principles and Practice.* 5th ed. Philadelphia: Lippincott Williams & Wilkins; 2011.)

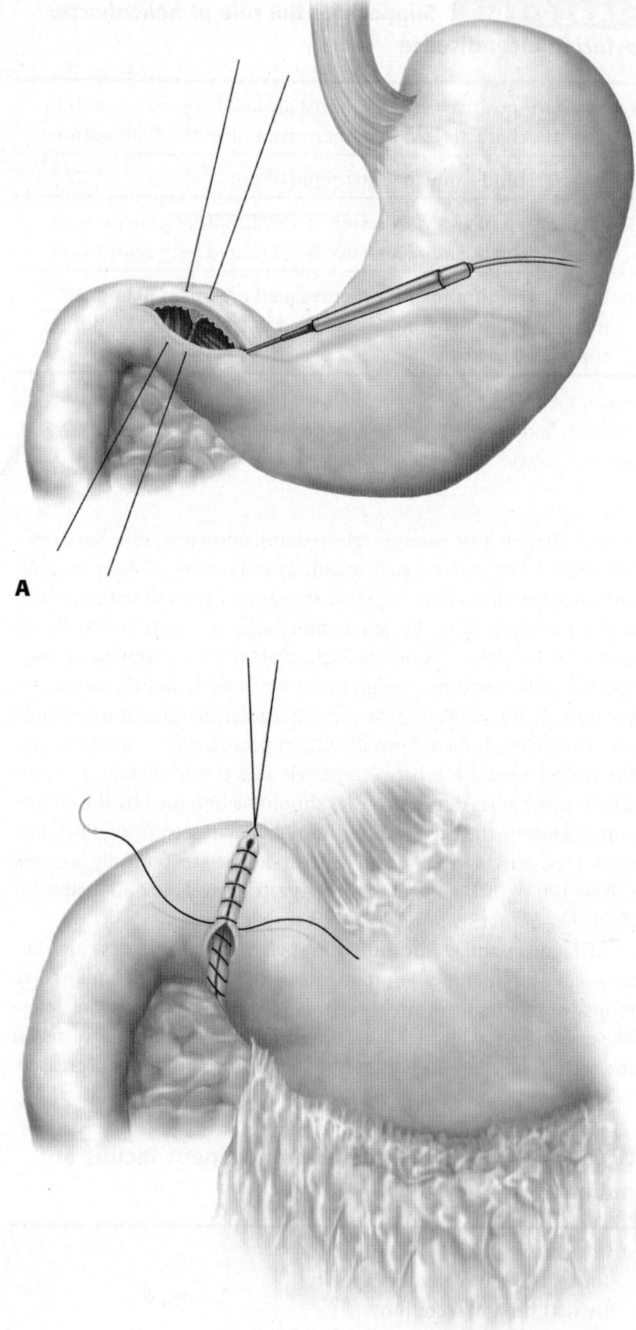

FIGURE 10.7 The Heineke–Mikulicz pyloroplasty enlarges the gastric outlet by closing a longitudinal pyloric incision **(A)** in a transverse fashion **(B)**. (From Etala E. *Atlas of Gastrointestinal Surgery*. Philadelphia: Lippincott–Raven Publishers; 1997:1085, with permission.)

an antrectomy or gastrojejunostomy (Fig. 10.7). Highly selective vagotomy involves division of the nerve fibers to the acid-secreting fundic mucosa while preserving the fibers to the antrum and the pylorus, thereby preserving gastric emptying (Fig. 10.8).

The choice of procedure should reflect the patient's clinical status and history. Since DUs are associated with hyperacidity, some acid-reducing procedure should be considered, even in an emergent operative setting. GUs, on the other hand, are variably associated with hyperacidity. The modified Johnson classification categorizes GUs according to their location and pathogenesis. Type I ulcers are usually found in the body of the stomach most often along the lesser curvature. Antral gastritis is always present, and in most cases, *H. pylori* infection is present. Type II ulcers are usually prepyloric and occur in association with DUs. Type III ulcers occur in the antrum and pyloric channel. Type IV ulcers occur high on the lesser curvature in the more proximal stomach, have a pathology similar to type I ulcers, and are similarly associated with decreased mucosal protection (Fig. 10.9). Type V ulcers are associated with NSAID use and can occur throughout the stomach. Traditionally, Johnson types II and III are due in part to hyperacidity. Surgical therapy should therefore include an acid-reducing procedure.

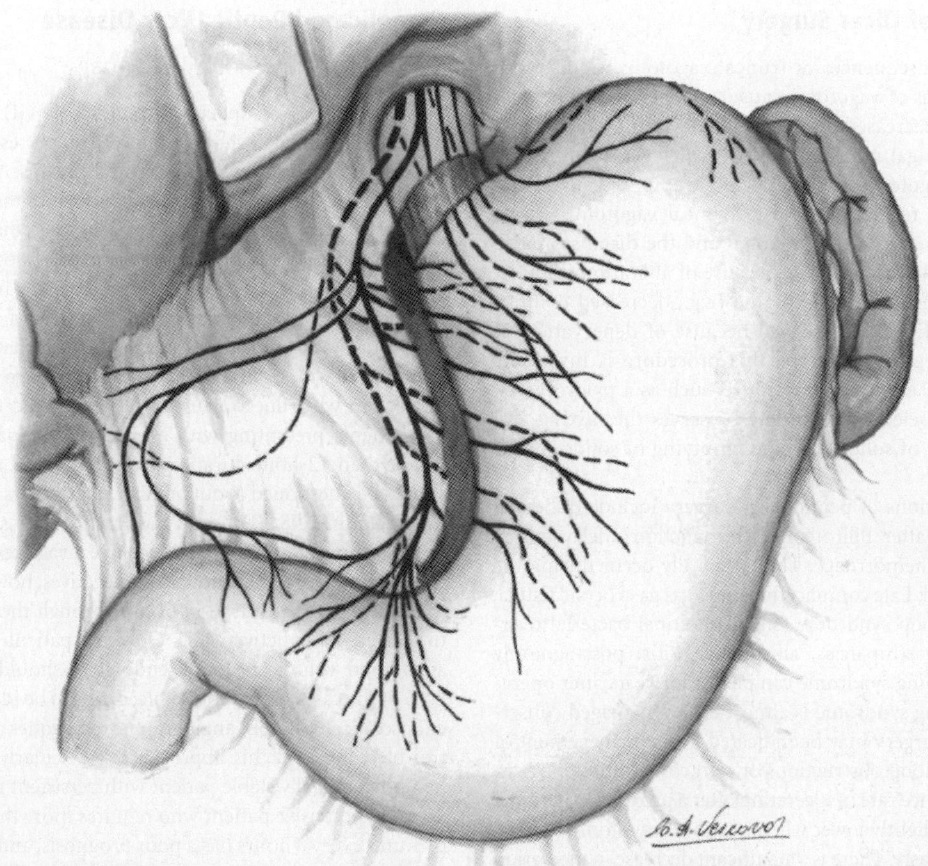

FIGURE 10.8 Unlike the truncal vagotomy, the proximal gastric vagotomy selectively denervates the lesser curvature of the stomach but spares the nerves to the pylorus and antrum. (From Etala E. *Atlas of Gastrointestinal Surgery*. Philadelphia: Lippincott–Raven Publishers; 1997:1047, with permission.)

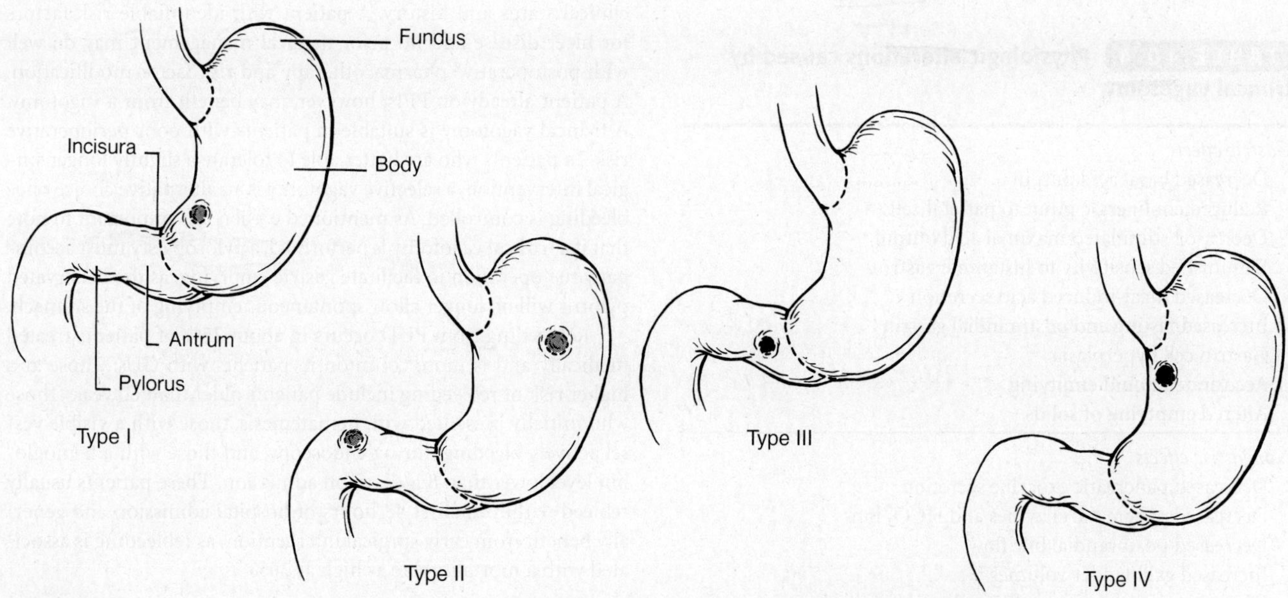

FIGURE 10.9 GUs can be classified into four types based on location and pathogenesis. (From Mulholland MW. Peptic ulcer disease. In: Bell RH, Rikkers LF, Mulholland MW, eds. *Digestive Tract Surgery: A Text and Atlas*. Philadelphia: Lippincott–Raven Publishers; 1996:190).

Complications of Ulcer Surgery

The physiologic consequences of truncal vagotomy are listed in Table 10.4. All forms of vagotomy cause postoperative hypergastrinemia owing to decreased luminal acid, loss of inhibitory feedback, and loss of vagal inhibition, all of which result in gastrin cell hyperplasia. Vagotomy also alters gastric emptying, as vagus-mediated receptive relaxation is lost. Truncal vagotomy affects the motor activity of both the proximal and the distal stomach. Liquids are emptied at a faster rate because of alteration in intraluminal pressure for any given volume (e.g., decreased compliance). Emptying of solids is delayed because of denervation of the pyloroantral region; therefore, this procedure is invariably accompanied by an emptying procedure, such as a pyloroplasty. Conversely, highly selective vagotomy preserves the mixing and triturating capacity of solid food, and emptying of solids is near normal.

Early complications of peptic ulcer surgery include duodenal stump dehiscence (after Billroth II reconstruction), delayed gastric emptying, and hemorrhage. These typically occur during the perioperative period. Late complications, such as gastrocolic fistula, roux stasis, blind loop syndrome (small intestinal bacterial overgrowth), chronic gastroparesis, alkaline gastritis, postvagotomy diarrhea, and dumping syndrome can persist for years after operation. While dumping syndrome is almost always managed conservatively, remedial surgery may be indicated in the management of afferent or efferent loop obstructions or refractory blind loop syndrome. The recurrence rate of ulceration after a proximal vagotomy is 10%; the rate is slightly lower when a truncal vagotomy is combined with pyloroplasty. There is a significant decrease in ulceration when truncal vagotomy is combined with antrectomy (1% to 2%). Ulcers almost always develop on the intestinal side of the anastomosis (also known as marginal ulcers). Patients classically complain of pain that is ameliorated by eating or by antacids. In some patients, pain is referred to the shoulder.

TABLE 10.4 Physiologic alterations caused by truncal vagotomy

Gastric effects
Decreased basal acid output
Reduced cholinergic input to parietal cells
Decreased stimulated maximal acid output
Diminished sensitivity to histamine gastrin
Decreased meal-induced acid secretion
Increased fasting and postprandial gastrin
Gastrin cell hyperplasia
Accelerated liquid emptying
Altered emptying of solids
Nongastric effects
Decreased pancreatic exocrine secretion
Decreased pancreatic enzymes and HCO_3 ions
Decreased postprandial bile flow
Increased gallbladder volumes
Diminished release of vagally mediated peptide hormones

From Mulholland MW. Duodenal ulcer. In: Greenfield LJ, Mulholland MW, Oldham KT, et al., eds. *Surgery: Scientific Principles and Practice*. 2nd ed. Philadelphia: Lippincott–Raven Publishers; 1997:768, with permission.

Complicated Peptic Ulcer Disease

Upper Gastrointestinal Hemorrhage

Common causes of upper gastrointestinal (GI) bleeding requiring hospital admission include peptic ulceration, esophageal or gastric bleeding from portal hypertension, and gastritis. An upper GI bleed is defined as bleeding that originates proximal to the ligament of Treitz. The presence of coffee-ground emesis indicates that blood has been in the stomach long enough for conversion of hemoglobin to methemoglobin. Melena (passage of black tarry stools) is a nonspecific sign that, in general, provides little insight into the rate of bleeding. The black color is due to *hematin*, the product of heme oxidation by bacterial and intestinal enzymes. *Hematochezia*, or the passage of bright red blood per rectum, when due to an upper GI source indicates massive bleeding.

Patients presenting with a history of hematemesis or melena of less than 12-hour duration require hospital admission. Patients should be questioned about predisposing factors for upper GI bleeding, including NSAID use. A nasogastric tube should be placed to check for intragastric blood; a positive lavage result can confirm an upper GI source of bleeding. False negatives, however, occur in 20% of bleeding DUs. Aspiration of bile through the tube may improve the negative predictive value. Once the patient has been stabilized and blood volume restored, endoscopy should be performed. In 80% of the cases, the source of bleeding can be identified and treated endoscopically. Rarely, angiographic techniques are required to control bleeding, and this approach is particularly well suited to the hemodynamically stable patient with persistent refractory bleeding.

A hypotensive patient who requires more than 4 units of blood or 1 unit every 8 hours has a poor prognosis, and surgical treatment is often indicated. In the operating room, a duodenotomy or gastroduodenotomy exposes the bleeding ulcer, allowing the surgeon to suture ligate points of active bleeding. This commonly entails three-point ligation of the gastroduodenal artery and its transverse branches. The decision of whether to concurrently perform an antisecretory procedure is a complex one that depends on the patient's clinical status and history. A patient with identifiable risk factors for ulcer disease and no prior medical management may do well with postoperative pharmacotherapy and risk factor modification. A patient already on PPIs, however, may benefit from a vagotomy. A truncal vagotomy is suitable in patients with poor perioperative risk. In patients who are better able to tolerate a slightly longer surgical intervention, a selective vagotomy is an alternative choice once bleeding is controlled. As mentioned earlier, it is important to note that if a truncal vagotomy is performed, a pyloroplasty must accompany the operation to facilitate gastric emptying, as the denervated pylorus will no longer allow spontaneous emptying of the stomach.

Rebleeding from PUD occurs in about 25% of patients treated medically and is more common in patients with GUs. Those at a higher risk of rebleeding include patients older than 60 years, those who initially presented with hematemesis, those with a visible vessel actively bleeding during endoscopy, and those with a hemoglobin level lower than 8 g/dL upon admission. These patients usually rebleed within the first 48 hours of hospital admission and generally benefit from early surgical intervention, as rebleeding is associated with a mortality rate as high as 30%.

Perforated Peptic Ulcer

The most common site of perforation for peptic ulcer is the anterior gastric or duodenal wall. Erosions of ulcers through the anterior wall tend to present with perforation rather than bleeding. The so-called *kissing ulcers* or posterior bleeding ulcers complicating an anterior perforation are rare and carry a high mortality rate. Following gastric perforation, patients present with sudden onset of severe upper abdominal pain. Pain may be referred to the shoulder or to the back. History of PUD is not a consistent finding. Classically, patients are severely distressed, lying still with the knees drawn up, and taking shallow breaths. There may be a temporary improvement of symptoms with the onset of bacterial peritonitis, as initial chemical peritonitis is diluted by peritoneal fluid. Patients are usually afebrile upon presentation with boardlike rigidity of the abdomen. The continual loss of air from the perforation can result in tympany and abdominal distention. Peristaltic sounds are usually reduced or absent. However, patients can present with abdominal pain without any classic physical findings, especially those taking chronic glucocorticoids. The initial diagnostic test is an upright chest film, which will demonstrate free intraperitoneal air. Duodenal leaks can track down the paracolic gutter and cause signs and symptoms that may be confused with appendicitis or colonic diverticulitis. Subclinical perforations can also be sealed off by the omentum or liver and present as a subdiaphragmatic or subphrenic abscess. Laboratory findings usually will include a mild leukocytosis (12,000/μL) in the early stages, which can rise during the course of the illness. Serum amylase levels are usually mildly elevated. If the diagnosis remains unclear, an abdominal computerized tomographic (CT) scan, which is very sensitive to free intraperitoneal air, can be obtained. Treatment is dictated by the overall condition of the patient but invariably begins with fluid resuscitation, intravenous antibiotics, PPIs, and a nasogastric tube. Surgical repair is often best achieved with an omental patch (Graham patch). Surgical treatment of ulcer disease with a truncal vagotomy or pyloroplasty is rarely necessary today given the efficacy of PPIs and directed *H. pylori* treatment. However, perforation in the presence of pyloric obstruction is best treated by pyloroplasty or a gastroenterostomy. Antrectomy combined with truncal vagotomy is another option. Nonoperative treatment with fluids and antibiotics is occasionally indicated but is associated with higher rates of peritoneal and subphrenic abscess. A conservative approach does not necessarily carry a higher mortality rate and has been shown to be effective if the risk of operative intervention is high. Delay in treatment, the presence of other systemic illnesses, and advanced age are associated with an increased mortality rate.

Pyloric Obstruction

Pyloric obstruction due to PUD is less common than perforation and is usually caused by DUs. Most patients have a long history of PUD, and up to one third have had some treatment for a previous obstruction or perforation. Anorexia and vomiting of undigested food without biliary staining is the usual presentation. A succussion splash can be elicited in some patients from gastric dilation and retained gastric contents, but a visible peristaltic wave in the abdominal wall is rare in adults. The usual laboratory studies reveal a metabolic alkalosis with hypochloremia, hypokalemia, hyponatremia, and increased HCO_3 ions. A large nasogastric tube should be passed into the stomach and gastric contents lavaged. Medical therapy consists of decompression of the stomach, which allows resolution of pyloric edema and muscular spasm. In most circumstances, improvement is seen within 72 hours of conservative management. Endoscopic evaluation is favored over an upper GI series because biopsy specimens can be obtained to exclude malignancy. Early surgical intervention is indicated if medical therapy and decompression do not relieve the obstruction within 1 week. Endoscopic-guided balloon dilatation can relieve symptoms in a subset of patients. The surgical treatment of choice in cases of chronic or recurrent obstruction is usually a truncal vagotomy and drainage procedure.

Zollinger–Ellison Syndrome

ZES is a rare cause of PUD caused by gastrin-secreting neuroendocrine tumors of the duodenum (80%) and pancreas (20%) called gastrinomas. While the majority of cases are sporadic, 20% occur in association with type I multiple endocrine neoplasia syndrome. Presentation usually includes symptoms of epigastric pain, heartburn, and diarrhea. Ulcers occurring in unusual locations such as the distal duodenum and jejunum, recurrent ulcers despite therapy, and PUD associated with diarrhea should always raise suspicion for ZES. Measurement of serum gastrin level and basal acid output (high serum gastrin despite a low gastric pH) is the initial diagnostic tests of choice, and a secretin stimulation test is positive in over 90% of affected patients. Somatostatin receptor scintigraphy and CT are used to localize lesions. Treatment varies between sporadic ZES and MEN-I–associated ZES. Due to the malignant potential of gastrinomas, it is recommended that patients with sporadic ZES undergo surgical exploration even when the gastrinoma is not localized preoperatively. In patients with MEN-I–associated ZES, gastrinomas are more likely to be located in the duodenum and to be multiple in number; subsequently, cure rates in this situation tend to be low. Generally, patients with gastrinomas (>2 cm) evident on imaging should undergo surgical resection. In patients with metastatic disease, most commonly to abdominal lymph nodes and the liver, treatment options include debulking surgery, systemic therapy, hepatic arterial embolization, and somatostatin analogue therapy.

GASTROESOPHAGEAL REFLUX DISEASE

Gastroesophageal reflux disease (GERD) is the most common GI disorder in the Western hemisphere, with a prevalence of approximately 5% to 10%. Its diagnosis is based upon symptoms or complications related to the reflux of stomach contents into the esophageal lumen. Patients principally note heartburn and regurgitation but may also complain of chest pain, wheezing, water brash, or dysphagia. In normal individuals, multiple physiologic mechanisms coincide to form a "high-pressure zone" within the lumen of the GE junction to prevent reflux. These mechanisms include the tonically contracted smooth muscle fibers of the distal esophagus known as the lower esophageal sphincter (LES), the sling fibers of the stomach and diaphragmatic crura, and the opposing intra-abdominal and intrathoracic pressures. Medical management of GERD includes lifestyle modifications and pharmacotherapy with PPIs. Antireflux surgery is reserved for GERD refractory to adequate medical management and for complications of the disease, such as severe esophagitis on endoscopy, benign stricture, Barrett metaplasia, or recurrent pulmonary manifestations. Typical preoperative evaluation includes endoscopy, manometry, pH monitoring, and esophagogram, all of which help identify those patients most likely to benefit from antireflux surgery. Multivariate analyses show a symptomatic improvement in up to 97% of those patients with typical symptoms, a documented response to acid suppression, and the presence of an abnormal 24-hour pH score.

There are several variations of the fundoplication; each has advantages and should be used rationally. Patients with early disease and normal esophageal length and motility should be treated with a laparoscopic or transabdominal *Nissen fundoplication*. If the patient is severely obese, a transthoracic approach may be the better procedure. For patients with decreased peristaltic amplitude in the distal esophagus, the *Belsey fundoplication*, which is characterized by a partial wrap (270 degrees), will result in fewer obstructive symptoms. If the esophagus is foreshortened because of chronic disease or the site of previous surgery, a *Collis gastroplasty* with a partial wrap is a reasonable option. In the presence of a nondilatable esophageal stricture, high-grade dysplasia, or esophageal carcinoma, a total esophagectomy should be performed. The essential principles of the fundoplication are identification and preservation of the vagus nerve and the anterior hepatic branch, dissection of the esophagus, crural repair, mobilization and division of the short gastric vessels, and, lastly, creation of a loose wrap enveloping the anterior and posterior wall of the fundus around the esophagus.

SURGICAL TREATMENT FOR MORBID OBESITY

The surgical treatment of morbid obesity has become more frequent in the United States, owing to the increasing disease burden. Over the past 40 years, the prevalence of morbid obesity has increased from 13% to 35%. Obesity is defined as having a body mass index (BMI) greater than 30 kg/m^2. Patients with severe obesity have a BMI greater than 35 kg/m^2, and patients classified as morbidly obese have a BMI greater than 40 kg/m^2. Potentially reversible complications related to obesity include obstructive sleep apnea, hypertension, coronary artery disease, nonalcoholic fatty liver disease, adult-onset diabetes mellitus, and pseudotumor cerebri. Bariatric surgery is recommended for patients who are severely obese with obesity-related complications or morbidly obese. Previous failure of medically supervised weight reduction, no active history of alcohol or other substance abuse, acceptable medical risk for surgery, and psychosocial stability (i.e., they are realistic in their expectations and are capable of a long-term commitment) are additional requirements.

Bariatric surgery has changed drastically in the last 2 decades. Vertical banded gastroplasty (VBG), adjustable gastric banding (AGB), jejunoileal bypass, and biliopancreatic diversion with duodenal switch (DS) have largely been supplanted by *Roux-en-Y gastric bypass* (RYGB) and vertical sleeve gastrectomy (VSG). Additionally, the majority of bariatric procedures are now being done in laparoscopic or robotic fashion, which affords comparable weight loss to open procedures.

RYGB is a combination restrictive and malabsorptive procedure that involves bypass of most of the stomach, the entire duodenum, and an additional 100 to 150 cm of the small intestine. It is the treatment of choice in most centers. Sleeve gastrectomy is restrictive procedure that reduces the size of the stomach to less than 25% of its original volume by resection of a large portion of the stomach along the greater curvature including the entire fundus. Data support use of sleeve gastrectomy in the extremely obese.

GI leak at anastomoses or staple lines is the most significant technical complication of bariatric surgery. Patients often present with tachycardia, tachypnea, fever, pain, or leukocytosis. Early reexploration and source control are paramount. Persistent leak after sleeve gastrectomy can sometimes require conversion to RYGB. Anastomotic stricture or stenosis can also complicate bypass and sleeve gastrectomy. Barium swallow evaluations can assist with diagnosis. Endoscopy and subsequent dilation are diagnostic and potentially therapeutic. Marginal ulceration is also a relatively common complication after RYGB occurring in approximately 10% of patients. PPI therapy and smoking cessation are mainstays of treatment. Internal herniation through mesenteric defects with risk of bowel compromise is a delayed complication after RYGB, especially in those who demonstrate good weight loss. Colicky abdominal pain is characteristic. Cross-sectional imaging is frequently equivocal and surgical exploration is indicated in the presence of clinical suspicion. Late complications of bariatric surgery include dumping syndrome, nutrient and vitamin deficiency, and failure to sustain weight loss sometimes requiring revision surgery.

GASTRIC CANCER

In the United States, in 2014, 22,200 new cases of gastric cancer are expected to result in 10,990 deaths. For reasons that are not entirely clear, the past 80 years have witnessed a steady decline in the incidence of gastric cancer in the United States; it is now the 15th most common cancer. Possible explanations are a relatively low prevalence of *H. pylori* infection and features of the American diet. The increasing predominance of proximal gastric carcinomas has been attributed to an epidemic of obesity and increasing prevalence of GERD.

Lauren described two histologic subtypes of gastric adenocarcinoma: intestinal and diffuse. The intestinal subtype, unlike the diffuse, is associated with precursor lesions and usually arises in the distal stomach. Indeed, one theory proposes a progression from atrophic gastritis to intestinal metaplasia, and finally gastric dysplasia. Therefore, conditions associated with atrophic gastritis, such as pernicious anemia, chronic *H. pylori* infection, autoimmune gastritis, and prior distal gastrectomy, are all risk factors for the development of intestinal-type gastric cancer. The adenomatous gastric polyps, which are typically found incidentally on endoscopy, represent another precursor lesion. Polyps greater than 2 cm in size carry a 10% to 20% risk of containing a focus of adenocarcinoma. Other risk factors include smoking, GUs, Epstein–Barr virus (EBV) infection, familial predisposition, and diet (high in dietary nitrates and salt and low in vitamin C and raw fruits and vegetables). No association with alcohol has been demonstrated. The diffuse subtype is not associated with precursor lesions, often arises in the cardia, and rarely forms a discrete mass or ulcer. It carries a worse prognosis.

Gastric adenocarcinoma has a variety of morphologic presentations including ulcerating carcinoma, polypoid carcinoma, superficial spreading carcinoma, and linitis plastica. *Linitis plastica* involves all the layers of the gastric wall. The stomach loses its pliability because of malignant infiltration. Most patients have metastatic disease at the time of presentation.

Patients with gastric cancer frequently present with new-onset epigastric discomfort in the setting of chronic dyspepsia. Anorexia develops early with concurrent weight loss. Vomiting is associated with pyloric obstruction, whereas involvement of the cardia is associated with dysphagia. A mass can be palpated in some patients. Occult blood can be detected in the stool of 50% of patients; frank anemia is less common. Unfortunately, symptoms often indicate advanced disease and most gastric cancer in the United States are diagnosed when it is locally advanced or metastatic. Physical signs of dissemination include a palpable *Virchow node* in the left supraclavicular space, indicating metastasis along the thoracic duct, and palpable ovarian metastases (*Krukenberg tumors*). "Drop" metastases can occasionally be palpated as a *Blumer shelf* on rectal examination. Distant metastasis can involve the liver, lungs, brain, or bone. Carcinoembryonic antigen level is usually elevated in the presence of metastatic disease.

The initial diagnostic procedure of choice is an upper endoscopy. At least four biopsies should be taken from polyps or ulcers that are suspicious for cancer. An endoscopic ultrasound (EUS) performed at that time increases the accuracy of both primary tumor and lymph node staging. CT can identify malignant ascites, bulky abdominal adenopathy, and visceral metastases greater than 5 mm. Unfortunately, CT occult metastases occur in nearly one third of cases. In the past, small intra-abdominal metastases less than 5 mm and peritoneal disease went undetected. In more recent years, diagnostic laparoscopy has emerged as a valuable and underutilized staging modality. Peritoneal washings for cytology at the time of diagnostic laparoscopy have substantial clinical yield as positive cytology denotes stage IV disease and is a powerful independent predictor of outcome. Positron emission tomography is an increasingly popular component of staging. While tumor markers (CEA, CA 19-9) are regularly measured as part of the initial workup, their greatest utility lies in gauging treatment response and monitoring for recurrent disease.

Surgical resection with negative margins and removal of regional lymph nodes. The location of the tumor dictates the extent of resection necessary. Antral tumors are treated with subtotal gastrectomy with *en bloc* resection of the omentum, the subpyloric lymph nodes, and the left gastric artery and lymph nodes. Bowel continuity is then reestablished, either with Billroth II or with Roux-en-Y reconstruction. Proximal and distal margins of 5 to 6 cm are traditionally sought, though this margin threshold is not supported by high-level evidence. Proximal gastric cancers almost always require total gastrectomy; there are no data demonstrating the superiority of esophagogastrectomy over total gastrectomy assuming sufficient negative margins. Siewert and colleagues proposed a classification scheme for GE junction tumors to guide surgical management (Table 10.5). Type I tumors are managed with subtotal esophagectomy. Type III tumors most often require total gastrectomy. Type II tumors are thought to behave more similarly to type III cancers and thus can be managed with transabdominal total gastrectomy, provided that appropriate margins and a tension-free anastomosis can be achieved.

Unresectable tumors causing bleeding or pyloric obstruction may require a palliative gastrojejunostomy or gastrectomy. The latter should be avoided when possible to limit complications

TABLE 10.5 Siewert classification of tumors of the esophagogastric junction

Type	Anatomic Criteria
I	Adenocarcinoma of the distal esophagus that may infiltrate the GE junction from above
II	Adenocarcinoma of the cardia proper arising at the GE junction
III	Adenocarcinoma of the subcardial stomach that infiltrates the GE junction from below

TABLE 10.6 "D" extent of lymphadenectomy

Extent	Area of Resection
D0	Anything less than D1
D1	All nodal tissue within 3 cm of primary tumor along greater and lesser curvature of the stomach
D2	D1 + celiac axis nodal tissue ± distal pancreatectomy/splenectomy
D3	D2 + nodal tissue in hepatoduodenal ligament and root of mesentery + distal pancreatectomy/splenectomy
D4	D3 + retroperitoneal para-aortic lymph nodes

(e.g., duodenal stump leak) that delay systemic therapy. Decompressive gastrostomy and feeding jejunostomy tubes can be used for symptom palliation in challenging cases.

The extent of lymphadenectomy required for curative resection is controversial. The "D" nomenclature system standardizes the extent of lymphadenectomy and is outlined in Table 10.6. Several Western studies have failed to reproduce the survival benefit previously observed with extended lymphadenectomy in the East. Most recently, long-term follow-up data from have suggested a disease-free survival advantage with extended lymphadenectomy. Many US centers now advocate a "modified" D2 resection with preservation of the tail of the pancreas and spleen in order to minimize the perioperative morbidity and mortality associated with traditional D2 resections. Notwithstanding extent of lymphadenectomy, examination of at least 15 lymph nodes is self-recommending and has been adopted as a part of consensus guidelines to allow for accurate staging and rational application of adjuvant therapy.

Adjuvant monotherapy for gastric cancer, including chemotherapy, radiation, and intraperitoneal chemotherapy, has not consistently proven efficacious. A randomized prospective trial (Intergroup Trial) demonstrated a survival advantage with combined adjuvant 5-FU and leucovorin and external beam radiation following curative resection. Perioperative (pre- and postoperative) chemotherapy-only protocols (MAGIC Trial) have also been shown to confer a survival benefit over surgery alone. Theoretical benefits of neoadjuvant therapy include potential tumor down-staging, assessment of tumor biology, and responsiveness to therapy, as well as better tolerance of chemotherapy or radiotherapy. The optimal sequence for administration of chemo- and radiotherapy in the management of gastric cancer remains an area of ongoing investigation. Unfortunately, despite advances in medical and surgical therapy, the overall 5-year survival rate for gastric adenocarcinoma in the United States is estimated at about 27%.

OTHER GASTRIC TUMORS

Gastric lymphoma is the second most common malignancy of the stomach and occurs as mucosal-associated lymphoid tissue lymphoma (MALT) or non-Hodgkin's lymphoma or (NHL). Risk factors include *H. pylori* and immunosuppression. Symptoms are similar to those seen with gastric adenocarcinoma, and only a minority of patients experience B-symptoms. Diagnosis is made by endoscopy with biopsy. CT and sometimes bone marrow biopsy are used for staging. In the absence of complications such as bleeding, obstruction, or perforation, gastric lymphomas are managed nonsurgically. Low-grade MALT lymphoma can be managed with *H. pylori* therapy alone. Lymphomas that are more advanced are treated with chemoradiotherapy.

The stomach is the most common location of gastrointestinal stromal tumors (GIST). These tumors are thought to arise from interstitial cells of Cajal, and diagnosis is confirmed by immunohistochemical staining for the tyrosine kinase receptor cKIT. While many GISTs are discovered incidentally on cross-sectional imaging, some present with symptoms secondary to mass effect. Preoperative biopsy is often unnecessary when the endoscopic or imaging features of the tumor suggest GIST. Due to the range of biologic aggressiveness, primary surgical resection is indicated in the absence of metastatic or locally advanced disease. The goal of surgery is resection with grossly negative margins, which can often be accomplished with nonanatomic gastric wedge resection. There is limited role for formal anatomic gastric resection or lymph node sampling. Patients with high-risk GISTs characterized by size greater than 10 cm or greater than 5 mitoses/hpf are often treated with the selective tyrosine kinase inhibitor imatinib (Gleevec) postoperatively. Very large GISTs or those that may necessitate multivisceral resections may be treated with neoadjuvant Gleevec following diagnostic biopsy.

Gastric carcinoids are rare tumors often discovered incidentally in an otherwise asymptomatic patient. Type I and II carcinoids are often small, multiple, and indolent. Both are associated with hypergastrinemia—type I with atrophic gastritis and type II with ZES. These lesions can often be managed with endoscopic resection. Rarely antrectomy to reduce gastrin production is indicated for progressive type I disease. Surgical management of a gastrinoma often leads to regression or stability of small type II lesions. Type III gastric carcinoids are larger and often biologically aggressive. In the absence of diffuse metastatic disease, formal gastrectomy with lymph node dissection is indicated. Metastatic disease can be managed with cytoreductive debulking surgery, and octreotide can be employed for treatment of the symptoms of carcinoid syndrome.

Suggested Readings

Baker RJ, Fisher JE, eds. *Mastery of Surgery*. 4th ed. Philadelphia: Lippincott Williams & Wilkins; 2001.

Cameron JL, ed. *Current Surgical Therapy*. 8th ed. St. Louis: Mosby; 2004.

Mulholland MW. Duodenal ulcer. In: Greenfield LJ, Mulholland MW, Oldham KT, et al., eds. *Surgery: Scientific Principles and Practice*. 2nd ed. Philadelphia: Lippincott–Raven Publishers; 1997.

Mulholland MW. Gastric anatomy and physiology. In: Greenfield LJ, Mulholland MW, Oldham KT, et al., eds. *Surgery: Scientific Principles and Practice*. 3rd ed. Philadelphia: Lippincott Williams & Wilkins; 2001.

CHAPTER

11 The Small Bowel

JANE J. KEATING AND STEVEN E. RAPER

KEY POINTS

- Small bowel obstruction: Both the diagnosis and management of small bowel obstruction are common problems for the general surgeon. Although often managed nonoperatively, it is important to recognize the need for immediate surgical intervention including closed loop obstruction and/or evidence of bowel ischemia. Additionally, when conservative management fails to alleviate the obstruction, surgery is often indicated.
- Small bowel Crohn's disease: Most patients with Crohn's disease will eventually require surgical intervention. Common indications for surgery include an acute Crohn's flare, obstruction, fistula formation, and intractability.
- Small bowel fistulas: The primary sources of morbidity and mortality from small bowel fistulas are malnutrition, electrolyte imbalance, and sepsis. Consequently, initial management focuses on providing optimal nutrition, correction of the fluid and electrolyte derangements, and control of sepsis with appropriate antibiotics and judicious surgical drainage.
- Visceral ischemia: The diagnosis of acute mesenteric ischemia should ideally be made before bowel infarction develops. Selective mesenteric angiography is considered the gold standard in diagnosis, but newer imaging modalities are changing the algorithm. If there are signs and symptoms of peritonitis, laparotomy is mandatory; however, even in this setting, angiography may assist in the identification of the cause of bowel ischemia.
- Small bowel neoplasms: Tumors of the small bowel are less common than are those of the colon or rectum. Benign tumors are more commonly asymptomatic but may manifest as lower GI hemorrhage or as the lead point for intussusception.

OVERVIEW

The small bowel is a highly specialized, hollow viscus, approximately 8 m in length; its major function is to absorb nutrients. Additionally, the small bowel has a variety of endocrinologic and immunologic functions.

ANATOMY AND PHYSIOLOGY

The anatomy of the small bowel is well adapted to its highly specialized function. The small bowel consists of three sections: the *duodenum* (approximately 40 cm in length), the *jejunum* (approximately 200 cm in length), and the *ileum* (approximately 300 cm in length). The jejunum and the ileum are covered by visceral peritoneum and are tethered to the posterior abdominal wall by a mesentery. The duodenum, a partially retroperitoneal organ, is composed of four portions. The first portion, the *duodenal bulb*, lies superior to the pancreatic head and anterior to the gastroduodenal artery (Fig. 11.1) and common bile duct (CBD). This portion of the duodenum is the only intraperitoneal portion and derives its blood supply from the supraduodenal branch of the hepatic artery and the gastroduodenal artery. Importantly, it is the site of 90% of duodenal ulcerations. The second portion of the duodenum abuts the head of the pancreas and is retroperitoneal. The ampulla of Vater, through which the major and minor pancreatic ducts enter the duodenum, is located within this portion. The third portion of the duodenum abuts the uncinate process of the pancreas and is also retroperitoneal, coursing between the superior mesenteric artery (SMA) and the aorta. The second and third portions of the duodenum receive their blood supply from the anterosuperior and posterosuperior pancreaticoduodenal branches of the gastroduodenal artery and the anteroinferior and posteroinferior pancreaticoduodenal branches of the SMA. The fourth, or ascending, portion of the duodenum receives its blood supply from the first jejunal branch of the SMA. The *ligament of Treitz* is a suspensory fold of peritoneum derived from the right crus of the diaphragm and serves as an anatomic landmark for the transition between the duodenum and the jejunum.

The small bowel may be differentiated from the remainder of the intestine both grossly and radiographically by the *valvulae conniventes*, circular folds of mucosa and submucosa that markedly increase absorptive surface area. Additional gross features allow differentiation of the jejunum from the ileum. The jejunum is of larger diameter and has a thinner mesentery compared to the ileum. Additionally, the mesenteric vessels of the jejunum form only one or two arterial arcades and send out long vasa recta. In contrast, the ileum is smaller in diameter and has a thicker mesentery, which contains multiple arterial arcades that give off short vasa recta.

Embryologically, the jejunum and the ileum are derived predominantly from the midgut and, as such, derive their blood supply from the SMA. Venous drainage is via the superior mesenteric vein (SMV). Additionally, the abundant lymphatic drainage of the small bowel allows for fat absorption, which is integral to the small bowel's role in digestion.

The bowel wall is composed of four layers: the mucosa, the submucosa, the muscularis, and the serosa. The innermost layer, the *mucosa*, lines the bowel lumen and is characterized by its many villi and crypts (crypts of Lieberkühn), which provide the small bowel

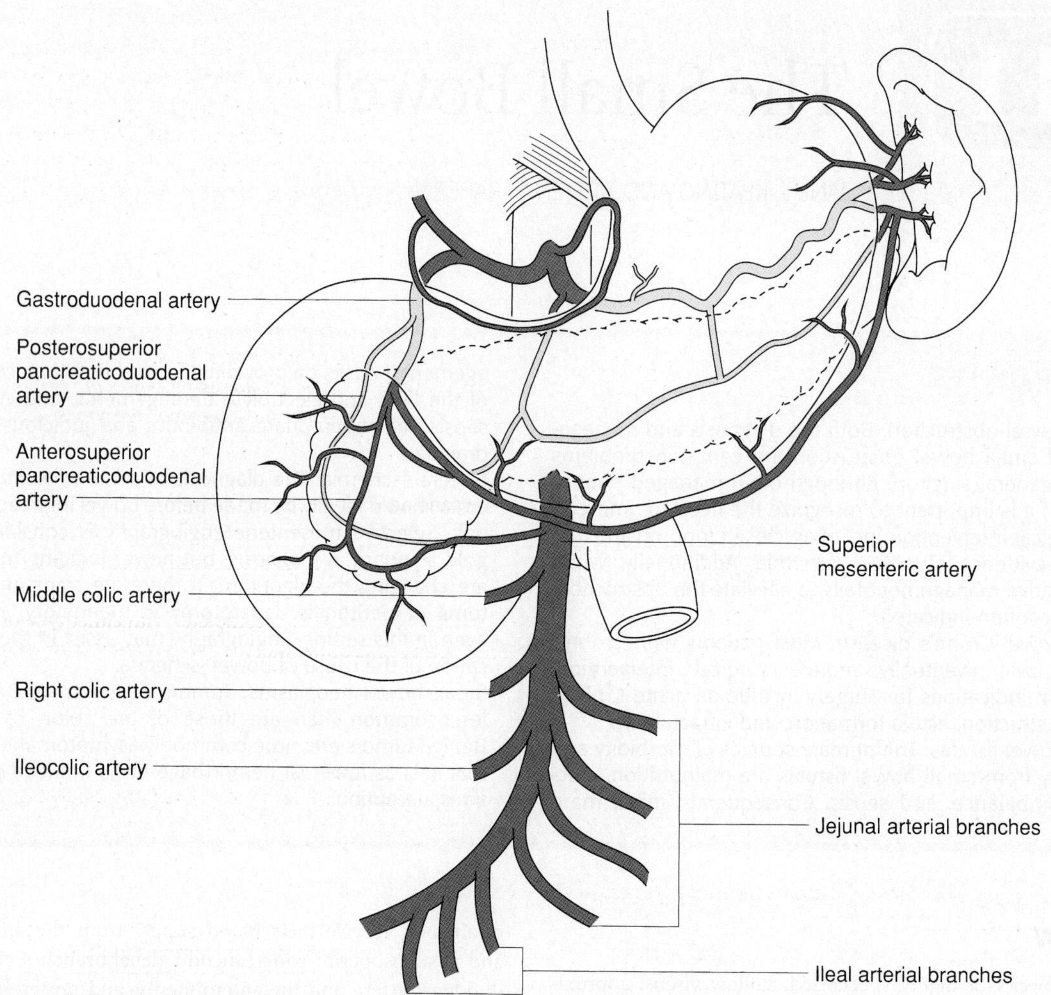

FIGURE 11.1 The distribution of the celiac artery, the SMA, and their branches. (From Greenfield LJ, Mulholland MW, Oldham KT, et al., eds. *Surgery: Scientific Principles and Practice*. 3rd ed. Philadelphia: Lippincott Williams & Wilkins; 2001:1693, with permission.)

with a massive surface area important to its secretory and absorptive roles (Figs. 11.2 and 11.3). The small bowel mucosa may be further subdivided into three layers: the muscularis mucosa, the lamina propria, and the epithelium. The outermost layer, the muscularis mucosa, is a thin layer of the muscle separating the mucosa from the submucosa. The middle mucosal layer, the lamina propria, is a continuous layer of connective tissue between the muscularis mucosa and epithelium and serves as a supportive base for the villi and a protective barrier against microorganisms. Cells of the immune system reside in this layer, including Peyer's patches. Peyer's patches are aggregates of lymphoid tissue containing immune cells including macrophages, dendritic cells, B lymphocytes, and T lymphocytes. They appear as elongated thickenings of the intestinal epithelium and are involved in immune surveillance of the intestinal ileum. The epithelium constitutes the innermost layer of the mucosa. The major functions of the epithelial lining of the villi and crypts of Lieberkühn are digestion, absorption, cell renewal, and secretion of hormones. The fibroelastic *submucosa* serves as a support and strength layer and contains blood vessels, lymphatics, and nerves. The *muscularis* is composed of an inner circular and an outer longitudinal layer. The muscle cells that constitute these layers have specialized gaps in their cell membranes, which allow the bowel to function as an electrical syncytium. Sandwiched between the layers are a group of ganglion cells that constitute the myenteric (Auerbach) plexus. The *serosa* is the outermost layer of the small bowel and is composed of flattened mesothelial cells.

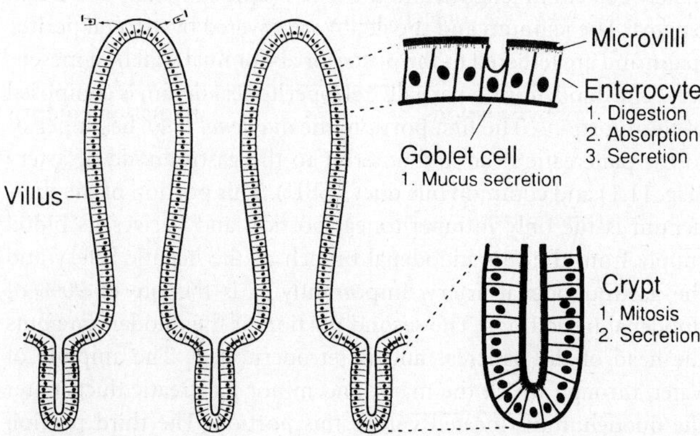

FIGURE 11.2 Microscopic anatomy of the small intestine mucosa. (From Johnson LR. *Essential Medical Physiology*. New York: Raven Press; 1992:508, with permission.)

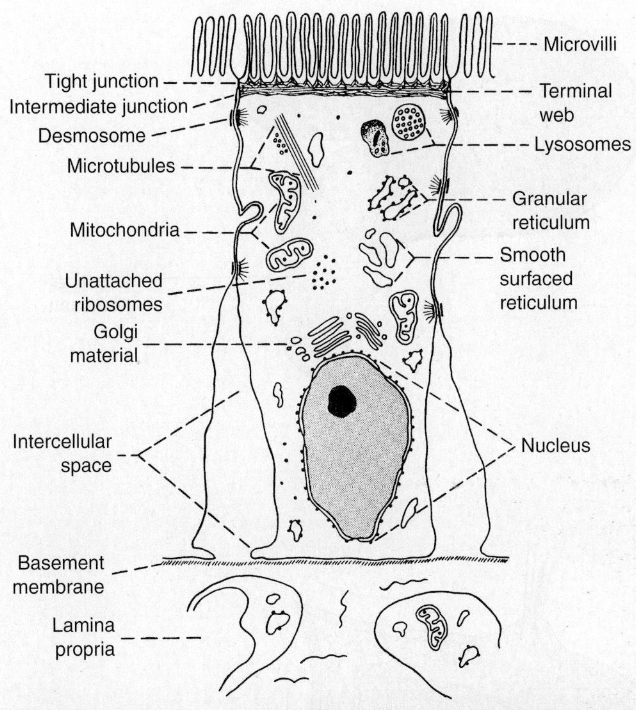

FIGURE 11.3 An intestinal epithelial cell. (From Trier JS, Rubin CE. Electron microscopy of the small intestine: a review. *Gastroenterology.* 1965;49:574, with permission.)

Innervation of the small bowel comes from both the sympathetic and parasympathetic nervous systems. Three sympathetic ganglia are located around the base of the SMA and control blood vessel tone and, to a lesser extent, gut secretory function and motility. Pain is mediated through visceral afferent fibers of the sympathetic nervous system. Parasympathetic nerve fibers are derived from the vagus nerve and primarily regulate gut secretory function and motility.

DISEASES OF THE SMALL BOWEL

Obstruction

Obstruction is one of the most common pathologic processes affecting the small bowel. There are many causes of small bowel obstruction (SBO), but the three most common are adhesive disease, hernias, and tumors (Table 11.1). Greater than 60% of SBOs result from adhesive disease. Lower abdominal and pelvic operations (appendectomy and adnexal procedures) appear to be associated with a higher incidence of adhesive obstruction than are upper abdominal procedures. In patients with no prior history of abdominal surgery, hernias are the most common cause of SBO (Fig. 11.4). SBOs may be further characterized as partial or complete. With either type of obstruction, all or part of the bowel wall may be incarcerated or strangulated.

Clinical Manifestations

Patients typically present with nausea, vomiting, crampy abdominal pain, distention, obstipation, and high-pitched or absent bowel

TABLE 11.1 Classification of adult mechanical intestinal obstructions

Intraluminal	Intramural	Extrinsic
Foreign bodies	Congenital	Adhesions
Barium inspissation (colon)	Atresia, stricture, or stenosis	Congenital
Bezoar	Web	Ladd or Meckel's bands
Inspissated feces	Intestinal duplication	Postoperative
Gallstone	Meckel's diverticulum	Postinflammatory
Meconium (cystic fibrosis)	Inflammatory process	Hernias
Parasites	Crohn's disease	External
Other (e.g., swallowed objects, enteroliths)	Diverticulitis	Internal
Intussusception	Chronic intestinal ischemia or postischemic stricture	Volvulus
Polypoid, exophytic lesions	Radiation enteritis	External mass effect
—	Medication induced (nonsteroidal anti-inflammatory drugs, potassium chloride tablets)	Abscess
—	Neoplasms	Annular pancreas
—	Primary bowel (malignant or benign)	Carcinomatosis
—	Secondary (metastases, especially melanoma)	Endometriosis
—	Traumatic	Pregnancy
—	Intramural hematoma of duodenum	Pancreatic pseudocyst

From Greenfield LJ, Mulholland MW, Oldham KT, et al., eds. *Surgery: Scientific Principles and Practice*. 3rd ed. Philadelphia: Lippincott Williams & Wilkins; 2001:800, with permission.

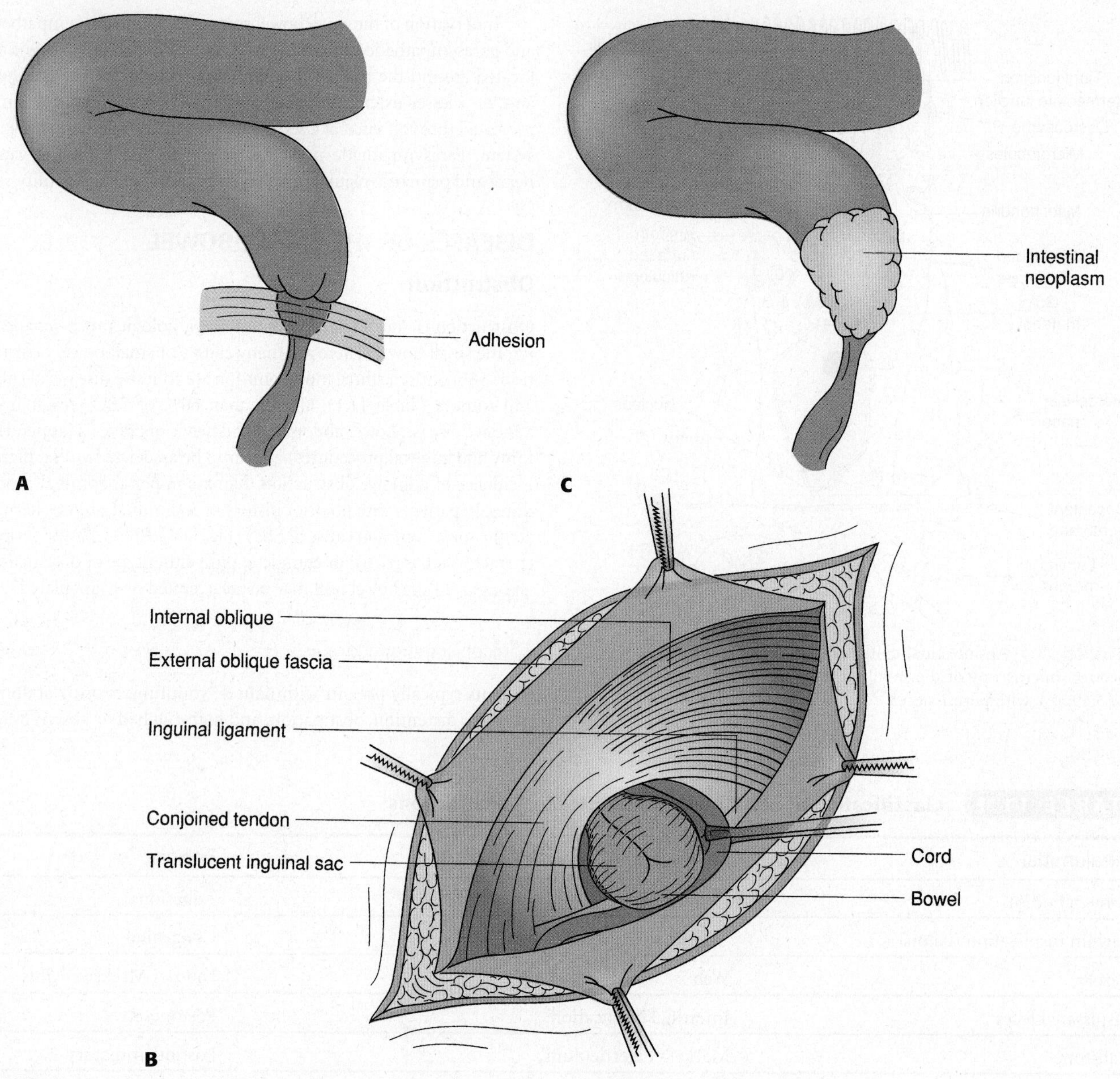

FIGURE 11.4 Schematic illustration of different forms of simple mechanical obstruction. Simple obstruction is most often due to adhesion **(A)**, groin hernia **(B)**, or neoplasm **(C)**. (From Mulholland MW, Lillemoe KD, Doherty GM, et al., eds. *Surgery: Scientific Principles and Practice*. 5th ed. Philadelphia: Lippincott Williams & Wilkins; 2011.)

sounds (Table 11.2). The pain may be intermittent, intense, and accompanied by prominent bowel sounds (the so-called *peristaltic rush*). Obstipation, severe and persistent constipation, is particularly concerning as it suggests high-grade or complete obstruction. Clinically relevant signs and symptoms include tachycardia, fever, localized pain or peritonitis, and leukocytosis, which may reflect strangulation of bowel. Hypokalemic, hypochloremic, metabolic alkalosis, or metabolic acidosis may also be observed. The hematocrit may be falsely elevated because of hemoconcentration resulting from volume depletion. The presence of anemia may indicate an underlying malignancy.

Patients with SBO should be evaluated for the presence of external or internal hernias, especially for obstruction in the absence of prior surgery. External hernias include those found in the inguinal canal, the femoral canal, and in previous incisions. Internal hernias include those related to the inadequate closure of mesenteric defects created by prior operations, congenital mesenteric defects, and obturator foramen hernias.

Radiographic Diagnosis

If SBO is suspected, an obstruction series (upright chest, supine and upright abdominal radiographs) may be obtained. Findings consistent with an SBO include dilated loops of bowel and air–fluid levels, often with a steplike appearance and a paucity of gas beyond the point of obstruction.

Computerized tomography (CT) scan of the abdomen and pelvis with intravenous and oral contrast (Gastrografin) is a frequently utilized diagnostic tool for obstruction and may delineate the cause of SBO. CT imaging can detect the specific location of a lesion (by visualization of a transition point between proximal dilated and distal collapsed small bowel) and may demonstrate signs of bowel

TABLE 11.2 Symptoms and signs of bowel obstructions

Symptom or Sign	Proximal Small Bowel (Open Loop)	Distal Small Bowel (Open Loop)	Small Bowel or Sign (Closed Loop)	Colon and Rectum
Pain	Colicky, often relieved by vomiting	Intermittent, sometimes constant	Progressive, intermittent, or constant, worsens quickly	Continuous
Vomiting	Frequent, bilious, large volume	Low volume, low frequency, becomes feculent with time	May be prominent (reflex)	Intermittent, not prominent; feculent when present
Tenderness	Epigastric or periumbilical, usually mild unless strangulation present	Diffuse and progressive	Diffuse and progressive	Diffuse
Distention	Absent	Moderate to marked	Often absent	Marked
Obstipation	May not be present	Present	May not be present	Present

From Greenfield LJ, Mulholland M, Oldham KT, et al., eds. *Surgery: Scientific Principles and Practice*. 2nd ed. Philadelphia: Lippincott–Raven Publishers; 1997:819, with permission.

infarction or perforation. CT scanning is approximately 95% sensitive and specific in making the correct diagnosis. Furthermore, in some cases, the oral contrast may provide a therapeutic effect. Gastrografin (diatrizoic acid) is a hyperosmolar gastrointestinal (GI) water-soluble agent, which has been shown to speed the resolution of partial SBO and has also been shown to reduce hospital length of stay. CT findings that require immediate surgical intervention include closed loop obstruction and strangulation. Radiographic findings of a closed loop obstruction include a C- or U-shaped section of bowel with dilation of the loop and proximal bowel and decompression of the distal bowel (Fig. 11.5). Strangulation is suggested by thickening of the bowel wall, *pneumatosis intestinalis*, ascites, or mesenteric hematoma.

Barium upper GI tract series with small bowel follow through (SBFT) may also be employed in the evaluation of the SBO, and has greater than 80% accuracy in delineating obstruction in subacute cases. Following the introduction of oral contrast, serial abdominal plain films are taken over time to follow the transit of contrast. This study is helpful in differentiating adynamic ileus from mechanical obstruction. The former is characterized by an overall delay in contrast transit time, whereas a discrete transition point may be noted in the case of the latter. Barium studies should be used judiciously in the setting of obstruction, as the presence of intraluminal barium adds significantly to the technical challenge associated with operative therapy.

Enteroclysis, a less frequently used study, involves the placement of a nasoenteric tube beyond the ligament of Treitz. Dilute barium (sometimes air and contrast) is then injected into the tube at a constant rate and radiographs are taken. This procedure is more sensitive and specific than an upper GI with SBFT because the injection of air and contrast allows for the more detailed evaluation of the mucosa. The test is particularly sensitive for the diagnosis of small bowel tumors and inflammatory bowel disease (IBD); however, it often causes patient discomfort.

Treatment

The initial management of an SBO should include intravenous fluid resuscitation, electrolyte correction, and if appropriate, the placement of a nasogastric tube and urinary catheter. The extent of intravascular volume depletion, owing to sequestration of large amounts of fluid in the bowel lumen, is often underestimated. Multiple factors contribute to this intraluminal fluid accumulation including decreased reabsorption and increased secretion of fluid resulting from increased intraluminal pressure and release of vasoactive agents such as vasoactive intestinal peptide (VIP) and

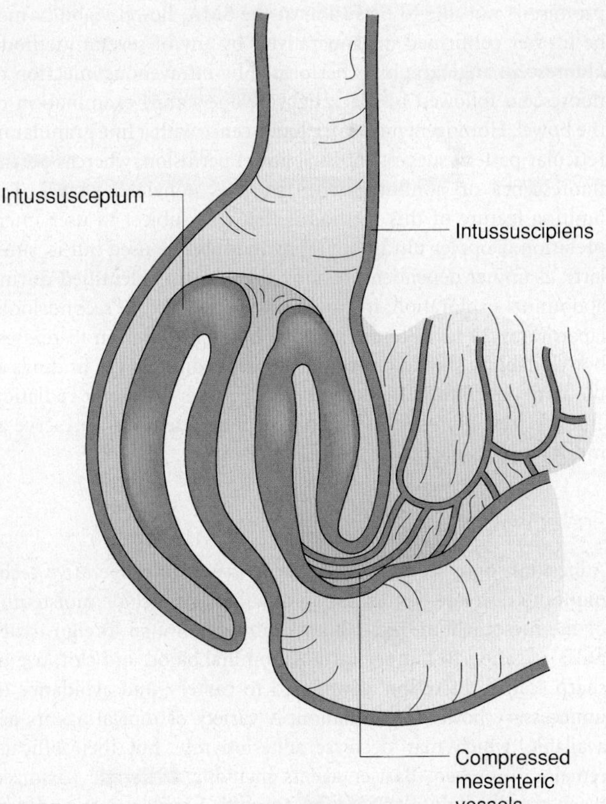

FIGURE 11.5 Anatomy of intussusception. The intussusceptum is the segment of bowel that invaginates into the intussuscipiens. (From Mulholland MW, Lillemoe KD, Doherty GM, et al., eds. *Surgery: Scientific Principles and Practice*. 5th ed. Philadelphia: Lippincott Williams & Wilkins; 2011.)

prostaglandins. Although initially increased, blood flow may be compromised when intraluminal pressures exceed intramural capillary and venous pressure. Intravenous antibiotics are generally not necessary unless operation is undertaken, and bowel resection is anticipated. In patients with partial SBO, treatment is initially nonoperative. If there is no or minimal improvement in 3 to 5 days, parenteral nutrition should be started. Timing of operation in such cases is individualized. If the patient's signs and symptoms worsen at any time, laparotomy should be performed. Patients who initially resolve a partial SBO but then recur are generally best served by surgical exploration. Patients with a complete SBO are at a high risk of strangulation, a surgical emergency. The risks of nonoperative therapy in complete SBO are compounded by the fact that only 60% to 70% of patients with strangulation will manifest the classic signs and symptoms. In general, once the decision to operate for an SBO has been made, there is little to gain by waiting. In some circumstances, a delay in operative management of between 6 and 8 hours may be warranted to allow resuscitation or to stabilize a comorbid condition (e.g., diabetic ketoacidosis or acute myocardial infarction). In patients who develop an early SBO soon after abdominal surgery, management requires case-by-case judgment. Observation and conservative management for up to 2 weeks may allow resolution.

Surgical treatment may include lysis of adhesions (LOA), resection of nonviable or diseased bowel with anastomosis, or intestinal bypass. These procedures can be done utilizing either laparoscopic or open approaches. First, one should palpate the root of the small bowel mesentery for a pulse in the SMA to be certain vascular compromise is not due to occlusion of the SMA. Bowel viability may be further confirmed intraoperatively by any of several methods. Fluorescein angiography is performed by intravenous injection of fluorescein followed by black light (Wood lamp) examination of the bowel. Homogeneous hyperfluorescence with a fine granular or reticular pattern suggests normal bowel perfusion, whereas patchy fluorescence or nonfluorescence suggests nonviable bowel. The limiting feature of this method is that it is subject to user interpretation. Doppler ultrasonography may also be used but is, similarly, examiner dependent. If nonviable bowel is identified during abdominal exploration, it should be resected and a "second-look" laparotomy 24 to 48 hours after the initial exploration to reassess bowel viability should be considered depending on the findings at the initial operation. In patients with Crohn's disease or radiation enteritis, resection should be limited in an attempt to preserve as much bowel as possible.

Prevention

Adhesions, once formed, are likely to recur. Intraoperative techniques to decrease the formation of adhesions include moistening of the mesothelium, reduction of intra-abdominal foreign materials, irrigation to remove intra-abdominal blood and clot, use of sharp scalpel dissection as opposed to cautery, and avoidance of unnecessary bowel manipulation. A variety of topical agents are available, which may decrease adhesion rate, but their efficacy remains unproven. Barrier agents including Intercede (oxidized regenerated cellulose), Seprafilm (modified hyaluronate and carboxymethylcellulose), Gore-Tex, and fibrin sheets have been used with limited evidence of success. Additionally, anti-inflammatory agents like polyethyleneglycol spray, hyaluronic acid gel, and glucose peritoneal instillates are under investigation. Plication of the small bowel (suturing of adjacent loops of small bowel and mesentery into an orderly pattern to prevent mechanical obstruction) may be considered in patients with multiple adhesive obstructions to promote the formation of nonobstructive adhesions. However, plication is associated with higher rates of enterocutaneous (EC) fistulas, abdominal abscesses, and wound infections. None of these techniques has been shown to consistently reduce postoperative adhesion formation.

Prognosis

SBO is associated with a 0.5% mortality rate. After LOA, approximately 10% of patients will have a recurrence of SBO. The incidence of recurrence increases further with each subsequent LOA. Strangulated bowel is associated with increased morbidity and mortality.

Other Causes of Small Bowel Obstruction

Several additional causes of SBO deserve special consideration. These include *gallstone ileus*, *intussusception*, and *volvulus*. Gallstone ileus is the development of a cholecystoduodenal fistula with distal propagation of a gallstone is an uncommon cause of SBO associated with considerable morbidity and mortality. It occurs more frequently in the elderly, in patients with severe concomitant disease, and in patients with gallstones 2 to 5 cm in diameter. Classical findings include intestinal obstruction (>70%), pneumobilia (>50%), a radiopaque gallstone in the right lower quadrant (>30%), or a change in position of a gallstone from previous studies. The progression and pathophysiology of the disease involves cystic duct obstruction, cholecystitis, cholecystoduodenal fistula formation, distal migration of the stone, and eventual trapping of the gallstone causing obstruction at a narrow part of the bowel, usually the ileocecal valve. Surgical intervention generally includes laparotomy, enterotomy, and removal of the stone. If the patient is stable enough, cholecystectomy may be performed; most commonly, this procedure is usually delayed until a second operation.

In adults, intussusception is caused by small bowel pathology approximately 80% of the time. The leading edge or intussusceptum is usually an intraluminal lesion (Fig. 11.5). The patient may present with crampy abdominal pain, nausea, vomiting, and heme-positive stools. The diagnosis is now usually made by CT scan. The CT finding most indicative of intussusception is an intraluminal soft tissue "mass" with high attenuation peripherally and low attenuation centrally, known as a *target sign*. It is a matter of some judgment as to whether an intussusception seen on CT scan is the source of symptoms. Unlike the pediatric population, hydrostatic reduction by barium enema is not recommended in adults. Surgical exploration is warranted in most instances because up to 40% of cases are caused by malignancy.

Volvulus is the twisting of a loop of bowel around the axis of a long narrow mesentery, often associated with malrotation or internal herniation (Fig. 11.6). Volvulus accounts for approximately 4% of SBOs with the incidence being equivalent in men and women. The clinical presentation usually includes acute abdominal pain and distention, nausea, and bilious vomiting. Leukocytosis is the only frequently associated laboratory abnormality. If the bowel appears viable upon exploration, a simple enterolysis, and in the case of malrotation, a Ladd procedure (counterclockwise reduction of the volvulus, division of Ladd bands/adhesions, and appendectomy)

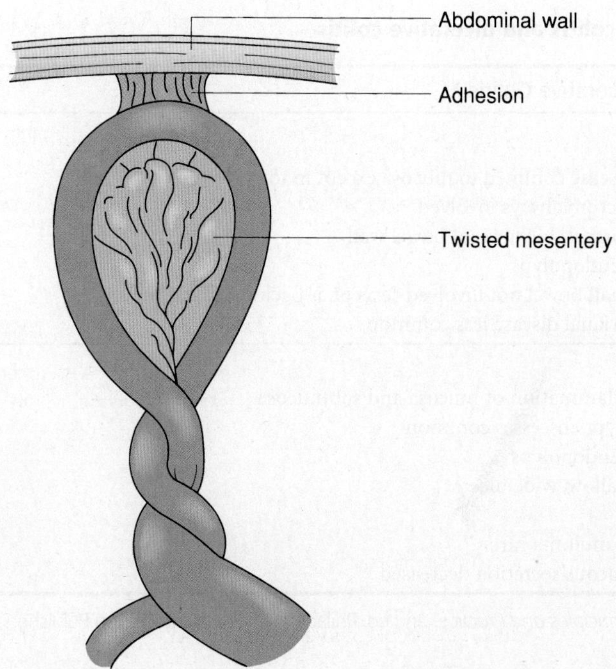

FIGURE 11.6 Closed-loop obstruction. The small intestine twists around its mesentery, compromising inflow and outflow of luminal contents from the loop. The vascular supply to the loop may also be compromised because of the twisting of the mesentery. (From Mulholland MW, Lillemoe KD, Doherty GM, et al., eds. *Surgery: Scientific Principles and Practice.* 5th ed. Philadelphia: Lippincott Williams & Wilkins; 2011.)

is adequate. The Ladd bands are fibrous stalks or peritoneal tissue connecting the cecum to the abdominal wall, which creates the site of duodenal obstruction in malrotation. If the bowel appears nonviable, then a Ladd procedure and bowel resection is required. This should be followed by a second-look laparotomy in most cases.

Intestinal pseudo-obstruction mimics the symptoms of SBO. It is a chronic, severe failure of intestinal propulsion. Symptoms include abdominal pain, distention, constipation, nausea, vomiting, and malnutrition. Patients may have a history of repeated surgical procedures in attempt to detect a mechanical cause of these symptoms. It is most commonly idiopathic but can be familial or associated with scleroderma, hypothyroidism, hypoparathyroidism, or celiac disease. The pathophysiology is not well understood but is thought to be from dysfunctional enteric neurons or smooth muscle cells. Radiographic evidence shows distended loops of bowel and air–fluid levels. Therapy usually includes nutritional support and symptomatic control. Approximately 30% of patients are unable to tolerate enteral nutrition and ultimately home parental nutrition. Surgical options are limited and usually only afford temporary relief, but include enterostomy creation, bypass procedure, and/or bowel resection.

INFLAMMATORY DISEASES

Crohn's Disease

Crohn's disease, or *regional enteritis,* is a chronic granulomatous disease of unknown cause. Any part of the GI tract from the mouth to the anus can be affected, although the terminal ileum is the most commonly involved site (approximately 70% to 90% of cases). The incidence is approximately 5 per 100,000 in the general population. It has a bimodal distribution, with an increased incidence in the second and third decades, and the sixth decade of life. There is a slight female predominance and a familial association has been demonstrated. The disease more commonly affects smokers, people who reside in industrial areas, and Ashkenazi Jews. The disease is characterized by periods of remission and exacerbations.

Etiology

The cause of Crohn's disease remains unclear. Autoimmune, infectious, and genetic factors have all been implicated. Humoral and cell-mediated immune reactions against gut cells have been identified in patients with Crohn's disease, suggesting an autoimmune pathogenesis, although there has been no direct correlation between this and the development of Crohn's disease. It has, likewise, been hypothesized that certain organisms, such as atypical mycobacterium or viruses, play a role. However, clinical trials in which these organisms were targeted using antimicrobial agents failed to demonstrate a benefit.

Pathology

Macroscopically, the affected bowel is usually thick, firm, and rubbery. Areas of thick grayish-white exudate or fibrosis and extension of the mesenteric fat around the circumference of the bowel (i.e., fat wrapping) may be present. The bowel proximal to the involved segment is usually dilated resulting from relative obstruction. Bowel perforation, abscess formation, or an enterovisceral fistula may be found at the time of surgical exploration. Microscopically, Crohn's disease is characterized by transmural involvement of the affected bowel with varying amounts of fibrosis and ulceration. Linear ulcerations with surrounding mucosal and submucosal edema create a "cobblestone" appearance. The edema may be sufficiently extensive to cause obstruction. The lesions are segmental, meaning that normal bowel is found in between areas of diseased bowel. Under the microscope, 60% to 70% of patients may have noncaseating granulomas with Langerhans giant cells.

Clinical Manifestations

Crohn's disease has an extremely diverse clinical presentation often characterized by periods of crampy or dull abdominal pain or diarrhea alternating with periods of remission. The onset of Crohn's disease is usually insidious, and during the course of the disease, intervals of remission may become progressively shorter, while episodes of symptomatic disease become longer and more severe. Bloody diarrhea is less frequent in patients with Crohn's disease when compared to patients with ulcerative colitis (Table 11.3), and frank lower GI bleeding is unusual. Other less common symptoms include fever, weight loss, malaise, and malnutrition. Extraintestinal manifestations such as arthralgias, iritis, uveitis, erythema nodosum, pyoderma gangrenosum, arthritis, hepatitis, and pericholangitis occur in approximately 30% of patients. Patients with Crohn's disease may develop a range of complications requiring surgical intervention including obstruction, perforation, fistula, abscess, and perianal disease. Obstruction occurs secondary to chronic inflammation, fibrosis, and progressive narrowing of the bowel lumen. Fistulas may form between diseased intestine and adjacent organs such as the bladder, vagina, other bowel segments, and the skin. Although toxic megacolon has been described in patients with

TABLE 11.3 Histopathologic differentiation of Crohn's colitis and ulcerative colitis

Crohn's Colitis	Ulcerative Colitis
Macroscopic	
Transmural involvement	Disease confined to mucosa except in toxic dilation
Segmental disease, fistulae	Rectum always involved
Thickened wall with "creeping fat"	Normal thickness of bowel wall
Occasional pseudopolyps	Pseudopolyps
Small bowel may be involved	Small bowel not involved (except as backwash ileitis)
Perianal disease common	Perianal disease less common
Microscopic	
Transmural inflammation and fibrosis	Inflammation of mucosa and submucosa
Crypt abscesses less common	Crypt abscesses common
Cobblestoning	Pseudopolyps
Narrow, deeply penetrating ulcers	Shallow, wide ulcers
Fissures, fistulae	—
Granuloma common	Granuloma rare
Mucous secretion increased	Mucous secretion decreased

From Greenfield LJ, Mulholland MW, Oldham KT, et al., eds. *Surgery: Scientific Principles and Practice*. 2nd ed. Philadelphia: Lippincott–Raven Publishers; 1997:835, with permission.

Crohn's disease, this diagnosis more often suggests ulcerative colitis. The incidence of colonic malignancy, although less common in patients with Crohn's disease than in patients with ulcerative colitis, is approximately six times greater than in the general population. Perianal disease has been known to precede intestinal disease by months to years; therefore, patients with recurrent perianal disease should be évaluated for Crohn's disease.

Diagnosis

The evaluation of a patient with suspected Crohn's disease usually includes endoscopy and biopsy (colonoscopy and esophagogastroduodenoscopy) as well as radiographic studies (CT scan/magnetic resonance imaging [MRI], upper GI and SBFT, and barium or Gastrografin enema). Stool cultures should be obtained to rule out infectious enteritis. Endoscopic findings suggestive of Crohn's disease include granular, discrete, aphthous ulcerations surrounded by normal tissue and a cobblestone-like appearance of the mucosa (i.e., linear ulcers, transverse sinuses, and clefts), diffuse narrowing of bowel lumen (most often the terminal ileum), and asymmetric involvement of the bowel wall leading to a nodular contour. Fistulas and abscesses may also be present.

Nutritional Considerations

Protein–calorie malnutrition occurs in 80% to 90% of patients with Crohn's disease at some point. Multiple factors contribute to this malnutrition, including abdominal pain, anorexia, nausea, and emesis. The cytokines interleukin-1 (IL-1) and tumor necrosis factor (TNF) may play a role as well. Total parenteral nutrition (TPN), total enteral nutrition (TEN), or elemental diets may help to correct nutritional derangements. In general, enteral formulas are preferred over parenteral nutrition, as they are more effective, easier to administer, less costly, and are associated with fewer complications.

Medical Treatment

Crohn's disease remains a chronic and incurable disease. The main goal of therapy is, therefore, symptomatic relief and control of inflammation with medical management until such time as a complication requires surgery. Anti-inflammatory and immunosuppressive medications that are commonly used to treat flares of Crohn's disease include steroids (intravenous and oral) and sulfasalazine. Other immunosuppressive agents such as azathioprine, 6-mercaptopurine, methotrexate, and cyclosporine have been shown to be effective as maintenance therapies. Antibiotics (most commonly metronidazole) are also prescribed during acute exacerbations and to treat anal disease. In recent years, a chimeric mouse–human antibody against TNF, infliximab, has emerged as an important therapy for Crohn's disease. In patients refractory to steroids or immunosuppression, infliximab infusion results in symptomatic improvement or remission in greater than 60% and 33% of patients, respectively.

Surgical Treatment

Most patients diagnosed with Crohn's disease require surgical intervention. The most common indications for surgery are intractability, obstruction, abscess, or fistula formation. The goal of an operation in a patient with Crohn's disease is to treat the complication or source of acute symptoms while conserving as much bowel as possible. Many patients with Crohn's will undergo more than one bowel resection during their lifetime, and multiple indiscriminate resections may lead to short gut syndrome, which afflicts a reported 2% to 13% of patients with Crohn's disease.

Fistula

The second most common indication for operation is fistula formation. EC fistulas are common in Crohn's patients and can develop spontaneously or as complications of bowel anastomoses or external drainage of an intra-abdominal abscess. Simple fistulas (i.e., those not complicated by sepsis or other complications) can be treated conservatively with bowel rest, TPN, and medication. Failure of conservative management and development of complications are indications for surgical management. Generally, EC fistulas are treated with resection of affected bowel and debridement of the fistula tract. Enteroenteric fistulas may be left alone if asymptomatic; however, if large segments are bypassed, significant malabsorption and fluid loss may ensue necessitating surgery. Surgery for enterovesical and enteroadnexal fistulas involves resection of the affected bowel and fistula tract and closure of the bladder or adnexal defect.

Obstruction

Another frequent indication for operation is obstruction. As discussed earlier in this chapter, partial obstruction is often treated conservatively with nasogastric tube decompression, bowel rest, intravenous hydration, and electrolyte correction. Obstruction that does not resolve requires operative treatment. Again, minimal resection is recommended. Healthy intervening segments of bowel flanked by diseased segments should only be resected if less than 5 cm in length. If a short stricture is the cause of the obstruction, then strictureplasty (Heineke–Mikulicz type) can be performed making a longitudinal incision through the stricture and closing it in a transverse fashion. Contraindications to strictureplasty include small bowel perforation, multiple strictures in a short segment, and concern for malignancy. Intestinal bypass is an alternative approach but is usually reserved for the patients at high risk for short-bowel syndrome (e.g., patients with multiple prior bowel resections) or other perioperative complications (e.g., the elderly).

Prognosis

There is no cure for Crohn's disease, and recurrences tend to increase in frequency and severity over time. The most common site of recurrence is the small bowel, just proximal to the prior site of resection. Many patients will ultimately undergo multiple procedures. The disease tends to recede gradually with increasing age.

DIVERTICULAR DISEASES

Meckel's Diverticulum

Meckel's diverticula are the most common true diverticula of the GI tract. Although more common in the pediatric population, such diverticula are found in adults as well. The overall incidence is approximately 2%; however, only a small percentage of these diverticula are symptomatic. Approximately 50% of symptomatic Meckel's diverticula contain ectopic gastric mucosal cells. Secretion of acid from these cells sometimes leads to ulceration of adjacent small bowel and bleeding, which is the most common clinical presentation in the pediatric population. In contrast, obstruction is the most common presenting symptom in adults. Acute inflammation (diverticulitis) is also common and can mimic appendicitis. A technetium-99 m (^{99m}Tc) pertechnetate scan is the investigation of choice for the diagnosis of Meckel's diverticula. All symptomatic Meckel's diverticula should be resected. Segmental ileal resection is necessary in the patient who presents with GI bleeding to eliminate the base of the diverticulum where ectopic gastric mucosa may be found and the adjacent small bowel (the typical site of hemorrhage). Although resection of incidental asymptomatic Meckel's diverticula is controversial, some surgeons resect lesions greater than 2 cm in individuals younger than 40 years of age. In children, a Meckel's diverticulum should be removed. It is often helpful to use the well-known "Rule of *2*'s" when remembering important characteristics about Meckel's diverticulum: approximately *2*% are symptomatic, *2* types of mucosa possible (small intestine and gastric), located within *2* feet of the ileocecal valve, *2* times more common in males, and commonly presents within first *2* years of life.

Duodenal Diverticula

Duodenal diverticula are the most common acquired or false diverticula of the small bowel. The true incidence is unknown but may be as high as 10% to 20% in the general population. Duodenal diverticula are more common in women and in individuals older than 50 years of age.

Greater than 95% of these diverticula are asymptomatic, and fewer than 5% require any surgical intervention. More than 60% of these diverticula are found in the periampullary region projecting from the medial wall.

Clinical Manifestation

Patients may present with obstruction, perforation, or bleeding into the small bowel. More frequently, these diverticula are asymptomatic. Periampullary diverticula may also be responsible for recurrent pancreatitis, cholangitis, and recurrent CBD stones even after cholecystectomy, resulting from mechanical distortion of the CBD.

Treatment

Asymptomatic diverticula do not require treatment. If they are symptomatic, treatment is aimed at controlling complications. If pancreatic and biliary structures are not involved, the most common and effective treatment is to perform a diverticulectomy. A *Kocher maneuver* (dissecting the lateral peritoneal attachments of the duodenum to allow access to the pancreas, duodenum, and other retroperitoneal structures) is performed, and a duodenotomy is made. The diverticulum is then excised, followed by closure of the defect in a transverse fashion to avoid narrowing of the lumen. If pancreatic and biliary structures are involved, a choledochoduodenostomy or a choledochojejunostomy to a Roux-en-Y limb may be indicated.

Jejunoileal Diverticula

Most jejunoileal diverticula are acquired pulsion pseudodiverticula associated with increasing age. Such diverticula are frequently a marker for an underlying dysmotility syndrome. Like colonic diverticula, most are located where blood vessels perforate the muscularis propria. They may be multiple and are usually asymptomatic but can be complicated by infection, obstruction, and perforation. Associated bacterial overgrowth occasionally leads to malabsorption. Enteroclysis is the study of choice for making the diagnosis. Complications of diverticulitis, obstruction, and perforation are treated similarly as with colonic diverticular disease. Jejunoileal diverticula are associated with an increased risk of lymphoma.

VASCULAR DISEASE

Acute Mesenteric Ischemia

Acute mesenteric ischemia may result from (i) SMA embolization (from a cardiac source), (ii) SMA thrombosis (a complication of underlying atherosclerotic disease), (iii) nonocclusive mesenteric ischemia (associated with a low cardiac output state), and (iv) acute mesenteric venous thrombosis (most often associated with dehydration or infection). Rarely, visceral ischemia may result from an aortic dissection. Therefore, a review of the patient's history is important, which may include known risk factors such as atrial fibrillation, congestive heart failure, atherosclerotic coronary, carotid, or peripheral vascular disease and a history of hypercoagulability.

Clinical Manifestations

Patients usually present with abdominal pain out of proportion to physical findings. The pain is typically periumbilical and may be accompanied by nausea, vomiting, or bloody diarrhea. Leukocytosis, hyperkalemia, metabolic acidosis, and elevated serum levels of lactate, lactate dehydrogenase (LDH), alanine aminotransferase (ALT), aspartate aminotransferase (AST), or creatine phosphokinase (CPK) may also be present. Changes in the mucosa can be detected under light microscopy within minutes of the onset of ischemia; these changes later develop into hemorrhagic necrosis, edema of the bowel wall, sloughing of the mucosa, and hemorrhage into the bowel lumen. This loss of mucosal integrity increases its permeability to luminal bacterial flora leading to peritonitis, bacteremia, and septicemia.

Diagnosis

The diagnosis of mesenteric ischemia is difficult because of its relative rarity, the nonspecific nature of the associated symptoms, and the frequent presence of significant comorbidities. If the diagnosis is delayed (beyond 24 hours), the disease is associated with higher mortality. Traditionally, consideration of visceral ischemia in patients with acute abdominal pain mandated visceral arteriography. Today, however, computed tomographic (CT) and magnetic resonance (MR) angiography/venography are used to aid in the diagnosis of mesenteric ischemia. These studies can also assist in differentiating between the main causes of arterial ischemia. (i) SMA embolism is characterized by emboli at the origin of the middle colic artery distal to the first few jejunal branches. (ii) SMA thrombosis is characterized by thrombus at the origin of the SMA proximal to the jejunal branches. (iii) Nonocclusive ischemia is characterized by segmental mesenteric vasospasm involving the branches of the SMA (Fig. 11.1).

Because of availability and lower cost, CT is often preferred over MR. Findings on CT associated with acute ischemia include bowel dilation, wall thickening, intestinal pneumatosis, portal venous gas, and mesenteric stranding. These findings, while sensitive, are not specific to ischemia. Additionally, lack of enhancement of the arterial or venous vasculature using timed contrast injections are suggestive of mesenteric occlusion.

Treatment

All patients with suspected mesenteric ischemia should be placed on bowel rest, intravenous fluid, broad-spectrum antibiotics, and if possible, preemptive intravenous heparin until a diagnosis is secure. Correction of metabolic derangements and acidosis is a goal of initial therapy and is facilitated by cardiac monitoring and placement of a Foley catheter. Surgical treatment varies, depending on the cause of ischemia, and in patients suspected of having intestinal infarction or perforation, surgery should not be delayed. If SMA embolus is suspected, traditional treatment has included surgical laparotomy and embolectomy. The bowel is then examined for areas of persistent ischemia requiring resection. Another approach to treatment is local infusion of thrombolytic therapy, which is an option only if the patient is a candidate for thrombolytic therapy and if there is no evidence of bowel infarction. This approach has been reviewed in several small series and case reports, which shows that a percentage of these patients may require additional surgical intervention, and long-term reocclusion rate has not been well studied. If SMA thrombus is suspected, a bypass graft or endovascular stent is often needed to reestablish flow to the affected bowel in conjunction with thrombectomy. Thrombectomy alone is not durable due to the presence of atherosclerotic plaques. Although a newer technique, recent reports suggest that endovascular repair may be as effective and durable as traditional bypass approaches to revascularization.

The treatment of nonocclusive mesenteric ischemia is usually nonoperative, which is managed by correcting the cause of the low flow state with appropriate volume resuscitation, vasopressors, or cardiac support. In general, restoration of adequate cardiac index will alleviate symptoms. Vasodilating agents such as papaverine and tolazoline may be used as an adjunct during arteriography to further enhance perfusion. Operative treatment is indicated for clinical deterioration despite optimal medical management.

Treatment of mesenteric venous thrombosis includes early anticoagulation and resection of any compromised bowel. If the patient lacks peritoneal signs and has adequate arterial blood flow demonstrated by imaging, he or she may be managed with anticoagulation alone. After the initial treatment, anticoagulation with warfarin is indicated for at least 6 months.

Chronic Mesenteric Ischemia

Chronic mesenteric ischemia usually is caused by atherosclerotic disease of the celiac axis, SMA, and IMA. Other causes include fibromuscular dysplasia, radiation enteritis, the autoimmune arteritides, and external compression. The atherosclerotic process usually begins with plaque formation, which occurs at the origins of the visceral arteries. The chronicity of the disease allows for the formation of collateral circulation, an important characteristic of the disease. The common collateral circuits are (i) the celiac artery and the gastroduodenal artery, (ii) the SMA and the pancreatic branches, (iii) the SMA and the inferior mesenteric artery (IMA) through the meandering mesenteric artery (most important) and the marginal artery of Drummond (Fig. 11.7), and (iv) the left colic and middle colic arteries. The meandering mesenteric artery is present only in occlusive disease. It is more tortuous, shorter in length, and more medial than the marginal artery of Drummond.

Diagnosis

Patients classically complain of postprandial abdominal pain starting approximately 20 minutes to 1 hour after a meal. The intensity of pain correlates with the amount of food ingested; chronic mesenteric ischemia has, therefore, also been referred to as *intestinal*

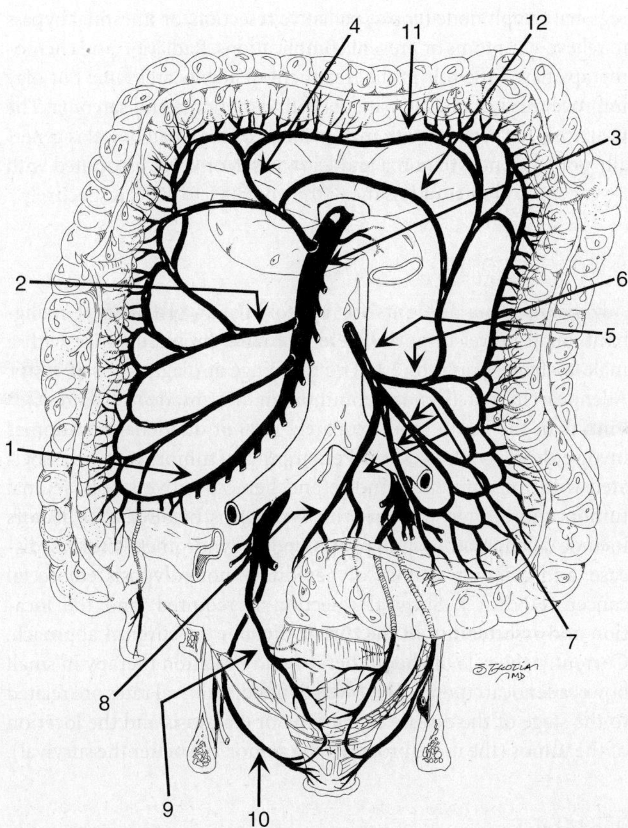

FIGURE 11.7 The arterial blood supply to the colon: (*1*) ileocolic artery, (*2*) right colic artery, (*3*) SMA, (*4*) middle colic artery, (*5*) IMA, (*6*) left colic artery, (*7*) sigmoidal artery, (*8*) superior hemorrhoidal artery, (*9*) middle hemorrhoidal artery, (*10*) inferior hemorrhoidal artery, (*11*) marginal artery of Drummond, (*12*) meandering artery of Gonzalez. (From Blackbourne LH, ed. *Surgical Recall.* 2nd ed. Philadelphia: Lippincott Williams & Wilkins; 1998, with permission.)

angina. Patients may also complain of weight loss secondary to "food fear." Patients are usually cachectic, with a midabdominal bruit, and have other clinical signs of atherosclerotic disease including carotid, femoral, and/or abdominal aortic bruits. Chronic mesenteric ischemia rarely occurs with occlusion of a single artery. The gold standard diagnostic study is arteriography, which may reveal occlusion or stenosis of the celiac axis, the SMA, and the presence of collateral vessels. CT/MR angiography as well as duplex ultrasonography have been used with increasing frequency for the detection of mesenteric occlusive disease. Occult GI bleeding is unusual; therefore, if occult blood is found, another diagnosis, such as acute ischemia or malignancy, must be sought.

Treatment

To prevent bowel infarction, revascularization is indicated in all symptomatic patients. Options for treatment include surgical reconstruction or percutaneous transluminal angioplasty (PTA) with or without a stent. Several factors dictate treatment choice including the number and severity of occluded vessels and the ease of vascular access to the compromised vessel. Surgery is often used in younger patients with fewer comorbidities, while endovascular approaches may be preferred for the elderly and infirm. A contraindication to endovascular therapy is extrinsic compression of the celiac axis by the median arcuate ligament because it has a high failure rate. Relative contraindications include bleeding disorders, renal insufficiency not requiring dialysis, and extensive aortoiliac vascular disease. Although PTA is a newer technique and surgical literature is limited, authors have reported comparable success rates of residual stenosis, restenosis, and symptomatic relief. Bypass grafting, endarterectomy, and reimplantation are all frequently described techniques of surgical reconstruction. The choice usually depends on surgeon experience, as no method has proven superiority.

Small Bowel Neoplasms

There are several possible explanations for the extremely low incidence of primary small bowel neoplasms. The rapid transit of material through the small bowel and low intraluminal pH may protect the mucosa from contact with carcinogens. Additionally, the small bowel is equipped with a highly evolved immune system, which may eliminate premalignant transformed cells. Small bowel neoplasms are usually asymptomatic but can present with obstruction, diarrhea, abdominal distention, obstipation, or anemia. Benign tumors include adenomas, leiomyomas, lipomas, hamartomas, and hemangiomas. Malignant tumors include adenocarcinomas, sarcomas, lymphomas, GIST (gastrointestinal stromal tumors), and carcinoids. Malignant and benign neoplasms occur in equal frequency, but malignant tumors are more likely to produce symptoms.

Benign Neoplasms

The majority of benign small bowel tumors are asymptomatic, and the diagnosis is often delayed or missed. Benign small bowel tumors are of epithelial or connective tissue origin. Benign tumors include adenomas (the most common benign tumor), leiomyomas (the most common symptomatic benign tumor), and lipomas. These neoplasms are usually slow growing but may become large enough to cause intraluminal obstruction. They may also be polypoid and cause intussusception or may twist axially, causing hemorrhage. When suspected, diagnostic studies including upper endoscopy, upper GI and SBFT, enteroclysis, and capsule endoscopy may be helpful. Though rarely performed, enteroclysis is superior to SBFT in detecting subtle mucosal lesions and has an approximate accuracy of 90% for the diagnosis of small bowel tumors. Surgical intervention is indicated because of the possibility of cancer and the risks of mechanical complications. Operation usually consists of segmental resection and primary anastomosis, though small lesions may be simply excised.

Adenoma

There are three types of true adenomas: tubular, villous, and Brunner's gland. Approximately 20% are located in the duodenum, 30% in the jejunum, and 50% in the ileum. Most are single and asymptomatic. They may also occur in association with familial polyposis syndromes. *Villous adenomas* in the small bowel are rare and are most commonly found in the duodenum. They can be quite large (i.e., >5 cm) and have significant malignant potential. *Brunner's gland adenomas* are also found in the duodenum and are caused by the hyperplastic proliferation of normal submucosal exocrine glands. Diagnosis is usually made by endoscopic biopsy. These tumors have no malignant potential; therefore, conservative local resection should be reserved for symptoms.

Leiomyomas

Leiomyomas are the most common symptomatic benign tumors of the small bowel. Histologically, these are smooth muscle tumors and are most commonly located in the jejunum. Leiomyomas may be single or multiple and have an equal male and female incidence. They can grow to a large size intramurally or extramurally. If they grow large enough, they can outgrow their blood supply, necrose, and bleed. The most common indication for operative management is bleeding. Angiography can be useful for diagnosis and temporary control of hemorrhage.

Lipoma

Lipomas are most often intramural and located in the ileum. They are usually single and small but may cause obstruction by acting as the lead point of an intussusception. Bleeding can also result from ulceration of the overlying mucosa. They have no malignant potential.

Hamartoma

Hamartomas commonly occur as part of the Peutz–Jeghers syndrome, an autosomal dominant inherited syndrome characterized by mucocutaneous melanotic pigmentation and GI polyps. The polyps are not true polyps and are, therefore, not premalignant; however, patients diagnosed with Peutz–Jeghers are at increased risk for the development of GI malignancies. Classically, patients have small, 1- to 2-mm brown-black spots on the circumoral region of the face, buccal mucosa, palms and soles, lips, digits, and the perianal area. The hamartomas are most frequently located in the jejunum and ileum. Approximately 50% of patients also have concomitant lesions in the colon and rectum, and about 25% have gastric polyps. If the colonic, rectal, or gastric polyps are found to be hamartomas, the small bowel should also be investigated for polyps. Patients may complain of colicky abdominal pain secondary to intermittent intussusception or obstruction and bleeding. Surgical resection is indicated for symptoms. Bowel resection should be limited to the symptomatic portion.

Hemangiomas

Hemangiomas are developmental malformations of proliferating submucosal blood vessels and account for 3% to 4% of all benign small bowel tumors. They are most commonly found in the jejunum but can occur anywhere in the GI tract. Most patients with hemangiomas are asymptomatic. The onset of GI bleeding may be the only presenting symptom. Diagnostic studies most useful in diagnosis are angiography and ^{99m}Tc-labeled red blood cell scanning, although diagnosis is usually difficult. If the lesion can be localized, conservative resection is recommended. If the lesion cannot be localized, intraoperative palpation or localization via intraoperative enteroscopy may be helpful.

Malignant Neoplasms

Adenocarcinoma, sarcoma, lymphoma, and carcinoid tumors are the most common malignant neoplasms of the small bowel. Patients most often present with weight loss, diarrhea, or obstructive symptoms such as nausea, vomiting, or abdominal pain. Anemia and melena are less common. Treatment options include wide surgical resection with regional lymph node biopsy, palliative resection, or intestinal bypass to relieve symptoms or prevent complications. Radiation and chemotherapy have little role in the treatment of adenocarcinoma but may improve survival rates in patients with lymphoma and sarcoma. The prognosis for patients with malignancies of the small bowel is generally poor. Adenocarcinoma and leiomyosarcoma are associated with 5-year survival rates of less than 20% and 30% to 40%, respectively.

Adenocarcinoma

Adenocarcinoma accounts for approximately one half of malignant small bowel tumors. There is a male preponderance with a male-to-female ratio of 2:1. The mean age at diagnosis is 50 years. Adenocarcinoma is more common in the duodenum and jejunum than the ileum. Approximately 50% of duodenal carcinomas involve the ampulla of Vater. Periampullary tumors may be associated with intermittent jaundice and heme-positive stools. Jejunal tumors more often present with symptoms of SBO. Risk factors include adenomatous polyps, polyposis syndromes, Crohn's disease, and a family history of hereditary nonpolyposis colorectal cancer (HNPCC). Surgical resection is required, and the location and resectability of the tumor dictates the surgical approach. Currently, the role of chemotherapy and radiation therapy in small bowel adenocarcinoma is not well defined. Survival rates are related to the stage of the disease at the time of diagnosis and the location of the tumor (the more proximal the tumor, the better the survival).

Sarcoma

These mesenchymal neoplasms account for 2% of malignant small bowel tumors, with the most common type being leiomyosarcoma. Other rare sarcomas include fibrosarcoma, Kaposi sarcoma, liposarcoma, and angiosarcoma. Sarcoma occurs with equal incidence in men and women, and the diagnosis is most often made in the sixth decade of life. Small bowel sarcoma spreads by several routes: direct invasion of adjacent tissues, hematogenous dissemination, and transperitoneal seeding leading to sarcomatosis. Obstruction, bleeding, or perforations are common presentations and indications for urgent operative management.

Lymphoma

Lymphoma accounts for 10% to 15% of small bowel malignancies. The ileum is the most common location, probably owing to the greater concentration of gut-associated lymphoid tissue in this portion of the bowel. Lymphoma of the small bowel may be part of a generalized lymphoma or conversely a primary local disease process. Features that distinguish primary from generalized disease include the absence of peripheral and mediastinal lymphadenopathy on chest x-ray, a normal white blood cell count and differential, a dominant small bowel mass as the principal tumor, and the absence of metastatic disease in the liver and spleen. More than 30% of patients with bowel lymphoma have generalized lymphoma.

Gastrointestinal Stromal Tumors

GISTs account for 10% to 20% of all small bowel malignancies. They are thought to originate from the interstitial cells of Cajal (intestinal pacemaker cell) and express a transmembrane tyrosine kinase receptor called KIT. GISTs most commonly occur in the stomach but can also occur anywhere in the GI tract including the small bowel where they are more commonly found in the jejunum and ileum. Most are asymptomatic and are most often found incidentally. They arise from the submucosa and are typically smooth and rounded lesions. They can become quite large, and when they do become symptomatic, they usually present with an abdominal mass, obstruction, abdominal pain, and weight loss. GISTs can also present with bleeding, owing to their vascularity. Two important prognostic factors associated with recurrence (aside from their location in the GI tract) include tumor size and mitotic index. Diagnosis is usually made with radiographic studies (upper GI and SBFT and CT scan). Surgical management is indicated for nonmetastatic lesions. Treatment is resection with primary anastomosis. Wide mesenteric resection is not indicated, as these tumors do not typically spread via lymphatics to the regional nodes. Metastatic or nonresectable tumors are treated with imatinib mesylate, a tyrosine kinase inhibitor, or other newer agents, which may also be considered in the adjuvant setting after resection of high-risk lesions.

Carcinoid

Small bowel carcinoid tumors account for less than one half of malignant small bowel neoplasms. Carcinoid tumors are derived from enterochromaffin (argentaffin) cells or Kulchitsky cells found in the crypts of Lieberkühn. About 50% of carcinoid tumors occur in the appendix and 25% occur in the ileum. Carcinoid tumors of the ileum are much more frequently metastatic than are appendiceal carcinoids. Small bowel carcinoid tumors are derived from multipotential cells and have the ability to secrete substances such as serotonin and substance P. Because of this, approximately 5% of patients with small bowel carcinoids present with episodes of cutaneous flushing, bronchospasm/asthma, diarrhea/malabsorption, vasomotor collapse, and right heart valvular disease, known together as *malignant carcinoid syndrome*. In most cases, malignant carcinoid syndrome is indicative of tumor metastasis beyond the small bowel or mesentery. With localized tumor, the liver will metabolize both serotonin and kallikrein, which are the breakdown products of the tumor responsible for these symptoms. Exceptions to this rule are carcinoid primaries of the ovaries and bronchus or disease with concomitant liver failure, which may result in carcinoid syndrome without metastasis. Malignant potential is predicted by the size, location, depth, and growth pattern of the tumor as characterized by its histologic differentiation and its mitotic or Ki67 index. Intraoperatively, carcinoids appear as slightly elevated, smooth, round, hard, submucosal lesions. When transected, they have a characteristic yellow-gray appearance. The mesentery may be severely fibrotic secondary to an intense desmoplastic reaction caused by expression of humoral agents secreted by the tumor (e.g., substance P). About 30% to 70% of carcinoid tumors of the GI tract are found to be metastatic at the time of diagnosis. The presence of a second primary tumor of different histology has been identified in as many as a quarter of patients. About one third of patients are found to have multiple carcinoid neoplasms upon surgical exploration.

Diagnosis

Seventy-five percent of patients with nonmetastatic carcinoid (as compared to 100% of patients with metastatic carcinoid) will have elevated urinary levels of 5-hydroxyindoleacetic acid (5-HIAA), a metabolite of serotonin. The localization of a carcinoid may be aided by radiographic studies such as CT scan and upper GI and SBFT. Somatostatin receptor scintigraphy is successful in localizing the primary carcinoids and metastases in 80% of cases, a higher rate than that associated with other imaging modalities.

Treatment

The surgical management of carcinoid is dictated by the size and site of the neoplasm as well as the presence of metastatic disease. Tumors up to 1 cm in the greatest dimension require segmental resection; those greater than 1 cm and those associated with regional lymph node metastases require wider segmental and mesenteric excision to remove the draining nodes; larger duodenal lesions often require pancreaticoduodenectomy. If the tumor is localized, surgical resection is curative. If carcinoid has metastasized, surgical resection may provide reasonable palliation. Chemotherapy (usually streptozotocin, doxorubicin, and 5-fluorouracil) may also be used for palliation. Long-term palliation is often possible as the tumors are slow growing and indolent. If the tumor is localized, the 5-year survival rate for small bowel carcinoids is approximately 65%, whereas appendiceal and rectal carcinoids have a better prognosis due to smaller size and rarity of metastasis upon detection.

Malignant Carcinoid Syndrome

The malignant carcinoid syndrome is found in only 6% to 9% of patients with metastatic carcinoid cancer. The primary tumor is most often in the small bowel, and the syndrome is seen only in the presence of functional liver metastases or if the primary tumor is in the lung, ovary, or testicle (allowing for serotonin to enter the systemic venous system bypassing liver metabolism). The syndrome is characterized by diarrhea, flushing, and hepatomegaly in approximately 80% of patients; right heart valvular disease in 50% of patients; and bronchospasm/asthma in 25% of patients. Diarrhea is caused by elevated serum serotonin levels and is often postprandial and episodic in nature. It may be accompanied by severe abdominal pain secondary to intestinal ischemia caused by mesenteric perivascular fibrosis and vasoconstriction induced by vasoactive substances secreted by the tumor. Flushing and asthma may result from secretion of serotonin, substance P, bradykinins, and prostaglandins E and F. Right heart valvular disease is the result of irreversible fibrosis of the endocardium. Only the right heart valves are affected (tricuspid and pulmonary valves), as vasoactive agents are cleared efficiently by the lungs. Repeatedly elevated levels of 5-HIAA (a metabolite of serotonin) in the urine are highly suggestive of carcinoid syndrome. Treatment may include tumor resection and debulking of the tumor in the liver, ablation of liver lesions, hepatic artery embolization, and chemotherapy (doxorubicin, cisplatin, 5-fluorouracil). Drug therapy (interferon, Sandostatin, somatostatin-14) may be used for prevention or relief of symptoms. Carcinoid crisis is a potentially catastrophic complication usually seen upon induction of anesthesia. Immediate administration of a somatostatin analog may be lifesaving.

MISCELLANEOUS SMALL BOWEL DISEASES

Ileus

Postoperative ileus is common and may result from dysregulation of autonomic stimulation to the gut after surgery. The basal motility pattern, or migrating motor complex (MMC), is typically disturbed for approximately 24 hours after laparotomy, owing in part to the anesthetic effects. Additionally, bowel resection temporarily blocks the MMC and peristalsis. Generally, small bowel function returns within hours of manipulation, but the return of stomach function requires about 48 hours, and the return of colon function requires about 72 hours. Return of bowel function is not always clinically apparent, as a recent prospective randomized trial found that many patients may be safely discharged from the hospital on a clear liquid diet before the passage of flatus or stool.

Small Bowel Fistulas

Fistulas are connections between two epithelialized structures. Small bowel fistulas may connect multiple segments of small bowel, small bowel and skin (i.e., EC fistulas), or small bowel and other organs (e.g., enterovesical fistulas). The most common cause of a small bowel fistula is a previous abdominal operation. Postoperative fistulas result principally from anastomotic leaks, unrecognized bowel injuries, or injury to the small bowel blood supply with resultant ischemia. The word "*FRIENDS*" is a popular mnemonic often used by students to remember the multiple risk factors of failed fistula closure (*F*: presence of a Foreign body, *R*: patient history of bowel Radiation, *I*: recent or active Infection and/or IBD, *E*: Epithelialization of the tract, *N*: presence of a Neoplasm, *D*: obstruction Distal to the fistula, *S*: Short tract <2 cm). Complications from fistulas include sepsis, fluid and electrolyte derangements, necrosis of the soft tissue at the drainage site, and malnutrition. Small bowel fistula mortality may be as high as 20%.

Diagnosis

Diagnosis of a fistula may be confirmed radiographically with studies including upper GI and SBFT, barium enema, CT scan, and contrast fistulogram. Oral administration of charcoal or nonabsorbable food coloring may also allow for confirmation of a fistula. It is important to determine whether the fistula is proximal (involving the stomach or small bowel) or distal, and whether it is high or low output. In general, a low-output fistula drains less than 200 mL/day. A moderate-output fistula drains between 200 and 500 mL/day, and a high-output fistula drains more than 500 mL/day. These factors dictate the prognosis and the treatment plan. Proximal fistulas tend to have a greater impact on fluid and electrolyte balance as well as nutrition.

Treatment

Management of an enteric fistula should focus on four life-threatening concerns, that is, sepsis, fluid and electrolyte imbalance, nutrition, and skin care. Fistulas may be associated with intra-abdominal infection, which may present either as contained abscess or as peritonitis. Peritonitis requires emergent laparotomy for source control. Contained abscesses are usually amenable to percutaneous or local drainage. Additionally, antibiotic therapy and debridement of devitalized tissue are employed when appropriate. Aggressive correction of hypovolemia should be addressed early. Electrolyte management and correction is also essential. Hypokalemia is the most common electrolyte abnormality, so potassium supplementation is often necessary. High-output proximal fistulas should be replaced with isotonic saline, and duodenal or pancreatic fistulas may cause metabolic acidosis and require bicarbonate replacement. Generally, nonoperative management consisting of bowel rest, TPN, and wound care should be attempted for up to 6 weeks if the patient is stable. During this conservative management, enteral feedings are preferable because of positive immunologic and hormonal effects on the gut; however, this can often be impossible because of high-output fistula losses or feeding intolerance. Operative treatment of a chronic fistula is best undertaken when the patient's condition has stabilized and sepsis is controlled. Operative management should include a careful exploration for factors contributing to the persistence of a fistula (e.g., obstruction, foreign body, or intrinsic bowel pathology), excision of the fistula tract, and resection of the affected bowel. A proximal enterostomy may be required to protect tenuous anastomoses or if primary repair cannot be performed.

Blind Loop Syndrome

Blind loop syndrome is rare and may present with diarrhea, steatorrhea, abdominal pain, vitamin deficiencies, neurologic symptoms, anemia, and weight loss. It is caused by bacterial overgrowth in a stagnant segment of small bowel. Stagnation of bowel may be caused by strictures, adhesive obstruction, defunctionalized segments (e.g., after jejunoileal bypass), or extensive jejunoileal diverticular disease. Vitamin B_{12} deficiency is caused by increased bacterial consumption and may result in megaloblastic anemia and neurologic symptoms related to demyelination of the posterior and lateral spinal columns. Other nutrient malabsorption may be secondary to direct injury to the mucosa. The diagnosis of blind loop syndrome is confirmed by decreased serum vitamin B_{12} levels. Alternatively, a Schilling test may be performed. Labeled vitamin B_{12} is orally administered and then measured in the urine. The test is repeated with addition of intrinsic factor. In true pernicious anemia, the urinary excretion of B_{12} is increased to normal levels by the addition of intrinsic factor; in blind loop syndrome, the urinary excretion is unchanged. The patient is then given a course of antibiotics (e.g., tetracycline or doxycycline), and the test is repeated. In blind loop syndrome, the urinary excretion of B_{12} should increase to normal levels following antibiotic therapy. Operative intervention is occasionally indicated for the treatment of blind loop syndrome and should include correction of the anatomic defect(s) or resection of the diseased segment of bowel.

Radiation Enteritis

Radiation therapy is employed for the treatment of many abdominal and pelvic malignancies. Despite its benefits, radiation-induced complications may lead to severe acute and chronic damage to the irradiated bowel. The degree of damage is dependent on the dose of radiation and is more common in the presence of certain comorbidities or exposure (e.g., previous abdominal surgeries, diabetes, hypertension, vascular disease, and chemotherapy). Bowel epithelium is highly sensitive to irradiation because of its high cellular turnover rate. Symptoms such as abdominal pain, diarrhea, and malabsorption are common but often self-limiting. Damage to the submucosa and its vessels may result in late symptoms of necrosis, perforation, fistula formation, stricture, and obstruction. Radiation injury to the submucosa progresses to submucosal fibrosis and obliterative arteritis, leading to bowel ischemia and necrosis. Radiation damage can be minimized or prevented by delivering the treatment to a limited field, either by adjusting the patient's position or by adjusting the equipment. If preradiation laparotomy is performed, the bowel can be protected by retroperitonealization, omental transposition, or placement of mesh slings to exclude the bowel from the pelvis (prior to irradiation of a pelvic malignancy).

Treatment should be conservative and geared toward improved nutritional status. Operative intervention should be avoided when possible but is required for symptomatic stricture, fistula, and obstruction. Primary anastomosis of irradiated bowel is associated with a higher rate of anastomotic leak and should be avoided; however, short-bowel syndrome must be avoided while obtaining adequate margins of resection. If the affected bowel is fixed and rigid making resection technically difficult, intestinal bypass or proximal enterostomy may be indicated. About one half of those patients undergoing their first operative procedure will require further surgical intervention.

Short-Bowel Syndrome

Short-bowel syndrome is caused by massive surgical resection of the small bowel. Common reasons for such resections include midgut volvulus, traumatic injury, and vascular occlusion. Clinical manifestations include diarrhea, malnutrition, and fluid and electrolyte abnormalities. Symptoms depend on the amount of small bowel resected, the state of the ileocecal valve, and whether the proximal or distal bowel is lost. If the ileocecal valve is intact, resection of approximately 70% of the small bowel may be well tolerated. Resection of the proximal small bowel is better tolerated than resection of distal small bowel, as distal bowel can undergo adaptation, thereby increasing absorptive capacity. This adaptation is characterized by hyperplasia of the remaining enterocytes, lengthening of the villi, wall hypertrophy, and increased caliber. Stimuli for bowel adaptation may include enteral feeding and gut hormones (e.g., insulin-like growth factor 1, glucagon-like peptide 2, growth hormone, and neurotensin).

Small Bowel Restoration

Intestinal transplantation has recently become a therapeutic option for patients with short-bowel syndrome. These patients often have received prolonged TPN and may have suffered serious complications including catheter-related sepsis, electrolyte disturbances, and/or cholestatic liver failure. Although long-term outcomes have improved in recent years following transplantation, this method of treatment is still used infrequently due to significant morbidity and mortality related to both the operation itself and postoperative immunosuppression.

Prior to consideration of transplantation, patients should undergo an intense multidisciplinary treatment program referred to as intestinal rehabilitation. This therapy aims to liberate the patient from parental nutrition by improving enteral nutrition through use of specialized diet, as well as pharmacologic and surgical techniques. After an initial period of stabilization with parental nutrition, enteral feeds may be introduced. Continuous enteral feeding via nasogastric or gastrostomy tube has been found to facilitate intestinal adaptation and may help accelerate the transition to oral feeding. Diets with higher protein and fat content, as opposed to carbohydrates, may be beneficial as this creates a lower osmotic load and may be better tolerated. High-fiber diets are often also useful, as are small frequent oral feedings.

A number of pharmacologic agents have been used to reduce GI looses in patients with high output. H2-blockers, proton pump inhibitors, and octreotide are useful in limiting gastric and pancreatic secretion, while loperamide decreases stool output. Glutamine and growth hormone in combination with a high-fiber diet have been suggested to hasten the time of intestinal adaptation and therefore decrease the time reliant on parental nutrition. Teduglutide is a glucagon-like peptide-2 growth factor that has been shown to reduce the number of days of parental nutrition required by patients with short-bowel syndrome, perhaps by enhancing mucosal growth. Other growth factors, including hepatocyte, keratinocyte, and epidermal growth factors, and IL-11 are being evaluated in experimental models of small bowel resection for their potential trophic and adaptive effects.

When performed by highly experienced surgeons, surgery may be used as a treatment for short-bowel syndrome. These bowel lengthening procedures include interspersing reversed segments of small bowel or colon in order to slow the progression of peristalsis. Also infrequently performed is serial transverse enteroplasty, which transects the bowel longitudinally creating a segment of bowel twice as long but half the diameter of the original bowel length. Like intestinal transplantation, these procedures should only be performed when more conservative measures have failed.

Small Bowel Hemorrhage

Patients with GI blood loss and anemia after unrevealing upper endoscopy and colonoscopy may benefit from wireless capsule endoscopy. During this procedure, a patient swallows a tiny wireless camera that takes pictures throughout the digestive tract, which allows for localization of pathology. This method is equally or more sensitive than traditional diagnostic tools, including enteroscopy, for the diagnosis of small bowel hemorrhage. Enteroscopy involves passing an enteroscope beyond the ligament of Treitz, but it is often limited by patient discomfort or looping of the scope. A primary advantage of capsule endoscopy is its less invasive approach as well as its ability to examine the entirety of the small bowel. The main disadvantage is that it does not allow tissue biopsy or intervention at the time of study. The diagnostic yield is highest when performed as soon as possible when bleeding is noted. A double-balloon technique may also be diagnostic.

Other radiographic techniques used to diagnose small bowel hemorrhage include small bowel series, enteroclysis, enterography, angiography, and radionuclide scan. Small bowel series involves oral dilute barium with serial fluoroscopic imaging, while enteroclysis is performed by injecting barium through a tube, which is passed into the proximal small bowel. Both techniques have largely been replaced by CT and MRI enterography/angiography, which combines low-density oral contrast and multiphase imaging to detect small bowel abnormalities. Additionally, radionuclide bleeding scans are more sensitive than angiography (detects bleeding at a rate of 0.1 to 0.5 mL/min), but less specific than either endoscopic or angiographic examination in detecting site of bleed. Angiography (with or without CT) may be used if the patient is bleeding enough to require a transfusion and may allow for embolization if a vascular lesion is visualized.

ACKNOWLEDGMENT

The authors would like to acknowledge Dr. Jin Lee Ra for her contribution to this chapter in the prior edition of *The Surgical Review*.

Suggested Readings

Behrns KE, Kircher AP, Galanko JA, et al. Prospective randomized trial of early initial and hospital discharge on a liquid diet following elective intestinal surgery. *Gastrointest Surg.* 2000;4:217–221.

Clavien PA, Richon J, Burgan S, et al. Gallstone ileus. *Br J Surg.* 1990;77:737–742.

Section 3: Small bowel. In: Cameron JL, Cameron AM, eds. *Current Surgical Therapy*. 11th ed. Philadelphia: Mosby Elsevier; 2014.

Cheifetz AS. Management of active Crohn disease. *JAMA.* 2013;309(20):2150–2158.

Megibow AJ. Bowel obstruction: evaluation with CT. *Radiol Clin North Am.* 1997;32(5):861–870.

Pickleman J, Lee RM. The management of patients with suspected early postoperative small bowel obstruction. *Ann Surg.* 1989; 210(2):216–219.

Roggo A, Ottinger LW. Acute small bowel volvulus in adults: a sporadic form of strangulating intestinal obstruction. *Ann Surg.* 1992;216(2):135–141.

Song HK, Buzby GP. Nutritional support for Crohn's disease. *Surg Clin North Am.* 2001;81(1):103–115.

Tavakkoli A, Ashley SW, Zinner MJ. Small intestine. In: Brunicardi FC, Andersen DK, Billiar T, et al., eds. *Schwartz's Principles of Surgery*. 10th ed. New York: McGraw-Hill Education; 2014.

Taylor MR, Lalani N. Adult small bowel obstruction. *Acad Emerg Med.* 2013;20:528–544.

CHAPTER 12

The Colon, Rectum, and Anus

KATHREEN P. LEE AND CARY B. AARONS

KEY POINTS

- The colon functions as a site for the absorption of water and sodium. Short-chain fatty acids are a key source of energy for colonic epithelia.
- Uncomplicated diverticulitis can be treated with IV antibiotics and bowel rest. Elective colectomy should be considered after an episode of complicated diverticulitis and/or recurrent uncomplicated diverticulitis
- Cancer is the leading cause of large bowel obstruction.
- Elective surgical treatment for ulcerative colitis includes total proctocolectomy with end ileostomy or total proctocolectomy with ileal pouch anal anastomosis. In cases of fulminant colitis, a staged approach is indicated starting with total abdominal colectomy and end ileostomy.
- Sigmoid volvulus is the most common form of intestinal volvulus. In the absence of peritonitis or strangulation, detorsion via sigmoidoscopy followed by bowel prep and then elective sigmoidectomy with primary anastomosis or a Hartmann's procedure is indicated.
- Squamous cell cancers of the anal canal are initially treated with chemoradiation therapy. APR is second-line therapy for residual or recurrent disease.
- Carcinoid tumors of the appendix are the most common tumor of the appendix. Surgical treatment (appendectomy vs. right hemicolectomy) is dependent on the tumor location, size of the tumor, and evidence of lymphovascular invasion.

ANATOMY

The gut arises from the endoderm and by the 3rd week of development divides into the foregut, midgut, and hindgut. Foregut-derived structures end at the second portion of the duodenum and rely on the celiac artery for blood supply. The midgut extends from the duodenal ampulla to the first two thirds of the transverse colon and is supplied by the superior mesenteric artery (SMA). The hindgut gives rise to the distal transverse and descending colon as well as the proximal rectum. Importantly, the inferior mesenteric artery (IMA) supplies this final portion of the colon and proximal rectum (via the superior rectal artery). Branches of the internal iliac artery supply the distal rectum, which is derived from the cloaca that also differentiates into the urogenital tract. The anus is formed by an invagination of the ectodermal anal pit and fuses with the distal rectum at the dentate line.

The colon is composed of four major layers: the mucosa (columnar epithelium), the submucosa (including the muscularis mucosa), the muscularis propria (inner circular and outer longitudinal smooth muscle), and serosa. The longitudinal muscular layer forms three distinct bands, the *teniae* coli, which run along the colon and then converge distally at the top of the rectum. These longitudinal bands produce sacculations or *haustra*, which give the colon its typical radiographic appearance (Fig. 12.1).

The colon is approximately 150 cm long, starting at the cecum in the right lower quadrant, and ending approximately 15 cm from the anal verge. The rectum is 12 to 15 cm long and extends from the peritoneal reflection to the dentate line, which lies 2 to 4 cm from the anal verge (Fig. 12.2).

With an average diameter of 7.5 cm, the cecum is the most capacious area of the colon. Acute dilation to greater than 12 cm can result in ischemic necrosis and perforation of the bowel wall; therefore, the cecum is the most common site of rupture secondary to obstruction or pseudo-obstruction. The appendix arises from the base of the cecum, within 2 to 3 cm of the ileocecal valve at the convergence of the three teniae coli. Its blood supply traverses its mesentery, the "mesoappendix." The position of the tip of the appendix is variable, most commonly (65%) coursing posterior to the cecum (retrocecal).

The right colon ascends to the hepatic flexure. The posterior surface is retroperitoneal and lies near the duodenum. The transverse colon is completely intraperitoneal and is suspended from a broad mesentery. The splenic flexure is more acutely angled and higher than is the hepatic flexure and is in close proximity to the spleen. The gastrocolic ligament, from the greater curve of the stomach, fuses with the peritoneal covering of the colon to form the *greater omentum*. The descending colon, like the ascending colon, is partially retroperitoneal and fixed. The intraperitoneal sigmoid is often redundant, occasionally residing in the right lower quadrant, where, if inflamed, it can mimic symptoms of appendicitis.

The teniae coli of the colon broaden and merge at the approximate level of the sacral promontory, marking the start of the rectum. The upper third of the rectum is covered anteriorly and laterally by peritoneum. The middle third is covered by peritoneum only anteriorly, and the remaining distal rectum is entirely extraperitoneal. The posterior rectum and the surrounding mesorectum abut the presacral fascia and are enveloped by a distinct mesothelial layer known as the *fascia propria*. Dissection in the plane between the fascia propria of the rectum and the sacrum preserves the integrity of the lymphatics contained within the mesorectum, which is particularly important in rectal cancer surgery. Finally, the fascia

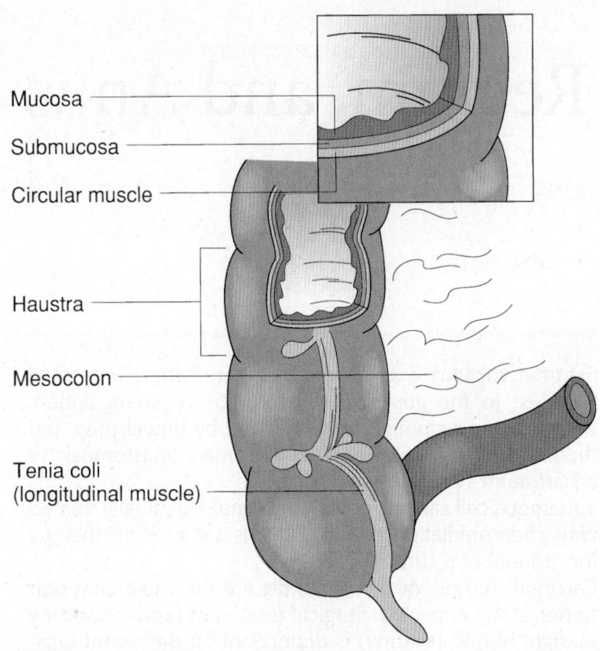

FIGURE 12.1 Layers of the colon. (From Mulholland MW, Lillemoe KD, Doherty GM, et al., eds. *Greenfield's Surgery: Scientific Principles and Practice*. 5th ed. Philadelphia: Lippincott Williams & Wilkins; 2010:1018, with permission.)

propria condenses anterolaterally into two rectal "ligaments." These contain the middle rectal artery and mixed autonomic nerves. Injury to these during dissection may result in erectile and bladder dysfunction.

The anus begins at the *dentate line* as traditionally described by anatomists, but clinically, the surgical anorectal junction begins at the level of the pelvic floor muscle. The mucosa at the dentate line forms longitudinal folds called the *columns of Morgagni*. Infection of glands at the base of these folds can result in anorectal abscesses and fistulas. Fecal continence is controlled by the muscles of the pelvic floor, together called the *levator ani*, as well as the *internal anal sphincter* (smooth muscle under involuntary control) and *external anal sphincter* (striated muscle under voluntary control) (Fig. 12.3).

The SMA branches from the aorta and supplies the right colon and first two thirds of the transverse via its branches, the middle colic, right colic, and ileocolic (in order of their origin from the SMA). The ileocolic branches into the appendiceal artery. The middle colic has left and right branches, supplying the proximal and middle thirds of the transverse colon. The right branch is typically ligated during traditional right colectomy leaving the left branch to supply the remaining transverse colon. The IMA branches from the aorta and supplies the left colon and proximal rectum via its branches, the left colic, sigmoidal, and superior rectal vessels. The middle rectal (arising from the internal iliac) and inferior rectal (arising from the internal pudendal) arteries supply the distal rectum and anus (Figs. 12.4 and 12.5).

These arterial distributions overlap to provide significant redundancy. The *marginal artery of Drummond* is a series of arterial arcades running along the mesenteric border of the entire colon. The *arc of Riolan* connects the proximal SMA and the IMA. Despite this, the splenic flexure is at risk for ischemia as it lies between the IMA and SMA distributions (i.e., a *watershed area*) (Fig. 12.6).

Venous drainage follows a similar pattern to the arterial supply. The inferior mesenteric vein drains into the splenic vein, which joins with the superior mesenteric vein to form the portal vein. The distal rectum and anus are drained by the middle and inferior rectal veins into the internal iliac veins, which becomes part of the systemic rather than the portal circulation. Lymphatics drainage follows the blood supply; therefore, tumors arising in the mid and distal rectum can metastasize to the iliac nodal basins. Colorectal

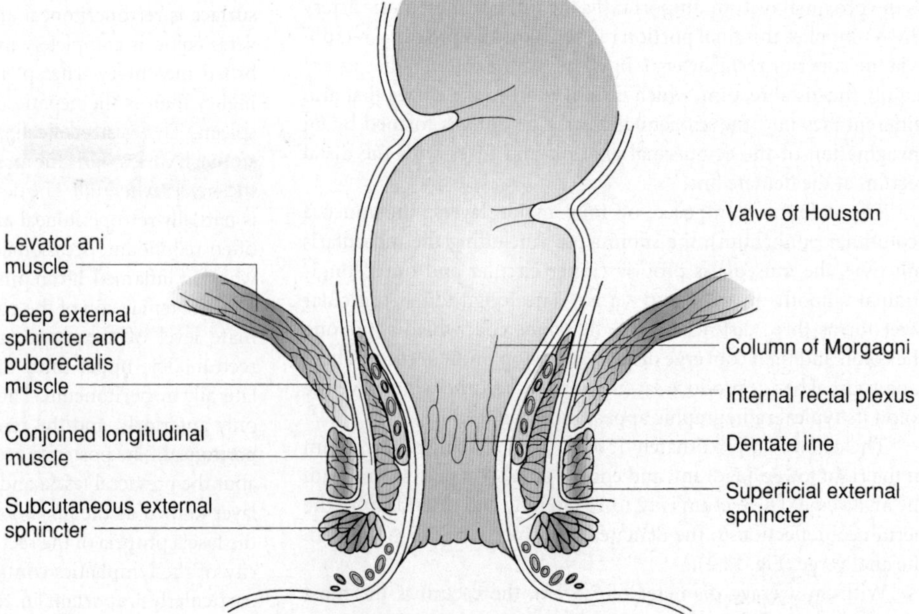

FIGURE 12.2 Distal rectum and anus. (From Mulholland MW, Lillemoe KD, Doherty GM, et al., eds. *Greenfield's Surgery: Scientific Principles and Practice*. 5th ed. Philadelphia: Lippincott Williams & Wilkins; 2010:1132, with permission.)

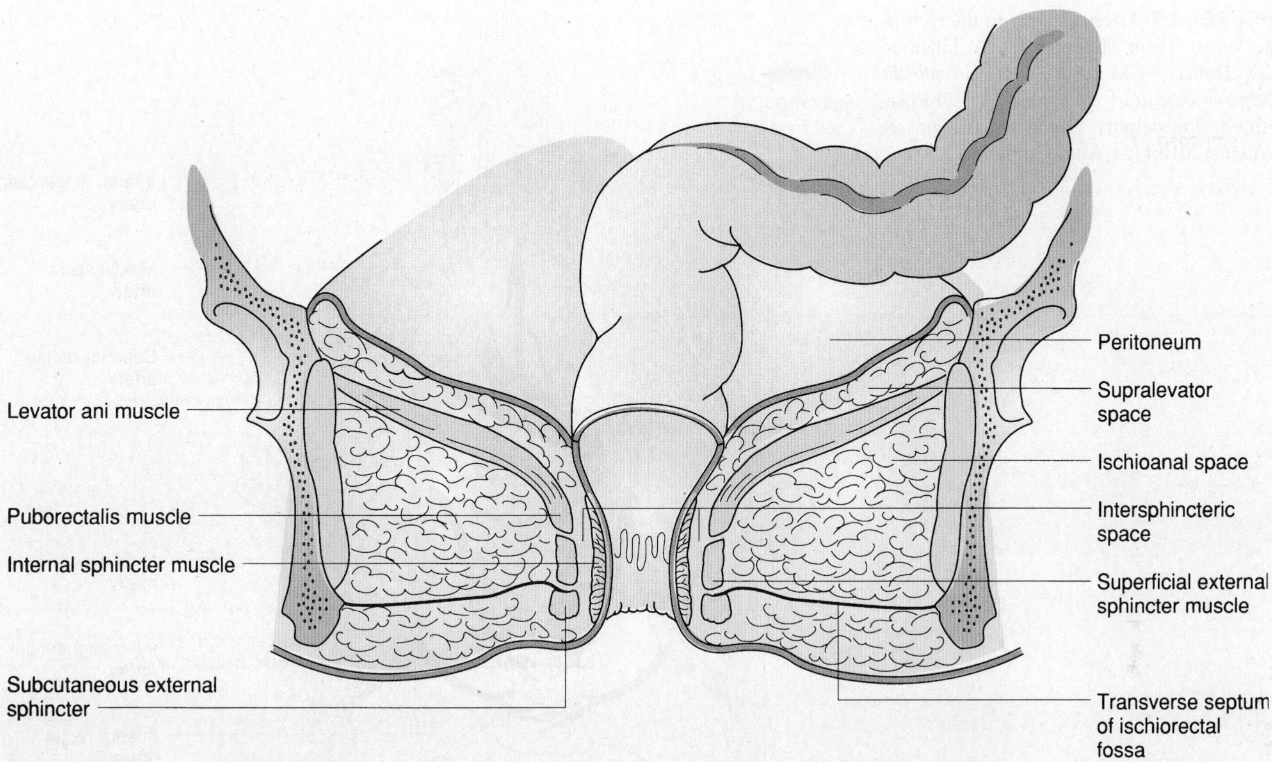

FIGURE 12.3 Anterior–posterior view of the anus, with perianal spaces and sphincters. (From Mulholland MW, Lillemoe KD, Doherty GM, et al., eds. *Greenfield's Surgery: Scientific Principles and Practice*. 5th ed. Philadelphia: Lippincott Williams & Wilkins; 2010:1133, with permission.)

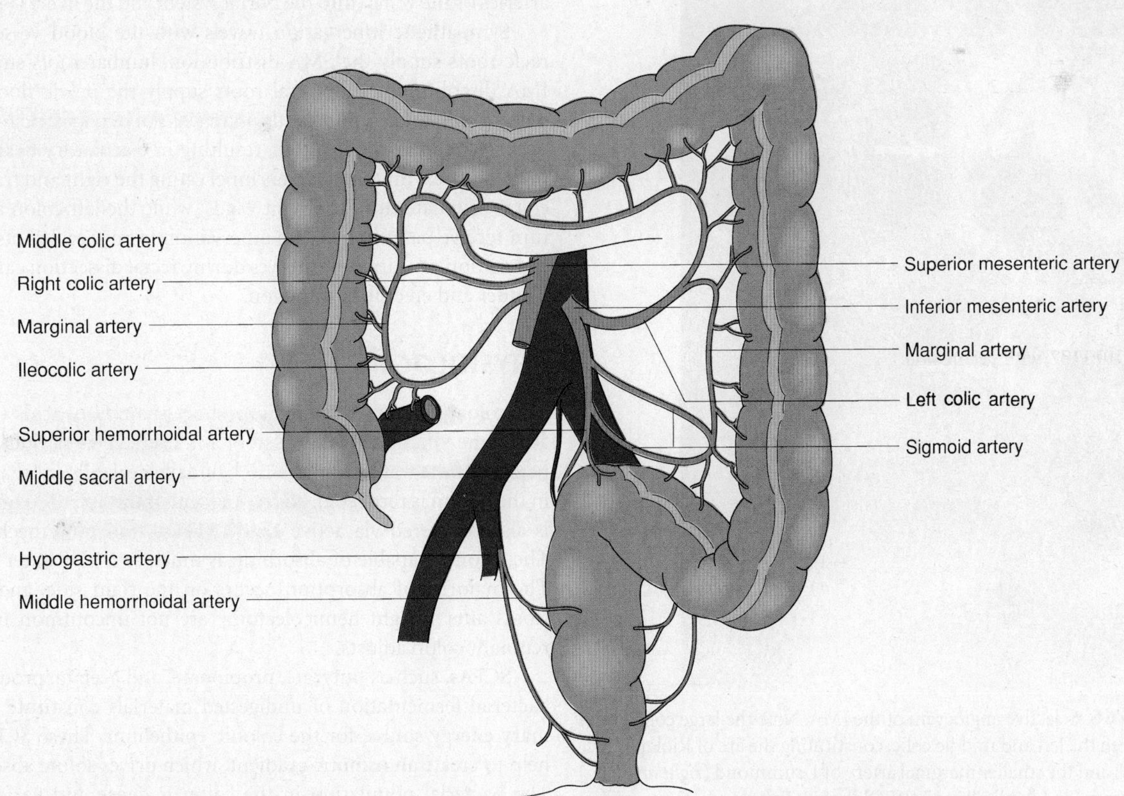

FIGURE 12.4 Arterial supply of the colon. (From Mulholland MW, Lillemoe KD, Doherty GM, et al., eds. *Greenfield's Surgery: Scientific Principles and Practice*. 5th ed. Philadelphia: Lippincott Williams & Wilkins; 2010:1020, with permission.)

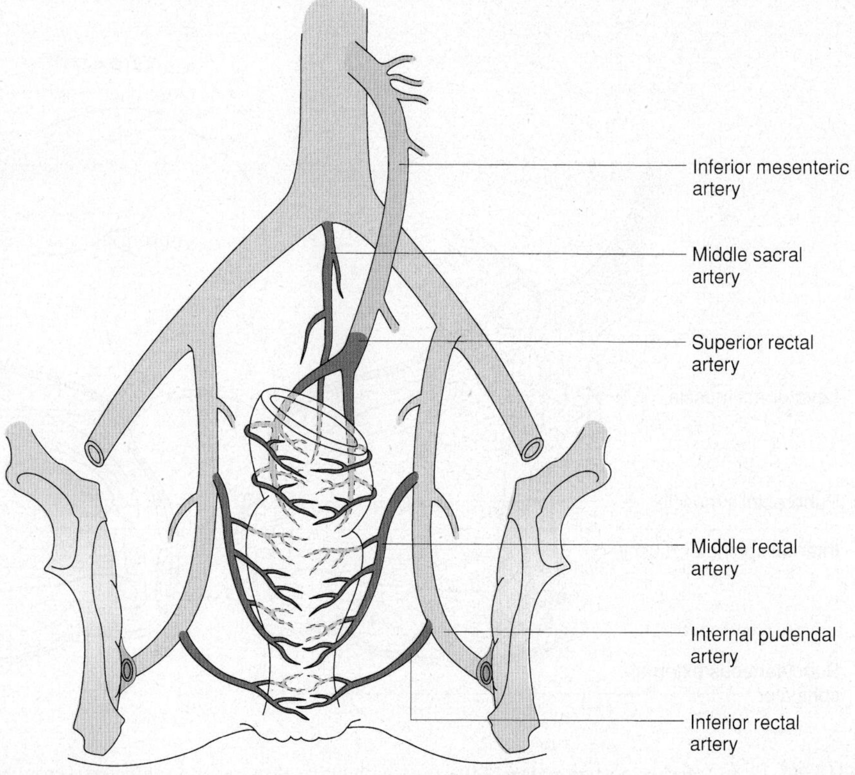

FIGURE 12.5 Arterial supply to the rectum and anus. (From Mulholland MW, Lillemoe KD, Doherty GM, et al., eds. *Greenfield's Surgery: Scientific Principles and Practice.* 5th ed. Philadelphia: Lippincott Williams & Wilkins; 2010:1134, with permission.)

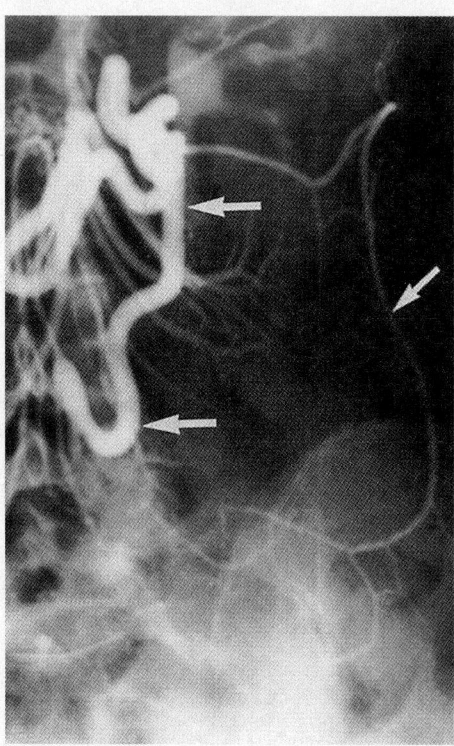

FIGURE 12.6 Selective angiogram of the IMA. Note the large collateral flow between the left and middle colic, constituting the arc of Riolan (*left two arrows*) and the smaller marginal artery of Drummond (*right arrow*). (From Greenfield LJ, Mulholland MW, Oldham KT, et al., eds. *Greenfield's Surgery: Scientific Principles and Practice.* 3rd ed. Philadelphia: Lippincott Williams & Wilkins; 2001:1694, with permission.)

cancers can additionally spread via lymphatics along the major arteries or the veins (into the portal system and the liver) (Fig. 12.7).

Sympathetic innervation travels with the blood vessels; thoracic roots supply the SMA distribution, lumbar roots supply the IMA distribution, and sacral roots supply the pelvic floor, distal rectum, and anus. Importantly, injury to the hypogastric nerve can occur when ligating the IMA, resulting in ejaculatory dysfunction in men. Parasympathetic fibers innervating the right and transverse colon originate from the right vagus, while the left colon and rectum receive parasympathetic innervation from sacral roots (S2-4). Disruption of autonomic nerves during rectal dissection can lead to bladder and erectile dysfunction.

PHYSIOLOGY

The colon extracts water, sodium, short-chain fatty acids (SCFAs), and some vitamins from the stool and excretes potassium. Ninety percent of the water from the 1.5 L of daily ileal effluent that arrives in the cecum is recovered. Ninety percent of the 300 mEq of sodium is also recovered via active Na–K ATPase transport mechanisms. The colon is capable of absorbing as much as 6 L of water per day. The majority of absorption occurs on the right side, and watery stools after a right hemicolectomy are not uncommon until the remnant colon adjusts.

SCFAs, such as butyrate, propionate, and acetate, produced by bacterial fermentation of undigested materials constitute the primary energy source for the colonic epithelium. These SCFAs also help to create an osmotic gradient, which drives solute absorption. The bacterial population in the colon is dense and varied composed of more than 400 different species and constituting greater than 50% of stool weight. *Bacteroides*, an anaerobe, is the most

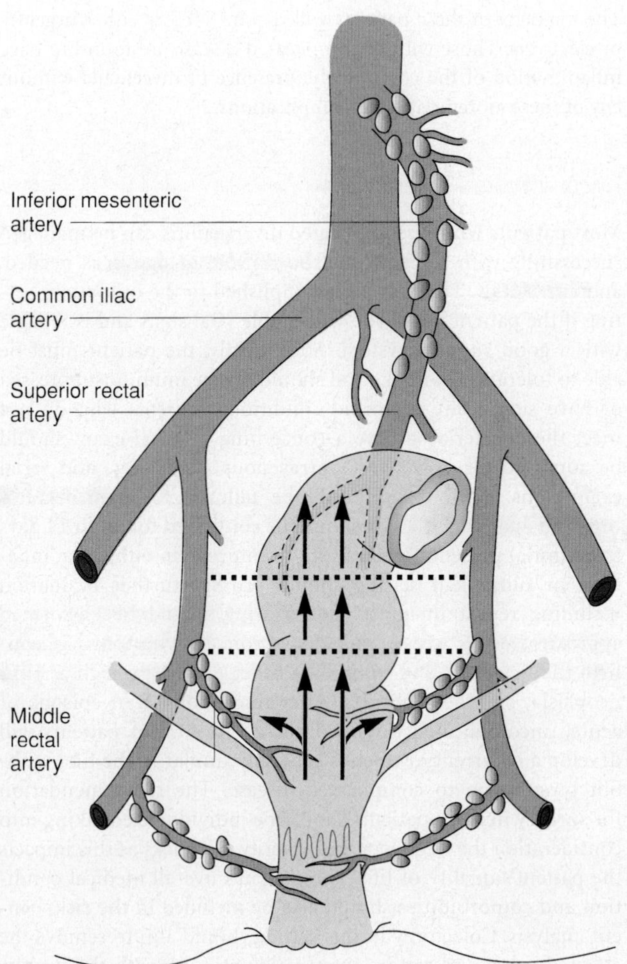

FIGURE 12.7 Lymphatic drainage of the rectum. Note the variable portal versus caval drainage (*arrows*) to approximately 10 cm above the dentate line, with gradual complete transition (*dotted lines*) to the portal circulation. (From Mulholland MW, Lillemoe KD, Doherty GM, et al., eds. *Greenfield's Surgery: Scientific Principles and Practice*. 5th ed. Philadelphia: Lippincott Williams & Wilkins; 2010:1135, with permission.)

common bacteria overall, and *Escherichia coli* is the most common aerobe. Previously, preoperative colonic washing and prep were recommended to address the bacterial abundance, but the practice has undergone a reappraisal as recent data suggest no difference in anastomotic leak rates or wound infection rates with colonic preparation.

There are three basic patterns of colonic motility. *Retrograde movements* are antiperistaltic contractions that start near the hepatic flexure and travel toward the cecum, resulting in slowing of the colonic transit and increasing fecal mixing. In the transverse and left colon primarily, *segmental contractions* propel stool forward over small distances and further increase stool mixing. Finally, there are long *mass movements*, which progress along the length of the colon and can move a column of stool up to one third of the length of the bowel. During these contractions, pressures can rise as high as 200 mm Hg and are highest in the sigmoid colon. Overall control of colonic motility involves both neuronal and hormonal factors. Parasympathetic and sympathetic neurons supply extrinsic control, stimulating and inhibiting motility, respectively. Intrinsic neurons within the wall of the colon form two plexuses. The myenteric (Auerbach) is at the junction between the longitudinal and circular layers of the muscularis propria, and the submucosal (Meissner) is a secondary plexus formed in the submucosa from the nerve fibers that perforate the circular muscle layer. Absence of these ganglion cells in the colon due to the failure of neural crest cells to migrate appropriately during embryonic development leads to functional obstruction of that segment of the colon in neonates, a gut motility disorder known as Hirschsprung disease. Ingestion of a meal results in increased colonic tone, termed the *gastrocolic reflex*.

The rectum functions as a reservoir for stool. Filling of this reservoir results in an urge to defecate as the internal anal sphincter relaxes. During normal defecation, the initial trigger is rectal distention, which results in relaxation of the internal anal sphincter and sampling of the rectal contents. When the decision to defecate is made, the puborectalis relaxes, resulting in straightening of the anorectal junction. The external anal sphincter is then relaxed, and the rectal contents are evacuated as the intra-abdominal pressure increases.

PATHOLOGY OF THE COLON AND RECTUM

Appendicitis

Appendicitis is caused by inflammation of its inner lining that can be due to obstruction of the lumen by a fecalith or due to infection. Classically, the presenting symptoms include periumbilical pain that migrates to the right lower quadrant, nausea, and anorexia. However, presentation can vary among patients, and many other pathologies such as inflammatory bowel disease (IBD), pelvic inflammatory disease, and neutropenic enterocolitis can present in a similar fashion. Therefore, a thorough history and physical examination are key in differentiating appendicitis from other possible etiologies that have significantly different treatment strategies.

Once a history and physical examination is complete, basic labs including liver function and pancreatic enzymes should be gathered. For the adult patient, the standard imaging modality has been CT scan of the abdomen and pelvis, which has both a high sensitivity and specificity for appendicitis and which has significantly reduced the incidence of negative laparotomies. For pediatric or pregnant patients, ultrasonography of the abdomen is the usual primary diagnostic tool. A noncompressible tubular structure on ultrasound is indicative of appendicitis, but if the US is inconclusive, MRI has also been shown to be a diagnostic alternative.

For patients with simple appendicitis, appendectomy is the definitive therapy. However, in those with an associated small abscess or phlegmon, initial therapy may consist of IV antibiotics followed by an interval appendectomy after 4 to 6 weeks once the inflammation and abscess are resolved. For those with a large abscess, a drainage catheter may have to be placed by interventional radiology in addition to antibiotic therapy in order to adequately treat the infection prior to interval appendectomy.

Diverticular Disease

Diverticular disease comprises a spectrum of symptoms and presentations related to the presence of diverticula in the colon wall. These diverticula are outpouchings of the colon wall, which occur most commonly due to high intraluminal pressure in the areas of relative anatomic weakness where the small arterioles traverse the colon wall (Fig. 12.8). As a result, the mucosa and submucosa are pushed through the muscular layer—termed a *pseudodiverticulum*. The sigmoid colon is the most common site for the development of diverticula. Diverticulosis was first described in the mid 19th century, and the incidence has been increasing. While the pathophysiology of diverticulosis has not been definitively established, it is commonly held that it is largely related to a diet low in dietary fiber. It has been well described that the incidence increases with age with an estimated 40% of people affected by the age of 65 years. Diverticulosis is usually asymptomatic, but approximately 10% to 20% will develop symptoms of diverticulitis, characterized by infection and inflammation resulting from perforation of a diverticulum. Diverticulosis is also a common cause of lower gastrointestinal (GI) bleeding, which resolves spontaneously in the majority of patients.

Evaluation

Patients with diverticulitis typically present with localized abdominal pain. As the sigmoid is the most commonly affected site, this pain is typically located in the left lower quadrant. Change in bowel habits, anorexia, nausea, fever/chills, and urinary urgency (resulting from bladder irritation) are also commonly associated symptoms. Physical findings may reveal localized peritonitis, and leukocytosis is a common laboratory finding. Prior to the advent of CT scans, barium enema studies were the primary imaging modality for the diagnosis of acute diverticulitis; however, these studies are limited as they only provide information of the colon and cannot be performed if perforation is suspected. CT scan of the abdomen is now considered the standard for the evaluation of acute diverticulitis with high studied sensitivity. CT scan also provides useful information on the extent and severity of disease as well as pathology outside of the colon, which may be useful in operative planning.

Management

Generally, the management of acute diverticulitis depends on the severity of disease at presentation. Acute diverticulitis is often clinically divided into *uncomplicated* and *complicated* disease. Patients with complicated diverticulitis are characterized by the presence of an abscess, fistula, obstruction, or free perforation. The majority of these patients will require surgery either urgently or electively. Those with uncomplicated disease are found to have inflammation of the colon in the presence of diverticula without any of these aforementioned complications.

Uncomplicated Diverticulitis

Most patients with uncomplicated diverticulitis can be managed successfully with a regimen of bowel rest, analgesia as needed, and antibiotics. This can be accomplished in the outpatient setting if the patient is afebrile with stable vital signs and is reliable with a good support system. Additionally, the patient must be able to tolerate oral intake and should not be immunosuppressed or have significant comorbid conditions. Patients who do not meet these criteria or have a concerning physical exam should be admitted for bowel rest, intravenous antibiotics, and serial evaluations. Antibiotics should be tailored to gram-negative rods and anaerobes, which should be continued for 10 to 14 days from initial presentation. Failure to improve in either the inpatient or outpatient setting should prompt further evaluation including repeat imaging. Colonoscopy should be performed approximately 6 weeks after resolution of symptoms to confirm the diagnosis and to exclude other pathology such as IBD, neoplasia, or other colitides. After resolution of an episode of acute, uncomplicated diverticulitis, up to 40% of patients will develop a recurrence, which is generally similar to the first without progression to complicated disease. The recommendation for surgery in these patients should be individualized taking into consideration the frequency and severity of attacks as this impacts the patient's quality of life. The patient's overall medical condition and comorbidities should also be included in the risk–benefit analysis. Colectomy in this setting should aim to remove the affected colon and restore intestinal continuity with the healthy remaining bowel. This can be managed either laparoscopically or with a conventional open approach. Following sigmoid colectomy, anastomosis should be made to the upper rectum in order to minimize recurrence.

Complicated Diverticulitis

Diverticulitis associated with a large (≥4 cm) pericolonic abscess can often be managed successfully with percutaneous drainage in order to reduce the inflammation and convert an otherwise urgent

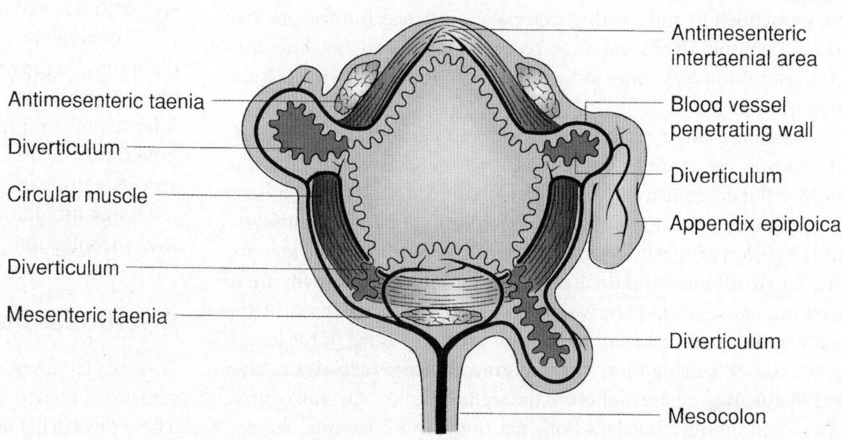

FIGURE 12.8 Diverticulosis. Diverticulum form where the blood vessels penetrate on the antimesenteric border of the tenia. (From Mulholland MW, Lillemoe KD, Doherty GM, et al., eds. *Greenfield's Surgery: Scientific Principles and Practice*. 5th ed. Philadelphia: Lippincott Williams & Wilkins; 2010:1121, with permission.)

problem to a semielective one. Smaller abscesses, which are typically not amenable to percutaneous drainage, can be managed with antibiotics and observation. Following resolution of diverticular disease with associated abscess, elective colectomy should typically be considered. Failure of percutaneous drainage or antibiotic therapy should mandate more urgent surgical management.

Abscesses caused by diverticulitis can erode into an adjacent organ, resulting in fistula formation. Colovesical fistulas are the most common type and typically present with pneumaturia or recurrent urinary tract infections. Other organs involved may include the vagina, small bowel, and skin (especially after percutaneous drainage). The diagnosis of a fistula can be confirmed with a CT scan. Air in the bladder without previous catheterization is pathognomonic for a colovesical fistula. A contrast study (fistulogram, barium enema, or small bowel follow-through) can also be helpful in further delineating the path of the fistula tract but are not as sensitive as is CT scan. Broad-spectrum antibiotics should be instituted until resolution of the inflammation, and then, elective resection of the involved colon and fistula tract is performed. If small bowel is involved, then resection with primary anastomosis may be required. Simple fistulas to the bladder may require primary repair with absorbable suture and almost always heal without extensive reconstruction.

Obstruction due to stricture formation is rarely associated with acute diverticulitis. However, this may occur due to chronic inflammation and scarring, which results in narrowing of the lumen. Most often, the obstruction is partial and insidious. Preoperative colonoscopy to exclude carcinoma is critical prior to appropriate elective resection.

The *Hinchey* classification is often used to stratify the severity of diverticular disease complicated by perforation.

Stage I: Small, confined pericolonic or mesenteric abscess
Stage II: Larger, walled-off pelvic abscess
Stage III: Generalized purulent peritonitis
Stage IV: Generalized fecal peritonitis

As discussed previously, Hinchey stages I and II are often initially managed with administration of antibiotics and percutaneous drainage, if feasible. If this strategy is successful, elective colectomy should be performed and a primary anastomosis can often be achieved. Hinchey III and IV generally constitute surgical emergencies that require immediate exploration. Patients often present with generalized peritonitis and signs and symptoms of sepsis. After resuscitation and stabilization, operative goals include washout of the abdomen and removal of the diseased colon. In the setting of a grossly contaminated field, primary anastomosis is often not safe. The strategy of choice in this setting should be the *Hartmann's procedure*: segmental resection, a proximal end colostomy, and closure of the rectal stump. The colostomy is usually temporary and can be reversed once the inflammation subsides; however, a substantial amount of patients will never have their colostomy reversed. Primary anastomosis with or without proximal diversion has been studied extensively and should be individualized based on patient and intraoperative factors.

Laparoscopic lavage has emerged recently as an attractive approach in the management of diverticulitis with purulent peritonitis as it mitigates much of the morbidity and mortality associated with standard colectomy. The procedure typically entails an initial diagnostic laparoscopy, which confirms purulent peritonitis followed by irrigation with 4 L of warm saline and placement of drains. While there have been good results noted in small series, the safety and efficacy of laparoscopic lavage has yet to be proven in a prospective, randomized fashion.

Immunocompromised and transplant patients are a unique subset who require special consideration with respect to management of acute diverticulitis. While diverticulitis is not more prevalent in this cohort, studies indicate that they are at greater risk of presenting with recurrent and complicated disease. Therefore, after the initial presentation of acute diverticulitis, providers should have a low threshold to offer elective colectomy. Prophylactic colectomy in pretransplant patients remains controversial.

Large Bowel Obstruction

Large bowel obstruction is a challenging clinical entity that can present with similar symptoms to that of small bowel obstruction (SBO), namely abdominal pain, distention, obstipation, and possibly nausea/vomiting. However, unlike obstructions of the small intestine, which are typically caused by adhesions, colonic obstructions are most commonly caused by neoplasms. Other etiologies of mechanical obstruction include diverticular disease, volvulus, IBD, and ischemic or anastomotic strictures. Colonic pseudo-obstruction is the most common cause for nonmechanical colonic obstruction.

In a patient with a competent ileocecal valve, colonic obstruction is particularly dangerous because it creates a closed-loop obstruction between the valve and the point of obstruction in the colon. The progressive distention of the bowel leads to vascular compromise and potentially perforation, particularly of the cecum. Prompt evaluation of these patients is of utmost importance. Signs of sepsis (fever, tachycardia, hypotension, leukocytosis) or peritonitis on physical exam should prompt urgent surgical exploration. Patients who are hemodynamically stable without an urgent indication for surgery should be evaluated further with radiographic imaging. A plain abdominal radiograph and upright chest x-ray can provide immediate information on free intra-abdominal air, but they also provide a general assessment of the degree of bowel distention. Profound dilation of the cecum (10 to 12 cm) may herald impending perforation. Dilation of the cecum and small bowel denotes an incompetent ileocecal valve, while dilation of the proximal colon with a paucity of air in the rectum typically signifies a left-sided obstruction. CT scans of the abdomen and pelvis are readily accessible and are very sensitive for diagnosis of most etiologies for colonic obstruction. If a diagnosis is not immediately obvious on CT scan, then a water-soluble contrast enema study may provide more information on the area of transition between decompressed and dilated colon. Finally, colonoscopy is an immensely useful tool for diagnosis and tissue biopsy in patients without a complete obstruction or severe abdominal pain.

Volvulus

Colonic volvulus is characterized by the twisting of a loop of colon around the axis of its mesentery, which essentially causes a closed-loop obstruction. This occurs most commonly in areas of the colon without fixed peritoneal attachments such as the sigmoid colon, the cecum, and the transverse colon.

The sigmoid is the most common location for volvulus and accounts for up to 65% of cases. Increased risk is noted in patients of advanced age, particularly those who are debilitated or institu-

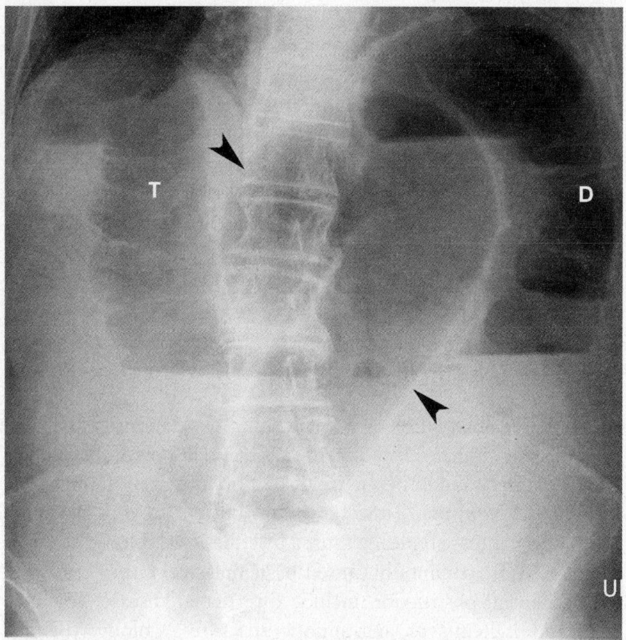

FIGURE 12.9 Abdominal radiograph demonstrating the "bent inner tube" of sigmoid volvulus. The excessive small bowel gas, in addition, indicates obstruction. (From Mulholland MW, Lillemoe KD, Doherty GM, et al., eds. *Greenfield's Surgery: Scientific Principles and Practice.* 5th ed. Philadelphia: Lippincott Williams & Wilkins; 2010:754, with permission.)

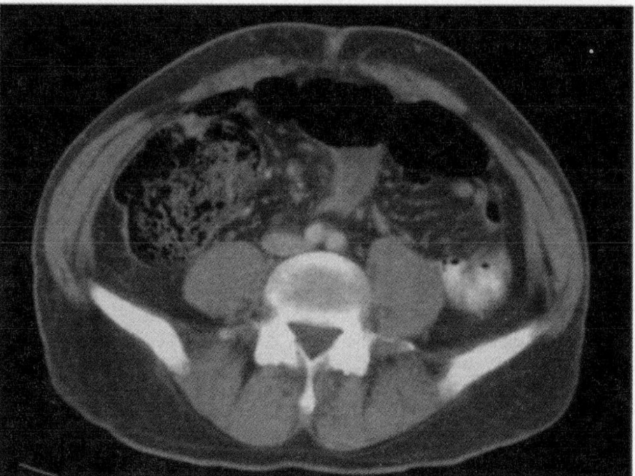

FIGURE 12.10 Abdominal CT scan demonstrating the "mesenteric whorl" often seen in cases of volvulus. (From Mulholland MW, Lillemoe KD, Doherty GM, et al., eds. *Greenfield's Surgery: Scientific Principles and Practice.* 5th ed. Philadelphia: Lippincott Williams & Wilkins; 2010:755, with permission.)

tionalized, as well as those with chronic constipation and on psychotropic medications. Patients with sigmoid volvulus typically present with acute or chronic abdominal pain, distention, and vomiting. Obstipation and diminished appetite are also common complaints. The traditional finding on plain radiograph is the "bent inner tube" sign with the dilated sigmoid pointing to the right upper quadrant (Fig. 12.9). In these cases, a contrast enema study would show a "bird's beak" as the retrograde contrast abruptly stops at the twisted segment of sigmoid colon. CT scan has largely supplanted these other studies for diagnosis of sigmoid volvulus and will reveal a characteristic mesenteric whorl (Fig. 12.10). Additionally, CT scan is able to give useful information on potential bowel compromise including wall thickening, free air or fluid, pneumatosis, or portal venous gas.

The initial management of sigmoid volvulus involves prompt IV resuscitation followed by detorsion of sigmoid. This can be accomplished via rigid proctoscopy or, preferably, with a flexible endoscope, which can be passed gently beyond the volvulus with minimal insufflation. Successful detorsion should prompt a rush of gas and stool from the dilated proximal colon, which can be further decompressed endoscopically. The colon should be inspected for ischemic changes, and a rectal tube should be placed. Endoscopic detorsion is successful in up to 80% of cases and facilitates continued resuscitation and evaluation. Recurrence is common; therefore, if endoscopic detorsion is successful, the patient should undergo resection of the sigmoid colon during the same admission. Urgent laparotomy is indicated if endoscopic detorsion is unsuccessful or if the patient exhibits signs of bowel ischemia on initial assessment.

The cecum is the second most common site of colonic volvulus. Similar to the sigmoid, a true cecal volvulus involves rotation of the cecum and terminal ileum around the mesentery, which can lead to vascular compromise. Another variant, known as a *cecal bascule*, occurs when the floppy cecum flips anteriorly and superiorly becoming fixed, which often does not result in vascular compromise. Patients with cecal volvulus typically present with abdominal pain, distention, and nausea/vomiting. A plain abdominal radiograph may show the classic "coffee bean sign" with the dilated cecum pointing to the left upper quadrant. A contrast enema study or CT scan is also sensitive for making the diagnosis. Unlike sigmoid volvulus, endoscopic detorsion is much less likely to be successful; therefore, surgical resection with a right colectomy is the primary treatment modality in these patients. Cecostomy and cecopexy have been described as nonresectional strategies but are fraught with morbidity and are associated with increased rates recurrence as compared to segmental resection.

Malignant Obstruction

Up to 29% of patients with colorectal cancer will initially present with either a partial or complete bowel obstruction. Therefore, a careful history regarding the signs and symptoms of colorectal cancer should be obtained at the time of initial evaluation. In addition to the initial assessments with plain radiographs, CT scans, or water-soluble contrast enema, colonoscopy provides direct visualization and biopsy of the obstructing lesion. Surgery is the mainstay of treatment for these malignancies causing obstruction.

In patients with proximal lesions, a right colectomy is the treatment of choice. An extended right colectomy can be performed for obstructing lesions of the proximal or mid transverse colon. Primary ileocolonic anastomosis has been found to be safe even in the emergent setting, but patient selection is important. High-risk patients may benefit from a resection with end ileostomy.

The surgical management of obstructing distal lesions has evolved over the years. A traditional approach includes proximal diversion with a loop colostomy, which is ideal for patients with unresectable colon cancers, rectal cancers, or those who are severely ill. Another option is a Hartmann's procedure, which entails resection of the colonic segment with the mass and creation of an end proximal colostomy. This is a useful strategy in cases of profound proximal colonic dilation or perforation in higher-risk patients. Definitive resection of the colonic mass and primary anastomosis is another safe and feasible option that has gained recent favor in properly selected patients. Increased risk of colo-colonic anastomotic leak has been identified in those with malnutrition, immunosuppression, and chronic renal failure.

Endoluminal stenting has become increasingly popular both for palliation and as a primary intervention for obstructing distal lesions. In cases that would otherwise require emergency surgery, endoluminal stents offers the benefit of decreased procedure time, decreased length of hospital stay, and decreased need for ostomy formation. The main risks include stent migration, perforation, and obstruction. In a recent Cochrane Review of five randomized trials, Sagar et al. concluded that while endoluminal stents were not as clinically successful, they seem to be safe and feasible with comparable morbidity and mortality.

Colonic Pseudo-obstruction

Ogilvie's syndrome, or colonic pseudo-obstruction, presents with similar symptoms to acute large bowel obstruction; however, this entity is characterized by marked dilation, primarily of the proximal colon, without a mechanical obstruction. The exact pathogenesis is unclear, but in the acute setting, the majority of cases are associated with secondary underlying causes. Nonoperative trauma, infection, orthopedic surgery, and cardiac disease are among the most commonly associated conditions. Additionally, electrolyte imbalance and narcotic use have been implicated.

A water-soluble enema study should be performed to exclude a mechanical etiology of obstruction in patients without evidence of impending bowel compromise. An initial trial of conservative management including nasogastric tube decompression, bowel rest, intravenous fluid resuscitation, cessation of narcotics and anticholinergics, and correction of electrolyte abnormalities should be employed. If pseudo-obstruction fails to resolve with a conservative approach, administration of neostigmine, an acetylcholinesterase inhibitor, and endoscopic decompression have been shown to be highly efficacious. The need for surgery is uncommon and should be reserved for those with peritoneal signs or those who have failed maximal medical management. Any colonic perforation should be resected. If the colon is viable without perforation, the use of decompressing cecostomy or colostomy has been described.

Infectious Colitides

Infections of the colon are common. Most do not require surgical intervention, but a few can occasionally develop into surgical emergencies.

Pseudomembranous colitis is an increasingly common and virulent infection caused by colonic overgrowth of the endogenous bacteria, *Clostridium difficile*, which can develop after the normal colonic flora is altered by antibiotic use. Transmission is via the fecal–oral route, and the bacteria are readily communicable either by direct person-to-person contact or via fomites such as clothes, bedding, and medical instruments. *C. difficile* produces two exotoxins: enterotoxin (A) and cytotoxin (B), which causes mucosal damage resulting in the characteristic exudative pseudomembrane seen on endoscopy. Presentations can vary greatly and range from self-limiting watery diarrhea and abdominal pain to fulminant colitis with marked leukocytosis and a clinical picture consistent with septic shock. Complications of fulminant colitis include toxic megacolon and bowel perforation. The diagnosis of C. Difficile colitis can be confirmed with enzyme-linked immunosorbent assay (ELISA), which tests for both A and B toxins as well as glutamate dehydrogenase (GDH), a constitutively expressed enzyme by *C. difficile* isolates. Discordant ELISA results should be resolved with confirmatory PCR. Initial therapy consists of oral metronidazole or oral vancomycin for 2 weeks. In more severe cases, oral vancomycin should be used over oral metronidazole as randomized trials have shown a higher cure rate with the former. Intravenous metronidazole or vancomycin enemas can be used if oral administration is not feasible; however, intravenous vancomycin is not recommended, as it is not excreted into the colon. In the setting of septic shock and documented colitis, mortality approaches 60%; therefore, immediate surgical intervention may be necessary. Traditionally, subtotal colectomy with end ileostomy has been the procedure of choice. A diverting loop ileostomy combined with antegrade colonic lavage with vancomycin flushes via the ileostomy may be an alternative colon-sparing procedure that has thus far shown promising results. Relapse rates up to 25% have been identified in patients with *C. difficile* infections treated with conventional antibiotic regimens; therefore, alternative strategies such as fecal transplantation are being studied. While this has been shown to be safe and efficacious in smaller series, widespread adoption has been hindered by the paucity of large, randomized data and the lack of standardized practices in preparation and administration.

Other infectious etiologies that may result in bloody diarrhea include *Shigella*, *Campylobacter jejuni*, enterohemorrhagic *E. coli* (EHEC), *Entamoeba histolytica*, and certain *Salmonella* species. Consuming food or water contaminated with cysts of *E. histolytica* can cause amebic colitis. Symptoms can mimic IBD and include crampy abdominal pain and bloody diarrhea. Diagnosis is usually through a combination of clinical history, stool studies, antigen testing, as well as endoscopy with biopsies typically showing ulcerations and trophozoites. Treatment consists of metronidazole plus a luminal agent, such as paromomycin. However, like *C. difficile* colitis, complications can include fulminant colitis, which could necessitate emergent surgical intervention. The liver is a frequent site of secondary infection (i.e., hepatic abscesses), and treatment usually consists of the same antiparasitics but can also include therapeutic aspiration or percutaneous drainage if necessary.

Shigellosis in the United States is usually spread via the fecal–oral route but can also be transmitted through contaminated food and water. Symptoms vary depending on the specific *Shigella* species, but infection by *S. flexneri* or *S. dysenteriae* presents with abdominal pain, fever, tenesmus, as well as bloody and mucoid diarrhea. Diagnosis is made by stool culture, and while the disease is usually self-limited, treatment with an antibiotic, such as a fluoroquinolone, is recommended to reduce the duration and severity of the disease.

Outbreaks of EHEC in the United States have mostly been through fecal contamination of foods such as raw produce. Hemorrhagic colitis is the most common symptom, often requiring hospital admission. Treatment is usually supportive with no clear role for antibiotic therapy at this time. Hemolytic uremic syndrome (HUS) is the major potential systemic sequela of EHEC infections affecting almost 10% of patients, with children under 10 years old having the highest risk. The onset of HUS is usually 5 to 10 days after the start of diarrheal symptoms and consists of acute renal failure, thrombocytopenia, and microangiopathic hemolytic anemia. Treatment for postdiarrheal HUS includes supportive therapy and often plasmapheresis if symptoms are severe.

Different salmonellae strains can cause a host of diverse infections in humans, but gastroenteritis caused by nontyphoidal salmonellae strains are the most common. Transmission is usually by the fecal–oral route or via ingesting improperly handled foods. The clinical manifestation of salmonellosis includes diarrhea, abdominal pain, fever, and vomiting, which can start between 1 and 3 days after exposure. Since symptoms are indistinguishable from other causes of gastroenteritis, stool culture is necessary for diagnosis. Salmonella gastroenteritis is self-limiting, and treatment is normally supportive.

Campylobacter enteritis is usually caused by either *C. jejuni* or *C. coli*, which can be found in the intestinal tract of different animal hosts, primarily poultry. Symptoms of this foodborne illness are similar to previously mentioned infectious gastroenteritis and include abdominal pain, fever, and watery or bloody diarrhea. Diagnosis is made by history and stool culture, and the infection is usually self-limited with antibiotic therapy reserved for severe cases. Preventive measures include avoiding ingesting raw poultry and unpasteurized dairy products.

Cytomegaloviral colitis affects 10% of patients with acquired immunodeficiency syndrome (AIDS) and can present with findings similar to appendicitis. Ganciclovir is the treatment of choice.

Neutropenic enterocolitis most commonly affects the cecum ("typhlitis") and most commonly affects immunosuppressed patients undergoing chemotherapy. While not technically an infection, the clinical presentation is often confused with appendicitis with acute localized abdominal pain. Unlike appendicitis, treatment is conservative with bowel rest and IV antibiotics, and surgery is only indicated in the setting of complications such as perforation or persistent bleeding.

Ischemia of the Colon

The colon is the most common site of bowel ischemia, occurring most commonly due to prolonged hypoperfusion of the colon secondary to hemodynamic instability. Other causes include thrombosis, atherosclerosis, embolism, or ligation of a major vessel. Colonic ischemia is often transient and may be difficult to diagnose. The disease pattern usually is segmental with the watershed areas, such as the splenic flexure, being most commonly affected. Classically, patients present with worsening abdominal pain (usually out of proportion to exam), bloody diarrhea, and abdominal distention. Lactic acidosis and leukocytosis are common laboratory findings, especially late in the presentation. Bowel wall edema, or pneumatosis of the intestinal wall on contrast CT scan, can suggest the diagnosis of ischemia with compromise of the bowel. Sigmoidoscopy or colonoscopy findings of patchy hemorrhagic areas with dusky mucosa are more definitive findings. Urgent segmental resection and creation of a stoma are indicated in the setting of full-thickness necrosis or perforation. In the presence of partial-thickness ischemia, antibiotics, bowel rest, and correction of hypoperfused state can often lead to resolution without necessitating resection. If symptoms continue for more than 2 weeks, segmental resection and creation of an ostomy are indicated (Fig. 12.11).

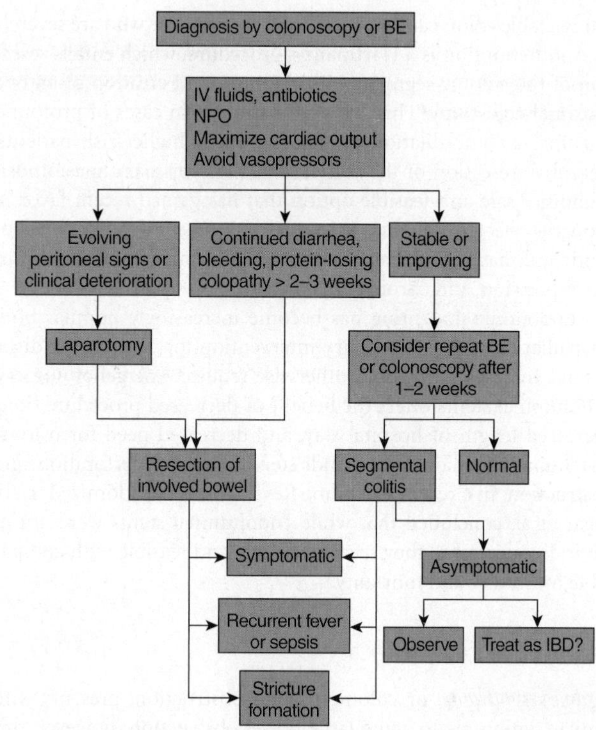

FIGURE 12.11 Treatment algorithm for ischemic colitis. BE, barium enema; NPO, nothing by mouth. (From Townsend CM, Beauchamp RD, Evers BM, et al., eds. *Sabiston Textbook of Surgery*. 19th ed. Philadelphia: WB Saunders; 2012:1336, with permission.)

Inflammatory Bowel Disease

IBD is a clinical entity composed of ulcerative colitis (UC) and Crohn's disease. The exact etiology of IBD is still unknown but likely includes a combination of genetic and environmental factors. It is four times more common in Caucasian populations and two times more in those of Jewish descent. The peak age of onset is 15 to 40 years; however, there may be a second peak in the sixth and seventh decade of life. The clustering of cases among patients with certain human leukocyte antigen (HLA) subtypes and elevated expression of antineutrophil cytoplasmic antibodies (pANCAs) and antibodies against tropomyosin in some patients with UC implicate autoimmune mechanisms as well.

Crohn's disease and UC share some common symptoms; however, differentiating between them is critically important, as the surgical treatment of the two diseases differs significantly. Crohn's disease can occur anywhere in the GI tract, from the mouth (aphthous ulcers) to the anus (fistulizing anal disease), with the terminal ileum being the most frequently involved area. In contrast, UC starts, and is the most severe, in the rectum and then progresses proximally in a continuous fashion. It does not generally involve the small bowel, although in the 10% of UC patients who have pancolitis, the terminal ileum is also secondarily inflamed (*backwash ileitis*). UC affects the bowel in a contiguous fashion, while Crohn's disease is characterized by patchy involvement (skip lesions). Importantly, Crohn's disease causes *transmural* inflammation, while UC involves *only the mucosa*. As a result, the gross appearance of the colon is frequently normal in UC, while segments of bowel affected by Crohn's disease appear grossly inflamed with a thickened mesentery and *creeping serosal fat*. Colonoscopic examination for UC typically reveals an extremely friable mucosa. Long *longitudinal ulcers* and erosions of the submucosa causing a nodular appearance known as *cobblestoning* are seen with Crohn's disease. The pathologic hallmarks of Crohn's disease include transmural infiltration with deep penetrating fissures through the muscularis propria and, most importantly, *noncaseating granulomas*. In UC, a denuded, but normal, muscularis propria may be seen. *Pseudopolyps*, clumps of regenerating mucosa, and *crypt abscesses*, inflammatory collections at the base of the crypts of Lieberkühn, can be seen in both UC and Crohn's disease.

Ulcerative Colitis

Clinically, UC most often presents with frequent bloody diarrhea. Patients also often report crampy abdominal pain, tenesmus, and urgency occasionally resulting in fecal incontinence. Disease severity can range from mild to severe and can be stratified using factors such as number of stools per day, degree of rectal bleeding, and presence of systemic symptoms. Patients with severe diarrhea (>10 stools per day) can also present with dehydration, hypotension, tachycardia, anemia, hypoalbuminemia, and weight loss. The diagnosis of UC requires a sharp clinical acumen and initial evaluation should include a complete history, including any recent travel, physical exam, basic labs, as well as stool studies for ova and parasites and stool cultures to exclude infectious etiologies of bloody diarrhea (e.g., *Shigella* sp., *E. coli.*, *Campylobacter* sp., *Salmonella* sp.). A colonoscopy should be performed to delineate the extent of disease, and multiple biopsies should be obtained. The remainder of the GI tract should also be evaluated radiographically to look for signs of Crohn's disease.

UC is associated with a variety of extracolonic manifestations. *Pyoderma gangrenosum* is a destructive inflammatory ulcerative disease of the skin commonly found around ostomy sites and on the arms and legs. Although it can be difficult to control medically, multiple immunosuppressive regimens have been found to be effective. Surgical excision should be avoided, because in 50% of patients with underlying colitis, the skin manifestations will resolve once active disease is effectively controlled. *Primary sclerosing cholangitis* (PSC) is an obliterating inflammatory disease of the small and large bile ducts and is the most common noninfectious indication for liver transplantation. Unfortunately, colectomy does not ameliorate sequelae of PSC. Arthritides, including *ankylosing spondylitis and sacroiliitis*, have been linked to UC and HLA-B27 carriers and are also not improved by colectomy.

Once the diagnosis of UC is made, medical management with sulfasalazine or its derivatives is generally initiated. Sulfasalazine is effective in 70% to 80% of patients with moderate disease and can also be used as maintenance therapy. In more severe cases, immunosuppressive medications are often indicated. Most patients receive corticosteroids, during periods of acute exacerbation, but other medications such as azathioprine (AZA) and 6-mercaptopurine (6-MP) have been used to induce and maintain remission for long periods in UC patients. Newer drugs targeting tumor necrosis factor-α (TNF-α) (e.g., infliximab and adalimumab) are increasingly utilized in the management of moderate-to-severe UC that is refractory to other therapies.

Approximately one third of patients with UC ultimately require operation. Disease that is refractory to medical therapy is the most common indication for surgery and includes severe persistent symptoms that compromise quality of life, complications of long-term steroid dependence, and malnutrition or growth retardation (in the pediatric population). Occasionally, severe colitis being treated with fluid resuscitation and IV steroids may progress to fulminant or toxic colitis, which requires emergent surgery. Fulminant colitis is clinically characterized by diffuse abdominal tenderness, tachycardia, fever, and leukocytosis. The procedure of choice in this setting is a total abdominal colectomy and ileostomy. Pelvic dissection should be avoided in this setting.

Patients with UC are at higher risk of developing colorectal cancer, which increases with the duration and/or extent of the disease. During the first 10 years of the disease, the absolute risk is 2% to 3%, but it rises by 2% per year after that with a lifetime risk of 35%. Close surveillance with annual colonoscopy starting 10 years after onset of the disease, or sooner if the patient has pancolitis, is indicated. Colonoscopic examination in patients with UC should include 4-quadrant biopsies every 10 cm to exclude dysplasia. High-grade dysplasia is associated with cancer 40% of the time and constitutes an absolute indication for surgery. Most surgeons recommend excision if low-grade dysplasia is found as well; however, this remains controversial.

Surgical therapy aimed at removing all mucosa at risk cures UC. Common surgical options include total proctocolectomy with end ileostomy or proctocolectomy with ileal pouch–anal anastomosis (IPAA). The choice of operation is guided by patient preference, patient age, functional status, and preoperative risk. The sphincter-sparing IPAA is generally preferred over permanent end ileostomy in appropriately selected patients and may be performed using an open or a laparoscopic approach with similar results.

During total proctocolectomy with IPAA, the entire colon and rectum are mobilized and removed. To partially compensate for the loss of rectal reservoir function, a J-pouch is constructed using the terminal ileum. The pouch is then anastomosed to the remnant distal rectum and anus (Fig. 12.12). Other pouch configurations have been described, but the J-pouch is the most common. A temporary diverting loop ileostomy is typically fashioned at the time of ileal pouch surgery to protect the anastomosis; however, a single stage approach without ileostomy has been described in specialized centers. A rectal mucosectomy may be performed in an effort to remove the remaining rectal mucosa. Routine mucosectomy with hand-sewn ileal anal anastomosis is often associated with an increased incidence of postoperative stool seepage but has similar, excellent long-term functional outcomes as the double-stapled approach. Additionally, there has been no difference identified in the rates of postoperative complications or dysplasia between the two techniques.

Complications include bleeding, infection, injury to the pelvic nerves controlling sexual and bladder function, infertility, and anastomotic leak. *Pouchitis*, or idiopathic inflammation of the ileal pouch, is seen in up to 50% of patients after an IPAA and is likely due to bacterial overgrowth. Symptoms may include increased frequency of stool and crampy abdominal pain. The diagnosis of pouchitis can be confirmed by pouchoscopy, and treatment consists of antibiotic therapy, which is highly effective.

Crohn's Disease

Crohn's disease often has an insidious onset. Moreover, the disease presentation is highly variable depending upon the portion of the GI tract affected. Eighty percent of patients have small bowel involvement, half of which have disease limited to the small bowel only. Thirty percent of patients have disease that involves both the colon and small bowel, and another 30% have isolated colonic disease, which, unlike UC, is usually rectal sparing. Approximately 30% of patients develop anal fistulas. The clinical presentation of Crohn's is more variable than in UC due to its more diverse disease distribution, but common symptoms usually include crampy abdominal pain, diarrhea with or without bleeding, fever, and weight loss.

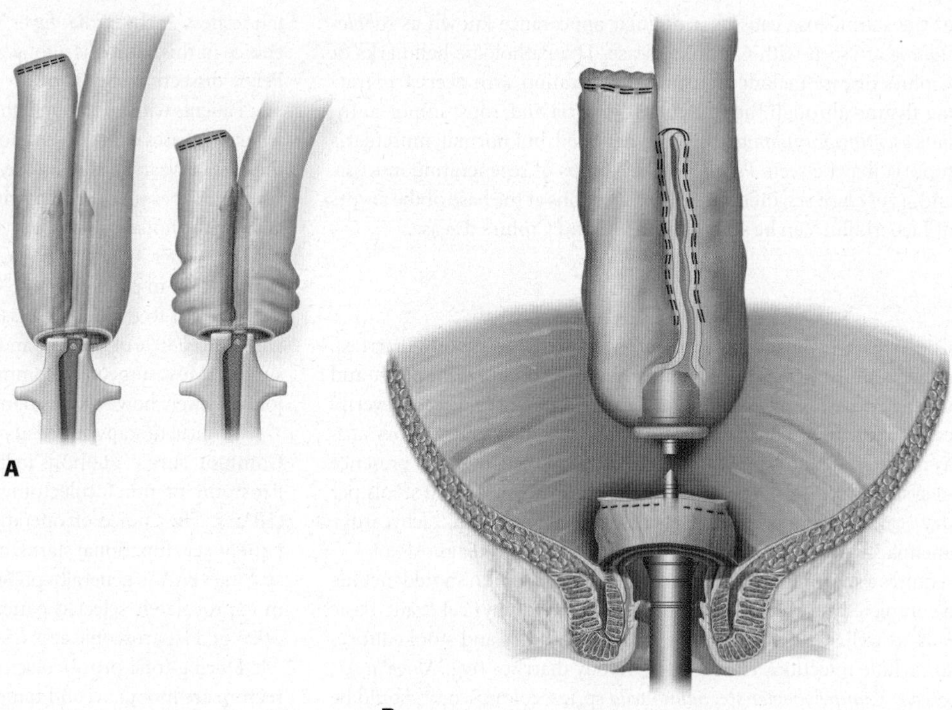

FIGURE 12.12 Formation of J-pouch **(A)** and advancement of shaft/trocar and creation of double-stapled anastomosis **(B)**. (Mulholland MW, ed. *Operative Techniques in Surgery*. Philadelphia: Wolters Kluwer Health; 2015; pp. 1234-1236.)

Diagnosis is typically made by clinical history, colonoscopy, and imaging of the small bowel, after exclusion of infectious or neoplastic processes. Granulomas seen on pathologic evaluation of biopsies strongly suggest Crohn's disease but are not always present. The colon cancer risk for patients with long-standing Crohn's colitis appears to approach that of UC patients as the duration and severity of their pancolitis increases. Therefore, patients with Crohn's disease also require close surveillance, including colonoscopy every 1 to 2 years beginning 10 years after the onset of disease.

The medical management of Crohn's disease is similar to that of UC. Sulfasalazine, immunosuppressives, and biologics are all useful. Although many surgeons advocate delaying surgery in Crohn's disease until absolutely necessary, patients with highly symptomatic focal disease may benefit from earlier intervention. The majority of patients with Crohn's disease will ultimately require surgery and indications for surgery include failure of medical therapy, obstruction (from inflammation, abscess, or stricture), intra-abdominal abscess, symptomatic fistulas, severe perianal disease, failure to thrive, and colorectal cancer. *Fulminant colitis*, which does not respond to medical management within 5 to 6 days, is treated with total abdominal colectomy and end ileostomy. Total proctocolectomy and IPAA are contraindicated in Crohn's disease because of the high associated rates of recurrence and complications involving the ileal pouch. If there is rectal sparing and no perianal disease, then reconstruction with an ileorectal anastomosis is feasible. Finally, benign stenoses are common, and when obstructive symptoms are present, surgery is recommended. Since patients with Crohn's may require multiple surgeries and bowel resections during their lifetime, conservation of bowel is paramount. In cases of short fibrotic strictures of the small bowel, a simple strictureplasty can be performed, obviating the need for any bowel resection; however, long, inflammatory stenosis should be resected. Strictures in the colon should be resected. Repeated resection of small bowel can result in *short-gut syndrome*, in which the remnant small bowel is of insufficient length to extract adequate nutrition (generally <200 cm).

Fistulas are a hallmark of Crohn's disease. One in three patients will develop an *internal fistula* (either small bowel to small bowel or small bowel to colon). Unless a substantial portion of bowel is bypassed, these may resolve with medical therapies and do not mandate surgical therapy. *Enterocutaneous fistulas* are classified as low output (<500 mL/day) or high output (>500 mL/day). Bowel rest, with total parenteral nutrition and aggressive medical treatment of the Crohn's disease (including biologics such as TNF-α inhibitors), allows fistulas to close spontaneously in some cases. Refractory fistulas require operation and resection of the diseased segment of bowel. Colovesical and colovaginal fistulas are often associated with intolerable symptoms. Although not surgical emergencies, they often require surgical repair.

In general, postoperative remission is not always durable with as few as 25% of patients remaining disease free 3 years after, and the reoperative rate approaches 5% per year.

Neoplasms of the Colon and Rectum

Six percent of Americans, the majority of whom will be over the age of 50, will be diagnosed with colorectal cancer, making it the third most common cancer in the United States. The pathogenesis of adenocarcinoma follows a stepwise progression from adenoma, through varying degrees of dysplasia, to frank invasive carcinoma. Several specific genetic mutations are known to occur during this progression in both sporadic and hereditary cases.

Polyps

Polyps in the colon are classified as neoplastic (adenomatous) or benign (hyperplastic, juvenile, and inflammatory). Hyperplastic polyps are the most commonly encountered type, are usually very small less than 3 mm, and usually have no malignant potential. Juvenile polyps are hamartomas and are seen throughout the GI tract. These polyps are associated with several polyposis syndromes and have no malignant potential but often bleed. Inflammatory polyps are

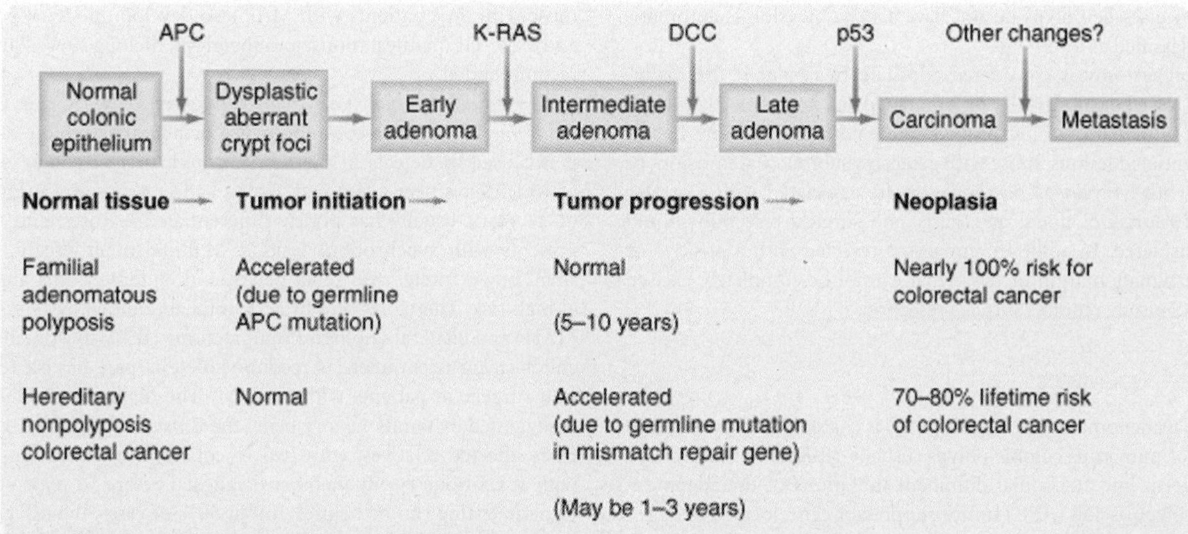

FIGURE 12.13 The Fearon–Vogelstein adenoma–carcinoma sequence. (From Townsend CM, Beauchamp RD, Evers BM, et al., eds. *Sabiston Textbook of Surgery*. 19th ed. Philadelphia: WB Saunders; 2012:1338, with permission.)

composed of layers of colonic mucosa, which form as a result of repetitive mucosal ulceration and regeneration, which can be seen with IBD and some erosive infections. Even polyps without malignant potential may harbor metaplastic or adenomatous components and should, therefore, be removed when encountered. Adenomas are the most common neoplastic polyps and are the precursors for nearly all colorectal cancers. The *Fearon–Vogelstein* model delineating the *adenoma–carcinoma sequence* is shown in Figure 12.13. The first step in the sequence is the formation of an adenomatous polyp, which is characterized by gross appearance as *pedunculated* (with a stalk) or *sessile* (flat). Histologically, they can be classified as *tubular* (i.e., with branching glands), *villous* (i.e., containing long finger-like glands), or *tubulovillous* (i.e., containing mixed features). Tubular, villous, and tubulovillous adenomas account for 65% to 80%, 5% to 10%, and 10% to 15% of adenomatous polyps, respectively. Size greater than 2 cm, villous features, and sessile appearance are all indicators of increased cancer risk. A tubular adenoma has a 5% risk of harboring a malignancy. Tubulovillous and villous adenomas are associated with a 22% and 40% risk of harboring a malignancy, respectively. The Haggitt criteria have been used to ascertain the prognostic significance of invasion at different levels and can be used to classify malignancies found within polyps as follows (Fig. 12.14):

Level 0: Carcinoma in situ. No invasion.
Level 1: Invasion limited to the head of the polyp.
Level 2: Invasion extends to the neck of the polyp at the junction of adenoma and stalk.
Level 3: Invasion into the stalk of the polyp.
Level 4: Invades into the submucosa of the bowel wall but above the muscularis propria.

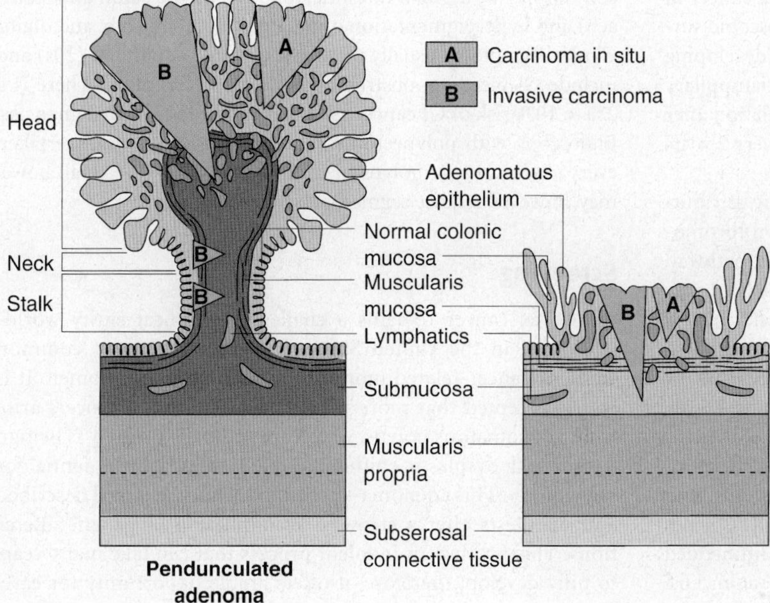

FIGURE 12.14 Adenomatous polyps. Note that invasive disease in a sessile lesion is unable to be less and constitutes at least Haggitt level 4. (From Mulholland MW, Lillemoe KD, Doherty GM, et al., eds. *Greenfield's Surgery: Scientific Principles and Practice*. 5th ed. Philadelphia: Lippincott Williams & Wilkins; 2010:1079, with permission.)

Since sessile polyps do not have a stalk, invasion is automatically classified as level 4.

Polypectomy is considered adequate treatment if the malignancy is well or moderately differentiated and is completely excised *en bloc* with margins of resection that are negative (>2 mm). Poorly differentiated lesions, those with extensive submucosal invasion, or those with lymphovascular invasion are associated with a greater than 10% risk of nodal metastasis, and surgical resection should be considered. In addition, any polyp resected with a positive or indeterminate margin or those that cannot be completely excised endoscopically requires surgical resection.

Familial Syndromes

Familial adenomatous polyposis (FAP) is characterized by development of numerous colonic polyps (usually >100) and is associated with germ-line autosomal dominant mutations of the adenomatous polyposis coli (APC) tumor suppressor gene, located on chromosome 5q. Although the majority of such mutations are inherited, approximately 20% of cases result from *de novo* mutations. As shown in Figure 12.13, the *APC* gene is an early contributor to the adenoma–carcinoma sequence. With a germ-line mutation in *APC*, patients with FAP develop hundreds to thousands of adenomatous polyps by the time they reach puberty, and cancer develops in all patients if left untreated by the age of 40. The severity and extent of disease, as well as the spectrum of associated extraintestinal tumors, are dependent upon the specific location and type of mutation within the *APC* gene. *Gardner syndrome* is characterized by polyposis and osteomas, sarcomas, and epidermoid inclusion cysts. Patients with *Turcot syndrome* develop polyposis and brain tumors. Screening of at-risk individuals should begin at the age of 10 years; sigmoidoscopy is usually sufficient for identifying emerging polyps. Alternatively, if a mutation has been identified in a family member, genetic analysis can be performed. Patients positive for the mutation require removal of the colon and rectum. This can be accomplished with a total proctocolectomy and permanent end ileostomy, a total proctocolectomy with IPAA, or a total abdominal colectomy with ileorectal anastomosis. The latter option should be reserved for patients with minimal disease in the rectum. Ileorectal anastomosis is associated with a 25% risk of developing cancer in the rectum over 20 years, and therefore, frequent endoscopic surveillance is imperative. All FAP patients are at risk of developing polyps in the stomach and near the duodenal papilla. Periampullary cancer is the second leading cause of death in this population after colon cancer; therefore, upper endoscopy surveillance every 2 years is recommended.

A subset (12%) of FAP cases have been found to be attributable to mutations of the *MutY homologue* (*MYH*) gene on chromosome 1, which is part of the DNA excision repair (DER) pathway. This has been termed MYH-associated polyposis (MAP). Large case series suggest that patients with two mutated alleles have a 2,000-fold increased risk of developing colon cancer compared with the general population. One mutant allele increases risk by at least 50% above baseline. Although MAP patients generally present with fewer polyps (dozens to a few hundred) and patients develop colon cancer at a slightly older age, they cannot be distinguished from FAP patients clinically. Therefore, all patients with numerous adenomatous polyps found to have normal *APC* genes should undergo sequencing of the *MYH* gene. Recommended treatment currently consists of removal of the entire colon. Like those with FAP, patients with MAP also develop duodenal polyps and extra-GI manifestations, and therefore, lifelong surveillance is recommended.

Hereditary nonpolyposis colorectal cancer (*HNPCC*) or *Lynch syndrome* is the most common cause of hereditary colon cancer. It is caused by defects in the *DNA mismatch repair* genes, several of which have been identified. Colon cancer arises at a mean age of 44 years, usually has poorly differentiated features, and often presents with synchronous lesions. Multiple other organs (e.g., small bowel, ureter and renal pelvis, and endometrium) are also at high risk. Therefore, prophylactic total abdominal hysterectomy (TAH) and bilateral salpingo-oophorectomy (BSO) in women after childbearing is complete is recommended as part of risk reduction surgery in patients with HNPCC. The diagnosis of HNPCC is suggested by family history using the *Amsterdam criteria*, that is, three affected relatives, with two in consecutive generations and with at least one family member diagnosed before 50 years of age. Genetic testing can be helpful, but in 50% of cases, the defect will not be identified. If a patient has HNPCC on the basis of family history, colonoscopic surveillance every 2 years between the ages 20 and 35 and then yearly after age 35 is recommended. If a cancer is identified, total abdominal colectomy and ileorectal anastomosis or conventional segmental colectomy with subsequent endoscopic surveillance can be offered. With either approach, surveillance with proctoscopy or colonoscopy is tremendously important to minimize metachronous disease.

Juvenile polyps can arise as part of *multiple polyposis coli or juvenile polyposis coli*, an autosomal dominant syndrome associated with the *SMAD4* gene mutation. These polyps are hamartomas and can bleed or act as lead points for an intussusception. In addition, adenomatous elements are present in 10% of polyps, and patients are at increased risk of developing gastric, pancreatic, and duodenal cancer as well. Therefore, both upper and lower endoscopy surveillance starting at ages 15 and 25, respectively, is recommended. Treatment consists of endoscopic polypectomy, with formal resection reserved for diffuse disease.

Peutz–Jeghers syndrome is a rare, autosomal dominant disease associated with mutations of the tumor suppressor gene *STK11*. Clinical features include multiple GI hamartomatous polyps (most commonly in the small intestine, followed by the colon and stomach) and hyperpigmentation of the lips, buccal mucosa, and digits. Clinical symptoms usually manifest by young adulthood (20s) and include GI bleeding, obstruction, and intussusception. There is a 2% to 10% risk of GI cancer as well as extraintestinal malignancies. Endoscopy with polypectomy as indicated should be undertaken every 2 years. Large polyps or multiple polyps in the small bowel may, however, require segmental bowel resection.

Screening

Colorectal cancer remains a challenging clinical entity worldwide, and in the United States, it is the third most common cause of cancer-related mortality in both men and women. It is widely accepted that more than 95% of colorectal cancers arise from adenomatous polyps, which are generally defined as benign lesions with dysplastic epithelium that have variable potential for malignancy. This adenoma–carcinoma sequence is well described and manifests after a stepwise accumulation of genetic alterations. This is often an indolent process that can take many years to fully develop; therefore, it offers ample opportunity for early

TABLE 12.1 Screening recommendations for patients at average, moderate, and high risk for colon cancer

Test	Age to Initiate	Interval
Average Risk		
FOBT plus sigmoidoscopy or colonoscopy	50 y	Every 5 y or every 10 y
Moderate risk (cancer in first-degree relatives >60 y)		
FOBT plus sigmoidoscopy or colonoscopy	40 y	Every 5 y or every 10 y
Moderate risk (cancer in first-degree relatives <60 y or >2 relatives with cancer)		
Colonoscopy	10 y before youngest relative's diagnosis	Every 5 y
High risk—FAP		
Sigmoidoscopy	10 y	Yearly until 40, if negative
High risk—HNPCC		
Colonoscopy	20 y	Every 2 y until 35, then yearly
High risk—IBD		
Colonoscopy	10 y after start of colitis	Every 1–2 y

FOBT, fecal occult blood testing; FAP, familial adenomatous polyposis; HNPCC, hereditary nonpolyposis colon cancer; IBD, inflammatory bowel disease.

intervention. The incidence of colorectal cancer is steadily declining in large part due to more prevalent educational and screening programs designed to detect early cancers and their precursor polyps. Screening guidelines are based on patient risk factors, and common modalities include colonoscopy, fecal occult blood testing, flexible sigmoidoscopy, double-contrast barium enema, and CT colonography (Table 12.1). Colonoscopy is considered the gold standard and is both diagnostic and therapeutic. Approximately 80% to 90% of adenomas are less than 1 cm and, therefore, more easily amenable to complete excision with conventional snare polypectomy.

Diagnosis and Staging

Patients with colorectal cancer are often asymptomatic; however, common symptoms include bleeding, anemia, weight loss, changes in bowel habits, and obstruction. Abdominal pain and a palpable abdominal mass are late findings. Colonoscopy is a common modality used for diagnosis of colorectal cancer, and it also provides useful information on the remainder of the colon, as ruling out synchronous polyps or malignancy is an important initial step in evaluation. Once the diagnosis of colorectal cancer has been made, staging usually begins with radiographic examination of the body for sites of potential distal spread. The most common site of spread within the abdomen is liver; therefore, CT scan of the abdomen is recommended. Any potential liver lesions may be further assessed with an MRI. Routine chest x-ray or CT scan of the chest can be used to evaluate the lungs and other thoracic structures. Positron emission tomography (PET) scans are being used more commonly and have been shown to detect occult disease not seen on CT scan in 20% of cases. Carcinoembryonic antigen (CEA) is an important prognostic tool and is commonly elevated in the setting of metastasis. As such, it is commonly used in surveillance following curative therapy. The overall stage for colorectal cancer is determined using the TNM system from American Joint Committee on Cancer (Table 12.2).

The evaluation of rectal cancers requires a slightly different approach. Given the distal location, useful clinical information can be derived from digital rectal examination, including size, location, fixation, and distance from the anal verge. Cancers in the mid and upper rectum are best assessed initially with rigid proctoscopy to determine the distance from the sphincter complex and anal verge. MRI of the pelvis and endorectal ultrasound (ERUS) supplement the local staging of rectal cancers by giving information on the degree of local invasion and any suspicious perirectal adenopathy.

Management

Colon Cancer

Surgical resection offers the only chance of achieving cure, but the management of colorectal cancer often requires a multidisciplinary approach, which has been pivotal in achieving better patient satisfaction and outcomes. Segmental colectomy should be offered to those patients who have resectable tumors without any evidence of distant metastasis. The extent of this segmental resection should be determined by the location of the tumor as well as the blood supply to that segment of colon. Appropriate margins (≥5 cm) should be achieved proximal and distal to the primary tumor and should include the associated mesentery containing the regional lymph nodes (Fig. 12.15). The current guidelines recommend a minimum of 12 lymph nodes that should be identified and assessed in the resected specimen. This can be accomplished with similar rates of morbidity and mortality without compromise of oncologic metrics by either a laparoscopic or conventional open approach. Tumors that are adherent to adjacent organs should be resected *en bloc* to ensure complete removal of the cancer with negative margins. Adjuvant chemotherapy is routinely offered to patients with evidence of spread of cancer cells to any regional lymph nodes. First-line therapy typically includes either 5-fluorouracil (5-FU) or leucovorin with either oxaliplatin (FOLFOX) or irinotecan (FOLFIRI).

TABLE 12.2 American Joint Commission on Cancer (AJCC) TNM classification for colon cancer

Primary tumor staging (T)	
T0	No evidence of primary tumor
Tis	Carcinoma in situ
T1	Tumor invades submucosa
T2	Tumor invades muscularis propria
T3	Tumor invades through the muscularis propria into the pericolonic tissue
T4a	Tumor penetrates to the surface of the visceral peritoneum (serosa)
T4b	Tumor invades and/or is adherent to other organs or structures
Regional lymph node staging (N)	
N0	No regional lymph node metastasis
N1a	Metastasis in 1 regional lymph node
N1b	Metastasis in 2–3 regional lymph nodes
N1c	Tumor deposits in subserosa, mesentery, or nonperitonealized pericolic or perirectal tissues without regional nodal metastases
N2a	Metastasis in 4–6 regional lymph nodes
N2b	Metastasis in 7 or more regional lymph nodes
Distant metastasis staging (M)	
M0	No distant metastasis
M1a	Metastasis confined to 1 organ or site
M1b	Metastasis in more than 1 organ/site or the peritoneum

Stage	*T*	*N*	*M*
0	Tis	N0	M0
I	1–2	N0	M0
IIA	T3	N0	M0
IIB	T4a	N0	M0
IIC	T4b	N0	M0
IIIA	T1-T2	N1–N1c	M0
	T1	N2a	M0
IIIB	T3–T4a	N1–N1c	M0
	T2–T3	N2a	M0
	T1–2	N2b	M0
IIIC	T4a	N2a	M0
	T3–T4a	N2b	M0
	T4b	N1–N2	M0
IVA	Any T	Any N	M1a
IVB	Any T	Any N	M1b

(Reprinted from Dis Colon Rectum 55(8), Chang, GJ et al., Practice parameters for the management of colon cancer, p. 834, 2012, with permission from Wolters Kluwer Health, Inc)

Rectal Cancer

The surgical decision-making process for rectal cancer is more complex owing to its unique location within the bony pelvis and often requires a multidisciplinary approach. In recent years, an improved understanding of the histopathology as well as patterns of recurrence has afforded significant strides in the treatment of rectal cancer. Ultimately, the management strategy hinges initially on the location of the tumor within the rectum and the depth of local invasion. Patients with evidence of locally advanced cancers (defined as stage IIA and beyond) are routinely referred for neoadjuvant chemoradiation (5-FU and leucovorin and radiation [5,040 cGy]), which has been shown to decrease rates of local recurrence. Patients with earlier staged cancers should be referred for surgery first.

Historically, local and radical resections for rectal cancers were associated with significant patient morbidity and high local recurrence rates. However, the concept of total mesorectal excision (TME) has drastically changed the surgical approach to rectal cancers resections. An appropriate TME requires sharp dissection in the areolar plane between the mesorectal envelope (fascia propria) and the adjacent pelvic structures. This allows complete removal of the rectal tumor and the regional lymph nodes while ensuring a negative circumferential margin, which has been shown to be important in achieving lower local recurrence rates. Proximal rectal tumors do not require a complete TME since lymphatic spread is generally limited to within a few centimeters of the tumor. In these cases, a partial mesorectal excision can be performed after ensuring an adequate distal margin. Based on the available data, a 2-cm distal margin is adequate for most rectal cancers, while smaller tumors that are very low in the rectum may be resected with an acceptable negative margin of 1 cm.

For tumors in the mid and upper rectum, a low anterior resection (LAR) with colorectal anastomosis is the standard approach. Tumors in the lower rectum can also be considered for this approach as long as a 1- to 2-cm distal margin can be obtained adequately. Intestinal continuity is then restored low in the pelvis using either a stapled or hand-sewn anastomosis.

Patients with preexisting fecal incontinence or with very low rectal cancers that are not amenable to a sphincter-preserving technique will ultimately require an abdominoperineal resection (APR). During the abdominal phase of the procedure, the TME dissection is carried out down circumferentially to the levator muscles and a permanent colostomy is created using the proximal colon. The perineal dissection involves the complete excision of the anus and the sphincter complex in continuity with the proximal specimen. This is done in a wide manner to ensure a negative circumferential margin.

In carefully selected patients, a transanal local excision may be considered as an acceptable treatment alternative for small, early (T1) cancers in the distal rectum that have favorable histologic features (well-differentiated, absence of lymphovascular invasion, superficial submucosal invasion). It may also be an alternative for patients who are unsuitable for radical surgery due to prohibitive comorbidities. Transanal excision of T1 and T2 tumors is associated with higher local recurrence rates of up to 8% and 20%, respectively.

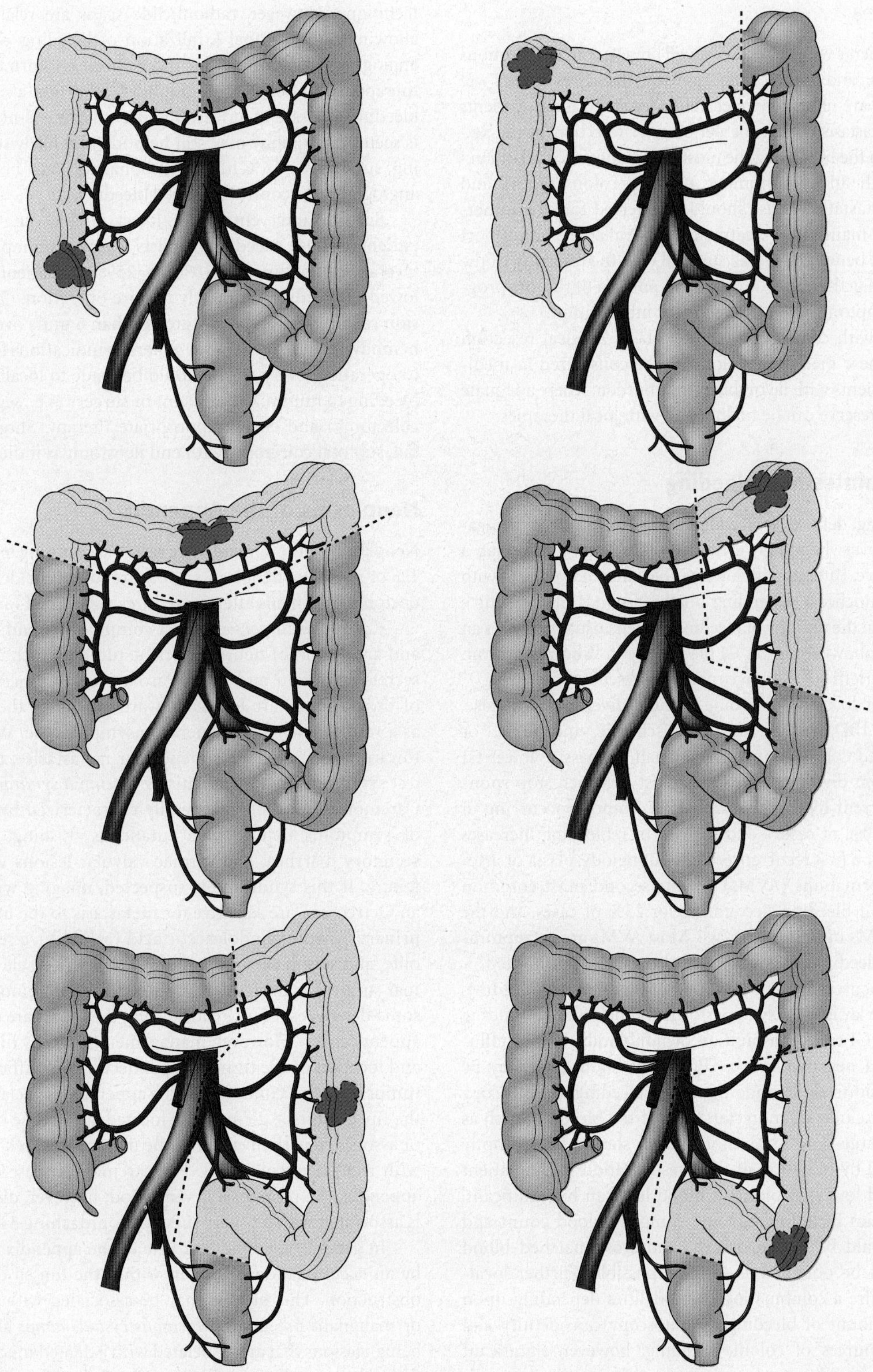

FIGURE 12.15 Segmental colon resections for colorectal cancer. (From Mulholland MW, Lillemoe KD, Doherty GM, et al., eds. *Greenfield's Surgery: Scientific Principles and Practice*. 5th ed. Philadelphia: Lippincott Williams & Wilkins; 2010:1110, with permission.)

Metastatic Disease

Up to 25% of patients with colon cancer will present with synchronous metastatic disease, and of these, only approximately 10% to 20% will have lesions that are ultimately resectable. More commonly, patients will develop metastasis during the period after resection of the primary tumor with the liver being the most commonly involved organ.

Patients with an asymptomatic primary colon tumors and unresectable metastatic disease should be referred for chemotherapy as this is the mainstay of treatment. The available data support that there is little benefit in overall survival with the resection of the primary tumor. Furthermore, only a small portion of tumors progress to cause symptoms that require urgent intervention.

In patients with colorectal liver metastasis, surgical resection or ablation of these metastatic lesions can be considered in medically suitable patients with favorable tumor burden, where adequate functional liver reserve can be maintained with local therapies.

Lower Gastrointestinal Bleeding

Lower GI bleeding, defined as bleeding originating distal to the ligament of Treitz, overwhelmingly arises from a colonic rather than a small bowel source. Patients with lower GI bleeding may present with melena or hematochezia depending on the distance of the source from the anus and the rapidity of bleeding. Melena usually implies an upper GI source; however, lower GI bleeding with slow transit from a small bowel or right colon source may also present with melena.

Etiologies of lower GI bleeding include diverticular disease, angiodysplasia, IBD, neoplasms, and ischemic, infectious, or radiation-induced colitis. Approximately half of massive lower GI bleeds result from diverticular disease, most of which stop spontaneously. Recurrent bleeding is relatively common (occurring in approximately 20% of cases), and the risk of rebleeding increases significantly after a first recurrence. Colonic angiodysplasia or arteriovenous malformations (AVMs) are the second most common cause of lower GI bleeding, accounting for 25% of cases, and the incidence of AVMs increases with age. Most AVMs are asymptomatic, and when bleeding occurs, they are also usually self-limited.

Diagnosis focuses on the localization of the source of bleeding. Nasogastric tube lavage is easy to perform and helpful in excluding an active upper GI source; aspiration of nonbloody, bilious effluent constitutes a negative lavage. Ultimately, endoscopy may be necessary to definitively exclude upper GI bleeding. Proctoscopy is indicated to exclude an anorectal cause of the bleeding, such as hemorrhoids. Large-bore intravenous access should be promptly secured followed by initiation of fluid resuscitation in the patient with a suspected lower GI bleed, as blood loss can be significant. Laboratory studies including baseline complete blood count and coagulation should be obtained early, and cross-matched blood products should be obtained as soon as possible. Further localization can require a combination of modalities depending upon the rate and amount of bleeding. Colonoscopy can identify and treat possible sources of colonic bleeding; however, significant active bleeding or inadequate bowel preparation may limit its utility. Radionuclide scan involves the injection of labeled colloid or autologous technetium-labeled "tagged" red blood cells (RBCs). Labeled colloid scans can identify bleeding at a rate as low as 0.1 to 0.5 mL/min but requires active bleeding at the time of injection. A tagged RBC scan requires bleeding at a rate of 1 mL/min. Because labeling of RBCs persists for up to 24 hours, intermittent bleeding can be identified with serial scanning, which is an advantage of this technique. However, radionuclide scans are relatively imprecise, allowing only regional localization of bleeding. Selective visceral angiography often provides more specific information and offers therapeutic options. Angiographic localization also requires active bleeding at a rate of at least 0.5 to 1 mL/min. If no active bleeding is seen, angiography may still help identify likely sources of bleeding, such as AVMs. Catheter embolization may be combined with angiography to control localized bleeding.

Surgical intervention for lower GI bleeding is reserved for patients whose bleeding persists despite nonoperative therapy. Overall, approximately 10% to 25% of patients with massive lower GI bleeding ultimately require operation. Ongoing transfusion requirement, typically greater than 6 units over 24 hours, and hemodynamic instability are generally indications for surgery. Prior to operation, every effort should be made to localize the source of bleeding to minimize the extent of surgery (i.e., segmental vs. total colectomy) and ensure appropriate therapy. Should such efforts fail, subtotal colectomy with end ileostomy is indicated.

Neoplasms of the Appendix

Neoplasms of the appendix are rare—accounting for approximately 1% of intestinal neoplasms. Most are found incidentally in appendectomy specimens after procedures performed for appendicitis.

Carcinoids tumors are most commonly found in the appendix and are a form of neuroendocrine tumor, which contain and can secrete serotonin and other vasoactive substances. The majority of these tumors are located toward the tip of the appendix, and as a result patients are generally asymptomatic. When they occur toward the base of the appendix or metastasize, they may manifest symptoms of appendicitis or *carcinoid syndrome*, respectively. Carcinoid syndrome is generally characterized by a constellation of symptoms that include cutaneous flushing, bronchospasm, secretory diarrhea, and cardiac valvular lesions with right heart failure. If this syndrome is suspected, imaging with CT scans or an Octreoscan are sensitive for metastasis to the liver. In addition, urinary 5-hydroxyindoleacetic acid (5-HIAA), a serotonin metabolite, and serum chromogranin A levels will be elevated. The optimal surgical management of appendiceal carcinoids still garners some debate, especially considering that most are discovered after appendectomy. However, management typically hinges on the size and location of the tumor. Appendectomy is sufficient for smaller tumors (<2 cm) contained to the appendix, especially those toward the tip. Tumors ≥ 2 cm, those located at the base of the appendix, or associated with invasion of the mesoappendix should be treated with right hemicolectomy. For carcinoid disease confined to the appendix, the prognosis is very good; however, distant metastasis is associated with a 5-year survival approaching 34%.

In general, a simple *mucocele* of the appendix is characterized by an accumulation of mucin within the lumen due to proximal obstruction. This process may be associated with either a benign or malignant precursor. *Mucinous cystadenomas* are histologically benign lesions that are associated with a dilated mucin-filled appendix and adenomatous epithelium. Its malignant counterpart, *mucinous cystadenocarcinoma, can* perforate causing a unique condition known as, *pseudomyxoma peritonei*, where the peritoneal cavity becomes seeded by cancer cells that continue to secrete mucin. If untreated, this condition, which is typically insensitive to systemic chemotherapy, is associated with a poor prognosis; therefore, the mainstay of treatment is surgical debulking. In select cases, hyperthermic intraperitoneal chemotherapy (HIPEC) is considered in addition to cytoreductive surgery with the goal of achieving more durable control of the disseminated peritoneal disease.

PATHOLOGY OF THE ANUS

Benign Anorectal Disorders

Abscess and Fistula-in-Ano

At the level of the dentate line, the anal glands lie in the intersphincteric plane and are associated with ducts that open into the crypts of Morgagni. Obstruction of these glands and ducts results in a local infection that manifests in the potential spaces around the anus. If such infections track downward toward the anal orifice, a *perianal abscess* forms, which is the most common form of anorectal abscess. Alternatively, the infection can remain with the intersphincteric plane, forming an *intersphincteric* abscess, penetrate laterally through the external sphincter to form an *ischiorectal* abscess, or it can track superiorly above the levator ani, forming a *supralevator* abscess (Figs. 12.3 and 12.16). In rare cases, infections that start in the postanal space and spread bilaterally in the ischiorectal spaces around the anus, forming a *horseshoe* abscess.

In all cases, abscesses typically present with anal pain, but there may be associated swelling or fever. On examination, a tender mass adjacent to the anal canal is usually palpable. A CT scan or MRI can be helpful in delineating the extent of disease but are often unnecessary except in cases of Crohn's disease or extensive, recurrent perianal sepsis. All abscesses should be incised and drained, either under local anesthesia or in the operating room, with emphasis on creating an adequate external opening that will promote complete drainage. Additionally, the external opening should be made on the anal side on the abscess to minimize the complexity of a fistula should one occur. The use of antibiotics is of little value in the primary management of anorectal abscesses except as an adjunct in immunocompromised patients or those with extensive cellulitis. Intersphincteric and postanal abscesses require special consideration as patients may present with symptoms of anorectal abscess without external signs on physical exams. Intersphincteric abscesses can be drained into the anal canal by performing a limited sphincterotomy. Postanal abscesses can be drained by incising between the

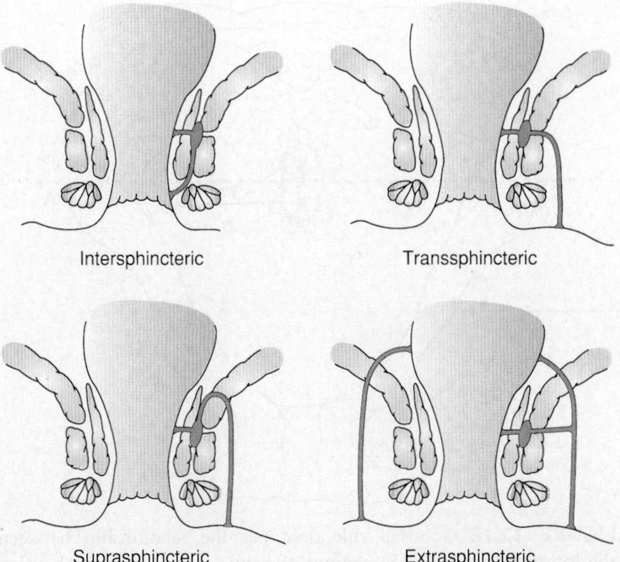

FIGURE 12.17 Parks classification of fistula-in-ano. (From Mulholland MW, Lillemoe KD, Doherty GM, et al., eds. *Greenfield's Surgery: Scientific Principles and Practice*. 5th ed. Philadelphia: Lippincott Williams & Wilkins; 2010:1148, with permission.)

coccyx and the anus—spreading the superficial external muscles and the anococcygeal ligament, which allows entry into the space. The *Hanley technique* for horseshoe abscesses involves drainage of the postanal space and additional lateral counter incisions to drain the lateral components of the horseshoe abscess. Full drainage is necessary, as neglected perirectal abscesses can progress to devastating necrotizing pelvic fascial infections.

Up to 50% of perirectal abscesses will progress to *fistula-in-ano*, either acutely or within 6 months of the initial infection. These fistulas are defined by the tissues they traverse—a classification system popularized by Parks and is still commonly used (Fig. 12.17). The general course of the tract of cryptoglandular fistulas can be predicted on the basis of the site of the external opening using *Goodsall's rule*. Tracts with external openings in the skin anterior to a line drawn

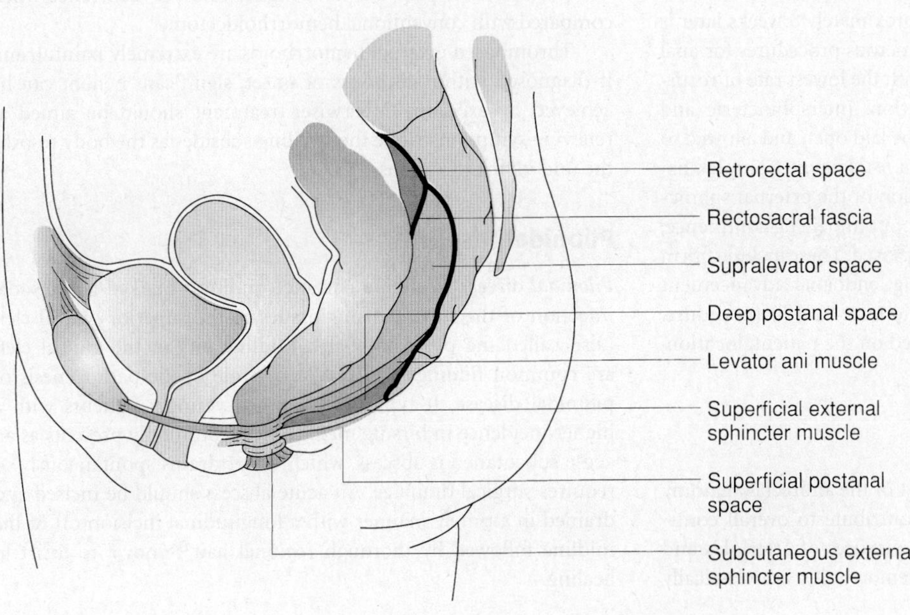

FIGURE 12.16 Lateral view of the perianorectal spaces. (From Mulholland MW, Lillemoe KD, Doherty GM, et al., eds. *Greenfield's Surgery: Scientific Principles and Practice*. 5th ed. Philadelphia: Lippincott Williams & Wilkins; 2010:1133, with permission.)

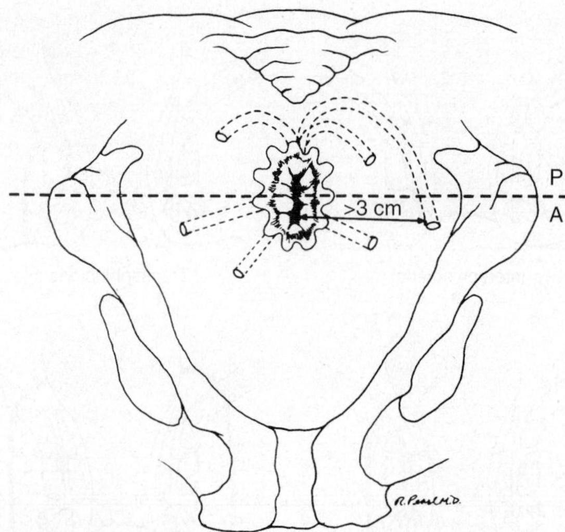

FIGURE 12.18 Goodsall rule describes the relationship between the internal and external openings of fistula-in-ano. (From Abcarian H. Surgical treatment of anal disorders. In: Nyhus LM, Baker RJ, eds. *Mastery of Surgery*. 2nd ed. Boston: Little, Brown and Company; 1992:1358, with permission.)

transversely through the midpoint of the anus will course directly to the anal canal, while those with posterior external openings will follow a curved path toward a posterior midline opening (Fig. 12.18). Exceptions to this rule include Crohn's fistulas and those with external openings greater than 3 cm from the anus.

Digital rectal exam and anoscopy may aid in the assessment of the internal opening as well as the quality of the surrounding anorectal tissues. While CT scan can be helpful for identifying perianal sepsis, it is not generally a useful modality for identifying anal fistulas. MRI and ERUSs (especially with the concomitant use of hydrogen peroxide through the tract) can be helpful in delineating complex tracts.

If identified in the setting of an abscess or inflammation, a seton should be placed in order to allow continued drainage of infection and maturation of the tract. Seton placement also facilitates the assessment of the amount of the sphincter muscles incorporated in the fistula tract. A staged procedure approximately 8 weeks later is frequently required. The goal of the numerous procedures for anal fistulas is to eliminate the fistula tract with the lowest rate of recurrence while preserving sphincter function. Intersphincteric and superficial transsphincteric fistulas can be laid open and allowed to heal by secondary intention, known as a *fistulotomy*. Complex fistulas that incorporate a significant portion of the external sphincter are not amenable to fistulotomy without impairing continence; therefore, other modalities should be employed. These include fibrin glue injection, bioprosthetic fistula plug, endoanal advancement flap, and ligation of the intersphincteric tract (LIFT) procedure. Treatment should be individualized based on the patient, location, and course of the tract.

Hemorrhoids

Anal vascular cushions are a normal part of the anorectal anatomy and are considered, in small part, to contribute to overall continence. These cushions are made up of plexuses of arterioles and veins supported by smooth muscle. Hemorrhoids are classically described in three positions: right anterior, right posterior, and left lateral. Engorgement of these tissues, often related to irregular bowel habits, constipation, and straining with bowel movements, is termed "*hemorrhoids*." Hemorrhoids above the dentate are classified as *internal*, and those below the dentate line are classified as *external*. Frequently, patients have both hemorrhoids simultaneously. Internal hemorrhoids typically present with bright red bleeding and prolapse, while external hemorrhoids cause acute discomfort, especially when associated with an underlying thrombus.

Internal hemorrhoids can be categorized by the extent of prolapse as follows:

First degree: Bulging within the lumen without prolapse below dentate line
Second degree: Prolapse with straining, but spontaneously reduces
Third degree: Prolapse that reduces only with digital manipulation
Fourth degree: Irreducible prolapse

Diagnosis requires anoscopy to determine the location and extent of disease. Asking the patient to strain while seated over a toilet may reproduce prolapsing internal hemorrhoids. Endoscopic evaluation in appropriately selected patients is also important to exclude other causes of bleeding, especially neoplasia.

Symptomatic patients should initially be treated conservatively with fiber supplementation and sitz baths. A large proportion of patients will see improvement with this strategy alone. First- and second-degree hemorrhoids can be treated with nonsurgical therapy such as rubber band ligation with good success. Although multiple treatments may be required, success rates up to 75% have been identified. Surgery may be considered for the treatment of symptomatic second-, third-, and fourth-degree hemorrhoids that have failed conservative management. In the classic hemorrhoidectomy, excision can be performed in the prone jackknife position. The hemorrhoidal bundles are carefully dissected free of the underlying sphincter and excised. The wounds are closed primarily or left open to heal by secondary intention. Care should be taken as extensive excision can lead to anal stenosis. Pain can be significant, and common complications include bleeding, infection, and urinary retention. Other surgical options include stapled hemorrhoidopexy and hemorrhoid artery ligation, which generally result in significantly less postoperative pain but have higher rates of recurrence when compared with conventional hemorrhoidectomy.

Thrombosed external hemorrhoids are extremely painful, and if diagnosed within 48 hours of onset, significant benefit can be achieved by excision. Otherwise, treatment should be aimed at relieving symptoms while the swelling subsides as the body resorbs the underlying thrombus.

Pilonidal Disease

Pilonidal disease is often a chronic condition marked by episodic infection of the subcutaneous tissues of the superior gluteal cleft (also called the postnatal cleft). Midline pits in the gluteal cleft are common findings and play a key role in the pathogenesis of pilonidal disease. It typically occurs in younger patients with a higher incidence in hirsute men. It most commonly presents as an acute subcutaneous abscess, which either drains spontaneously or requires surgical drainage. An acute abscess should be incised and drained in a timely manner with a longitudinal incision off of the midline followed by thorough regional hair removal to assist in healing.

Complex tunneling sinuses are characteristic of chronic pilonidal disease resulting in recurrent infections, which usually requires definitive surgical resection to resolve completely. Most frequently, this is approached with a midline excision with or without primary closure of the defect. It is important to probe all of the sinus tracts to ensure complete excision. An open wound that heals by secondary intention is associated with a low recurrence and a low rate of recurrent infection but can be a morbid process that requires months to heal completely. The skin at the wound edge can be sutured to the base, *marsupialization*, in order to eliminate overhanging edges and make the wound smaller. Primary closure is associated with slightly higher rates of infection, but it avoids the morbidity of an open wound. It is important to close the wound off of midline to promote optimal healing. Alternatively, after cyst excision, a rotational, pedicle flap (e.g., the *Limberg flap*) may be used to cover the defect (Fig. 12.19). This technique is associated with low recurrence rates and good healing.

Anal Fissure

Anal fissures are linear tears in the anoderm distal to the dentate line. Ninety percent occur at the posterior midline, but it is possible to have a fissure anteriorly as well. Lateral fissures should raise concern for other anorectal processes such as Crohn's disease, infectious conditions (i.e., tuberculosis, HIV/AIDS, and syphilis), and, in rare cases, carcinoma. A history of constipation is common in these patients, and fissures are commonly believed to be caused by the passage of hard stools. Patients frequently complain of intense pain with defecation as well as bleeding. This condition results from mucosal ischemia secondary to hyperplasia and hypertonicity of the internal anal sphincter. A chronic fissure is classically associated with heaped up epidermis, called a *sentinel tag*, which is a marker of chronic inflammation. Diagnosis is often made by history and inspection with gentle eversion of the buttocks. Anoscopy is frequently not tolerated in the acute setting.

Initial treatment is generally conservative, aiming at changing bowel consistency and bowel habits. Fiber supplementation and sitz baths combined with locally administered calcium channel blockers or nitroglycerin cream can heal up to 70% of fissures in 4 to 6 weeks. Injection of botulinum toxin in order to achieve muscle relaxation has also been studied with good results, but there is not enough consensus on the site for injection or the ideal dose. Refractory cases will often require surgery, and a tailored *lateral internal sphincterotomy* (Fig. 12.20) is the procedure of choice. The rate of recurrence after surgery is low as is the rate of fecal incontinence.

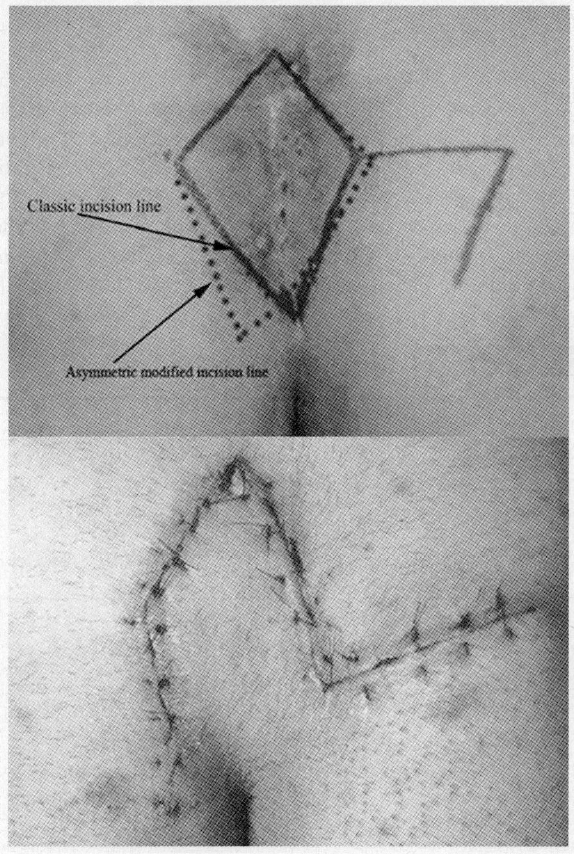

FIGURE 12.19 Modified Limberg flap for pilonidal disease. **Top:** Diagram of the classic and modified flaps. **Bottom:** Completed modified Limberg flap. (From Cihan A, Ucan BH, Comert M, et al. Superiority of asymmetric modified Limberg flap for surgical treatment of pilonidal disease. *Dis Col Rectum.* 2006;49(2):245-6, with permission.)

Rectal Prolapse

Rectal prolapse is most common in women older than 50 years. Most have a constellation of findings including a patulous anus, diastasis of the pelvic floor muscles, a deep cul-de-sac, redundant sigmoid colon, and loss of inherent sacral attachments. Full-thickness rectal prolapse can be visualized on physical examination when the patient bears down. It is characterized by extrusion of rectal mucosa from the anus, forming concentric folds; this can help differentiate it from prolapsing hemorrhoids, which forms radial mucosal folds. Defecography is often unnecessary but can help confirm the diagnosis of internal intussusception when examination findings are equivocal. Prior to surgery for prolapse, a colonoscopy should be performed to exclude other colonic pathology.

Rectal prolapse can generally be managed via transabdominal procedures or perineal procedures based on patient surgical history and comorbidities. A transabdominal approach includes a rectopexy with or without resection of the redundant sigmoid colon. During this procedure, the rectum is elevated from the pelvis and secured to the presacral fascia in the midline. This can be approached laparoscopically or with a conventional open lower abdominal incision. The use of mesh for rectopexy has been described but should not be used if a resection is performed.

The *Altemeier procedure, or perineal proctosigmoidectomy*, is the most common perineal approach described. This technique involves full-thickness circumferential incision of the prolapsed rectum starting just proximal to the dentate line. The peritoneum is entered, and the rectum and sigmoid colon are pulled through the anus until no redundancy remains. The excess is removed, and an anastomosis is fashioned between the colon and the anal canal. Recurrence rates are higher with this repair than the transabdominal approach; however, it is often better tolerated.

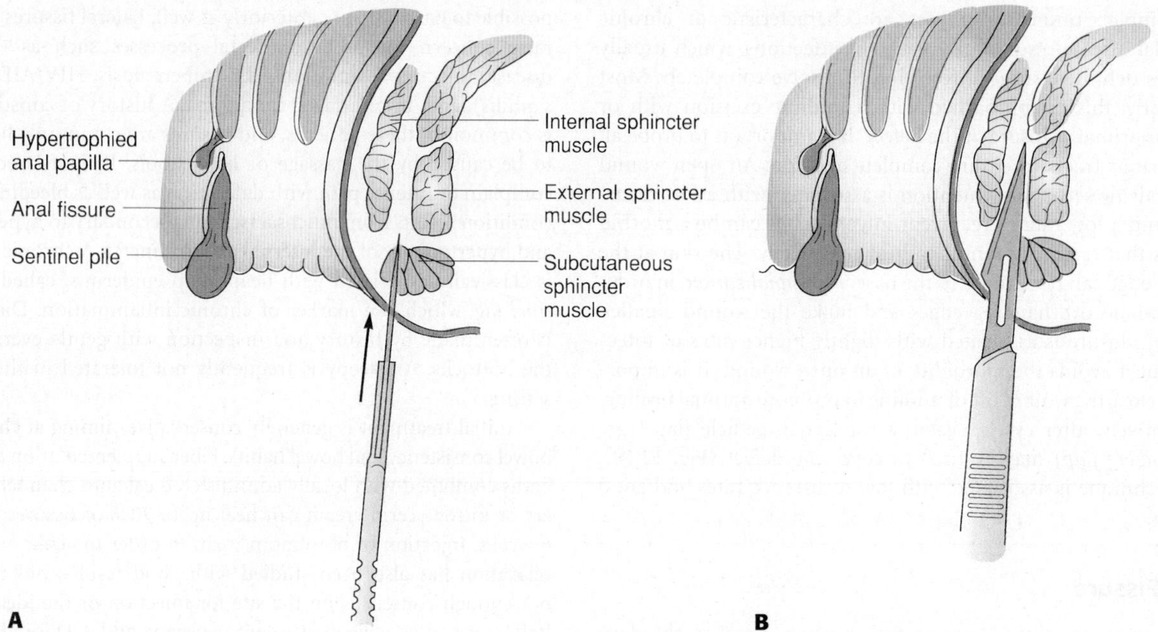

FIGURE 12.20 Technique for closed lateral sphincterotomy in the treatment of anal fissure. (From Mulholland MW, Lillemoe KD, Doherty GM, et al., eds. *Greenfield's Surgery: Scientific Principles and Practice.* 5th ed. Philadelphia: Lippincott Williams & Wilkins; 2010:1146, with permission.)

Neoplasia of the Anus

Tumors of the anus are rare, constituting only 1.5% of GI malignancies; however, the incidence has been increasing over the past several decades. The TNM system is used for staging and differs from colorectal cancer as it is, in part, based on the size of the cancer (see Tables 12.3 and 12.4).

When discussing the anatomy of the anus, a distinction must be made between the *anal margin* and the *anal canal*. The anal margin surrounds the anus beyond the anal verge. The anal canal begins at the verge and extends cephalad. By convention, the term anal cancer refers to those arising from the anal canal, while as those arising from the anal margin are referred to as perianal skin cancers or anal margin cancers.

Anal Margin

Bowen's disease is an indolent in situ squamous cell carcinoma of the anal verge. Its appearance is extremely varied, but is generally plaque-like, and can be asymptomatic or present with pruritis and burning. Treatment consists of *wide local excision* with adequate margins; intraoperative frozen sections are helpful in guiding the extent of resection. A flap may be needed for coverage and closure. Invasion is found in 5% of cases, and APR is recommended in such cases.

Paget disease is a shallow intraepithelial adenocarcinoma, which, like Bowen's disease, presents as a plaque. More common in older patients, Paget disease is associated with a poor prognosis. It can arise primarily, perhaps from Langerhans cells, or can represent a metastasis from an underlying rectal carcinoma. Wide local excision is the treatment of choice for noninvasive disease. APR is indicated for underlying invasive disease. Adjuvant chemotherapy and radiation are used in some cases.

Condyloma acuminatum is perianal wart disease secondary to human papillomavirus (HPV) infection and is the most common perianal sexually transmitted disease (STD). Symptoms include itching, bleeding, pain, and anal discharge. Preoperative *anoscopy* is required, since some cases extend into the anal canal. Medical therapies are often inadequate and ultimately fulguration with electrocautery and/or direct excision is required. Recurrence is very common; therefore, surveillance is important. Some HPV

TABLE 12.3 TNM scores for anal cancer

Tumor (T)	
T1	Tumor <2.0 cm
T2	Tumor 2.0–5.0 cm
T3	Tumor >5.0 cm
T4	Any-sized tumor invading adjacent extradermal structures
Regional lymph nodes (N)	
N0	No regional nodes involved
N1	Perirectal nodal involvement
N2	Tumor involving unilateral internal iliac or inguinal lymph nodes
N3	Tumor involving unilateral perirectal and inguinal nodes or bilateral inguinal or internal iliac nodes
Distant metastasis (M)	
M0	No distant metastasis
M1	Distant metastasis

From Edge S, Byrd DR, Compton CC, et al. *The AJCC Cancer Staging Manual.* 7th ed. New York: Springer-Verlag; 2010, with permission.

TABLE 12.4 Staging schema for anal carcinoma

Stage	TNM Scores
I	T1, N0
II	T2–3, N0
IIIA	T4, N0, or T1–4, N1
IIIB	T4, N1, or Tany, N2-3
IV	M1

From Edge S, Byrd DR, Compton CC, et al. *The AJCC Cancer Staging Manual*. 7th ed. New York: Springer-Verlag; 2010, with permission.

strains are more aggressive and may lead to *verrucous carcinomas* (*Buschke–Lowenstein tumors*)—large, invasive derivatives of condyloma. These slow-growing tumors are large and friable and can become infected or fistulize. Transformation to frank squamous cell carcinoma is not uncommon. Treatment includes radical wide local excision or APR, and the addition of radiation and chemotherapy, if carcinoma is found.

Squamous cell carcinoma of the anal verge can be treated with wide local excision. Recurrence or locally advanced disease very rarely warrants an APR. Lymphadenectomy is rarely required. *Basal cell carcinoma* is rare in the anus and presents with characteristic pearly borders and a central depression. Wide local excision is adequate treatment, but one third of patients recur and therefore close follow-up is recommended.

Anal Canal

Tumors of the anal canal vary in histologic appearances (e.g., *squamous, cloacogenic*, and *mucoepidermoid*) but share an aggressive natural history. Nearly 75% are invasive, 25% have spread to local lymph nodes, and 10% have metastasized at the time of diagnosis. Treatment consists of a combined multimodal regimen of radiation and chemotherapy referred to as the Nigro protocol, which consists of radiotherapy given concurrently with 5-FU and mitomycin infusions. Surgical intervention is not indicated as initial therapy, but salvage surgery with APR may be necessary if there is evidence of persistent disease after chemoradiation or if there is evidence of posttreatment recurrence.

Melanoma of the anal canal is rare, frequently amelanotic, and very aggressive. Local excision is indicated for smaller lesions, as long-term survival appears to be similar to APR. For larger, more invasive anorectal melanomas, APR is the procedure of choice. Prophylactic superficial inguinal lymph node dissection is not recommended, although sentinel lymph node biopsy may be considered. *Adenocarcinoma* of the anal canal is likewise extremely rare. These tumors arise in the anal ducts that form a communication between the intersphincteric anal glands and the crypts of Morgagni. As a result, these cancers are often extramucosal. Prognosis is poor, but APR, preceded usually by radiation and chemotherapy, is recommended.

The anorectum is the fourth most common site of *carcinoid tumors*. Tumors less than 2 cm should be locally excised. Those greater than 2 cm in size require APR.

ACKNOWLEDGMENTS

The authors would like to acknowledge and thank Robert Lewis, MD, and Robert Fry, MD, for their contribution to the prior edition of this chapter.

Suggested Readings

Aarons CB, Mahmoud NN. Current surgical considerations for colorectal cancer. *Chin Clin Oncol.* 2013;2(2):14.

Bauer VP. Emergency management of diverticulitis. *Clin Colon Rectal Surg.* 2009;22(3):161–168.

Cameron JL. *Current Surgical Therapy*. 9th ed. St. Louis: Mosby; 2007.

Edge S, Byrd DR, Compton CC, et al. *AJCC Cancer Staging Manual.* 7th ed. New York: Springer-Verlag; 2010.

Feingold D, Steele SR, Lee S, et al. Practice parameters for the treatment of sigmoid diverticulitis. *Dis Colon Rectum.* 2014;57(3):284–294.

Fleshman JW, Wolff BG. *The ASCRS Textbook of Colon and Rectal Surgery*. New York: Springer; 2007.

Frago R, Ramirez E, Millan M, et al. Current management of acute malignant large bowel obstruction: a systematic review. *Am J Surg.* 2014;207(1):127–138.

Gordon PH, Nivatvongs S. *Principles and Practice of Surgery for the Colon, Rectum, and Anus*. New York: Informa Healthcare; 2007.

Greenfield LJ, Mulholland MW, Oldham KT, et al., eds. *Greenfield's Surgery: Scientific Principles and Practice*. 3rd ed. Philadelphia: Lippincott Williams & Wilkins; 2001.

Hensgens MP, Goorhuis A, Dekkers OM, et al. All-cause and disease-specific mortality in hospitalized patients with Clostridium difficile infection: a multicenter cohort study. *Clin Infect Dis.* 2013;56(8):1108–1116.

Kassam Z, Lee CH, Yuan Y, et al. Fecal microbiota transplantation for *Clostridium difficile* infection: systematic review and meta-analysis. *Am J Gastroenterol.* 2013;108(4):500–508.

Kumar V, Abbas AK, Fausto N, eds. *Robbins and Cotran: Pathologic Basis of Disease*. 7th ed. St. Louis: Elsevier Saunders; 2005.

Mulholland MW, Lillemoe KD, Doherty GM, et al., eds. *Greenfield's Surgery: Scientific Principles and Practice*. 5th ed. Philadelphia: Lippincott Williams & Wilkins; 2010.

Sagar J. Colorectal stents for the management of malignant colonic obstructions. *Cochrane Database Syst Rev.* 2011;(11):CD007378.

Shankar S, Ledakis P, El Halabi H, et al. Neoplasms of the appendix: current treatment guidelines. *Hematol Oncol Clin North Am.* 2012;26(6):1261–1290.

Sieber OM, Lipton L, Crabtree M, et al. Multiple colorectal adenomas, classic adenomatous polyposis, and germ-line mutations in *MYH*. *N Engl J Med.* 2003;348(9):791.

Townsend CM, Beauchamp RD, Evers BM, et al., eds. *Sabiston Textbook of Surgery*. 19th ed. Philadelphia: WB Saunders; 2012.

CHAPTER

13

The Hepatobiliary System

ELIJAH W. RIDDLE AND PAIGE M. PORRETT

KEY POINTS

- Hepatic arterial anatomic variation is extremely prevalent: an accessory/replaced left hepatic artery frequently branches from the left gastric artery and an accessory/replaced right hepatic artery usually arises from the superior mesenteric artery.
- Both focal nodular hyperplasia and hepatic adenoma affect young women but are treated differently: FNH is usually managed nonoperatively, while adenomas should be resected due to risk of rupture.
- Treatment for parasitic liver abscesses varies depending on etiologic organism. *Entamoeba histolytica* (amebic liver abscess) is treated medically with metronidazole, while hydatid cyst disease (*Echinococcus granulosus*) often requires operation.
- Colorectal metastases to the liver are aggressively treated surgically.
- Hepatic resection is the preferred treatment for hepatocellular carcinoma in noncirrhotic patients, but liver transplantation should be considered in cirrhotic patients.

ANATOMY OF THE LIVER AND BILIARY SYSTEM

The liver and gallbladder are digestive organs located in the right upper quadrant (RUQ) of the abdominal cavity. Bile produced by the liver and stored in the gallbladder is critical for the absorption of fats; cholecystokinin (CCK) released by the intestine in response to ingested fats (see Chapter 4) causes the gallbladder to contract and propel bile through the cystic duct, into the common bile duct (CBD), and eventually into the duodenum (Fig. 13.1). The liver also plays a central role in nutrient and drug metabolism, synthesis of coagulation proteins, and detoxification of the blood.

In most people, arterial blood from the aorta reaches the hepatobiliary system via the right and left hepatic arteries, which are terminal branches of the proper hepatic artery (Fig. 13.1). Blood to the gallbladder is supplied by the cystic artery, which commonly arises from the right hepatic artery; the cystic artery courses through the triangle of Calot, an anatomic construct composed of the inferior border of the liver, the common hepatic duct, and the cystic duct. However, hepatic arterial anatomy is extremely variable, and all surgeons must be well acquainted with the *common anatomic variants* that are frequently encountered during pancreatic, gastric, or other foregut procedures (Fig. 13.2). Importantly, both cadaveric dissections and angiographic studies have confirmed that one out of five people have replaced or recurrent hepatic arteries. A replaced or recurrent left hepatic artery commonly courses from the left gastric artery through the hepatogastric ligament, and a replaced or recurrent right hepatic artery branching off the superior mesenteric artery frequently travels to the right of the CBD in the lateral hepatoduodenal ligament.

The liver receives 70% of its blood supply via the portal vein, which is the most posterior structure in the porta hepatis (Fig. 13.1). Deoxygenated blood from the liver is drained by three large intraparenchymal hepatic veins (right, middle, and left) that empty into the inferior vena cava (IVC). Veins from the gallbladder penetrate the hepatic parenchyma in the vicinity of the gallbladder fossa.

Two distinct classification schemes are commonly used to describe the anatomy of the liver. The *morphologic* classification system divides the liver into four lobes; these lobes are separated by external fissures or ligaments (Fig. 13.3). The dominant right lobe is separated from the left lobe by the falciform ligament, while the smaller quadrate and caudate lobes are located on the inferior surface of the liver adjacent to the porta hepatis. Alternatively, the *functional* classification system as described by *Couinaud* (Fig. 13.4) divides the liver into eight segments that are supplied by distinct branches of the arterial and portal blood supply. These segments are separated by the vertically oriented *portal scissurae* containing the hepatic veins and the transversely oriented *portal pedicles* containing the portal vein branches within the hepatic parenchyma. This classification scheme is of practical utility to the surgeon, as the dissection planes involved in major liver resections follow this internal segmental anatomy (Table 13.1). Segments 5, 6, 7, and 8 constitute the right hemiliver (resected in a formal right hepatectomy), while segments 2, 3, and 4 compose the left hemiliver (resected during a formal left hepatectomy). Segment 1 (also known as the caudate lobe) represents a functionally distinct lobe and drains directly into the IVC. The internal division of the liver into right and left hemilivers follows an imaginary line between the gallbladder bed anteriorly and the IVC posteriorly known as *Cantlie's line*. This line also approximates the location of the *main portal scissura*, which envelops the middle hepatic vein.

LABORATORY AND RADIOGRAPHIC EVALUATION OF THE HEPATOBILIARY SYSTEM

Common signs and symptoms of hepatobiliary pathology (Table 13.2) should prompt laboratory (Table 13.3) and radiographic (Tables 13.4 and 13.5) evaluation of the hepatobiliary system. The chronicity of symptoms and a history of alcohol use, occupational exposures, or viral hepatitis infection help to differentiate different disease processes. Physical exam findings including stigmata of portal

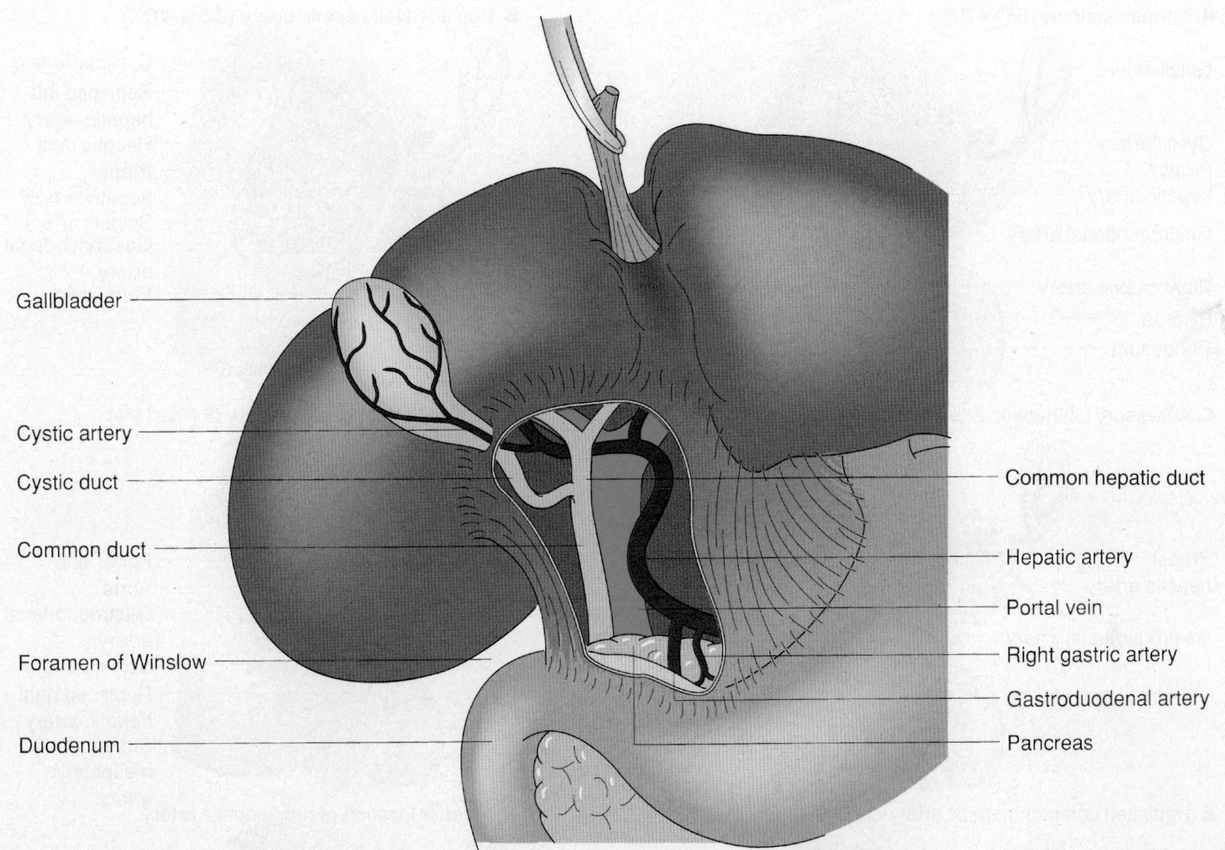

FIGURE 13.1 Anatomic relations of hepatic artery, portal vein, and CBD. (From Mulholland MW, Lillemoe KD, Doherty GM, et al., eds. *Greenfield's Surgery: Scientific Principles and Practice*. 5th ed. Philadelphia: Lippincott Williams & Wilkins; 2010:1018, with permission.)

hypertension (e.g., splenomegaly, caput medusa, etc.) or Murphy's sign (RUQ pain with palpation on inspiration) can further help narrow the differential diagnosis and direct further workup. When evaluating the patient with hepatobiliary disease, the surgeon's initial priority is to determine whether the patient has necrotic or infected tissue (i.e., a gangrenous gallbladder), if biliary obstruction with infection is present (i.e., cholangitis), or if there is acute liver failure. These conditions can be life threatening and sometimes require urgent surgical intervention. The serum bilirubin level and a hydroxyiminodiacetic acid (HIDA) or DISIDA scan (see Table 13.4) are frequently utilized diagnostic modalities in the patient who is acutely ill in order to determine if infection, a bile leak or biliary obstruction is present. Ultrasound, transaminase levels (i.e., serum AST/ALT), and cross-sectional imaging (MRI, CT scan) are also useful adjuncts, but these tests are more often used to evaluate less urgent hepatobiliary pathology (e.g., cholelithiasis, cirrhosis, viral hepatitis, and hepatic masses). The role of these examinations in the diagnosis of specific pathology is discussed further in the following text.

BENIGN SURGICAL DISEASE OF THE GALLBLADDER AND BILIARY TREE

Gallstones and Their Complications

Gallstones are extremely prevalent in the United States; 10% to 15% of the general population has gallstones (*cholelithiasis*), but only a minority of these patients (5% to 10%) becomes symptomatic. Risk factors for the development of symptomatic gallstone disease include obesity, rapid weight loss or gain, and estrogen exposure (i.e., women, especially pregnant women or women taking oral contraceptives), as estrogen increases the cholesterol saturation of bile.

Gallstones are classified by their composition as *cholesterol stones* or *pigment stones*; cholesterol stones are the more common type. Under normal circumstances, cholesterol, bile salts, and lecithin remain in aqueous solution as bile salt–lecithin micelles; however, when the concentration of bile salts or lecithin decreases, cholesterol may precipitate out of solution to form cholesterol stones (Fig. 13.5). The pathophysiology of pigment stone formation is similar; these stones are further subdivided into *black* or *brown pigment stones*. Patients with hemolytic blood dyscrasias may have increased concentrations of insoluble unconjugated bilirubin in the bile that predispose to black stone formation within the gallbladder. *Brown pigment stones* may form under infectious conditions when calcium concentrations within the bile increase resulting in precipitation. These stones, therefore, more frequently form in the bile duct primarily.

Gallstones become symptomatic when they obstruct ductal structures. Gallstones can intermittently obstruct the cystic duct and cause *biliary colic* (*symptomatic cholelithiasis*). Patients with biliary colic present with RUQ pain, nausea, and vomiting that commonly begins a few hours after a fatty meal but ultimately regresses spontaneously once the gallstone dislodges from the cystic duct. If cholelithiasis is confirmed by ultrasound in a symptomatic, at-risk patient, elective cholecystectomy is the treatment of choice.

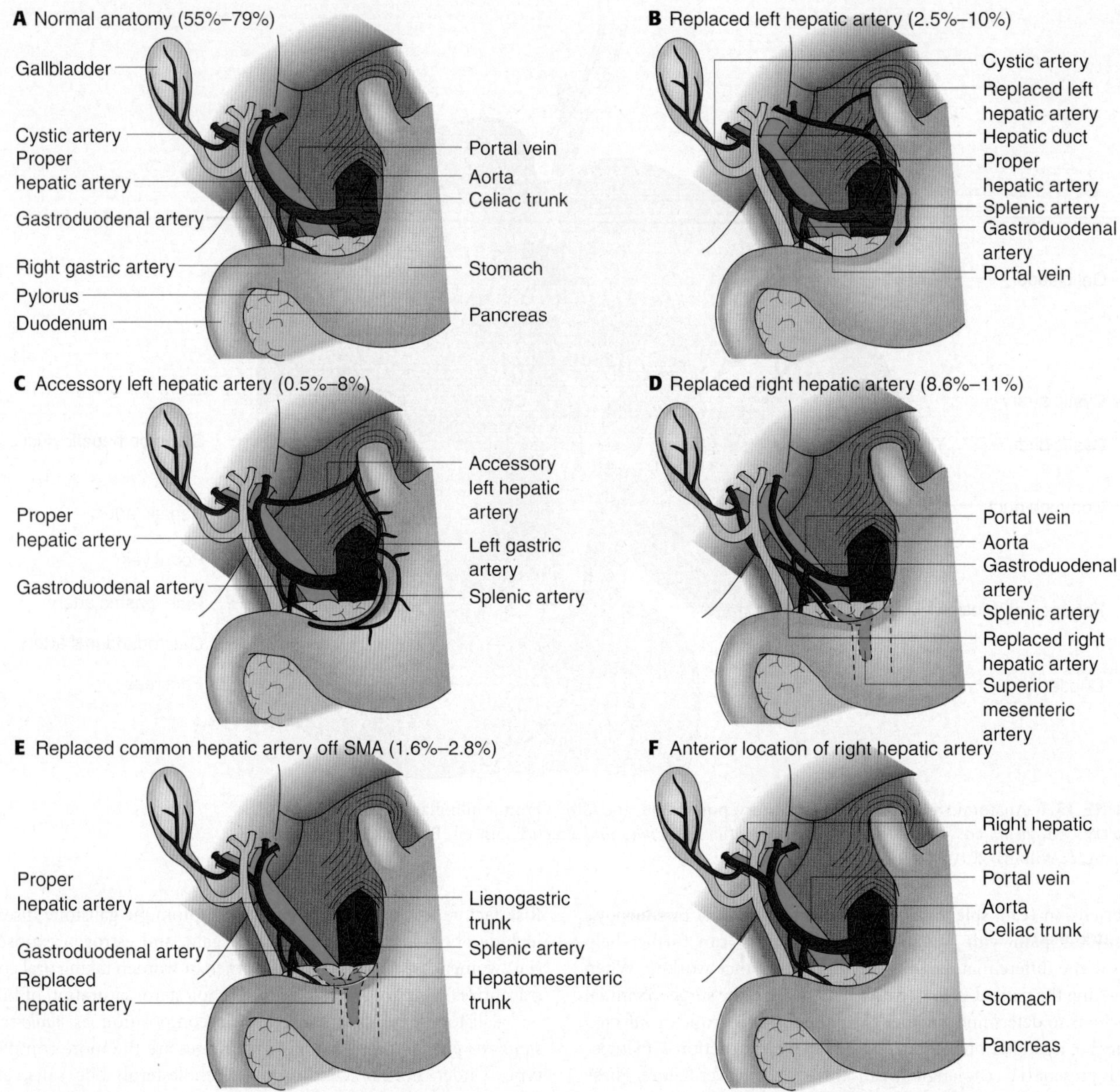

FIGURE 13.2 Variations in hepatic arterial anatomy. Additional described variations include accessory right hepatic artery from SMA (3.3%–7%), common hepatic artery from left gastric artery (0.5%) or aorta (0.3%), replaced right hepatic artery with replaced left hepatic artery (1%), and accessory right hepatic artery with accessory left hepatic artery (1%). (From Mulholland MW, Lillemoe KD, Doherty GM, et al., eds. *Greenfield's Surgery: Scientific Principles and Practice*. 5th ed. Philadelphia: Lippincott Williams & Wilkins; 2010:1018, with permission.)

Acute cholecystitis develops when bile flow from the gallbladder is persistently obstructed, usually from a gallstone in the cystic duct (calculous cholecystitis). Acute cholecystitis can also result from biliary sludging (acalculous cholecystitis) in very ill patients or in patients who are on TPN. Symptoms of cholecystitis initially resemble those of biliary colic (e.g., RUQ pain); however, unlike biliary colic, the pain persists for hours to days without resolution. On physical examination, patients are tender upon palpation of the RUQ with deep inspiration (i.e., *Murphy's sign*) and may be febrile or have a leukocytosis. Ultrasonographic findings can be helpful and are often diagnostic (Table 13.4). Although ultrasound is often used as the first test for cholecystitis given its lower cost and wider availability, calculous cholecystitis is most definitively diagnosed by HIDA scanning. During this examination, a nuclear tracer administered to the patient is taken up by the hepatocytes and excreted into the bile. Normally, the gallbladder and intestine can be visualized as the bile passes through the biliary tree and ampulla of Vater (Fig. 13.6). In acute calculous cholecystitis, however, obstruction of the cystic duct prevents reflux of bile into, and visualization of, the gallbladder. Unfortunately, HIDA scan is frequently falsely negative in acalculous cholecystitis; this entity is much more difficult to diagnose, and a high degree of clinical suspicion in at-risk patient populations is warranted.

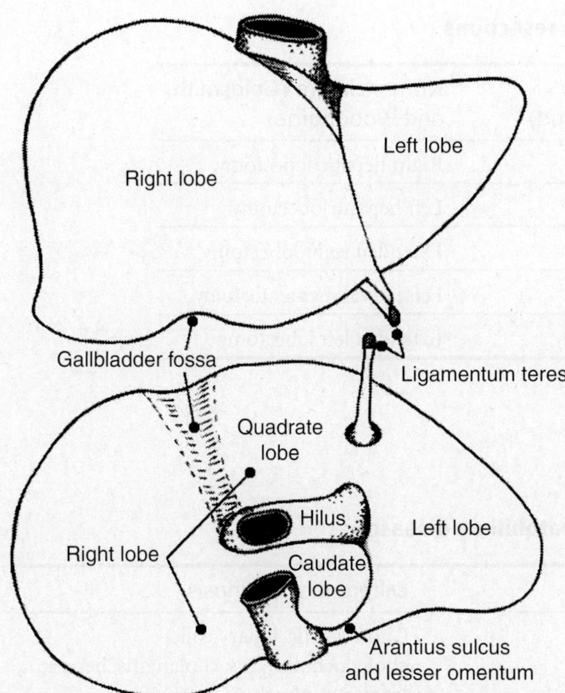

FIGURE 13.3 Lobar anatomy of the liver. (From Baker RJ, Fischer JE, eds. *Mastery of Surgery*. 4th ed. Philadelphia: Lippincott Williams & Wilkins, 2001:1048, with permission.)

Whether caused by gallstones or not, persistent cystic duct obstruction leads to increased intraluminal pressure in the gallbladder, which can lead to ischemia of the gallbladder wall with subsequent perforation or necrosis (i.e., *emphysematous cholecystitis*); this condition is life threatening and a surgical emergency. In contrast, the timing of laparoscopic cholecystectomy in stable patients with uncomplicated cholecystitis remains somewhat controversial. Generally, laparoscopic cholecystectomy should be performed within 24 to 72 hours of hospital admission. The *cooling off* period advocated in the past for patients who present after several days of symptoms is not supported by a robust literature. Conversely, complication rates appear to increase with greater delays before cholecystectomy. In the inoperable patient, cholecystostomy drainage may allow for temporization of acute infection. This is a particularly good option in acalculous disease, where it may serve as definitive therapy.

Occasionally, the severe inflammation that accompanies cholecystitis results in an *enterobiliary fistula*. Such fistulas may allow for passage of large diameter gallstones directly from the gallbladder into the intestine and, rarely, obstruction of the bowel lumen (*gallstone ileus*). A plain radiograph demonstrating small bowel obstruction and air in the biliary system is pathognomonic for gallstone ileus and should prompt exploratory laparotomy. An enterolithotomy to remove the gallstone or resection of the affected intestinal segment should be performed. Cholecystectomy to treat the fistula is often delayed until the patient has stabilized physiologically, although individual case reports suggest that in stable patients, cholecystectomy can be performed at the time of enterolithotomy.

Gallstones can also cause complications when they migrate into the CBD. *Choledocholithiasis* may cause common duct obstruction and ascending infection (*cholangitis*), or pancreatic ductal obstruction and *gallstone pancreatitis*. In cases of suspected choledocholithiasis, common duct stones may be retrieved via urgent endoscopic retrograde cholangiopancreatogram (ERCP), which is the initial intervention of choice if a skilled endoscopist trained in ERCP is available. Alternatively, the surgeon may explore the bile duct at time of either laparoscopic or open cholecystectomy.

Laparoscopic cholecystectomy has revolutionized the treatment of gallbladder disease. Extensive study of this procedure over the 1990s confirmed the safety of this approach and its advantages over open cholecystectomy: specifically shorter length of hospital stay and convalescence. The safety of laparoscopic cholecystectomy

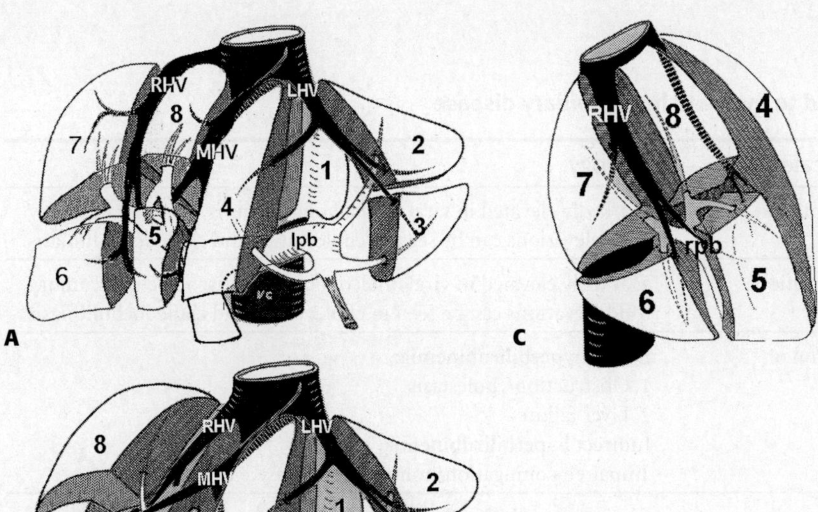

FIGURE 13.4 Couinaud's segmental anatomy of the liver. **A.** Couinaud's classic drawing of the liver in the autopsy or "bench" position. This depiction does not accurately portray the anterior–posterior dimension of the hepatic segments in relation to the IVC. **B.** A representation of the true anatomic position of the hepatic segments *in vivo*. Note the difference compared to **(A)**. **C.** Lateral schema of the *in vivo* lobar anatomy. Note the posterior position of segments 6 and 7. (From Mulholland MW, Lillemoe KD, Doherty GM, et al., eds. *Greenfield's Surgery: Scientific Principles and Practice*. 5th ed. Philadelphia: Lippincott Williams & Wilkins; 2010:1018, with permission.)

TABLE 13.1 Anatomy of common hepatic resections

Segments Resected	Nomenclature (Couinaud)	Nomenclature (Goldsmith and Woodburne)
V, VI, VII, VIII	Right hepatectomy	Right hepatic lobectomy
II, III, IV	Left hepatectomy	Left hepatic lobectomy
IV, V, VI, VII, VIII[a]	Right lobectomy	Extended right lobectomy
II, III	Left lobectomy	Left lateral segmentectomy
II, III, IV, V, VIII[b]	Extended left hepatectomy	Extended left lobectomy

[a]Also known as right trisegmentectomy.
[b]Also known as left trisegmentectomy.

TABLE 13.2 Common signs and symptoms of surgical hepatobiliary disease

Sign/Symptom	Underlying Etiology	Differential Diagnosis
RUQ pain[a]	1. Biliary obstruction 2. Biliary inflammation	Cholecystitis, biliary colic, choledocholithiasis, cholangitis, hepatic infection, tumor
Jaundice[a]	Hyperbilirubinemia[b] (direct or indirect)	Biliary obstruction (i.e., choledocholithiasis or biliary/pancreatic tumor), hepatic failure (i.e., cirrhosis).
Caput medusa/splenomegaly/varices	Portal hypertension	Cirrhosis, mesenteric venous thrombosis
Ascites	Liver failure and/or portal hypertension	Cirrhosis, mesenteric venous thrombosis
Fever[a]	Infection/inflammation	Cholecystitis, cholangitis, hepatic abscess

[a]The combination of RUQ pain, jaundice, and fever is known as *Charcot's triad* and is highly suggestive of underlying cholangitis. A patient with *Reynold's pentad* (Charcot's triad + mental status changes + hypotension) has cholangitis with signs of systemic sepsis and must be treated immediately.
[b]Surgeons primarily treat direct causes of hyperbilirubinemia (i.e., biliary obstruction, tumor, etc.) as indirect hyperbilirubinemia is caused by RBC lysis or hematologic disorders that are treated medically.

TABLE 13.3 Serologic tests performed to evaluate hepatobiliary disease

Test	Abnormality Indicates:	Etiology
Serum AST	Hepatocyte inflammation and/or necrosis	Markedly elevated in viral or alcoholic hepatitis, or ischemic injury Mild elevations can be seen in cholecystitis and choledocholithiasis
Serum ALT	Hepatocyte inflammation and/or necrosis	Markedly elevated in viral or alcoholic hepatitis, or ischemic injury Mild elevations can be seen in cholecystitis and choledocholithiasis
Serum bilirubin	Impaired conjugation or excretion	**Direct hyperbilirubinemia:** 1. Obstruction/cholestasis 2. Liver failure **Indirect hyperbilirubinemia:** Impaired conjugation/nonsurgical disease
Serum alkaline phosphatase	Cholestasis or obstruction	Choledocholithiasis Cholangitis Compression by tumor
PT/PTT/INR	Poor hepatic synthetic function	Liver failure
Albumin	Poor hepatic synthetic function	Liver failure

TABLE 13.4 Radiographic evaluation of the hepatobiliary tree

Exam:	Best Evaluates:	Useful in Diagnosis of:	Notes:
Ultrasound	1. Gallstones in gallbladder 2. Intrahepatic ductal dilatation	1. Cholelithiasis 2. Biliary obstruction 3. ± Cholecystitis[a]	Sensitivity for stones in gallbladder >95%. Sensitivity for cholecystitis ≈85%[a]
CT scan/MRI	Hepatic parenchyma	1. Tumor 2. Cyst 3. Abscess	Contrast phases useful in delineating pathology (see Table 13.5)
Cholangiography	Intra- or extrahepatic ductal obstruction	1. Choledocholithiasis 2. Tumor compression 3. Choledochal cysts 4. Ductal agenesis/atrophy	Can be performed fluoroscopically (ERCP/PTC/IOC)[b] or via MRCP
Cholescintigraphy (HIDA or DISIDA)[c]	Patency of cystic and/or CBDs	1. Cholecystitis[a] 2. CBD[d] obstruction 3. CBD leak	Test of choice for diagnosis of cholecystitis

[a]The specificity of U/S for cholecystitis is greatest when the quatrad of gallstones within the gallbladder, gallbladder wall thickening >3 mm, pericholecystic fluid, and sonographic Murphy's sign (pain with direct pressure over the sonographically visualized gallbladder) are all concomitantly present. However, the sensitivity of U/S for detecting three of the four parameters is reportedly 80% in patients with cholecystitis. Hence, the greater sensitivity of HIDA/DISIDA for cholecystitis (>90%) makes cholescintigraphy a more definitive test in patients with suspected cholecystitis.

[b]ERCP, endoscopic retrograde cholangiopancreatogram. An endoscope is inserted orally and passed into the duodenum where the ampulla of Vater can be visualized and cannulated. Contrast dye is then injected in retrograde fashion into the biliary tree, which can be visualized fluoroscopically (i.e., with an external, real-time x-ray source).

PTC, percutaneous transhepatic cholangiogram. A needle is passed through the skin and into the hepatic parenchyma to allow contrast to be injected into the biliary tree. This allows antegrade visualization of the biliary tree.

IOC, intraoperative cholangiogram. The biliary tree can be cannulated intraoperatively during open or laparoscopic procedures via the cystic duct or less commonly, the CBD. Contrast is injected, and the biliary tree anatomy is imaged fluoroscopically.

[c]HIDA, hepatic 2,6-dimethyl iminodiacetic acid; DISIDA, diisopropyl iminodiacetic acid. DISIDA scan has now predominantly replaced HIDA scanning; the techniques are very similar and vary only with regard to nuclear tracer. Specifically, DISIDA has higher hepatic extraction and is thus more useful in patients with liver disease.

[d]CBD, common bile duct.

relies on correct identification of the ductal and arterial anatomy. Many surgeons advocate obtaining the "critical view of safety" prior to division of any structures, which includes dissection to completely expose and delineate the hepatocystic triangle (of Calot), identification of a single duct and single artery entering the gallbladder, and complete dissection of the lower part of the gallbladder away from the cystic plate. Intraoperative cholangiography may be useful in cases with complex ductal anatomy and to evaluate for choledocholithiasis and bile duct injury or pathology. When the delineation of ductal anatomy is difficult, or if significant bleeding develops, conversion to the traditional open approach is recommended. In experienced hands, conversion rates from laparoscopy to laparotomy during elective cholecystectomy are less than 10%. However, conversion rates increase dramatically in the setting of acute cholecystitis as a result of the marked inflammation that can obscure anatomy in this condition; rates as high as 30% are commonly reported in the literature.

Though laparoscopic cholecystectomy is generally associated with excellent outcomes, complications of the procedure may result in significant morbidity. *Cystic duct stump leaks* with resulting *bilomas* complicate 0.3% of laparoscopic cholecystectomies. Leaks may occur when the surgical clip on the cystic duct stump slips off. Patients typically present 3 days after the procedure with abdominal pain, fever, and/or vomiting. A HIDA scan or ERCP will confirm the diagnosis. Cystic duct stump leak can often be managed successfully with ERCP stenting of the CBD as well as percutaneous drainage of the resulting biloma(s). Recent reviews of this approach indicate that over 90% of cystic duct stump leaks seal after CBD stenting and do not require additional operative intervention.

A more serious surgical complication of cholecystectomy than cystic duct leak, however, is iatrogenic injury to surrounding ductal structures. Cystic duct anatomy is highly variable (Fig. 13.7), and inflammation or bleeding at the time of surgery can obscure biliary anatomy. Published data suggest that *injury to the CBD* occurs more frequently during laparoscopic cholecystectomy versus the open approach, though ductal injury remains rare (0.6% of cases). Electrocautery injuries that occur during ductal dissection may lead to ductal stricture formation, and inadvertent ligation of the common bile or hepatic duct may result from misidentification of the anatomy. If the surgeon recognizes ductal injury intraoperatively, termination of the procedure and transfer of the patient to a tertiary care center for definitive management is generally recommended. Ductal injuries unrecognized at the time of initial surgery may lead to postoperative symptoms and can be confirmed

TABLE 13.5 Radiographic characteristics of primary solid hepatic masses

Tumor	Ultrasound	CT	MRI
Hemangioma	Hyperechoic solid lesion	*Unenhanced:* Hypodense lesion *Enhanced:* Peripheral nodular enhancement with centripetal filling on delayed images	*T1 images:* Hypointense *T2 images:* Hyperintense *After gadolinium:* Similar to CT scan Diagnostic modality of choice
FNH	May or may not be visible. FNH has no specific characteristic features on ultrasound.	*Unenhanced:* Homogeneous and hypo/isodense to the liver *Enhanced:* Characteristic pattern of early enhancement with washout on delayed images. **Central scar** noted in 50% of cases	*T1 images:* Hypo/**isointense** *T2 images:* Iso/**hyperintense** After gadolinium: Similar to CT scan
Hepatic adenoma	Nonspecific. Use of color Doppler technology may help distinguish from FNH.	*Unenhanced:* Heterogeneous hypodense lesion *Enhanced:* Early variegated enhancement, well-defined border because of capsule	*T1 images:* Heterogeneous and hyperintense *T2 images:* **Hyperintense** *After gadolinium:* Similar to CT scan
HCC	May be hypoechoic or hyperechoic. Insensitive in screening studies in cirrhotic livers.	*Unenhanced:* Hypodense lesion *Dual-phase enhancement:* Enhancement in arterial phase 20 s after contrast administration Portal phase washout 60 s after administration Iodized oil more sensitive modality	*T1 images:* Hypo/hyperintense *T2 images:* Also variable *After gadolinium:* Similar to CT scan

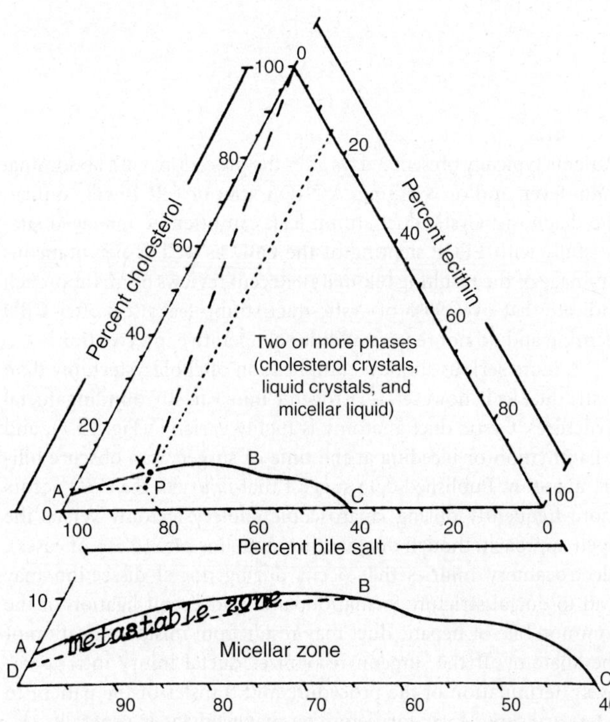

FIGURE 13.5 Cholesterol solubility decreases with decreasing bile salt or lecithin concentration. (From Schoenfield LJ, Marks JW. Formation and treatment of gallstones. In: Schiff L, Schiff ER, eds. *Diseases of the Liver*. 6th ed. Philadelphia: JB Lippincott Co.; 1987:1268, with permission.)

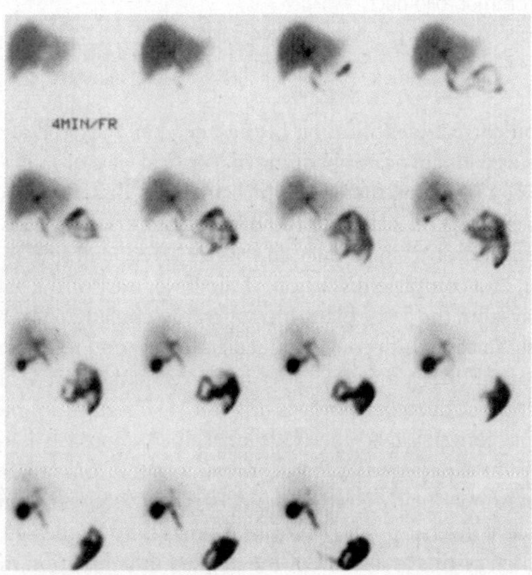

FIGURE 13.6 Normal HIDA scan. The nuclear tracer is concentrated in the bile after being taken up from the blood by the hepatocytes. As bile passes antegrade through the biliary tree, the gallbladder (high signal, bottom left of lower panels) and the intestine (high signal, bottom right of lower panels) become visible. (From Cacciarelli AG, Naddaf SY, el-Zeftawy HA, et al. Acute cholecystitis in AIDS patients: correlation of Tc-99m hepatobiliary scintigraphy with histopathologic laboratory findings and CD4 counts. *Clin Nucl Med.* 1998;23(4):226, with permission.)

by ERCP (Fig. 13.8). In contrast to the conservative management of cystic duct stump leak, almost 90% of bile duct injuries require operative bile duct reconstruction. *Roux-en-Y hepaticojejunostomy* remains the procedure of choice in most cases.

Gallbladder Polyps

Epidemiologic studies have revealed that 5% to 10% of the population have polypoid lesions of the gallbladder. While the vast majority of gallbladder polyps are benign cholesterol polyps (70%), approximately 8% are malignant. Polypoid lesions are commonly detected with ultrasound; asymptomatic lesions are managed expectantly with ultrasonographic surveillance performed every 3 to 6 months for several years to ensure stability of polyp size. As the probability of malignancy correlates with polyp size, laparoscopic cholecystectomy is recommended for any patient who has a gallbladder polyp that is greater than 10 mm in size. Open cholecystectomy is recommended for the removal of larger lesions to avoid dissemination of malignancy.

Choledochal Cysts

Though more common in children, *choledochal cysts* may manifest in adulthood. Choledochal cysts are rare congenital anomalies (incidence = 1:100,000 live births) but are more common in patients of Asian ethnicity. Only a minority of patients present with the classic triad of abdominal pain, jaundice, and an RUQ mass. More commonly, choledochal cysts present in adults with complications such as cholangitis or pancreatitis. Choledochal cysts are classified according to their location in the biliary tree (Fig. 13.9). While imaging modalities such as ultrasonography, CT scan, and ERCP may aid in the diagnosis of choledochal cysts, magnetic resonance cholangiopancreatography (MRCP) has emerged as the imaging modality of choice. Cyst excision with hepaticoenterostomy is indicated in most cases given the risks of complications and malignant degeneration of the cysts. Type III disease and type V disease require special therapeutic consideration. As the intrahepatic cysts of *Caroli's disease* (type V) may not be amenable to resection, these patients may require liver transplantation. In light of recent

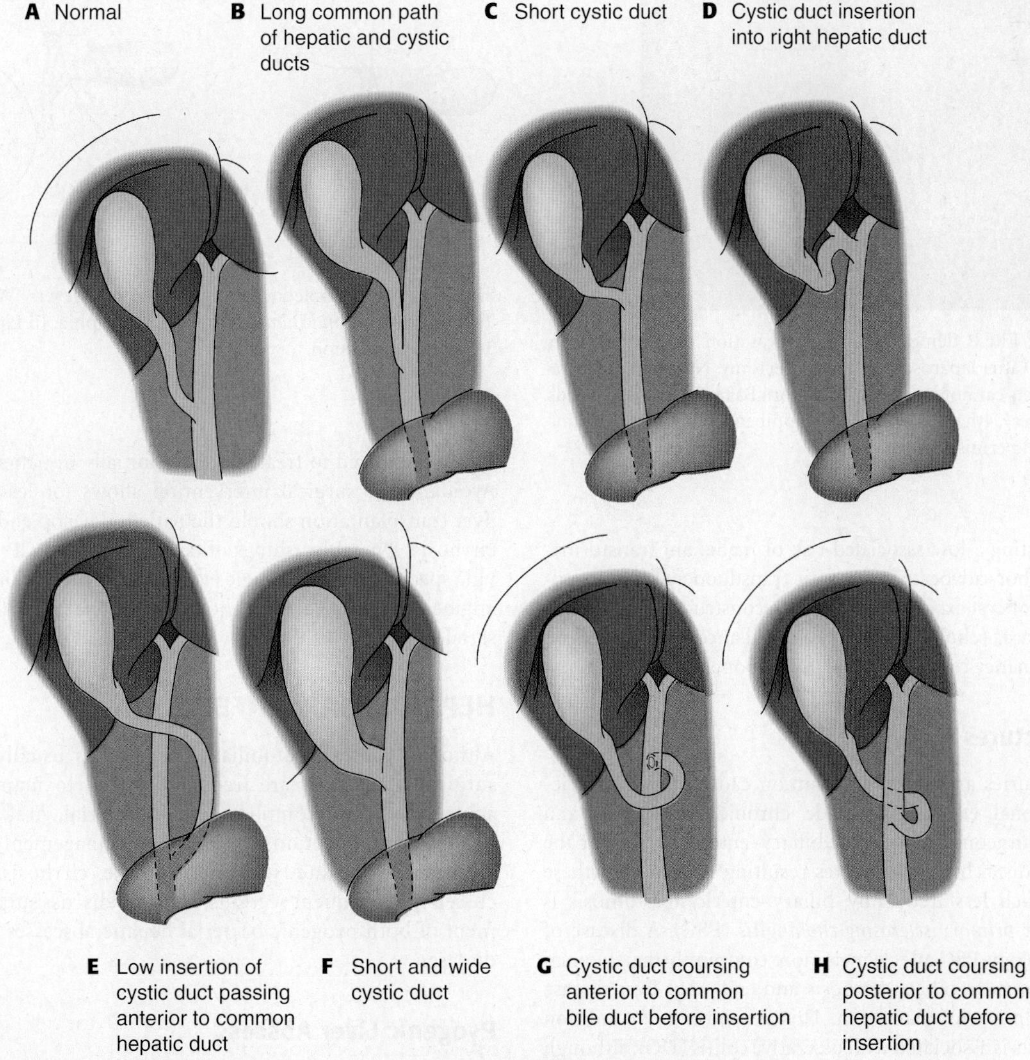

FIGURE 13.7 Anatomic variants of the cystic duct. (From Mulholland MW, Lillemoe KD, Doherty GM, et al., eds. *Greenfield's Surgery: Scientific Principles and Practice*. 5th ed. Philadelphia: Lippincott Williams & Wilkins; 2010:1018, with permission.)

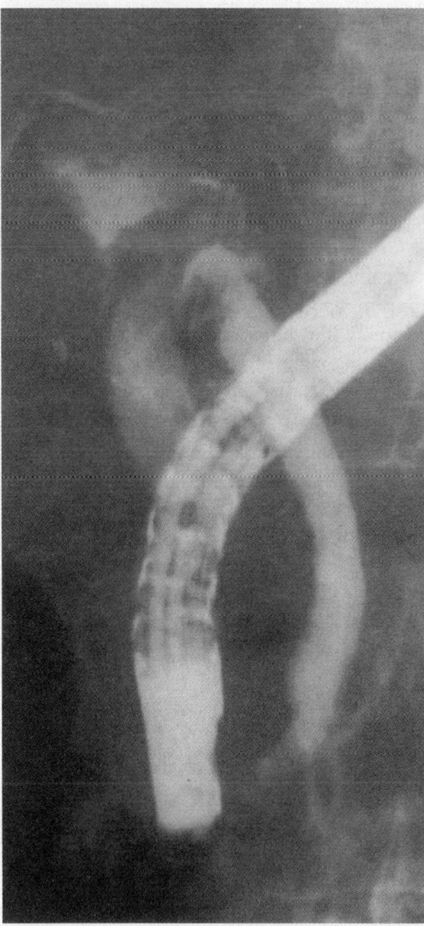

FIGURE 13.8 ERCP demonstrating extravasation of contrast from transected CBD after laparoscopic cholecystectomy. Note that the intrahepatic bile ducts cannot be visualized. (From Baker RJ, Fischer JE, eds. *Mastery of Surgery*. 4th ed. Philadelphia: Lippincott Williams & Wilkins, 2001:1063, with permission.)

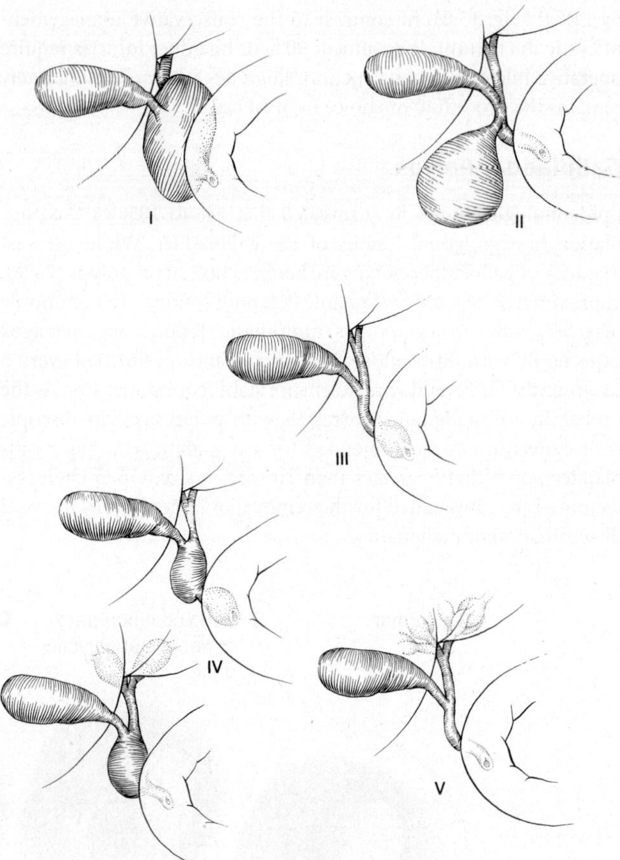

FIGURE 13.9 Choledochal cysts. (From Meyers WC, Jones RS. *Textbook of Liver and Biliary Surgery*. Philadelphia: JB Lippincott; 1990; 313, with permission.)

reports suggesting a low associated risk of malignant transformation, some authors advocate therapeutic transduodenal sphincteroplasty instead of cyst excision and biliary reconstruction in patients with type III cysts (choledochoceles). Surveillance for the development of malignancy remains critical in this population.

Biliary Strictures

Iatrogenic injuries are the most common cause of biliary strictures. Additional etiologies include chronic pancreatitis and malignancy. Surgeons may employ biliary–enteric bypass for the treatment of distal biliary strictures resulting from any of these etiologies. Much less frequently, biliary–enteric anastomosis is performed for *primary sclerosing cholangitis* (PSC). A disease of unknown etiology, PSC affects men more commonly than women and may progress to biliary cirrhosis and end-stage liver disease necessitating liver transplantation. This inflammatory condition of the bile ducts is associated with ulcerative colitis (UC), although the majority of patients with PSC do not have UC. Patients with PSC are at elevated risk for the development of cholangiocarcinoma. Currently, either ERCP or percutaneous biliary stenting is typically utilized to treat strictures initially in patients with PSC. Avoidance of surgical intervention allows for less complicated liver transplantation should the patient develop end-stage biliary cirrhosis. Ductal brushings obtained during ERCP can also provide specimens for cytologic evaluation and surveillance for cholangiocarcinoma. Patients should additionally be followed with serial serum CA 19-9 levels.

HEPATOBILIARY INFECTION

Although acute hepatobiliary infection is usually not treated surgically, surgeons are frequently asked to manage the subacute and chronic complications of bacterial, viral, and parasitic hepatobiliary infections. The surgical management of long-term sequelae of HBV and HCV infections (i.e., cirrhosis, HCC) is discussed in subsequent sections. Here, we discuss surgical management of both pyogenic bacterial hepatic abscesses and parasitic disease.

Pyogenic Liver Abscess

Patients with *pyogenic hepatic abscess* frequently present with nonspecific signs and symptoms; most will have fever, but only half of patients will have abdominal pain, and jaundice is infrequent.

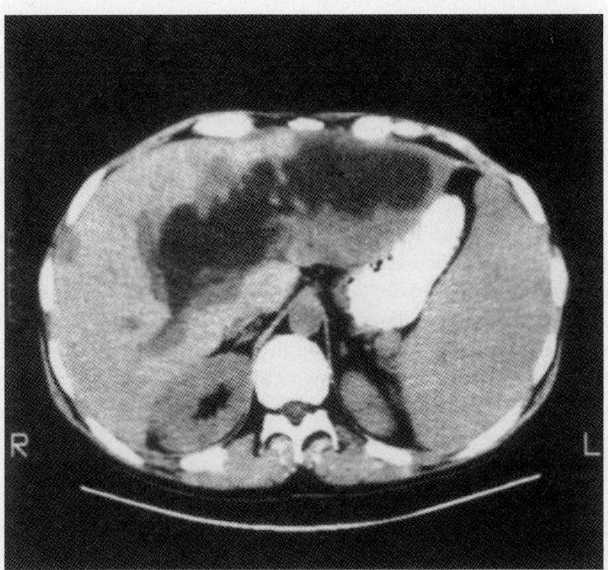

FIGURE 13.10 Computed tomogram of the abdomen demonstrating a hepatic abscess. (From Greenfield LJ, Mulholland MS, Oldham KT, et al., eds. *Surgery: Scientific Principles and Practice*. 2nd ed. Philadelphia: Lippincott-Raven Publishers; 1997:958, with permission.)

CT scan is the most sensitive and specific test for the diagnosis (Fig. 13.10). Importantly, neither the radiographic appearance nor clinical symptoms reliably distinguish pyogenic bacterial abscesses from parasitic abscesses. Nonetheless, this distinction must be made as treatment varies significantly with abscess etiology. Serologic testing employing indirect hemagglutination or ELISA assay provides valuable information, as elevated antibody titers in cases of amebic abscess or hydatid cyst disease can distinguish these lesions from pyogenic abscesses.

Figure 13.11 illustrates the various causes of pyogenic hepatic abscesses. Bacterial abscesses result from ascending cholangitis or from portal venous seeding from intra-abdominal infections such as diverticulitis and appendicitis. Iatrogenic pyogenic liver abscesses can develop following therapeutic interventions such as radiofrequency ablation (RFA) or hepatic artery chemoembolization and can also complicate liver transplantation should hepatic artery thrombosis occur. Abscesses are usually polymicrobial; *Klebsiella pneumoniae*, *Escherichia coli*, streptococci, and *Bacteroides fragilis* are frequently sampled in abscess fluid. Treatment consists of image-guided percutaneous drainage coupled with appropriate broad-spectrum antibiotic therapy. Open surgical drainage of pyogenic abscess is reserved for septic patients who fail percutaneous drainage or for cases of free intraperitoneal rupture and contamination.

Parasitic Liver Disease

Entamoeba histolytica, an ameba that infects 10% of the global population (most commonly alcoholic patients or homosexuals in developed countries) may cause *amebic liver abscesses*. The inciting trophozoites are released by ingested cysts and migrate from the intestine to the liver. Medical management consisting of a 10- to 14-day course of metronidazole usually provides adequate treatment. There is no role for surgical management.

In *hydatid liver disease* (*Echinococcus granulosus*), however, surgical resection of the hydatid cyst constitutes definitive therapy, as only 50% of these cysts resolve with antiparasitic albendazole treatment. While dogs are the definitive hosts for this tapeworm, humans become intermediate hosts after ingesting the eggs of *E. granulosus* that are passed from sheep or cattle. The eggs penetrate the small bowel wall and migrate via the portal bloodstream to the liver, where they hatch into larval scoleces. The scoleces are contained within the hydatid cyst until the cyst ruptures into the chest or abdomen.

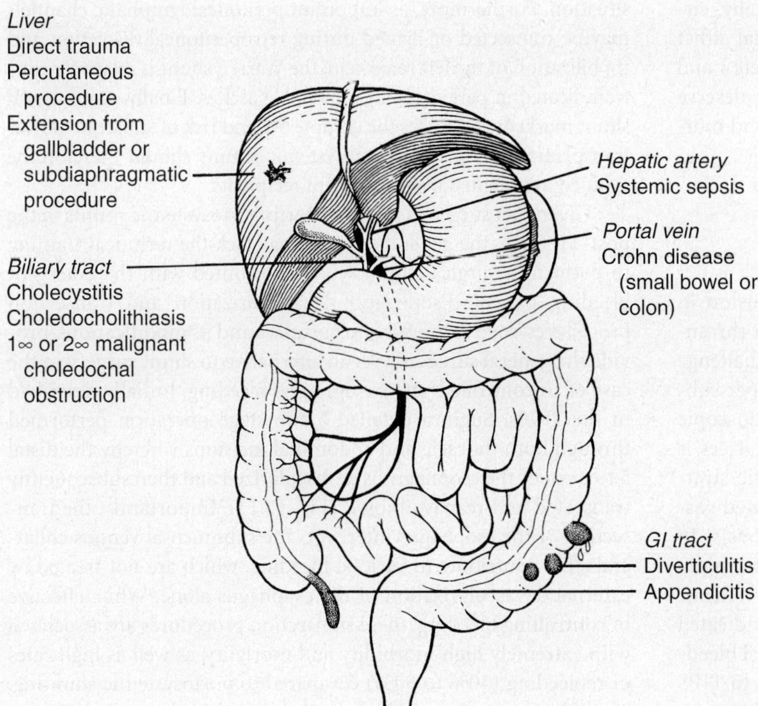

FIGURE 13.11 Etiology of pyogenic hepatic abscesses. (From Baker RJ, Fischer JE, eds. *Mastery of Surgery*. 4th ed. Philadelphia: Lippincott Williams & Wilkins, 2001:1073, with permission.)

As the fluid within the hydatid cyst is highly immunogenic, cyst rupture may result in anaphylactic shock. Great care must therefore be taken intraoperatively to avoid inadvertent rupture of the cyst with spillage of fluid and infective scoleces, which can adhere to other intra-abdominal serosal surfaces. Some authors advocate decompression of the cyst followed by irrigation of the cyst cavity by a scolicidal agent such as hypertonic saline and subsequent drainage of the pericystic cavity. Other experts recommend against puncture of the cyst and instead advocate total cystopericystectomy, whereby the entire cyst is carefully dissected from the hepatic parenchyma and removed *in toto*. Alternatively, the intact cyst may be removed by partial or complete hepatic lobectomy, depending on its anatomic location.

CIRRHOSIS AND PORTAL HYPERTENSION

Cirrhosis of the liver is a diagnosis characterized by the replacement of normal functioning hepatocytes with fibrous connective tissue and regenerative hepatic nodules. It represents the pathologic common end point of severe hepatic injury. Common causes of cirrhosis include chronic HBV or HCV infection, exposure to hepatotoxins such as alcohol, and a variety of metabolic derangements including $\alpha 1$-antitrypsin deficiency, hemochromatosis, and Wilson's disease. Cirrhosis has a range of clinical presentations; patients may be relatively well compensated and asymptomatic, or they may suffer from encephalopathy, jaundice, and coagulopathy indicative of frank hepatic failure. Complications of *portal hypertension*, such as gastroesophageal varices and ascites, may also afflict the cirrhotic patient.

Although cirrhosis, its underlying causes, and its complications are most frequently managed medically, surgeons are still asked to intervene on behalf of cirrhotic patients under a number of circumstances. First, surgeons provide the only curative and definitive therapy for end-stage cirrhotic patients: liver transplantation. Second, surgeons may be asked to manage complications of portal hypertension including bleeding varices and ascites. Finally, cirrhotic patients may develop any of the surgical diseases that afflict noncirrhotic patients (cholecystitis, appendicitis, cancer, etc.) and management of general surgical disease in the cirrhotic deserve special attention given the increase in surgical morbidity and mortality in these patients.

Surgical Management of Gastroesophageal Variceal Bleeding

Bleeding *gastric varices* can result from portal hypertension in a cirrhotic patient, or they may occur from splenic vein thrombosis. Gastric varices provide a greater therapeutic challenge than do esophageal varices (see below) due to their deeper submucosal position, which may preclude effective endoscopic therapy. Knowledge of the specific etiology of gastric varices is important in the development of an effective therapeutic strategy. *Splenectomy* is the best option in patients with isolated gastric variceal bleeding secondary to splenic vein thrombosis. In patients with gastric varices secondary to portal hypertension, however, insertion of a *transjugular intrahepatic portosystemic shunt* (TIPS) provides effective decompression. TIPS is indicated in virtually all cases of refractory gastroesophageal variceal bleeding secondary to portal hypertension. Contraindications to TIPS include right-sided heart failure with increased central venous pressure, severe hepatic failure, portal vein thrombosis, severe hepatic encephalopathy, and active local or systemic infection.

Gastroesophageal variceal bleeding is a major source of morbidity and mortality in the cirrhotic population. Twenty-five to thirty-five percent of cirrhotic patients will develop gastroesophageal variceal bleeding, and as many as 30% of initial bleeding episodes are fatal. Moreover, patients who survive an initial bleeding episode are at high risk for recurrent bleeding. In stark contrast to the treatment of gastric varices, endoscopic band ligation (EBL) will terminate bleeding in 80% to 90% of patients with bleeding gastroesophageal varices, and serial endoscopy with banding should be performed until varices are eradicated. TIPS should be attempted for bleeding that fails to resolve with EBL. Importantly, TIPS placement in bleeding patients is associated with a 3% to 30% mortality. Massive acute bleeding may require control with a Sengstaken–Blakemore tube prior to the initiation of more definitive therapy.

While TIPS and EBL are frequently successful in the treatment of gastroesophageal varices, *surgical portosystemic shunts* may be emergently required in the unusual event that TIPS fails to stop bleeding or is unavailable. It should be emphasized that these surgical procedures are rarely performed, as TIPS is associated with less perioperative mortality than are surgical shunts. *Nonselective portosystemic shunts*, such as the portacaval or mesocaval shunts, decompress the entire portal system (Fig. 13.12). Side-to-side portacaval shunts not only shunt portal blood away from the liver but also result in retrograde decompression of the liver into the vena cava. Thus, hepatic encephalopathy and even hepatic failure may develop after the placement of such a shunt. Given the relative technical ease with which portacaval shunting is performed and its efficacy, the portacaval shunt is the surgical shunt of choice. *Selective* surgical shunts such as the distal splenorenal (Warren) shunt decompress the gastroesophageal bed only (Fig. 13.12). This shunt maintains portomesenteric flow through the liver and therefore results in less encephalopathy and a decreased risk of hepatic failure as compared to nonselective shunts; however, technical complexity may prevent the use of this shunt in the emergent situation. Furthermore, as important peritoneal lymphatic channels may be transected or ligated during retroperitoneal dissection and mobilization of the left renal vein, the Warren shunt is relatively contraindicated in patients with intractable ascites. Finally, any surgical shunt markedly increases the complexity and risk of subsequent liver transplantation. Surgical portosystemic shunts should therefore be avoided in potential liver transplant recipients.

Given that surgeons rarely perform portosystemic shunts in the post-TIPS era, the general surgeon may lack the technical training to perform a surgical shunt when confronted with the emergent bleeding patient. Esophageal devascularization and transection procedures, such as the *Sugiura operation* and its modifications, provide the general surgeon with an alternative to shunt surgery in the case of uncontrolled gastroesophageal bleeding. Initially described in the 1970s, Sugiura detailed a two-stage operation performed through both thoracic and abdominal incisions whereby the distal 5 to 8 cm of the esophagus is devascularized and then subsequently transected and reanastomosed (Fig. 13.13). Importantly, the transection of the esophagus interrupts the submucosal venous collaterals that contribute to variceal bleeding, which are not treated by external devascularization of the esophagus alone. While effective in controlling bleeding, these transection procedures are associated with extremely high morbidity and mortality, as well as high rates of rebleeding (30% to 50%) compared to portosystemic shunting. Thus, the Sugiura procedure is rarely indicated in the post-TIPS era.

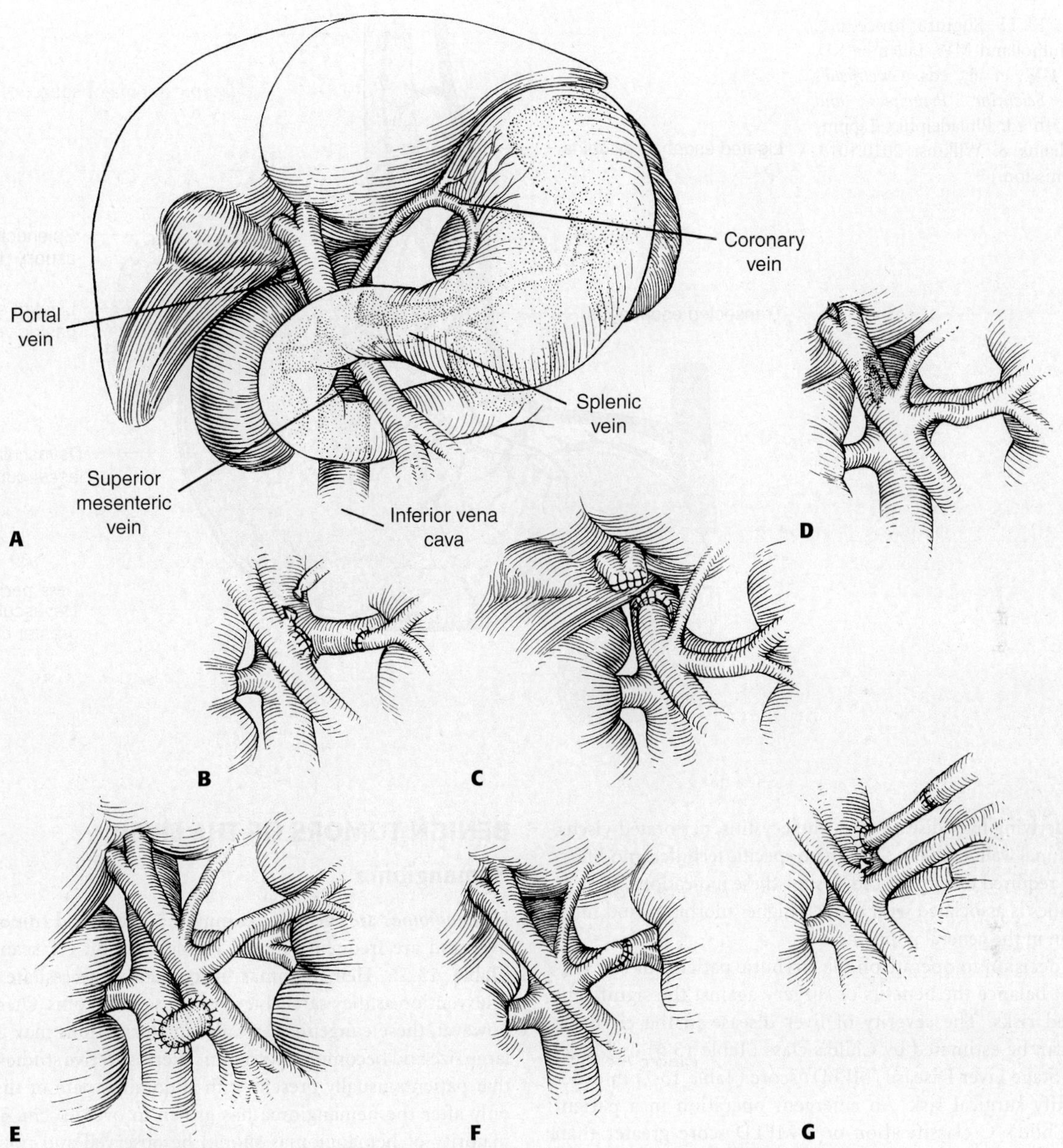

FIGURE 13.12 Portosystemic shunts. **A.** Intact portal venous anatomy. **B.** Distal splenorenal (Warren) shunt. **C.** End-to-side portacaval shunt. **D.** Side-to-side portacaval shunt. **E.** Mesocaval (H) shunt. **F.** Proximal splenorenal shunt. **G.** Coronary–caval shunt. (From Meyers WC, Jones RS. *Textbook of Liver and Biliary Surgery*. Philadelphia: JB Lippincott: 1990;184, with permission.)

Surgical Management of Ascites

Though usually treated medically with diuretics, large-volume paracentesis, or TIPS placement, refractory ascites may also be treated with the surgical placement of a *LeVeen shunt*. This extra-anatomic peritoneovenous shunt drains ascitic fluid from the peritoneal cavity directly into the internal jugular vein (Fig. 13.14). Significant complications include infection of the shunt or coagulopathy and bleeding secondary to systemic fibrinolysis. Fibrinolysis can develop because the ascitic fluid contains high concentrations of tissue plasminogen activator (TPA), which is then directly infused into the bloodstream via the shunt and may result in a severe consumptive coagulopathy. Though an effective treatment for ascites, the LeVeen shunt does not confer a survival benefit to cirrhotic patients with ascites as many patients undergoing the procedure succumb to the aforementioned complications. It is therefore not a recommended therapy in this patient population. In patients with refractory ascites who do not have hepatic encephalopathy, TIPS should be strongly considered.

General Surgery in the Cirrhotic Patient

While the complications of cirrhosis are less frequently treated surgically given the success of less invasive techniques, cirrhotic patients continue to require surgical therapy for indications unrelated to

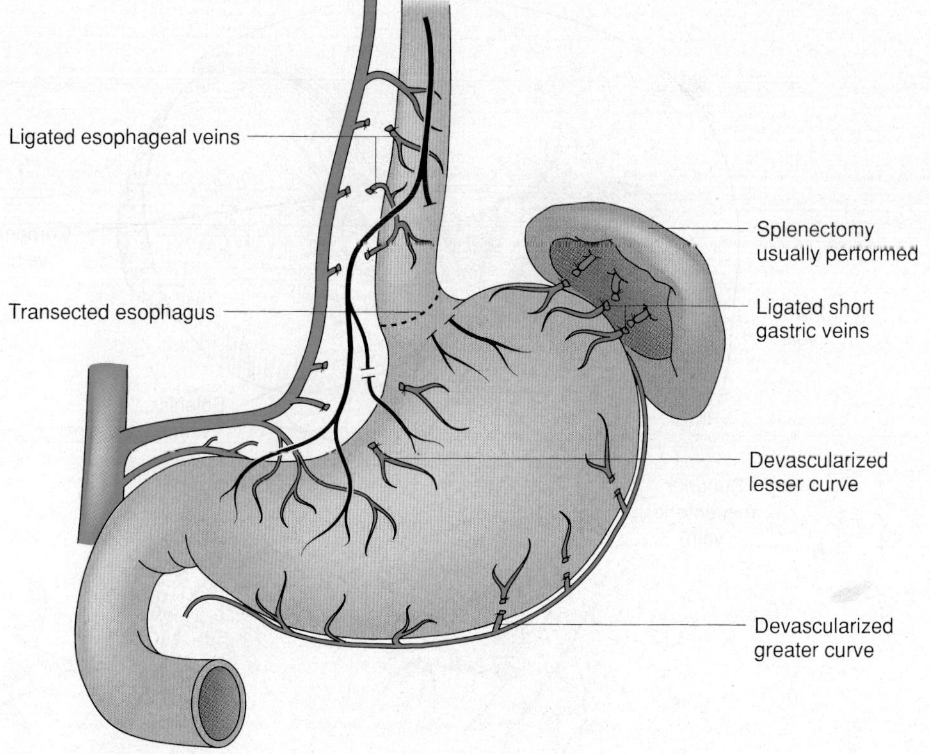

FIGURE 13.13 Sugiura procedure. (From Mulholland MW, Lillemoe KD, Doherty GM, et al., eds. *Greenfield's Surgery: Scientific Principles and Practice*. 5th ed. Philadelphia: Lippincott Williams & Wilkins; 2010:1018, with permission.)

their underlying liver disease (e.g., cholecystitis, perforated viscus, or abdominal wall hernias). Though no specific technical modifications are required during procedures for these indications, surgery in cirrhotics is associated with a much higher morbidity and mortality than in the general population.

The decision to operate on the cirrhotic patient for any reason must balance the benefits of surgery against the significant associated risks. The severity of liver disease in the cirrhotic patient can be estimated by Child's class (Table 13.6) or Model for End-Stage Liver Disease (MELD) score (Table 13.7) in order to quantify surgical risk. An emergent operation in a patient with a Child's C classification or a MELD score greater than 25 is associated with the worst perioperative survival—over 80% of these patients will die within 30 days of surgery. Death results primarily from sepsis, rapid decompensation of hepatic function, and severe coagulopathy. Recent data suggest that even under the best of circumstances, 10% to 25% of relatively well-compensated patients with MELD scores of 10 to 15 will die within 30 days of elective surgery (Table 13.8). Hence, the decision to operate on any cirrhotic patient, even well-compensated cirrhotics with retained hepatic reserve who undergo uncomplicated elective procedures, must not be entered into lightly. Such surgical intervention should only be performed in a center capable of supporting the cirrhotic patient through an anticipated difficult perioperative course; the center should be staffed with surgical, anesthetic, and critical care personnel versed in the care of these complicated patients. If elective surgery must be performed, a preoperative evaluation for liver transplantation should be considered, as emergent liver transplantation may be required to salvage the cirrhotic patient who decompensates after surgery.

BENIGN TUMORS OF THE LIVER

Hemangioma

Hemangiomas are the most common benign solid tumors of the liver and are frequently noted incidentally on CT scan or MRI (Table 13.5). Hemangiomas infrequently necessitate surgical intervention as they rarely bleed or cause symptoms. On occasion, however, these congenital vascular malformations may grow to a large size and become symptomatic. Retrospective studies indicate that patients usually present with abdominal pain or discomfort only after the hemangioma has grown to over 10 cm. The great majority of hemangiomas should be observed and not resected unless there are significant symptoms. When surgical intervention is warranted, the hemangioma can be enucleated; this is facilitated by the presence of an outer rim of fibrous tissue surrounding these tumors. The thrombocytopenia and consumptive coagulopathy that heralds *Kasabach–Merritt syndrome* is an additional indication for hemangioma resection. While more common in children, this syndrome can occasionally affect adults and is associated with high mortality.

Hepatic Cysts

Simple *hepatic cysts* occur in 7% of the population and are commonly identified during radiographic evaluation of the abdomen for other indications. They require no intervention but must be distinguished from *cystadenomas*, which can undergo malignant degeneration. Internal septations within a cyst on ultrasound or CT scan suggest cystadenoma; such lesions should be evaluated for resectability. If not resectable, open or laparoscopic biopsy of the cyst wall should be considered.

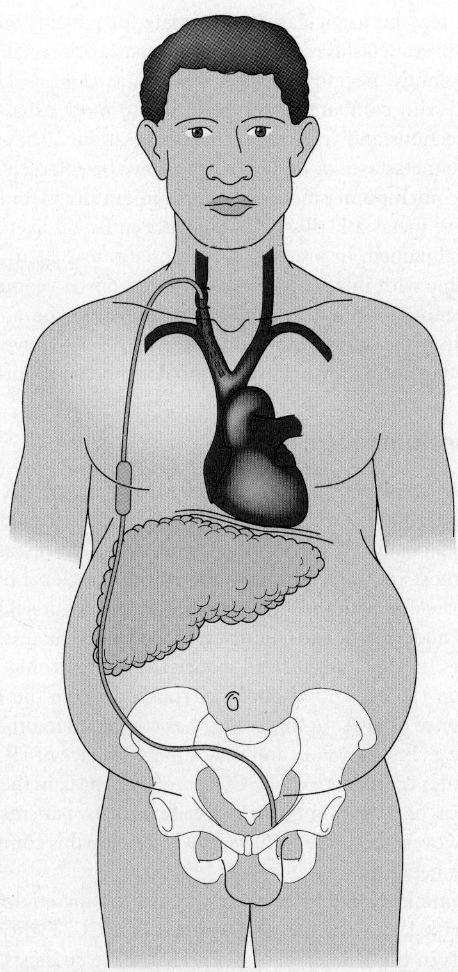

FIGURE 13.14 LeVeen peritoneovenous shunt. (From Mulholland MW, Lillemoe KD, Doherty GM, et al., eds. *Greenfield's Surgery: Scientific Principles and Practice*. 5th ed. Philadelphia: Lippincott Williams & Wilkins; 2010:1018, with permission.)

Focal Nodular Hyperplasia and Hepatic Adenomas

Discriminating *focal nodular hyperplasia* (*FNH*) from *hepatic adenoma* (*HA*) remains challenging despite advances in modern imaging techniques, as both these tumors afflict young women of reproductive age and are associated with similar CT scan findings; FNH is sometimes associated with a classic central scar on CT scan (Table 13.5; Fig. 13.15). The distinction is nonetheless important as HA usually requires surgical resection, while FNH is treated nonsurgically (see below). Currently, published studies indicate that MRI most reliably distinguishes between these lesions, though technetium-99m sulfur colloid scan may be used as a confirmatory study. The Kupffer cells of FNH will take up the radionuclide and are "hot" on scintigraphy. In contrast, HAs do not contain such reticuloendothelial cells and do not enhance. If a definitive diagnosis cannot be achieved with imaging, resection or core biopsy is indicated.

As its name implies, FNH is a hyperplastic nodule formed by normal hepatocytes and Kupffer cells that congregate around a solid central artery without associated portal veins. The nodule forms in response to increased arterial flow and can change in size over time. These nodules do not hemorrhage, are not hormonally responsive, and are not associated with malignant change. In contrast, histopathologic examination of HAs demonstrates that 40% of these tumors do contain intraparenchymal hemorrhage. Moreover, rare cases of malignant degeneration of HA to HCC have been reported. HA usually causes more symptoms than does FNH and may enlarge upon exposure to higher levels of circulating hormone (e.g., during pregnancy or with the use of oral contraceptive pills [OCPs]). Cessation of OCPs sometimes results in regression of HA tumor size and improvement of symptoms. Importantly, spontaneous intra-abdominal hemorrhage of HAs is not associated with larger size and is fatal in 5% to 10% of cases. Therefore, HAs should be resected if feasible. Arterial embolization of the tumor during an episode of spontaneous bleeding may prevent life-threatening hemorrhage until definitive surgical resection can be performed. Arterial embolization has also been used to reduce the size of the adenoma prior to resection or in the case of multiple adenomas when not all lesions can be resected.

TABLE 13.6 Child's classification of liver failure (one modification)

Criterion	Class A (Good Risk)	Class B (Modest Risk)	Class C (Poor Risk)
Serum bilirubin (mg/100 mL)	<2.0	2.0–3.0	>3.0
Serum albumin (g/100 mL)	>3.5	3.0–3.5	<3.0
Ascites	None	Easily controlled	Not easily controlled
Encephalopathy	None	Minimal	Advanced
Nutrition	Excellent	Good	Poor

From Meyers WC, Jones RS. *Textbook of Liver and Biliary Surgery*. Philadelphia: JB Lippincott: 1990;213, with permission.

HEPATOBILIARY MALIGNANCY

Treatment of Metastatic Disease

Metastatic tumors to the liver from the GI tract, breast, or lung constitute *the most common malignant hepatic neoplasms*. Metastatic liver disease often represents advanced systemic cancer and precludes surgical intervention; palliative resection of liver metastases is only rarely indicated. However, *liver metastases from colorectal cancer* represent an important exception. Data indicate that approximately 20% of patients with resectable lesions who undergo

TABLE 13.7 MELD score calculation

$$\begin{aligned} \text{MELD score} = {} & 9.57 \times \log_e(\text{creatinine [mg/dL]}) \\ & + 3.78 \times \log_e(\text{bilirubin [mg/dL]}) \\ & + 11.2 \times \log_e(\text{INR}) \\ & + 6.43 \end{aligned}$$

TABLE 13.8 Pre- and postsurgical mortality associated with cirrhosis

MELD Score	90-d Mortality (Preoperative)[a]	30-d Mortality (Postoperative)	90-d Mortality (Postoperative)
0–7	5%–10%	6%	10%
8–11	5%–10%	10%	18%
12–15	5%–10%	25%	32%
16–20	5%–10%	45%	56%
21–25	10%–20%	55%	66%
≥26	20%–100%[b]	90%	>90%

[a]Ninety-day mortality in patients who do not have surgical disease and do not require surgical intervention (as predicted by MELD score).
[b]Increases according to specific MELD score above 26 (25–40).

hepatic metastasectomy may be cured of their disease, and multiple studies have documented prolonged disease-free survival of 5 or even 10 years postoperatively. Such survival data have encouraged an aggressive surgical approach to the treatment of metastatic colorectal cancer in recent years (Table 13.9). Many questions remain regarding the specific procedure that provides the best disease-free survival and the optimal timing of surgery for the 20% to 30% of patients with colorectal cancer who present with synchronous hepatic metastases.

Traditionally, many patients with resectable synchronous lesions have undergone staged resection. This procedure is performed with or without perioperative chemotherapy, which may allow for an assessment of disease biology and responsiveness to systemic therapy. Simultaneous hepatic and colon resection is appropriate in selected cases. Older patients, patients who require hemihepatectomy and patients with rectal primaries may be less well suited for this *combined approach.* In recent years, several centers have reported good outcomes with the *reverse approach*—resecting liver metastases prior to the colorectal primary. Such an approach may be particularly appropriate for patients with more extensive liver metastases and an asymptomatic colorectal primary.

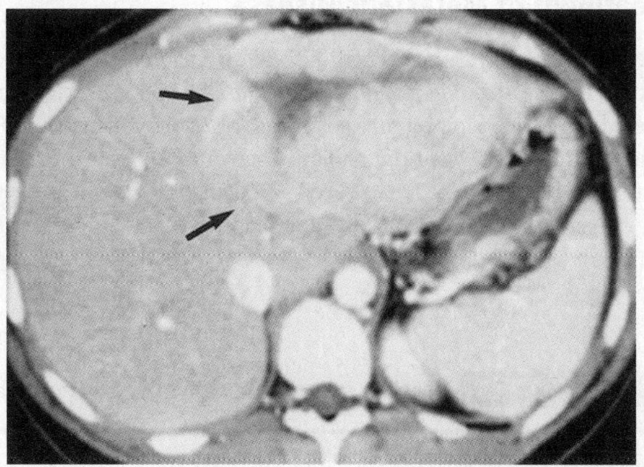

FIGURE 13.15 Enhanced CT scan demonstrating FNH. *Arrows* indicate large mass in left hepatic lobe. Note the hypodense central scar characteristic of FNH. (From Leconte I, Van Beers BE, Lacrosse M., et al. Focal nodular hyperplasia: natural course observed with CT and MRI. *J Comput Assist Tomogr.* 2000;24(1):61–66, with permission.)

Importantly, negative surgical margins as close as 1 mm are associated with comparable survival rates to more extensive anatomic resections and traditional contraindications such as greater than three metastases or bilobar disease have been largely discredited. The contemporary management paradigm allows for resection of extensive metastatic disease as long as a sufficient liver remnant can be maintained. In practice, this translates to 20% of the total liver volume with intact hepatic arterial and portal venous inflow, hepatic venous outflow, and biliary drainage, in the absence of intrinsic liver disease or liver injury. In patients who have received extensive chemotherapy, a 30% threshold is more appropriate.

Hepatocellular Carcinoma

The incidence of primary *hepatocellular carcinoma* (HCC) of the liver in the United States in 2005 is 4.9 cases per 100,000 persons annually. Globally, HCC is a much more prevalent disease and is the fifth most common cancer in the world; the global burden of disease correlates with the high carriage rate of hepatitis B infection (HBV) in underdeveloped countries. In the United States, however, most cases of HCC are instead associated with chronic hepatitis C infection (HCV) and alcoholic cirrhosis. Despite the relatively low incidence of HCC in this country as compared to other malignancies (e.g., breast, colon, and lung), the incidence of HCC in the United States is on the rise. The CDC projects a peak in the number of new cases of HCC over the next decade, as many patients infected with HCV over the last 10 to 20 years will develop this complication of chronic hepatitis.

Epidemiologically, cirrhosis of the liver of any etiology is the primary risk factor for the development of HCC. Eighty percent of patients in the United States with HCC have cirrhosis, and the risk of developing HCC for a cirrhotic patient is 2% to 6% per year. Those at highest risk for developing HCC include men over the age of 40 with HCV cirrhosis. Despite the clear association of cirrhosis with the development of this cancer, researchers cannot yet fully explain how cirrhosis resulting from metabolic, viral, or toxic injury to the liver progresses to frank carcinoma. Importantly, the risk of HCC development is higher in patients who are coinfected with both HCV and HBV, as well as in patients infected with either virus who also consume alcohol.

HCC may present as an RUQ mass, or more commonly, is discovered incidentally on cross-sectional imaging performed for another indication. The diagnosis of HCC can be made without biopsy if the patient has a liver mass and an elevated alpha-fetoprotein (AFP) level. However, AFP is not an extremely sensitive marker for HCC, and a significant percentage of patients with HCC do not have an elevated AFP level. As technology has improved, CT and MRI have become increasingly sensitive and specific for the diagnosis of HCC (Table 13.5).

Given the known association of HCC with cirrhosis of the liver, many physicians have maintained an interest in the development of screening programs targeting cirrhotic patients. A number of prospective surveillance studies employing both ultrasonography and AFP levels at 6-month intervals have reported successful detection of HCC, but no randomized controlled trials have established a reduction in mortality from HCC following the institution of such screening protocols. Based on the paucity of quality data regarding screening for HCC, the NCI does not

TABLE 13.9 Criteria for hepatic resectability for metastatic colorectal cancer

Resectable:	
1. Metastasis confined to the liver a. Unilobar OR bilobar disease b. Single OR multiple metastases c. Remnant liver = 20%–30% of original volume (equivalent to 2 segments)	1. Concomitant extrahepatic disease a. Liver mets in the presence of resectable or ablatable pulmonary disease b. Liver mets in the presence of resectable isolated extrahepatic disease (e.g., spleen, adrenal) c. Liver mets in the presence of resectable invasion of adjacent structures (e.g., diaphragm, adrenal)
Unresectable:	
1. Untreatable primary tumor 2. Widespread pulmonary disease 3. Untreatable locoregional recurrence of primary tumor 4. Distant peritoneal disease 5. Extensive nodal disease (retroperitoneal, mediastinal, distant nodes) 6. Bone or CNS metastases	

Adapted from Lochan R, White SA, Manas DM, et al. Liver resection for colorectal cancer metastasis. *Surg Oncol.* 2007;16(1):33–45.

recommend a standard screening protocol in any population for this disease. Debate continues regarding this issue, however, and most hepatologists as well as a number of consensus conferences have strongly recommended screening in high-risk cirrhotic populations with AFP levels every 3 to 6 months and imaging with CT or MRI every 6 to 12 months.

Just as the optimal screening for HCC remains controversial, uncertainty persists regarding the optimal surgical treatment of HCC. Since current regimens employing chemotherapeutics as primary treatment for HCC provide very limited survival benefit, surgical resection of the disease has been the standard of care. The indications for primary resection of the cancer versus transplantation, however, remain controversial. Patients who meet the *Milan criteria* (Table 13.10) and receive liver transplants have impressive long-term survival that rivals that achieved with transplantation for nonmalignant disease, and these criteria have been adopted by the United Network of Organ Sharing (UNOS) in order to expedite the transplant process in patients with HCC. Since the publication of the Milan criteria, multiple studies have confirmed that 5-year disease-free survival is superior in HCC patients who undergo transplantation compared to resection; however, limited organ availability coupled with the aggressive nature of HCC precludes this treatment option for many patients. Candidates who will tolerate limited hepatic resection (i.e., Child's A cirrhotics with preserved liver function and small peripheral solitary nodules) are, therefore, typically considered for resection. Child's B or C cirrhotics benefit most from liver transplantation provided they meet the Milan criteria, and living-donor liver transplantation in addition to cadaveric liver transplantation should be considered for these patients. In the noncirrhotic patient with HCC, aggressive anatomic resection should be performed so long as the liver remnant will provide adequate hepatic mass to physiologically support the patient.

TABLE 13.10 The milan criteria for transplantation of patients with HCC

One tumor ≤5 cm
OR
Three or fewer tumors, each ≤3 cm in size AND no extrahepatic manifestations or macrovascular involvement

Importantly, the vast majority of patients with HCC (>80%) are neither transplant candidates nor do they have resectable disease due to the size or location of the primary tumor. For these unresectable patients, locally ablative therapies such as RFA (Fig. 13.16), percutaneous ethanol injection (PEI), cryotherapy, transarterial chemoembolization (TACE), or combinations thereof constitute the main surgical treatment options. While these ablative therapies hold promise for patients who have unresectable HCC, a recent review of these procedures concluded that despite the abundance of case series in the literature that utilize these therapies, it is unclear whether these treatments provide any overall survival benefit. However, there is conflicting literature regarding this subject,

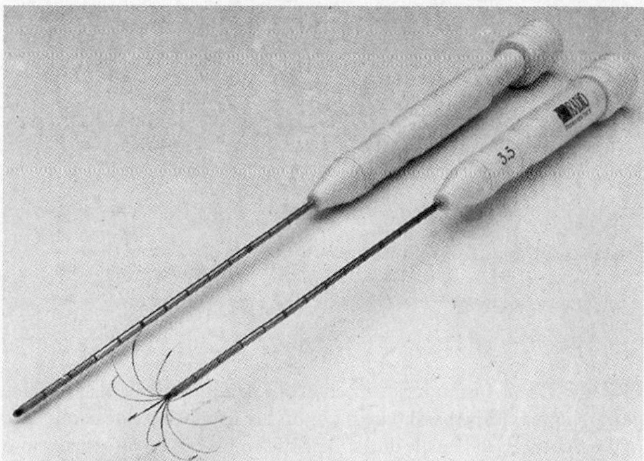

FIGURE 13.16 RFA probe. The probe is inserted into the hepatic lesion to be ablated, and the radial prongs are deployed. The surrounding tissue is superheated and necroses. (From Curley SA, Izzo F, Delrio P, et al. Radiofrequency ablation of unresectable primary and metastatic hepatic malignancies: results in 123 patients. *Ann Surg.* 1999;230(1):3, with permission.)

in particular with respect to TACE, and additional data are needed. Despite the relative paucity of data to indicate improved survival in treated patients, locoregional ablative therapies are widely employed, are generally well tolerated (except in those with severe liver disease), and are relatively safe.

Cholangiocarcinoma and Klatskin Tumors

Cholangiocarcinoma is an adenocarcinoma that arises from biliary ductal epithelium. With an incidence of 8 cases per 1,000,000 U.S. citizens, this cancer is relatively rare in the United States, but its incidence is on the rise. Known risk factors for its development include congenital choledochal cysts, PSC, and infection with the liver fluke *Clonorchis sinensis*. Cholangiocarcinoma can be subdivided into intrahepatic or extrahepatic disease; this anatomic distinction influences presentation of disease, resectability, and overall survival.

Intrahepatic cholangiocarcinoma (ICC), also known as *peripheral cholangiocarcinoma*, constitutes 10% of primary hepatic malignancies. Of the primary hepatic malignancies, it is second only to HCC in prevalence and is frequently confused with HCC because of its similar appearance on cross-sectional imaging. By virtue of its location, ICC does not commonly result in obstructive jaundice, and patients therefore usually present late in the disease. Advanced disease at presentation results in poor outcomes in these patients, with published 3-year survival rates of 15% to 40% postresection. Resection provides the only chance for long-term survival, but only approximately two thirds of patients are resectable at presentation, and most patients ultimately develop recurrent disease.

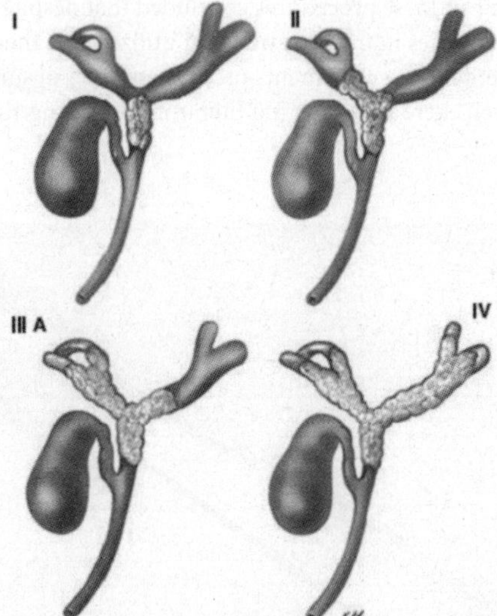

FIGURE 13.17 Bismuth classification of Klatskin tumors (hilar cholangiocarcinoma). Type I and type II tumors are confined to the confluence of the right and left hepatic ducts. Type III tumors extend proximally into the intrahepatic segmental ducts. Type IV tumors involve both intrahepatic ductal systems. Most type II tumors, as well as all type III and type IV tumors, necessitate hilar resection in combination with hemihepatectomy. (From Van Gulik TM, Dinant S, Busch OR, et al. Original article: new surgical approaches to the Klatskin tumour. *Aliment Pharmacol Ther.* 2007;26(Suppl 2):127–132, with permission.)

Extrahepatic cholangiocarcinoma, also known as *hilar cholangiocarcinoma* or a *Klatskin tumor*, presents earlier with obstructive jaundice owing to its location at the confluence of the hepatic ducts (Fig. 13.17). Despite the typically earlier presentation, survival also remains poor with this cholangiocarcinoma as a result of its association with the major vascular structures of the liver at the hilum. Resection represents the only curative modality, and patients fortunate enough to be diagnosed early with this disease have a chance of long-term cure provided they have resectable disease. Data published in small retrospective series confirm the importance of negative margins and suggest that increasing surgical radicality by extending the resection into the hepatic parenchyma instead of limiting it to the biliary ductal confluence improves median survival. Interestingly, studies also demonstrate that radical resection with negative surgical margins influences overall survival more than does the absence of regional lymph node involvement.

Orthotopic liver transplantation has been performed for certain patients with small, unresectable cholangiocarcinoma, usually in the presence of cirrhosis from PSC. Unfortunately, it has demonstrated poor outcomes compared to transplantation for HCC. However, there have been reported series of long-term survival posttransplantation for patients with limited disease, and some centers are utilizing a protocol of preoperative radiotherapy and exploratory staging laparotomy prior to transplantation for patients with small cholangiocarcinomas. Thus, improved patient selection criteria and the development of more effective neoadjuvant therapies may improve outcomes following liver transplantation for cholangiocarcinoma in the future.

Gallbladder Cancer

Although it remains an extremely rare tumor in the United States with an incidence of approximately 2 per 100,000 people, *gallbladder adenocarcinoma* is the most common cancer of the biliary tree. Primary risk factors include female gender and gallstones. Other risk factors include certain infections, such as *Salmonella* or *Helicobacter* in the bile, as well as adenomatous polyps of the gallbladder. Polyp size is correlated with neoplastic transformation, and any patient with a gallbladder polyp greater than 1 cm should undergo cholecystectomy for this reason.

Tumor stage (T stage) significantly influences prognosis and the treatment strategy; ultrasound and CT scan are the most useful radiographic studies to determine T stage. Resection of very early-stage tumors is associated with a high cure rate; this most commonly occurs when gallbladder cancer is found incidentally in a cholecystectomy specimen. Unfortunately, the majority of patients in whom gallbladder cancer is detected have advanced, unresectable disease and a very poor prognosis. The poor 5-year survival rates reported in patients with T2 disease treated with cholecystectomy alone is a testament to the aggressive biology of this cancer; however, a more radical surgical approach including *en bloc* hepatic resection improves 5-year survival rates to 60% to 80% in node-negative patients. Hence, an extensive hepatic *en bloc* resection in addition to regional lymphadenectomy is recommended for any patient with T2 or resectable T3 disease. Given that aggressive resection of this tumor with negative margins provides the only opportunity to cure this malignancy, reconstruction of the CBD and portal vein resection with reanastomosis may be warranted in selected cases.

Hepatic Angiosarcoma and Hepatoblastoma

Angiosarcomas constitute a subset of primary hepatic sarcomas. Primary sarcomas involving the liver are exceedingly rare, and angiosarcomas have been associated with environmental exposure to vinyl chloride, Thorotrast contrast material, or arsenic. Cirrhosis is not a primary risk factor for this malignancy. Surgical resection remains the only curative treatment, but prognosis remains uniformly poor because of the late presentation of the majority of these tumors.

Hepatoblastomas are the most common primary malignant liver tumors afflicting children and have a peak incidence before the age of 2 years. Most children present with some combination of abdominal pain, mass, bloating, nausea, or vomiting. Jaundice is rare. Initial treatment includes chemotherapy; however, resection or transplantation remains the primary modality of therapy, even in children with pulmonary metastases that are responsive to chemotherapy. Neoadjuvant or adjuvant chemotherapy with cisplatin and doxorubicin regimens have resulted in cure rates of 60% to 70% and are considered standard of care in the perioperative setting. Serum AFP is usually massively elevated in children with this malignancy and is useful for both diagnosis and follow-up, since elevation of this tumor marker postresection is frequently the first indication of recurrent disease. The liver and lung are the most common sites of disease recurrence.

Suggested Readings

Blumgart LH. *Surgery of the Liver, Biliary Tract and Pancreas.* 4th ed. Philadelphia: Saunders; 2007.

Knight SR, Friend PJ, Morris PJ, et al. Role of transplantation in the management of hepatic malignancy. *Br J Surg.* 2007;94: 1319–1330.

Koops A, Wojciechowski B, Broering DC, et al. Anatomic variations of the hepatic arteries in 604 selective celiac and superior mesenteric angiographies. *Surg Radiol Anat.* 2004;26:239–244.

Lochan R, White SA, Manas DM, et al. Liver resection for colorectal cancer metastasis. *Surg Oncol.* 2007;16:33–45.

Low JK, Barrow P, Owera A, et al. Timing of laparoscopic cholecystectomy for acute cholecystitis: evidence to support a proposal for an early interval surgery. *Am Surg.* 2007;73:1188–1192.

Teh SH, Nagorney DM, Stevens SR, et al. Risk factors for mortality after surgery in patients with cirrhosis. *Gastroenterology.* 2007;132:1261–1269.

Van Gulik TM, Dinant S, Busch OR, et al. Original article: new surgical approaches to the Klatskin tumour. *Aliment Pharmacol Ther.* 2007;26(Suppl 2):127–132.

Zorzi D, Mullen JT, Abdalla EK, et al. Comparison between hepatic wedge resection and anatomic resection for colorectal liver metastases. *J Gastrointest Surg.* 2006;10:86–94.

CHAPTER

14

The Pancreas

JASHODEEP DATTA AND CHARLES M. VOLLMER JR

KEY POINTS

- The pancreas contains numerous cell types with discrete exocrine and endocrine functions, all of which can degenerate into malignancy.
- Acute pancreatitis is usually self-limiting but may be associated with serious complications including infection, pulmonary edema, hemorrhage, renal failure, and circulatory collapse.
- Chronic pancreatitis is characterized by pain as well as endocrine and exocrine dysfunction. Properly selected patients may benefit from surgery; however, the underlying cause should always be addressed.
- Most pancreatic pseudocysts usually resolve without an operation. Endoscopic or surgical intervention is reserved for symptomatic pseudocysts or those incurring complications.
- Treatment of pancreatic leaks usually consists of simple drainage.
- Pancreatic ductal adenocarcinoma is the most common malignancy of the pancreas. Multimodality therapy offers the best chance for cure. A palliative operation may be useful to resolve biliary or duodenal obstruction in advanced cases of unresectable cancer.
- Pancreatic cystic neoplasms are increasing in incidence; surgery is typically recommended for mucin-producing subtypes including mucinous cystic neoplasm, main duct IPMN, and selected side-branch IPMN.
- Tumors of the endocrine pancreas are exceedingly rare and are usually associated with specific symptoms relating to the type of hormone produced.

EMBRYOLOGY

The pancreas develops from two endodermal tissues, the dorsal and ventral pancreatic buds (Fig. 14.1). Formation of these portions of the developing foregut begins during the 4th week of gestation. The dorsal bud is larger and slightly more cranial than is the ventral bud and gives rise to the majority of the fully formed gland. The ventral bud develops in close proximity with the bile duct and migrates dorsally as the foregut and duodenum rotate to the right. In fact, the ventral bud ultimately ends up lying posterior to the dorsal bud. The ventral bud gives rise to the uncinate process and a portion of the head of the pancreas.

Two pancreatic ducts are typically formed during development. The main duct (duct of Wirsung) is formed by the fusion of the ventral bud duct and distal portion of the dorsal bud duct. This main duct joins with the common bile duct in an intrapancreatic location and drains into the duodenum via the major duodenal papilla. The accessory duct (duct of Santorini) is derived from the proximal portion of the dorsal bud duct and empties via the minor papilla. The main and accessory ducts usually communicate; however, variations occur. In just under 10% of the population, the ducts are completely separate, and the accessory duct drains into the second portion of the duodenum via a minor papilla, proximal to the ampulla of Vater (Fig. 14.2).

The authors would like to acknowledge Joshua Fosnot and Ernest F. Rosato for their contribution to the previous iteration of this chapter.

The anatomy of the gland itself is also somewhat variable. Several important embryologic malformations of the pancreas are summarized in Table 14.1.

ANATOMY

The pancreas lies in the retroperitoneum, posterior to the stomach at the level of the first and second lumbar vertebrae (Fig. 14.3). The organ is composed of the head, uncinate process, neck, body, and tail. The head of the pancreas rests within the C-loop of the duodenum to the right of the midline. It constitutes roughly 30% of the adult organ. The uncinate process is an inferior projection off the head, which curves posterior to the superior mesenteric vessels and anterior to the inferior vena cava. The neck is the portion of the pancreas that lies anterior to the portal vein (PV) and superior to mesenteric vessels. To the left of these vessels, the body lies superior to the fourth portion of the duodenum and forms the floor of the lesser sac. The tail is the smallest portion of the pancreas and lies in proximity to the splenic hilum.

The blood supply of the pancreas is extensive and complex. The anterior and posterior superior and inferior pancreaticoduodenal arteries supply the vast majority of blood flow to the head and uncinate process. The superior pancreaticoduodenal artery(s) branches off the gastroduodenal artery (GDA), which emanates from the celiac axis. The inferior pancreaticoduodenal arteries arise from the superior mesenteric artery (SMA). These systems anastomose within the pancreatic head and run parallel to the medial wall of the duodenum. The blood supply to the body and tail of the pancreas is more variable. Branches of the splenic and left gastroepiploic arteries supply the distal body and tail of the pancreas, the largest of these being the dorsal pancreatic and transverse pancreatic arteries. Within the posterosuperior

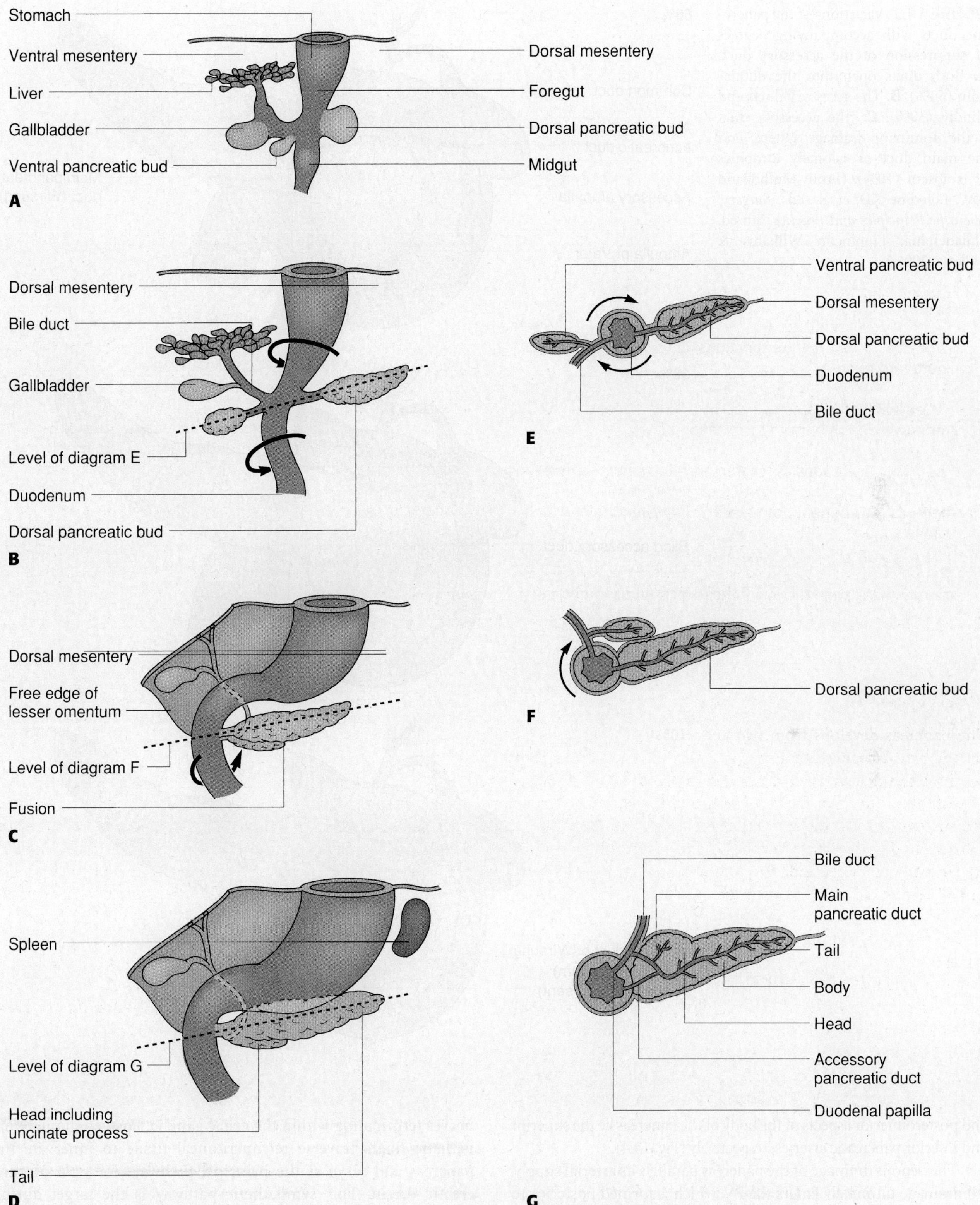

FIGURE 14.1 Development of the pancreas from the 5th through the 8th weeks. The smaller ventral pancreas rotates clockwise in a dorsal direction. The ventral pancreas is connected to the common bile duct and enters the duodenum at the major papilla. The dorsal pancreas enters the duodenum at the minor papilla. (From Mulholland MW, Lillemoe KD, et al., eds. *Surgery: Scientific Principles and Practice*. 5th ed. Philadelphia: Lippincott Williams & Wilkins; 2001.)

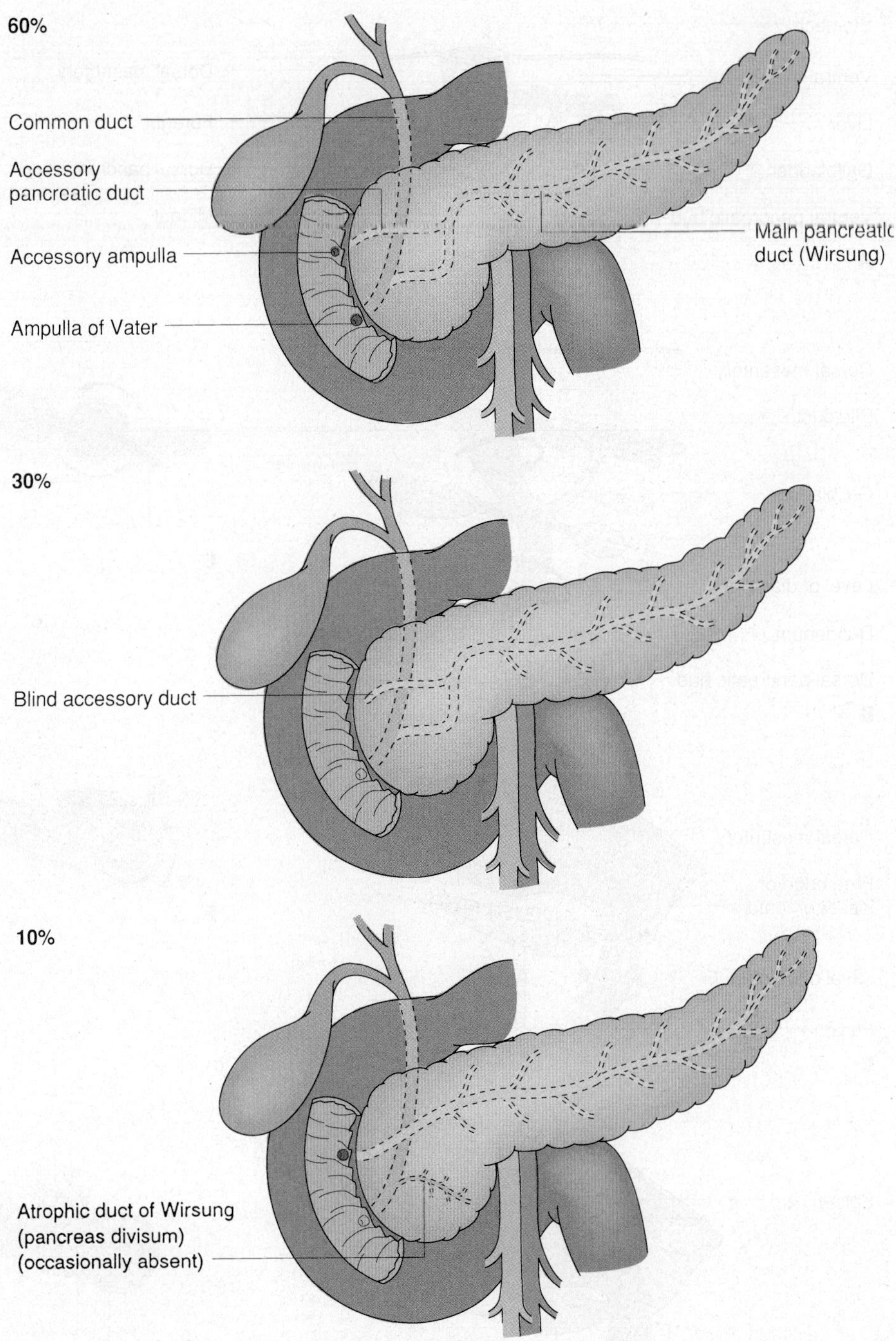

FIGURE 14.2 Variations of the pancreatic ducts with accompanying degrees of suppression of the accessory duct. **A.** Both ducts open into the duodenum (60%). **B.** The accessory ducts end blindly (30%). **C.** The accessory duct is the dominant drainage system, and the main duct occasionally atrophies or is absent (10%). (From Mulholland MW, Lillemoe KD, et al., eds. *Surgery: Scientific Principles and Practice*. 5th ed. Philadelphia: Lippincott Williams & Wilkins; 2001.)

and posteroinferior aspects of the body of the pancreas lie the superior and inferior pancreatic arteries, respectively (Fig. 14.4).

The venous drainage of the pancreas parallels its arterial supply. All drainage ultimately enters the PV, which is formed posterior to the neck of the pancreas by the confluence of the splenic and superior mesenteric veins (SMV).

Multiple lymph node groups drain the pancreas (Fig. 14.5). The extensive distribution and drainage pattern of the pancreas contribute to the rapidly progressive nature of many pancreatic malignancies.

Both sympathetic and parasympathetic fibers innervate the pancreas. Preganglionic sympathetic axons arise from cell bodies within the thoracic sympathetic ganglia and travel as splanchnic nerves terminating within the celiac ganglia. Postganglionic sympathetic fibers traverse retroperitoneal tissue to innervate the pancreas and serve as the principal pathways for pain of pancreatic origin. This sympathetic pathway is the target during splanchnicectomy for the relief of pain of pancreatic origin. The parasympathetic innervation of the pancreas includes preganglionic fiber cell bodies that reside within the vagal nuclei and travel through the posterior vagal trunk. These axons traverse the celiac plexus and terminate in parasympathetic ganglia within the pancreatic parenchyma. Short postganglionic parasympathetic fibers then innervate the pancreatic islets, acini, and ducts, serving an exclusively efferent function.

TABLE 14.1 **Embryologic variations**

Embryologic Malformation	Description	Clinical Presentation	Treatment
Heterotopic pancreas	Pancreatic tissue is found in anatomic locations other than the pancreas.	• Intussusception • Obstruction • Ulceration • Hemorrhage	Surgical excision if symptomatic
Pancreas divisum	The 2 ductal systems fail to fuse. The majority of organ is drained by duct of Santorini. The ventral pancreas is drained by duct of Wirsung.	• Usually asymptomatic • May be associated with recurrent pancreatitis	ERCP, sphincterotomy, and/or stenting if a stenosed minor papilla causes pancreatitis
Annular pancreas	Normal pancreatic tissue completely surrounds the second portion of the duodenum.	• Duodenal obstruction • Often associated with Down syndrome, intracardiac defects, or intestinal malrotation in children	If symptomatic, duodenojejunostomy to bypass the annulus

HISTOLOGY

The cellular components of the pancreas are numerous but fall into two general categories, exocrine or endocrine. Early in development, clusters of pancreatic parenchymal cells called acini—the primary exocrine units of the pancreas—develop. Acinar cells constitute roughly 80% of the total organ. These cells are connected to each other by a network of tubules and ducts, which eventually drain into the duodenum. The acinar cells contain zymogen granules, which when released aid in enteric digestion.

Islets, by contrast, are groups of endocrine cells including, but not limited to, α, β, and Δ cells. Islets account for only 2% of the adult pancreatic mass and weigh approximately 1 g in total. Each islet consists of a *core*, composed of β cells, and a *peripheral mantle*, composed of α, Δ, and pancreatic polypeptide (PP) cells. There is regional variation in the distribution of islet cell subtypes within the pancreas. For example, the head of the pancreas is rich in PP cells, while α cells predominate in the body and tail. In contrast, β and Δ cells are evenly distributed throughout the pancreas.

Historically, islet cells were believed to be derived from migrating neural crest cells; however, this theory has since fallen out of favor. A complex array of signaling pathways controlled by a multitude of genes work in concert to carry out the functions of the pancreas. The best characterized of these genes are Pdx1 and Ptf1. The relative expression of Pdx1 and Ptf1a appears to help control the conversion of progenitors to mature endocrine and exocrine cells.

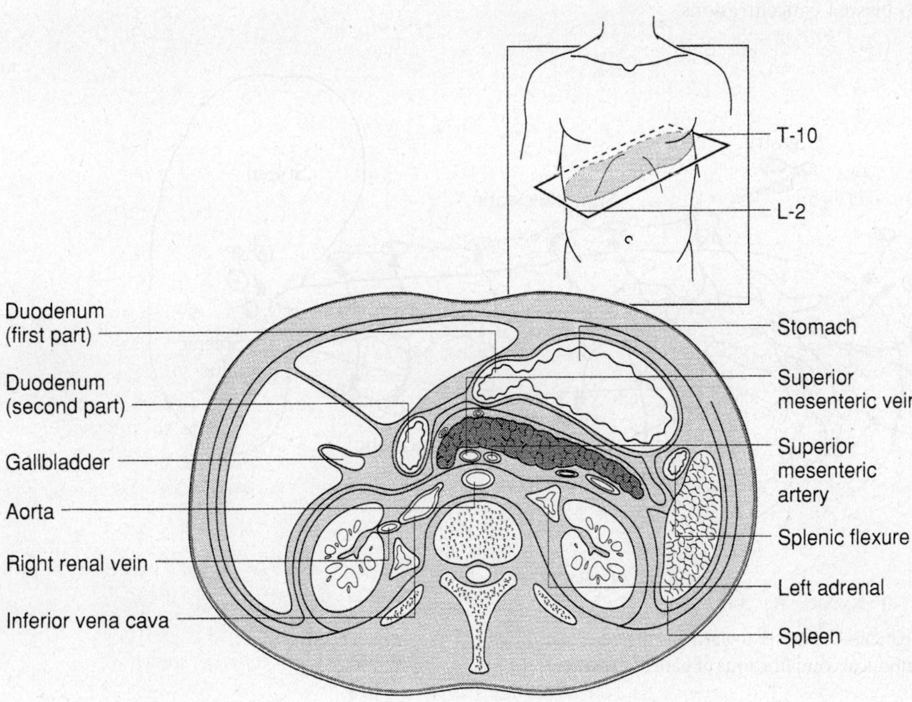

FIGURE 14.3 Relationship of the pancreas to other abdominal organs and viscera. (From Mackie CR, Moosa AR. Surgical anatomy of the pancreas. In: Moosa AR, ed. *Tumors of the Pancreas.* Baltimore: Williams & Wilkins; 1980, with permission.)

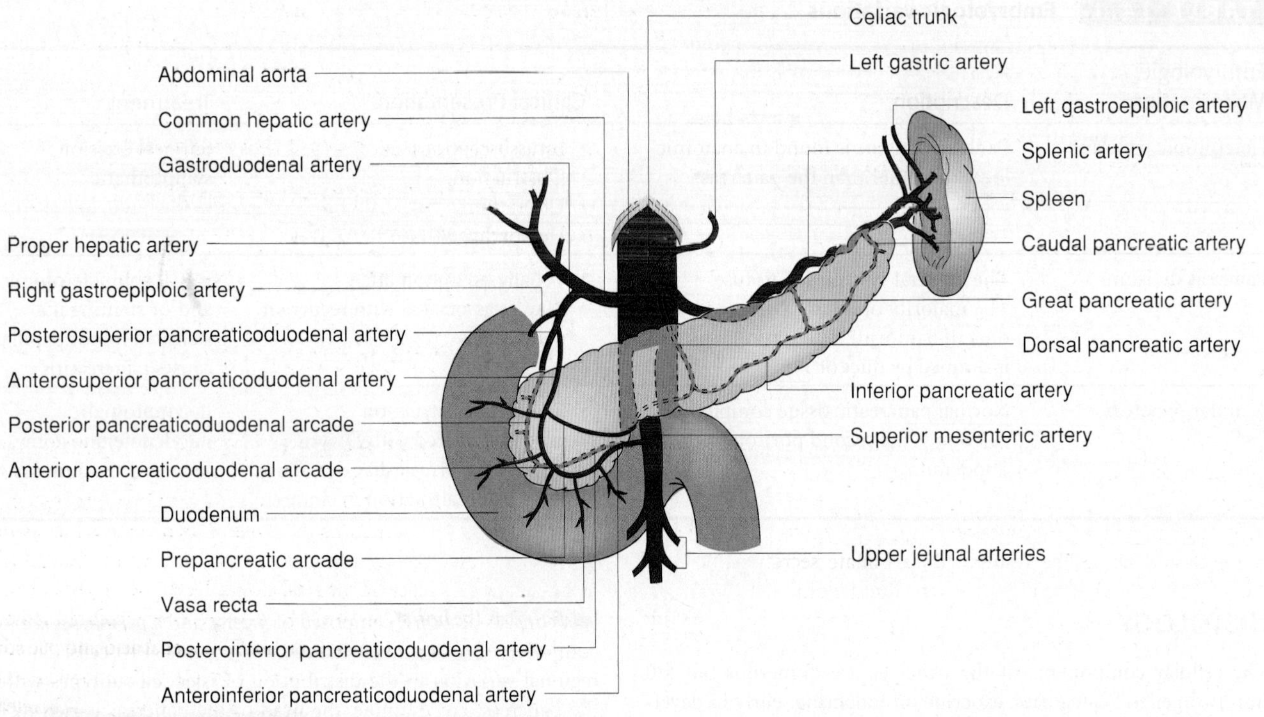

FIGURE 14.4 Arterial supply to the pancreas. (From Mulholland MW, Lillemoe KD, et al., eds. *Surgery: Scientific Principles and Practice*. 5th ed. Philadelphia: Lippincott Williams & Wilkins; 2001.)

EXOCRINE PHYSIOLOGY

The exocrine pancreas produces up to 20 g of digestive enzymes and 2.5 L of bicarbonate-rich fluid each day. The acinar cells are responsible for the production of enzymes, while ductal cells secrete fluid and electrolytes under both vagal and humoral control. The sodium and potassium concentrations of pancreatic secretions remain constant and are approximately equivalent to plasma concentrations. In contrast, the anion concentration of pancreatic exocrine secretion is dependent on secretory rate. At low secretory rates, the concentrations of chloride and bicarbonate ions are equivalent to those in plasma, but with neurohumoral stimulation, the bicarbonate concentration increases and the chloride concentration decreases. Secretin is the most potent endogenous stimulant of pancreatic bicarbonate secretion. Secretin is synthesized in the mucosal S cells

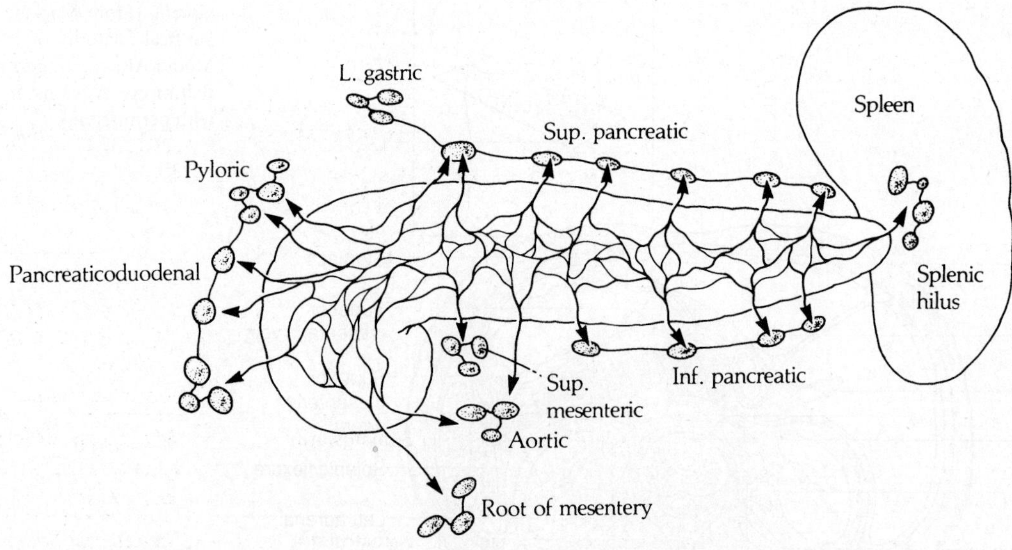

FIGURE 14.5 Lymphatic drainage of the pancreas. Flow is toward the nearest margin of the pancreas. (From Skandalakis JE, Gray SW, Rowe JS Jr, et al. Anatomical complications of pancreatic surgery. *Contemp Surg*. 1979;15:17, with permission.)

TABLE 14.2 Enzymes of the exocrine pancreas and their functions

Pancreatic Enzyme	Active Form	Function
Trypsinogen	Trypsin (activated by enterokinase in the duodenum)	Protease; activates other pancreatic proenzymes for protein digestion (chymotrypsin, elastase, carboxypeptidase A and B)
Lipase	Excreted in active form	Cleaves fatty acids in preparation for gut absorption
Colipase	Excreted in active form	Prevents lipase inactivation by bile acids in duodenum
Cholesterol esterase	Excreted in active form	Cleaves cholesterol ester bonds in preparation for fatty acid and cholesterol absorption
Amylase	Excreted in active form	Cleaves complex carbohydrates in preparation for sugar absorption

of the crypts of Lieberkühn of the proximal small bowel and is released in the presence of luminal acid and bile. Secretin circulates in the blood and binds to secretin receptors on pancreatic ductal cells, effecting signal transduction through the intracellular adenylate cyclase system. The resultant bicarbonate secretion serves to neutralize stomach acid that enters the duodenum.

The other components of exocrine pancreatic juice include digestive enzymes, which aid in amino acid, lipid, and complex carbohydrate breakdown. These enzymes are formed from proteins produced in the ribosomes of pancreatic acinar cells. These proteins combine to form proenzymes in the rough endoplasmic reticulum and are subsequently packaged in the Golgi apparatus. The resultant zymogen granules are exocytosed into the ductal system. Some of these enzymes are immediately active, whereas others require activation in the duodenum (Table 14.2).

The contribution of the pancreas to digestion is classically divided into three phases. During the *cephalic* phase, stimuli (smell and taste) activate vagal efferent signals, which stimulate pancreatic enzyme release. The net effect of cephalic phase stimulation is the secretion of an enzyme-rich, bicarbonate-poor fluid. During the *gastric* phase, antral distention and protein delivery stimulate the release of gastrin. Gastrin promotes gastric acid secretion from parietal cells and, because of the sequence homology between gastrin and cholecystokinin (CCK), also serves as a weak stimulant for pancreatic enzyme secretion. Acidification of the duodenum in turn leads to secretin release, which stimulates pancreatic bicarbonate secretion. This can be thought of as a "brake" for gastric acid in the small bowel. During the *intestinal* phase of digestion, the hormones secretin and CCK serve a major function in mediating pancreatic exocrine secretion. Duodenal acid and bile stimulate secretin release, in turn stimulating pancreatic bicarbonate secretion from ductal cells. Duodenal fat and protein stimulate CCK release, stimulating the secretion of pancreatic enzymes from acinar cells.

ENDOCRINE PHYSIOLOGY

In contrast to the exocrine function of the pancreas, which is primarily involved in nutrient digestion and absorption, the endocrine function of the pancreas serves a broader purpose—one of whole body metabolism and energy utilization. Insulin and glucagon work in concert to maintain appropriate serum and intracellular glucose levels and energy storage. Table 14.3 summarizes the functions of select pancreatic hormones.

TABLE 14.3 Hormones produced by the endocrine pancreas

Cell Type	Endocrine Hormone	Stimulants for Release	Inhibitor	Primary Functions
Alpha (α)	Glucagon	Hypoglycemia, arginine, alanine	Hyperglycemia, insulin, somatostatin	Glycogenolysis, gluconeogenesis, lipolysis; increase blood sugar
Beta (β)	Insulin	Hyperglycemia, glucagon, CCK, GIP, cholinergic, β-adrenergic input	Somatostatin, amylin, pancreatin, α-adrenergic input	Glucose uptake at cellular level, protein synthesis
Delta (Δ)	Somatostatin	Acid in duodenum	None	General inhibitor of acid production, pancreatic and biliary secretion; helps regulate pancreatic endocrine function in paracrine manner
PP	Pancreatic PP	Food, vagal stimulation; ghrelin	Somatostatin	Decreases gallbladder and pancreatic secretion; inhibits food intake
Delta 2 ($\Delta 2$)	Vasoactive intestinal peptide (VIP)	Fat in diet, acetylcholine	Somatostatin	Increases gut motility and secretion

GIP, gastrin inhibitory protein.

PATHOLOGY

Acute Pancreatitis

Presentation

Acute pancreatitis is characterized by diffuse inflammation of the pancreas and encompasses a wide spectrum of clinical disease. Eighty percent of cases of pancreatitis, while symptomatic, resolve without complication; however, 20% of patients progress to more severe disease with complications including hemorrhage, pancreatic necrosis, infection, shock, and multisystem organ failure. The goals of management, therefore, include early diagnosis, supportive therapy, and treatment of the underlying cause.

Pancreatitis classically presents with sudden onset of epigastric pain that radiates to the back, usually accompanied by nausea and vomiting. In fact, the absence of vomiting suggests an alternative diagnosis. On physical examination, epigastric tenderness is typically elicited and may be pronounced with rebound and guarding. Retroperitoneal hemorrhage, while rare, may manifest as Turner's sign (flank ecchymosis), Cullen's sign (periumbilical ecchymosis), or Fox's sign (ecchymosis below the inguinal ligament and/or involving the scrotum). Jaundice is unusual in acute pancreatitis, barring those cases caused by gallstones. A left pleural effusion may be present. The systemic inflammatory response can lead to tachycardia, edema, and hypovolemic shock. Early complications of pancreatitis are usually related to massive fluid sequestration and include pulmonary edema, circulatory collapse, and renal failure. Late complications usually result from infection or hemorrhage.

Etiology

The causes of acute pancreatitis are numerous; however, the vast majority of cases (80% to 90%) are caused by gallstones or alcohol (Table 14.4). Gallstone pancreatitis is not always caused by impacted stones. The migration of stones through the biliary system alone may cause ductal inflammation and reflux of bile salts into the pancreatic duct. Small stones (<5 mm) are more likely to lead to pancreatitis than are large ones. It is estimated that 3% to 8% of patients with symptomatic cholelithiasis will ultimately develop pancreatitis. The exact mechanism of alcohol-related pancreatitis is unknown. Potential mechanisms include alcohol-related ampullary obstruction or spasm, alcohol-induced enzyme release and ductal plugging, hypertriglyceridemia related to alcohol ingestion, and oxygen-derived free radical–mediated injury.

Pathophysiology

Pancreatitis results from autodigestion and inflammation caused by unregulated release of pancreatic enzymes within the organ. Activation of trypsinogen *within* the acinar cells results in the accumulation of trypsin. This in turn leads to a cascade of enzyme activation (e.g., elastase and phospholipase A2) coupled with the release of proinflammatory mediators such as interleukin (IL)-1, IL-6, IL-8, and tumor necrosis factor (TNF)-α. The degree of pancreatic inflammation and injury is directly related to the level of enzymatic autodigestion. Organ edema, peripancreatic inflammation with severe fluid loss, and multiorgan dysfunction secondary to circulating toxins are end points of this process.

TABLE 14.4 Etiology of acute pancreatitis

Causes of Acute Pancreatitis	Comments
Alcohol	Along with gallstones, the most common cause of pancreatitis worldwide; the exact mechanism unknown
Gallstones	Physical migration of stones, with or without outlet obstruction of the pancreatic duct
Pancreatic or biliary mass	Causing outlet obstruction
Trauma	Physical trauma, surgery including laparotomy, cardiac surgery, post-ERCP
Hypercalcemia	Usually from hyperparathyroidism
Hyperlipidemia	
Infection	Mumps, coxsackievirus, hepatitis B, CMV, chickenpox, herpes; salmonella, mycoplasma, legionella; ascaris, cryptosporidium, toxoplasma
Duodenal or distal intestinal obstruction	Tumor, previous surgery, annular pancreas
Pancreas divisum	From aberrant ductal drainage
Medications	Examples include lasix, steroids, azathioprine, 6MP, tetracycline, sulfasalazine, mesalazine, HCTZ, sulindac, valproic acid, enalapril, erythromycin
Pregnancy	
Autoimmune	SLE, Sjögren syndrome
Genetic	*PRSS1, SPINK1, CFTR* mutations
Idiopathic	No identifiable cause of pancreatitis found in 10%–15% of all cases

CMV, cytomegalovirus; HCTZ, hydrochlorothiazide; SLE, systemic lupus erythematosus. ERCP: Endoscopic retrograde cholangiopancreatography.

TABLE 14.5 Causes of hyperamylasemia

Intra-Abdominal	Extra-Abdominal
Biliary tract disease	Salivary gland inflammation
Intestinal disorders including esophageal inflammation, obstruction, and ischemia	Renal failure
Peritonitis	Pneumonia
Appendicitis	Trauma
Cholecystitis	Burns
Peptic ulcer	Diabetic ketoacidosis
—	Pregnancy
—	Drugs

Diagnosis

Amylase and lipase are released into the serum during pancreatitis and are the primary diagnostic markers of pancreatitis. An elevated serum amylase in the absence of signs and symptoms of pancreatitis is inconsistent with the disease. An estimated 30% of people with elevated amylase levels do not have pancreatitis (i.e., peptic ulcer disease [PUD], bowel perforation, etc.). In addition, 10% of people with pancreatitis do not have an elevated amylase (see Table 14.5). Amylase levels peak early in the disease process and do not stay elevated beyond 5 days of ongoing inflammation. The absolute level of serum amylase does not correlate with the degree of injury. Lipase on the other hand peaks later, but remains elevated for a longer period of time. In addition, other biomarkers may correlate with severity of disease such as serum C-reactive protein, IL-2 and IL-6, procalcitonin, and urinary trypsin activating peptide, although these are rarely used in clinical practice.

Imaging is helpful in diagnosing pancreatitis. Plain films of the abdomen are often nonspecific but may show a dilated, air-filled duodenal loop in the right upper quadrant, suggesting a focal ileus. Likewise, a focal jejunal ileus (*sentinel loop sign*) or transverse colonic ileus (*colon cutoff sign*) may be evident. Abdominal ultrasound is very helpful in the diagnosis of cholelithiasis or cholecystitis with a sensitivity of over 95%; however, in the setting of acute pancreatitis, the sensitivity is as low as 70% due to surrounding inflammation and dilated bowel. Computerized tomographic (CT) scanning is the imaging modality of choice for the diagnosis of pancreatitis and should be performed with intravenous contrast for better visualization of inflammation, assessment of pancreatic perfusion (to demarcate necrosis), and evaluation for rim-enhancing collections.

Treatment

In up to 80% of all patients with clinical pancreatitis, the disease is self-limiting and resolves without complication. The remainder of patients may, however, progress to a more severe form of complicated pancreatitis, with significant associated morbidity and mortality. Multiple grading systems have been described to predict pancreatitis severity. The Ranson criteria—albeit more for historic interest—encompass 11 prognostic signs that are predictive of morbidity and mortality from pancreatitis (Table 14.6). Table 14.7 correlates mortality with the number of Ranson criteria present. Other contemporary scoring systems based on multiple laboratory and radiographic criteria have been described. These include the APACHE II, the Sequential Organ Failure Assessment (SOFA) score, the Marshall score, and the Balthazar score, among others. No one scoring system is universally accepted in clinical practice, and their implementation is institution and provider specific.

TABLE 14.6 Ranson criteria

Admission	Pancreatitis	Gallstone Pancreatitis
Age (y)	>55	>70
WBC count (per mm^3)	>16,000	>18,000
Glucose (mg/dL)	>200	>220
LDH (IU/L)	>350	>400
AST (IU/L)	>250	>250
During initial 48 h	—	—
Hematocrit decrease (%)	>10	>10
BUN increase (mg/dL)	>5	>2
Serum calcium (mg/dL)	<8	<8
PaO_2 (mm Hg)	<60	<60
Base deficit (mEq/L)	>4	>5
Fluid requirement (L)	>6	>4

AST, aspartate aminotransferase; BUN, blood urea nitrogen; LDH, lactate dehydrogenase; WBC, white blood cell.

The Atlanta classification (developed in 1992 and revised in 2012) identifies three grades of severity based on the presence and timing of complications—mild, moderately severe, and severe. The overarching emphasis in this classification is on the presence and persistence of organ failure. A recent international "determinant-based" classification has been proposed encompassing both local (i.e., presence of (peri)pancreatic necrosis) and systemic (i.e., organ failure) determinants of severity.

In the majority of cases of *mild* acute pancreatitis, the mainstay of therapy includes fluid resuscitation. Acute pancreatitis is commonly associated with massive fluid sequestration secondary to paralytic ileus, peripancreatic edema, third-space fluid losses from inflammation, and emesis. The degree of resuscitation needed is

TABLE 14.7 Mortality associated with Ranson criteria

Presenting Criteria	Mortality
<3	1%
3–4	15%
5–6	50%
≥7	Nearly 100%

often underappreciated; aggressive fluid resuscitation with crystalloid solutions is essential to restore and maintain circulating plasma volume. Metabolic and electrolyte derangements—particularly magnesium and potassium deficits—should be corrected. An indwelling urinary catheter may be indicated in more severe cases to assess volume status and insure adequate urine output. Analgesia is often necessary for symptomatic relief. Although narcotic (e.g., morphine) use was historically discouraged due to concerns for sphincter of Oddi spasm, little evidence supports this contention. Percutaneous splanchnic nerve blocks and epidural analgesia can also be used.

At least in the initial phase of mild-to-moderate acute pancreatitis, oral intake should be restricted. If an ileus is present, nasogastric tube placement should be considered. As pain improves and serum levels of markers of inflammation decrease, an oral diet should be reinitiated. A subset of patients—up to 15%—may develop "refeeding" pancreatitis; withholding oral diet for a short duration is typically successful in these patients. If prolonged inflammation or complications arise, supplementary nutrition should be provided. Traditionally, this has been provided in the form of total parenteral nutrition (TPN); however, more recent evidence indicates that total enteral nutrition (TEN) may lead to more rapid recovery, fewer infectious complications, and better glycemic control.

A variety of other specific therapies have been studied. Suppression of pancreatic enzyme secretion has been attempted with nasogastric suction and administration of H2-blockers, anticholinergics, glucagon, calcitonin, somatostatin, peptide YY, and CCK receptor antagonists such as proglumide. None of these therapies are effective in shortening the duration of the disease, reducing complications, or reducing mortality. H2 receptor antagonists or antacids are indicated as prophylaxis against upper gastrointestinal tract hemorrhage in critically ill patients. Octreotide, a long-acting somatostatin analogue, has not consistently been shown to influence morbidity and mortality. Steroids are also contraindicated, and cytokine mediators have thus far been shown to be ineffective.

In all cases of gallstone pancreatitis and most cases of idiopathic pancreatitis, early cholecystectomy is recommended—preferably during the same hospitalization—following resolution of acute inflammation and subjective patient-reported pain. In the absence of intervention, early recurrence rates approach 35%. Endoscopic retrograde cholangiopancreatography (ERCP) with sphincterotomy may be "definitive" therapy in patients considered too infirm to tolerate cholecystectomy.

Treatment priorities in *severe* acute pancreatitis focus on early identification and amelioration of organ failure. Certain unique treatment considerations are entertained in this disease entity. Fluid resuscitation remains of utmost importance and should be guided by end-organ perfusion. A low threshold should be applied for invasive monitoring, including central venous catheters and arterial lines. The *prophylactic* use of intravenous antibiotics is not currently supported by randomized data, although these studies are criticized for being underpowered in order to detect a meaningful difference. Documented infections (e.g., bloodstream, urinary, etc.) should be treated with discrete end points. If infected pancreatic necrosis is strongly suspected or documented, antibiotic therapy should be initiated. Many antibiotics do not achieve adequate pancreatic tissue penetration. Antimicrobials thought to be effective include imipenem, third-generation cephalosporins, piperacillin, mezlocillin, fluoroquinolones, and metronidazole, but not aminoglycosides, amino penicillins, and first-generation cephalosporins.

Pancreatic Infection

Pancreatic abscess, infected pancreatic pseudocyst, and infected pancreatic necrosis are three life-threatening infectious complications of acute pancreatitis that may require surgical intervention. They occur in up to 5% of patients with acute pancreatitis, and their incidence increases proportionally with increasing severity of acute pancreatitis and extent of pancreatic necrosis. Most infections are polymicrobial and may arise from transmural migration of bacteria from adjacent inflamed bowel or from hematogenous seeding. Fungal infection is uncommon, and antifungal agents are rarely indicated. However, patients subjected to long courses of powerful antibiotics are susceptible to fungal superinfection. The development of septic complications should be suspected in patients with severe pancreatitis, documented bacteremia, clinical deterioration, or failure of resolution of pancreatitis within 7 to 10 days. Clinical manifestations may include fever, tachycardia, abdominal pain, and abdominal distention. Associated laboratory abnormalities include persistent hyperamylasemia, elevations of liver function tests, and leukocytosis.

Plain films of the abdomen may show extraluminal retroperitoneal air (the *soap bubble sign*). Contrast-enhanced CT scanning is the most widely used and accurate modality for evaluating pancreatic septic complications. A CT-guided fine needle aspiration (FNA) may diagnose infected peripancreatic necrosis; however, no indication currently exists for routine FNA—a relatively high false-negative rate (12% to 25%) is associated with this approach.

The treatment of pancreatic infectious complications includes antibiotics and judicious intervention. Although open operative debridement/necrosectomy is the classic approach, recent evidence suggests that a nuanced approach involving less invasive therapeutic strategies may be of benefit in selected patients. These strategies involve percutaneous drainage followed by minimally invasive retroperitoneal debridement (the so-called "step-up" approach, espoused by the randomized Dutch PANTER trial), laparoscopic and/or transgastric debridement, or endoscopic necrosectomy. Regardless of the intervention strategy, the basic principles of pancreatic debridement should be followed—optimal timing (preferably >4 weeks, allowing for organization of necrotic tissue), thorough debridement, wide drainage, establishing durable enteral access, and addressing underlying etiology (e.g., gallbladder) in the same setting. For necrosis that is *not* limited to the lesser sac (i.e., more widespread involving paracolic gutters), open necrosectomy with wide drainage is still considered standard of care.

Chronic Pancreatitis

Presentation

Chronic pancreatitis occurs with an incidence of 4 cases per 100,000 individuals per year. Whereas acute pancreatitis is characterized by inflammation of the organ, chronic pancreatitis is characterized by acinar loss, glandular atrophy, proliferative fibrosis, calcification, and ductal stricturing. Histologically, chronic pancreatitis is characterized by collagen and fibroblastic proliferation within the parenchyma. Patients present with recurrent or persistent epigastric abdominal pain in conjunction with exocrine and endocrine pancreatic insufficiency; the pain may radiate to the back. Nausea and vomiting are typical. Patients are often hyperglycemic due to endocrine dysfunction and experience steatorrhea and weight loss related to exocrine dysfunction. Many patients present with a history of narcotic overuse/abuse, typically in an effort to control their refractory abdominal pain.

TABLE 14.8 Causes of chronic pancreatitis

Alcohol abuse
Hyperlipoproteinemia
Hypercalcemia, i.e., hyperparathyroidism
Cystic fibrosis
Pancreas divisum
Pancreatic trauma
Idiopathic
Autoimmune disease (PSC, Sjögren's, PBC)
Hereditary pancreatitis

Etiology

The most common cause of chronic pancreatitis in industrialized countries is alcohol abuse (60% to 80%); however, many of the other causes of acute pancreatitis eventually lead to chronic disease as well (see Table 14.8). Idiopathic chronic pancreatitis has been associated with social drinking, analgesic abuse, autoimmune diseases (e.g., primary sclerosing cholangitis [PSC], Sjögren syndrome, primary biliary cirrhosis [PBC]), and genetic abnormalities.

Various mechanisms may play a role in the pathogenesis of chronic pancreatitis. These include hypersecretion of protein from acinar cells, plugging of the pancreatic ducts with protein precipitates, and pancreatic ductal hypertension. The genetic abnormalities found in cystic fibrosis (*CFTR* gene mutations) and hereditary pancreatitis (mutations in the cationic trypsinogen gene) are found in up to 10% of patients with idiopathic pancreatitis.

Diagnosis

Besides a detailed history and physical examination, the most important tests for the evaluation of chronic pancreatitis are CT scan, MRI, magnetic resonance cholangiopancreatography (MRCP), and ERCP. Routine laboratory tests are rarely helpful. Pancreatic calcifications on plain films of the abdomen are at least 95% specific for chronic pancreatitis but are less sensitive. Pancreatography (MRCP or ERCP) can document ductal abnormalities not demonstrated by CT scan and plays an essential role in guiding surgical therapy. Early changes observed by pancreatography include ductal dilation and filling of secondary and tertiary branches, which are not ordinarily visualized. Uniform ductal dilatation is the most common finding; the characteristic "chain-of-lakes" pancreatogram is often described but less common. An entirely normal pancreatogram in a patient with abdominal pain essentially excludes the diagnosis of chronic pancreatitis.

A simple test to evaluate exocrine pancreatic function is the measurement of fecal fat excretion with a Sudan stain. Elevated fecal elastase levels are very sensitive and specific for the diagnosis of exocrine dysfunction. Pancreatic endocrine function can be assessed with the glucose tolerance test. More than two thirds of all patients with chronic pancreatitis have abnormal results; however, a minority of patients actually progress to insulin dependence.

Treatment

The nonoperative management of chronic pancreatitis requires control of abdominal pain as well as the treatment of endocrine and exocrine insufficiencies. Interventions that aid in the control of abdominal pain include abstinence from alcohol, dietary modification favoring small meals, and substitution of medium-chain triglycerides for long-chain fatty acids. Pain control often necessitates the early use of nonnarcotic and narcotic analgesics. Celiac plexus blocks have had mixed results.

Endogenous enzyme secretion must be decreased by 90% to produce malabsorption. In such advanced cases, treatment includes a low-fat diet and exogenous pancreatic enzyme supplementation. Proton pump agents are given to prevent the acid-induced degradation of exogenous enzyme preparations. Alternatively, enteric-coated enzyme supplement preparations, particularly enteric-coated microspheres, may be used.

Various endoscopic techniques have been utilized in the management of diverse clinical problems associated with chronic pancreatitis. These techniques include pancreatic sphincterotomy, pancreatic duct stenting, stricture dilation, and pancreatic stone extraction or lithotripsy. These techniques have not been associated with durable benefit.

Operative Management

The goal of operation for chronic pancreatitis is relief of pain with maximum preservation of endocrine and exocrine function. Approaches to achieving this include ampullary procedures, ductal drainage procedures, denervation procedures, and ablative procedures. Ablative procedures are usually considered the last step in surgical treatment for patients with chronic pancreatitis because of the associated risks including, but not limited to, a significant rate of iatrogenic insulin-dependent diabetes mellitus.

Ampullary Procedures

The indications for ampullary procedures are limited. Transduodenal sphincteroplasty and pancreatic duct septoplasty may be indicated for patients with focal obstruction of the ampullary orifice. Transduodenal minor papilloplasty is somewhat successful in patients with pancreas divisum associated with recurrent acute pancreatitis but is less effective in chronic pancreatitis. With the increasing availability of ERCP, these procedures are less frequently performed operatively.

Ductal Drainage Procedures

The longitudinal side-to-side Roux-en-Y pancreaticojejunostomy (PJ; Puestow procedure) is the most commonly applied pancreatic ductal drainage procedure and is recommended for patients with a dilated pancreatic duct in need of operative therapy for chronic pancreatitis (Fig. 14.6). It has widely replaced the end-to-end caudal PJ of Duval since it relieves ducts with numerous strictures better. In patients with early disease, this procedure may delay the progression of functional impairment of the pancreas. However, the Puestow is associated with increased risk of pain recurrence; this has been hypothesized to be related to inadequate drainage of proximal pancreatic tissue. The Frey procedure is a modification of the Puestow and adds a localized pancreatic head resection ("coring" out) to allow for better drainage. Another variation—the Beger procedure—involves a duodenum-preserving resection of the pancreatic head combined with Roux-en-Y drainage of the main pancreatic duct in the neck of the gland.

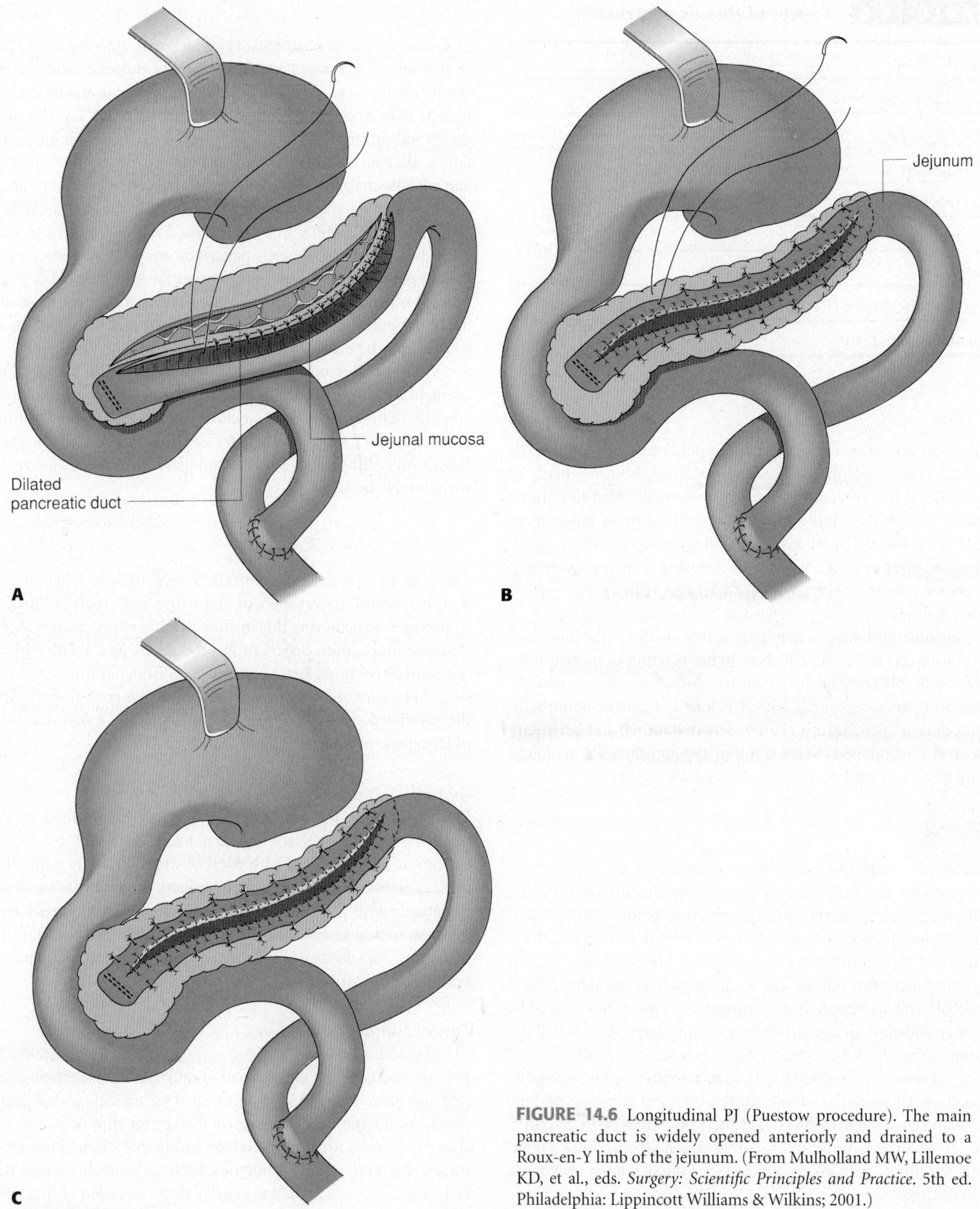

FIGURE 14.6 Longitudinal PJ (Puestow procedure). The main pancreatic duct is widely opened anteriorly and drained to a Roux-en-Y limb of the jejunum. (From Mulholland MW, Lillemoe KD, et al., eds. *Surgery: Scientific Principles and Practice*. 5th ed. Philadelphia: Lippincott Williams & Wilkins; 2001.)

Resection Procedures

The treatment of chronic pancreatitis with surgical resection of the pancreas is associated with variable success rates (60% to 80% of patients obtain adequate pain relief). Left-sided procedures, such as limited distal pancreatectomy (with or without splenectomy), may be indicated in patients with disease in the body and tail of the pancreas. Right-sided procedures such as pylorus-preserving pancreaticoduodenectomy (i.e., modified Whipple operation) are indicated if the head of the pancreas is primarily affected. The modified Whipple procedure has the advantage of also relieving associated biliary or duodenal obstruction and preserving a substantial mass of islet cell tissue in the body and tail of the gland.

In some patients with debilitating pain from chronic pancreatitis, there is increasing enthusiasm in utilizing total pancreatectomy (TP) with or without islet cell autotransplantation. Candidates for TP include those with diffuse small duct pancreatitis, who have failed lesser procedures, and those with hereditary pancreatitis. However, the significant problems associated with labile insulin sensitivity (despite innovations such as the insulin pump), steatorrhea, and weight loss dictate that TP be applied in carefully selected patients. The advent of islet autotransplantation (IAT) has energized efforts to apply the TP paradigm to this patient population. Pain relief is reportedly 80% to 85% after TP-IAT, and insulin independence is seen in up to 40% of patients on short-term follow-up.

Denervation Procedures

Neuroablation for the treatment of pancreatic pain can be achieved using one of several approaches. These include celiac ganglionectomy, thoracic splanchnicectomy, and chemical splanchnicectomy through infiltration of the celiac ganglion either at the time of open operation or as an isolated percutaneous procedure.

Disruption of the Pancreatic Duct

A broad category of complicated pancreatic disease involves disruption of the drainage of pancreatic fluid. The most frequent etiologies include acute and/or chronic pancreatitis, recent surgery with pancreatic resection, and iatrogenic injury or trauma. The resultant pathology and management depend on the route of fluid egress. These disease processes are summarized in Table 14.9.

Pancreatic Pseudocyst

A pancreatic pseudocyst is an organized fluid collection of pancreatic secretions that develops in the setting of ductal disruption secondary to pancreatitis, necrosis, or trauma. Pseudocysts are enclosed by nonepithelialized tissues and by surrounding structures such as the stomach, transverse mesocolon, gastrocolic omentum, spleen, or the pancreas itself. Most pseudocysts communicate with the pancreatic ductal system and contain high concentrations of digestive enzymes.

Pancreatic pseudocysts account for 75% to 80% of all cystic lesions of the pancreas. They develop in up to 10% of patients after an attack of acute alcoholic pancreatitis. Pseudocysts can also develop in the setting of other causes of acute or chronic pancreatitis, pancreatic trauma, and, rarely, pancreatic neoplasms. By convention, collections of fluid containing pancreatic enzymes that occur within the first 3 weeks after an episode of acute pancreatitis are termed acute fluid collections; those that persist beyond 4 weeks are termed pseudocysts. Imaging may help discern pseudocysts from walled-off pancreatic necrosis (WOPN) to allow for decision making in these complicated clinical settings.

Via mass effect, pseudocysts can cause symptoms such as abdominal pain, early satiety, nausea, and vomiting. Other sequelae include jaundice secondary to common bile duct obstruction, gastric variceal bleeding (i.e., related to sinistral hypertension) secondary to either splenic vein or PV obstruction, sepsis secondary to pseudocyst infection, and intra-abdominal hemorrhage secondary to bleeding from a pseudoaneurysm (from erosion of adjacent visceral vessels bathed in pancreatic secretions).

Asymptomatic pseudocysts are managed without intervention; endoscopic or surgical intervention is reserved for persistent abdominal pain or early satiety, pseudocyst enlargement, or pseudocyst complications. Serial follow-up with CT or ultrasonography is performed to assess the progression of the pseudocyst. Spontaneous resolution is observed in a majority of patients. Pseudocyst size still correlates with the eventual need for intervention; over half of patients with pseudocysts greater than 6 cm will

TABLE 14.9 Pancreatic ductal leaks or aberrant ductal drainage

Process	Description	Treatment
Pancreatic ascites	Drainage of pancreatic fluid into the peritoneal cavity in the setting of underlying ascites. Fluid is not walled off or contained.	Control of underlying cause of ascites.
Pancreatic pleural effusion	Drainage of pancreatic fluid into the pleural cavity via fistulous tract.	Diagnostic thoracentesis. Usually observation, NPO, and supplemental nutrition. Consideration of ampullary decompression with ERCP.
Pancreaticocutaneous fistula	Drainage of pancreatic fluid from the pancreas out through a well-defined tract communicating with the skin.	Usually observation. Can be controlled with reduced oral intake and supplemental nutrition. Consideration of ampullary decompression with ERCP. Octreotide may decrease output but rarely rate of closure. Rarely pancreatic resection.
Pancreaticoenteric fistula	Drainage of pancreatic fluid through a fistulous tract connecting the pancreas with bowel, usually transverse colon.	No treatment necessary unless complicated by bleeding.
Pancreatic pseudocyst	Drainage of pancreatic fluid is walled off, usually by surrounding structures including stomach; collection surrounded by fibrous/granulomatous tissue and *not* lined by epithelium.	Initial course of observation. NPO and supplemental nutrition, percutaneous drainage, endoscopic drainage, and internal drainage.

eventually require a definitive endoscopic or surgical procedure. A trial of at least 6 weeks of observation without intervention should be attempted since many pseudocysts regress.

Since traditional operative drainage carries a morbidity rate of 10% and mortality rate of 1%, radiologic and endoscopic interventions have evolved and now compete with surgery as first-line therapy. Endoscopic drainage can be transpapillary (e.g., reserved for smaller pseudocysts in communication with the main pancreatic duct) or transmural (transgastric or transduodenal; reserved for large pseudocysts without obvious ductal communication).

The preferred operative approach is internal drainage via either cyst jejunostomy (using a Roux-en-Y conduit) or cyst gastrostomy (Fig. 14.7). Surgical intervention should always include a biopsy of the pseudocyst wall to exclude a cystic neoplasm. Surgical resection of pancreatic pseudocysts is generally reserved for lesions within the tail. External drainage of pancreatic pseudocysts is indicated for unusual indications: infected pseudocysts and unstable patients. A pancreaticocutaneous fistula occurs after external drainage but usually closes spontaneously. Some persist and may be rectified by interventional radiology techniques that reroute drainage into the gastrointestinal tract. Rarely, surgical bypass of the fistulous tract is necessary.

Pancreatic Trauma

Pancreatic trauma is a relatively uncommon occurrence—less than 2% of patients with abdominal trauma have pancreatic injuries—largely due to the protected position of the pancreas within the depths of the abdominal cavity. Roughly two thirds of pancreatic injuries are from penetrating, as opposed to blunt, injury; other visceral injuries are often present. Mortality rates range from 5% to 60% depending on injury severity and location. The most common cause of early death following pancreatic injury is uncontrolled hemorrhage. Pancreatic leaks and resultant intra-abdominal sepsis result in a second, later peak in mortality. Blunt trauma can result in pancreatic neck transection because of the proximity of the pancreas to the vertebral column.

Diagnosis

CT scan is the imaging modality of choice for identifying blunt pancreatic injury; however, penetrating injuries may be missed, especially if scanned early. Plain films, ultrasound, and diagnostic peritoneal lavage have no role in diagnosing pancreatic trauma given the retroperitoneal location of the organ. ERCP may play a role in evaluating ductal injury in a delayed setting, but should not be part of the acute evaluation. Laboratory studies are generally insensitive and nonspecific. Elevated amylase is present in 90% of patients with blunt pancreatic injury, but in only a minority of patients with penetrating pancreatic injury. In addition, hyperamylasemia is seen in 50% of patients with blunt abdominal trauma without a pancreatic injury.

Treatment

The goals of operative therapy for pancreatic injury include control of hemorrhage, debridement of nonviable tissue with maximal

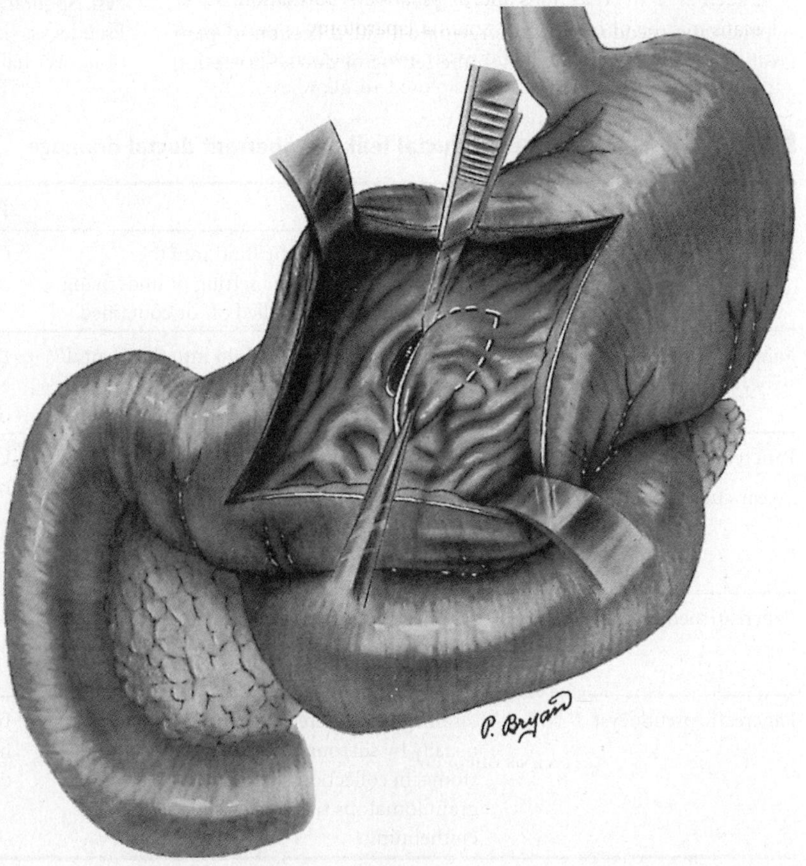

FIGURE 14.7 Drainage of pancreatic pseudocyst into the stomach. Once an incision has been made through the posterior wall of the stomach, through the cyst wall, and into the pseudocyst, a continuous locking suture is placed through the posterior wall of the stomach and the cyst wall. (From Bradley EL. Pancreatic cystenterostomy. In: Baker RJ, Fischer JE, eds. *Mastery of Surgery*. Philadelphia: Lippincott Williams & Wilkins; 2001, with permission.)

TABLE 14.10 Pancreatic trauma classification (1990 AAST guidelines)

Injury Grade	Description	Treatment
I	Minor pancreatic contusion or superficial laceration *without* main ductal injury.	Observation and/or external drainage depending on whether laparotomy is indicated for other injuries.
II	Major contusion or major laceration without main ductal injury.	Observation and/or external drainage depending on whether laparotomy is indicated for other injuries. If encountered, devitalized tissue is debrided. The capsule is closed if possible. An omental patch may be considered.
III	Severe parenchymal injury or main distal ductal disruption. Distal pancreatic transection.	Body and tail injuries are treated with distal pancreatectomy. Inferior head/uncinate process injuries are treated with external drainage or PJ. Central head injuries adjacent to duodenum are treated like class IV injuries.
IV	Severe parenchymal injury with a proximal pancreatic ductal injury involving the ampulla.	Debridement and external drainage. Discrete duodenal injuries may be closed primarily. Duodenal decompression with G tube and retrograde and anterograde J tubes. Consider pyloric exclusion and gastrojejunostomy.
V	Massive disruption of the pancreatic head.	As with class IV; consider Whipple procedure.

preservation of viable pancreatic tissue, and adequate drainage of pancreatic leaks. Several classification systems for pancreatic injuries exist and are useful in guiding therapy. For the sake of simplicity, the American Association for the Surgery of Trauma (AAST) guidelines are included in Table 14.10. Stable patients with no other indication for laparotomy can be managed conservatively. Such patients are followed clinically for the development of complications such as fluid collections and/or pseudocyst formation. Serial CT scans may be of benefit. If a trauma laparotomy is performed, complete assessment of the pancreas is always indicated. All peripancreatic hematomas should be explored to allow exclusion or repair of major vascular injuries.

Neoplasms of the Exocrine Pancreas

Pancreatic ductal adenocarcinoma (PDAC; representing 90% of all exocrine malignancies) remains one of the most lethal solid tumors, owing largely to early systemic dissemination of malignant cells. It is the fourth leading cause of cancer-related death in the United States, accounting for roughly 37,000 deaths per year. At diagnosis, most patients are advanced (metastatic) with only 15% to 20% of patients being candidates for a potentially curative surgical resection. Resection offers the best possibility for cure (particularly when margin negative and node negative), with 5-year survival rates around 20% when performed at specialized high-volume centers. Nevertheless, median survival after resection is only about 2 years, and, for all stages, 5-year survival is an abysmal 3%.

Inherited forms account for a small minority (under 5%) of all PDAC cases. Data from the National Familial Pancreas Tumor Registry (NFPTR) indicate that individuals with a positive family history have a 16- to 33-fold increased risk of the development of pancreatic cancer. The tumor suppressor genes *p16*, *p53*, *DPC4/SMAD4*, and *BRCA2* as well as oncogenes K-*ras*, *AKT*, *BRAF*, and *MYB* have all been implicated in the pathogenesis of pancreatic cancer. Table 14.11 summarizes the risk factors for pancreatic cancer.

Presentation

Pancreatic head masses classically present with painless jaundice. Abdominal pain, weight loss, pruritus, malaise, changes in bowel habits, and anorexia may also be present. Roughly 10% of patients present with new-onset diabetes mellitus. On physical examination, the gallbladder may be palpable (*Courvoisier sign*). It is not uncommon for patients to present with advanced disease (i.e., distant lymphadenopathy or metastases). Findings may include left supraclavicular adenopathy (*Virchow's node*), periumbilical lymphadenopathy (*Sister Mary Joseph nodes*), and drop metastases in the pelvis (*Blumer shelf*) palpable on rectal examination.

Distal pancreatic masses may be much more insidious in onset and often have no or few associated symptoms (usually change in appetite, weight loss, or vague left upper quadrant pain). For this reason, distal masses tend to be larger and more advanced at initial presentation.

TABLE 14.11 Risk factors for pancreatic cancer

Risk Factors for Development of Pancreatic Cancer
Increasing age
African American descent
Male gender
Cigarette smoking
HNPCC Type II (hereditary nonpolyposis colorectal cancer)
Peutz–Jeghers syndrome
Ataxia-telangiectasia syndrome
FAMMM (familial atypical multiple mole melanoma syndrome)
Hereditary pancreatitis
Chronic pancreatitis
Cystic fibrosis

Diagnostic Evaluation

Multidetector-row CT (MDCT) with three-dimensional reconstruction is the preferred noninvasive imaging modality for the diagnosis and staging of PDAC. MDCT utilizes dual-phase imaging in the arterial and venous phases of enhancement, acquiring sub-3-mm slices during one 20-second breath hold. PDAC typically appears as a hypodense mass—although it can appear isodense—in the parenchyma and is best seen on the portal venous phase of enhancement. MDCT also provides a comprehensive view of tumor abutment or encasement of the major peripancreatic vascular structures (celiac axis, SMA and vein, splenic artery, and PV) as well as peripancreatic lymphadenopathy and hepatic or omental metastasis. Finally, it provides the best spatial road map for the anatomic relationships between the primary tumor and the local vasculature.

Other imaging modalities utilized in PDAC detection include MRI, ERCP, and endoscopic ultrasound (EUS). ERCP can be useful in the evaluation of patients with presumed pancreatic cancer and obstructive jaundice or symptoms without evidence of a mass on CT. The particular benefit of EUS is realized in the clarification of small (<2 cm) lesions in the setting of negative or equivocal CT findings, evaluation of malignant lymphadenopathy, detection of vascular involvement, and the ability to obtain a tissue diagnosis when combined with FNA. However, unless protocol-based neoadjuvant therapy is planned or the patient is a poor operative candidate, a tissue diagnosis is not necessary or routinely recommended in acceptable-risk patients with resectable lesions on noninvasive axial imaging (CT or MRI).

While the only FDA-approved biomarker in PDAC—CA 19-9—is not sensitive enough for screening, it may be useful for postoperative (or posttreatment in case of unresectable tumors) surveillance. Increasing CA 19-9 levels after surgical resection typically indicate recurrence or disease progression, whereas stable or declining levels postoperatively indicate absence of recurrence and improved overall prognosis. It can also be used to monitor response to neoadjuvant therapy and therefore assist in decisions to perform surgery or not. CEA has little to no additive value in securing a diagnosis of PDAC.

Pathology

PDAC accounts for almost 90% of all primary pancreatic malignancies. Approximately 65% of ductal adenocarcinomas arise in the head, neck, or uncinate process of the pancreas; 15% originate in the body and tail; and 20% involve the gland diffusely. At the time of diagnosis, most PDACs have metastasized to the peripancreatic lymph nodes. Precursor lesions such as intraductal papillary mucinous neoplasms (IPMNs) or mucinous cystic neoplasms (MCNs) can progress to infiltrating ductal adenocarcinoma (see Table 14.12 for a list of pancreatic lesions).

TABLE 14.12 Benign and malignant lesions of the pancreas

Malignancy	Description
Ductal adenocarcinoma	The most common subtype.
Adenosquamous carcinoma	A rare variant with a very poor prognosis
Giant cell carcinoma	An extremely aggressive tumor, which grows rapidly. It often has necrotic or hemorrhagic components.
Acinar cell carcinoma (ACC)	Thought to result from malignant degeneration of acinar cells of the pancreas, ACC can present with subcutaneous fat necrosis, an erythema nodosum–like rash, eosinophilia, or polyarthralgia.
IPMN	Generally considered a precursor lesion to adenocarcinoma (particularly main duct), IPMN is characterized by genetic mutations such as k-*ras* and *p53*. IPMNs are mucin producing, with cellular atypia. ERCP may demonstrate mucinous secretion from the ampulla of Vater. Cyst aspiration demonstrates high CEA levels.
Solid pseudopapillary tumor (SPT)	SPTs have a low malignant potential, but can grow as large as 30 cm, leading to significant compressive symptoms. They are more common in females than males (10:1) and occur primarily in patients in their midtwenties.
Mucinous cystic neoplasm (MCN)	Cystic mucin-secreting tumor, not in continuity with the duct. MCNs will likely degenerate to cystadenocarcinoma if not resected early. They have a female predominance, age 40 to 50 years.
Mucinous cystadenocarcinoma	Malignant degeneration of an MCN
Intraductal oncocytic and papillary neoplasm (IOPN)	Intraductal neoplasm similar to an IPMN with slightly more malignant potential. Oncocytic cells on histology
Serous cystadenoma	Benign cystic lesion cured by resection. Sometimes difficult to differentiate from a pseudocyst. Resection for symptoms or size >4 cm
Pancreatic lymphoma	Non-Hodgkin–type lymphoma with primary involvement of the gland. Treated with chemotherapy, not surgery unless small lesion
Metastatic lesions	Unusual location for metastatic lesions, but renal cell carcinoma is the most common.

Surgical Resection of a Pancreatic Mass

Pancreaticoduodenectomy for Tumors of the Head of the Pancreas (Whipple Procedure)

The Whipple procedure is used to resect masses in the head of the pancreas or other periampullary tumors. In experienced hands, the perioperative mortality rate is as low as 1% to 2%, and studies have shown that higher operative volume at specialized pancreatic centers is associated with a reduced risk of perioperative complications and improved survival. Although mortality remains low, morbidity approaches 50% in some studies (see "Postoperative Considerations" below).

Unfortunately, prognosis following a pancreaticoduodenectomy for cancer leaves much room for improvement. Roughly 80% to 85% of all patients will have a recurrence following operation for resectable disease. Factors that determine overall prognosis include clinicopathologic stage, biologic features of the tumor, and the use of postoperative adjuvant therapy. Tumor characteristics found to be important predictors of survival include tumor size, lymph node status, and resection margin status.

Determination of surgical resectability is an important preoperative step in the workup of these patients. PDAC of the pancreatic head, neck, or uncinate process is stratified into the following: (a) *resectable*, defined as no radiographic evidence of extrapancreatic disease, a patent SMV-PV confluence, and no evidence of tumor extension to the celiac axis or SMA; (b) *borderline resectable*, defined as nonmetastatic tumor with SMA abutment (≤180 degrees), abutment or encasement of the GDA up to or around a short, reconstructable segment of the common hepatic artery (CHA), or complete occlusion of the SMV-PV confluence, with suitable, uninvolved vein above and below to allow venous reconstruction. As a general rule, tumors encasing up to 2 cm of the SMV and/or PV for up to 180 degrees circumference are considered technically possible; (c) *locally advanced*, defined as encasement (>180 degrees) of the celiac axis or SMA or occlusion of SMV-PV confluence without an option for venous resection and reconstruction; (c) *metastatic*, defined as distant metastatic spread to the liver, peritoneum, or rarely the lung.

After determination of resectability, planning for pancreaticoduodenectomy is undertaken. An open pancreaticoduodenectomy may be performed through a bilateral subcostal or midline laparotomy. Upon entering the abdomen, attention should first be directed toward assessing resectability and looking for locally advanced disease. Distant metastasis to the peritoneum or liver and local extension to the mesenteric vessels precludes resection. Next, access to the head of the pancreas is obtained through mobilization of the hepatic flexure of the colon and extensive mobilization (Kocher maneuver) of the duodenum and the head of the pancreas. The gallbladder is removed, and the portal structures are dissected. The bile duct is transected proximal to the cystic duct insertion. The GDA is ligated and the distal stomach or proximal duodenum is divided, while preserving or resecting the pylorus depending on surgeon preference. The jejunum is divided 6 to 10 cm beyond the ligament of Treitz. The pancreatic dissection is performed by developing a plane between the pancreas and the SMV. The pancreas is then transected at the plane of the pancreatic neck; the resection margin should be tumor free on frozen section if possible. Finally, the interface of the uncinated process with the SMA is transected as close to the SMA as possible.

Following resection of the specimen, three anastomoses are created to complete the reconstruction. The PJ is performed first, followed by the hepaticojejunostomy. The third anastomosis is the duodenojejunostomy or gastrojejunostomy (depending on whether the pylorus is preserved), typically performed 40 to 50 cm downstream from the hepaticojejunostomy (Fig. 14.8).

The pylorus-preserving modification of the Whipple procedure is now more commonly performed than is the originally described procedure, which involved a distal gastrectomy. The pylorus-preserving procedure leaves behind the entire gastric reservoir and

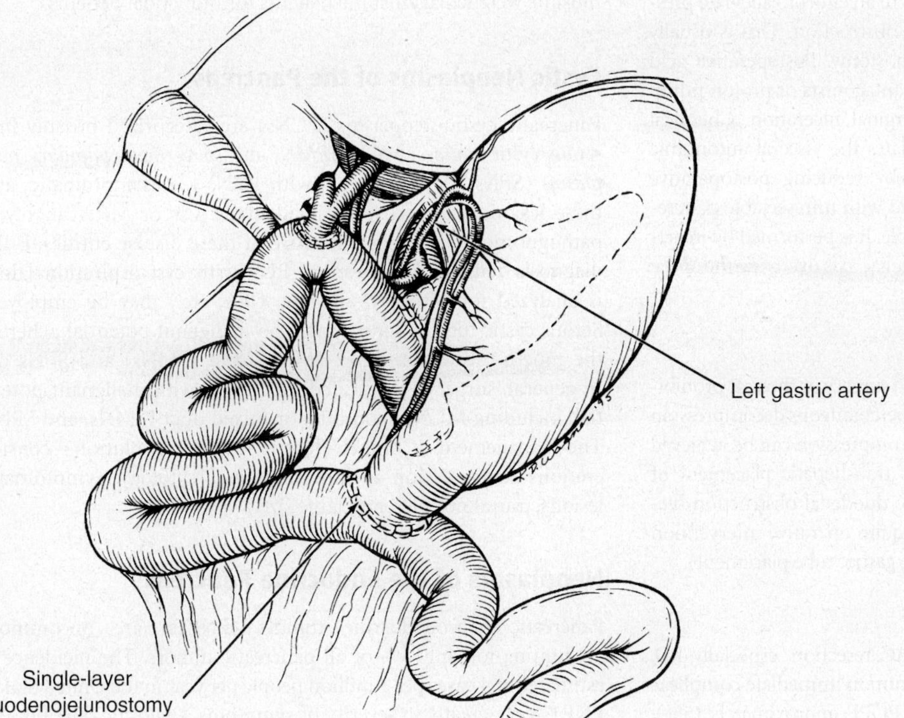

FIGURE 14.8 Whipple procedure. After the end-to-end PJ and the end-to-side hepaticojejunostomy, the duodenum is anastomosed to the jejunum in an end-to-side fashion. (From Evans DB, Lee JE, Pisters PW. Pancreaticoduodenectomy (Whipple operation) and total pancreatectomy for cancer. In: Baker RJ, Fischer JE, eds. *Mastery of Surgery*. Philadelphia: Lippincott Williams & Wilkins; 2001, with permission.)

pyloric sphincter maintaining more normal gastric acid secretion and hormone release, does not appear to be associated with additional complications, reduces operative time and blood loss, and does not compromise oncologic outcomes (negative margin rate or overall survival). Some reports have suggested longer hospital stays due to persistent delayed gastric emptying (DGE).

Extended or radical pancreaticoduodenectomy was initially reported in Japan. Adjacent structures were added to the resection margin including retroperitoneal lymph nodes and nerve plexi. Four randomized studies suggest that extended lymphadenectomy increases the morbidity without significantly improving median or 5-year survival.

Minimally invasive (laparoscopic or robotic) approaches to pancreaticoduodenectomy are growing in popularity, but the learning curve for these techniques is considerable. Consequently, these minimally invasive approaches lack widespread acceptance because matched comparative trials and long-term outcomes comparing them to the open approach are currently lacking.

Distal Pancreatectomy for Tumors of the Body and Tail

Adenocarcinomas of the body and tail of the pancreas account for up to one third of all PDAC. Tumors in this location often present as large tumors with a much higher incidence of metastatic disease at initial diagnosis. Patients undergoing resection for PDAC of the body and tail of the pancreas have a median survival between 7 to 13 months, with 5-year survival rates in the range of 10%. Resection with curative intent typically includes splenectomy.

Palliative Surgery

As mentioned earlier, most patients with PDAC are not candidates for curative resection. Palliative operation for PDAC aims to relieve biliary and/or gastric outlet obstruction. In addition, splanchnic nerve blocks may be used to treat pain.

Biliary obstruction may be bypassed with a hepaticojejunostomy. This is usually performed with a Roux-en-Y reconstruction. Gastrojejunostomy is generally recommended in patients who are undergoing operative palliation of PDAC in an effort to alleviate present or future gastric outlet or duodenal obstruction. This is usually achieved with a side-to-side gastrojejunostomy. Postoperative acid suppression with histamine H2 receptor antagonists or proton pump inhibitors may be used to prevent marginal ulceration. Chemical splanchnicectomy with 50% alcohol ablates the visceral autonomic innervation to the celiac plexus, thereby reducing postoperative abdominal and back pain often associated with unresectable pancreatic cancer, but its durability is questionable. It is performed by injecting 20 mL of alcohol on either side of the celiac axis overlying the aorta.

Nonoperative Management

Patients deemed to be unresectable prior to surgery or those at prohibitively high surgical risk may benefit from percutaneous decompression if obstructed. In these patients, biliary decompression can be achieved with either endoscopic or percutaneous transhepatic placement of stents or drains. Patients with high-grade duodenal obstruction secondary to pancreatic cancer generally require operative intervention (e.g., gastrojejunostomy or decompressive gastric tube placement).

Postoperative Considerations

The overall complication rate after PDAC resection, especially PD, continues to approach 40%. The most common immediate complications are postoperative pancreatic fistula (POPF; approximately 15%), DGE (approximately 10%), hemorrhage (approximately 5%), and wound infection (approximately 20%). A gradation of POPF—*A* (biochemical, with no clinical impact) through *C* (rendering a life-threatening, major deviation from clinical recovery)—was developed by a consensus panel (ISGPF) in 2005. There is *no* unequivocal evidence to suggest that anastomotic route (PJ vs. pancreaticogastrostomy), anastomotic technique (duct to mucosa vs. invagination vs. single-layer end-to-side PJ), pancreatic duct stenting, or use of long-acting somatostatin analogues alters the incidence of POPF formation.

Intense investigations have recently focused on strategies to mitigate the morbidity from POPF. Intraoperative drain placement is one such strategy that has been extensively explored. Based on the contemporary literature, it would appear that routine drainage is associated with lower rates of overall morbidity and mortality; however, the decision to drain should be made after an intraoperative assessment of the individual patient's perceived risk for developing a clinically relevant POPF. This assessment should incorporate factors such as intraoperative blood loss, gland texture, and pancreatic duct diameter and the patient's pathology—these factors have been weighted and are available as a risk stratification system known as the Fistula Risk Score.

Multimodality Therapy

Because of the early microscopic spread and aggressive biology of pancreatic cancers, additional treatment modalities such as external beam radiation and chemotherapy have been explored. Overall, *adjuvant* therapy, supported by a large body of evidence, is a critical part of the postoperative management of PDAC. Chemotherapeutic agents include 5-fluorouracil (5-FU), gemcitabine, nab-paclitaxel, and FOLFIRINOX. There is now particular interest in applying a *neoadjuvant* approach to PDAC, especially in borderline resectable disease, and for some locally advanced tumors. The palliative use of radiotherapy and chemotherapy may improve median survival time. The toxicity of this therapy and influence on quality of life must be weighed against the benefits for individual patients.

Cystic Neoplasms of the Pancreas

Pancreatic cystic neoplasms (PCNs) are categorized broadly into *serous cystic tumors*, *MCN*, *IPMN*, and *solid pseudopapillary neoplasms (SPNs)*. Most patients with PCNs are asymptomatic, and these lesions are discovered incidentally. CT or MRI can reveal pathognomonic findings indicative of these disease entities; if the diagnosis remains in question, EUS with cyst aspiration (fluid is analyzed for cytology, amylase, CEA, etc.) may be employed. Serous cystic tumors have almost no malignant potential, whereas the mucin-producing PCNs (MCNs and IPMNs) and SPNs do. In general, surgery is indicated for lesions with malignant potential, including MCN, main duct or mixed duct IPMNs, and SPNs. The management of branch-duct IPMN is in evolution—considerations for resection include abnormal cytology, symptomatic lesions, mural nodules, and large size.

Neoplasms of the Endocrine Pancreas

Pancreatic neuroendocrine tumors (PNETs) are uncommon, accounting for only 1% of all pancreatic tumors. The incidence is estimated at 4 cases per 1 million people per year in the United States. PNETs vary greatly in severity of symptoms, anatomic distribution,

TABLE 14.13 Pancreatic neuroendocrine tumors

Tumor Type	Islet Cell Type	Malignant Potential	Anatomic Distribution	MEN-1 (capitalize) Association	Extrapancreatic
Insulinoma	β	Rare (10%)	Evenly distributed	5%–8%	Rare
Gastrinoma	G	Most (>50%)	Gastrinoma triangle	15%–35%	>30%
Glucagonoma	α	75%	Body/tail	Rare	Rare
VIPoma	$\Delta 2$	Most (>50%)	Body/tail	Rare	10%
Somatostatinoma	Δ	Most	Pancreatic head	Rare	Rare

and malignant potential. Whereas only 10% of insulinomas are malignant, a majority of glucagonomas and somatostatinomas are. Table 14.13 summarizes the various PNETs and their characteristics.

PNETs can occur sporadically or as a component of inherited genetic syndromes, such as multiple endocrine neoplasia type1 (MEN-1), von Hippel–Lindau (VHL), and neurofibromatosis (NF) type 1. MEN-1 is an autosomal dominant genetic syndrome characterized by the development of 4-gland parathyroid hyperplasia, PNETs, and pituitary adenomas. The association of various PNETs with MEN-1 is also detailed in Table 14.13.

Although recent evidence suggests that a majority of PNETs are nonfunctional, the functional subtypes are still of academic interest and are discussed below.

Insulinoma

Presentation

Insulinomas are the most common functioning tumors of the pancreas. Whipple first described a triad of symptoms pathognomonic for the disease: hypoglycemia while exercising or fasting, a plasma glucose level lower than 50 mg/dL, and resolution of symptoms with administration of IV glucose. Patients may present with headaches, confusion, lethargy, seizures, obtundation, irritability, or even coma. Without proper treatment, persistent and profound hypoglycemia can lead to permanent brain injury.

Diagnosis

The definitive test used for diagnosis of insulinoma is a closely monitored 72-hour inpatient fast, with measurement of serial blood glucose and insulin levels. Alternatively, the insulin to glucose ratio may be measured and, in fact, is more sensitive. Almost all patients will have inappropriately elevated insulin levels in the setting of hypoglycemia. Other entities that should be excluded in the evaluation of a suspected insulinoma include adrenal insufficiency, carcinoid, sepsis, hepatic insufficiency, and iatrogenic administration of insulin. Factitious hyperglycemia can be distinguished from endogenous hyperinsulinemia by lower concentrations of C-peptide and proinsulin. In addition to blood tests, CT scanning should be obtained to visualize the pancreas. Most PNETs will enhance during early arterial-phase administration of contrast. Insulinomas, unlike other PNETs, do not express somatostatin receptors and cannot be visualized on somatostatin receptor scintigraphy ("octreoscan"). EUS is a sensitive study for the localization of insulinomas. Even if the tumor is localized preoperatively, intraoperative ultrasound is helpful and should be utilized during operation to confirm tumor location and adequate resection. Other studies that are largely of historic interest include portal venous sampling and arteriography with selective arterial stimulation using secretin or calcium. These rare diagnostic modalities are usually reserved for cases in which operation has failed to identify and remove the tumor.

Treatment

While preparing for operation, patients should eat more frequent meals to avoid hypoglycemia. The medication diazoxide is helpful in about two thirds of patients but should be discontinued at least a week before operation because it may cause intraoperative hypotension. Patients may need to be admitted to the hospital preoperatively to be maintained on IV dextrose while fasting after midnight. The long-acting somatostatin analogue octreotide, although helpful in children with nesidioblastosis, is not usually effective in adults. Most insulinomas are benign—while enucleation may be entertained in select cases, if malignancy is suspected, tumors should be resected with wide margins either with a distal pancreatectomy or pancreaticoduodenectomy depending upon location. If bulky metastatic disease is present, attempts should be made to debulk the tumor. Persistent hyperinsulinemia after surgical resection may be managed with diazoxide or streptozotocin and fluorouracil.

Hyperinsulinism in infants is caused by nesidioblastosis, a nest-like increase in islet cells. Prolonged hypoglycemia leads to mental retardation in most of these children. A near-total (95% to 98%) pancreatectomy appears to offer the best results, with octreotide therapy reserved for preoperative preparation and those children with persistent hypoglycemia after operation.

Gastrinoma (Zollinger–Ellison Syndrome)

Presentation

Gastrinoma is the second most common islet cell tumor. The presenting symptoms may include epigastric pain, complications of peptic ulcers, diarrhea, and reflux esophagitis. The diagnosis of gastrinoma should be suspected in patients with recurrent gastroduodenal PUD who have failed medical management with acid suppression as well as patients who have PUD associated with diarrhea. Seventy-five percent of gastrinomas are sporadic, while 25% are associated with MEN-1 syndrome. A majority arise in the duodenum rather than pancreas. Patients with the MEN-1 syndrome typically have multiple tumors, often microadenomas, scattered throughout the pancreas.

Diagnosis

The evaluation of a suspected gastrinoma should include measurement of the serum gastrin level. Elevated levels are highly suggestive, and levels greater than 1,000 pg/mL are virtually diagnostic in the setting of gastric pH <5.0. Not all patients with elevated gastrin

TABLE 14.14 Differential diagnosis of hypergastrinemia broken down by the presence of ulcerative pathology

Normal Acid Secretion (No Ulcers)	Elevated Acid Secretion (Ulcers)
Renal failure	Zollinger–Ellison syndrome
Atrophic gastritis	Retained antrum
Pernicious anemia	Gastric outlet obstruction
Previous vagotomy	Antral hyperplasia
Short gut syndrome	

levels, however, have a gastrinoma (Table 14.14), and patients should be studied off of all suppressive medications (proton pump inhibitors) to confirm overproduction. Finally, a secretin stimulation test can be used to confirm the diagnosis. An increase in gastrin levels following a secretin bolus constitutes a positive test.

The majority of gastrinomas are found within the so-called gastrinoma triangle (Passaro's triangle) as shown in Figure 14.9. Attempts to localize gastrinomas by means of ultrasonography, arteriography, enhanced CT, and MRI should be attempted preoperatively; however, these modalities are not always helpful. As opposed to insulinomas, gastrinomas are fairly sensitive to localization with somatostatin receptor scintigraphy, which is also helpful in the evaluation for metastatic disease. If these methods fail, intraoperative ultrasound and direct visualization are usually successful.

Treatment

The initial treatment of gastrinoma includes acid suppression with H2-blockers or proton pump inhibitors; however, every patient should be evaluated for surgical resection. Resection is indicated in

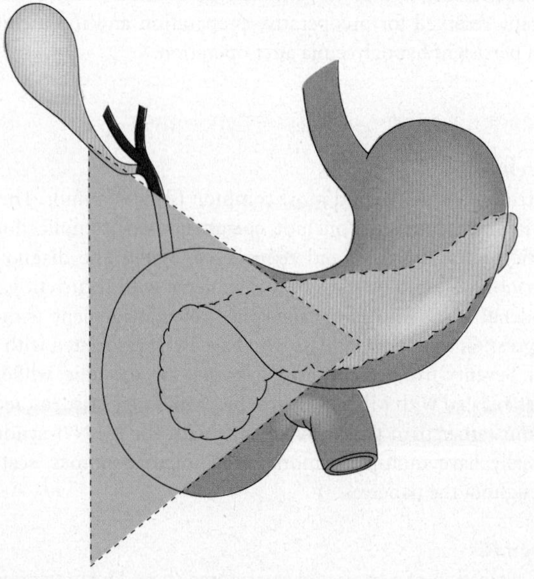

FIGURE 14.9 The gastrinoma triangle. (From Stabile BE, Morrow DJ, Passaro E. The gastrinoma triangle: operative implications. *Am J Surg.* 1984;147:26, with permission.)

cases of localized disease and can usually be accomplished by full-thickness excision and primary closure of the duodenum or pancreatic resection. A Whipple procedure may be necessary for resection of larger lesions or those involving the ampulla. Most gastrinomas are malignant (30% to 90%). Liver metastases are not uncommon and have a major influence on overall survival. Gastrinomas are usually slow growing, and some patients may live for many years with metastatic disease.

Over 90% of all patients with successful resection will experience immediate resolution of symptoms; however, 50% of these patients will recur within 5 years. Debulking may have some clinical benefit in these patients.

VIPoma (Verner–Morrison Syndrome)

Verner–Morrison syndrome is characterized by profound watery diarrhea, hypokalemia, and achlorhydria and is caused by a tumor that secretes vasoactive intestinal peptide (VIP). The diarrhea is secretory in nature and is not affected by eating. Approximately 50% of patients have metastatic disease by the time of diagnosis; however, surgical resection should be considered if the disease is localized. In patients with unresectable tumors, octreotide is helpful for amelioration of symptoms.

Glucagonoma

Glucagonomas are endocrine tumors derived from α cells in the pancreas and are characterized by secretion of glucagon. They are exceptionally rare. Symptoms include erythematous skin eruptions, which become necrotic (necrolytic migrating erythema) and are associated with mild diabetes mellitus, anemia, weight loss, and elevated circulating levels of glucagon. Treatment consists of complete surgical resection if possible. As with other PNETs, debulking is usually very helpful for symptomatic relief and long-term survival. The skin lesions are responsive to a high-protein diet, zinc, control of diabetes, and, in severe cases, TPN. Symptomatic relief can be achieved with octreotide and chemotherapy.

Somatostatinoma

Somatostatinomas are very rare lesions. They are usually found in the pancreas or, infrequently, in the duodenum. The clinical features relate to the general inhibitory nature of somatostatin and include steatorrhea, bloating, nausea, vomiting, and gallstones. Surgical resection is indicated, and debulking often results in clinical improvement.

Nonfunctioning Endocrine Tumors

While the overwhelming majority of nonfunctioning PNETs are incidentally identified, some patients may present with symptoms from mass effect. Such tumors are usually malignant and have metastasized by the time of diagnosis. Surgical resection is recommended given the typically slow progression of these tumors.

Resection of Metastatic Disease

Hepatic neuroendocrine metastases are commonly multifocal and are often not amenable to complete resection. Given the indolent nature of the disease, however, resection (with or without microwave or radiofrequency ablation) has been employed for the cytoreduction of metastatic foci. Liver-directed therapies such as transarterial chemoembolization or radioembolization are reserved for multifocal unresectable lesions. Obviously, resection of the primary tumor is also recommended in these scenarios.

Systemic Therapy

Systemic therapy for PNETs has typically been restricted to somatostatin analogs (e.g., octreotide, lanreotide) and cytotoxic chemotherapy (e.g., 5-FU, streptozocin, doxorubicin). Recent randomized data suggest delayed progression with somatostatin analog therapy, everolimus, and sunitinib in patients with metastatic disease.

Suggested Readings

Bakker OJ, Issa Y, van Santvoort HC, et al. Treatment options for acute pancreatitis. *Nat Rev Gastroenterol Hepatol.* 2014;11(8):462–469.

Datta J, Vollmer CM Jr. Investigational biomarkers for pancreatic adenocarcinoma: where do we stand? *South Med J.* 2014;107(4):256–263.

Lewis R, Drebin JA, Callery MP, et al. A contemporary analysis of survival for resected pancreatic ductal adenocarcinoma. *HPB (Oxford).* 2013;15(1):49–60.

Murtaugh LC. Pancreas and beta-cell development: from the actual to the possible. *Development.* 2007;134(3):427–438.

Partelli S, Maurizi A, Tamburrino D, et al. GEP-NETS update: a review on surgery of gastro-entero-pancreatic neuroendocrine tumors. *Eur J Endocrinol.* 2014;171(4):R153–R162.

Ryan DP, Hong TS, Bardeesy N. Pancreatic adenocarcinoma. *N Engl J Med.* 2014;371(11):1039–1049.

SECTION

III

Endocrine System and Oncology

Tumor Biology

ARJUN N. JEGANATHAN AND JEFFREY A. DREBIN

KEY POINTS

- Malignant transformation results from the accumulation of genetic mutations within a cell. Ultimately, the transformed cell will acquire the ability to become self-sufficient and no longer rely on the normal temporal sequences of programmed cell growth.
- The tumor microenvironment plays an important role in tumor growth and development by supporting cell–cell and cell–matrix interactions that drive growth, invasion, and metastasis. These interactions alter the response to growth factors, decrease rates of apoptosis, and stimulate angiogenesis.
- Due to the diverse biology of cancer, the clinical treatment mandates a multimodal approach, with surgery, medical oncology, and radiation oncology as the mainstays.
- Gene therapy and nanotechnology are areas of active investigation that have not yet reached standard practice; however, targeted therapies and immunotherapies continue to develop for various cancers and are increasingly used in clinical care.

INTRODUCTION

Cancer is a widely prevalent disease, affecting people of all ages and races as well as economic and geographic extremes. In 2010, malignant cancers accounted for 23.3% of all deaths in the United States, second only to heart disease. In 2013, excluding basal and squamous cell skin cancer and *in situ* carcinomas, it is estimated that more than 1.6 million new cases of cancer will be diagnosed and over 580,000 people will die from cancer. In the United States, the three most common cancers in men are prostate, lung, and colorectal and in women, breast, lung, and colorectal (Fig. 15.1). Although the incidence of many cancers has increased in past years, scientific advances in cancer biology have permitted more effective diagnosis and treatment.

The progression to cancer, or carcinogenesis, is a complex process generating changes in cellular identity at the microscopic level with macroscopic consequences. Malignant transformation results from the accumulation of genetic mutations within a cell, leading to the dysregulation of mechanisms governing cellular growth, differentiation, and death. As an example, the process of carcinogenesis has been particularly well characterized in colon cancer. The progression from normal colonic epithelium to invasive cancer typically develops over decades and appears to require at least seven rather discrete genetic events for completion (Fig. 15.2).

Following malignant transformation within the cell, a series of tumor initiation pathways are enacted, leading to growth, invasion, and metastasis. During this time, tumor cells continue to accumulate genetic alterations, resulting in a heterogeneous population of tumor cells. Carcinogenesis will continue to be driven via alterations in growth and angiogenesis factors, as well as changes in cell surface adhesion molecules.

The following chapter focuses on three main areas of tumor biology. The first section identifies the factors contributing to malignant transformation. The second section reviews elements of the cancer phenotype, including tumor growth and the microenvironment. Finally, in the third section, the range of current treatment modalities are highlighted.

MALIGNANT TRANSFORMATION

The process of malignant transformation results from the accumulation of genetic defects within a cell, thereby releasing the cell from normal mechanisms that regulate cell growth, differentiation, and death. Numerous genetic, environmental, and host factors contribute to this process. In 2000, Hanahan and Weinberg characterized the six hallmarks of cancer acquired during the multistep development of human tumors (Fig. 15.3). They included (i) sustaining proliferative signaling, (ii) evading growth suppressors, (iii) resisting cell death, (iv) enabling replicative immortality, (v) inducing angiogenesis, and (vi) activating invasion and metastasis.

Genetic Factors

Oncogenes

Oncogenes are mutated forms of normal cellular genes generally conferring uninhibited cell growth. The first description of the role of oncogenes in carcinogenesis was described by Peyton Rous in the early 1900s. He demonstrated that sarcomatous tumors were transmissible between chickens via the injection of virus-containing tumor extract. This oncogenic retrovirus, later termed Rous sarcoma virus (RSV), became the foundation for years of study. It was the first demonstration of how an alteration in a normal cellular gene could result in a gene with transforming activity.

Several mechanisms for the activation of oncogenes have been identified, including point mutation, chromosomal translocation, and gene amplification. Examples of oncogenes that are activated by point mutation include the *Ras* family. The *ras* oncogenes encode guanosine triphosphate (GTP)-binding proteins that are involved in signal transduction. A single point mutation has been identified between the proto-oncogene and the oncogene responsible for transforming cellular activity. Of note, mutant *ras* genes are found in a significant fraction of colon, pancreas,

Cancer statistics, 2013

Estimated New Cases*

Males			Females		
Prostate	238,590	28%	Breast	232,340	29%
Lung & bronchus	118,080	14%	Lung & bronchus	110,110	14%
Colorectum	73,680	9%	Colorectum	69,140	9%
Urinary bladder	54,610	6%	Uterine corpus	49,560	6%
Melanoma of the skin	45,060	5%	Thyroid	45,310	6%
Kidney & renal pelvis	40,430	5%	Non-Hodgkin lymphoma	32,140	4%
Non-Hodgkin lymphoma	37,600	4%	Melanoma of the skin	31,630	4%
Oral cavity & pharynx	29,620	3%	Kidney & renal pelvis	24,720	3%
Leukemia	27,880	3%	Pancreas	22,480	3%
Pancreas	22,740	3%	Ovary	22,240	3%
All Sites	**854,790**	**100%**	**All Sites**	**805,500**	**100%**

Estimated Deaths

Males			Females		
Lung & bronchus	87,260	28%	Lung & bronchus	72,220	26%
Prostate	29,720	10%	Breast	39,620	14%
Colorectum	26,300	9%	Colorectum	24,530	9%
Pancreas	19,480	6%	Pancreas	18,980	7%
Liver & intrahepatic bile duct	14,890	5%	Ovary	14,030	5%
Leukemia	13,660	4%	Leukemia	10,060	4%
Esophagus	12,220	4%	Non-Hodgkin lymphoma	8,430	3%
Urinary bladder	10,820	4%	Uterine corpus	8,190	3%
Non-Hodgkin lymphoma	10,590	3%	Liver & intrahepatic bile duct	6,780	2%
Kidney & renal pelvis	8,780	3%	Brain & other nervous system	6,150	2%
All Sites	**306,920**	**100%**	**All Sites**	**273,430**	**100%**

FIGURE 15.1 Ten leading cancer types for the estimated new cancer cases and deaths by sex, United States, 2013. Estimates are rounded to the nearest 10 and exclude basal cell and squamous cell skin cancers and *in situ* carcinoma except urinary bladder. (From Siegel R, Naishadham D, Jemal A. Cancer statistics, 2013. *CA Cancer J Clin.* 2013;63:11–30, with permission.)

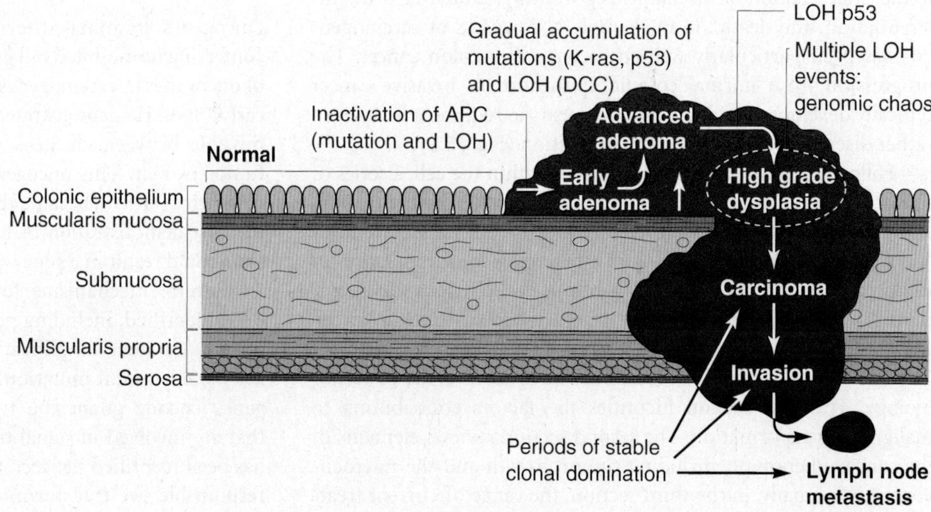

FIGURE 15.2 Model of genetic events mediating neoplastic progression in the colon. LOH, loss of heterozygosity. (From Greenfield, LJ, Mulholland MW, Lillemoe KD, et al. *Surgery: Scientific Principles and Practice.* 4th ed. Philadelphia: Lippincott Williams & Wilkins; 2006:1106.)

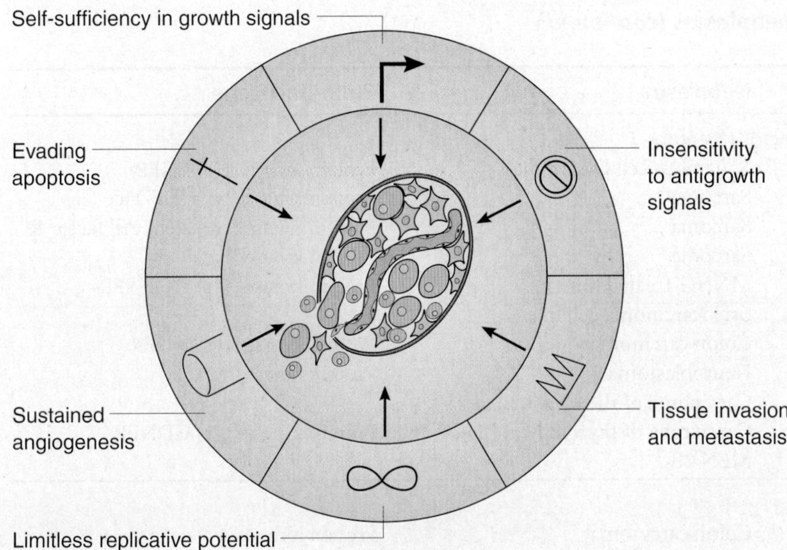

FIGURE 15.3 Acquired capabilities of cancer. (From Greenfield, LJ, Mulholland MW, Lillemoe KD, et al. *Surgery: Scientific Principles and Practice.* 4th ed. Philadelphia: Lippincott Williams & Wilkins; 2006:294.)

and lung cancers. A well-described chromosomal translocation resulting in activation of an oncogene is the Philadelphia chromosome in chronic myelogenous leukemia (CML). A translocation of *c-abl* from chromosome 9 to chromosome 22 leads to the fusion protein *bcr-abl*. Through enhanced tyrosine kinase activity, the Philadelphia chromosome, designated t(9;22)(q34;q11), plays a critical role in the development of CML. An example of an oncogene that is activated by amplification is the *N-myc* oncogene in neuroblastoma. Amplification of this gene has been shown to correlate with tumor progression, recurrence, and resistance to chemotherapy.

A wide variety of oncogenes have been identified that are involved in different steps of cell growth, differentiation, and death. One form of classification of oncogenes is according to cellular location or mechanism of action as growth factors, tyrosine, serine, or threonine kinases, regulatory GTPases, and nuclear transcription factors to name a few. See Table 15.1 for a list of oncogenes and associated neoplasms.

Tumor Suppressor Genes

In contrast to oncogenes, in which mutations to normal cellular genes lead to a gain of function, mutations in tumor suppressor genes (TSGs) result in a loss of function. Therefore, a single wild-type copy of the gene is sufficient for normal cellular function, and, in humans, only a loss of both copies of the gene results in a cancer phenotype. Similar to oncogenes, TSGs are involved in a diverse range of cellular activities, including cell differentiation, adhesion, and death.

The discovery of TSGs came from two concurrent lines of research. Initially, it was found that growth of tumor cells could be suppressed following the fusion of malignant cells with normal cells. However, when these cells were cultured for extended periods of time, many reverted back to the malignant state. It was noted that reversion to the cancer phenotype was associated with the loss of chromosomal fragments. The second line of research was a genealogic study by Alfred Knudson in patients with retinoblastoma (Rb).

TABLE 15.1 Oncogenes and associated neoplasms

Oncogene	Lesion	Neoplasm	Proto-oncogene
Growth factors			
v-sis	—	Glioma/fibrosarcoma	B-chain PDGF
int 2	Proviral insertion	Mammary carcinoma	Member of FGF family
KS3	DNA transfection	Kaposi sarcoma	Member of FGF family
HST	DNA transfection	Stomach carcinoma	Member of FGF family
int-l	Proviral insertion	Mammary carcinoma	Possible growth factor
Receptors lacking protein kinase activity			
mas	DNA transfection	Mammary carcinoma	Angiotensin receptor

(*continued*)

TABLE 15.1 Oncogenes and associated neoplasms (*continued*)

Oncogene	Lesion	Neoplasm	Proto-oncogene
Tyrosine kinases: integral membrane proteins, growth factor receptors			
EGFR	Amplification	Squamous cell carcinoma	Protein kinase (tyr) EGFR
v-fms	—	Sarcoma	Protein kinase (tyr) CSF-1R
v-kit	—	Sarcoma	Protein kinase (tyr) stem cell factor R
v-ros	—	Sarcoma	Protein kinase (tyr)
MET	Rearrangement	MNNG-treated human osteocarcinoma cell line	Protein kinase (tyr) HGF/SFR
TRK	Rearrangement	Colon carcinoma	Protein kinase (tyr) NGFR
NEU	Point mutation	Neuroblastoma	Protein kinase (tyr)
	Amplification	Carcinoma of the breast	
RET	Rearrangement	Carcinoma of thyroid MEN 2A, MEN 2B	Protein kinase (tyr) GDNFR
Tyrosine kinases: membrane associated			
scr	—	Colon carcinoma	Protein kinase (tyr)
v-yes	—	Sarcoma	Protein kinase (tyr)
v-fgr	—	Sarcoma	Protein kinase (tyr)
v-fps	—	Sarcoma	Protein kinase (tyr)
v-fes	—	Sarcoma	Protein kinase (tyr)
Bcr/abl	Chromosome translocation	CML	Protein kinase (tyr)
Membrane-associated G proteins			
H-RAS	Point mutation	Colon, lung, pancreatic carcinoma	GTPase
K-RAS	Point mutation	Acute myelogenous leukemia thyroid carcinoma, melanoma	GTPase
N-RAS	Point mutation	Carcinoma, melanoma	GTPase
gsp	Point mutation	Carcinoma of the thyroid	$G_6\alpha$
gip	Point mutation	Ovarian, adrenal carcinoma	$G_1\alpha$
GEF family of proteins			
Dbl	Rearrangement	Diffuse B-cell lymphoma	GEF for Rho and Cdc42Hs
Ost	—	Osteosarcomas	GEF for RhoA and Cdc42Hs
Tiam-1	Metastatic and oncogenic	T lymphoma	GEF for Rac and Cdc42Hs
Vav	Rearrangement	Hematopoietic cells	GEF for Rho
Lbc	Oncogenic	Myeloid leukemias	GEF for Rho
Serine/threonine kinases: cytoplasmic			
v-mos	—	Sarcoma	Protein kinase (ser/thr)
v-raf	—	Sarcoma	Protein kinase (ser/thr)
pim-1	Proviral insertion	T-cell lymphoma	Protein kinase (ser/thr)
Cytoplasmic regulators			
v-crk	—	—	SH-2/SH-3 adaptor
Nuclear protein family			
v-myc	—	Carcinoma myelocytomatosis	Transcription factor
N-MYC	Gene amplification	Neuroblastoma, lung carcinoma	Transcription factor
L-MYC	Gene amplification	Carcinoma of the lung	Transcription factor
v-myb	—	Myeloblastosis	Transcription factor
v-fos	—	Osteosarcoma	Transcription factor API
v-jun	—	Sarcoma	Transcription factor API
v-ski	—	Carcinoma	Transcription factor
v-rel	—	Lymphatic leukemia	Mutant NF-κB
v-ets	—	Myeloblastosis	Transcription factor
v-erbA	—	Erythroblastosis	Mutant thioredoxin receptor

EGFR, epidermal growth factor receptor; PDGF, platelet-derived growth factor; CSF-1R, macrophage colony–stimulating factor-1 receptor; FGF, fibroblast growth factor; GEF, guanine nucleotide exchange factor; GDNR, glial-derived neurotropic factor receptor; HGF/SFR, hepatic growth factor/scatter factor receptor; NGF, nerve growth factor.

From Park M. Oncogenes. In: Volgelstein B, Kinzler KW, eds. *The Genetic Basis of Human Cancer*. 2nd ed. New York: McGraw-Hill; 2002:181, with permission.

Mechanism of inactivating p53	Typical tumours	Effect of inactivation
Amino-acid-changing mutation in the DNA-binding domain	Colon, breast, lung, bladder, brain, pancreas, stomach, oesophagus and many others	Prevents p53 from binding to specific DNA sequences and activating the adjacent genes
Deletion of the carboxy-terminal domain	Occasional tumours at many different sites	Prevents the formation of tetramers of p53
Multiplication of the MDM2 gene in the genome	Sarcomas, brain	Extra MDM2 stimulates the degradation of p53
Viral infection	Cervix, liver, lymphomas	Products of viral oncogenes bind to and inactivate p53 in the cell, in some cases stimulating p53 degradation
Deletion of the p14ARF gene	Breast, brain, lung and others, especially when p53 itself is not mutated	Failure to inhibit MDM2 and keep p53 degradation under control
Mislocalization of p53 to the cytoplasm, outside the nucleus	Breast, neuroblastomas	Lack of p53 function (p53 functions only in the nucleus)

FIGURE 15.4 The many ways in which p53 may malfunction in human cancers. (Reprinted by permission from Macmillan Publishers Ltd: Vogelstein B, Lane D, Levine AJ. Surfing the p53 network. *Nature.* 2000;408:307–310.)

He found that in certain families, there was an autosomal dominant inheritance of Rb. From his observation, Knudson generated the two-hit hypothesis—in order for the cancer phenotype to occur in humans, both copies of the gene had to be lost secondary to mutation. In those families with autosomal dominant Rb, a germ-line mutation in the Rb gene was present and, therefore, only a single additional somatic mutation was necessary to result in the cancer phenotype.

Arguably, the most significant gene in cancer research due to its mutation in the majority of human cancers is the TSG p53. The gene was first described in 1979 but originally thought to be an oncogene. A decade later, p53 was shown to be a TSG. See Figure 15.4 for the many ways in which p53 may malfunction in human cancers.

TSGs can be categorized into two broad groups, termed *gatekeepers* and *caretakers* by Vogelstein and Kinzler. Gatekeepers are TSGs that directly regulate cell growth and death. Examples of gatekeepers include the adenomatous polyposis coli (APC) gene and the Rb gene. On the other hand, caretakers are generally involved in the maintenance of genomic stability. Alterations to caretaker genes lead to the accumulation of mutations in other genes, including the activation of oncogenes or loss of gatekeeper TSGs. Examples of caretaker TSGs include mismatch repair genes in hereditary nonpolyposis colon cancer (HNPCC) and nucleotide excision repair (NER) genes in xeroderma pigmentosum (XP).

Inheritance of mutations in TSGs predisposes to the development of cancer phenotypes. As such, numerous familial cancer syndromes have since been identified that result from germ-line mutations; examples are listed in Table 15.2.

Environmental Factors

Multiple environmental factors have been shown to increase risk of cancer development in humans. These exogenous factors include physical, chemical, viral, and dietary carcinogens.

Physical Carcinogens

Radiation, in the form of either ionizing radiation or ultraviolet (UV) light, is a clinically significant environmental carcinogen. The toxicity of ionizing radiation was recognized after noting a high incidence of leukemia in radiation workers. Subsequent studies have demonstrated a clear role of ionizing radiation as a "universal carcinogen" capable of inducing tumor formation in a variety of human tissues. Exposure to ionizing radiation occurs from naturally occurring radioisotopes as well as man-made sources. Not to be minimized is the contribution from medical intervention, and it must be considered in the clinical decision-making process.

The induction of double-stranded DNA breaks (DSBs) is the principal mechanism for the mutagenic effects of ionizing radiation. Patients with ataxia-telangiectasia (A-T) are extremely sensitive to the effects of ionizing radiation due to a defect in their DNA repair mechanism. These patients often develop fatal complications after conventional radiation doses and are prone to developing lymphoreticular malignancies at a young age. The genetic defect in A-T is in the ataxia-telangiectasia mutated (ATM) gene that senses DSBs and is responsible for facilitating the DNA repair mechanism. The result is lack of DNA repair prior to initiation of the next cell cycle and propagation of genetic defects.

Striking examples of the impact of ionizing radiation on cancer rates and genetic mutation can be seen in epidemiologic studies of populations who have been exposed to large doses of radiation, including inhabitants of the areas surrounding Chernobyl and survivors of the atomic bombs in Hiroshima and Nagasaki. Studies of children born in Belarus following the Chernobyl accident demonstrate an increased frequency of germ-line mutations that was directly related to the amount of parental radiation exposure. Ionizing radiation has also been shown to be a risk factor in the development of several other malignancies including papillary thyroid cancer, sarcoma, breast cancer, and lymphoma.

UV light has also been implicated in carcinogenesis, contributing to the development of nonmelanocytic skin cancers. UVA, UVB, and UVC light have all been shown to induce DNA damage by via pyrimidine dimerization. Support for an association between UV light and skin cancer comes from studies of patients with XP. Patients with XP have a defect in nucleotide excision repair (NER) genes that prevents excision of UV-induced pyrimidine dimers and, thus, have a significantly increased incidence of skin cancers.

TABLE 15.2 Germ-Line and somatic mutations in TSGs and functions of the tumor suppressor proteins

Gene	Associated Inherited Cancer Syndrome	Cancers with Somatic Mutations	Presumed Function of Protein
RB1	Familial Rb	Rb, osteosarcoma, SCLC, breast, prostate, bladder, pancreas, esophageal, others	Transcriptional regulator E2F binding
TP53	Li–Fraumeni syndrome	~50% of all cancers (rare in some types, such as prostate carcinoma and neuroblastoma)	Transcription factor; regulates cell cycle and apoptosis
P16/INK4A	Familial melanoma, familial pancreatic carcinoma	25%–30% of many different cancer types (e.g., breast, lung, pancreatic, bladder)	Cyclin-dependent kinase inhibitor (i.e., cdk4 and cdk6)
P14^{Arf}(p19^{Arf})	Familial melanoma?	~15% of many different cancer types	Regulates Mdm-2 protein stability and hence p53 stability; alternative reading frame of *p16/INK4A* gene
APC	FAP coli, Gardner syndrome, Turcot syndrome	Colorectal, desmoid tumors	Regulates levels of *b*-catenin protein in the cytosol; binding to microtubules
WT-1	WAGR, Denys–Drash syndrome	Wilms tumor	Transcription factor
NF-1	Neurofibromatosis type 1	Melanoma, neuroblastoma	p21 ras-GTPase
NF-2	Neurofibromatosis type 2	Schwannoma, meningioma, ependymoma	Juxtamembrane link to cytoskeleton
VHL	von Hippel–Lindau syndrome	Renal (clear cell type), hemangioblastoma	Regulator of protein stability (e.g., HIF-α)
BRCA1	Inherited breast and ovarian cancer	Ovarian (~10%), rare in breast cancer	DNA repair; complexes with Rad 51 and BRCA2; transcriptional regulation
BRCA2	Inherited breast (both female and male), pancreatic cancer, others?	Rare mutations in pancreatic, others?	DNA repair; complexes with Rad 51 and BRCA1
MEN-1	Multiple endocrine neoplasia type 1	Parathyroid adenoma, pituitary adenoma, endocrine tumors of the pancreas	Not known
PTCH	Gorlin syndrome, hereditary basal cell carcinoma syndrome	Basal cell skin carcinoma, medulloblastoma	Transmembrane receptor for sonic hedgehog factor; negative regulator of smoothened protein
PTEN/ MMAC1	Cowden syndrome; sporadic cases of juvenile polyposis syndrome	Glioma, breast, prostate, follicular thyroid, carcinoma, and head and neck squamous carcinoma	Phosphoinositide 3-phosphatase; protein tyrosine phosphatase
DPC4	Familial juvenile polyposis syndrome	Pancreatic (~50%), 10%–15% of colorectal cancers, rare in others	Transcriptional factor in TGF-β signaling pathway
E-CAD	Familial diffuse-type gastric cancer	Gastric (diffuse type), lobular breast carcinoma, rare in other types (e.g., ovarian)	Cell–CAM
LKB1/STK1	Peutz–Jeghers syndrome	Rare in colorectal, not known in others	Serine/threonine protein kinase
EXT1	Hereditary multiple exostoses	Not known	Glycosyltransferase; heparan sulfate chain elongation
EXT2	Hereditary multiple exostoses	Not known	Glycosyltransferase; heparan sulfate chain elongation
TSC1	Tuberous sclerosis	Not known	Not known; cytoplasmic vesicle localization
TSC2	Tuberous sclerosis	Not known	Putative GTPase-activating protein F or Rap1 and rab5; Golgi localization
MSH2, MLH1, PMS1, PMS2, MSH6	Hereditary nonpolyposis colorectal cancer	Colorectal, gastric, endometrial cancer	DNA mismatch repair

From Butel JS. Viral carcinogenesis: revelation of molecular mechanisms and etiology of human disease. *Carcinogenesis.* 2000;21:415, with permission.

Chemical Carcinogens

Numerous chemical carcinogens have been identified, with tobacco being one of the most well known. Tobacco consumption has clearly been shown to be a risk factor for lung cancer, with approximately 90% of lung cancers in men and 80% in women attributed to its use. The duration and amount of tobacco use have been shown to affect the risk of developing lung cancer, with cessation of smoking resulting in a considerable decrease in mortality from lung cancer. Numerous carcinogens are present in tobacco smoke, so it is difficult to determine the relative potency of each of these agents; they include polycyclic aromatic hydrocarbons, nitrosamine 4-(*N*-nitrosomethyl-amino)-1-(3-pyridyl)-1-butanone, and free radicals. Other malignancies associated with tobacco use include cancers of the oropharynx, esophagus, pancreas, kidney, and bladder.

Occupational chemical exposures have also been shown to be carcinogenic including exposure to asbestos, benzene, and aromatic amines. The association between pleural mesothelioma and asbestos exposure has been demonstrated following both occupational and household exposure. Recent estimates predict that mortality from mesothelioma will be approximately 250,000 in the next 35 years. Although the use of asbestos in developed countries has decreased considerably, there continues to be a significant use of this material in developing countries.

Dietary Carcinogens

Dietary constituents and nutrition have also been implicated in carcinogenesis. Alcohol consumption has been shown to be associated with multiple cancers, including those of the oropharynx, esophagus, and liver. This increased cancer risk is directly related to the amount of alcohol intake. An example of a dietary toxin, aflatoxin is produced by *Aspergillus parasiticus* and *Aspergillus flavus* and can be found as contaminants in food. These toxins are most prevalent in Southeast Asia and sub-Saharan Africa and have been shown to induce hepatocellular carcinoma. Additionally, high salt intake is associated with an increased risk of nasopharyngeal cancer and gastric cancer. In gastric cancer, high doses of salt may disrupt the protective mucin layer in the stomach, thereby exposing the underlying epithelial cells to damage. This leads to increased epithelial proliferation in the stomach, which increases the potential for mutation. In addition, salted foods are often also smoked, which increases their carcinogenicity. Nitrosamines, which are present in foods as preservatives or generated in the stomach from nitrites, have been found to be associated with cancers of the esophagus, stomach, bladder, and colon. More recently, heterocyclic amines (HCAs) have been identified in meat and other proteinaceous foods that have been exposed to open flames. HCAs are known carcinogens that can induce cancers of the breast, colon, liver, prostate, skin, and lymphoid tissue.

In addition to the carcinogenic effects of dietary constituents, the amount and type of food consumed also influence the development of cancer. Diets high in animal fats have been linked to an increased risk of breast and colon cancers. Additionally, low intake of fruits and vegetables has been associated with cancers of the upper digestive tract, stomach, and lung. Conversely, diets rich in antioxidant vitamins may be associated with decreased cancer risk, although this remains controversial.

Viral Carcinogens

Although a causal role for viruses in human cancer was initially rejected, several human cancers have since been shown to be induced by viral pathogens. Viral carcinogenesis in humans generally results from infection with either non-transforming retroviruses, such as human T-lymphotropic virus 1 (HTLV-1), or DNA tumor viruses, such as hepatitis B virus (HBV), Epstein–Barr virus (EBV), human herpesvirus 8, human papillomavirus (HPV), and polyomavirus. For example, through transcriptome analysis, a polyomavirus was recently linked to Merkel cell carcinoma, a rare but highly aggressive cutaneous malignancy. Additionally, the RNA tumor virus hepatitis C virus (HCV) has also been implicated in hepatocellular carcinoma. In fact, approximately 15% of all human cancers are virally induced with the majority represented by cervical and hepatocellular carcinomas. These cancers are seen with increased frequency in developing countries where the incidence of HPV, HBV, and HCV infection remains high. Table 15.3 summarizes properties of accepted and potential human tumor viruses.

Host Factors

Immune Dysregulation

The increased incidence of malignancies in patients following bone marrow or solid organ transplantation, as well as in patients with inherited or acquired immune deficiencies, that is, AIDS, suggests a role for the immune system in the destruction of cancerous cells. Of note, several of these cancers appear to be due to virally-mediated carcinogenesis and respond to decreases in immunosuppressive therapy. Posttransplantation lymphoproliferative disorders (PTLDs) and Hodgkin's disease are related to EBV infection in the majority of cases. In addition, HHV-8 also appears to be a causative agent in the development of Kaposi sarcoma in patients following solid organ transplantation, with an incidence up to 500 times the general population. Although there is also an increased incidence of other solid tumors in patients following transplantation including skin, oropharyngeal, and bone cancers, the role of the immune system in preventing them remains elusive.

Patients with HIV and AIDS have a significantly increased risk of developing several malignancies. In fact, three malignant conditions are now considered AIDS-defining illnesses in an HIV+ individual: Kaposi sarcoma, non-Hodgkin's lymphomas (NHLs), and invasive cervical cancer. Virally mediated carcinogenesis is heavily implicated in the pathogenesis of all three malignancies. As noted earlier, HHV-8 has been shown to be a causative agent for all forms of Kaposi sarcoma. The majority of large B-cell and primary central nervous system lymphomas in HIV-infected patients are associated with EBV infection. In addition, persistent HPV infection is found in a greater number of HIV-infected women, which may account for the increased incidence of invasive cervical cancer in this population.

Hormonal Dysregulation

Several malignancies can be categorized as partially influenced by endogenous hormones, including carcinomas of the breast, endometrium, ovary, testicle, prostate, and thyroid. These tumors share a common mechanism of carcinogenesis in which elevated or unopposed hormone levels induce cellular proliferation, eventually leading to the development of a malignant phenotype.

Hormone-mediated mechanisms appear to play an important role in the development of breast and prostate cancers, the most

TABLE 15.3 Properties of accepted and potential human tumor viruses

Characteristic	HBV	EBV	HPV	HTLV-1	HCV	HHV-8 (KSHV)	SV40	MCV
Genome								
Nucleic acid	dsDNA[a]	dsDNA	dsDNA	SsRNA → dsDNA	ssRNA	dsDNA	dsDNA	dsDNA
Size (kb/kbp)	3.2	172	8	9.0	9.4	165	5.2	190
No. genes	4	≈90	8–10	6	9	≈90	6	≈180
Cell tropism	Hepatocytes, white blood cells	Oropharyngeal epithelial cells, B cells	Squamous epithelial cells (mucosal, cutaneous)	T cells	Hepatocytes	Vascular endothelial cells, lymphocytes	Kidney epithelial cells, others	Epidermal cells
Unique biology	May cause chronic infection and inflammation	Immortalizes B cells	Highly species and tissue specific, replication dependent on cell differentiation	Immortalizes T cells, encodes trans-acting factor	High rate of chronic infection and inflammation	Contains many cellular genes	Stimulates cell DNA synthesis	Species and tissue specific
Prevalence of infection	Chronic infections common— Asia, Africa	Common	Common	Common—Japan, Caribbean	Common	Not ubiquitous	—	—
Transmission	Vertical, parenteral, horizontal, venereal	Saliva	Venereal, skin abrasions	Breast milk, parenteral	Parenteral, horizontal	Horizontal, venereal	Urine?	Contact, venereal
Human diseases	Hepatitis, cirrhosis	IM, oral hairy leukoplakia	Skin warts, EV, genital warts, LP	HAM/TSP	Hepatitis, cirrhosis	—	—	—
Human cancers	HCC	BL[b], NPC[c], HD, lymphomas	Cervical, skin, oropharynx	ATL	HCC	KS, PEL, Castleman disease	Brain, bone, mesothelioma	MC
Transforming genes	HBx	LMP-1	E6, E7	Tax	NS3, NS4B, NS5A	—	Large T antigen, small t antigen	—
Viral genome integrated in human tumors	Usually		Usually	Yes (provirus)	No	—	—	No

[a]Partially double-stranded (ds) and partially single-stranded (ss) in virion.

[b]Equatorial Africa—endemic; elsewhere—sporadic.

[c]Southeast Asia—common.

HBV, hepatitis B virus; EBV, Epstein–Barr virus; HPV, human papilloma virus; HTLV-1, human T lymphotropic virus 1; HCV, Hepatitis C virus; HHV-8, human herpes virus 8; SV40, simian virus 40; MCV, molluscum contagiosum virus; EV, echo virus; HD, Hodgkin's disease; IM, infectious mononucleosis; KS, Kaposi sarcoma; LP, laryngeal papilloma; MC, molluscum contagiosum; PEL, primary effusion lymphoma; HAM/TSP, HTLV-1-associated myelopathy/tropical spastic paraparesis; BL, Burkitt lymphoma; NPC, nasopharyngeal carcinoma.

From Butel JS. Viral carcinogenesis: revelation of molecular mechanisms and etiology of human disease. *Carcinogenesis.* 2000;21:415, with permission.

TABLE 15.4 Summary of the strength of epidemiologic evidence for association between physical activity or obesity and cancer risk

	Sedentary Lifestyle	Obesity
Breast, postmenopausal	+++	+++
Colon	+++	+++
Endometrium	+	+++
Esophagus, adenocarcinoma	?	+++
Kidney, renal cell	?	+++
Pancreas	?	++
Gallbladder	?	++
Non-Hodgkin's lymphoma	?	+
Prostate, aggressive	++	+
Lung	+	?
Ovary	?	?

From DeVita VT, Lawrence TS, Rosenberg SA, eds. *Cancer: Principles and Practice of Oncology*. 8th ed. Philadelphia: Lippincott Williams & Wilkins; 2008:243.

common malignancies in women and men in the United States, respectively. The role of estrogens in breast cancer has been established in epidemiologic and clinical studies. Increased exposure to estrogen may result from early menarche, late menopause, nulliparity, obesity, alcohol consumption, and hormone replacement therapy. Epidemiologic studies have demonstrated that postmenopausal women who develop breast cancer have mean estradiol serum concentrations that are 15% higher than those in unaffected women. In addition, hormone replacement therapy in postmenopausal women has been shown to increase the risk of breast cancer. Similarly, elevated levels of testosterone have been shown to increase the risk of developing prostate cancer in men.

Obesity and Physical Activity

Convincing evidence is accumulating for the increased association of obesity and sedentary lifestyle with cancer. Although an interdependent relationship exists, the two factors must not be considered as one entity. The steroid hormone and insulin-like growth factor (IGF) pathways are two global mechanisms implicated in the role of carcinogenesis. Not to be understated, the prevalence of obesity, defined as body mass index (BMI) greater than 30 kg/m^2, is at epidemic levels in the United States. Epidemiologic evidence for the role of physical activity or obesity in relation to cancer exists for carcinomas of the breast, colon, endometrium, esophagus, and kidney. See Table 15.4 for the strength of epidemiologic evidence for association between physical activity or obesity and cancer risk.

TUMOR PHENOTYPE

Although many genetic, environmental, and host factors influence the process of carcinogenesis, not every cell exposed to these insults will become transformed and proliferate. In fact, the majority of transforming events are lethal to the cell. Of those that do survive, a large number of cells will undergo terminal differentiation. Tumors are only able to develop after a transformed cell results in a clonal population. Transformed cells acquire phenotypic, biochemical, and immunologic characteristics that distinguish them from wild-type cells (Fig. 15.5). These characteristics include changes in cell

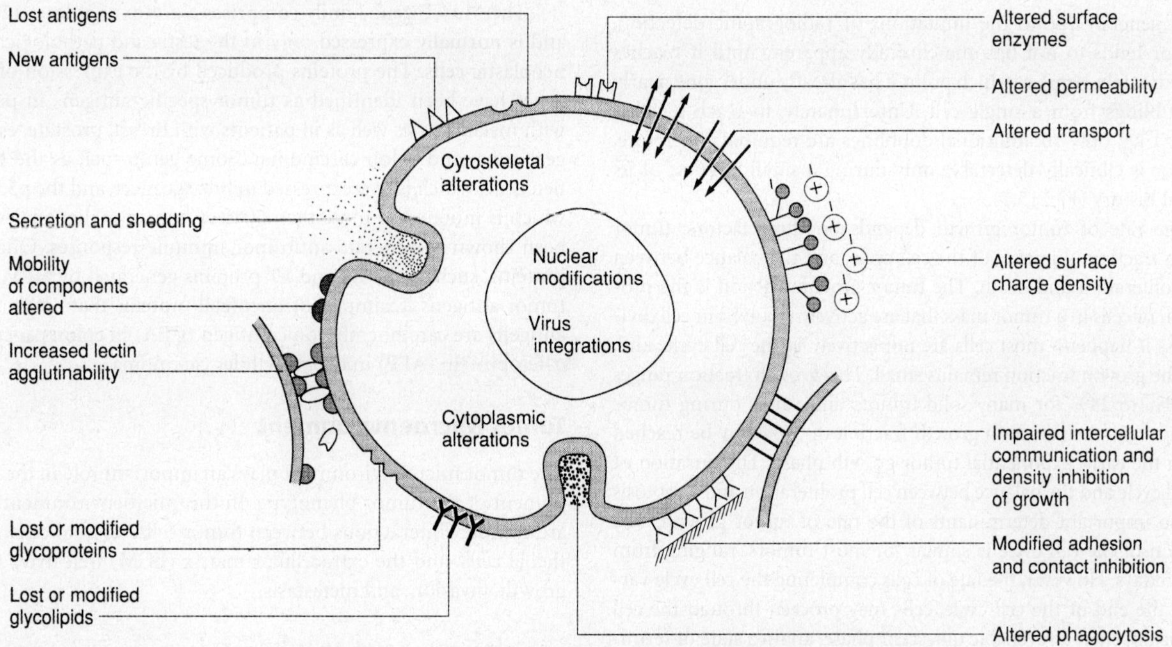

FIGURE 15.5 Alterations of cell structure and function that have been noted with neoplastic transformation. (From Ellis LM, Jones Jr DV, Chiao PJ, et al. Tumor biology. In: Greenfield, LJ, Mulholland MW, Oldham KT, et al. *Surgery: Scientific Principles and Practice*. 2nd ed. Philadelphia: Lippincott–Raven Publishers; 1997:465; Figure 4-3.)

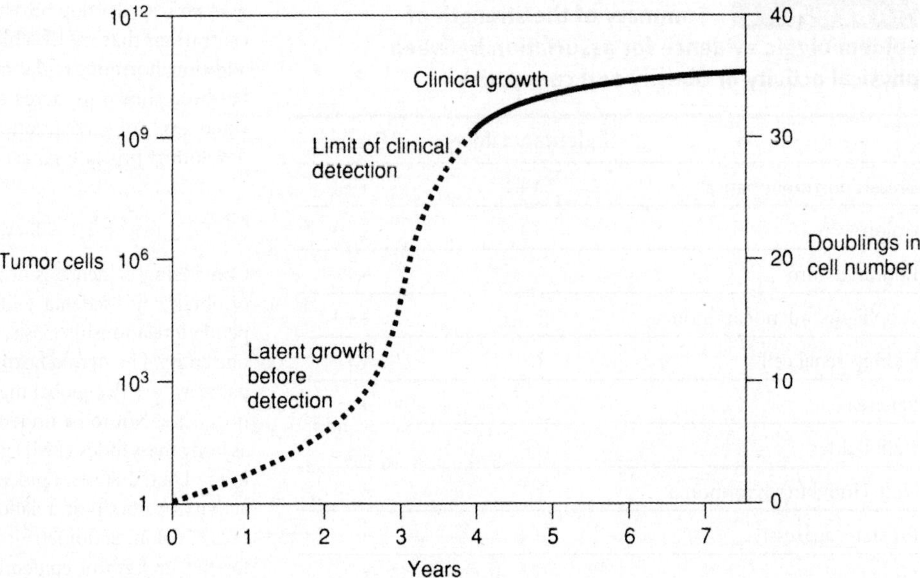

FIGURE 15.6 Theoretical growth curve for human tumors. Growth rates slow as tumors approach lethal mass. (From Ellis LM, Jones Jr DV, Chiao PJ, et al. Tumor biology. In: Greenfield, LJ, Mulholland MW, Oldham KT, et al. *Surgery: Scientific Principles and Practice*. 2nd ed. Philadelphia: Lippincott–Raven Publishers; 1997:467.)

surface receptors and antigens, disordered cytoskeletal arrangements, nuclear and cellular polymorphism, karyotypic changes, and increased antigenicity.

Growth Characteristics

In the 1960s, A.K. Laird modeled the growth of a tumor as a Gompertz function—portraying tumor growth as exponential with a shortening of the doubling time as the tumor grows. However, it must be noted that exponential growth only occurs when nutrients do not play a limiting factor. As a tumor grows, it outstrips its blood supply and nutrition, therefore, displaying a deceleration of growth (Fig. 15.6).

In general, due to the limitations of radiographic detection, a tumor tends to not become clinically apparent until it reaches approximately 1 cm^3, at which point it has already undergone nearly 30 doublings from a single cell. Unfortunately, to reach a lethal size of 1 kg, only 10 additional doublings are required. Therefore, a tumor is clinically detectable only during a small fraction of its natural history (Fig. 15.7).

The rate of tumor growth depends on three factors: tumor growth fraction, duration of the cell cycle, and the balance between cell proliferation and death. The tumor growth fraction is the proportion of cells in a tumor mass that are actively involved in cell division. As it happens, most cells are not actively in the cell cycle, and, thus, the growth fraction remains small. This growth fraction ranges from 4% to 24% for many solid tumors and varies during tumor development. A maximum growth fraction of 37% may be reached during the early, exponential tumor growth phase. The duration of the cell cycle and the balance between cell proliferation and apoptosis are also important determinants of the rate of tumor growth. The duration of the cell cycle is similar for most tumors, ranging from 2 to 4.5 days. However, the fate of cells completing the cell cycle varies. At the end of the cell cycle, cells may proceed through the cell cycle again, enter a reversible quiescent phase, attain a state of terminal differentiation, or undergo programmed cell death. In neoplastic tissues, an imbalance between continued proliferation and cell loss or terminal differentiation occurs leading to continued tumor growth.

Tumor Antigens

Numerous types of tumor antigens have been identified and can be grouped into several categories: (i) antigens that are expressed in both normal and neoplastic cells derived from the same tissue but that elicit a host immune response only when expressed in tumor cells; (ii) antigens that are expressed only in immune-privileged areas of the testis and in certain neoplastic cells; (iii) antigens that are derived from the overexpression of certain genes or from gene mutations; (iv) antigens that are generated from oncoviral proteins; and (v) oncofetal proteins that are overexpressed in neoplastic tissues. Immunotherapy strategies that target these specific tumor antigens are being developed in an effort to generate high levels of specific antitumor reactivity.

The MAGE gene family comprises a group of at least 12 genes and is normally expressed only in the testis and pathologically by neoplastic cells. The proteins produced by the expression of these genes have been identified as tumor-specific antigens in patients with melanoma as well as in patients with breast, prostate, esophageal, lung, and colon carcinomas. Some genes such as the HER2/neu gene, which is overexpressed in breast cancer, and the p53 gene, which is mutated in more than 50% of human malignancies, have been shown to generate antitumor immune responses. Oncoviral proteins, such as the E6 and E7 proteins generated by HPV, act as tumor antigens. Examples of oncofetal proteins that act as tumor antigens are carcinoembryonic antigen (CEA) in colon cancer and α-fetoprotein (AFP) in hepatocellular carcinoma.

Tumor Microenvironment

The tumor microenvironment plays an important role in the development of the tumor phenotype. In this microenvironment, there are complex interactions between tumor cells, stromal cells, endothelial cells, and the extracellular matrix (ECM) that drive tumor growth, invasion, and metastasis.

Growth Factors and Apoptosis

The uncontrolled cellular proliferation of tumor cells results from a combination of activation of growth stimulatory signals and

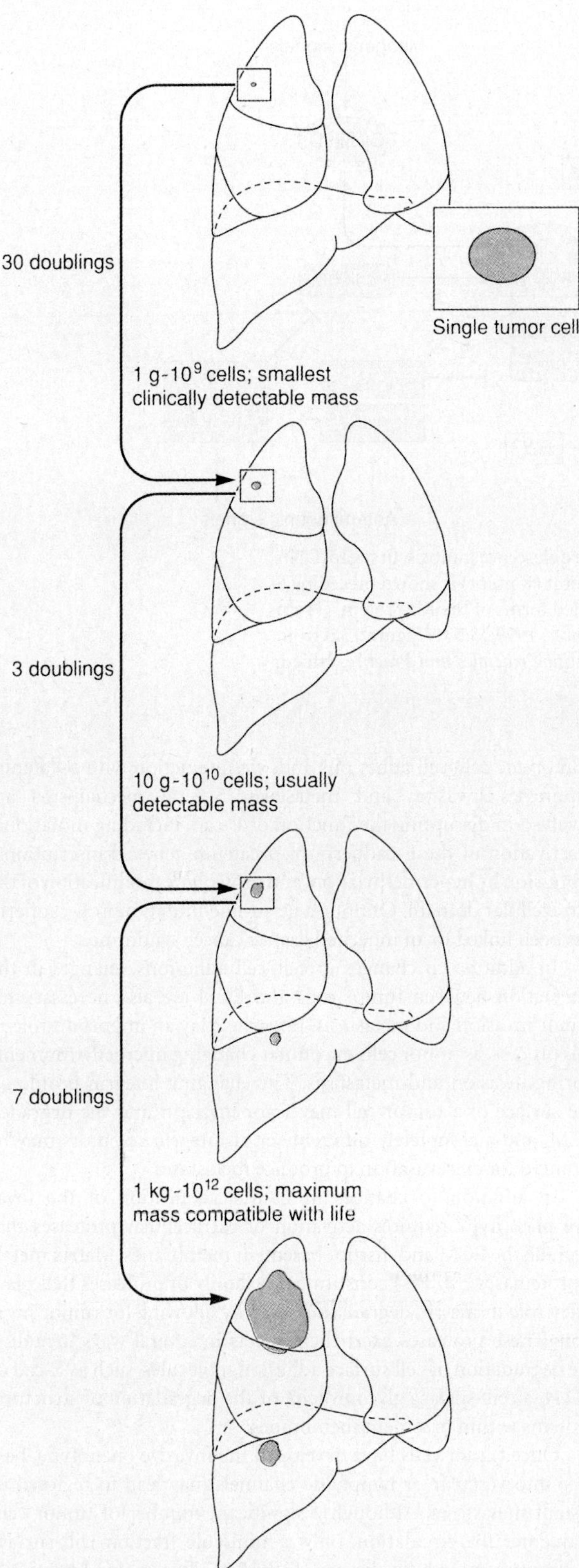

FIGURE 15.7 Growth of a solid tumor from a single transformed cell into a lethal tumor mass. (From Ellis LM, Jones Jr DV, Chiao PJ, et al. Tumor biology. In: Greenfield, LJ, Mulholland MW, Oldham KT, et al. *Surgery: Scientific Principles and Practice*. 2nd ed. Philadelphia: Lippincott–Raven Publishers; 1997:466.)

evasion of growth inhibitory signals. Tumor cells develop autonomous growth signaling mechanisms that circumvent normal growth checkpoints. Many oncogene products have been identified that are involved in growth signaling pathways including growth factors, growth factor receptors, or mitogenic signal transduction molecules. These oncogenes induce cellular proliferation by autonomous production of growth factors with autocrine stimulation, overexpression of growth factor receptors, and deregulation of mitogenic signal transduction pathways. One example of this is the HER2/neu growth factor receptor that is overexpressed in breast cancer and ovarian cancer.

In addition to growth stimulatory signals, tumor cells develop mechanisms that block growth inhibitory and differentiation signals. The most commonly affected growth inhibitory pathway is the phosphorylated retinoblastoma (pRb) pathway, which controls the majority of cellular antiproliferative signals. When Rb is in a hypophosphorylated state, cell progression from G1 to S phase is blocked by interaction of Rb with the E2F transcription factor, thereby preventing cellular proliferation (Fig. 15.8). As it so happens, the pRb pathway may be affected in multiple ways including direct mutation of the Rb gene, sequestering of pRb by viral oncoproteins, mutations in the expression of cyclin-dependent kinases that phosphorylate Rb, and decreased production of transforming growth factor-β (TGF-β) receptors that block phosphorylation of Rb. In addition, cells may downregulate cell surface receptors such as integrins that produce growth inhibitory signals, favoring cell proliferation.

Although normal tissue growth is controlled through balanced cell proliferation and death, tumor cells develop mechanisms to evade apoptosis in response to intracellular and extracellular abnormalities such as DNA damage, activation of oncogenes, and hypoxia. These mechanisms include increased expression of antiapoptotic proteins, such as members of the Bcl-2 family, and mutations in genes involved in the apoptotic pathway, such as p53. The p53 TSG is involved in apoptosis through up-regulation of proapoptotic proteins in response to DNA damage.

Angiogenesis

The importance of angiogenesis in tumor growth and metastasis was elucidated by Judah Folkman in the 1970s, following the observation that the delivery of nutrients and growth factors is required to sustain tumor growth. Without neovascularization, tumors fail to grow beyond a few millimeters. Numerous endogenous proangiogenic and antiangiogenic factors have been identified, and it is the balance between these factors that is thought to be important in controlling angiogenesis (Tables 15.5 and 15.6). At some point during tumor development, an "angiogenic switch" occurs, favoring proangiogenic factors. This may result from an increase in proangiogenic factors such as vascular endothelial growth factor (VEGF) or basic fibroblast growth factor (bFGF) or from a decrease in antiangiogenic factors such as thrombospondin-1 (TSP-1). Regardless, the end result is neovascularization leading to tumor growth and metastasis.

Due to the dependence of tumor growth on angiogenesis, numerous targeted therapies have developed revolving around inhibition of blood vessel formation. These agents function by either inhibiting proangiogenic factors (e.g., anti-VEGF antibodies) or increasing antiangiogenic factors (e.g., angiostatin and endostatin). The first and one of the more well-known angiogenesis inhibitors

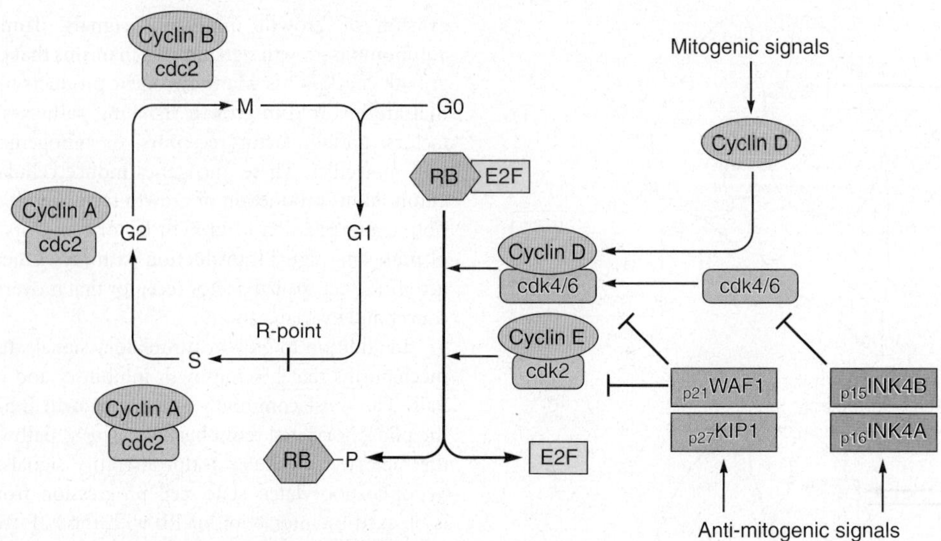

FIGURE 15.8 The cell cycle clock machinery. G0, M, G1, S, and G2 refer to the quiescence, mitosis, first gap, DNA synthesis, and second gap phase of the cell cycle, respectively. The restriction point (R point) is shown preceding S phase entry. RB and RB-p represent unphosphorylated and hyperphosphorylated forms of the RB protein. (From Lundberg AS, Weinberg RA. Control of the cell cycle and apoptosis. *Eur J Cancer*. 1999;35:531. Figure 13.6 from Greenfield, LJ, Mulholland MW, Lillemoe KD, et al. *Greenfield's Surgery: Scientific Principles and Practice*. 4th ed. Philadelphia: Lippincott Williams & Wilkins; 2006:298.)

is bevacizumab, a monoclonal antibody that specifically recognizes and binds to VEGF. When VEGF is attached to bevacizumab, it is unable to activate the VEGF receptor. It has been approved to be used alone for glioblastoma that has not responded to other treatments and to be used in combination with other drugs to treat metastatic colorectal cancer, some non-small cell lung cancers, and metastatic renal cell cancer.

Invasion and Metastasis

Tumors consist of heterogeneous populations of cells that vary in their growth rates, production of growth factors, stimulation of angiogenesis, and receptor expression. In addition, these heterogeneous cell populations have different propensities to metastasize. The hallmark of the invasive phenotype is the ability to cross the basement membrane. To develop this ability, several additional characteristics must be acquired by tumor cells that result in changes in cell–cell adhesions and cell–ECM interactions. In a well-described biologic process known as epithelial–mesenchymal transition (EMT), a polarized epithelial cell with basal attachment to the basement membrane acquires mesenchymal traits, including migratory capacity, invasiveness, and production of stromal elements. Pathologic adaptation of this pathway can result in aggressive metastatic capability. For instance, perturbations in *Slug* and *Snail*, known modulators of EMT, are associated with aggressive metastases in transformed melanocytes.

Several classes of cell surface proteins are involved in cell–cell adhesions and cell–ECM interactions including the cell adhesion molecules (CAMs) of the cadherin, immunoglobulin, and integrin superfamilies. Changes in cell surface expression of these receptors enable tumor cells to invade the stromal compartment and to eventually metastasize. One important cell surface receptor that loses its function in numerous epithelial cancers is epithelial cadherin (E-cad). E-cad is a transmembrane glycoprotein that mediates homotypic cell–cell adhesions and, via interaction with β-catenin, suppresses invasion and metastasis. Several mechanisms are involved in disrupting the function of E-cad, including mutational inactivation of the E-cadherin or β-catenin genes, transcriptional repression by hypermethylation, and proteolytic modification of the extracellular domain. Of note, a germ-line mutation in E-cadherin has been linked to an inherited gastric cancer syndrome.

In addition to changes in cell–cell adhesions, changes in the interaction between tumor cells and ECM are also necessary for tumor invasion and metastasis. Integrins play an important role in this process, as tumor cells encounter changing microenvironments during invasion and metastasis. The changing integrin profile on the surface of a tumor cell may favor invasion into the degraded ECM, and a completely different set of integrin receptors may be required for extravasation to produce metastases.

In addition to changes in CAMs, acquisition of the invasive phenotype requires activation of extracellular proteases that degrade the ECM and disrupt basement membranes. Matrix metalloproteinases (MMPs) constitute one family of proteases that plays a key role in matrix degradation, thereby allowing for tumor invasion. These proteases exert their effects in several ways including the degradation of cell surface adhesion molecules, such as E-cad or CD44, a cell–surface glycoprotein, or the degradation of structural proteins within basement membranes.

Once tumor cells have developed the invasive phenotype, passage into vascular or lymphatic channels may lead to regional or distant metastases. Although a significant number of tumor cells may enter the circulation, only a miniscule fraction will survive to produce metastatic disease (Fig. 15.9). Two major hypotheses attempt to explain the organ distribution of metastases for various malignancies. The first hypothesis was proposed by J. Ewing who attributed the distribution mainly to mechanical and anatomic factors such as the structure of the vascular system. The second notion is the "seed and soil" theory proposed by Paget in 1889. On the basis

TABLE 15.5 **Proangiogenic growth factors**

Factor	Properties	Receptor	Study
VEGF—vascular permeability factor	Endothelial mitogen, survival factor, and permeability inducer produced by many types of tumor cells	Flk-1/KDR (VEGFR-2), Flt-1 (VEGFR-1) (both present on activated endothelium)	Veikkola et al. (2000)
Placental growth factor	Weak endothelial mitogen	Flt-1 (VEGFR-1)	Veikkola et al. (2000)
Basic fibroblast growth factor (bFGF/FGF-2)	Endothelial mitogen, angiogenesis inducer, and survival factor; inducer of Flk-1 expression	FGF-R1–4	Baird and Klagsbrun (1991), Gimenez-Gallego and Cuevas (1994)
Acidic fibroblast growth factor (aFGF/FGF-1)	Endothelial mitogen and angiogenesis inducer	FGF-R1–4	Baird and Klagsbrun (1991), Gimenez-Gallego and Cuevas (1994)
Fibroblast growth factor-3 (FGF-3/*int*-2)	Endothelial mitogen and angiogenesis inducer	FGF-R1–4	Baird and Klagsbrun (1991), Gimenez-Gallego and Cuevas (1991)
Fibroblast growth factor-4 (FGF-4/*hst*/K-FGF)	Endothelial mitogen and angiogenesis inducer	FGF-R1–4	Baird and Klagsbrun (1991), Gimenez-Gallego and Cuevas (1991)
TGF-α	Endothelial mitogen and angiogenesis inducer; inducer of VEGF expression	Epidermal growth factor-R	Schmitt and Soares (1999)
Epidermal growth factor (EGF)	Weak endothelial mitogen; inducer of VEGF expression	Epidermal growth factor-R	Mooradian and Diglio (1990)
Hepatocyte growth factor/ scatter factor (HGF/SF)	Endothelial mitogen, mitogen, and angiogenesis inducer	c-Met	Lamszus et al. (1999)
TGF-β	*In vivo*—acting angiogenesis inducer; endothelial growth inhibitor; inducer of VEGF expression	TGF-β–RI, II, III	Pepper (1997)
Tumor necrosis factor-α (TNF-α)	*In vivo*—acting angiogenesis inducer; endothelial mitogen (low concentrations) or inhibitor (at high concentrations); inducer of VEGF expression	TNF-R55	Yoshida et al. (1997)
Platelet-derived growth factor	Mitogen and motility factor for endothelial cells and fibroblasts; *in vivo*—acting angiogenesis inducer	Platelet-derived growth factor-R	Kuwabara et al. (1995)
Granulocyte colony–stimulating factor	*In vivo*—acting angiogenesis inducing factor with some mitogenic and mitogenic activity for endothelial cells	Granulocyte colony–stimulating factor	Bussolino et al. (1991)
IL-8	*In vivo*—acting, possibly indirect angiogenesis inducer	IL-8R present on endothelial cells remains uncertain.	Desbaillets et al. (1997)
Pleiotropin	Angiogenesis-inducing pleiotropic growth factor	Proteoglycan	Choudhuri et al. (1997)
Thymidine phosphorylase (TP)–platelet-derived endothelial cell growth factor (PD-ECGF)	*In vivo*—acting angiogenesis factor	Unknown	Takahashi et al. (1996)
Angiogenin	*In vivo*—acting angiogenesis inducer with RNAse activity	170-kDa angiogenin receptor	Hartmann et al. (1999)
Proliferin	35-kDa angiogenesis-inducing protein in mouse	Unknown	Jackson et al. (1994)

From Fidler IJ, Kerbel RS, Ellis LM. Biology of cancer: angiogenesis. In: DeVita VT, Hellman S, Rosenberg SA, eds. *Cancer: Principles and Practice of Oncology*. 6th ed. Philadelphia: Lippincott Williams & Wilkins; 2002:141, with permission.

TABLE 15.6 Endogenous inhibitors of angiogenesis

Name	Description	Study
TSP-1 and internal fragments of TSP-1	Large, modular (180-kDa) ECM protein	Tolsma et al. (1993)
Angiostatin	38-kDa fragment of plasminogen involving either kringle domains 1–3 or smaller kringle 5 fragments	O'Reilly et al. (1994)
Endostatin	20-kDa zinc-binding fragment of type XVIII collagen	O'Reilly et al. (1997)
Vasostatin	NH_2 terminal fragment (amino acids 1–80) of calreticulin	Pike et al. (1998)
VEGF inhibitor	174-amino acid protein with 20%–30% homology to tumor necrosis factor superfamily	Zhai et al. (1999)
Fragment of platelet factor-4	N-terminal fragment of platelet factor-4	Gupta et al. (1995)
Derivative of prolactin	16-kDa fragment of prolactin	Clapp et al. (1993)
Restin	NC10 domain of human collagen XV	Ramchandran et al. (1999)
Proliferin-related protein	Protein related to the proangiogenic molecule proliferin	Jackson et al. (1994)
SPARC cleavage product	Fragments of *s*ecreted *p*rotein, *a*cidic and *r*ich in *c*ysteine	Vasquez (1999)
Osteopontin cleavage product	Thrombin-generated fragment containing an RGD sequence	Sage (1999)
Interferon-α, interferon-β	Well-known antiviral proteins, may downregulate angiogenic factor expression	Ezekowitz et al. (1992)
METH-1 and METH-2	Proteins containing metalloprotease and thrombospondin domains and disintegrin domains in NH_2 terminus	Vasquez (1999), Sage (1999)
Angiopoietin-2	Antagonist of angiopoietin-1 that binds to Tie-2 receptor	Davis and Yankopoulos (1999), Maisonpierre et al. (1997)
Antithrombin III fragment	A fragment missing the carboxy-terminal loop of antithrombin III (a member of the serpin family)	O'Reilly et al. (1999)
Interferon-inducible protein-10	Up-regulated by interferon-γ and whose mechanism of antiangiogenic effect is unknown	Moore et al. (1998)

From Fidler IJ, Kerbel RS, Ellis LM. Biology of cancer: angiogenesis. In: DeVita VT, Hellman S, Rosenberg SA, eds. *Cancer: Principles and Practice of Oncology*. 6th ed. Philadelphia: Lippincott Williams & Wilkins; 2002:141, with permission.

of the organ distribution of specific metastases, Paget concluded that metastatic disease does not occur by chance and that specific tumors metastasize to specific organs where the microenvironment is favorable. Both ideas appear to have merit as colorectal cancer generally metastasizes to the regional lymph nodes first and then to the liver because of the organization of the draining vasculature and lymphatics of the colon. In contrast, ocular melanoma metastases are generally found in the liver without a clear lymphatic or hematogenous relationship.

TREATMENT MODALITIES

Historically, surgical resection was the only option in the treatment of cancer. Therefore, surgeons would perform extremely morbid, radical surgical procedures in an effort to completely eradicate disease. However, with an increasing understanding of cancer biology and the recognition of residual microscopic disease, the focus of cancer therapy has shifted from radical surgical options in favor of multimodal therapy. Included in the spectrum of treatment modalities are chemotherapy, radiotherapy, immunotherapy, biotherapy, cancer vaccines, gene therapy, and nanotechnology. The multimodal approach to oncologic therapy has generally resulted in improved survival while minimizing the morbidity and mortality.

Principles of Surgical Oncology

The role of surgical oncologists in the diagnosis and staging of malignancies has decreased with the development of more sensitive cross-sectional and nuclear imaging techniques, as well as minimally invasive diagnostic techniques such as core biopsy. For example, core biopsy of breast masses and soft tissue tumors has largely supplanted operative incisional biopsy. Surgical oncologists may still play a role in the prevention of cancer particularly in conditions with exceedingly high risk of malignancy. Examples include colectomy for familial adenomatous polyposis (FAP) or bilateral mastectomy for familial breast cancer syndromes. Additional conditions in which prophylactic surgery can prevent cancer are listed in Table 15.7. However, the principal role of surgical oncologists remains resection of primary cancers. In addition to providing local control, resection allows for tissue diagnosis and more accurate

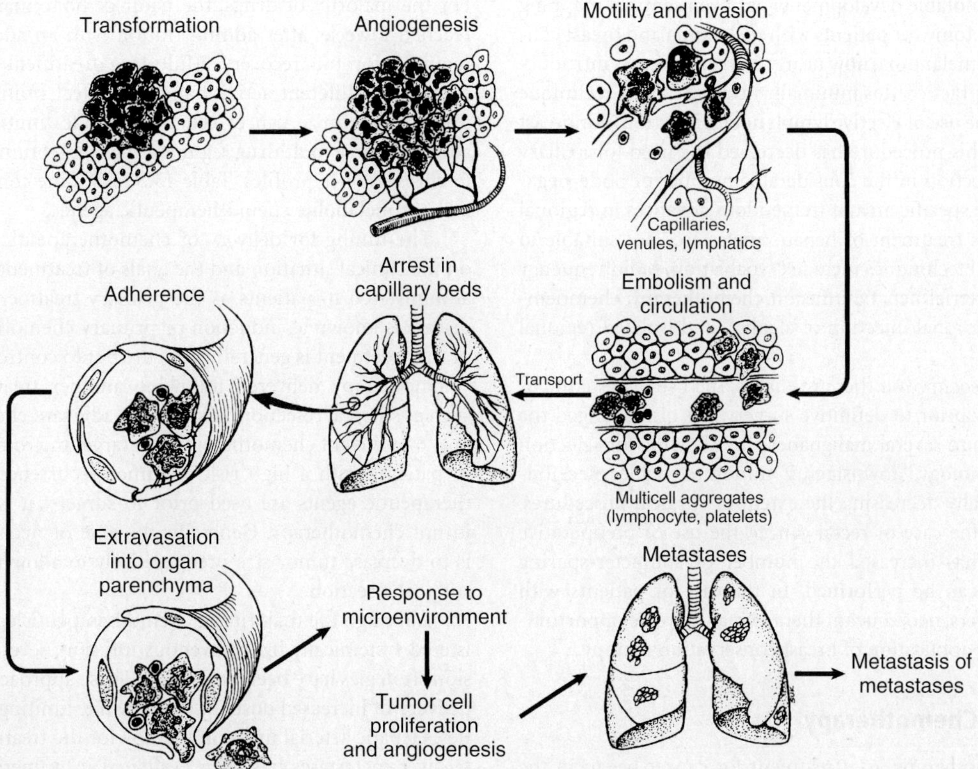

FIGURE 15.9 The pathogenesis of cancer metastasis. To produce metastases, tumor cells must detach from the primary tumor, invade the extracellular membrane and enter the circulation, survive in the circulation to arrest in the capillary bed, adhere to subendothelial basement membrane, gain entrance into the organ parenchyma, respond to paracrine growth factors, proliferate and induce angiogenesis, and evade host defenses. The pathogenesis of metastasis is, therefore, complex and consists of multiple sequential, selective, and interdependent steps, the outcome of which depends on the interaction of tumor cells with homeostatic factors. (From Stetler-Stevenson WG. Invasion and metastases. In: DeVita VT, Hellman S, Rosenberg SA, eds. *Cancer: Principles and Practice of Oncology*. 7th ed. Philadelphia: Lippincott Williams & Wilkins; 2005:117.)

TABLE 15.7 Conditions in which prophylactic surgery can prevent cancer

Underlying Condition	Associated Cancer	Prophylactic Surgery
Cryptorchidism	Testicular	Orchiopexy
FAP	Colon	Colectomy
HNPCC/Lynch syndrome	Colon	Colectomy
Ulcerative colitis	Colon	Colectomy
Multiple endocrine neoplasia types 2 and 3	Medullary cancer of the thyroid	Thyroidectomy
Familial breast cancer	Breast	Mastectomy
Familial ovarian cancer	Ovary	Oophorectomy

FAP, familial adenomatous polyposis; HNPCC, hereditary nonpolyposis colorectal cancer.

From DeVita VT, Lawrence TS, Rosenberg SA, eds. *Cancer: Principles and Practice of Oncology*. 8th ed. Philadelphia: Lippincott Williams & Wilkins; 2008:290.

staging of cancers. On many occasions, surgical intervention may be the only treatment indicated. Examples include wide local excision for thin melanoma and partial colectomy for early-stage colon cancer. In other cases, surgical resection may reveal metastasis to regional lymph nodes, for which the use of adjuvant chemotherapy may be recommended.

Operative indications may also include surgery for the resection of metastatic disease (metastasectomy) as well as palliative procedures. For example, hepatic resection for isolated colorectal liver metastases has been associated with significantly improved 5-year survival rates and the resection of pulmonary sarcoma metastases has been associated with long disease-free intervals in up to 30% of patients. Considerations for metastasectomy include number and size of metastatic lesions, location, histology and grade of the tumor, disease-free interval from treatment of the primary, and suitability of the patient for surgery. Surgical oncologists may also be able to provide palliative surgical options in cases of tumors causing bleeding or pain through a debulking or resection. For obstructions, entero-enteric or biliary-enteric bypasses can be performed to minimize symptoms.

Numerous advances in technology and surgical technique have been made in the field of surgical oncology in the last few decades. These advances include the use of diagnostic laparoscopy, intraoperative ultrasonography, and local therapies for metastatic disease.

One of the most notable developments has been sentinel mapping and lymphadenectomy for patients with melanoma and breast cancer. In the case of melanoma, now nearly 25 years since its introduction into clinical practice, this minimally invasive staging technique has supplanted the use of elective lymph node dissection. For breast cancer patients, this procedure has decreased the need for axillary lymph node dissection in the considerable number of node-negative patients. One specific area of tremendous advances in regional therapies involves treatment of hepatic metastases not suitable to resection. Utilized techniques include cryoablation, radiofrequency ablation, intra-arterial hepatic infusion chemotherapy, chemoembolization, intralesional injection of alcohol, and isolated regional perfusion.

The use of *neoadjuvant* therapy, that is, the use of systemic or radiation therapy prior to definitive surgery, has also changed the surgical approach to several malignancies by allowing for selection based on tumor biology, "downstaging" tumors to enable resectability, and occasionally decreasing the extent of surgical procedures. For example, in the case of rectal cancer, the use of preoperative chemoradiation has increased the number of sphincter-sparing procedures that can be performed. In the case of patients with larger breast cancers, neoadjuvant therapy may increase opportunities for successful application of breast conservation therapy.

Principles of Chemotherapy

The use of chemotherapy as a treatment for cancer began in the 1940s. During both world wars, it was observed that exposure to mustard gas resulted in myelosuppression. Consequently, nitrogen mustard was selected as the first clinical chemotherapy for non-Hodgkin's lymphoma. The use of these alkylating agents in patients with lymphoid and hematologic malignancies resulted in dramatic clinical response. Complete cancer cures using chemotherapy alone were first noted in the 1960s with childhood leukemias and Hodgkin's disease. Very quickly, the use of chemotherapeutic agents was approved for solid tumors.

With time, a variety of limitations of chemotherapy have emerged due to the toxic side effects. Chemotherapeutic agents target actively proliferating tumor cells; however, most cells within a solid tumor are quiescent. Thus, only a small fraction of tumor cells are susceptible to chemotherapy at any given time. In addition, although tumors start out as a clonal proliferation of a transformed cell, mutations during tumor growth lead to subpopulations of tumor cells that are variably sensitive to differing agents. Numerous mechanisms of acquired drug resistance have been described including the expression of the multidrug resistance gene, which encodes a membrane glycoprotein that extrudes various chemotherapeutic agents from the cell. Even under optimal conditions, with a 100% tumor growth fraction and no drug resistance, elimination of greater than 99.9% of a tumor, a 5-log kill, may leave behind enough viable tumor cells to cause a cancer recurrence. Lastly, since chemotherapeutic agents are not selective for neoplastic cells, normal proliferating cells are also exposed to the toxicities of chemotherapy. The cells most affected are those with the highest growth rates and turnover, namely, the gut mucosa, hair follicles, and bone marrow.

Most chemotherapeutic agents have well-defined dose–response curves. These agents are dosed to maximize the therapeutic effect while minimizing toxicity. The interval between doses is determined by the amount of time necessary for recovery of normal tissues. For the majority of drugs, the nadir of bone marrow function is reached 2 weeks after administration with an additional 2 weeks required for full recovery. Multidrug treatment regimens using drugs with different activity and side effect profiles are generally used to maximize cancer cell death while limiting toxicities. In addition, these multidrug regimens may target tumor cells with different resistance profiles. Table 15.8 lists some common alkylating and antimetabolite chemotherapeutic agents.

The timing for delivery of chemotherapeutic agents depends on the clinical situation and the goals of treatment. Chemotherapy administered to patients as the primary treatment for metastatic disease is known as induction or primary chemotherapy. The goal of this treatment is generally not cure but to control tumor growth. Chemotherapy delivered following another treatment modality, such as surgical resection, is known as adjuvant chemotherapy. The goal of adjuvant chemotherapy is to target micrometastatic disease in patients with a high risk of tumor recurrence. When chemotherapeutic agents are used prior to surgery, it is termed neoadjuvant chemotherapy. Generally, the goal of neoadjuvant therapy is to decrease tumor size preoperatively to allow for a less radical surgical resection.

Although the majority of chemotherapeutic agents are administered systemically by intravenous infusion, several regional infusion strategies have been developed. These approaches allow for the delivery of increased doses of a drug while limiting systemic toxicities. Hepatic arterial infusion therapy for the treatment of colorectal liver metastases has been evaluated in numerous studies, and while response rates are significantly higher than are those with systemic chemotherapy, the overall survival benefit has been marginal. Another example is the use of regional chemotherapy in the form of isolated limb perfusion (ILP) or isolated limb infusion (ILI) for locally advanced melanoma of the extremity.

Principles of Radiation Therapy

Ionizing radiation is one of the primary treatment modalities for cancer. Ionization of molecules in the tissue has directly as well as indirectly toxic effects on tumor cells. The direct effects of ionizing radiation occur through induction of double-stranded breaks in DNA. Indirect effects are seen through the generation of free radical species that further damage DNA and other intracellular molecules.

The two principal methods by which radiation is delivered to patients are internal radiotherapy (brachytherapy) and external beam radiotherapy (teletherapy). With brachytherapy, the source of radiation is placed within or adjacent to the target tissues. The dose delivered is inversely proportional to the distance squared from the source of the radiation; therefore, normal tissues are largely spared. Examples of brachytherapy include the use of intrauterine devices for cervical cancer and seeds for prostate cancer. With teletherapy, the source of radiation is outside the patient and is delivered as a high-energy electromagnetic beam. Delivery of radiation by this method can be modified through the use of filters and collimators that focus the radiation source on the target tissue while sparing surrounding tissues. More recently, the use of *proton* beam therapy is gaining increasing application in the treatment of sold malignancies, offering the potential advantage of more targeted treatment of the tumor while minimizing exposure of the nearby normal tissue to the toxic side effects of radiation.

Tumor cells are variably sensitive to the effects of ionizing radiation according to their oxygen status and stage in the cell cycle

TABLE 15.8 **Chemotherapeutic agents (alkylating agents and antimetabolites)**

Drug	Indication	Toxicities
Alkylating agents: Transfer alkyl groups to nucleic acids and other biologically important molecules		
Busulfan	CML, myeloproliferative disorders	Myelosuppression, pulmonary fibrosis, gonadal dysfunction, marrow failure
Chlorambucil	Chronic lymphocytic leukemia, Waldenström macroglobulinemia	Myelosuppression, gonadal dysfunction, secondary leukemia
Cyclophosphamide	Hematologic malignancies, Hodgkin's disease, NHLs, carcinomas of the breast and ovary, sarcomas, small cell lung cancer, pediatric malignancies	Leukopenia, cystitis, nausea and vomiting, alopecia, cardiac necrosis, gonadal dysfunction, SIADH
Ifosfamide	Carcinomas of the breast, ovaries, lung, testicles; lymphomas; sarcomas	Myelosuppression, cystitis, nephrotoxicity, hepatotoxicity, lethargy, and confusion
Dacarbazine	Hodgkin's disease, NHLs, melanoma, sarcomas	Nausea and vomiting, flulike syndrome, myelosuppression, hepatotoxicity
Cisplatin	Carcinomas of the ovary, testis, cervix, head and neck, bladder, lung (small and non-small cell), esophagus; lymphomas	Nausea and vomiting, nephrotoxicity, neurotoxicity, hearing loss, electrolyte imbalance
Carboplatin	Carcinoma of the ovary; bone marrow transplantation	Myelosuppression, nausea and vomiting
Oxaliplatin	Carcinoma of the colon and rectum	Nausea and vomiting, neurotoxicity, myelosuppression, electrolyte imbalance
Melphalan	Multiple myeloma, ovarian cancer	Myelosuppression, anorexia, nausea and vomiting
Mechlorethamine	Lymphomas, Hodgkin's disease	Myelosuppression, secondary leukemia, severe vesicant, nausea and vomiting, alopecia, rash, gonadal dysfunction, neurotoxicity
Nitrosoureas (carmustine or lomustine)	Lymphomas, Hodgkin's disease, brain cancer, bone marrow transplantation	Myelosuppression, secondary leukemia, hepatotoxicity, pulmonary fibrosis, nausea and vomiting, nephrotoxicity, confusion
Streptozocin	Neuroendocrine tumors	Nephrotoxicity, nausea and vomiting, myelosuppression, hepatotoxicity, hypoglycemia
Procarbazine	Hodgkin's disease, lymphomas, brain cancer	Myelosuppression, monoamine oxidase inhibition, nausea and vomiting, lethargy, myalgias, arthralgias, neurotoxicity, dermatitis
Mitomycin C	Carcinomas of the breast, lung, gastrointestinal tract, cervix, bladder	Myelosuppression, severe vesicant, weakness, anorexia, hemolytic anemia, renal insufficiency, nausea and vomiting
Antimetabolites: Interfere with nucleic acid synthesis and are cell cycle specific		
Cytosine arabinoside	Acute myelogenous leukemia, leptomeningeal carcinomatosis, lymphomas	Myelosuppression, ischemic bowel, stomatitis, nausea and vomiting, hepatotoxicity, cerebellar toxicity
5-Fluorouracil	Carcinomas of the breast, cervix, head and neck, gastrointestinal tract; nonmelanoma skin cancer	Mucositis, diarrhea, myelosuppression, dermatitis, hepatotoxicity (intra-arterial therapy), nausea and vomiting
Floxuridine	Hepatic arterial therapy	Mucositis, biliary sclerosis, nausea and vomiting, abdominal pain
6-Mercaptopurine	Acute lymphoblastic leukemia	Myelosuppression, cholestasis, rash, anorexia, nausea and vomiting
Methotrexate	Carcinomas of the breast, head and neck, esophagus; choriocarcinoma; leptomeningeal carcinomatosis; osteogenic sarcoma	Myelosuppression, stomatitis, diarrhea, intestinal bleeding and perforation, arachnoiditis, hepatic dysfunction, cirrhosis, radiation recall, pneumonitis, renal dysfunction
Gemcitabine	Carcinomas of the lung, pancreas, breast, and bladder	Myelosuppression, weakness
Pentostatin	Hairy cell leukemia, T-cell lymphomas	Nephrotoxicity, risk of severe infections without neutropenia, lethargy, hepatotoxicity, mild myelosuppression
Fludarabine	B-cell chronic lymphocytic leukemia	Myelosuppression, tumor lysis syndrome, weakness, neurotoxicity, edema, pneumonitis, nausea and vomiting, anorexia, gastrointestinal bleeding, stomatitis, diarrhea

SIADH, syndrome of inappropriate antidiuretic hormone secretion.

From Ellis LM, Jones Jr DV, Chiao PJ, et al. Tumor biology. In: Greenfield, LJ, Mulholland MW, Oldham KT, et al. *Surgery: Scientific Principles and Practice.* 2nd ed. Philadelphia: Lippincott–Raven Publishers; 1997:501, with permission.

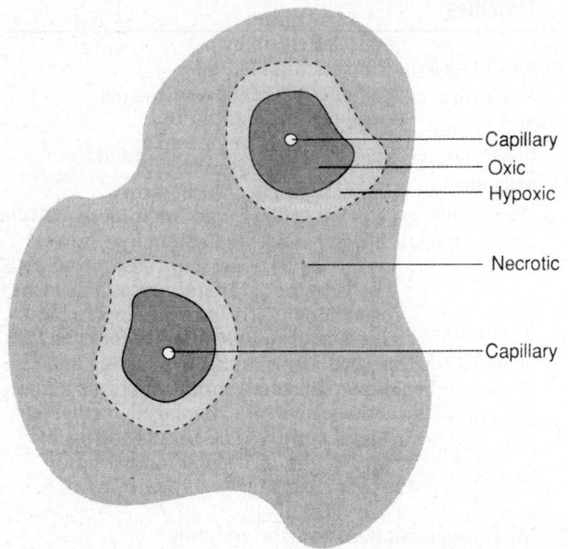

FIGURE 15.10 Tumors contain regions that are anoxic, hypoxic, and well oxygenated and that vary in distance from capillaries. The response to ionizing radiation varies with the degree of tissue oxygenation. (From Ellis LM, Jones Jr DV, Chiao PJ, et al. Tumor biology. In: Greenfield, LJ, Mulholland MW, Oldham KT, et al. *Surgery: Scientific Principles and Practice.* 2nd ed. Philadelphia: Lippincott–Raven Publishers; 1997:465.)

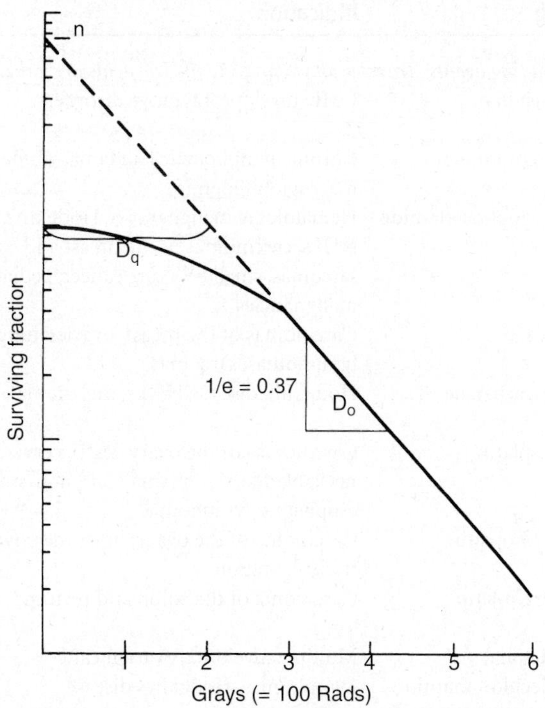

FIGURE 15.11 Idealized radiation survival curve. D_o, dose required to reduce the survival fraction to 37% on the exponential curve; D_q, the quasithreshold dose; 1/e, dose energy divided by dose loss. (From Hellman S. Principles of cancer management: radiation therapy. In: DeVita VT, Hellman S, Rosenberg SA, eds. *Cancer: Principles and Practice of Oncology.* 6th ed. Philadelphia: Lippincott Williams & Wilkins; 2002:272.)

(Fig. 15.10). Those tumor cells that are well oxygenated are more susceptible to the effects of ionizing radiation, since the generation of oxygen free radicals is one way ionizing radiation produces its effects. Pharmacologic modifiers have been used to increase the sensitivity of cells to ionizing radiation. For example, nitroimidazole compounds can substitute for oxygen and sensitize hypoxic cells. Additionally, halogenated pyrimidines when incorporated into DNA increase the sensitivity of cells to radiation. Hyperbaric oxygen treatment has also been used to increase the sensitivity of tumor cells. In addition to varying susceptibilities based on oxygen status, it has also been shown that those cells that are in the mitotic phase of the cell cycle are more susceptible to the effects of ionizing radiation.

Radiation survival curves are used to describe the sensitivity of cells to ionizing radiation (Fig. 15.11). These curves have a shallow initial slope, which reflects the ability of the cell to recover from sublethal doses of radiation. Clinical doses of radiation generally target the steeper slope of the radiation survival curve. Ionizing radiation is usually delivered in a series of smaller doses known as fractionation. This method of delivery has two main advantages over delivery of a larger single dose. First, normal tissues have time to recover from sublethal doses of radiation. Second, since only a small proportion of tumor cells will be sensitive to ionizing radiation at a given time, fractionation allows for targeting of multiple subpopulations of tumor cells.

Immunotherapy

The goal of immunotherapy is to generate antitumor immune responses by stimulating or bolstering the host immune system. Both active and passive immunotherapy approaches have been utilized for cancer therapy.

Active immunotherapy approaches include those in which a host antitumor immune response is elicited following the delivery of either nonspecific or specific stimulants of the immune system. Examples of nonspecific stimulants include microorganisms, such as bacille Calmette–Guérin (BCG), levamisole, and cytokines. Some clinical efficacy has been demonstrated with the use of BCG for melanoma metastases and superficial bladder cancer; levamisole, when used in concert with 5-fluorouracil, to decrease colon cancer recurrence and improve survival; and interferons, when used for hematologic malignancies and certain epithelial carcinomas. It was the use of interleukin-2 (IL-2) in patients with metastatic melanoma, renal cell carcinoma, and NHL that first demonstrated that manipulation of the immune system could lead to regression of bulky solid tumors and metastatic disease. In these initial studies, systemic delivery of IL-2 led to clinical responses in 15% to 20% of patients, with durable complete responses in approximately one half of those patients. Specific active immunotherapy strategies using vaccines derived from tumor cell preparations or antigen-presenting cells (APCs) have also been utilized.

Passive immunotherapy strategies include the delivery of agents that already possess antitumor activity such as monoclonal antibodies and immune cells. The two most widely studied passive immunotherapy strategies are those that have utilized nonspecific lymphokine–activated killer (LAK) cells and tumor-infiltrating lymphocytes (TILs).

Several important developments have been critical to continued progress in the field of immunotherapy. The first of these was the initial identification and isolation of T-cell growth factor (TCGF), now known as IL-2, which could be utilized for the *in vitro* expansion of lymphocytes. It was found that the incubation of lymphocytes with IL-2 led to the development of nonspecific cytotoxic cells, or LAK cells. A second important discovery was the identification of TILs that had specific antitumor activity. The identification of TILs was a clear indication that the immune system did play a role in fighting cancer and that there were specific tumor antigens that could be recognized and targeted by the immune system. This finding led to the identification of numerous tumor antigens that are recognized by the cellular immune system and provide immunotherapeutic targets. Recently, two new immunotherapeutic agents targeting negative regulators of the immune response have been approved for clinical use in the treatment of metastatic melanoma: ipilimumab, an inhibitor of CTLA4 (cytotoxic T-lymphocyte–associated antigen 4), and pembrolizumab, which targets the programmed cell death-1 (PCD-1) receptor. These immunomodulators have shown promising results in a subset of patients, although can occasionally be associated with severe autoimmune side effects.

Finally, the development of methods to genetically manipulate lymphocytes, tumor cells, and APCs *in vitro* to enhance their *in vivo* antitumor activity has had a considerable impact on immunotherapy. Genetic manipulation of these cells has included insertion of genes that express cytokines, costimulatory molecules, and tumor antigens. The importance of APCs in stimulating the immune system has been recognized, and attempts have been made to use these cells for cancer vaccines. APCs have been pulsed with antigens, lysates, or peptides from tumor preparations to generate highly specific antitumor immune responses.

Gene Therapy

The introduction of cancer gene therapy more than a decade ago was greeted with considerable optimism. Although numerous preclinical studies and clinical trials have been initiated since that time with variable results, multiple limitations still exist in the field. Increasing knowledge of the molecular basis of malignant transformation, however, and a more complete understanding of tumor biology, including the tumor microenvironment and host–tumor interactions, have led to the identification of an increasing number of potential targets for cancer gene therapy.

Successful gene therapy strategies require delivery of vectors that are safe, efficient, and selective. Both nonviral and viral vectors have been developed and utilized. Examples of nonviral gene delivery methods include the injection of naked DNA and DNA complexed to cationic carriers. The advantages of nonviral gene delivery methods are that they are less immunogenic than viral vectors and can be produced in higher titers *in vitro*. Viral vectors that have been used frequently in cancer gene therapy include delivery vectors based on adenovirus, retrovirus, and herpes simplex virus (HSV). These viral vectors vary in their size, DNA-carrying capacity, ability to transduce cells, potential for long-term gene expression, and in the titers that can be generated *in vitro*. The advantages of viral vectors are that they have higher transduction efficiencies as compared to nonviral vectors and that some have the potential for long-term gene expression.

Gene therapy strategies are generally divided into five main categories: mutation compensation, molecular chemotherapy, immunopotentiation, antiangiogenic therapy, and viral-mediated oncolysis. Mutation compensation gene therapy approaches attempt to correct the genetic alterations that occurred during malignant transformation by restoring the function of a TSG or by inactivating an oncogene. One area of focus in mutation compensation therapy has been the restoration of p53 function, as it is mutated in the majority of human cancers. The goal of molecular chemotherapy is to produce high concentrations of cytotoxic metabolites locally, thereby circumventing the dose-limiting toxicities of systemic chemotherapy. This is accomplished by transducing cells with an enzyme that leads to the conversion of an inactive prodrug to a cytotoxic metabolite. The two most frequently utilized enzyme–prodrug combinations are HSV thymidine kinase with ganciclovir and *Escherichia coli* cytosine deaminase with 5-fluorocytosine. Immunopotentiation gene therapy strategies attempt to enhance antitumor immune responses. Numerous approaches have been evaluated including delivery of cytokines, development of vaccines based on tumor antigens, up-regulation of costimulatory molecules, and inhibition of immunosuppressive molecules. Antiangiogenic gene therapy strategies have focused on blocking proangiogenic factors or increasing inhibitors of angiogenesis. Combination gene therapy approaches as well as gene therapy in concert with radiation therapy and chemotherapy have been evaluated. Although preclinical studies have produced promising results, only limited responses have been observed in clinical trials.

Molecular Diagnostics and Therapeutics

As our understanding of the specific genetic alterations that are necessary for malignant transformation has increased, potential new targets for cancer therapy have been identified. Identification of these targets has been facilitated by the development of technologies that allow for rapid transcription and molecular profiling of individual cancers. Gene expression and protein microarrays are examples of these emerging technologies and can provide a significant amount of information about genetic perturbations within cancer cells. The identification of genetic and epigenetic alterations in cancer cells may improve the characterization of cancers beyond what is currently possible, allowing oncologists to tailor therapy to the individual patient.

The use of molecular diagnostics to identify genetic mutations in cancer cells has led to the development of inhibitors that target specific signaling pathways in cancer cells. The first successful example of targeted molecular therapy was the tyrosine kinase inhibitor imatinib mesylate for the treatment of patients with chronic myeloid leukemia (CML) and gastrointestinal stromal tumors (GISTs). The principal genetic defect in 95% of patients with CML is a reciprocal translocation between chromosomes 9 and 22, which leads to the *bcr-abl* fusion protein that functions as a constitutively active tyrosine kinase. In the case of GISTs, the majority of tumors have a gain-of-function mutation in the c-kit proto-oncogene, which leads to a constitutively active tyrosine kinase receptor. In CML, up to 95% of chronic-phase patients who failed interferon therapy had a clinical response to imatinib mesylate with approximately one-half exhibiting molecular remission. The use of imatinib mesylate has also revolutionized the treatment of patients with metastatic GISTs, and the efficacy of this agent as adjuvant therapy is currently being evaluated.

Following the success of imatinib mesylate, several additional molecular therapies have been developed. The overexpression of EGFRs in numerous cancers has led to the development of agents that target these receptors. Overexpression of the HER2/neu receptor in 25% to 30% of patients with breast cancer leads to an aggressive form of the disease. Trastuzumab, a monoclonal antibody against

TABLE 15.9 Nanodevices in cancer diagnosis and therapy

Device	Development Stage	Cancer Application	Current State
Dendrimer	*In vivo* (mouse)	Imaging Drug delivery	1. 10–50× increase in chemotherapeutic efficiency with decreased toxicity 2. Diagnostic MRI enhancement 3. Apoptosis sensing
Liposomes	Human clinical trials	Imaging Drug delivery	Liposomal-encapsulated chemotherapeutics presently under study in a wide variety of malignancies
Buckyballs/nanotubes	*In vivo* (mouse)	Diagnostic and therapeutic	Conjugation to antibodies and chemotherapy Delivery of siRNA
Quantum dots	*In vivo* (mouse)	Imaging	Capable of imaging tumors with defined DNA sequences as well as lymphatic mapping in animal models
Nanoshells	*In vivo* (mouse)	Imaging Photothermal ablation Drug delivery	Preferential migration to tumor with imaging and treatment capability via photothermal ablation Targeted drug delivery via antibody and chemotherapeutic conjugation

MRI, magnetic resonance imaging; siRNA, small interfering RNA.

From DeVita VT, Lawrence TS, Rosenberg SA, eds. *Cancer: Principles and Practice of Oncology*. 8th ed. Philadelphia: Lippincott Williams & Wilkins; 2008:3032.

the HER2/neu receptor, has been shown to slow disease progression and improve overall survival when administered in combination with chemotherapy. Vemurafenib, an inhibitor of the mutated BRAF tyrosine kinase (mutated in 50% to 60% of melanomas), and dabrafenib, an MEK inhibitor, have recently been approved for the treatment of metastatic melanoma. While these targeted therapies show high response rates initially, resistance to therapy is almost uniformly seen with continued treatment. Efforts to overcome these resistance mechanisms remain areas of active investigation.

Nanotechnology

By strict definition, nanotechnology refers to devices less than 100 nanometers (nm). As a frame of reference, a human cell on average measures 10,000 to 20,000 nm. Nanomedicine has developed as a subset of the technology specifically to examine the role in medical therapy. This field merges the expertise of medicine, biology, mathematics, and engineering. While the possible applications of nanotechnology in medicine appear limitless, the area of greatest interest includes the development of specific targeted therapies. See Table 15.9 for a list of nanodevices in cancer diagnosis and therapy.

Dendrimers, or dendritic polymers, are spherical nanostructures used as a backbone for the attachment of biologic materials. Functional attachments have included iron oxide for targeted imaging. Engineered for biologic compatibility, liposomes are spherical vesicles with a biologic phospholipid membrane, and buckyballs, or nanotubules, are solely carbon-based structures. Utilized for drug delivery, liposomes and buckyballs sequester therapeutic agents that would not normally be able to enter the intracellular compartment. Quantum dots are crystals capable of emitting variable wavelengths of light when exposed to UV light. Quantum dots are conjugated to variety of targeting agents for purposes of cancer imaging. Lastly, nanoshells are beads with gold that can absorb specific wavelengths of light, converting this energy to heat. These devices can be used for imaging as well as selective cell destruction.

CONCLUSIONS

Cancer remains a major concern in the public health realm. More than 50% of patients with malignancies still succumb to metastatic disease that cannot be controlled by standard treatment modalities. Although advances in tumor biology have markedly increased our understanding of malignant transformation and the cancer phenotype, they have also highlighted the complexity and heterogeneity of carcinogenesis that make prevention and treatment so difficult. Surgery, chemotherapy, and radiation therapy continue to be the standard treatment modalities. However, molecular diagnostic techniques and targeted molecular therapies will likely play an increasing role in cancer detection and treatment in the future as therapies are tailored for specific genetic mutations in individual patients.

ACKNOWLEDGMENTS

The authors wish to thank Paul J. Foley and Susan B. Kesmodel for their contributions to prior editions.

Suggested Readings

DeVita VT, Lawrence TS, Rosenberg SA, eds. *Cancer: Principles and Practice of Oncology*. 8th ed. Philadelphia: Lippincott Williams & Wilkins; 2008.

Greenfield LJ, Mulholland MW, Lillemoe KD, et al., eds. *Surgery: Scientific Principles & Practice*. 4th ed. Philadelphia: Lippincott Williams & Wilkins; 2006.

Hanahan D, Weinberg RA. Hallmarks of cancer: the next generation. *Cell.* 2011;144(5):646–674.

Howlader N, Noone AM, Krapcho M, et al., eds. *SEER Cancer Statistics Review, 1975–2010*. Bethesda, MD: National Cancer Institute; 2013.

Kinzler KW, Vogelstein B. Lessons from hereditary colorectal cancer. *Cell.* 1996;87(2):159–170.

Lundberg AS, Weinberg RA. Control of the cell cycle and apoptosis. *Eur J Cancer*. 1999;35:531–539.

Rosenberg SA. Progress in human tumour immunology and immunotherapy. *Nature.* 2001;411:380–384.

Shih T, Lindley C. Bevacizumab: an angiogenesis inhibitor for the treatment of solid malignancies. *Clin Ther.* 2006;28(11):1779–1802.

Siegel R, Naishadham D, Jemal A. Cancer statistics, 2013. *CA Cancer J Clin.* 2013;63:11–30.

Vogelstein B, Lane D, Levine AJ. Surfing the p53 network. *Nature.* 2000;408:307–310.

Vogelstein B, Kinzler KW. *The Genetic Basis of Human Cancer*. 2nd ed. New York: McGraw-Hill; 2002.

Vogelstein B, Sur S, Prives C. p53: the most frequently altered gene in human cancers. *Nat Educ.* 2010;3(9):6.

CHAPTER

16

Melanoma, Sarcoma, Lymphoma, and the Spleen

EDMUND K. BARTLETT AND GIORGOS C. KARAKOUSIS

KEY POINTS

- The recommended resection margin for melanomas of 1 mm thickness or less is 1 cm; for those between 1 and 2 mm thickness, it is 1 to 2 cm, and for those of greater than 2 mm thickness, it is 2 cm.
- Sentinel lymph node status is the most important predictor of overall survival in patients with localized melanoma.
- Sentinel lymph node biopsy is recommended for all patients with melanomas of more than 1 mm thickness. In patients with less than or equal to 1-mm melanomas, sentinel lymph node biopsy is recommended selectively (thickness >0.75 mm, present mitoses, elevated Clark level, and present ulceration are all considered risk factors).
- Core needle biopsy is the preferred diagnostic modality for the evaluation of suspected extremity sarcomas. Incisional biopsy, when necessary, should be performed using a longitudinal skin incision.
- Wide radical excision, with pre- or postoperative radiation therapy for high-risk tumors, allows for low rates of local recurrence and limb preservation in over 90% of patients with extremity soft tissue sarcomas.
- Retroperitoneal sarcomas carry a worse prognosis than do extremity sarcomas because they are frequently diagnosed at a relatively advanced stage and because complete gross resection can only be achieved in approximately 75% of patients.
- Gastric mucosa–associated lymphoid tissue (MALT) lymphoma is associated with *Helicobacter pylori* infection in over 90% of cases, and most resolve with treatment of the infection alone.
- Hereditary spherocytosis, a type of familial hemolytic anemia, is characterized by defective erythrocyte membranes resulting from a defect in spectrin. Splenectomy is typically curative.
- Idiopathic thrombocytopenic purpura (ITP) is characterized by immunoglobulin (Ig) G antibodies directed at platelets. Steroids are the first-line therapy, but splenectomy is indicated for patients in whom steroids are ineffective or contraindicated.

This chapter reviews a diverse set of topics; each is important in its own right to the general surgeon. Melanoma and sarcoma are malignancies for which surgical resection provides the only potentially curative treatment and, in advanced cases, can provide palliation. Surgical treatment for lymphoma is now limited primarily to obtaining tissue for diagnosis and in treating complications, particularly those affecting the gastrointestinal (GI) tract. The final section deals with the spleen and the disease processes that may necessitate splenectomy.

MELANOMA

In 2013, there were nearly 76,690 cases of melanoma diagnosed in the United States, making it the fifth most common cancer type. Although melanoma accounts for only 1.6% of all cancer deaths overall, an estimated 9,480 patients died from melanoma in 2013 making it the most deadly form of skin cancer. From 1975 to 2010, the incidence of melanoma has increased more rapidly than any other cancer type. The death rate from melanoma, however, has remained constant over this period. As a result, the overall 5-year survival has increased from 82% to 91% across all patients. Simultaneously, the average thickness of melanoma has fallen, such that 70% of melanomas are now diagnosed with a thickness of less than 1 mm. Both the improved survival and the decreasing thickness are likely a reflection of earlier detection, perhaps due to increased awareness and surveillance.

Pathogenesis

Melanoma arises from the malignant transformation of epidermal melanocytes and as such can occur at any anatomic site where melanocytes are present. The pathogenesis is multifactorial, but a number of genetic mutations have now been identified in a substantial portion of melanomas. Gain-of-function mutations are of particular interest recently due to the development of targeted therapies. *BRAF* mutation is most common (approximately 60% of melanomas), followed by *NRAS* (15% to 20%) and *KIT* (2% to 20%). Additionally, loss-of-function mutations such as in *PTEN* (60% to 70% of melanomas) and *CDKN2A* (50%) are prevalent.

History and Physical Examination

The evaluation of patients with pigmented lesions should include a thorough *history* directed at identification of *risk factors* for melanoma. Important elements of the history include the following:

- *Age*: The median age of diagnosis is 61 years, but the range is wide. In particular, among woman aged 20 to 30 years, melanoma is the most commonly diagnosed malignancy.
- *Race*: White individuals are nearly 30-fold more likely to develop melanoma compared to black individuals. Freckles, fair-complexion, blue eyes, and red or blond hair are associated with increased risk even among whites.

- *History of the lesion*: Lesions that have recently developed or changed are more suspicious than are long-standing nevi that have not changed. In particular, changes in size, shape, color, and any history of itching or bleeding are worrisome for malignant transformation.
- *Personal history of melanoma*: Patients who have had a prior melanoma have a nine-fold increased risk of developing a second primary melanoma compared with patients without a history of melanoma.
- *Family history of melanoma*: A familial melanoma syndrome is typically defined when a patient has two or more first-degree relatives with melanoma, and this accounts for approximately 2% of melanoma diagnoses. Currently, two genes are known to be associated with familial melanoma (*CDKN2A* and *CDK4*). Additionally, patients with xeroderma pigmentosum or BRCA2 mutations are at increased risk of developing melanoma.
- *Environmental risk factors*: Exposure to *ultraviolet radiation*, even a history of a single blistering sunburn, has been shown to increase the risk of developing melanoma. The increased exposure of the population to ultraviolet radiation from decreased ozone shielding of solar radiation and from increased use of tanning booths is thought to be contributing to the increasing rates of melanoma and other skin cancers.

Physical exam should include a thorough survey of the skin for other lesions, as early detection of melanoma can improve survival. Patients with a large number of benign nevi (>50) are at increased risk for developing melanoma, and synchronous lesions may be present. Individual lesions should be examined to identify those features suggestive of melanoma: *asymmetry*, irregular *borders*, variegated *color*, large *diameter*, and *elevated* surface (i.e., the *ABCDEs*). Importantly, the absence of these features does not exclude melanoma—amelanotic (nonpigmented) melanoma accounts for approximately 1% of melanomas. Palpation of regional nodal basins (cervical, axillary, inguinal, epitrochlear, or popliteal) is critical as clinically palpable nodal metastases will change management.

Diagnosis

The differential diagnosis for pigmented lesions is extensive, and the vast majority of these lesions are benign (Table 16.1). Most melanomas arise *de novo*; however, they can develop in precursor lesions such as dysplastic or congenital nevi. Dysplastic nevi are differentiated based upon the extent of dysplasia, which is determined following biopsy. Lesions with mild dysplasia may be observed, whereas the presence of moderate-to-severe dysplasia warrants an excision with negative margins. Congenital nevi are rare (approximately 1% of children), and the risk of melanoma correlates with both the size and number of nevi. Giant nevi (>20 cm) are associated with a 10% lifetime risk of melanoma, and therefore, excision is recommended when feasible. *Acquired nevi* appear after the first few months of life and can be divided into *junctional nevi*, *compound nevi*, and *intradermal nevi*.

TABLE 16.1 Pigmented lesion, differential diagnosis

Melanocytic	Nonmelanocytic
Congenital nevus	Hemangioma
Acquired nevus	Kaposi sarcoma
Atypical nevus	Pyogenic granuloma
Melanosis of the genitalia	Dermatofibroma
Blue nevus	Angiokeratoma
Solar lentigo	

Suspicious lesions should be *biopsied*. Excisional biopsy is ideal as it reliably allows determination of tumor thickness, and minimal margins are usually adequate since the majority of these lesions will be benign. The biopsy incision should be oriented so that it can be incorporated into a subsequent wide local excision if necessary. With large lesions in critical locations (such as above joints or on the face), an incisional or punch biopsy may be the only practical option. Although frequently performed, shave biopsies may preclude accurate assessment of tumor thickness and should be avoided.

Melanomas can be classified into four main types according to their appearance and clinical behavior:

- *Superficial spreading melanoma* is the most common type and accounts for 70% of cases. These lesions are initially characterized by a radial growth phase. Over a variable period of time, they transition to a phase of vertical growth.
- *Nodular melanoma* is the second most common type and accounts for 15% to 30% of cases. These tumors are characterized by a vertical growth phase without radial growth. They are more aggressive than is the superficial spreading type and more frequently present with adverse prognostic features.
- *Lentigo maligna melanoma* constitutes 4% to 10% of cases and develops in older patients in sun-exposed areas. They are more common in women than in men and typically are large (>3 cm in diameter) at the time of diagnosis. These lesions characteristically develop over many years from a precursor macular brown nevus, the so-called *Hutchinson freckle*, and tend to be less aggressive than are other melanomas.
- *Acral lentiginous melanoma* is relatively uncommon. This lesion accounts for 2% to 8% of melanoma in white patients but 35% to 60% of melanomas in patients with dark skin. Typically, these lesions occur on the palms or soles and are highly aggressive.

Rarely, melanoma may also arise in noncutaneous sites. Ocular melanoma is the most common noncutaneous melanoma. Treatment of localized disease typically requires enucleation and/or brachytherapy, which have been associated with similar results. Primary melanoma may also occur in the mucous membranes of the genitalia, anus, oropharynx, and GI tract. Noncutaneous melanomas are associated with a poor prognosis.

Staging

Melanoma is staged using the American Joint Committee on Cancer (AJCC) staging system (Tables 16.2 and 16.3). T stage is dependent on *tumor thickness* (*Breslow scale*) and by the presence of *tumor ulceration* or *mitoses*. Thickness cutoffs are 1 mm or lesser, 1.01 to 2 mm, 2.01 to 4 mm, and greater than 4 mm. N stage is determined by the number of positive nodes and by the presence of microscopic versus macroscopic nodal metastases. In-transit and satellite metastases are considered equivalent to nodal disease. M stage is dependent on the site of metastasis, with distant skin,

TABLE 16.2 AJCC 7th edition TNM classification for melanoma

Tumor (T) classification	
T1	a. Primary melanoma ≤1 mm without ulceration and mitosis <1/mm^2
	b. Primary melanoma with ulceration or mitoses ≥1/mm^2
T2	a. Primary melanoma 1.01–2.0 mm without ulceration
	b. Primary melanoma 1.01–2.0 mm with ulceration
T3	a. Primary melanoma 2.01–4.0 mm without ulceration
	b. Primary melanoma 2.01–4.0 mm with ulceration
T4	a. Primary melanoma >4 mm without ulceration
	b. Primary melanoma >4 mm with ulceration
Node (N) classification	
N1	a. One positive lymph node with micrometastasis[a]
	b. One positive lymph node with macrometastasis[b]
N2	a. Two to three positive lymph nodes with micrometastasis
	b. Two to three positive lymph nodes with macrometastasis
	c. In-transit/satellite metastases without positive lymph nodes
N3	Four or more positive lymph nodes, matted lymph nodes, or in-transit metastasis with metastatic node(s)
[a]Micrometastases diagnosed after sentinel and completion lymphadenectomy; [b]Macrometastases diagnosed on clinical examination or when nodal metastasis exhibits gross extracapsular extension.	
Metastasis (M) classification	
M1a	Distant skin, subcutaneous, or lymph node metastases with normal LDH level
M1b	Lung metastases with normal LDH level
M1c	All other visceral metastases with normal LDH level or any distant metastases with elevated LDH level

LDH, lactate dehydrogenase.

TABLE 16.3 AJCC 7th edition pathologic staging classification for melanoma

IA	T1a, N0, M0
IB	T1b, N0, M0 T2a, N0, M0
IIA	T2b, N0, M0 T3a, N0, M0
IIB	T3b, N0, M0 T4a, N0, M0
IIC	T4b, N0, M0
IIIA	Any Ta, N1a, M0 Any Ta, N2a, M0
IIIB	Any Tb, N1a, M0 Any Tb, N2a, M0 Any Ta, N1b, M0 Any Ta, N2b, M0 Any Ta, N2c, M0
IIIC	Any Tb, N1b, M0 Any Tb, N2b, M0 Any Tb, N2c, M0 Any T, N3, M0
IV	Any T, Any N, M1

subcutaneous, and lymph node metastases being more favorable than lung metastases, which, in turn, are more favorable than are other visceral organ metastases. In addition, elevated lactate dehydrogenase (LDH) level is associated with a worse prognosis in patients with disseminated melanoma.

Surgical Management of Melanoma

Primary Tumor

Surgical resection via wide local excision remains the mainstay of curative treatment for patients with melanoma. The recommended margins of resection are dictated by the thickness of the primary tumor. Consensus guidelines have been proposed based upon a number of clinical trials. Current recommended margins are 0.5 to 1 cm for *in situ* melanoma, 1 cm for melanomas less than or equal to 1 mm thick, 1 to 2 cm for melanomas with a thickness 1.01 to 2 mm, and 2 cm for melanomas greater than 2 mm thick. The benefits in reducing the risk of local recurrence with adequate margins must be weighed against potential functional deficits, particularly in patients with thick (>4-mm primary tumors) melanoma in whom the risk of both local and distant recurrence remains high. Some interest, particularly in the dermatologic community, has been given to *Mohs surgery* for the resection of melanoma. This practice of obtaining minimal margins with repeated frozen sections until margins are negative does not have any evidence to support its practice in melanoma. While there may be a select few cases, particularly in sensitive areas of the face, in which

Mohs may be considered, the value of frozen section margins for melanoma is very limited, and oncologic outcomes in these patients are not well described.

Primary closure is achievable for most excision sites, as long as adequate skin flaps are raised on either side of the resection site. In the event that primary closure is not possible, a split-thickness skin graft or a rotational flap is an option for wound closure. On the face, full-thickness skin grafts are preferred for cosmetic and functional reasons.

Regional Lymph Nodes

The *regional lymph nodes* are the most common site of first metastasis for melanoma. *Sentinel lymph node biopsy* is now the standard procedure for detecting subclinical metastatic to the regional nodes. Alternatively, patients with clinically detectable lymph node metastases are candidates for *therapeutic lymphadenectomy*, provided that they have no other metastatic disease. This therapy is curative in a subset of patients and provides palliation in patients who ultimately develop metastatic disease because it improves locoregional tumor control.

Sentinel lymph node biopsy was pioneered by Morton in 1991 and has rapidly become the standard of care for the assessment of regional lymph node metastases. It involves the selective removal of the primary node or nodes that receive lymphatic drainage from the tumor site. Sentinel lymph node biopsy is recommended for all patients with primary tumors of greater than 1 mm. The use of *sentinel lymph node biopsy* in patients with tumors 1 mm or less in thickness remains controversial. Currently, it is recommended for patients with tumor thickness of 0.76 to 1 mm who have T1b lesions (e.g., present ulceration or mitotic rate ≥1 per mm^2), it can be considered in patients with tumor thickness of 0.76 to 1 mm who have T1a lesions, and it is not recommended for patients with tumor thickness less than 0.76 mm. High-risk features (e.g., high mitotic rate, lymphovascular invasion, microsatellites, Clark level IV, and/or ulceration) are rare in thin lesions but when present may warrant *sentinel lymph node biopsy* in selected individuals in whom it is not otherwise recommended. The status of the sentinel node is considered the single strongest prognostic factor for patients with clinically localized melanoma.

Optimal identification of the sentinel node(s) involves preoperative lymphoscintigraphy for which the primary tumor is injected with technetium-99m–labeled sulfur colloid, and the regional nodal basins are then imaged for uptake of the tracer in the sentinel node(s). Preoperative imaging is particularly useful in head and neck and trunk lesions, which may drain to multiple nodal basins. The accuracy of the procedure is maximized by the additional intraoperative injection of isosulfan blue dye into the tumor site, which allows both visualization of the blue sentinel node and detection with a handheld gamma probe.

Several studies have confirmed the accuracy of this technique—less than 5% of positive nodes go undetected by sentinel lymph node biopsy. Given this high rate of success, patients found to have a negative sentinel lymph node can avoid a complete lymph node dissection. In those patients with a positive sentinel node, completion lymph node dissection remains the standard of care, although the impact of completion dissection in this group is poorly defined. The Multicenter Sentinel Lymphadenectomy Trial II (MSLT2) is an ongoing randomized trial investigating this question.

In patients with stage III disease, either at time of presentation or by virtue of a positive sentinel node, a workup for distant metastases should be considered prior to nodal dissection. In the absence of distant metastases, *therapeutic lymph node dissection* is recommended. In the axilla, node dissection involves removal of level I to III nodes (the nodes that are lateral, underlying, and medial to the pectoralis minor muscle). In the inguinal region, the superficial femoral nodes, which reside in the triangle between the sartorius muscle laterally; the adductor muscles medially; and the inguinal ligament superiorly, are removed (Fig. 16.1). The femoral vein serves as the deep margin for this lymph node basin, and *en bloc* resection requires ligation of the saphenous vein. Dissection of the deeper iliac and obturator nodes is recommended only if (a) the deeper nodes clinically appear to be involved based on preoperative imaging or intraoperative assessment, (b) there are three or more positive nodes in the superficial group, or (c) a Cloquet node is involved. Primary melanomas of the head and neck have a somewhat predictable pattern of lymph node drainage depending on their specific location. Parotid, submandibular, submental, jugular, and posterior triangle lymph nodes drain areas anterior to the ear and superior to the mouth. Anterior lesions inferior to the mouth drain to cervical nodes and posterior lesions drain to

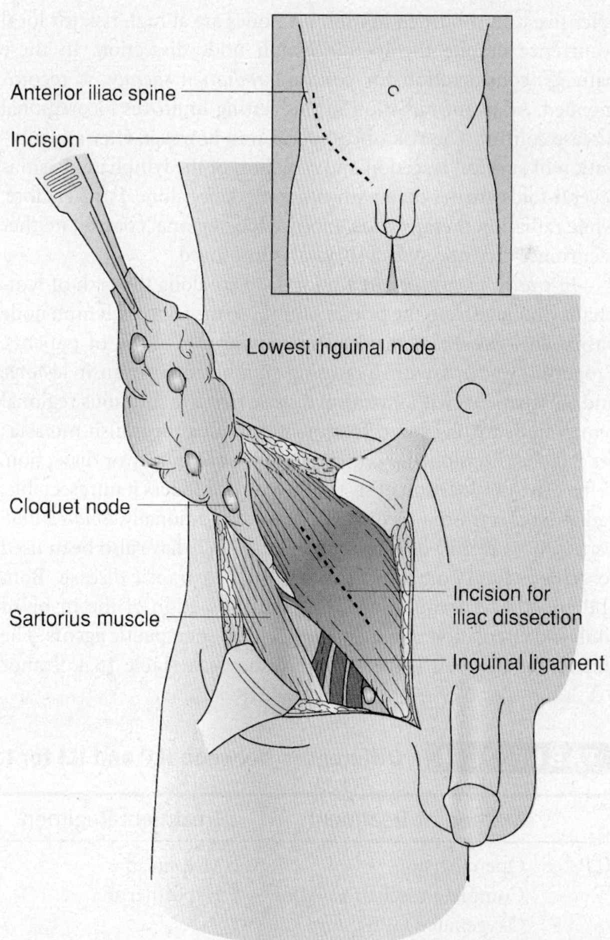

FIGURE 16.1 Technique of groin dissection. (From Mulholland MW. *Greenfield's Surgery: Scientific Principles and Practice*. 5th ed. Philadelphia: Lippincott Williams & Wilkins; 2011.)

occipital, postauricular, posterior triangle, and jugular nodes. A radical neck dissection is generally performed in the presence of clinically apparent nodal involvement.

Complications of lymph node dissection include infection, wound dehiscence, seroma, and lymphedema. Axillary and neck dissections are associated with substantially lower rates of complication than are inguinal dissections. The incidence of infection may be reduced by administration of perioperative antibiotics as well as avoidance of overly thin skin flaps. For inguinal lymph node dissection in particular, additional surgical techniques such as saphenous vein preservation, prophylactic sartorius transposition, omental flap, and fascial preservation have all been described with inconclusive results. The incidence of clinically significant lymphedema may be decreased by protecting the extremity from trauma, burns, venipuncture, and blood pressure measurements. Patients who develop lymphedema can be treated with limb elevation, application of compression stockings, gentle diuresis, or physical therapy. The possibility of recurrent disease should always be considered since extremity swelling may be indicative of lymphatic recurrence.

Advanced Lymphatic and In-Transit Metastases

Patients with lymph node metastases that grow through the capsule of the lymph node (extracapsular extension) and those with extensive tumor burden in multiple nodes are at high risk for local recurrence despite therapeutic lymph node dissection. In these patients, consideration for adjuvant *radiation therapy* is recommended. Adjuvant radiation in this setting improves locoregional disease control. The risk of complications, however, after a combination of surgical resection and radiation of the lymphatic basin is several-folds greater than with either modality alone. Furthermore, while radiation therapy does improve locoregional control, neither recurrence-free nor overall survival is improved.

In-transit metastases are tumor deposits along the path of lymphatic drainage from the primary tumor to the regional lymph node basin. This pattern of metastasis occurs in 2% to 3% of patients. Prognosis worsens with increasing number of in-transit lesions, and 66% patients with in-transit disease have synchronous regional lymph node involvement. Treatment of limited in-transit metastases includes excision and sentinel lymph node biopsy or dissection. If the extent or location of in-transit disease renders it unresectable, radiation therapy may provide palliation. Additionally, *isolated limb perfusion* (ILP) and *isolated limb infusion* (ILI) have also been used to achieve local control in patients with in-transit disease. Both ILP and ILI techniques involve vascular isolation of the involved limb and circulation of high doses of chemotherapeutic agents. The differences between ILP and ILI are shown in Table 16.4. Tumor necrosis factor-α (TNF-α) was used in ILP regimens in an attempt to improve response rates; however, on the basis of results of the ACOSOG Trial Z0020, the use of TNF-α during ILP was not shown to be beneficial. TNF-α is currently no longer available in North America for clinical use. Intralesional injection of nonspecific immunostimulatory agents such as bacille Calmette–Guérin (BCG) has also been used with occasional success.

Treatment of Local Recurrences

Local recurrence is defined as regrowth of tumor within 5 cm of the primary resection site. Malignant melanoma is associated with an approximately 4% rate of *local recurrence*, overall. Recurrence occurs more frequently in patients with thick (>4 mm) primary lesions (13%) and ulcerated tumors (11.5%) and in lesions of the foot, hand, scalp, and face (5% to 12%). Initial local recurrences of low-risk tumors are treated with wide excision. Excision and/or ILP should be considered for the treatment of multiple recurrences or recurrence of high-risk tumors. Radiation therapy may be used as an alternative to ILP.

Distant Metastases

Melanoma is capable of metastasizing to nearly any site in the body. Metastases to the lung, liver, brain, and bone (in decreasing order of frequency) are most common. Cardiac, adrenal, pancreatic, visceral, and renal metastases are less common. Brain metastases can lead to hemorrhage in approximately 50% of cases, and strong consideration should be given to radiation and/or resection, particularly given that a percentage of patients with solitary brain metastases who undergo resection and radiation therapy survive for more than 5 years. As a rule, however, distant metastases are associated with a poor prognosis. Median survival after diagnosis is 15 to 20 months, with improved prognosis associated with subcutaneous or lymph node metastases only and a normal LDH. Treatment options for systemic melanoma are shown in Table 16.5. After many years of ineffective treatment for systemic disease, the past few years have witnessed a remarkable number of new agents for the treatment of advanced melanoma. The optimal sequencing and combination of these new therapies remains an area of active investigation.

Prognosis

Multiple patient- and tumor-related factors influence the prognosis of melanoma. Women have a better prognosis than do men, although when matched for stage survival among men and women is similar. In addition, age and survival are inversely correlated.

TABLE 16.4 Differences between ILP and ILI for treatment of in-transit melanoma

	Method of Treatment	Treatment Regimen	Complete Response Rates (%)	Overall Response Rates (%)
ILP	Open incision Complete vascular isolation Oxygenated CPB pump	Melphalan Hyperthermia	50–60	80–90
ILI	Percutaneous access Hypoxic infusion	Melphalan Actinomycin D	30–40	60–90

CR, complete response; CPB, cardiopulmonary bypass.

TABLE 16.5 Treatment options for patients with systemic melanoma

Observation	• Often warranted for asymptomatic patients in poor medical condition
Surgical resection of metastases	• For select patients, resection can provide effective palliation of symptoms and a 5-y survival of up to 29%
Radiation therapy	• Palliative treatment of symptomatic lesions and brain metastases
Chemotherapy	• Combination regimens including dacarbazine (DTIC) are used predominately but are now reserved for patients failing other options
Targeted therapy	• BRAF inhibitors (vemurafenib, dabrafenib) target the activating mutation in BRAF (present in 60% of melanomas). Response rates of 50%, but resistance develops after a median of 9 mo • MEK inhibitor (trametinib) often in combination with BRAF inhibition
Biologic therapy	• Interleukin-2 results in a 10%–20% response rate (some responses are dramatic) but largely supplanted by ipilimumab • Anti-CTLA-4 antibody (ipilimumab) is associated with modest response rates, but substantially improves overall survival • Anti-PD-1 antibody (pembrolizumab) recently demonstrated improved response rates and overall survival compared to ipilimumab in a phase III trial

Older patients generally present with thicker melanomas and, accordingly, do worse, although for unexplained reasons, the incidence of lymph node metastases in the elderly is decreased.

Both anatomic site (head/neck, trunk, or extremity) and histologic subtype (superficial spreading, nodular, acral lentiginous, or lentigo maligna) have prognostic significance, but when other factors are accounted for, these tend not to be independent risk factors.

Thickness of the primary melanoma is a powerful prognostic factor. The Breslow scale divides melanoma into thickness groups; thickness is inversely correlated with survival. The other common measure of depth (the Clark system) is also highly predictive of prognosis. Figure 16.2 outlines the Clark system, which classifies tumors by anatomic level of invasion. Accurate determination of Clark level requires an experienced pathologist, a disadvantage of the Clark level compared to the Breslow scale. In most cases, including the staging criteria, Breslow depth has supplanted Clark level as more predictive of outcome.

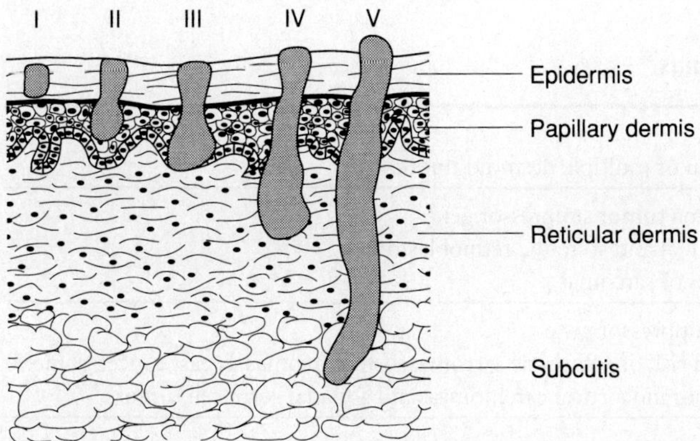

FIGURE 16.2 Clark levels of invasion. (From Chang AE, Johnson TM, Rees RS. Cutaneous neoplasms. In: Greenfield LJ, Mulholland MW, Oldham KT, et al., eds. *Surgery: Scientific Principles and Practice.* 2nd ed. Philadelphia: Lippincott–Raven Publishers; 1997:2233, with permission.)

Ulceration is another important prognostic factor. The presence of ulceration confers the risk of a nonulcerated melanoma of the next highest T stage. For example, for a patient with a T2b ulcerated lesion (1.01 to 2 mm thickness), the 5-year survival is 82%, which is comparable to the 79% 5-year survival of a patient with a T3a lesion (2 to 4 mm thickness, nonulcerated). Thus, ulcerated lesions are upstaged accordingly in the current staging system. Ulceration remains prognostic in stage III lesions, particularly those with microscopic lymph node metastases. In patients with a single microscopic lymph node metastasis and no ulceration, the 5-year survival is 82% compared to 52% if ulceration is present.

Additional factors such as lymphovascular invasion and microsatellitosis are rare but strongly associated with adverse outcomes. The presence of tumor infiltrating lymphocytes and regression of the primary lesions are typically reported but have been associated with variable prognostic significance. Analyses of large series examining multiple factors have consistently underscored the importance of thickness, ulceration, and nodal status as key independent prognostic factors in patients with melanoma, whereas other primary tumor factors such as age, mitotic rate, and Clark level may only impact on prognosis in select patients.

SOFT TISSUE SARCOMA

Soft tissue *sarcomas* are malignant tumors of mesenchymal origin, arising in tissues such as fat, muscle, and connective tissue. Sarcomas include a diverse group of neoplasms including over 50 separate histologic subtypes. Clinically, extremity sarcomas (approximately 50% of tumors) are distinguished from those arising in the abdominal cavity or retroperitoneum (approximately 30%) (Fig. 16.3). Sarcomas have an age-adjusted incidence of 3.3 per 100,000 and represent approximately 1% of adult malignancies and 20% of pediatric malignancies. Each year in the United States, there are approximately 12,000 new cases of soft tissue sarcomas, with cases divided equally between men and women, and approximately 4,700 deaths from soft tissue sarcomas.

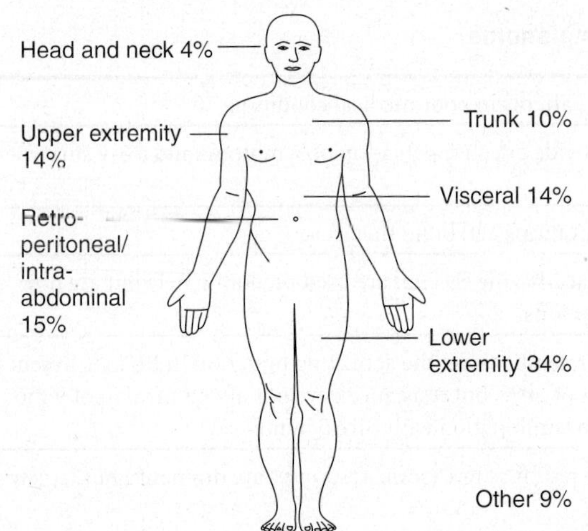

FIGURE 16.3 Anatomic distribution of the site of soft tissue sarcoma.

Etiology

Both genetic and environmental factors appear to play a role in the pathogenesis of sarcomas. Several *genetic syndromes* are associated with the development of sarcomas. These are summarized in Table 16.6. Additional genetic abnormalities are common but tend to be specific to certain histologic subtypes, for example, CDK4 and MDM2 amplifications are frequently identified in well-differentiated liposarcomas. *Environmental factors*, including exposure to herbicides, arsenic, vinyl chloride, and radiation, are also associated with an increased incidence of sarcoma. Generally, the onset of disease follows exposure to radiation by 10 or more years. *Stewart–Treves syndrome* is characterized by the development of a lymphangiosarcoma in the setting of lymphedema, classically in patients with breast cancer following mastectomy, axillary lymph node dissection, and external beam radiation. Lymphangiosarcomas can also develop in patients who have long-standing lymphedema from other causes.

Histology

Although not incorporated into the staging system, the importance of histologic subtype is increasingly appreciated. Table 16.7 summarizes the most common histologic subtypes. Specific histologic subtypes have characteristic biology and may dictate the role for additional radiation or chemotherapy. For example, both rhabdomyosarcoma and Ewing sarcoma tend to respond favorably to chemotherapy, whereas no evidence of responsiveness exists for gastrointestinal stromal tumor (GIST), clear cell sarcoma, or alveolar soft part sarcoma.

Extremity Sarcomas

Diagnosis

Diagnosis begins with a comprehensive history and physical examination. During the early course of the disease, clinical manifestations are unusual, and a mass is the most common presenting complaint. Frequently, an incidental traumatic event may initially draw attention to the tumor.

The ratio of benign to malignant soft tissue tumors is approximately 100:1. Fixation to underlying structures, variation in consistency, and larger size should raise concern for malignancy. When a suspicious mass is discovered, *a tissue sample must be obtained for diagnosis.* Core needle biopsy is generally the diagnostic procedure of choice. Alternatively, open biopsy can be performed and is specifically indicated when a core needle biopsy is nondiagnostic. Incisional biopsies are preferable, with care taken to avoid raising tissue flaps, disturbing tissue planes, and creating hematomas to minimize dissemination of malignant cells. Excisional biopsy, particularly for lesions greater than 2 cm is discouraged, as the contamination of the surrounding tissue may necessitate a more extensive definitive excision. Biopsy incisions should be chosen to allow for subsequent incorporation into the definitive resection. Incisional biopsies on the extremities are therefore performed utilizing longitudinal skin incisions. Fine needle aspiration is generally not used as the initial diagnostic procedure because of the small amount of material obtained and the low diagnostic accuracy.

Staging

Imaging studies provide invaluable information for defining the extent of a tumor for staging purposes and for planning a resection. Imaging is typically obtained early in the diagnostic workup, as it may help differentiate benign from malignant etiologies. The most commonly used imaging modalities for evaluation of soft tissue

TABLE 16.6 Genetic syndromes associated with sarcomas

Gardner syndrome	• Mutations in APC gene • Associated with formation of multiple desmoid tumors
Retinoblastoma	• Mutation in retinoblastoma tumor suppressor gene • Responsible for both familial and sporadic retinoblastoma • Increased risk for all types of sarcomas
Li–Fraumeni syndrome	• Mutation in p53 tumor suppressor gene • Associated with increased risk of soft tissue sarcomas, osteosarcomas, breast cancer, acute leukemia, brain tumors, adrenocortical carcinomas, and gonadal germ cell tumors
Neurofibromatosis I (von Recklinghausen disease)	• Mutation in NF1 tumor suppressor gene • Associated with multiple neurofibromas and café au lait spots, and ~10% lifetime risk of developing sarcoma • Nearly all sarcomas are neurofibrosarcomas

APC, adenomatous polyposis coli.

TABLE 16.7 Most common histologic subtypes of soft tissue sarcoma

Histology	Frequency	Description
Leiomyosarcoma	24%	50% arise in retroperitoneum/abdominal cavity
Pleomorphic undifferentiated sarcoma[a]	17%	Diagnosis of exclusion
Liposarcoma	12%	Most commonly arise in retroperitoneum or thigh
Dermatofibrosarcoma	11%	Indolent, rare distant metastases
Rhabdomyosarcoma	5%	Most common childhood sarcoma
Angiosarcoma	4%	Frequently cutaneous and follow prior irradiation or lymphedema
Malignant peripheral nerve sheath tumor (MPNST)	4%	Arise in the major nerves of extremity and body wall
Fibrosarcoma	4%	Frequently in the thigh or trunk, rare metastases
Other	19%	Over 40 other subtypes are described

[a]Previously malignant fibrous histiocytoma.

sarcomas are computed tomographic (CT) scan and magnetic resonance imaging (MRI) with or without magnetic resonance angiography (MRA). Although MRI is widely considered to provide better resolution of soft tissues, a prospective observational study of 133 soft tissue sarcoma patients demonstrated no difference between CT and MRI in predicting tumor involvement of muscle, bone, joints, or neurovascular structures. Because hematogenous spread to the lungs is the most common site of distant failure for extremity and body wall sarcomas, chest imaging is indicated as part of the staging evaluation. Particularly for patients with high-grade lesions or those with tumors greater than 5 cm, chest CT (rather than x-ray) should be considered. Pulmonary metastases occur in fewer than 10% of patients with low-grade tumors.

A combination of pathologic and radiographic information is used to stage sarcomas. In addition to the classic TNM staging system, sarcoma staging also incorporates *pathologic grade* (G). *Pathologic grade*, rather than histologic type, is considered a more significant prognostic parameter and is more reproducible among pathologists. Pathologic grade is based on differentiation of cells, degree of necrosis, and number of mitoses per high-power field. A number of different grading systems have been employed over time, but currently, a 3-tier system is considered the standard. T stage is further divided into Ta and Tb based upon the depth of the tumor, with tumors either involving or deep to the superficial fascia considered "deep," although the ultimate pathologic stage is no longer influenced by tumor depth. The current (revised in 2009) AJCC staging system is shown in Table 16.8. Importantly, the current staging system specifically excludes *GIST* as a distinct entity with a separate staging system.

Surgical Treatment

Resection is the mainstay of treatment, although other modalities are useful as adjuvants. Sarcomas are characterized by a *pseudocapsule*, which cannot be used as a plane of dissection. Microscopic disease extends beyond the pseudocapsule, and dissection along this plane will lead to local recurrence in 75% of patients. Local recurrence rates decreased dramatically once this fact was recognized and *radical resection* (i.e., amputation or excision of entire muscle groups and compartments) was adopted. More recently, *limb-sparing surgery* has become the standard, with high-volume centers reporting amputation rates of less than 10%.

Wide radical excision is key to successful limb-sparing surgery, and involves the removal of all gross tumor with a wide margin of normal tissue. Generally, a 2-cm resection margin of normal tissue is obtained (Fig. 16.4). To obtain a negative margin, resection of high-grade tumors using wide radical excision may require resection and reconstruction of involved vascular structures and occasionally

TABLE 16.8 AJCC sarcoma staging system

G	Histologic grade of malignancy
G1	Well differentiated
G2	Intermediate
G3	Undifferentiated
T	Primary tumor size[a,b]
T1	Tumor ≤5 cm
T2	Tumor >5 cm
N	Regional lymph nodes
N0	Absent regional lymph node involvement
N1	Present regional lymph node involvement
M	Distant metastasis
M0	Absent distant metastasis
M1	Present distant metastasis
Pathologic staging classification	
I	G1, T1a-b, N0, M0
	G1, T2a-b, N0, M0
II	G2-3, T1a-b, N0, M0
	G2, T2a-b, N0, M0
III	G3, T2a-b, N0, M0
	Any G, any T, N1, M0
IV	Any G, any T, any N, M1

[a]Tumor entirely superficial to the superficial fascia.

[b]Tumor deep to or involving the fascia, also includes retroperitoneal, mediastinal, and pelvic sarcomas.

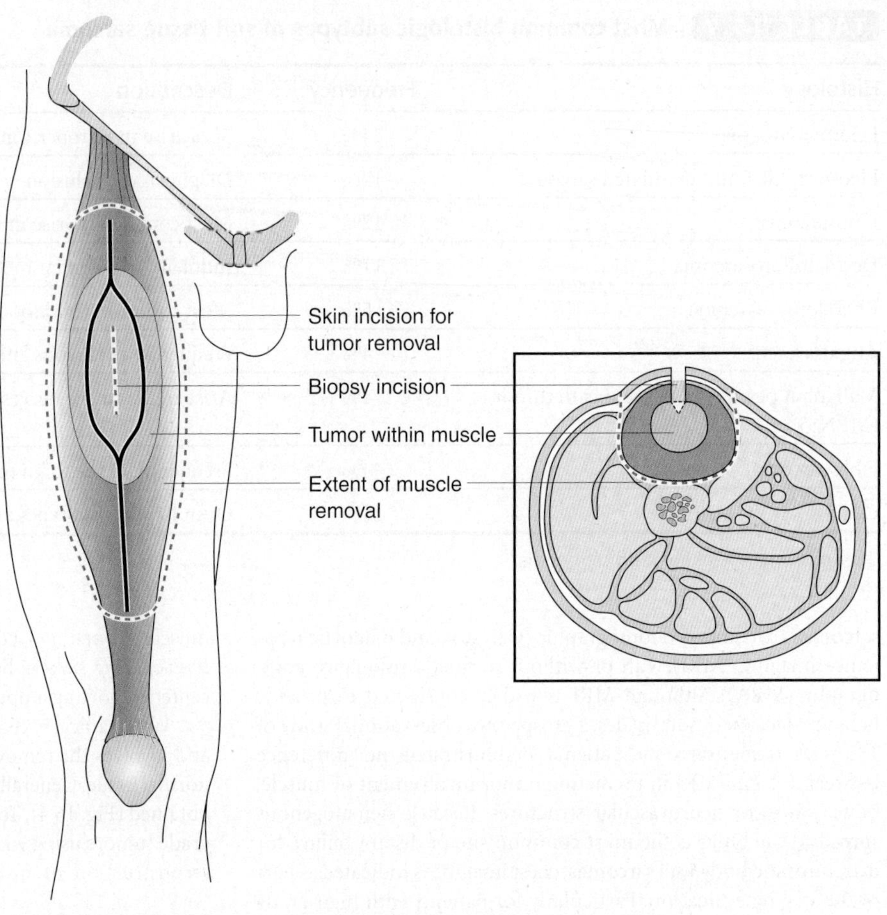

FIGURE 16.4 Surgical diagnosis and treatment of sarcoma. A longitudinal biopsy incision and definitive resection spares limb function. (From Mulholland MW. *Greenfield's Surgery: Scientific Principles and Practice*. 5th ed. Philadelphia: Lippincott Williams & Wilkins; 2011.)

resection of nerves. However, close margins are tolerated in order to preserve major neurovascular structures. If resection margins are found to be positive postoperatively, considerations should be given to reexcision if functionality will not be significantly impaired as positive margins are associated with dramatically increased rates of local recurrence. Amputation is indicated for patient preference or if gross total resection would leave the limb nonfunctional.

Sarcomas spread hematogenously, and lymph node metastases are seen in only 2% to 3% of cases. Since regional lymph node involvement is unusual, sentinel lymph node biopsy is not indicated. A possible exception is in a few rare histologic subtypes such as epithelioid, clear cell, or rhabdomyosarcomas where regional lymph node metastases are found in more than 20% of such cases. Nodal metastases are also seen approximately in 10% of synovial sarcomas.

Neoadjuvant and Adjuvant Therapy

Radiation therapy can be given before, after, or during surgery and can be administered in the form of external beam radiation or brachytherapy. Radiation therapy plays an important role for sarcomas with close margins, high grade, and/or larger (>5 cm) size. Multiple trials have now demonstrated decreased local recurrence following adjuvant radiotherapy. A more recent trial by O'Sullivan et al. compared neoadjuvant to adjuvant radiation therapy and found similar efficacy although with differing complication profile. Neoadjuvant therapy was associated with an increased incidence of operative wound complications, but on long-term follow-up, adjuvant therapy was associated with decreased functional outcomes such as joint stiffness, fibrosis, and edema.

Systemic chemotherapy has also been used in patients with sarcoma. Trials of adjuvant chemotherapy have generally demonstrated no survival benefit. A meta-analysis of data from clinical trials utilizing doxorubicin-based regimens did reveal a small statistically significant improvement in local recurrence-free, distant recurrence-free, and overall survival in patients who received adjuvant chemotherapy. In most cases, when used, systemic chemotherapy is paired with radiotherapy. Sequential or concurrent use of chemotherapy and radiation therapy has demonstrated promising short-term results with improvements in local control, disease-free survival, and overall survival. However, the modest therapeutic benefits must be weighed against the substantial toxicity of these regimens. Currently, no systemic therapy is recommended for stage I sarcomas. The role for systemic therapies and the appropriate sequence with radiotherapy in stage II/III disease remains poorly defined. Theoretically, the use of neoadjuvant chemotherapy is appealing, as the tumor remains in place to assess response; if a tumor is resistant to therapy, further adjuvant systemic therapy (and its associated toxicity) can then be avoided.

Finally, localized therapy in the form of ILP can be used in cases where local control or limb salvage is particularly challenging or for locally advanced cases that would otherwise require amputation. ILP with the combination of TNF-α and chemotherapeutic agents such as melphalan has demonstrated limb salvage rates of greater than 80%. Furthermore, ILP using TNF-α and chemotherapy may be used in patients with stage IV disease that is advanced at the site of origin. ILP may preserve both the function of the affected limb and quality of life over the anticipated short period of survival of these patients. However, in North America, TNF-α is not available for clinical use, and ILP using chemotherapeutic agents alone is associated with minimal benefit.

Treatment of Local Recurrences

At least one third of patients develop local recurrence, most within 2 to 3 years after treatment. Any lesions suspicious for recurrence should be biopsied. The surgical principles for recurrence are similar to primary tumors, and multimodality therapies should be considered since such therapies may be curative in the absence of synchronous distant disease. Even if the site has been irradiated previously, brachytherapy or intraoperative radiotherapy may be options for additional treatment. Chemotherapy should be also considered for patients with local recurrences.

Distant Metastases

Patients who die from extremity sarcoma generally succumb to *distant metastases*. Tumors with higher histologic grade and size greater than 5 cm have a greater propensity to metastasize. Longer intervals from the treatment of the primary tumor to the occurrence of metastatic disease are associated with a better prognosis. The lungs are the most common site of metastasis and represent the only distant site of disease in approximately 50% of patients. Pulmonary lesions should be resected provided the patient can tolerate the operation and has adequate pulmonary reserve. Survival at 5 years in highly selected patients with completely resected pulmonary metastases ranges from 15% to 30%. Patients who have metastatic lesions outside of the lungs or who have unresectable lung metastases are generally treated with chemotherapy and have a poor prognosis.

Follow-Up

After resection of a primary sarcoma, patients with no evidence of disease should be followed with a history and physical examination and chest radiograph (either x-ray or CT) every 3 to 6 months for the first 2 to 3 years. Imaging of the primary site by MRI, CT, or ultrasound should also be considered depending on the risk of locoregional recurrence. Follow-up every 6 months for the subsequent 2 years is recommended, then yearly.

Retroperitoneal Sarcomas

Retroperitoneal sarcomas are considerably less common than are extremity sarcomas; they account for approximately 15% of all sarcomas. These tumors carry a poorer prognosis because they are frequently asymptomatic and undiagnosed until relatively advanced stages. Because of this, and the location adjacent to multiple vital organs, complete resection is often more difficult to achieve. Approximately half of patients with retroperitoneal sarcomas eventually develop local recurrences, and local recurrence (rather than distant metastasis) is the leading cause of death for these patients.

Diagnosis

Common presentations include an abdominal mass (80%), lower extremity neurologic symptoms (42%), and pain (37%). Most tumors are greater than 10 cm in diameter at the time of presentation, about two thirds are intermediate to high grade, and about two thirds are either liposarcomas or leiomyosarcomas.

Evaluation of a suspected retroperitoneal sarcoma should include CT scanning to delineate the extent of disease. It is important to distinguish a sarcoma from a *lymphoma* or a *germ cell tumor*, both of which are treated primarily with chemotherapy. If the diagnosis is in question or preoperative therapy is considered, an image-guided fine needle aspiration biopsy and, if that is inadequate, a core needle biopsy may be obtained. In addition, α-fetoprotein and β-human chorionic gonadotropin levels should be obtained since elevated levels are consistent with the presence of a germ cell tumor. An abdominal/pelvic MRI and/or MRA may be necessary to delineate the involvement of adjacent vascular structures. The metastatic workup should include a CT scan of the chest, abdomen, and pelvis as the lung and liver are the most common sites for distant metastasis.

Treatment of Primary Tumor, Local Recurrence, and Distant Metastasis

Chemotherapy has not been shown to be effective for these tumors, and the role for *radiation* remains poorly defined. Resection is the only modality that offers the possibility of cure. The goal of surgical resection is to achieve complete gross resection with microscopically negative margins. Given the proximity of adjacent viscera as well as the poorly defined tissue plans posteriorly in the retroperitoneum, attaining microscopically negative margins can be quite difficult (Fig. 16.5). Importantly, *complete gross resection* has been shown to be critical for long-term disease-free survival. Complete gross resection is possible in 55% to 85% of all initial cases. Surgeons must often decide whether to widely resect adjacent viscera *en bloc* with the sarcoma or whether to dissect near the pseudocapsule and risk leaving microscopically positive margins. Most series report at least one additional organ resected in 75% of cases. Approximately 25% of patients who undergo complete gross resection are found to have positive microscopic margins.

For patients with close resection margins, adjuvant radiotherapy may be used; however, the data for the use of radiotherapy in

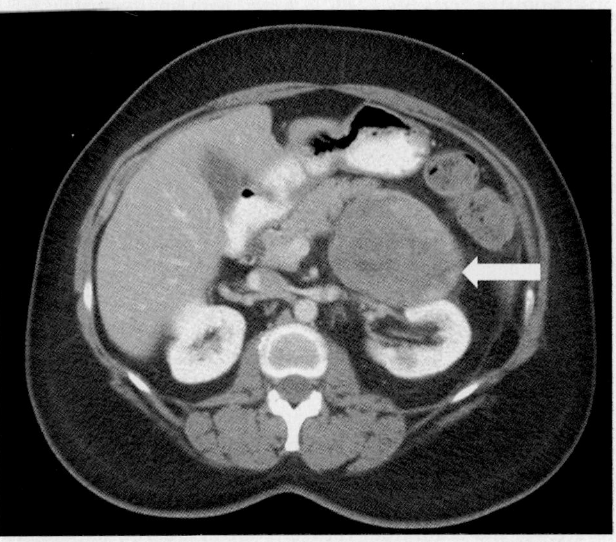

FIGURE 16.5 A large retroperitoneal sarcoma demonstrated on CT scan.

retroperitoneal sarcoma are not as strong as in the extremity setting. Given the proximity of many radiosensitive organs, adjuvant radiation therapy is frequently limited by toxicity. As such, most experts prefer neoadjuvant radiation if possible. Additionally, patients who have unresectable tumors on the basis of radiologic studies may be candidates for neoadjuvant chemoradiation in an attempt to decrease tumor size and render the tumor resectable. In the absence of multimodality therapy, surgery for patients with unresectable tumors has been associated with an equivalent survival to biopsy alone in some series. Particularly for aggressive histologies or high-grade tumors, surgeons should be very hesitant to operate on tumors felt to be unresectable. Cases requiring these multimodality approaches are best handled in centers that have a significant experience in dealing with these rare tumors.

A number of single institution surgical series have identified histologic subtype, grade, complete gross resection, and in some cases, the receipt of perioperative radiation as prognostic factors in patients with retroperitoneal sarcoma. Isolated local recurrence as the first site of recurrence occurs in approximately 40% of patients, although the timing of recurrence varies widely and can occur up to 10 years after resection in patients with low-grade malignancies such as well-differentiated liposarcomas. About half of these recurrences are amenable to complete gross re-resection, and resection represents the best option for therapy in recurrent disease. Distant recurrence develops in approximately 20% of resected patients with the liver and lung being the most frequent sites. As with extremity sarcoma, resection may be considered since long-term survival is possible following metastasectomy. Overall, however, patients with metastatic disease have only an 11-month median survival.

After resection of a primary retroperitoneal sarcoma, patients with no evidence of disease should be followed with a history and physical examination and abdominal CT every 3 to 6 months for the first 2 years. Chest imaging should also be considered during follow-up. Follow-up every 6 months for the subsequent 2 years is recommended, then yearly.

TABLE 16.9 AJCC gastric GIST staging system[a]

T	Tumor size
T1	Tumor is 2 cm or less
T2	Tumor is >2 cm but not larger than 5 cm
T3	Tumor is >5 cm but not larger than 10 cm
T4	Tumor is larger than 10 cm
N	Regional lymph nodes
N0	Absent regional lymph node involvement
N1	Present regional lymph node involvement
M	Distant metastasis
M0	Absent distant metastasis
M1	Present distant metastasis
Mitotic rate	
Low	Mitotic rate not >5/50 per high-power field
High	Mitotic rate >5/50 per high-power field
Pathologic staging classification	
IA	T1-2, N0, M0, low mitotic rate
IB	T3, N0, M0, low mitotic rate
II	T1-2, N0, M0, high mitotic rate
	T4, N0, M0, low mitotic rate
IIIA	T3, N0, M0, high mitotic rate
IIIB	T4, N0, M0, high mitotic rate
IV	Any T, N1, M0, any mitotic rate
	Any T, any N, M1, any mitotic rate

[a]The TNM classification is the same for nongastric GISTs, although there are slight differences in the pathologic staging classifications.

Gastrointestinal Stromal Tumors

GISTs are rare neoplasms of the GI tract with an estimated incidence of 4,000 to 6,000 a year in the United States. GISTs are thought to arise from the *interstitial cells of Cajal*, with approximately 60% located in the stomach, 30% in the small intestine, and the remainder throughout the rest of the GI tract, although omental GISTs can rarely occur. GISTs are molecularly characterized by overexpression of the receptor tyrosine kinase KIT (CD117) in 95% of tumors; 80% have a mutation leading to constitutive activation of KIT. Additionally 5% to 10% of GISTs overexpress PDGFRA, which is more frequent in tumors that do not overexpress KIT. Although GISTs were historically included in the sarcoma staging system, their unique biologic behavior and molecular classification have led to an independent staging classification shown in Table 16.9 for gastric GISTs. In GISTs, mitotic rate alone is used in place of tumor grade.

Surgical resection is the mainstay of therapy for localized GISTs. The goal is complete resection. Additional wide margins and regional lymphadenectomy are not necessary. Both laparoscopic and open approaches have been successfully utilized, so the approach to resection should be based upon surgeon expertise as well as anatomic considerations of the individual tumor. Disease recurrence and death from GIST are rare in low-risk tumors that are completely resected.

The prognosis associated with high-risk GISTs has been substantially altered with the development of imatinib—a tyrosine kinase inhibitor that targets both KIT and PDGFRA overexpression. Imatinib is now recommended for 3 years in the adjuvant setting for high-risk tumors. Although the precise definition of high-risk continues to be refined, tumors greater than 10 cm, a mitotic count greater than 10/50 high-power fields, tumors greater than 5 cm with a mitotic rate greater than 5/HPF, or a ruptured tumor have been used in trials showing benefit for adjuvant therapy. Neoadjuvant imatinib is reserved for patients with unresectable or borderline resectable tumors in order to decrease tumor size and allow for resection. Consideration for neoadjuvant imatinib may also be given for rectal GISTs. In the metastatic setting, imatinib is first-line therapy. Cytoreductive surgery may be considered in patients with potentially resectable disease if the disease has responded or only shown very focal disease progression with treatment.

LYMPHOMA

Hematologic malignancies are the most common malignancies in children younger than 15 years but constitute only 9% of adult cancers. Although the primary treatment of lymphomas is rarely surgical, surgeons are often asked to assist in obtaining a diagnosis, provide intravenous access for the administration of chemotherapy, or treat complications of this diverse group of malignancies.

Lymph Node Biopsy

Surgical biopsy, rather than fine needle aspiration or core needle biopsies, is frequently required to confirm the diagnosis of lymphoma since tissue architecture factors heavily in the pathologic classification of lymphomas. Additionally, a considerable amount of tissue is often needed for the genetic and molecular phenotyping that is now routinely used to characterize the various types of lymphoma. The evaluation of a recurrence is an exception, and a core needle biopsy is often sufficient. Additionally, when lymphadenopathy is only in regions where a lymph node biopsy would be a high-risk procedure, then core needle biopsy may be considered as an initial approach. Generally, larger and more accessible lymph nodes should be sampled during surgical biopsy. Cervical or axillary lymph nodes generally are preferred over inguinal nodes as wound complication is less frequent as is false-positive nodal enlargement caused by reactive inflammation.

Hodgkin Lymphoma

Hodgkin lymphoma constitutes approximately 10% of all lymphomas. It is a malignancy of B cells and can be characterized pathologically by the presence of Reed–Sternberg cells. It presents in a bimodal age distribution with the first peak at approximately 20 years of age and a second peak at age 65. Painless lymphadenopathy is the most common presentation. Cervical/supraclavicular lymph node basins are the most commonly involved sites (60% to 80%) at presentation followed by the axillary (10% to 20%) and inguinal (6% to 12%) nodal basins. Alternatively, Hodgkin lymphoma can present as an incidentally discovered mass on imaging—most commonly a mediastinal mass with retroperitoneal adenopathy seen less frequently. Patients may report the presence of other symptoms such as fever (>38°C), night sweats, or weight loss of more than 10% of body weight over a 6-month period. These are designated as *B symptoms*; the incidence is low (20%) in early-stage disease but increases to approximately 50% in patients with advance disease.

In addition to a complete history focusing on the duration of lymph node enlargement as well as recent injury to sites drained by that lymphatic basin, the evaluation of patients referred for *lymph node biopsy* should include a physical examination with detailed evaluation of all accessible lymphatic tissue. This includes palpation of all superficial lymph node basins and abdominal palpation for hepatic or splenic enlargement. Diagnostic laboratory studies should include a complete blood count with differential and peripheral blood smear examination.

Staging in Hodgkin lymphoma is based on the extent of disease and the presence or absence of B symptoms (Table 16.10). Staging workup includes laboratory evaluation of liver function, LDH, and erythrocyte sedimentation rate, and radiographic studies including chest radiographs, CT scan (typically neck, chest, abdomen, and pelvis), and PET scan. Bone marrow biopsies provide additional information regarding the extent of disease and are recommended for stage IB, IIB, and III to IV disease. Historically, *staging laparotomy* played an important role in the evaluation of patients with Hodgkin lymphoma localized clinically to above the diaphragm. Staging laparotomy involved examination of the liver, small bowel, colon, and mesentery. Splenectomy and wedge biopsies of the liver were also performed with additional core needle biopsies of deeper hepatic tissue. Major nodal groups were then dissected including nodes associated with the hepatic artery, celiac axis, porta hepatis, and inferior mesenteric artery. If there were any nodes that were considered suspicious on the basis of evaluation at laparotomy or preoperative lymphangiography, these would also be removed with concomitant oophoropexy in anticipation of radiation to the pelvis (Fig. 16.6). This procedure has now fallen out of favor as salvage chemotherapy was found to adequately treat patients who were understaged clinically. In fact, after accounting for procedure-related complications, the overall survival was found to be lower in patients undergoing staging laparotomy.

TABLE 16.10 Staging in Hodgkin lymphoma[a]

Stage I	Disease limited to single lymph node region or single extralymphatic site
Stage II	Involvement of 2 or more lymph node regions on the same side of the diaphragm or 1 extralymphatic site with only adjacent lymph nodes involved
Stage III	Involvement of lymph nodes on both sides of the diaphragm with or without involvement of an extralymphatic site and/or the spleen (denoted with S)
Stage IV	Diffuse or disseminated involvement of one or more extralymphatic sites with or without associated lymph node involvement

[a]Absence or presence of constitutional symptoms is denoted with A or B, respectively.

Chemoradiation is the treatment modality of choice for all patients with stage I–II Hodgkin lymphoma, with chemotherapy with or without radiation used for more advanced stages. Advances in chemotherapy have turned what was once a highly lethal disease into one with a cure rate of 75% across all stages.

Non-Hodgkin Lymphoma

Non-Hodgkin lymphoma is increasing in incidence in the United States and now accounts for approximately 8% of malignancies. The presentation of these diverse malignancies can vary widely from an indolent course over years to an acute presentation that can be fatal within weeks. Tumors are classified by their cell of origin (B cell, T cell, or rarely natural killer cells), with most cases of B-cell descent (80%).

More than two thirds of patients with non-Hodgkin lymphoma present with lymphadenopathy. The surgeon is typically called upon to obtain *tissue for diagnosis* and to *treat extranodal lymphomas in the gastrointestinal tract.* Suspicion of an aggressive non-Hodgkin lymphoma is one of the few indications for the urgent performance of a lymph node biopsy.

Gastric Mucosa–Associated Lymphoid Tissue Lymphoma

Gastric *mucosa–associated lymphoid tissue* (MALT) *lymphoma* is a clonal B-cell neoplasm typically associated with an indolent course but prone to local recurrence and occasionally capable of distant metastatic spread or degeneration into a high-grade B-cell lymphoma. MALT lymphoma is classically associated with *Helicobacter pylori* infection, which is present in over 90% of cases. For early disease, treatment of *H. pylori* alone serves as a highly effective treatment for MALT lymphoma. For those with advanced disease or in

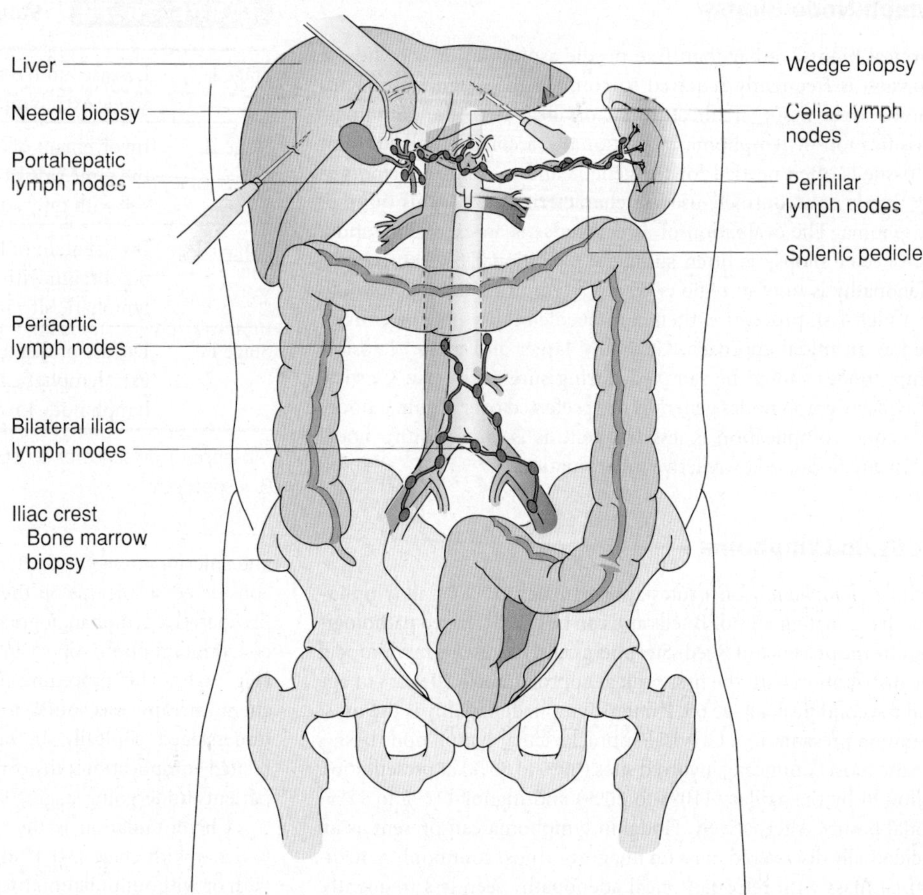

FIGURE 16.6 Biopsy sites for staging laparotomy. (From Mulholland MW. *Greenfield's Surgery: Scientific Principles and Practice*. 5th ed. Philadelphia: Lippincott Williams & Wilkins; 2011.)

whom *H. pylori* therapy fails, radiation therapy is typically highly effective, with surgical resection reserved for cases in which radiation is contraindicated. Additionally, if the diagnosis is in question, surgical resection may serve as both diagnostic and therapeutic. Typically, if negative margins after surgical resection are achieved, close surveillance without additional therapy is recommended.

Gastric Lymphoma

The GI tract is the most common site of involvement for extranodal non-Hodgkin lymphoma, and primary lymphoma of the GI tract represents a clinical entity managed distinctly from other lymphomas. The majority of GI lymphomas arise in the stomach (75%), and gastric lymphomas represent the second most common gastric malignancy in the United States. Gastric lymphomas typically present with nonspecific symptoms such as abdominal pain, weight loss, nausea/vomiting, or bleeding; rarely, perforation can occur.

Surgical resection is now rarely employed for these malignancies. Chemotherapy as the therapy of choice was established by a randomized trial comparing patients receiving surgery alone, surgery and radiation, surgery and chemotherapy, or chemotherapy alone. The overall survival differences were striking, with a 54% 10-year survival in patients receiving surgery alone compared to 96% in those receiving chemotherapy alone. Additionally, delayed toxicities were increased in those who received both surgery and chemotherapy compared to chemotherapy alone. Surgery is now reserved for those rare patients who develop complications from the disease or during therapy.

Other Gastrointestinal Lymphomas

Lymphomas of the small bowel are uncommon in the United States but are the most common extranodal lymphoma in the Middle East. These tumors have a higher incidence in patients with *celiac disease* and are most often found in the proximal jejunum. Patients may present with obstruction, intussusception, or bleeding. Like other GI lymphomas, chemotherapy is the mainstay of therapy; however, obtaining a tissue diagnosis in small bowel lesions can be challenging. As such, surgical resection is employed for this reason as well as for the treatment of symptomatic lesions. Following resection, adjuvant chemotherapy is indicated even in the absence of additional disease. Radiation therapy has been advocated by some, but its utility is limited by the incidence of radiation enteritis.

Colonic lymphomas are rare, although they are the most common noncarcinomatous tumors of the large bowel. They managed similarly to small bowel lymphomas with the exception that tissue diagnosis can typically be obtained via colonoscopy so surgical resection is reserved for refractory or symptomatic lesions.

SPLEEN

Surgical intervention is frequently required for *splenic trauma* and less frequently in patients with *splenic complications of hematologic disorders*. This section considers the normal anatomy and function of the spleen and discusses the surgical care of patients with splenic manifestations of systemic disease.

Anatomy and Normal Function

The normal adult *spleen* weighs between 100 and 200 g and extends in the left upper quadrant from the ninth to the eleventh rib. The blood supply is predominantly via the splenic artery, which classically arises from the celiac trunk, although in rare cases may be a direct branch off of the aorta or can be duplicated. The anatomy of the splenic artery is highly variable as it enters the spleen. In approximately 70% of patients, the artery branches proximally forming many small arteries distributed over a wide hilum; in the remainder of patients, the artery divides more distally and is associated with only a few branches in a relatively narrow hilum. Collaterals with the splenic artery include the left gastroepiploic artery as well as the short gastric arteries. The venous drainage of the spleen typically runs parallel and posterior to the arterial anatomy.

The spleen is attached to surrounding structures by *ligaments* including the gastrosplenic (containing the short gastric arteries), the splenorenal (containing the splenic vessels as well as the tail of the pancreas), the splenocolic (containing the left gastroepiploic vessels), and the splenophrenic ligaments. Knowledge of these ligamentous attachments is important to avoid inadvertent traction injury to the spleen or pancreas when operating in the left upper quadrant.

The parenchyma of the spleen is divided into *red pulp* and *white pulp*. Blood is carried into the spleen from the hilum via trabecular arteries, which branch to form the central arterioles. Central arterioles are surrounded by white pulp over much of their course and empty either into the red pulp from open-ended penicillary arterioles or into venules through a closed circulation without being directly exposed to the red pulp. After entering venous sinusoids, blood drains into trabecular veins and exits via the splenic vein (Fig. 16.7).

The red pulp contains a large numbers of macrophages that function to remove aged or defective red blood cells and to also remove cellular inclusions such as *Heinz bodies* (denatured hemoglobin), *Howell–Jolly bodies* (nuclear remnant), or *Pappenheimer bodies* (iron granules). In autoimmune hemolytic anemia, these macrophages recognize and destroy red blood cells coated with autoantibodies. The spleen is a *secondary lymphoid organ*, with the majority of lymphoid activity occurring in the white pulp. Serum and foreign antigens contained within blood extravasate through the splenic vasculature and are filtered through the white pulp and sinusoids. These antigens may then be taken up, processed, and presented by macrophages or dendritic cells.

The spleen has other functions including production of the opsonins *properdin* and *tuftsin*, production of monocytes and lymphocytes, and storage of 30% to 40% of the body's platelets. It also serves as a site of hematopoiesis during early development and in some pathologic conditions. Properdin plays an important role in activating the alternative pathway of complement and causing the subsequent destruction of bacteria and foreign cells. Tuftsin is important in augmenting the activity of phagocytic cells.

Splenomegaly and Hypersplenism

An absolute size criterion to define splenomegaly has not been defined. A palpable spleen on physical exam represents a spleen that has enlarged by at least 40%, but this finding is neither sensitive nor specific for any specific pathologic condition. The differential diagnosis of *splenomegaly* includes infectious, hematologic, neoplastic, congestive, inflammatory, and infiltrative processes. Splenomegaly may be associated with symptoms including shortness of breath, early satiety, and weight loss secondary to mass effect. Hypersplenism is often coincident with splenomegaly but refers to functional hyperactivity rather than simply enlarged size.

Splenectomy

General indications for *splenectomy* include severely symptomatic splenomegaly, splenic vein thrombosis, hypersplenism refractory to medical management, for diagnostic purposes (e.g., suspected lymphoma), and in some cases of *splenic trauma* as discussed in Chapter 23 (Management of Specific Traumatic Injuries).

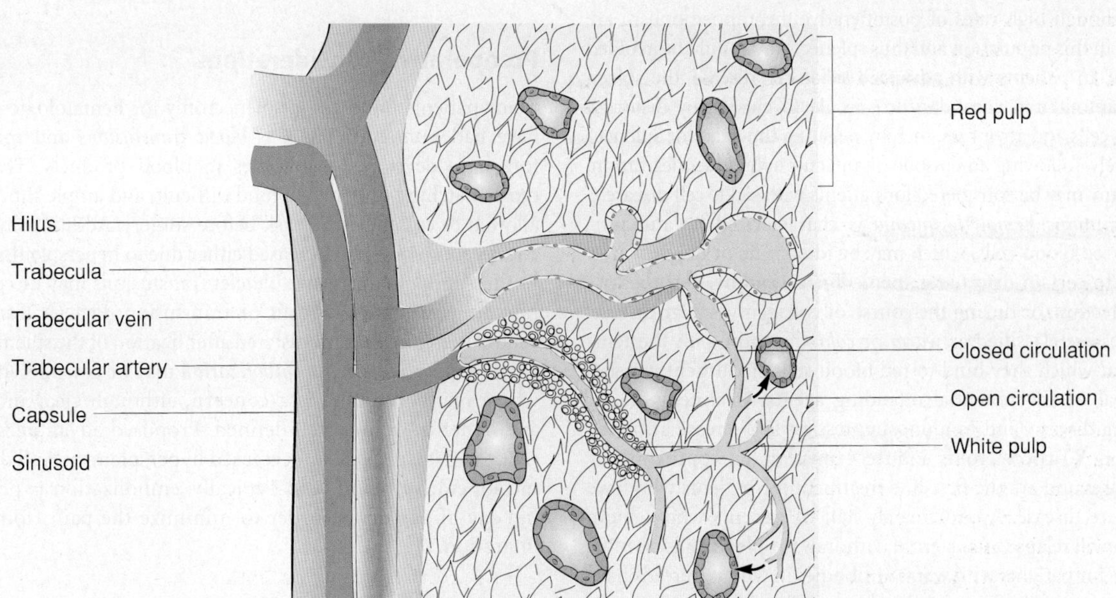

FIGURE 16.7 The splenic microcirculation is shown with depictions of both open and closed circulations. (From Meyer AA. Spleen. In: Greenfield LJ, Mulholland MW, Oldham KT, et al., eds. *Surgery: Scientific Principles and Practice*. 2nd ed. Philadelphia: Lippincott–Raven Publishers; 1997:1265, with permission.)

Congestion within the portal venous system, which may be due to primary hepatic disease, thrombosis of hepatic, portal, or splenic veins or right ventricular dysfunction, can result in splenomegaly. Pancreatitis is the most common cause of splenic vein thrombosis, and particularly in this setting, patients may present with bleeding gastric varices. Splenectomy is indicated to remove the source of gastric hypertension.

A number of *inflammatory* or *autoimmune conditions* may result in reactive hyperplasia of the spleen and splenomegaly. This is seen in a variety of disorders including infectious mononucleosis, autoimmune hemolytic anemia, and systemic lupus erythematosus. Rheumatoid arthritis, when accompanied by splenomegaly and neutropenia, is known as *Felty syndrome.* This condition is associated with antibodies against granulocytes, and splenectomy may be indicated for severe neutropenia or neutropenia resistant to the medical treatment of the underlying rheumatoid arthritis.

Some *hematologic diseases* respond well to splenectomy. *Hereditary spherocytosis*, the most common symptomatic familial hemolytic anemia, is characterized by defective erythrocyte membranes owing to defects in spectrin or ankyrin. In this disorder, red blood cells are relatively fragile and are destroyed after only a few passes through the splenic cords, resulting in anemia, jaundice, intractable leg ulcers, and an increased incidence of pigmented gallstones. Splenectomy typically resolves the symptoms and sequelae of the disease, although frequently a mild anemia persists. The optimal age for splenectomy remains undefined, but current recommendations recommend waiting until age 6 if possible and do not recommend splenectomy prior to age 3. The practice of prophylactic cholecystectomy at the time of splenectomy is controversial but may be considered on an individual basis. *Hereditary elliptocytosis* is a similar, though less severe, disorder of red blood cell membranes. Splenectomy may be indicated in symptomatic patients with this disorder. *Thalassemia major* and *sickle cell disease* are red blood cell disorders characterized by abnormal hemoglobin biosynthesis and increased red blood cell destruction. Occasionally splenectomy is required in thalassemia patients with persistent transfusion requirements, although high rates of postoperative thromboembolism are described in this population and thus splenectomy should be avoided if possible. In patients with advanced sickle cell disease, the spleen typically autoinfarcts secondary to vascular occlusion by distorted red blood cells and atrophies, thereby negating the need for splenectomy. Rarely, following an episode of an acute splenic sequestration, splenectomy may be considered for patients with sickle cell disease.

Autoimmune hemolytic anemia is characterized by autoantibodies to red blood cells, which may be idiopathic or develop after exposure to certain drugs (e.g., penicillin, quinidine, and methyldopa), infection, or during the course of collagen vascular disease. Antibodies are classified as *warm* or *cold*, depending on the temperature at which they bind to red blood cells. Treatment consists of removal of any potential offending agents, treatment of any underlying disease, and immunosuppression to decrease antibody production. Corticosteroids induce remission in approximately 70% of cases and are the first-line treatment for patients who have more severe disease. Approximately half of patients who achieve remission will relapse after steroid withdrawal. Splenectomy is indicated only for patients with warm antibodies in whom steroids have failed or are contraindicated. Splenectomy will achieve remission in approximately 70% of these patients.

Hematologic disorders may also result in *increased platelet destruction*, and splenectomy is often an effective treatment. ITP (also called immune thrombocytopenia) is characterized by IgG antibodies directed at platelets. The spleen contributes both to the production of these antibodies and to the destruction of antibody-coated platelets. ITP is a diagnosis of exclusion based upon isolated thrombocytopenia in the absence of another identifiable cause. ITP is more prevalent in children; in adults, women are more commonly afflicted. The presentation is widely variable in severity but is associated with prolonged bleeding times but normal clotting times. *The spleen is generally not enlarged.* Easy bruising, petechiae, epistaxis, bleeding from the gums, and menorrhagia are commons, whereas visceral hematomas or intracranial hemorrhage are rare. Treatment is recommended for symptomatic patients or any adult patient with a platelet count below 30,000/μL. Steroids are the first-line therapy; however, they are ineffective in the majority of patients and even when effective relapse can occur following discontinuation of the therapy. Splenectomy has the highest rate of long-term remission of any second-line therapy for patients in whom steroid therapy fails. Two thirds of patients undergoing splenectomy will experience a complete response with an additional 20% of patients experiencing an improvement in thrombocytopenia. Younger patients in particular have improved outcomes following splenectomy. In those who cannot tolerate splenectomy, rituximab (anti-CD20 antibody) is an additional second-line therapy. Newer thrombopoiesis-stimulating agents are available but serve only to raise the platelet count and do not induce remission. Persistence of symptoms may indicate the presence of an *accessory spleen. Technetium scanning* is a sensitive method of detecting accessory spleens, which should be removed if they are found.

Thrombotic thrombocytopenic purpura (TTP) is a microangiopathic hemolytic anemia. Small vessel thrombi result in activation or destruction of multiple blood components, resulting in anemia, thrombocytopenia, and thrombosis. This typically presents with neurologic derangement and renal failure and was highly fatal prior to the institution plasma exchange for these patients. Prior to the establishment of plasma exchange as the standard therapy, splenectomy was a mainstay of treatment although mostly ineffective. Splenectomy is now rarely, if ever, indicated for TTP.

Preoperative Considerations

Many patients undergoing splenectomy for hematologic disorders have had numerous *previous blood transfusions* and may therefore have developed antibodies to blood products. This makes cross-matching of banked blood difficult, and ample time must be allowed to complete this task before surgery. Additionally, platelet counts are frequently decreased either due to hypersplenism or ITP. In this setting preoperative platelet transfusions may be consumed rapidly negating the benefit of transfusion. Platelet transfusions should therefore be administered after ligation of the splenic vessels.

Preoperative *splenic embolization* may be considered in cases where major bleeding is a concern, although clear indications and benefits are not well defined. Proposed advantages include reduction in spleen size, decreased hypersplenism, and decreased intraoperative blood loss. Typically, embolization is performed the day of surgery in order to minimize the pain from splenic infarction.

Technical Considerations

Laparoscopic splenectomy is now widely utilized and is the preferred initial approach in many patients. Relative contraindications to laparoscopic resection include traumatic injury, those with severe portal hypertension, ascites, or coagulopathy, or extreme splenomegaly. Additionally, particular care must be taken with the laparoscopic approach to thoroughly search for *accessory spleens*, which are detected in approximately 15% of patients undergoing splenectomy. Care must be taken to avoid splenic rupture, as *splenosis* can result in potentially hundreds of small implants of splenic tissue being distributed throughout the abdomen. Particularly in the setting of ITP, the failure to resect all splenic tissue has been associated with disease recurrence and need for an additional operation.

Laparoscopic splenectomy is typically performed using a lateral approach with the patient in *right lateral decubitus position*. Alternatively, an anterior approach can be used with the patient typically placed in lithotomy. Port placement is variable but typically includes a 10- to 12-mm camera port and three to five other ports for placement of instruments and retractors. The search for accessory spleens should be the initial step, as detection may be difficult after intra-abdominal blood loss. The vast majority of accessory spleens are found along the vascular pedicle into the splenic hilum or by the pancreatic tail, but approximately 10% may be found more distantly in the greater omentum. After exploration, the left gastroepiploic and short gastric vessels are divided. The splenic hilum is then dissected. The pancreatic tail is in proximity to the splenic hilum, and care must be taken to avoid injuring the pancreas. Once isolated, the splenic artery and vein are either clipped individually (possible when patients have many small arterial branches in the hilum) or divided using an endoscopic stapling device. The spleen can then be removed either by enlarging one of the port-site incisions to allow for removal or by morcellation within a plastic retrieval bag placed into the peritoneal cavity.

Open splenectomy is generally approached through a *midline or left subcostal incision*. The ligamentous attachments to the spleen are divided to mobilize the spleen. These normally avascular attachments may contain collateral vessels in myeloid metaplasia and secondary hypersplenism. The short gastric vessels (within the gastrosplenic ligament) are ligated. The hilar vessels are then dissected and ligated. During elective splenectomy, the hilar dissection may be completed before mobilization of the ligamentous attachments. Initial ligation of the splenic artery serves to decrease the size of the spleen and facilitates complete mobilization.

No randomized data are available to support the use of laparoscopic versus open splenectomy. As such, all the series comparing the two approaches are limited by selection bias. In general, the laparoscopic approach has been associated with longer operative times, equivalent complication rates, and decreased hospital length of stay.

Complications of Splenectomy

Splenectomy is generally well tolerated in both elective and emergent cases. Overall, the morbidity rate following elective splenectomy is 12% to 20% and the mortality rate is approximately 1%, although these numbers vary widely depending on the indication for the procedure. Respiratory complications (atelectasis and pneumonia) and bleeding are the most common complications. Although less common, concern for *subphrenic abscess* should be raised if a patient develops hiccups postoperatively as this is frequently a sign of diaphragmatic irritation. Portal vein thrombosis is a complication that appears to have been underreported in the early splenectomy literature. In series of patients prospectively imaged following splenectomy, 8% to 50% of patients have been found to have portal vein thrombosis, although most patients remain asymptomatic. The mechanism for this complication appears to be propagation of clot in the splenic vein stump. A high index of suspicion must be maintained for patients presenting with atypical abdominal pain, anorexia, ileus, or ascites postoperatively as in rare cases this can be a fatal complication.

Leukocytosis and *thrombocytosis* are frequently observed in the postsplenectomy patient. These elevations generally occur 1 to 2 days after surgery and may persist for several weeks. These laboratory abnormalities are generally not clinically significant; however, antiplatelet agents such as aspirin should be considered if the platelet count increases over 1 million/μL. Delayed complications may also arise from splenectomy. These include *pseudoaneurysm formation* of the splenic artery and *pancreatic fistula* or *pseudocyst formation* resulting from iatrogenic injury to the pancreas.

Patients who have undergone a splenectomy are more susceptible to *infections* compared with the general population. Although this increase has been reported to be as high as 200 to 600 times the normal risk, this translates into an estimated incidence of approximately 0.2%. The risk is somewhat higher in the pediatric population with an estimated incidence of 0.6%. The indication for splenectomy appears to affect risk with posttraumatic splenectomy engendering the least risk. The first 2 years after splenectomy are considered the most dangerous in both the adult and pediatric populations, but cases of *overwhelming postsplenectomy infection* (OPSI) have been reported over 20 years after splenectomy.

Encapsulated bacteria are the most frequent infectious agents responsible for OPSI. *Streptococcus pneumoniae* infections account for between 50% and 90% of cases. *Haemophilus influenza* and more rarely nonencapsulated bacteria, such as *Streptococcus* type B, *Staphylococcus aureus, Salmonella, Escherichia coli*, constitute the vast majority of the remaining cases. The clinical course of OPSI may be fulminant; characteristically, patients develop fever and mild symptoms of infection followed rapidly by severe sepsis. Progression from good health to death can occur in less than 24 hours, and overall mortality has been reported at 40% to 70%. Treatment of patients with suspected OPSI must be prompt and aggressive.

Vaccines against three encapsulated organisms (*S. pneumonia, H. influenza*, and *Neisseria meningitidis*) are widely available and should be given at least 2 weeks before elective splenectomy. Following emergent cases, vaccines are ideally administered 14 days postoperatively; however, particularly in the trauma population where follow-up may be sporadic, many centers administer vaccines prior to discharge regardless of postoperative day.

Prophylactic antibiotics are not recommended in adults. Given the increased incidence of OPSI in the pediatric population, however, daily prophylactic penicillin is recommended for children until at least 5 years of age for at least 1 year following splenectomy. The data to support this came from a study of patients treated in 1995 and earlier, and the development of penicillin resistance since that time has likely negated some of the benefits of prophylaxis. Additionally, in all patients, antibiotics (extended-spectrum fluoroquinolones in adults) should be prescribed so that the patient can self-administer an immediate dose at the onset of a fever or rigors.

ACKNOWLEDGMENTS

The authors would like to acknowledge and thank Dale Han, MD; Robert J. Canter, MD; Francis R. Spitz, MD; and Mark B. Faries, MD, for their contributions in the prior editions of this book.

Suggested Readings

Avilés A, Nambo MJ, Neri N, et al. The role of surgery in primary gastric lymphoma: results of a controlled clinical trial. *Ann Surg.* 2004;240(1):44–50.

Bartlett E, Yoon SS. Current treatment for the local control of retroperitoneal sarcomas. *J Am Coll Surg.* 2011;213(3):436–446.

Carde P, Hagenbeek A, Hayat M, et al. Clinical staging versus laparotomy and combined modality with MOPP versus ABVD in early stage Hodgkin's disease: the H6 twin randomized trials from the European Organization for Research and Treatment of Cancer Lymphoma Cooperative Group. *J Clin Oncol.* 1993;11(11):2258–2272.

Kingham TP, Karakousis G, Ariyan C. Randomized clinical trials in melanoma. *Surg Oncol Clin N Am.* 2010;19(1):13–31.

Kojouri K, Vesely SK, Terrell DR, George JN. Splenectomy for adult patients with idiopathic thrombocytopenic purpura: a systematic review to assess long-term platelet count responses, prediction of response, and surgical complications. *Blood.* 2004;104(9):2623–2634.

Wargo JA, Tanabe K. Surgical management of melanoma. *Hematol Oncol Clin North Am.* 2009;23(3):565–581.

CHAPTER 17

Thyroid, Parathyroid, and Adrenal Glands

HEATHER WACHTEL AND DOUGLAS L. FRAKER

KEY POINTS

- The thyroid is derived from endoderm except for the calcitonin-secreting parafollicular cells (C cells), which are of ectodermal neural crest origin.
- Complications of thyroid or parathyroid surgery include recurrent laryngeal nerve (RLN) injury, which manifests as hoarseness of voice (if unilateral) or airway obstruction (if bilateral), hypoparathyroidism, and neck hematoma. The latter may require emergent evacuation at the bedside if there is evidence of airway compromise.
- A new or enlarging palpable thyroid nodule or thyroid nodule larger than 1.5 cm usually warrants FNA.
- Papillary cancers are characterized histologically by psammoma bodies and frequently spread via the lymphatics in contrast to follicular carcinomas, which spread hematogenously. Patients with well-differentiated thyroid cancers (i.e., papillary and follicular carcinomas) should generally undergo total thyroidectomy with postoperative radioactive iodine ablation therapy.
- Medullary thyroid cancer (MTC) is derived from parafollicular or C cells. It is associated with familial syndromes in about one third of the cases (MEN 2A or 2B), which frequently are associated with mutations of the *RET* protooncogene. Serum calcitonin levels can be helpful in the diagnosis, screening, and follow-up of patients with MTC.
- The most common cause of primary hyperparathyroidism is parathyroid adenoma. Most patients are asymptomatic, and the diagnosis is confirmed by elevated serum calcium levels with elevated PTH levels.
- *Hypercalcemic crisis* is a serious condition that can result from hyperparathyroidism and is characterized by elevated serum calcium levels, nausea and vomiting, weight loss, lethargy, and coma. Therapy is initially aimed at reducing calcium levels and includes hydration and loop diuretic administration. Hypercalcemia may manifest clinically with positive *Chvostek* and *Trousseau* signs.
- Incidentalomas are incidentally detected asymptomatic adrenal masses. Workup should include testing to exclude Cushing syndrome, hyperaldosteronism, and pheochromocytoma. Lesions larger than 5 cm should be resected because of the increased risk of adrenocortical carcinoma.
- Low- and high-dose dexamethasone suppression tests can help to establish the diagnosis of Cushing syndrome and differentiate between etiologies.
- Pheochromocytomas are neuroendocrine tumors of the adrenal medulla, and the characteristics of these tumors are summarized by the "rule of 10s": 10% of the tumors are (i) bilateral, (ii) extra-adrenal (commonly organ of Zuckerkandl-aortic bifurcation), (iii) familial, (iv) malignant, (v) present in children, or (vi) multicentric.
- Patients with pheochromocytomas are treated preoperatively with phenoxybenzamine (an α-blocker) and a β-blocker if tachycardia is present. Other preoperative pharmacologic agents include calcium channel blockers, and metyrosine, a tyrosine hydroxylase inhibitor that inhibits the rate-limiting step of catecholamine synthesis.

THYROID

Embryology

The thyroid gland is derived from *endoderm* and develops between the 3rd and 4th weeks of gestation. Originating from the first two pairs of pharyngeal pouches, the native thyroid develops from a diverticulum at the base of the tongue, the *foramen cecum*. The gland then descends along the thyroglossal duct anterior to the hyoid bone, and laryngeal cartilages, to arrive at its final position ventral to the trachea at about the 7th gestational week. As the gland matures in its descent, two lateral lobes form, which are connected at the midline by a bridge of tissue, the *isthmus*. The *parafollicular cells* or *C cells* of the thyroid, which secrete calcitonin, originate from *neural crest cells* that migrate into the ultimobranchial body. It is these cells that give rise to medullary cancer of the thyroid. By the 10th week of gestation, the thyroid gland can concentrate iodine and synthesize iodothyronines; by 18 to 20 weeks of gestation, fetal production of thyroxine (T_4) has reached a clinically significant level.

An appreciation of the normal embryology of the thyroid gland is helpful in understanding variations in thyroid anatomy and anomalies in thyroid development. By approximately the 8th week of gestation, the thyroglossal duct has lost its patency and involutes. A remnant of the distal duct remains in approximately 50% of the population as a midline structure extending superiorly from the isthmus, known as the *pyramidal lobe*. Failure of the duct to involute completely can also result in the formation of a *thyroglossal duct cyst*, which can present as a midline neck mass. Although these cysts may develop anywhere along the course of the thyroglossal duct, the majority (50% to 75%) are found inferior to the hyoid bone. Ruptured cysts may result in thyroglossal duct sinuses or fistulas. Thyroglossal duct cysts may be the source of infection or even malignancy (usually papillary thyroid cancer), and their excision is therefore generally recommended. To prevent cyst recurrence, full excision of the cyst along the ductal tract to the base of the tongue, with excision of the central portion of the hyoid bone (the *Sistrunk procedure*), is generally indicated.

Complete failure of the thyroid gland to descend results in a *lingual thyroid* at the base of the tongue, a condition more common in women. Autopsy series have demonstrated lingual masses in up to 10% of the population, but not all contain functional thyroid tissue. Up to 70% of patients with lingual thyroid have no thyroid tissue elsewhere in the neck. Management of this condition is frequently medical and includes suppression of the lingual thyroid with exogenous thyroid hormone, although operation is indicated in instances of bleeding, dysphagia, or dyspnea. Ectopic thyroid tissue in the lateral neck is rare because the lateral thyroid anlagen fuse with the median thyroid anlage during development. The presence of such aberrant tissue should, therefore, raise the suspicion for well-differentiated metastatic thyroid carcinoma.

Anatomy

The thyroid can vary considerably in size and weight, reflecting, in part, dietary iodine intake; however, in the American population the gland typically weighs between 10 and 20 g. The thyroid is encapsulated by a fibrous capsule, which is in turn invested by a false capsular layer arising from the deep cervical fascia (pretracheal fascia). This fascial attachment between the gland and the upper two or three tracheal rings is also known as the *ligament of Berry*. The strap muscles (sternothyroid and sternohyoid) reside anterior to the lobes of the gland and are innervated by the ansa cervicalis. These muscles can be divided or resected if necessary during thyroid surgery with little consequence. The thyroid itself wraps around the trachea and the esophagus, which define the posteromedial borders of the gland. Lateral to each lobe of the thyroid lie the common carotid artery, the internal jugular vein, and the vagus nerve. The recurrent laryngeal nerve (RLN) typically lies posteromedial to each thyroid lobe, in the cleft between the trachea and esophagus, and beneath or embedded in the ligament of Berry.

The thyroid is highly vascularized, receiving its blood supply predominantly from the paired superior and inferior thyroid arteries (Fig. 17.1). The superior thyroid artery is the first branch of the external carotid artery and descends toward the superior pole of the thyroid lobe, where it divides into anterior and posterior branches. These branches join with branches of the inferior thyroid artery just deep to the pretracheal fascia. The inferior thyroid artery is a branch of the thyrocervical trunk and travels posterior to the carotid sheath before it reaches the posterior surface of the midportion of the gland. This artery is closely associated with the RLN during part of its course, and great care must be taken in its dissection. The inferior thyroid artery also provides the principal blood supply to all four parathyroid glands in approximately 80% of people. During thyroid surgery, the inferior thyroid artery should, therefore, be ligated close to the thyroid gland to preserve the blood supply to the parathyroid glands. *Thyroid ima arteries*, present in 5% to 10% of the population, arise from the brachiocephalic trunk or directly from the aortic arch and can provide additional blood supply to the thyroid.

The venous drainage of the thyroid gland is supplied primarily by three pairs of veins: the superior, middle, and inferior thyroid veins. The superior and middle veins drain the superior poles and lateral aspects of the thyroid, respectively, and drain into the internal jugular veins. The middle thyroid veins are frequently the first vessels ligated during thyroidectomy, as the thyroid lobes are

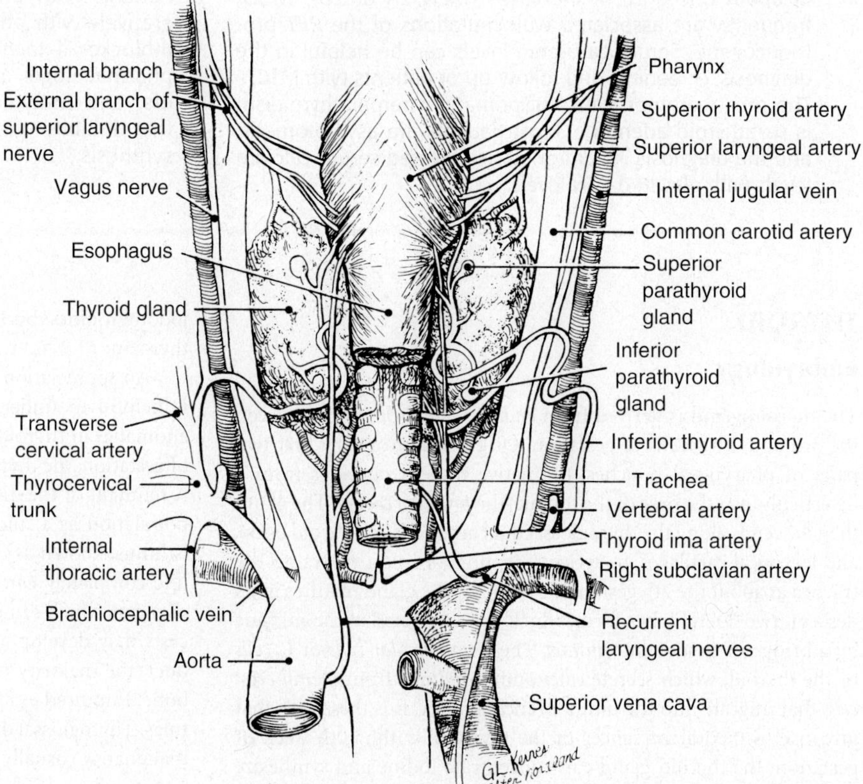

FIGURE 17.1 Posterior view of the larynx, trachea, thyroid, parathyroid glands, and the RLN. (From Black S. Surgical anatomy of the thyroid gland. In: Nyhus LM, Baker RJ, eds. *Mastery of Surgery*. 2nd ed. New York: Little, Brown and Company; 1992:193, with permission.)

retracted anteriorly and medially. The inferior thyroid veins arise from the inferior poles of the thyroid and course anterior to the trachea, draining into the brachiocephalic veins.

The thyroid gland has a rich and complex lymphatic drainage. Interlobular subcapsular lymphatics connect the two lobes of the gland through the isthmus explaining, in part, the relatively high frequency of multifocal tumors. Interlobular lymphatics communicate with intracapsular lymphatics, which in turn drain into various regional nodal beds, including the pretracheal lymph nodes, paratracheal lymph nodes, and the tracheoesophageal lymph nodes along the recurrent laryngeal chain. The supraisthmic pretracheal lymph nodes that run alongside the pyramidal lobe are also known as the *delphian nodes*. The regional nodal basins are a frequent site of metastatic thyroid cancer. Cancers of the upper thyroid gland typically drain into the nodes anterior and lateral to the internal jugular vein, whereas those of the mid and lower thyroid may drain beyond the regional nodes to the nodes of the middle and lower jugular veins and brachiocephalic veins in the anterior mediastinum.

The thyroid is innervated by postganglionic fibers that originate from the cervical sympathetic ganglia and travel alongside the arteries supplying the gland. A thorough appreciation of the anatomy of two other nerves, the RLN and the external branch of the superior laryngeal nerve, is essential for the safe performance of a thyroidectomy. The RLN innervates all the intrinsic laryngeal muscles except for the cricothyroid muscle. Injury to one RLN results in hoarseness and difficulty in phonation secondary to paralysis of the ipsilateral vocal cord. Bilateral RLN injury can result in abduction of both vocal cords with complete airway obstruction, necessitating emergent intubation or tracheostomy. The RLN is typically found in the tracheoesophageal groove. Less commonly, it may lie lateral or even anterolateral to the trachea. On the right side, the RLN branches from the vagus nerve and loops around the origin of the right subclavian artery to ascend in the tracheoesophageal groove. The left RLN branches from the vagus nerve and loops around the aortic arch near the ligamentum arteriosum. The RLN can pass anterior, posterior, or between branches of the inferior thyroid artery. In approximately 50% of cases, the RLN is embedded within the ligament of Berry. A nonrecurrent laryngeal nerve on the right side is present in approximately 1% of the population and is often associated with an aberrant subclavian artery. A nonrecurrent left laryngeal nerve is much less common but, when present, may be associated with a right-sided aortic arch.

The external branch of the superior laryngeal nerve travels in proximity to the superior thyroid artery for part of its course, and great care must, therefore, be taken when ligating this artery. Typically, the artery is ligated close to the superior pole of the gland to avoid injuring the nerve. The external branch of the superior laryngeal nerve innervates the cricothyroid muscle, and injury to this nerve may result in loss of vocal projection and volume, particularly at higher pitches.

Physiology

The thyroid gland synthesizes and secretes two groups of metabolically active hormones: *thyroid hormones* (triiodothyronine [T_3] or T_4) and *calcitonin*, which are discussed in more depth in the subsequent section on calcium metabolism.

Thyroid hormone is synthesized at the apical border of the follicular cell and is important for normal growth and development. *Iodine* is essential for the formation of thyroid hormone. Ingested iodine is converted to iodide and absorbed in the upper gastrointestinal (GI) tract. It reaches the thyroid gland via the bloodstream, where it is trapped by the thyroid follicular cells through an adenosine active (adenosine triphosphate [ATP] dependent) transmembrane transport mechanism. Approximately 90% of the total body iodine is stored in the thyroid gland in organic form.

In the follicular cell, iodide is rapidly oxidized to a free radical form by thyroid peroxidases. This activated form of iodine binds to tyrosine in the *thyroglobulin* molecule (a glycoprotein, which is the predominant component of colloid), forming either monoiodotyrosine (MIT) or diiodotyrosine (DIT). MIT and DIT molecules then combine with each other to form T_3 or T_4.

T_4 is the iodothyronine found in highest concentration in the plasma but is the less biologically active form of hormone. Because there is no conversion of T_3 to T_4 in the periphery, T_4 arises exclusively from secretion from the thyroid gland. Conversely, peripheral T_3 is largely derived by cleavage of the 5′-iodine from the outer ring of T_4 by 5′-monodeiodinase in the liver, muscle, and kidney. Direct T_3 secretion from the thyroid gland normally accounts for approximately 20% of T_3 present in the periphery, although this may be increased in certain hyperthyroid conditions. Only a small amount of thyroid hormone (<1%) circulates unbound in the plasma in a metabolically active form. Most thyroid hormones are bound to thyroxine-binding globulin (TBG), with the remainder bound to prealbumin and albumin. Pregnancy and oral contraceptives increase the levels of TBG and, therefore, the levels of total T_3 and T_4 but not the levels of free T_3 or free T_4. Androgens and anabolic steroids decrease serum levels of TBG and total T_4. Free thyroid hormone levels remain within normal limits.

The cellular effects of thyroid hormone are dependent on binding of thyroid hormone to an intracellular receptor, which migrates to the nucleus to regulate transcription and translation. Excess thyroid hormone up-regulates the activity and number of ATP-dependent sodium pumps, which increases the basal metabolic rate and oxygen consumption of most cells. Mitochondrial oxidative phosphorylation is up-regulated as well, the combined effects leading to increased heat production. T_3 may increase or decrease fat formation depending on the caloric status of the individual, although, overall, the lipolytic effect of thyroid hormones predominates.

Thyroid hormone production is regulated by the hypothalamic–pituitary–thyroid axis. Thyroid-stimulating hormone (TSH) is secreted by the anterior pituitary gland and leads to increased production of thyroid hormone (Fig. 17.2). TSH regulates iodine trapping by the thyroid gland and stimulates the synthesis of iodothyronines, acting via a second messenger cyclic adenosine monophosphate (cAMP) system. TSH also causes proteolytic separation of T_3 and T_4 from thyroglobulin, thereby stimulating the release of thyroid hormones into the circulation. Secretion of TSH is stimulated by thyrotropin-releasing hormone (TRH), a tripeptide that is synthesized by the hypothalamus and carried to the anterior hypophyseal lobe via the hypophyseal portal system. Increased plasma levels of free T_3 or T_4 decrease secretion of TSH directly and also inhibit the action of TRH. Large amounts of ingested iodine can also decrease thyroid hormone production.

Thyroid hormone production can be inhibited in hyperthyroid states by the thionamide class of drugs, which include propylthiouracil (PTU), methimazole (Tapazole), and carbimazole, which is converted *in vivo* to the active metabolite methimazole. These drugs act by inhibiting the oxidation of iodide to iodine, through

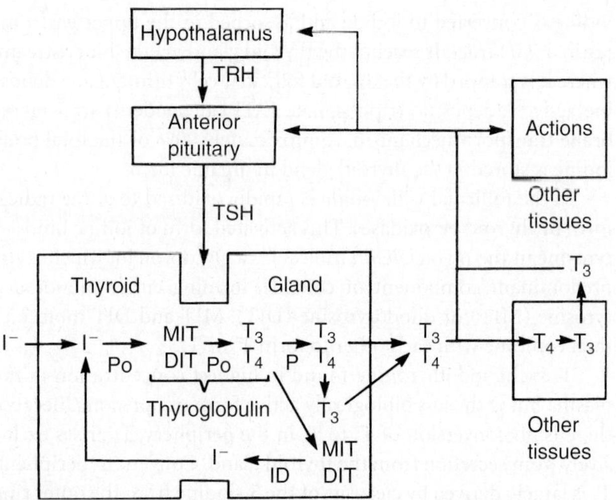

FIGURE 17.2 The regulation and feedback pathway of the hypothalamic–pituitary–thyroid system and intrathyroidal thyroid hormone synthesis and release. DIT, diiodotyrosine; I, inorganic iodide; ID, iodotyrosine deiodinase; MIT, monoiodotyrosine; P, proteolytic enzymes; Po, thyroid peroxidase; T_3, triiodothyronine; T_4, thyroxine; TRH, thyrotropin-releasing hormone; TSH, thyroid-stimulating hormone. (From Utiger RD. Disorders of the thyroid gland. In: Kelley WN, ed. *Textbook of Internal Medicine*. 3rd ed. Philadelphia: Lippincott–Raven Publishers; 1997:2205, with permission.)

inhibition of thyroid peroxidases, and thereby preventing the incorporation of iodine into the tyrosine residues of thyroglobulin. PTU also blocks the peripheral conversion of T_4 to T_3 by decreasing the activity of 5′-monodeiodinase. Methimazole can cross the placenta, and its use is generally restricted in pregnant women. A serious but rare side effect of the thionamides is agranulocytosis. Patients using these agents who have a rash, fever, or sore throat should be evaluated with measurement of white blood cell count.

Thyroid Function Tests

Measurement of *serum TSH* level is the single most useful test for assessing thyroid function. A normal TSH level in a healthy ambulatory patient essentially excludes the possibility of thyroid dysfunction. Unlike total T_4 or T_3 levels, which vary depending on the plasma levels of TBG, albumin, and prealbumin, serum TSH levels are independent of the concentration of carrier proteins in the circulation. Free (unbound) T_4 levels can be measured, but this test is generally more expensive, and TSH levels are thought to be the most sensitive indicator of thyroid dysfunction in mild or early stages of disease. TSH levels can also be used to titrate thyroid hormone replacement therapy or suppression. Because the half-life of T_4 is approximately 1 week, serum TSH measurement should be delayed for at least 4 to 8 weeks following adjustment of an oral T_4 dosage. TSH levels are not reliable indicators of thyroid dysfunction in patients who have neuropsychiatric disorders or diseases of the pituitary gland (e.g., pituitary adenomas).

The *TRH stimulation test* determines the functional status of anterior pituitary TSH secretion, although its role has diminished owing to the increased sensitivity of TSH assays. It is performed by checking a baseline TSH level, administering synthetic TRH intravenously, and measuring TSH level again after 30 and 60 minutes. Normally, a rise in TSH from the baseline is observed after TRH administration. Patients with hypothyroidism have a blunted response or no rise in TSH. This test can also determine whether TSH secretion is decreased in patients with pituitary tumors.

Thyroid Imaging

Ultrasonography of the thyroid is a noninvasive and inexpensive technique for differentiating between solid and cystic lesions. It provides excellent anatomic definition and is typically the imaging study of choice for suspected thyroid pathology. Ultrasound is particularly useful for detection and guidance of fine needle aspiration (FNA) of nodules that cannot be palpated, recurrent tumor in the thyroid bed, and regional lymph nodes. *High-resolution ultrasound* can detect areas of calcification, and *ultrasonography with Doppler* can identify regions of increased vascularity. Both of these sonographic features are associated with malignancy. *Computerized tomographic* (CT) scanning and *magnetic resonance imaging* (MRI) can detect subclinical cervical lymphadenopathy and substernal goiters. These studies cannot differentiate benign from malignant thyroid lesions and, therefore, play only a limited role in the evaluation of thyroid nodules. These studies may be used preoperatively in patients with anaplastic tumors to assess involvement of adjacent structures and also, occasionally, after treatment of patients with thyroid carcinoma to exclude recurrent disease. They should be obtained after radionuclide imaging studies because the iodine in the contrast blocks the uptake of radionuclides by the thyroid for at least 6 weeks.

A functional assessment of the thyroid gland can be achieved using *radionuclide imaging*. This modality allows for localization of thyroid tissue, detection of functional metastatic lesions from thyroid cancer, and an estimation of the size of the thyroid gland. Over the last decade, use of thyroid scintigraphy has become less common. Technetium-99m (^{99m}Tc) pertechnetate is the radioisotope most commonly used for thyroid scanning. Any defect in tracer uptake represents a nonfunctional or hypofunctional ("cold") nodule, whereas areas of increased tracer uptake represent functional ("hot") nodules. Cold nodules are associated with an approximately 12% to 15% incidence of thyroid cancer, although this incidence may be even higher in younger patients and patients with calcified nodules. Nuclear medicine scans are less reliable at diagnosing hypofunctional than autonomously hyperfunctional nodules. An iodine-123 (^{123}I) scan permits assessment of the trapping and organification capacity of the thyroid gland. The study is more expensive and less convenient to obtain compared with ^{99m}Tc. Iodine-131 (^{131}I) administration results in much higher exposure of the patient to radiation, and the images obtained are inferior to those obtained with ^{99m}Tc or ^{123}I. ^{131}I scanning is, however, the study of choice for assessing the distribution of functioning metastatic thyroid tumors, which concentrate radioiodine, and predicting the effectiveness of cancer therapy with ^{131}I.

Benign Conditions of the Thyroid

Hyperthyroid Conditions

Hyperthyroidism results from excess plasma thyroid hormone. Three causes that more commonly require surgical intervention are Graves disease (or toxic diffuse goiter), which accounts for more than 80% of cases; toxic nodular goiter; and solitary toxic nodule.

Other rarer causes of hyperthyroidism include postpartum thyroiditis, iodine-induced hyperthyroidism, drug-induced thyrotoxicosis, iatrogenic hyperthyroidism, struma ovarii, TSH-secreting pituitary tumors, and functioning metastatic carcinoma. Regardless of etiology, patients with hyperthyroidism may be accompanied by tachycardia, weight loss, tremors, increased anxiety, and sleep disturbances.

Graves disease is an autoimmune disorder characterized by the presence of antibodies directed against the TSH receptor on the follicular cell. Antibody–receptor binding leads to increased thyroid hormone production and secretion. Graves disease is six to seven times more common in women than in men. Various human leukocyte antigen (HLA) alleles have been associated with the disease, suggesting that genetic factors play a role in its pathogenesis. Clinical manifestations of Graves disease include those associated with hyperthyroidism, specifically, fatigue, heat intolerance, weight loss, diarrhea, hair loss, irritability, tremor, arrhythmias, hypertension, osteoporosis, amenorrhea, and sweating. In up to 15% of cases, dermopathy with pretibial myxedema and ophthalmopathy with periorbital edema, proptosis, and upper lid twitching can be seen. This manifestation is thought to be autoimmune mediated, and controversy persists regarding the effect of thyroid ablation on the risk of progressive eye disease. Graves ophthalmopathy is exacerbated by ^{131}I treatment, which is therefore contraindicated in the setting of active disease.

Older patients may initially present with atrial fibrillation or congestive heart failure. If left untreated, one third of patients with Graves disease will improve to euthyroidism or even develop hypothyroidism, one third will remain chronically hyperthyroid, and one third will progress to thyroid storm, a serious condition characterized by tachycardia, fever, and even death. On examination, the thyroid gland is typically diffusely enlarged, symmetric, and smooth. The presence of nodularity warrants investigation, as there is about a 5% incidence of concomitant carcinoma in patients with Graves disease. Laboratory testing typically reveals elevated levels of T_4 or T_3 and a suppressed serum TSH level. Diffuse, increased uptake of ^{131}I within a symmetrically enlarged gland is diagnostic.

There are three principal treatment options for patients with Graves disease: medical therapy, radioactive iodine thyroid ablation, and surgical thyroid ablation. The optimal treatment choice for a given patient depends upon age, health, severity of disease, size of the gland, and patient preference. *Medical therapy* is aimed at reducing thyroid hormone levels and is the first-line therapy for most patients with Graves disease. Thionamide therapy must be continued for a prolonged period to control thyroid levels and allow for spontaneous remission. Medical therapy is associated with high rates of persistent disease (up to 90% of patients) upon discontinuation of medications and with low success rates, particularly among patients with large goiters, a high T_3 level, or high T_3–T_4 ratio. An advantage of thionamide therapy is that there is no risk of hypothyroidism when the drug is dosed appropriately. β-Blocking agents such as propranolol may be used as adjuvants, particularly when symptoms of tachycardia are present in the hyperthyroid state.

Radioactive iodine (^{131}I) therapy induces long-standing remission in most patients, with relatively few side effects, and is the definitive treatment used for most adult patients with Graves disease in the United States. The primary advantage of this method is that it does not require an invasive procedure. The disadvantage is a high incidence of hypothyroidism, which is an expected complication following effective therapy, and can be easily diagnosed and effectively treated with lifelong hormone replacement therapy. Pregnant women, patients with concomitant thyroid nodules, and those with very large glands are not considered candidates for ^{131}I therapy. Additionally, radioactive iodine is generally avoided in children. Because of the success of nonoperative therapy, *operative intervention* is generally reserved for patients who are noncompliant with, or intolerant to, antithyroid drug therapy, those who are refractory to medical therapy, those with contraindications to ^{131}I therapy (such as pregnancy), those with large glands ($\geq$80 g) or symptomatic compression, and those with concern for malignancy. Patients who are younger than 20 years with large goiters are unlikely to become euthyroid with drug therapy and often require thyroidectomy. Preoperatively, a euthyroid state should be achieved medically to minimize the risk of intraoperative or postoperative thyroid storm. Administration of PTU in combination with propranolol is typically initiated 4 to 8 weeks before operation and continued during and after the operation. Lugol solution (a combination of potassium iodide and iodine) can be given to patients to decrease the vascularity of the gland and make it firmer and easier to resect. Some surgeons believe that propranolol results in the same decrease in gland vascularity, making the use of Lugol solution unnecessary. The extent of thyroidectomy for Graves disease remains controversial. Operative approaches include subtotal thyroidectomy, near-total thyroidectomy, and total thyroidectomy. The former two approaches do not completely eliminate the risk of postoperative thyrotoxicosis. With total thyroidectomy, there is virtually no incidence of persistent hyperthyroidism; however, patients require lifelong thyroid replacement. With increased extent of thyroid surgery, there is concern for increased risk of injury to the RLN or of transient or permanent hypoparathyroidism.

By definition, *autonomously functioning thyroid nodules* function and grow independent of TSH. Such nodules appear hot on radionuclide studies, and the function of surrounding thyroid tissue is frequently suppressed with nodules that are large in size. The majority of these nodules enlarge, develop central necrosis, and become nonfunctional; however, the risk of developing hyperthyroidism is increased with larger nodules. Patients can have either solitary or multiple autonomously functioning nodules. *Solitary toxic nodules* have a peak incidence during the fifth decade of life and are much more common in women. *Toxic multinodular goiter* (Plummer disease) accounts for approximately 20% of patients with hyperthyroidism and is most common in women older than 50 years. Patients usually have a nodular goiter for some time before they develop symptoms of hyperthyroidism. Patients with a nodular goiter and subclinical hyperthyroidism may develop thyrotoxicosis after receiving iodine-containing medication or iodine-containing contrast media.

Treatment of solitary functional nodules is influenced by size and degree of function, as well as by the patient's age and overall health. Toxic nodules that exceed 3 cm in diameter should usually be treated surgically with a thyroid lobectomy. Alternatively, radioiodine can be used; however, a prolonged treatment regimen may be required, as nodules persist in approximately 20% of patients. Many surgeons recommend prophylactic excision of nontoxic large solitary nodules with secretory function in the upper range of normal in elderly patients. The standard treatment for toxic multinodular goiter is antithyroid drug therapy, followed by thyroidectomy. ^{131}I may be used as an alternative in high-risk surgical patients who have no evidence of airway compression. Operation typically entails subtotal thyroidectomy, with removal of all autonomous nodules. Conservation of adequate remnant thyroid tissue is usually not a concern, as patients are typically placed on thyroid hormone postoperatively for thyroid suppression.

Hypothyroidism: Hashimoto Thyroiditis

Hypothyroidism results from deficient levels of thyroid hormone and may result from a variety of etiologies including iatrogenic (e.g., postsurgical ablation of the thyroid or following irradiation therapy), autoimmune disorders (e.g., Hashimoto thyroiditis), and endemic goiters. Hypothyroid patients may present with fatigue, weight gain, brittle nails, coarse hair, constipation, and neurocognitive disturbances, such as depression, irritability, or impaired memory. Typically, laboratory evaluation reveals decreased thyroid hormone levels with an elevation in TSH levels.

Hashimoto thyroiditis (also known as "chronic lymphocytic thyroiditis" or "struma lymphomatosa") is the most common inflammatory condition of the thyroid and the most frequent cause of spontaneous hypothyroidism. It is an *autoimmune disease* and is most common in middle-aged women, in geographic areas with a high dietary iodine intake, and in patients who received radiation during infancy or childhood. Characterized by high levels of circulating antibodies against the microsomal fraction of the thyroid cell, and lymphocytic infiltration of the thyroid, Hashimoto disease results in impaired thyroid hormone synthesis owing to thyrocyte destruction. Low T_4 and T_3 levels cause increased TSH secretion, which may result in goiter formation. During the acute phase of the disease, transient hyperthyroidism may be seen. Clinically, patients may present with signs and symptoms of hypothyroidism. Pain is not typically a manifestation of Hashimoto thyroiditis but may occur at the time of initial onset. On palpation, the gland is usually firm and rubbery with a lobulated surface. An elevated antimicrosomal antibody titer, along with a suggestive clinical examination, is usually sufficient to make the diagnosis. Treatment with thyroid hormone usually causes regression of the goiter. In some patients, the gland continues to grow despite thyroid suppression therapy. In these patients, partial thyroidectomy is indicated, particularly if symptoms are present. If a solitary nodule is found in a patient with Hashimoto disease, it should be fully evaluated. Likewise, rapid enlargement of the thyroid gland in a patient with a history of Hashimoto thyroiditis needs to be carefully evaluated because the incidence of *lymphoma*, including the mucosa-associated lymphoid tissue (MALT) type, is increased in these patients. FNA and cytologic evaluation should be undertaken if lymphoma is suspected. Hashimoto thyroiditis is also associated with a slightly increased risk of papillary thyroid cancer.

Other Thyroiditis Conditions

Thyroiditis is generally classified on the basis of rapidity of onset as acute, subacute, or chronic. *Acute thyroiditis* is an infectious disorder, which is more common in women. Bacteria such as *Streptococcus pyogenes*, *Staphylococcus aureus*, and *Pneumococcus pneumoniae* account for most cases and usually spread via the lymphatics from local infectious sources. The risk of developing acute thyroiditis is increased in patients with nodular goiters or anatomic defects such as thyroglossal ducts. This condition presents with acute onset of neck pain and fever. Patients are typically euthyroid. The treatment of acute thyroiditis usually entails appropriate intravenous antibiotic therapy and surgical drainage if an abscess is present.

Subacute thyroiditis (granulomatous thyroiditis or *de Quervain thyroiditis*) is a disease that typically occurs in middle-aged women within weeks of an upper respiratory or other viral infection. Symptoms may include weakness, depression, easy fatigability, anterior neck pain, or referred pain to the ear or angle of the jaw. On examination, the patient is usually febrile, and the thyroid is firm and extremely tender to palpation. The thyroid may be swollen unilaterally, and the overlying skin is occasionally erythematous. Laboratory evaluation and biopsy are usually not necessary. Transient mild hyperthyroidism can be observed during the initial phase of the disease in about half of patients. This is thought to be caused by a release of preformed thyroid hormone from the inflamed gland into the circulation. The later course of disease can be complicated by hypothyroidism, and some patients may require hormone replacement therapy. The disease is typically self-limited and usually resolves within a few months. The discomfort can be managed with salicylates, nonsteroidal anti-inflammatory drugs (NSAIDs), or corticosteroids. Surgical therapy is indicated only rarely if the disease is persistent despite several months of steroid therapy.

Riedel struma, or "invasive fibrous thyroiditis," refers to a very rare chronic inflammatory proliferative disorder in which the thyroid tissue and frequently the adjacent strap muscles and carotid sheaths are replaced by dense fibrous tissue. Its pathogenesis is largely unknown, although the disease is often associated with other fibrotic processes at other body sites, such as the retroperitoneum, mediastinum, periorbital area, and intrahepatic biliary tree (sclerosing cholangitis), as well as with autoimmune conditions. Similar to other forms of thyroiditis, Riedel struma is most commonly seen in middle-aged women. Patients with Riedel struma are most often euthyroid, although hypothyroidism may be seen in up to 30% of patients. An open biopsy should be obtained to rule out the presence of thyroid carcinoma or lymphoma. The disease is often self-limiting but may result in considerable localized pain and compression of adjacent tissues. Treatment with steroids or tamoxifen is sometimes beneficial, although no randomized control trials exist due to the rarity of the disease. If airway compromise is present, surgical therapy with isthmusectomy is indicated, but operative intervention should be limited to the minimum necessary in order to reduce the risk of damage to perithyroidal structures.

Thyroid Nodules

Clinically apparent thyroid nodules are present in approximately 5% of adult women and 1% of men in iodine-sufficient areas of the world. Both benign and malignant thyroid nodules are associated with prior radiation exposure. The incidence of malignancy is approximately 10% in patients with palpable solitary thyroid nodules who have no history of neck irradiation. This incidence is increased several-fold in patients with prior radiation exposure. Men and patients at the extremes of age are also at a higher risk for malignancy. A solitary nodule is more worrisome than a thyroid with multiple nodules; however, any nodule within a multinodular goiter that increases in size needs to be evaluated to exclude carcinoma. The appearance of a new nodule, a rapid increase in the size of an existing nodule, and a painful nodule are worrisome for malignancy. New onset of hoarseness or the development of a Horner syndrome may indicate local invasion of neural structures. On physical examination, adherence to adjacent structures and presence of palpable adenopathy are suggestive of carcinoma.

Evaluation of a newly identified thyroid nodule has evolved significantly over the past decade. Current guidelines recommend serum TSH testing in all patients. In patients with a low TSH, radionuclide scanning with ^{123}I or ^{99m}Tc is recommended to evaluate for hyperfunctioning nodules, which are rarely associated with malignancy. Patients with hyperfunctioning nodules identified on radionuclide scanning can be worked up for hypothyroidism. Higher serum TSH, even within the high normal range, is associated with elevated risk of malignancy in a nodule. Therefore, in patients with normal or elevated TSH, thyroid ultrasound is required, with FNA of any identified nodules. Patients with no nodules on ultrasound may require further evaluation for hyperthyroidism based upon TSH levels. For patients with visualized nodules, further evaluation is based upon FNA findings.

FNA is safe, minimally invasive, inexpensive, and accurate in the diagnosis of thyroid nodules. It can be performed with ultrasonographic guidance for nonpalpable nodules. All cervical lymphadenopathy should undergo FNA. Recommended size cutoffs for FNA of thyroid nodules are based upon a combination of sonographic features and clinical risk factors. FNA is recommended in nodules greater than 5 mm in high-risk patients (history of radiation exposure, or personal or family history of thyroid cancer, familial endocrinopathy, or 18FDG avid nodule on PET scan), or nodules with suspicious sonographic features; in moderate-risk nodules (solid nodules or those with microcalcifications present) greater than 1 cm; and in low-risk nodules (mixed cystic–solid nodules, or spongiform nodules) greater than or equal to 1.5 to 2 cm. FNA is not indicated for purely cystic nodules, which, although rare, are highly unlikely to be malignant.

Historically, the four diagnostic categories of FNA included (i) benign or negative, (ii) suspicious or indeterminate, (iii) malignant, and (iv) insufficient. This classification was expanded in 2007, and the current system, termed the *Bethesda criteria*, encompasses six categories: (i) nondiagnostic or unsatisfactory, (ii) benign, (iii) atypia of undetermined significance or follicular lesion of undetermined significance, (iv) follicular neoplasm or suspicious for follicular neoplasm, (v) suspicious for malignancy, and (vi) malignant.

Bethesda level I pathology is associated with a 1% to 4% risk of malignancy and requires repeat FNA under ultrasound guidance. For patients with a benign (Bethesda II) FNA biopsy, cancer is present in 0% to 3%, and such patients can generally be followed by physical examination or ultrasonography, which is more precise at delineating changes in size.

Patients with atypia or a follicular neoplasm of undetermined significance (FLUS) present a particular clinical challenge. One of the major limitations of FNA is its inability to distinguish between benign follicular cell adenomas and follicular cell carcinomas. On permanent pathologic specimens, follicular carcinoma can be distinguished from follicular adenoma by the presence of *capsular or vascular invasion*. The risk of malignancy in patients with FLUS on FNA is 5% to 15%, and although some clinical features (male gender, older age, nodule size >4 cm, or atypia on cytology) increase the likelihood of malignancy, it remains low overall. Repeat FNA may therefore be required in these patients. Several prospective studies have demonstrated the ability of molecular markers to improve the predictive value of FNA in the setting of indeterminate lesions. A combination panel screening for BRAF, Ras, RET/PTC, and PAX8/PPAR-γ mutations has recently become commercially available for this patient population but has yet to be uniformly adopted.

FNA biopsies of follicular neoplasms or those with extensive Hürthle cell changes were previously characterized as suspicious or indeterminate; these now are categorized as follicular neoplasm or suspicious for follicular neoplasm under the Bethesda criteria. Because 15% to 30% of these nodules are found to be malignant, they must be surgically resected. A thyroid lobectomy is generally recommended to patients with a follicular neoplasm; a completion thyroidectomy is performed if final pathology reveals carcinoma. A total thyroidectomy may be recommended initially in a select group of patients (e.g., those requiring thyroid replacement hormone for preexisting hypothyroidism). The implied risk of malignancy for Bethesda V and VI pathology is 60% to 75% and 97% to 99%, respectively. As a result, thyroidectomy is recommended for either of these findings; the management of thyroid cancer is discussed in more detail below.

Thyroid Carcinoma

The reported incidence of thyroid carcinoma varies significantly worldwide by geography in the United States, it is approximately 9 per 100,000 (accounting for <1% of all malignancies). The incidence has increased dramatically in recent decades, from 3.6 per 100,000 in 1973; approximately half of this increase has been in small (<1 cm) tumors and may reflect increased detection and earlier diagnosis.

The mortality rate is less than 1 per 100,000, indicating that most thyroid cancers carry a favorable prognosis. Thyroid cancers are more common in females than in males (approximately 3:1 ratio), although the mortality ratio is significantly lower than the incidence ratio (1.2–2:1, female to male). The incidence of thyroid cancer increases with age, and various environmental and genetic influences appear to be involved in the pathogenesis of the different tumor types. Thyroid malignancies are derived from either thyroid follicular cells (*papillary*, *follicular*, and *anaplastic carcinomas*) or parafollicular cells (*medullary carcinoma*). Thyroid cancers can be further classified on the basis of differentiation (e.g., well-differentiated, intermediate differentiation, and undifferentiated).

Well-Differentiated Thyroid Carcinoma (Papillary and Follicular Carcinoma)

Well-differentiated thyroid cancers include papillary and follicular types. Thyroid tumors with papillary and follicular features are generally classified as a follicular variant of papillary carcinoma because pure papillary and mixed papillary–follicular tumors have similar biology. Papillary carcinoma comprises approximately 80% to 90% of thyroid cancer in countries with sufficient dietary iodine intake. Histologically, papillary cancers are distinguished by nuclear features including large size, pale-staining appearance, inclusion bodies, and deep "grooving." *Psammoma bodies*, which are laminated calcified bodies, are found in approximately one half of specimens of this tumor type. Variants of papillary cancer include follicular, tall cell, columnar, and diffuse sclerosis. Papillary carcinomas frequently spread via lymphatics to regional lymph nodes (approximately 30% to 40% of cases at presentation). The sclerosis variant has a 100% incidence of lymph node metastasis at the time of diagnosis.

Follicular carcinomas are defined as tumors with only follicular elements. Pure follicular thyroid carcinomas are rare, making up only 5% to 10% of thyroid malignancies in areas of the world where goiter is not endemic. Follicular thyroid carcinomas are usually unifocal and well encapsulated, with areas of invasion into or through the capsule and frequent vascular invasion. Lymph node involvement is rare (1% to 10%).

Radiation exposure to the thyroid has been shown to increase the incidence of benign thyroid nodules and of well-differentiated thyroid carcinoma, particularly of the papillary type; however, previous radiation exposure accounts for less than 10% of cases in the United States. Intrachromosomal translocations of the *RET protooncogene* (which encodes a tyrosine kinase receptor) have been identified in some studies in more than 50% of papillary thyroid cancers. Other genetic mutations, including those affecting *Trk*, *BRAF*, *APC*, and *N-ras*, have been implicated in the development of papillary thyroid cancer as well. The fusion *PAX8/PPAR gamma1* oncogene has been implicated in the pathogenesis of follicular carcinoma, although it is present in some follicular adenomas as well.

Well-differentiated thyroid carcinoma typically presents with an asymptomatic thyroid nodule. Less commonly, patients present with palpable cervical lymphadenopathy without an identifiable thyroid primary. Symptomatic lesions may present with hoarseness, dyspnea, and dysphagia, reflecting local invasion of the RLN, the trachea, and the esophagus, respectively. Most of these neoplasms are nonfunctional, and patients are typically euthyroid.

Papillary and follicular cancers tend to be relatively indolent neoplasms and are associated with a favorable long-term prognosis. In contrast to other solid neoplasms, the presence of lymph node metastases has a marginal, if any influence on overall survival. The overall 10-year survival rate for papillary cancer ranges from 74% to 93%, compared with 43% to 94% for follicular cancer. One of the most important prognostic factors for well-differentiated thyroid cancer is age at diagnosis. The presence of distant metastases and size are also important predictors of outcome. Use of the American Joint Commission on Cancer (AJCC) is recommended in all thyroid cancers and required for all cancer registries. The AJCC staging system risk stratifies patient outcomes in terms of mortality based upon tumor, node, metastasis (TNM) staging, with separate classifications for patients less than 45 years and 45 years of age or older. A number of other classification systems have been developed to risk stratify patients. The Lahey Clinic developed the AMES (age, metastases, extent of primary cancer, and size of tumor) criteria to stratify patients into prognostically discreet risk categories. In this system, low-risk patients have a long-term overall survival of 98%, whereas high-risk patients have a long-term overall survival of 54%. The Mayo Clinic group devised a similar scoring system called the AGES (age, grade of tumor, extent of tumor, and size of tumor) system. A modification of this system is MACIS (metastasis, age, completeness of resection, invasion, and size). The survival rates for patients based on these prognostic factors are shown in Table 17.1.

Procedures for a thyroid neoplasm include thyroid lobectomy, subtotal thyroidectomy, near-total thyroidectomy, and total thyroidectomy. A *subtotal thyroidectomy* leaves a rim of 2 to 4 g of tissue in the region of the ligament of Berry of the contralateral lobe. This decreases the risk of injury to the RLN and helps preserve the blood supply to the upper parathyroid glands. A *near-total thyroidectomy* typically leaves less than 1 g of tissue adjacent to the ligament of Berry. Some specialized centers have utilized *video-assisted* approaches in combination with less conspicuous incisions in the lateral neck, the axilla, or below the clavicle. Prospective randomized trials have shown these techniques to be safe in small volume benign thyroid disease and low-risk thyroid cancers, but they are associated with significantly longer operative duration and have yet to be widely embraced in the United States.

TABLE 17.1 Survival rates in patients with well-differentiated thyroid cancer based on various prognostic classification schemes

AMES Risk Group		Low		High
Overall survival rate (%)		98		54
Disease-free survival rate (%)		95		45
Dames Risk Group	**Low**	**Intermediate**	**High**	
Disease-free survival rate (%)	92	45	0	—
AGES PS	<4	4–5	5–6	>6
20-y survival rate (%)	99	80	33	13
MACIS PS	<6	6–7	7–8	>8
20-y survival rate (%)	99	89	56	24

DAMES, AMES system modified by DNA content; PS, prognostic score.

The extent of resection for well-differentiated thyroid malignancies has been a point of significant controversy. Current recommendations from the American Thyroid Association call for total thyroidectomy in the setting of tumors greater than 4 cm in diameter, in patients with a personal history of radiation exposure or a family history of thyroid cancer, and those with FNA biopsy demonstrating marked atypia or Bethesda level V or VI pathology. Near-total or total thyroidectomy is recommended for tumors greater than 1 cm in size. For unifocal tumors less than or equal to 1 cm with no evidence of nodal metastases in the absence of a history of irradiation, a thyroid lobectomy alone may be sufficient treatment. For patients who undergo lobectomy alone, completion thyroidectomy should be offered if final surgical pathology is consistent with a diagnosis that would have required near-total or total thyroidectomy had it been known preoperatively.

Controversy also exists over the surgical management of *cervical lymph node metastases from well-differentiated thyroid carcinoma.* Regional lymph node metastases are present in 20% to 90% of patients with papillary carcinoma, and a smaller proportion of other histologic subtypes of thyroid cancer. Some surgeons perform selective resection for grossly involved nodes, pointing to retrospective studies that do not demonstrate any survival difference in patients treated with this approach compared with more radical neck dissections. Others advocate prophylactic modified radical neck dissections in an attempt to remove occult metastatic disease. Because lymph node involvement is a marker for more aggressive papillary carcinoma, a formal therapeutic central neck dissection (level VI) is generally recommended along with total thyroidectomy in patients with clinically evident adenopathy. In the setting of biopsy-proven carcinoma in lymph nodes of the central compartment, a complete lateral neck dissection (level II–IV) is indicated.

Radioiodine therapy (RAI) may be used after surgical resection for well-differentiated carcinomas. Administration of ^{131}I concentrates in and ablates residual thyroid tissue. RAI may achieve multiple clinical goals, including therapeutic management of known persistent disease, adjuvant therapy to decrease recurrence and mortality in the setting of suspected metastatic disease, and remnant ablation to facilitate early detection of recurrence by serum thyroglobulin measurement. RAI is generally recommended for all patients with known distant metastases, those with gross extrathyroidal extension, and for tumors greater than 4 cm in size. ^{131}I ablation is generally performed at 6 weeks after near-total or total thyroidectomy and requires TSH stimulation to optimize ^{131}I uptake. Radioiodine treatment is typically continued until there is no further ^{131}I uptake or serum thyroglobulin is in the athyrotic range. Serious side effects of ^{131}I are relatively uncommon. Women treated with RAI should generally avoid pregnancy for 6 to 12 months after receiving therapy, although conflicting literature exists about the risks of infertility, miscarriage, and fetal malformation.

Distant metastases from well-differentiated thyroid carcinoma are found in approximately 10% to 15% of patients overall and portend a worse prognosis. Papillary carcinomas are less frequently associated with remote metastases at the time of diagnosis than are follicular carcinomas; common sites of metastasis include the lung and bone. Less commonly, patients with well-differentiated thyroid cancer develop cerebral metastases. Radioiodine avid metastases may be treated with RAI.

Postoperative or post ablation TSH suppression has been shown to improve outcomes in high-risk patients. Long-term suppression of TSH levels to 0.1 to 0.5 mU/L is therefore recommended in patients who are considered high risk. After definitive therapy, patients should also undergo routine testing of serum thyroglobulin levels every 6 to 12 months to monitor for recurrent disease. Patients who have had less than a total thyroidectomy performed should also undergo periodic neck ultrasonography.

There is no demonstrated benefit to chemotherapy in patients with well-differentiated thyroid cancer. The use of external beam radiation therapy is generally reserved for palliative treatment of patients with locally advanced unresectable disease or for patients who are not considered candidates for RAI.

Intermediate Differentiation Thyroid Carcinomas (Hürthle Cell, Insular, and Medullary)

The *intermediate differentiation tumors* of the thyroid include Hürthle cell carcinoma, insular carcinoma, and medullary thyroid carcinoma (MTC). *Hürthle cell tumors* account for less than 5% of all thyroid carcinomas. They are considered to be variants of follicular tumors and cannot be classified as benign or malignant based on FNA. Compared with follicular tumors, Hürthle cell tumors are more often bilateral and multifocal and are more likely to spread to regional lymph nodes. Hürthle cell tumors do not take up radioiodine. Similar to the management of follicular tumors, patients who are found to have Hürthle cell neoplasm by FNA should undergo an ipsilateral lobectomy and isthmectomy. Total completion thyroidectomy is indicated if the final pathology reveals a carcinoma. *Insular carcinomas* are tumors that histologically resemble pancreatic islets and contain small follicles that stain positively for thyroglobulin. Treatment of insular carcinoma consists of surgical resection and radioiodine ablation.

MTC accounts for 5% to 10% of thyroid cancers and arises from the calcitonin-producing parafollicular or C cells. Unlike papillary carcinoma, radiation exposure is not associated with the development of MTC. MTC is sporadic or nonfamilial in 60% to 70% of cases and is associated with a familial syndrome in the remainder of the cases (either multiple endocrine neoplasia [MEN] 2A or MEN 2B or non-MEN familial MTC). Sporadic tumors are usually unilateral and involve regional lymph nodes, whereas familial tumors are generally multifocal. Patients with non-MEN familial MTC have the least aggressive form of this tumor, and MEN 2B is associated with the most aggressive variant. The characteristics of sporadic and familial forms of MTC are shown in Table 17.2.

TABLE 17.2 Characteristics of sporadic and various familial forms of medullary thyroid

		Familial		
	Sporadic	Non-MEN	MEN 2A	MEN 2B
Age at diagnosis (y)	42–45	43–45	24–27[a]	15–20
Gender	M = F	M = F	M = F	M = F
Associated diseases	None	None	1. Pheochromocytoma 2. Hyperparathyroidism	1. Pheochromocytoma 2. Marfanoid body habitus 3. Oral and eye mucosal neuromas 4. GI ganglioneuromas
Disease extent	Unilateral	Bilateral	Bilateral	Bilateral
Lymph nodes involved (%)	40–50	10–20	14	38 at diagnosis
Distant metastases at diagnosis (%)	12	0	0–3	20
Cured of MTC (%)	14–30	70–80	56–100	0
Dead due to MTC (%)	30	0	0–17	50
Mutations in RET on chromosome 10	MET 918 → Thr (33%) Glu 768 → Asp	Mutations in cysteines in extracellular domain near membrane	Mutations in cysteines in extracellular domain near membrane	MET 918 → Thr

[a]The age at diagnosis at centers doing genetic screening can be at or even before birth. Numbers reported reflect series based on biochemical screening of families at risk.

MTC, medullary thyroid cancer; Thr, thyroid.

MTC can secrete various peptide hormones, including adrenocorticotropic hormone (ACTH) and serotonin, and can also produce mucin or melanin.

It is important that family members of patients with medullary carcinoma (particularly multifocal tumors) be screened early for disease. Defects in the *RET protooncogene* on chromosome 10 have been found to be responsible for MEN and non-MEN familial forms of MTC. Gene carriers can be identified by a blood test and are candidates for prophylactic thyroidectomy. Patients with medullary carcinoma should also be evaluated for pheochromocytomas because of the relatively high concurrent incidence of these tumors.

Patients with sporadic MTC typically present with a mass in the thyroid. Some patients present with advanced cases with local invasion and symptoms of hoarseness, dysphagia, or cough. Those with extremely high levels of calcitonin may have severe secretory diarrhea. The basal and stimulated *serum calcitonin test* is an important tool for confirming the diagnosis of MTC. The test involves administering calcium gluconate and measuring serum calcitonin before and at multiple times after stimulation. An increase to more than 1,000 pg/mL (normal serum level 250 to 300 pg/mL) is abnormal and pathognomonic for MTC. Measurement of serum calcitonin levels can be useful as a screening tool for MTC and for following patients for recurrent disease posttreatment. Because MTC does not concentrate iodine, ^{131}I scans have no utility.

Surgical therapy is the only effective therapy for MTC. Chemotherapy and external beam radiation have not proven to be beneficial. Patients who present with MTC should undergo total thyroidectomy and central lymph node dissection. If there is evidence of metastatic spread in the central neck nodes, a formal modified radical neck dissection is performed. There is a direct correlation between lesion size and incidence of nodal metastases; lesions greater than 2 cm are associated with a 60% incidence of lymph node metastases. Therefore, some surgeons advocate a modified radical neck dissection for all lesions greater than 2 cm. The incidence of distant metastases at the time of diagnosis is lowest in patients with familial non-MEN MTC and MEN 2A (<5%) and highest in patients with MEN 2B (20%). Recent series show a 5-year survival rate between 80% and 90% and a 10-year survival rate between 70% and 80% for all MTCs. Persistently elevated calcitonin levels following resection are managed by close follow-up and reoperation only when clinically apparent disease is present.

Undifferentiated Thyroid Carcinoma (Anaplastic)

Anaplastic thyroid cancer (ATC) accounts for 1% to 2% of thyroid cancers in the United States and is one of the most aggressive and lethal malignancies. A recent decline in incidence likely reflects reclassification of some of these tumors as lymphomas. The median survival is 4 to 5 months, with a 5-year survival rate of approximately 5%. ATC is most common in the seventh decade of life and has an equal incidence in men and women. ATC has been associated with iodine deficiency in regions with endemic goiter, where ATC may account for as many as 10% of all thyroid cancers. Patients with ATC commonly have a prior or concurrent diagnosis of well-differentiated thyroid cancer or benign thyroid disease. Some evidence suggests that ATC can arise from the dedifferentiation of well-differentiated thyroid cancer. Patients with ATC typically present with a palpable mass that is growing or with symptoms of dyspnea or hoarseness. Synchronous pulmonary metastases are observed in up to 50% of patients. Most patients with ATC die from aggressive local–regional disease, most often from upper airway obstruction. A definitive tissue diagnosis should be made by FNA or biopsy whenever possible. The role of operation is generally palliative, preventing airway obstruction or securing a surgical airway via tracheostomy. Doxorubicin-based chemotherapy has been shown to prolong survival. External beam radiation has been used with limited success in patients with recurrent ATC. Anaplastic carcinoma cells do not concentrate iodine, and there is no role for ^{131}I imaging or therapy.

Thyroid Lymphoma and Metastatic Disease to the Thyroid

Lymphoma of the thyroid constitutes approximately 4% of thyroid cancers and represents only 1% of all lymphomas and 2% of extranodal non-Hodgkin lymphoma cases. Thyroid lymphoma is usually seen in older women with Hashimoto thyroiditis. Patients virtually never have hyperthyroidism and frequently have hypothyroidism. Treatment consists of radiation therapy and chemotherapy; typically, there is no role for surgical resection. Clinically apparent metastases to the thyroid from other sites account for less than 1% of all diagnosed thyroid malignancies, although autopsy studies identify metastases to the thyroid in 2% to 26% of people. In these series, the most predominant primary sites are the breast, lung, melanoma, renal cell carcinoma (most common), and GI tract malignancies. Surgery plays a limited role in the management of these patients and is generally reserved for the palliation of symptoms, although prolonged survival has been documented after resection in well-selected patients with oligometastatic disease.

PARATHYROID GLANDS

Embryology and Anatomy

The parathyroids are small, yellowish brown, usually flat and ovoid glands, typically 5 to 7 mm in greatest dimension and weighing on average 30 to 50 mg. Usually, there are four glands, two *superior* and two *inferior*, although 5% to 15% of the population has supernumerary glands (often within the thymus). The location of the glands, particularly the inferior parathyroids, can vary considerably and is better understood through an appreciation of their embryologic development. The parathyroid glands develop around the 5th to 6th weeks of gestation (Fig. 17.3). The superior glands are derived from the fourth pharyngeal pouch along with the lateral thyroid lobes. They migrate a shorter distance, and their final resting location is, therefore, less variable, typically on the extracapsular posteromedial surface of the thyroid lobes just below the level of the cricoid cartilage. The inferior glands originate from the third pharyngeal pouch along with the thymus. Although they often can be found near the inferior poles of the thyroid, their location can vary depending on the extent of their migration from the pharynx to the mediastinum. The parathyroid glands are typically located deep to the pretracheal fascia just outside the thyroid capsule, although they are sometimes intracapsular, embedded within the thyroid gland itself.

The blood supply to all the parathyroid glands is principally from the *inferior thyroid artery*, although additional blood supply may be provided by superior thyroid artery or the *thyroid ima*. The venous and lymphatic drainage of the glands are typically shared with those of the thyroid gland and thymus. The innervation to the parathyroid glands is from cervical sympathetic ganglia.

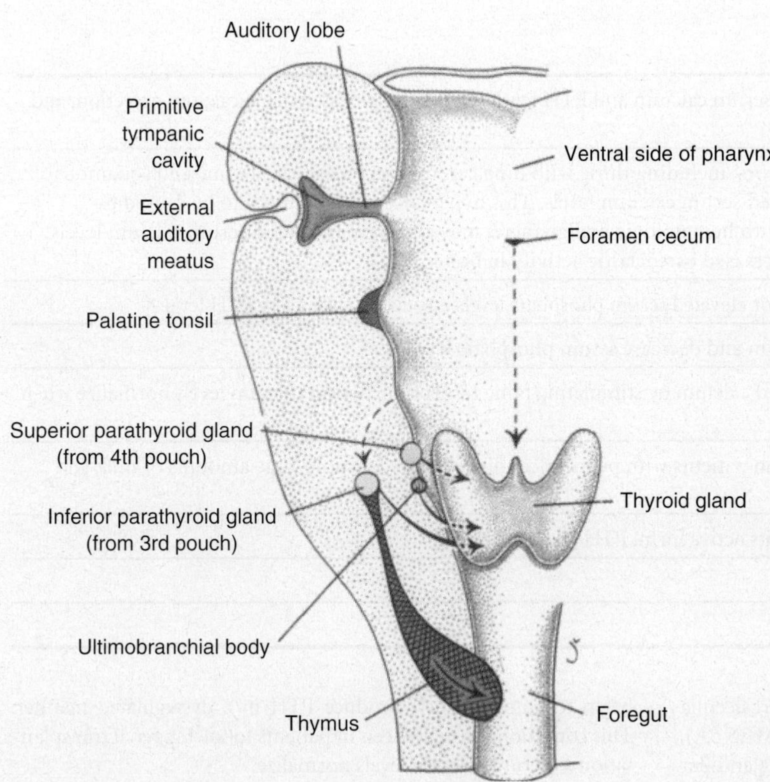

FIGURE 17.3 Schematic representation of the migration of the parathyroid glands. Although the inferior parathyroid glands arise from the third pharyngeal pouch, they migrate along with the thymus and end their descent inferior to the superior parathyroid glands, which arise from the fourth pharyngeal pouch. (From Sadler TW. *Langman's Medical Embryology*. 5th ed. Baltimore: Williams & Wilkins; 1985:289, with permission.)

Physiology

The parathyroid gland's primary physiologic role is the regulation of calcium and phosphate metabolism. The normal range of serum calcium is 9 to 10.5 mg/dL, although the normal range may vary between different laboratories. About half of the total serum calcium is in an ionized, biologically active form. Forty percent is bound to serum protein (albumin), and the remaining 10% is complexed with citrate. Calcium is absorbed in its inorganic form from the duodenum and proximal jejunum in a regulated fashion, reflecting calcium balance. Approximately 99% of calcium in the glomerular filtrate is reabsorbed by the kidney under normal conditions.

Phosphate is also an important component of many biologic systems, including the pathways of glycolysis. The normal range of serum phosphate ranges from 2.5 to 4.3 mg/dL, and the level varies inversely with that of the serum calcium. Phosphate absorption from the diet is relatively constant, and excretion provides the major mechanism for the regulation of phosphate balance.

The primary hormonal regulators of calcium and phosphate homeostasis are parathyroid hormone (PTH), vitamin D, and calcitonin. Regulation depends on three organ systems: the GI tract, the skeletal system, and the renal system.

PTH is the most important regulator of calcium and phosphate metabolism. It is synthesized by the *chief cells* of the parathyroids as a precursor of preproparathyroid hormone, which is then cleaved to form pre-PTH and ultimately PTH. Secretion of PTH is regulated by plasma calcium levels through a negative feedback mechanism. Secreted PTH is cleaved by the Kupffer cells of the liver into its biologically active form. In target tissues, PTH binds to membrane receptors, activating the cAMP pathway to regulate intracellular enzymes. In bone, PTH stimulates osteoclasts and inhibits osteoblasts, thereby stimulating bone resorption and the release of calcium and phosphate. In the kidney, PTH increases the reabsorption of extracellular calcium throughout the nephron, but particularly in the distal nephron. PTH also increases renal phosphate excretion. It acts indirectly on the GI tract by stimulating the hydroxylation of 25-hydroxy vitamin D to 1,25-dihydroxy vitamin D in the kidney.

Vitamin D has two major sites of action. It increases intestinal absorption of calcium and phosphate and enhances PTH-mediated mobilization of calcium and phosphate from bone. Vitamin D_3 is produced normally by the action of sunlight on 7-dehydrocholesterol in the skin. It then binds to plasma proteins and is transported to the liver where 25-hydroxylation occurs. In turn, 25-hydroxy vitamin D_3 undergoes a second hydroxylation in the renal tubular epithelial cell to form the active calcitriol or 1,25-dihydroxy vitamin D_3.

Calcitonin is a 32-amino acid peptide, which is secreted in its proprotein form by the parafollicular or C cells of the thyroid gland. Increased serum calcium levels stimulate secretion of calcitonin, which inhibits bone resorption and increases urinary calcium and phosphate excretion, both of which are mediated through cAMP pathways. Although G protein–coupled calcitonin receptors are located throughout the body, the absence of calcitonin (e.g., following total thyroidectomy) or its overexpression (e.g., in MTC) do not result in significant changes in serum calcium levels and have little clinical impact.

Pathophysiology: Hyperparathyroidism

Clinical Presentation

Increased secretion of PTH can be seen with *primary*, *secondary*, or *tertiary hyperparathyroidism*. *Primary hyperparathyroidism* is the most common cause of hypercalcemia in nonhospitalized patients,

TABLE 17.3 Causes of hypercalcemia

• Hyperparathyroidism. Typically patients have elevated serum calcium and PTH levels, normal or elevated urine calcium excretion, and low or normal plasma concentration of phosphate.
• Hypercalcemia of malignancy. Patients with solid tumors, including those with lung carcinoma, breast carcinoma, and squamous cell carcinoma of the head and neck, often have elevated serum calcium levels. This hypercalcemia is thought to be caused by PTH-related protein secreted by the tumor. Patients with hematologic malignancies may also have increased serum calcium levels, probably resulting from cytokine secretion causing increased osteoclastic activity in bone.
• Excess vitamin D and vitamin A. Patients have normal or elevated serum phosphate levels associated with a low PTH level.
• Thiazide diuretics. Thiazides may increase serum calcium and decrease serum phosphate levels.
• Hyperthyroidism. Hyperthyroidism may cause increased calcium by stimulating bone resorption. Serum calcium levels normalize when the patient becomes euthyroid.
• Milk–alkali syndrome. This syndrome typically occurs in patients with peptic ulcer disease who consume large amounts of milk and absorbable antacids. PTH levels are low.
• Sarcoidosis. Granulomas convert inactive vitamin into its active form. PTH levels are low.
• Paget disease (osteitis deformans).
• AI.

accounting for more than one half of cases (causes of hypercalcemia are listed in Table 17.3). In familial disease (e.g., MEN 1 or MEN 2A), primary hyperparathyroidism is usually caused by multiglandular disease. In nonfamilial disease, primary hyperparathyroidism is caused by a single adenoma in 85% to 90% of cases, a "double" adenoma in 5% to 10% of cases, hyperplasia in 3% to 4% of cases, and parathyroid cancer in less than 0.1% of cases. Approximately 50,000 to 100,000 cases of primary hyperparathyroidism are seen annually, and the disease is most commonly seen in postmenopausal women. Although the etiology of primary hyperparathyroidism is not completely understood, genetic influences seem to contribute at least to some degree to the development of this condition. Mutations in the *PRAD1/cyclinD1* oncogene are commonly seen (up to 40%) in patients with parathyroid adenoma. Parathyroid hyperplasia may also be seen in conjunction with familial syndromes, including MEN 1 (mutations in *menin*) or MEN 2A (mutations in *RET*), *familial isolated hyperparathyroidism* (FIH), and *familial hypocalciuric hypercalcemia (FHH)*. In patients with FHH, an autosomal dominant disease affecting the calcium-sensing receptor (CASR), urinary calcium levels are relatively low, and parathyroidectomy is seldom helpful in reducing serum calcium levels.

Secondary hyperparathyroidism is associated with disease states such as chronic renal failure or severe vitamin D deficiency, in which decreased levels of serum-ionized calcium result in parathyroid hyperplasia and a physiologic elevation in PTH levels. These patients may benefit from restricted dietary intake and dialysate phosphate and aluminum, dietary supplementation of calcium, vitamin D, and administration of phosphate-binding resins. *Cinacalcet*, a calcium mimetic agent that binds to the CASR in the parathyroid gland, was approved for use in 2004. Cinacalcet prevents PTH secretion and has become the standard of care in the management of secondary hyperparathyroidism. Patients who fail medical management may require surgical intervention; these patients undergo subtotal parathyroidectomy, with resection of three and a half glands, typically with cryopreservation or reimplantation of a gland remnant. *Tertiary hyperparathyroidism* results when the overstimulated hyperplastic parathyroid glands of secondary hyperparathyroidism begin to autonomously produce PTH in a dysregulated manner. This condition is usually seen in patients following renal transplantation as serum calcium levels normalize.

Patients with primary hyperparathyroidism are most commonly asymptomatic at the time of presentation and do not have any notable physical examination findings. The diagnosis is usually established by elevated serum calcium levels in the setting of elevated levels of PTH. Twenty-four-hour urinary calcium levels are typically increased and can be measured to exclude the diagnosis of FHH. Other laboratory abnormalities may include an elevation in alkaline phosphatase, a decrease in serum phosphate levels, and a hyperchloremic metabolic acidosis. Patients may present with symptoms of hypercalcemia, which may be remembered from the mnemonic "painful bones, stones, abdominal groans, and psychic moans." Radiographic manifestations of hypercalcemia are rare in adults but may include subperiosteal resorption on the middle phalanges, bone cysts of the skull and long bones, and in more advanced cases, *osteoclastomas* or brown tumors. Bone densitometric studies, or DEXA scans, are frequently obtained in hyperparathyroid patients. Nephrolithiasis occurs more frequently in patients with primary hyperparathyroidism secondary to increased calcium and phosphate excretion and from increased urinary pH. GI sequelae of hypercalcemia range from nonspecific complaints (e.g., nausea, vomiting, and constipation) to pancreatitis, gallstones, and peptic ulcer disease. Hypercalcemia can also result in a wide variety of neurocognitive symptoms including anxiety, depression, psychosis, memory impairment, fatigue, lethargy, and coma. Less commonly, patients present with *hypercalcemic crisis*, a serious and rapidly progressive condition characterized by elevated serum calcium levels, nausea and vomiting, polyuria, polydipsia, weight loss, lethargy, and coma. Initial treatment is aimed at reducing serum calcium levels with hydration (typically with normal saline) and loop diuretics. If these measures are unsuccessful, other strategies include the use of diphosphonates, calcitonin, or mithramycin. Ultimately, when calcium levels have been lowered to a safe range, therapy is aimed at eliminating the etiology of primary hyperparathyroidism, usually with operative intervention.

Preoperative Assessment of Patients with Hyperparathyroidism

Routine preoperative imaging and localization studies for patients with primary hyperparathyroidism were not traditionally advocated because the success rate of surgical treatment via bilateral neck exploration approached 95% in experienced hands. With the advent of minimally invasive parathyroidectomy (MIP), however, preoperative imaging has become more common; on a survey of American endocrinologists, 90% of those surveyed typically obtained preoperative imaging studies prior to making surgical referral. Localization studies also play an integral role in reoperative surgery for either persistent or recurrent disease. Sestamibi–^{99m}Tc imaging, which has largely replaced the thallium–technetium scan, has a sensitivity as high as 90% in identifying parathyroid adenomas and has emerged as the single most useful localizing study. Ultrasonography is a relatively inexpensive and rapid modality, which allows for the identification of lesions in approximately 50% to 60% of reoperative candidates and the acquisition of pathologic information through FNA. CT scan has similar sensitivity, although it is more expensive and is limited in differentiating thyroid and parathyroid tissue. This modality is particularly helpful in identifying ectopic parathyroids in the mediastinum. MRI is even more expensive but is more sensitive than is CT scan.

In general, surgical intervention is recommended for patients with primary hyperparathyroidism and clinical symptoms. The surgical management of patients with documented primary hyperparathyroidism in the absence of symptoms is somewhat controversial. The 2002 NIH Consensus Development Conference Statement on Diagnosis and Management of Asymptomatic Primary Hyperparathyroidism outlines guidelines for potential surgical intervention among these patients. Surgery is recommended for asymptomatic patients with (i) serum calcium levels greater than 1.0 mg/dL, the upper limit of normal; (ii) reduced creatinine clearance (>30% compared with age-matched controls); (iii) elevated 24-hour urinary calcium level (>400 mg/day); (iv) reduced bone mass (T score $\leq$ 2.5); (v) age below 50 years; and (vi) unsuitability for routine surveillance, including patients with poor medical compliance and patients requesting surgery. An increasing number of endocrinologists and surgeons offer operative intervention even for supposedly asymptomatic patients who do not meet these criteria, as neurocognitive symptoms in particular may be underappreciated in hyperparathyroid patients, but have been demonstrated to improve markedly after parathyroidectomy.

Surgery for Hyperparathyroidism

Parathyroidectomy provides definitive treatment for patients with primary hyperparathyroidism and is associated with high initial success rates of greater than 95% and morbidity typically less than 1%. Traditionally, experienced endocrine surgeons have advocated for bilateral neck exploration at the time of initial surgery with identification of all four parathyroid glands because of the possibility of multiglandular disease. With the introduction of highly sensitive sestamibi scans (often in conjunction with ultrasonography), many endocrine centers have moved toward MIP through small (2 to 4 cm) incisions with unilateral neck dissections, frequently under local anesthesia. Advocates of this method quote similar cure rates, reduced operative times, improved cosmetic outcomes, decreased cost, and, theoretically, lower morbidity with more limited dissection. Key components of this approach are the preoperative localization of the abnormal gland and the intraoperative measurement of serum PTH using a rapid PTH ELISA-based assay. A drop of greater than 50% with normalization of PTH levels upon excision of the abnormal gland, suggests that the patient has a single adenoma, and bilateral exploration can safely be omitted. Minimally invasive radioguided parathyroidectomy (MIRP) is similar to MIP but also involves the use of an intraoperative radioguided probe to detect ^{99m}Tc radiotracer injected prior to the procedure, which is taken up preferentially by the abnormal parathyroid gland(s).

In the event that a bilateral neck exploration is undertaken, the superior parathyroids are usually identified in their typical location. Identification of the abnormal inferior gland(s) is sometimes more difficult. Frequently, ectopic inferior parathyroid glands are found in the thyrothymic ligament or in the thymus itself. If the inferior glands cannot be localized, the thymic pedicle should be carefully inspected and mobilized, and a transcervical thymectomy should be performed. If the gland is not located by this method, then mobilization of the thyroid lobe ipsilateral to the missing parathyroid gland is indicated, as a small percentage (2% to 5%) of glands are intrathyroidal. Intraoperative ultrasonography may be helpful in identifying these parathyroid glands, but thyroid lobectomy is sometimes indicated if the abnormal gland cannot be localized. Intraoperative selective venous sampling with measurement of PTH levels may also be helpful in some instances to localize an ectopic gland. If all these methods prove to be unsuccessful, it is generally recommended that the procedure be aborted and further localization studies be obtained prior to reexploration.

The surgical procedure indicated for primary hyperparathyroidism depends upon the etiology of the disease. Simple excision of parathyroid adenomas is sufficient. Success of the procedure depends upon careful visual inspection of the size of the glands by an experienced surgeon and by histologic confirmation by frozen sections. Care should be taken not to rupture the capsule of the adenoma, as this may potentially lead to seeding of the neck and recurrent hyperparathyroidism due to *parathyromatosis*. Other methods, such as intraoperative PTH measurements can also help to ensure curative outcome. The recommended surgical treatment of parathyroid hyperplasia or four-gland disease is either subtotal parathyroidectomy (removal of 3.5 of the 4 glands) or total parathyroidectomy with immediate autotransplantation of parathyroid tissue, typically in the forearm muscle bed. The incidence of hypoparathyroidism is similar (approximately 5%) with these two surgical approaches. The incidence of recurrent disease is significantly higher in patients with MEN 1 or other familial parathyroid hyperplasia syndromes, and, therefore, total parathyroidectomy with cryopreservation and autotransplantation of parathyroid tissue is generally preferred in these patients, because it simplifies reoperation, if necessary.

Complications of operation for primary hyperparathyroidism are relatively rare. Persistent disease occurs in less than 5% of cases and usually results from a missed adenoma. Recurrent disease, characterized by a period (6 months) of normocalcemia followed by a return of hypercalcemia, is also uncommon and is frequently the result of unrecognized hyperplasia, an incompletely excised adenoma or spillage of tumor at the time of surgery. Reoperation should be performed only after exhaustive localization studies

TABLE 17.4 Causes of hypocalcemia

• Postoperative hypoparathyroidism most commonly occurs after total thyroidectomy for malignancy. The low calcium level probably results from contusion or transient ischemia of the parathyroids; the hypocalcemia is usually self-limited and not treated unless significant symptoms develop.
• Idiopathic hypoparathyroidism occurs in both sporadic and familial forms and may have an autoimmune basis. DiGeorge syndrome is a congenital disorder involving the branchial pouches and produces agenesis of the thymus and parathyroids.
• Vitamin D deficiency may result from a dietary deficiency or lack of exposure to sunlight. There is a decrease in calcium absorption and an increased secretion of PTH.
• Pseudohypoparathyroidism is a familial disease characterized by an unresponsiveness of the kidney to PTH. Elevated PTH levels cause bone resorption, but patients remain hypocalcemic and hyperphosphatemic.
• Hypomagnesemia with secondary hypocalcemia (HSH) is an autosomal recessive genetic disorder resulting in decreased magnesium absorption from the GI tract and, secondarily, decreased PTH secretion.
• Malabsorption.
• Pancreatitis.

have been performed. The incidence of bleeding and neck hematoma is less than 1%, and the incidence of injury to the RLN is approximately 1% during an initial procedure and 5% to 10% upon reexploration. Permanent hypoparathyroidism is relatively uncommon following an initial procedure but may occur in up to 20% of patients following reoperation.

Careful examination of patients postoperatively for the signs and symptoms of hypocalcemia that may result from hypoparathyroidism is important. Decreased plasma-ionized calcium levels, which may also be seen in other conditions (Table 17.4), result in increased neuromuscular excitability. Patients may complain of circumoral tingling or numbness, or tingling in the fingers and toes. They may also present with more vague psychiatric symptoms of confusion or anxiety. On physical examination, hypocalcemia may be revealed by tapping anterior to the facial nerve to elicit contraction of the facial muscles (*Chvostek sign*) or applying a blood pressure cuff for 3 minutes to occlude blood flow to the forearm to elicit carpal spasm (*Trousseau sign*). An electrocardiogram may reveal a prolonged QT interval. Generally, therapy is aimed at maintaining serum calcium levels greater than 8.0 mg/dL, which can usually be achieved with oral calcium supplementation. In some cases, administration of calcitriol may be indicated if oral calcium supplementation alone is unsuccessful. Following parathyroidectomy, particularly in patients with preexisting metabolic bone disease, *hungry bone syndrome*, characterized by hypocalcemia, hypophosphatemia, hypomagnesemia, and increased bone mineralization, may develop. Severe cases of hypocalcemia may result in convulsions and tetany. Rapid infusion of intravenous calcium solutions is warranted.

Parathyroid Carcinoma

Parathyroid carcinoma is an extremely rare functioning neoplasm, occurring in less than 0.1% of patients with primary hyperparathyroidism. There does not appear to be a gender predilection for this malignancy, which is more common in patients older than 30 years. Although the etiology is unknown, mutations in the retinoblastoma (RB) tumor suppressor gene and the *HRPT-2* gene (also associated with a particular type of familial hyperplasia) have been observed with higher frequency in patients with this cancer. Patients with parathyroid carcinoma often present with extremely high serum calcium levels and significantly elevated PTH levels. In some patients, an elevated serum human chorionic gonadotropin (hCG) level is also seen. Approximately one half of patients will present with a palpable firm neck mass, and many patients may have an affected voice from RLN involvement. If parathyroid carcinoma is suspected, initial treatment should include radical resection of the involved gland, the ipsilateral thyroid lobe, and regional lymph nodes. Management of parathyroid carcinoma that is metastatic is frequently oriented toward control of the resulting hypercalcemia, as chemotherapy and radiation have not been shown to provide any significant benefit.

ADRENAL GLANDS

Embryology

The *adrenal cortex* is derived from *coelomic mesoderm*, adjacent to the urogenital ridge. Aberrant adrenocortical tissue may be found near the kidney or in the pelvis, possibly along the bladder. The *adrenal medulla* is derived from the *neural crest*; consequently, the medulla and sympathetic nervous system develop together. During the 5th week of gestation, the neural crest cells migrate toward the adrenocortical cells and situate themselves within a capsule of mesodermal cortex.

Anatomy

The adrenal glands are paired retroperitoneal structures, located at the superior medial aspect of the upper portion of each kidney. They are firm in texture, and their dark-yellow hue distinguishes them from retroperitoneal fat. The right adrenal gland lies in proximity to the inferior vena cava, the right posterior liver, and the right diaphragmatic crus. The left adrenal gland is adjacent to the aorta, the tail of the pancreas, and the spleen (Fig. 17.4). The glands receive their blood supply from the inferior phrenic arteries, the aorta, and the renal arteries. Arterial branches form a subcapsular plexus, explaining the substantial bleeding that can result from

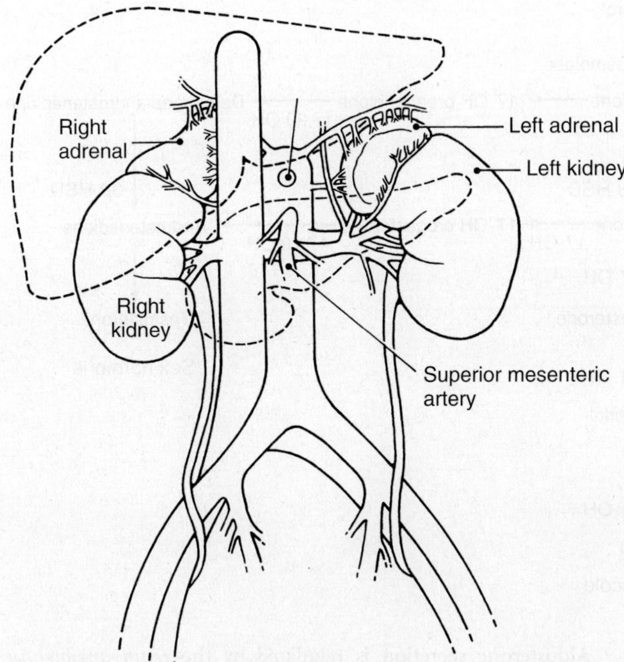

FIGURE 17.4 The right adrenal gland is situated near the inferior vena cava, the liver, and the right diaphragmatic crus. The left adrenal gland is situated near the aorta, the tail of the pancreas, and the spleen. (From Scott-Conner C, Dawson DL, eds. *Operative Anatomy*. Philadelphia: J.B. Lippincott; 1993:499, with permission.)

capsular injuries. A number of small vessels run from the cortex (outer layers) to the medulla, constituting what some refer to as the adrenal "portal venous" circulation. This relationship allows for the fundamental catecholamine–glucocorticoid interactions. Venous blood drains via the central veins into the inferior vena cava on the right side and the renal vein on the left side.

Functionally, the adrenal gland is divided into the adrenal cortex and the adrenal medulla. The cortex is organized into three distinct layers: the *zona glomerulosa*, the outer layer, which constitutes approximately 15% of the cortex; the *zona fasciculata*, the middle and largest layer accounting for 75% of the cortex; and the *zona reticularis*, the innermost layer of the cortex. The three zones are the sites of production of mineralocorticoids, glucocorticoids, and sex steroids, respectively. The adrenal medulla is similar to a peripheral sympathetic ganglia. It is the site of catecholamine production, primarily epinephrine.

Biologically Active Adrenal Products

All adrenal steroids have a 17-carbon structure comprising three hexane rings and single pentane rings. Cortisol and aldosterone have an additional two-carbon side chain. *Cortisol* regulates the intermediary metabolism of carbohydrates, proteins, and lipids. It stimulates the release of glucagon and lactate from muscle and down-regulates the sensitivity of insulin. Upon cortisol stimulation, muscle cells undergo proteolysis and adipocytes undergo lipolysis. The resulting amino acids and glycerol molecules are channeled to the liver for gluconeogenesis. In addition, cortisol acts directly on hepatic enzymes involved in gluconeogenesis. The combined effect of these processes is hyperglycemia.

In addition to the effect on intermediate carbohydrate metabolism, cortisol regulates the intravascular volume and modulates the immune system. It has positive chronotropic and inotropic effects on the heart and helps maintain blood pressure by stimulating angiotensin release and inhibiting the synthesis of prostaglandin I_2 (a potent vasodilator). Glucocorticoids retard wound healing by decreasing interleukin-2 production and release and lymphocyte activation, as well as by making mononuclear cells less responsive and less efficient for chemotaxis and phagocytosis. Osteoblast cell development necessary for bone growth and strength and fibroblast activity for collagen formation are also adversely affected. Finally, chronic corticosteroid excess can cause emotional and psychologic disturbances.

Aldosterone is a mineralocorticoid that controls intravascular volume by stimulating the distal convoluted tubules (DCTs) of the kidney to reabsorb sodium, and, indirectly, free water and to excrete potassium and hydrogen ion. The half-life of the mineralocorticoid is relatively short (15 minutes), and it is bound to transcortin and albumin much like cortisol. The majority (90%) of this steroid is cleared from the plasma after a single pass via the liver.

The major adrenal *androgens* are dehydroepiandrosterone, androstenedione, and testosterone. Estrogen is produced from androstenedione in the peripheral tissue. In adults, androgens promote the development of secondary sex characteristics such as deepening of the voice, male hair distribution, coarsening of the skin, and protein deposition in muscles. Estrogen has the opposite effects. In the fetus, androgens stimulate wolffian duct development, which results in male external genitalia. The lack of androgens in the female fetus allows the genital tubercle, labial folds, and urethral opening to remain in the normal female position. Adrenal androgen production and release is stimulated by ACTH and not by gonadotropins.

Cells of the adrenal medulla secrete *biologically active amines*, including dopamine, norepinephrine, and epinephrine, in response to sympathetic nerve innervation. Catecholamines bind with different affinities to specialized receptors (α_1, α_2, β_1, and β_2) found in different concentrations throughout many groups of cells. In contrast to steroids, catecholamines elicit physiologic responses in minutes, using cAMP as a secondary messenger molecule.

Biosynthetic Pathways

The early steroid synthesis pathways are common to all adrenal hormones and steroids. Cholesterol is converted to pregnenolone by a desmolase enzyme in the cell mitochondria (Fig. 17.5). Pregnenolone is shuttled either via a pathway for the synthesis of testosterone or via a pathway for the conversion to progesterone, which is an intermediate substrate for cortisol, aldosterone, and additional testosterone synthesis.

The adrenal medulla is the area of catecholamine synthesis, storage, and release as well as reuptake of released steroids. Sympathetic stimulation of the chromaffin cells increases the activity of the tyrosine hydroxylase, which converts the amino acid tyrosine into dihydroxyphenylalanine (DOPA) and ultimately leads to the sequential production of dopamine, norepinephrine, and epinephrine.

Regulatory Mechanisms for Hormone Secretion

Various regulatory mechanisms control the release of glucocorticoids, mineralocorticoids, and catecholamines. The production of cortisol is regulated by the hypothalamic–pituitary axis (Fig. 17.6).

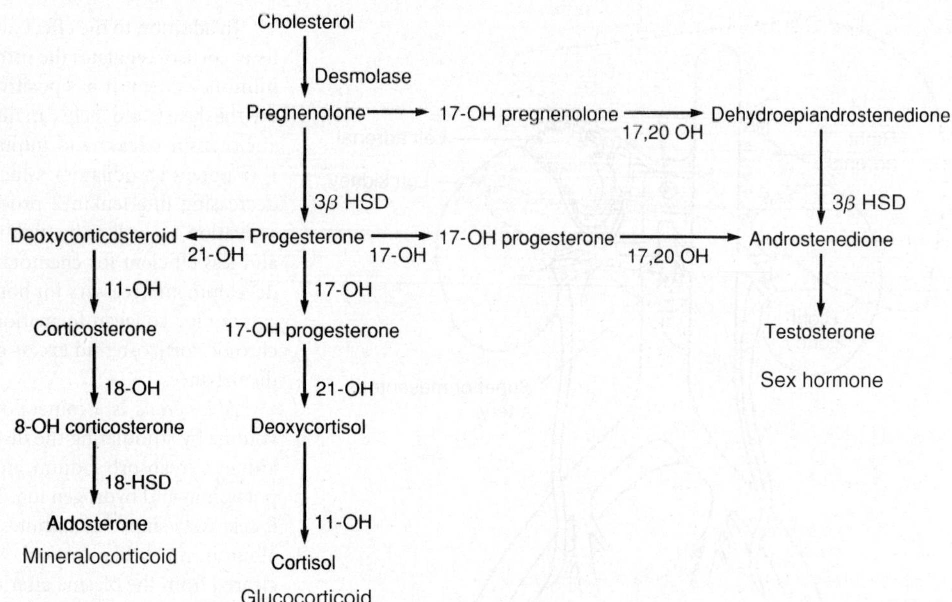

FIGURE 17.5 Steroidogenic pathways of the adrenal cortex. A deficiency of 21-hydroxylase is the most common cause of congenital adrenal hyperplasia. This condition results in decreased cortisol and aldosterone production as well as an excess of progesterone, which leads to increased androgen production. (From Newsome HH. Adrenal glands. In: Greenfield LJ, Mullholland MW, Oldham KT, et al., eds. *Surgery: Scientific Principles and Practice.* 2nd ed. Philadelphia: Lippincott–Raven Publishers; 1997: 1334, with permission.)

The central and peripheral nervous systems signal the hypothalamus during periods of emotional and physical stress to release corticotrophin-releasing hormone (CRH). CRH is delivered to the anterior pituitary, and, in response, the pituitary releases ACTH, and the adrenal glands synthesize and release cortisol. The resulting high level of cortisol antagonizes secretion of CRH and ACTH by the hypothalamus and pituitary, respectively.

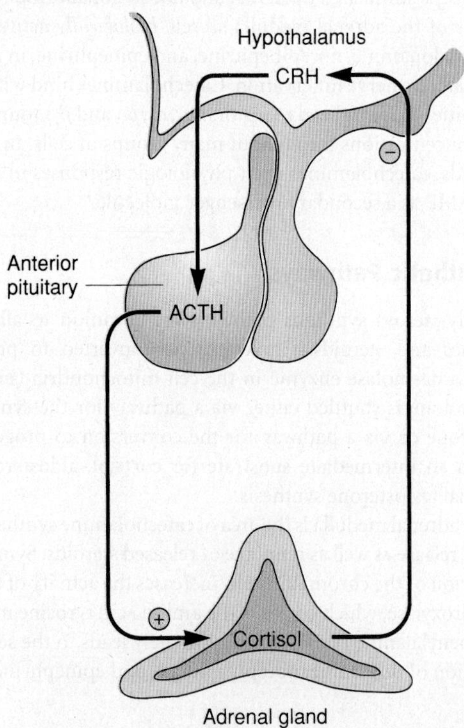

FIGURE 17.6 Feedback loop between the hypothalamus, the anterior pituitary, and the adrenal. (From Mulholland MW. *Greenfield's Surgery: Scientific Principles and Practice.* 5th ed. Philadelphia: Lippincott Williams & Wilkins; 2011.)

Aldosterone secretion is regulated by the *renin–angiotensin system* and plasma sodium concentration. The juxtaglomerular apparatus of the kidney and the macula densa—a grouping of cells located near the afferent arteriole—detect decreased renal blood flow and low plasma sodium concentration (Fig. 17.7). In response, the juxtaglomerular apparatus releases renin that converts angiotensinogen to angiotensin I, a decapeptide derived from a large hepatic protein. Angiotensin I is converted to angiotensin II in the lung by angiotensin-converting enzyme (ACE), the target of the pharmacologic category of antihypertensives termed *ACE inhibitors.* The newly formed protein signals aldosterone release. Two other minor factors that affect aldosterone release are plasma potassium concentration and ACTH. This hormone signals the adrenal glands to convert cholesterol into steroid products that are common to the mineralocorticoid and glucocorticoid synthesis pathway, but it favors the latter.

Catecholamine release is controlled by the *sympathetic nervous system.* The adrenal medulla is supplied by preganglionic sympathetic nerves from the greater splanchnic nerve and the celiac ganglion. Stimulation of the chromaffin cells results in transit of secretory granules to the cell membrane for release via exocytosis. The released catecholamines can be taken up by the chromaffin cells, enter the systemic circulation or neuronal cells, and undergo degradation or be excreted in the urine. The neuronal cells metabolize epinephrine and norepinephrine into vanillylmandelic acid (VMA) with monamine oxidase. Another enzyme, carboxy-*O*-methyltransferase converts extraneuronal epinephrine and norepinephrine into metanephrine and normetanephrine, respectively. A small portion will bind to specific receptors and elicit a physiologic response.

Adrenal Imaging

CT scan is the diagnostic study of choice to evaluate the adrenal gland. Simple cysts and myelolipomas can usually be identified by their CT characteristics (i.e., fluid and fat density, respectively). Intravenous contrast is not required. Benign and malignant lesions can often be distinguished on the basis of Hounsfield units (<20 and >30, respectively). MRI is an accurate alternative to CT scan and

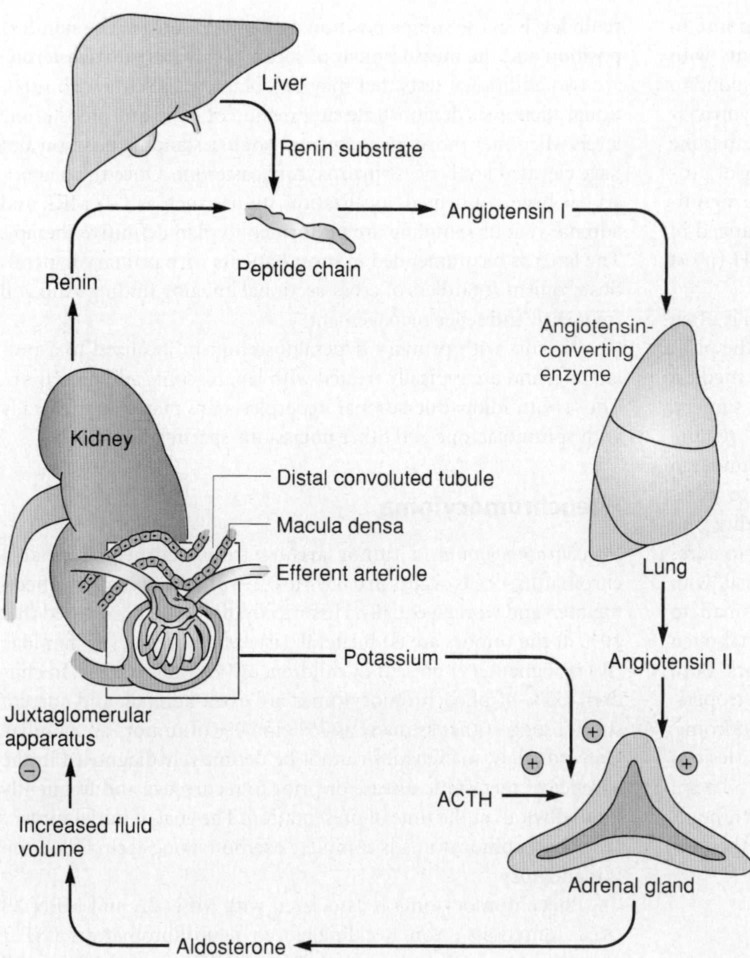

FIGURE 17.7 The renin–angiotensin–aldosterone system, including their sites of production. (From Mulholland MW. *Greenfield's Surgery: Scientific Principles and Practice.* 5th ed. Philadelphia: Lippincott Williams & Wilkins; 2011.)

unique enhancement characteristics allow for the distinction between benign and malignant lesions; the former are isointense in relation to the liver, while the latter and pheochromocytomas are hyperintense in relation to the liver on T2-weighted imaging. Radioisotope scans using iodocholesterol-labeled agents can help localize functional lesions such as aldosterone-producing adenomas; however, such studies are not widely available. Metaiodobenzylguanidine (MIBG) can be helpful if adrenal pheochromocytoma and neuroblastoma are suspected, as ^{131}I-MIBG and ^{123}I-MIBG are concentrated in catecholamine storage vesicles. Positron emission tomography (PET) can be useful in identifying extra-adrenal pheochromocytoma.

Pathophysiology

The production, release, and metabolism of the glucocorticoids and mineralocorticoids are tightly regulated to maintain body homeostasis. However, both benign and malignant adrenal and extra-adrenal tumors, adrenal hyperplastic states, and congenital enzymatic deficiencies can cause the overproduction and insufficiency of glucocorticoids and mineralocorticoids and result in pathologic conditions.

Cushing Syndrome

Patients with an excess of cortisol develop a syndrome characterized by moon facies, truncal obesity, striae, glucose intolerance, hypertension, polycythemia, hirsutism, osteoporosis, menstrual irregularity, muscle weakness, and pulmonary infections. There is also an increased incidence of peptic ulcer disease and pancreatitis in these patients. The most common cause is the excessive administration of exogenous glucocorticoid steroids. The most common cause of endogenous hypercortisolism is excessive pituitary ACTH secretion (Cushing disease) associated with a pituitary adenoma. Other causes include ectopic ACTH production, adrenal adenoma or carcinoma, and micronodular pigmented hyperplasia.

The evaluation of suspected *hypercortisolism* begins with 24-hour urinary-free cortisol and 17-hydroxycorticoid levels to determine whether hypercortisolism is indeed present. Once hypercortisolism is confirmed, a *dexamethasone suppression test* is administered to determine whether the process is ACTH dependent or ACTH independent. Finally, a localizing study (CT scan or MRI) is obtained to localize a lesion radiographically. The dexamethasone test involves administration of a single dose of steroid the night (11 o'clock) before and a morning (8 o'clock) measurement of cortisol levels in plasma and urine. In the presence of a normal hypothalamic–pituitary axis, cortisol production is suppressed by even low-dose dexamethasone; therefore suppression typically rules out the presence of Cushing disease. A high-dose dexamethasone suppression test can help to establish whether the source is from the pituitary or elsewhere, as higher doses of dexamethasone will typically suppress cortisol secretion in Cushing disease but not in ectopic ACTH-producing tumors. A patient may also be given CRH to help determine whether the hypercortisolism is dependent on the pituitary. ACTH and cortisol levels increase in response to CRH in patients with Cushing disease. In contrast, patients with adrenal or ectopic sources of cortisol production do not respond to the administration of CRH. Measurement of urinary 17-hydroxysteroid levels after administration of a high-dose of dexamethasone (8 mg/day) can also help to determine the source of cortisol production. The urinary levels of 17-hydroxysteroid decrease significantly in patients with Cushing disease and remain unchanged in patients with adrenal or with ectopic production of ACTH (most commonly from small cell lung cancers).

Treatment of many of the causes of Cushing syndrome is often surgical. In Cushing disease, transsphenoidal resection of the pituitary adenoma is the treatment of choice. Radiation or medical therapy may be used if the symptoms persist or recur after surgery. Likewise, patients with adrenal adenoma or carcinoma require adrenalectomy. Patients with adrenal adenomas typically undergo laparoscopic adrenalectomy. The laparoscopic approach to adrenalectomy has resulted in decreased length of stay, morbidity, and time to return to a normal diet and activity. The approach to adrenal carcinomas and metastatic lesions remains controversial, with some authors advocating a laparoscopic approach for small to moderately sized tumors and others preferring a traditional open procedure for all suspected or confirmed malignant tumors. Both approaches can be performed transperitoneally or via the retroperitoneum. Lastly, for those patients with ectopic ACTH syndrome, the primary lesion must be surgically removed. Unresectable lesions or tumor recurrences may be debulked with or without bilateral adrenalectomy to provide palliation. Drugs including metyrapone, aminoglutethimide, and mitotane can be used to suppress the production of cortisol.

Hyperaldosteronism

Hypersecretion of mineralocorticoids can cause a syndrome characterized by hypertension and hypokalemia. Insulin sensitivity and hyperglycemia may also be present. *Primary hyperaldosteronism* is generally caused by autonomously functioning adrenal cortex tumors (Conn syndrome). Causes of *secondary hyperaldosteronism* include renal artery stenosis, cirrhosis, congestive heart failure, and normal pregnancy. Treatment or resolution of the underlying conditions usually corrects the hyperaldosteronism. The diagnosis of primary hyperaldosteronism is established by the presence of diastolic hypertension without edema, hyposecretion of renin despite low intravascular volume, and hypersecretion of aldosterone. The diagnosis is confirmed by a plasma aldosterone–renin ratio of greater than 20 in the setting of an elevated plasma aldosterone level of greater than or equal to 15 ng/dL ($\geq$416 pmol/L). Hypokalemia is present in the majority, but not all, patients with hyperaldosteronism. Captopril, an angiotensin-converting enzyme (ACE) inhibitor may be given to the patient before measuring aldosterone and renin levels. In healthy patients, the ACE inhibitor decreases aldosterone production and increases renin production, thereby lowering the aldosterone–renin ratio. In contrast, patients with primary hyperaldosteronism will have a persistently high level of aldosterone and an aldosterone–renin ratio of more than 50. Twenty-four-hour urinary aldosterone secretion of more than 14 μg following 5 days of high-sodium diet is highly suggestive of primary hyperaldosteronism. Measuring urinary sodium and aldosterone levels after intravenous saline infusion may also be helpful in the diagnosis of primary hyperaldosteronism. The measurement of plasma aldosterone and renin levels in the supine position and 2 hours later in the standing position and the measurement of serum 18-hydroxycorticosterone are two additional tests that may be obtained. Patients with functional adenomas demonstrate suppression of renin and aldosterone levels when they move from a recumbent to a standing position and have elevated levels of 18-hydroxycorticosterone. Once the diagnosis has been confirmed, localization studies such as CT, MRI, and adrenal venous sampling are performed to plan definitive therapy. The latter is recommended in most patients with primary hyperaldosteronism regardless of cross-sectional imaging findings and will frequently influence management.

Patients with primary hyperaldosteronism localized to a unilateral gland are typically treated with laparoscopic adrenalectomy. Those with idiopathic adrenal hyperplasia are managed medically with spironolactone and other potassium-sparing diuretics.

Pheochromocytoma

Pheochromocytoma, a tumor arising from neuroectodermal—chromaffin—cells occurs in 0.05% to 0.1% of the population, affecting men and women equally. Historically, the rule of 10s stated that 10% of the tumors are (i) bilateral, (ii) extra-adrenal, (iii) familial, (iv) malignant, (v) present in children, or (vi) multicentric. In children, 35% of pheochromocytomas are extra-adrenal, and current studies suggest that as many as 25% to 30% of tumors are familial. Unfortunately, malignancy cannot be definitively diagnosed in the absence of metastatic disease or prior to recurrence and frequently is not obvious at the time of presentation. The goal of initial surgery for pheochromocytoma is complete excision. Long-term follow-up is mandatory.

Pheochromocytoma is associated with MEN 2A and MEN 2B (*RET* mutations), von Recklinghausen neurofibromatosis (*NF 1* mutations), von Hippel–Lindau disease (VHL mutations), as well as mutations of *succinate dehydrogenase* subunit B and D. Most tumors secrete norepinephrine, either continuously or episodically. Patients classically present with episodes of headaches, sweating, and palpitations, often described as anxiety attacks. The evaluation of a suspected pheochromocytoma consists of 24-hour urine catecholamines and metabolites, including dopamine, VMA, and metanephrine, and plasma measurements of epinephrine and norepinephrine. Because catecholamine secretion is often episodic, repeated 24-hour urinary tests may be necessary. Plasma fractionated metanephrines have been demonstrated to have increased sensitivity compared to urine testing. If the urinary and plasma measurements are equivocal for the diagnosis of pheochromocytoma, clonidine, a centrally acting antihypertensive, may be given. In normal patients, clonidine suppresses plasma concentrations of catecholamines; this is not the case in patients with pheochromocytomas. As with other functional tumors, following confirmation of the diagnosis, pheochromocytomas must be localized using CT scan, MRI, MIBG, and/or venous sampling.

Patients with pheochromocytomas require surgical excision. Today, most pheochromocytomas are treated with laparoscopic adrenalectomy. In preparation for operation, patients are given phenoxybenzamine, an α-blocker, to reduce blood pressure and to restore intravascular volume for at least 1 to 4 weeks. After adequate α-blockade has been achieved, a β-blocker may be added if the patient has evidence of tachycardia. β-Blockers can precipitate malignant hypertension and cardiac failure in patients with pheochromocytomas who are not adequately α-receptor blocked and therefore should never be started prior to the establishment of α-blockade. An additional preoperative medication is metyrosine, a tyrosine hydroxylase inhibitor that blocks the rate limiting step in catecholamine production. This decreases blood pressure fluctuations that occur with the manipulation of the tumor during operative resection.

Adrenocortical Carcinoma

Adrenocortical carcinoma is a highly lethal and rare malignancy. Patients commonly present with metastatic or locally advanced disease. The majority of patients present with an endocrinopathy, either Cushing syndrome or virilization. There is a bimodal distribution of disease by age with relatively high incidences in first 4 years and fourth to fifth decades of life. Women develop functional adrenocortical carcinomas more commonly than men. Adrenocortical carcinomas are usually larger than 6 cm in greatest dimension and weigh between 100 and 5,000 g. Several studies have demonstrated that metastasizing or recurring tumors are associated with high mitotic activity, nuclear DNA ploidy, and production of abnormal amounts of androgens and 11-deoxysteroids. The only hope for cure is complete excision. Often this is not possible, but aggressive local resection is appropriate. The overall prognosis is poor.

Congenital Adrenal Hyperplasia

Enzyme deficiencies of the steroid synthesis pathway in the adrenal gland can result in overproduction of sex steroids. These enzymatic deficiencies result in a syndrome known as "congenital adrenal hyperplasia." It is the most common adrenal disorder of infancy and childhood. The syndrome results in decreased cortisol production, accumulation of intermediate steroid metabolites, and increased androgen production. Peripheral tissues convert the androgen to testosterone, which can cause virilization. Prenatal congenital adrenal hyperplasia in girls results in ambiguous external genitalia (female pseudohermaphroditism), but the reproductive organs develop normally. Postnatal congenital adrenal hyperplasia can cause virilization of girls. Congenital adrenal hyperplasia in both sexes is associated with short stature, premature closure of bone epiphyses, and advanced bone age.

The most common cause of congenital adrenal hyperplasia is 21-hydroxylase deficiency (Fig. 17.5). This enzyme is responsible for the conversion of progesterone to 11-deoxycorticosterone and subsequently to corticosterone and aldosterone. Without the enzyme, there is an accumulation of progesterone and δ-5-pregnenolone, which are converted to androgen by 17α-hydroxylase, as well as a decreased production of aldosterone that results in dehydration, hyponatremia, and hyperkalemia. Other less common causes of the hyperplasia include 11β-hydroxylase and 3β-hydroxylase deficiencies.

Adrenal Insufficiency

Primary adrenal failure is caused by an inherent disease of the adrenal gland, whereas secondary failure is caused by disorders of the pituitary or hypothalamus. Primary adrenal insufficiency (AI) is typically caused by autoimmune disease (Addison disease), infectious disease (e.g., tuberculosis and histoplasmosis), adrenal hemorrhage, metastases, or surgical resection. The most common cause of secondary AI is exogenous steroid exposure. The symptoms of low cortisol are nonspecific and include nausea, vomiting, weight loss, weakness, and lethargy. Rarely, hypocortisolism can produce a sudden hypotension or shock (crisis) that is life threatening. AI may also be accompanied by hyponatremia and hyperkalemia.

A short cosyntropin stimulation test can be performed to establish the diagnosis of primary and secondary adrenal failure. Cosyntropin (ACTH) (250 μg intravenous or intramuscular) is administered, and plasma cortisol is measured 30 minutes later. Patients with adrenal failure will not respond to this stimulation with an increase in cortisol levels. An ACTH level can also help to distinguish between primary and secondary adrenal failure. In primary failure, patients will have elevated levels of ACTH but insufficient levels of glucocorticoids. Serum potassium and sodium levels may also be helpful in making the diagnosis.

The treatment of adrenal failure consists of exogenous glucocorticoids given twice daily with a higher morning dose. In primary failure, the treatment also includes mineralocorticoids (Florinef) because all adrenal hormone synthesis is impaired. The treatment of an Addisonian crisis includes volume resuscitation and intravenous glucocorticoids. Patients who use glucocorticoids or recently discontinued them require increased doses of the exogenous glucocorticoids during illness, injury, or surgery, as well as in the postoperative period (i.e., *stress dose steroids*), though the need for this has been questioned recently.

Incidentaloma

The widespread use of diagnostic cross-sectional imaging studies has increased the detection of asymptomatic adrenal masses or *incidentalomas*. Incidentalomas are seen in 0.6% to 5.0% of abdominal CT scans. The approach to an incidentaloma should take into account three basic questions: (i) Is the lesion functional, (ii) is it malignant, and (iii) is it metastatic?

Patients should undergo a thorough history and physical examination focusing on signs and symptoms of Cushing syndrome, aldosteronism, and pheochromocytoma. Traditionally, 24-hour collections of urine for cortisol, VMA, metanephrines, and catecholamines have been performed along with serum potassium levels. If the potassium levels are low and the patient is hypertensive, serum aldosterone and renin levels should be collected. More recent NIH guidelines suggest a 1-mg dexamethasone suppression test and a measurement of plasma-free metanephrines in addition to the measurement of serum potassium and plasma aldosterone–plasma renin activity ratio in hypertensive patients.

All functional tumors and all tumors larger than 5 cm are treated with unilateral laparoscopic adrenalectomy. Some authors advocate unilateral adrenalectomy for tumors larger than 4 cm. In addition, if the patient has a history of cancer, particularly lung cancer, and a negative biochemical workup, an FNA may be performed to help detect suspected metastatic disease to the adrenal or lymphoma. An alternative test to FNA in evaluating an incidentaloma in a patient with prior malignancy is a PET scan. In general, FNA should not be routinely performed, because it typically cannot distinguish between benign and malignant tumors. Masses that are smaller than 4 cm or are nonfunctional can be followed with serial CT scans every 6 months. Enlargement of the lesion warrants surgical resection.

Suggested Readings

Adrenal. *Selected Readings in General Surgery*. Vol 26, No. 7. Dallas, Texas: University of Texas, Southwestern Medical Center of Dallas; 1999.

Baker RJ, Fischer JE, eds. *Mastery of Surgery*. 4th ed. Philadelphia: Lippincott Williams & Wilkins; 2001:477–488.

Cooper DS, Doherty GM, Haugen BR, et al. Revised American Thyroid Association management guidelines for patients with thyroid nodules and differentiated thyroid cancer. *Thyroid*. 2009;19(11):1167–1214.

DeVita VT Jr, Hellman S, Roseberg SA, eds. *Cancer: Principles and Practice of Oncology*. 7th ed. Philadelphia: Lippincott Williams & Wilkins; 2005:1629–1652.

Norton J, Bollinger R, Chang AE, et al., eds. *Essential Practice of Surgery: Basic Science and Clinical Evidence*. New York: Springer-Verlag; 2003:369–399.

Parathyroid disease. *Selected Readings in General Surgery*. Vol 23, No. 4. Texas: University of Texas, Southwestern Medical Center of Dallas; 1996.

CHAPTER

18 The Breast

NIAMEY P. WILSON AND BRIAN J. CZERNIECKI

KEY POINTS

- Fibroadenoma is the most common tumor of the breast in women younger than 30 years of age and typically presents as a solitary painless mass.
- Most phyllodes tumors are benign, and treatment is excision with negative margins. There is generally no role for axillary staging in the management of these tumors.
- Atypical ductal hyperplasia and atypical lobular hyperplasia are associated with a four- to fivefold increased risk of subsequent breast cancer.
- LCIS is a risk factor for the subsequent development of invasive breast cancer in either the affected or the contralateral breast.
- Tumor size and lymph node involvement are the major determinants of prognosis in invasive breast cancer, with genetic profiling and hormonal receptor status adding to the decision-making process.
- Contraindications to breast-conserving therapy for breast cancer include large tumor burden in a small breast, multicentric disease, and contraindications to radiation therapy.
- Contraindications to sentinel lymph node biopsy include clinically positive nodes, tumor size greater than 5 cm, locally advanced cancer, and prior axillary surgery.
- Chemotherapy is generally the initial treatment modality for inflammatory breast cancer and is often followed by mastectomy and radiation therapy.

EMBRYOLOGY

The breast develops from a ridge of ectodermal tissue known as the *milk line*, which extends from the base of the forelimb to the region of the hind limb in early gestation. By the 9th week of gestation, this milk line involutes except in the thoracic region, where it persists as the *mammary ridge*. During the 3rd month of gestation, mesenchymal cells differentiate into the smooth muscle of the areola and nipple. Epithelial cells penetrate the underlying mesenchyme to form epithelial buds, which branch to form secondary buds. During late gestation, these primary and secondary epithelial buds undergo canalization eventually developing into the lactiferous ducts and small ducts leading to the secretory alveoli, respectively. Aberrant persistence of the milk line may lead to *polythelia* (accessory nipples) or *polymastia* (accessory mammary glands). Such accessory tissue is most often found in the axilla. Conversely, the breast may fail to develop completely (*hypomastia* or *micromastia*) or not develop at all (*amastia*). Amastia associated with hypoplasia of the ipsilateral pectoralis muscle and chest wall is referred to as *Poland syndrome*.

ANATOMY AND PHYSIOLOGY

Microscopic Anatomy and Physiology

The breast is composed of glandular epithelium, supporting stroma, and fat. The relative proportion of these components changes with age. In youth, epithelial and stromal components predominate; in old age, these components are increasingly replaced by fat. The glandular tissue of the breast constitutes a branching system of ducts. Breast lobules, the milk-forming glandular units of the breast, are made up of acini (milk-forming glands) and their small efferent ducts. These small ducts join others to form successively larger ducts that coalesce to form the lactiferous sinuses, which empty at the nipple–areolar complex (Fig. 18.1).

Changes in the hormonal milieu have a significant influence on the microscopic architecture of the breast. Stimulation of epithelial and stromal elements during the menstrual cycle results from relatively high levels of estrogen in the follicular phase and progesterone in the luteal phase. These cyclical changes are often accompanied by breast fullness (edema) and discomfort in late menses. More dramatic changes accompany pregnancy and include a characteristic lobular hyperplasia (i.e., *adenosis of pregnancy*) accompanied by diminution of stromal elements. As pregnancy progresses, placental lactogen, estrogen, and progesterone maintain the mammary epithelium in a presecretory phase. The abrupt withdrawal of placental hormones upon delivery leaves the breasts predominantly under the influence of pituitary-derived prolactin, which induces lactation. Finally, in premenopause, increasing irregularity of the menstrual cycle can be accompanied by nodularity of the breast. Later, as ovarian function declines, the lobular units disappear and are replaced by fat.

Surgical Anatomy of the Breast

The boundaries of the breast on the unilateral chest wall include the sternal edge medially, the anterior border of the latissimus dorsi muscles laterally, the second rib superiorly, and the seventh rib inferiorly; however, ductal tissue may extend to the clavicle, below the inframammary crease and over the sternum. The breast tissue is most dense in the upper outer quadrant, where it extends into the axilla as the axillary tail of Spence. The breast is contained within a fascial envelope that is continuous with Camper's fascia below and

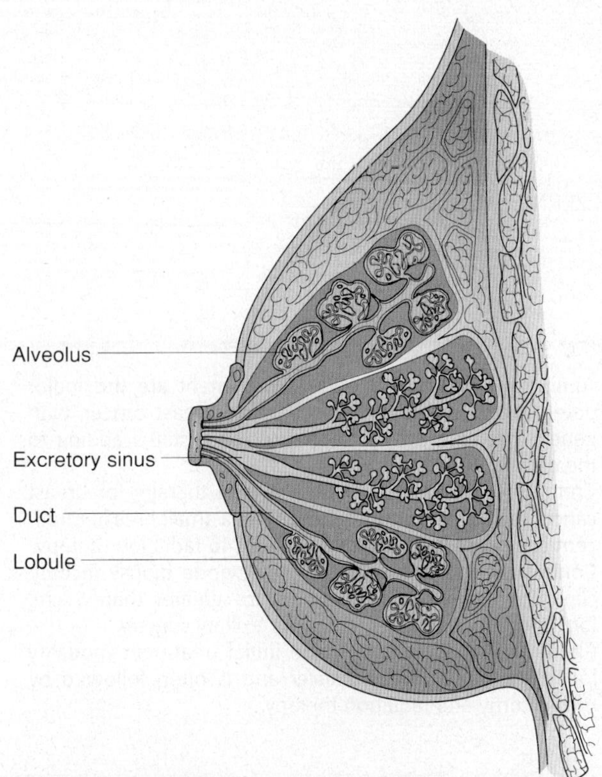

FIGURE 18.1 The ductolobular anatomy of the breast. (From Mulholland MW. *Greenfield's Surgery: Scientific Principles and Practice*. 5th ed. Philadelphia: Lippincott Williams & Wilkins; 2011.)

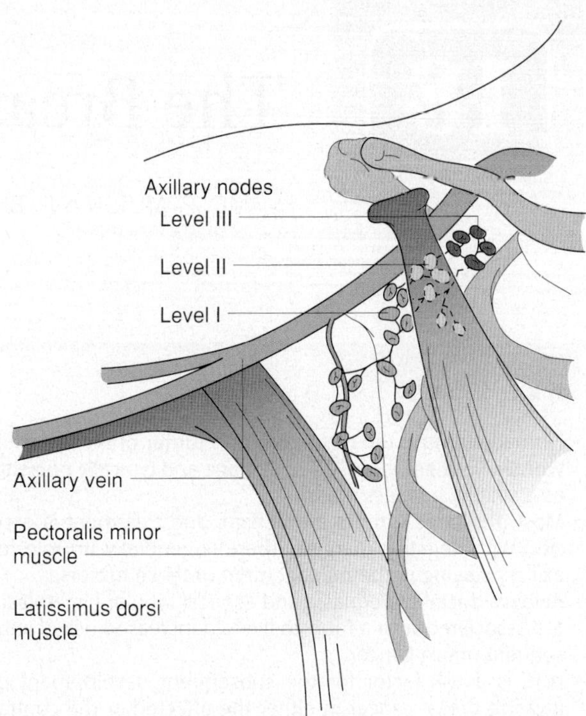

FIGURE 18.2 Axillary anatomy and distribution of axillary lymph nodes. (From Mulholland MW. *Greenfield's Surgery: Scientific Principles and Practice*. 5th ed. Philadelphia: Lippincott Williams & Wilkins; 2011.)

the superficial cervical fascia above. Posteriorly, this fascia is separated from the superficial fascia of the pectoralis major muscle by a loose areolar plane known as the retromammary space. A deep fascial layer, the clavipectoral fascia, represents a fusion of layers that attach to the clavicle, the subclavius muscle, the pectoralis minor muscle, and suspensory ligaments of the axilla. Laterally, this layer fuses with the fascia of the pectoralis major muscle and, inferiorly, with the axillary fascia. The suspensory ligaments of the breast, known as Cooper's ligaments, are contiguous with the superficial fascia deep to the dermis, the interlobular fascia within the breast parenchyma, and the pectoralis fascia that lies beneath the breast.

The breast receives the majority of its blood supply from the internal mammary and lateral thoracic arteries, with minor contributions from branches of the thoracodorsal, subscapular, and intercostal arteries. Venous drainage of the breast parallels the arterial supply. Medially, perforating veins join the internal mammary vein. Laterally, the pectoral branches from the breast join the axillary vein. The majority of the abundant lymphatic channels within the breast parenchyma and overlying dermis drain to the axilla; a small minority drain to the internal mammary chain. The axillary lymph nodes are divided into three levels based on their anatomic relationship to the pectoralis minor muscle. Level I nodes are those lateral, level II are those deep, and level III are those medial to the pectoralis minor muscle (Fig. 18.2). Within the breast, the lymph flows from the skin to the subareolar plexus (Sappey plexus) and then into the interlobular lymphatics of the breast parenchyma.

Several major nerves may be identified during procedures that involve dissection of the axillary lymph nodes. The lateral pectoral nerve, so named because of its origin in the lateral cord of the brachial plexus, innervates the lower portion of the pectoralis major muscle. It courses medial to the pectoralis minor muscle before branching out to innervate the lower portion of the pectoralis major muscle. The medial pectoral nerve arises from the medial cord of the brachial plexus and innervates the pectoralis minor muscle and the lateral border of the pectoralis major muscle. Importantly, the course of the medial pectoral nerve is lateral to that of the pectoralis minor muscle and the lateral pectoral nerve. The long thoracic nerve of Bell, which lies superficial and lateral to the serratus anterior muscle, arises from the posterior roots of the brachial plexus and innervates the serratus anterior and subscapularis muscles. Because the serratus stabilizes the scapula on the chest wall, transection of the long thoracic nerve results in a winged scapula deformity. The thoracodorsal nerve arises from the posterior cord of the brachial plexus and supplies the latissimus dorsi muscle. It lies on the subscapularis muscle, where it is accompanied by the thoracodorsal artery and vein. Division of the thoracodorsal nerve results in paralysis of the latissimus dorsi muscle, which manifests with weakened internal rotation and adduction of the arm. The intercostobrachial nerve arises from the second intercostal nerve, traverses the axillary contents, and supplies sensory fibers to the skin of the axilla, medial aspect of the upper arm and upper lateral breast.

EVALUATION OF BREAST DISEASE

The evaluation of a breast complaint focuses on obtaining a diagnosis and identifying risk factors for the development of breast cancer. This may be achieved through the combination of a thorough history and physical examination, imaging studies, and biopsy.

Mammography

Standard mammography consists of craniocaudal (CC) and mediolateral (ML) oblique views and is utilized in breast cancer screening to identify women with radiographic abnormalities. Tomosynthesis, or 3D mammography, has been approved by the FDA since February of 2011. This method of mammography utilizes multiple images of the breast to produce a three-dimensional reconstruction, while administering an increased but acceptable dose of radiation. The proposed benefits of tomosynthesis include earlier detection rate of small cancers, better detection rate for dense breast tissue, decreased call-back rates, and fewer biopsies. There is debate over the age at which breast cancer screening with mammography should begin. Currently, the American Cancer Society (ACS) recommends annual mammography for women aged 40 years and older. Annual mammography for women aged 50 years or older is recommended by the U.S. Preventative Task Force Services (USPTFS), with other individualized considerations for women younger than 50 years. *Diagnostic mammography*, which should be distinguished from screening mammography, is obtained to further evaluate a breast abnormality recognized on physical examination or screening mammography and may include additional magnification and compression views. Such imaging may help to establish a diagnosis in patients with a breast abnormality, although the specificity of mammographic findings is generally low. Mammographic features associated with malignancy include densities (e.g., masses or architectural distortions) and microcalcifications. Mammographic findings can be classified using the BI-RADS (Breast Imaging Reporting and Data System) (Table 18.1).

Additional diagnostic modalities sometimes utilized in the evaluation of breast lesions include *ultrasound* and *MRI* (magnetic resonance imaging). Ultrasound is helpful in distinguishing solid from cystic masses. MRI is highly sensitive in detecting invasive breast cancers, although the increased rate of detection comes with a false-positive biopsy rate of approximately 11%. A role is emerging for the use of MRI in screening high-risk patients for occult breast cancers. Indeed, recent data suggest that MRI can detect cancer in the contralateral breast that is missed by mammography and clinical examination at the time of an initial breast cancer diagnosis at a rate of approximately 3%. The ACS has now recommended annual MRI screening for women with *BRCA1* or *BRCA2* mutations, a lifetime risk of breast cancer of 20% to 25% or greater based on one of several scoring systems, a history of radiation to the chest between the ages of 10 and 30, Li–Fraumeni syndrome, Cowden syndrome, or Bannayan–Riley–Ruvalcaba syndrome. In addition, breast MRI may be used for the assessment of silicone implant integrity, diagnosis of occult primary breast cancers, determination of disease extent in newly diagnosed breast cancer patients, documentation of response to neoadjuvant chemotherapy, diagnosis of recurrence, or clarification of inconclusive clinical or mammographic findings. It has been shown that the increased use of MRI has led to increased rates of biopsies and more aggressive surgery, despite no apparent benefit in locoregional recurrence or mortality.

TABLE 18.1 Breast imaging reporting and data system

Category	Definition
0	Incomplete assessment; need additional imaging evaluation
1	Negative; routine mammogram in 1 y recommended
2	Benign finding; routine mammogram in 1 y recommended
3	Probably benign finding; short-term follow-up suggested
4	Suspicious abnormality; consider biopsy
5	Highly suggestive of malignancy

TABLE 18.2 Indications for surgical biopsy after core needle biopsy

Inconclusive histology
Inadequate sampling of mammographic abnormality
Discordance between imaging and pathology
Atypical hyperplasia (ductal or lobular)
LCIS
Complex sclerosing adenosis or radial scar
Papilloma
Flat epithelial atypia

Breast Biopsy

A variety of biopsy techniques are utilized in evaluating breast lesions, the two most common being core needle biopsy and needle localization breast biopsy. *Core needle biopsy* is generally the preferred initial approach. Mammographic (stereotactic) or ultrasound guidance may be utilized for the biopsy of nonpalpable, radiographically detected lesions. A definitive diagnosis of malignancy is obtained in 25% of women following core needle biopsy. Sixty-five percent of women are found to have a benign diagnosis. In the remaining 10%, the diagnosis is inconclusive, and surgical biopsy is required. Specific examples of inconclusive histologic findings include the presence of atypical cells suggesting atypical ductal hyperplasia (ADH) versus ductal carcinoma *in situ* (DCIS), lobular carcinoma *in situ* (LCIS), and increased cellularity within a fibroadenoma suggesting a possible phyllodes tumor. Additionally, inadequate sampling of the abnormality (e.g., calcifications not sampled or histology inconsistent with mammographic findings) is an additional indication for surgical biopsy (Table 18.2). Surgical biopsies for nonpalpable findings are facilitated by preoperative imaging-guided placement of a localizing wire (needle localization) and specimen radiographic confirmation at surgery.

BENIGN BREAST DISEASES AND THEIR MANAGEMENT

Breast Cysts

Simple breast cysts are fluid-filled, epithelial-lined cavities that are generally in continuity with a duct. Palpable cysts develop in approximately 7% of women and may occur at any age. They are most common in premenopausal women older than 35 years of age. Cysts tend to be firm, mobile, and well circumscribed and fluctuate in size predictably with the menstrual cycle. Aspiration of cyst fluid is generally indicated in most cases to confirm the diagnosis. In patients with large cysts, aspiration may also relieve symptoms. Routine submission of cystic fluid for cytologic evaluation is rarely indicated, as the incidence of malignancy is less than 1%. In contrast, aspiration of bloody fluid, persistence of a mass following aspiration, or rapid recurrence following aspiration justify a cytologic evaluation and, frequently, surgical excision.

Fibrocystic Condition

The terms "fibrocystic condition" (FCC) or "fibrocystic disease" describe a spectrum of clinical, histologic, and mammographic findings. Cyclical premenstrual mastalgia is the most common symptom of FCC. Clinical findings range from mild alterations in texture to cyst formation. Mammographic densities are common, and in up to 30% of women between 35 and 50 years of age, breast cysts are detectable by ultrasound. In addition to cysts, histology may demonstrate adenosis, sclerosis, apocrine metaplasia, stromal fibrosis, epithelial metaplasia, and hyperplasia.

Fibroadenoma

Fibroadenomas are benign tumors composed of epithelial and stromal elements. They are the most common tumors of the breast in women younger than 30 years of age and generally present as solitary painless masses. Grossly, they appear encapsulated with smooth or slightly lobulated borders. In most cases, when a fibroadenoma is suspected, excisional biopsy is undertaken to confirm the diagnosis, although close follow-up with imaging is also acceptable. This strategy is most frequently taken for younger asymptomatic patients with typical physical examination findings. Symptomatic lesions may be surgically excised or treated with cryoablative techniques. Core biopsy is followed by observation if the pathology is consistent with a fibroadenoma.

Hamartomas

Like fibroadenomas, *hamartomas* are composed of epithelial and stromal elements. They present as well-defined nodules and are characterized histologically by densely packed lobules and prominent extralobular ducts. Excision is curative.

Mondor Disease

Mondor disease is a variant of thrombophlebitis involving the superficial veins of the anterior chest wall and breast. Patients typically present with localized pain and a tender, palpable subcutaneous cord or skin dimpling. Mondor disease is often self-limited; however, anti-inflammatory agents and warm compresses may alleviate symptoms. Rarely, excision is performed for refractory symptomatic disease.

Inflammatory/Infectious Breast Disease

Mammary duct ectasia is an inflammatory condition characterized by dilation of the lactiferous sinuses. Most common in perimenopausal and postmenopausal women, mammary duct ectasia may be associated with nipple inversion. Periductal mastitis is a similar condition, seen more frequently in younger women, particularly those who are heavy smokers. This condition is characterized by episodes of periareolar inflammation, sometimes with accompanying nipple retraction and purulent discharge. Generalized *mastitis* results from an ascending infection that begins in the subareolar ducts. Most common during lactation, the characteristic erythema and induration may not be accompanied by abscess formation and frequently resolve with conservative measures (e.g., use of a mechanical breast pump and application of heat packs) and/or antibiotic therapy. Abscesses, particularly those that arise during lactation, are often amenable to aspiration. Larger abscesses, or those in patients with diabetes, require incision and drainage.

Papillomas

Intraductal papillomas are polyps of the epithelial lining of the breast ducts. Subareolar papillomas often present with bloody nipple discharge; indeed, papilloma is the most common cause of this symptom. Alternatively, large papillomas may present as a mass. Treatment consists of excision due to a 1% to 4 % risk of malignancy.

Sclerosing Lesions

Sclerosing adenosis is characterized by the proliferation of terminal ductules or acini and stromal elements. Calcium deposition may result in mammographic findings suggestive of intraductal cancer. *Radial scar* and *fat necrosis* represent two additional benign sclerosing lesions that may mimic infiltrating cancer. The former has been associated with an elevated risk of subsequent breast cancer, although the lesion itself is not premalignant, and the treatment is surgical excision.

MALIGNANT BREAST DISEASES AND THEIR MANAGEMENT

Incidence and Risk Factors for Breast Cancer

Breast cancer is the most common cancer and the leading cause of cancer deaths in women worldwide. It is also the most common cancer among American women, with an annual incidence of greater than 230,000 cases. Risk factors for the development of breast cancer are summarized in Table 18.3. The incidence of breast cancer increases with advancing age. Breast cancer is unusual in individuals younger than 20 years of age; thereafter, the incidence increases steadily. By age 80, 15% of women suffer from breast cancer. Reproductive factors that increase estrogen exposure, including menarche before 12 years of age, first live childbirth after age 30, nulliparity, and menopause after age 55, are also associated with an increased risk of breast cancer. Likewise, exogenous hormone exposure increases breast cancer risk; combination hormone replacement with both estrogen and progesterone is associated with a 20% increased incidence after 5 years. A prior history of unilateral breast cancer increases the likelihood of a cancer in the contralateral breast by a factor of 3 to 4 (Table 18.3). Finally, prior chest irradiation (e.g., from childhood lymphomas) is also a risk factor.

TABLE 18.3 Breast cancer risk factors

Age
Nulliparity
Age at first birth (>30)
Age at menarche (<12) and menopause (>55)
Exogenous hormone use or exposure
Alcohol consumption
Family history
History of previous breast cancer

A variety of histologic abnormalities are associated with an increased risk of subsequent breast cancer (Table 18.4). Benign proliferative diseases of the breast may be divided into those with atypical epithelial hyperplasia (atypia) and those without atypia. All hyperplastic lesions are associated with an increased breast cancer risk; however, this risk is more significant in lesions with atypia such as ADH and atypical lobular hyperplasia (ALH). Both of these entities are associated with a four- to fivefold increased risk of subsequent breast cancer. ADH is generally believed to place the patient at increased risk for cancer within the affected quadrant of the breast, whereas ALH places the patient at an increased risk for cancer in either the affected or the contralateral breast. Clinically, all patients with a core biopsy identifying atypical hyperplasia require excisional biopsy, as cancer has been found in 14% to 31% of biopsy specimens. Additionally, a role for tamoxifen therapy for patients diagnosed with ADH and ALH was demonstrated in the National Surgery Adjuvant Breast and Bowel Project (NSABP) P-1 Prevention Trial; 5 years of tamoxifen use was associated with an 86% reduction in subsequent breast cancer risk in this patient group.

LCIS is characterized by the presence of neoplastic cells that distend the breast acini (blind sacs that empty into the ductal system of the breast) without disrupting the breast's lobular architecture. Because it does not form a palpable mass and is not associated with radiographic abnormalities, LCIS is typically diagnosed by pathologic analysis of a biopsy performed for another indication. Although some controversy persists regarding the malignant potential of LCIS, it is generally not considered to be a preinvasive lesion. LCIS is, however, a risk factor for the subsequent development of invasive breast cancer in either the affected or the contralateral breast. This risk is estimated at approximately 1% per year. Close clinical follow-up consisting of biannual breast examinations by a physician and annual mammography is indicated following diagnosis. Bilateral prophylactic mastectomies may be an appropriate alternative option, particularly in women with a strong family history of breast or ovarian cancer or a mutation of the *BRCA1* or *BRCA2*. As in patients with ADH and ALH, a role for tamoxifen therapy for patients diagnosed with LCIS was demonstrated in NSABP P-1 Prevention Trial; 5 years of tamoxifen use was associated with a 56% reduction in the risk of breast cancer.

Inherited Causes of Breast Cancer

The risk of breast cancer is increased by a factor of 2 to 3 in first-degree relatives (mothers, sisters, and daughters) of patients with breast cancer. In families with multiple affected members with bilateral and early-onset cancers, the absolute risk to first-degree relatives approaches 50%. Genetic factors are responsible for an estimated 5% to 10% of breast cancers and may account for 25% of breast cancers in women younger than 30 years of age. *BRCA1* mutations account for up to 40% of familial breast cancer syndromes. It has been suggested that *BRCA1* plays a role in the differentiation (characterized by expression of estrogen receptor [ER]) of breast cancer precursors. This finding may explain why invasive breast cancers in patients with *BRCA1* mutations are typically of the so-called triple negative or basal phenotype (i.e., they do not express ER, progesterone receptor [PR], or HER-2/neu). In addition to an increased breast cancer risk, *BRCA1* mutations are also associated with a 15% to 45% lifetime risk of ovarian cancer. *BRCA2* mutations account for up to 30% of familial breast cancers and are associated with an increased risk of breast cancer in males. Women with a mutation in *BRCA2* have a 20% to 30% lifetime risk of ovarian cancer. Mutations in *BRCA1* or *BRCA2* are rare, with an estimated frequency of 1 in 1,000 people in the American population. The penetrance of BRCA1 and BRCA2 (i.e., the likelihood that carriers of these mutations will develop breast cancer) is between 40% and 85%.

TABLE 18.4 Benign breast disease classified by relative risk of subsequent breast cancer

No Increased Risk	Slightly Increased (1.5–2 Times)	Moderately Increased (5 Times)
Apocrine metaplasia	Hyperplasia, solid or papillary	ADH
Cysts	Papilloma with fibrovascular core	ALH
Duct ectasia	Sclerosing adenosis	—
Fibroadenoma	—	—
Fibrosis	—	—
Hyperplasia, mild	—	—
Mastitis	—	—

Source: From Morrow M, Jordan VC, eds. *Managing Breast Cancer Risk*. Ontario: BC Decker; 2000:7, with permission.

PREINVASIVE BREAST CARCINOMA

Ductal Carcinoma *In Situ*

DCIS is characterized by the clonal proliferation of malignant-appearing epithelial cells that are contained by the mammary duct basement membrane. DCIS is generally considered a preinvasive lesion; however, there is significant heterogeneity among DCIS lesions. Low-grade lesions progress slowly, if at all, to invasive cancer. High-grade lesions progress more rapidly to invasive cancer, frequently over the course of years. The traditional histologic classification system for DCIS includes five subtypes: comedo, cribriform, micropapillary, papillary, and solid. Alternative classification schemes are based on nuclear grade (i.e., high, intermediate, and low grade) and the presence or absence of necrosis. Comedo-type lesions tend to be characterized by high-grade nuclei, architectural distortion, and necrosis; therefore, DCIS is sometimes also referred to as comedo type or noncomedo type (Fig. 18.3).

The incidence of DCIS has increased 10-fold over the past 2 decades owing largely to the widespread implementation of screening mammography. DCIS now accounts for more than 20% of mammographically detected breast carcinomas. Nearly 90% of DCIS lesions are diagnosed mammographically, with microcalcifications (76%), soft tissue densities (11%), or both (13%) being common associated findings. Prevention of progression to invasive cancer and local recurrence are the goals of treatment for DCIS. Treatment options include mastectomy, partial mastectomy with radiation, and partial mastectomy alone. Overall survival following these approaches is very good and largely equivalent; however, local recurrence rates are lowest after mastectomy at 1.4% in a large meta-analysis. Another large meta-analysis from 2009 evaluated the addition of radiotherapy (RT) to breast conservation for DCIS; the addition of RT reduced the risk of recurrence by 49% (95% CI: 0.41 to 0.58, $p < 0.0001$). The recurrence risk is likely lower in patients with more favorable tumor characteristics such as low tumor grade or lack of comedonecrosis. Current research aims to identify those patients who can safely forgo RT. Most recurrences following partial mastectomy and radiation occur at or near the site of the original tumor. One half of these recurrences are DCIS, and the remaining half are invasive tumors.

Theoretically, confinement of DCIS lesions by the mammary duct basement membrane precludes metastasis to regional lymph nodes. Nonetheless, a small percentage of patients who carry the diagnosis of DCIS, even following pathologic evaluation of definitive surgical specimens, are diagnosed with nodal metastases. A much larger number of patients (10% to 30%) are ultimately found to have foci of synchronous invasive disease following definitive surgery. In part, this high incidence is related to the increasing dependence on core needle biopsy to achieve tissue diagnoses and associated sampling errors. Nonetheless, tumor-related factors such as high nuclear grade, the presence of comedonecrosis, and large tumor size may be associated with the presence of occult invasive disease. Sentinel lymph node biopsy (SLNB) may be considered and performed in patients at higher risk of occult invasive cancer, such as those with extensive or high-grade DCIS. Patients undergoing mastectomy for DCIS, in particular, benefit from SLNB because this procedure is no longer feasible following mastectomy if invasive cancer is identified.

INVASIVE BREAST CANCER

Invasive breast cancer is defined by the penetration of malignant cells through the basement membrane that surrounds the ductolobular system of the breast. Two major histologic subtypes, invasive ductal carcinoma (IDC) and invasive lobular carcinoma (ILC), account for the vast majority of infiltrating breast cancers (Fig. 18.4). IDC is the most common form of invasive breast cancer. Though most often unifocal, IDC encompasses a variety of disease patterns ranging from gland-forming to solid undifferentiated

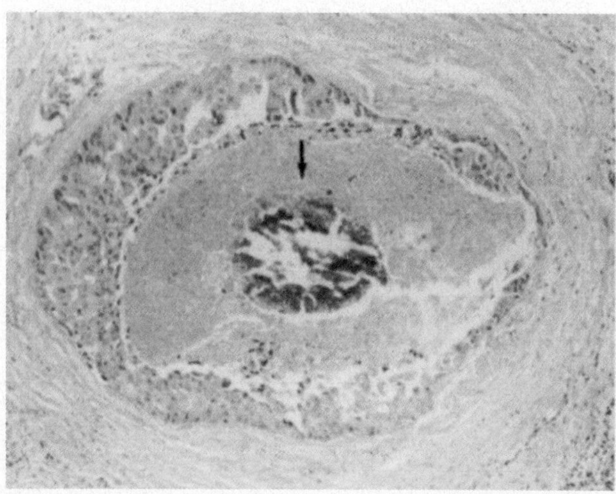
A

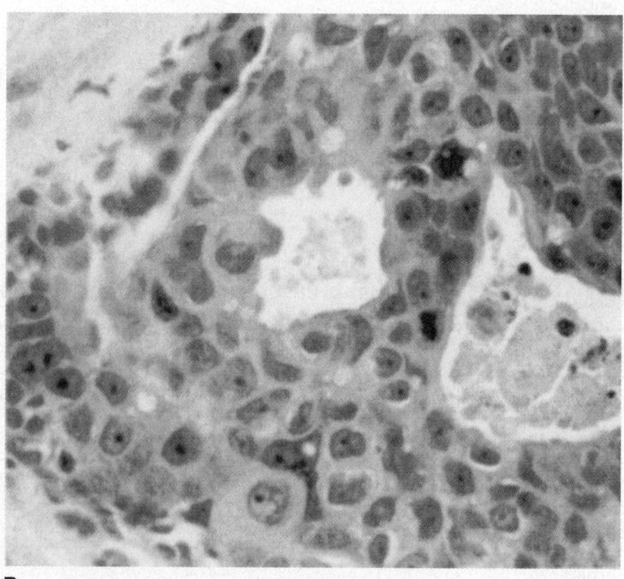
B

FIGURE 18.3 A. Comedo-type DCIS with central necrosis and dense calcification. **B.** Nuclear atypia and pleomorphism consistent with poorly differentiated DCIS. (From Harris JR, Lippman ME, Morrow M, et al., eds. *Diseases of the Breast.* 2nd ed. Philadelphia: Lippincott Williams & Wilkins; 2000:384 (1A) and 387 (4C), with permission.)

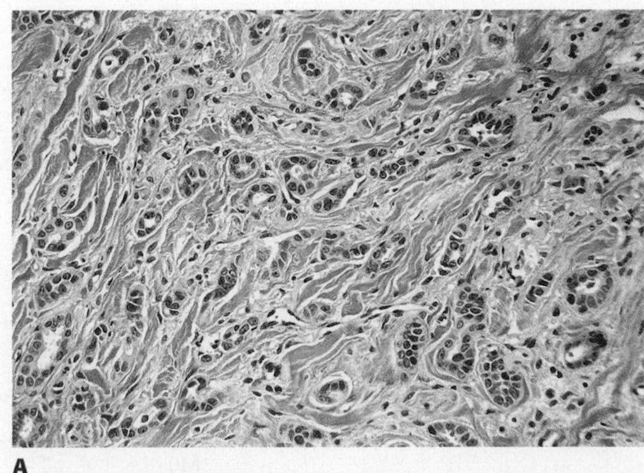

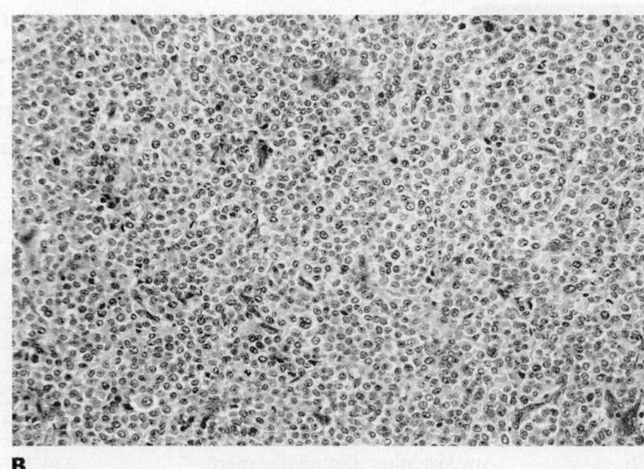

FIGURE 18.4 **A.** Infiltrating ductal carcinoma. **B.** Infiltrating lobular carcinoma. (From Harris JR, Lippman ME, Morrow M, et al., eds. *Diseases of the Breast*. 3rd ed. Philadelphia: Lippincott Williams & Wilkins; 2004:543 (34.2A) and 545 (34.4), with permission.)

tumors. ILC accounts for 5% to 10% of invasive breast cancers and is characterized by the presence of malignant cells interspersed between the normal glandular structures of the breast. In contrast to IDC, which tends to produce a significant desmoplastic reaction, ILC induces little inflammation. ILC is associated with a similar, or slightly better, prognosis than is IDC.

Other less common subtypes include tubular, medullary, mucinous, and metaplastic carcinomas. *Tubular carcinoma* accounts for approximately 2% of IDC. Characterized by the formation of neoplastic tubules that resemble breast ductules, these well-differentiated cancers are typically small (<1.0 cm) and are associated with a favorable prognosis. *Medullary carcinoma* accounts for 1% to 7% of IDC. These well-circumscribed, poorly differentiated tumors more frequently affect younger women and are, paradoxically, associated with a favorable prognosis. *Mucinous carcinoma* accounts for 2% of IDC and is characterized by grossly and microscopically visible extracellular mucus. Largely a disease of older women, mucinous carcinomas tend to have a slow growth rate and are associated with a favorable prognosis. *Metaplastic carcinomas* are so named because of the mesenchymal differentiation that characterizes these tumors. Several different neoplasms (e.g., those with spindle, squamous, or osseous elements) constitute the group of metaplastic carcinomas. Metaplastic differentiation appears to have little effect on prognosis.

Natural History and Staging of Breast Cancer

Carcinoma of the breast may spread by direct extension through the breast parenchyma, via the lymphatics to regional lymph nodes, and hematogenously to remote sites. Tumor size and lymph node involvement are the major determinants of prognosis (Table 18.5). As the size of the primary tumor increases, so too does the frequency of regional and remote metastases. The axillary nodes (ANs) are the most common site of regional metastases, with internal mammary nodes (IMNs) being the next most common site. Approximately 50% of patients with breast cancer detectable on physical examination will have AN involvement at the time of diagnosis. Twenty percent of patients with tumors smaller than 1 cm are found to have nodal metastases, indicating that even smaller tumors are associated with a considerable incidence of nodal disease. Common sites of distant metastasis include bones (40% to 50%) and lung (20%), followed by the liver, brain, and spine.

In 2010, the American Joint Committee on Cancer (AJCC) revised its recommendations for breast cancer staging (Table 18.6). The newest (7th) edition in the 2010 staging guidelines has minor changes related to tumor size definition, node classification, metastasis classification, and special issues in patients who received neoadjuvant chemotherapy. Within the pathology categories, only DCIS, LCIS, and isolated Paget disease of the nipple are classified as pTis. Atypical ductal or lobular hyperplasia (ADH, ALH) are no longer included. *In situ* lesions have also been called T1a. In addition, there is a new cM0(i+) category defined for the presence of circulating tumor cells. Lastly, stage I breast tumors have now been subdivided into stage IA and stage IB, with stage IB including small tumors (TI) with lymph node micrometastases (N1mi).

Although not incorporated into the current staging guidelines, several additional histopathologic features influence prognosis. Markers of tumor cell proliferation such as Ki67 proliferation index,

TABLE 18.5 **Five-year breast cancer survival rates according to tumor size and AN involvement.**

Tumor Size (cm)	Negative Nodes (%)	1–3 Positive Nodes (%)	>3 Positive Nodes (%)
<0.5	99	95	59
0.5–0.9	98	94	54
1.0–1.9	96	87	67
2.0–2.9	92	83	63
3.0–3.9	86	79	57
4.0–4.9	85	70	53
>5.0	82	73	46

Source: From Harris JR, Lippman ME, Morrow M, et al., eds. *Diseases of the Breast*. 2nd ed. Philadelphia: Lippincott Williams & Wilkins; 2000:415, with permission.

TABLE 18.6 TNM classification of breast cancer (AJCC, 7th edition)

TNM	Tumor Size	Nodal Status	Metastasis
	In situ	N0	M0
Stage Ia	<2 cm	N0	M0
Ib	<2 cm	N1 micro	M0
IIa	<2 cm 2–5 cm	1–3 AN or IMN detected by SLN N0	M0 M0
IIb	2–5 cm Or >5 cm	1–3 AN or IMN detected by SLN N0	M0 M0
IIIa	Any size	Metastasis in 4–9 AN or clinical IMN	M0
IIIb	Any size plus skin involvement (edema, *peau d'orange*, satellite skin nodules, ulcers) or chest wall involvement; inflammatory cancer	Any N	M0
IIIc	Any size (any T)	Metastasis in 10+ AN or infraclavicular node	M0
IV	Any size	Any N	Distant metastasis

S-phase fraction, and thymidine labeling index (TLI) have been used to predict early relapse. Expression of ER is associated with a longer disease-free survival and improved overall survival. Although PR status appears to have a less significant influence on prognosis, tumors that are both ER and PR positive appear to be more responsive to endocrine therapies than are tumors that are ER positive and PR negative. Overexpression of the tyrosine kinase growth factor receptor, HER-2/neu, is associated with an increased rate of metastases, poorer overall survival, and refractoriness to chemotherapy. Additionally, overexpression of HER-2/neu predicts responsiveness to trastuzumab (Herceptin), a HER-2/neu-targeted monoclonal antibody.

Recent DNA microarray profiling studies have established the existence of invasive breast cancer subtypes that correlate with HER-2/neu, ER, and PR expression patterns. These subtypes, classified using a system proposed by Perou and colleagues, are associated with distinct clinical outcomes and include the following: luminal (ER^{pos} or PR^{pos}), basal-like (ER^{neg}, PR^{neg}, and HER-2/neu^{neg}, cytokeratin $5/6^{pos}$ or $HER1^{pos}$), HER-2/neu positive (ER^{neg}, PR^{neg}, and HER-2/neu^{pos}), and unclassified. The luminal group may be further divided into lower-risk and higher-risk lesions, the so-called luminal A and luminal B tumors. The latter is sometimes characterized by coexpression of HER-2/neu with ER or PR. Clinical outcomes, including risk of recurrence and overall survival, are poorest among patients with basal-like and HER-2/neu-positive tumors. Luminal B tumors are associated with an intermediate prognosis, and luminal A tumors have a favorable prognosis.

Treatment of Breast Cancer

Surgery

The management of breast cancer has undergone a dramatic transformation over the past several decades. Until the mid-1970s, *radical mastectomy*, a procedure that involved *en bloc* excision of breast tissue, the underlying pectoralis muscles, and regional ANs, was the procedure of choice for the treatment of breast cancers. This operation was subsequently replaced by the *modified radical mastectomy* (MRM), which spares the pectoralis muscles (Fig. 18.5), and the *total or simple mastectomy*, a pectoralis-sparing mastectomy without axillary lymphadenectomy. Over the past two decades, breast-conserving therapy (BCT) consisting of *partial mastectomy* (lumpectomy) and radiation therapy has assumed a prominent role in the treatment paradigm for increasing numbers of breast cancers. More recently, *SLNB* has greatly reduced the number of axillary lymph node dissections (*ALND*) performed on patients without clinically evident nodal metastases.

A variety of largely synonymous terms have been applied to breast-conserving procedures for the treatment of breast cancer; these include lumpectomy, wide excision, segmental mastectomy, and partial mastectomy. Irrespective of the terminology used, the goal of breast-conserving procedures is to completely excise the lesion; currently, no tumor seen on ink has been proposed as adequate resection margins although most surgeons will still aim to achieve greater than 0.2 cm as an appropriate margin. Total mastectomy is generally reserved for instances in which the anatomic distribution of cancer does not allow breast conservation (e.g., large tumor burden in a small breast or multicentric disease). Additionally, contraindications to radiation therapy (e.g., pregnancy or prior radiation therapy) preclude breast conservation (Table 18.7).

While there is no convincing evidence that axillary dissection improves survival, AN involvement remains the dominant prognostic variable in patients with invasive breast cancer. The development of SLNB has allowed for the more limited, selective treatment of regional lymph nodes and has decreased the number of complete regional dissections performed in patients without nodal metastases. This procedure, as it is currently performed, maps the lymphatic drainage from the breast to a primary lymph node or nodes using a vital blue dye and/or a radioisotope-labeled tracer. Surgical excision and pathologic evaluation of these nodes for metastases allow for reliable staging and the prediction of additional lymph node metastases with a false-negative rate of approximately 7%. SLNB also allows a more meticulous histologic evaluation of multiple sections

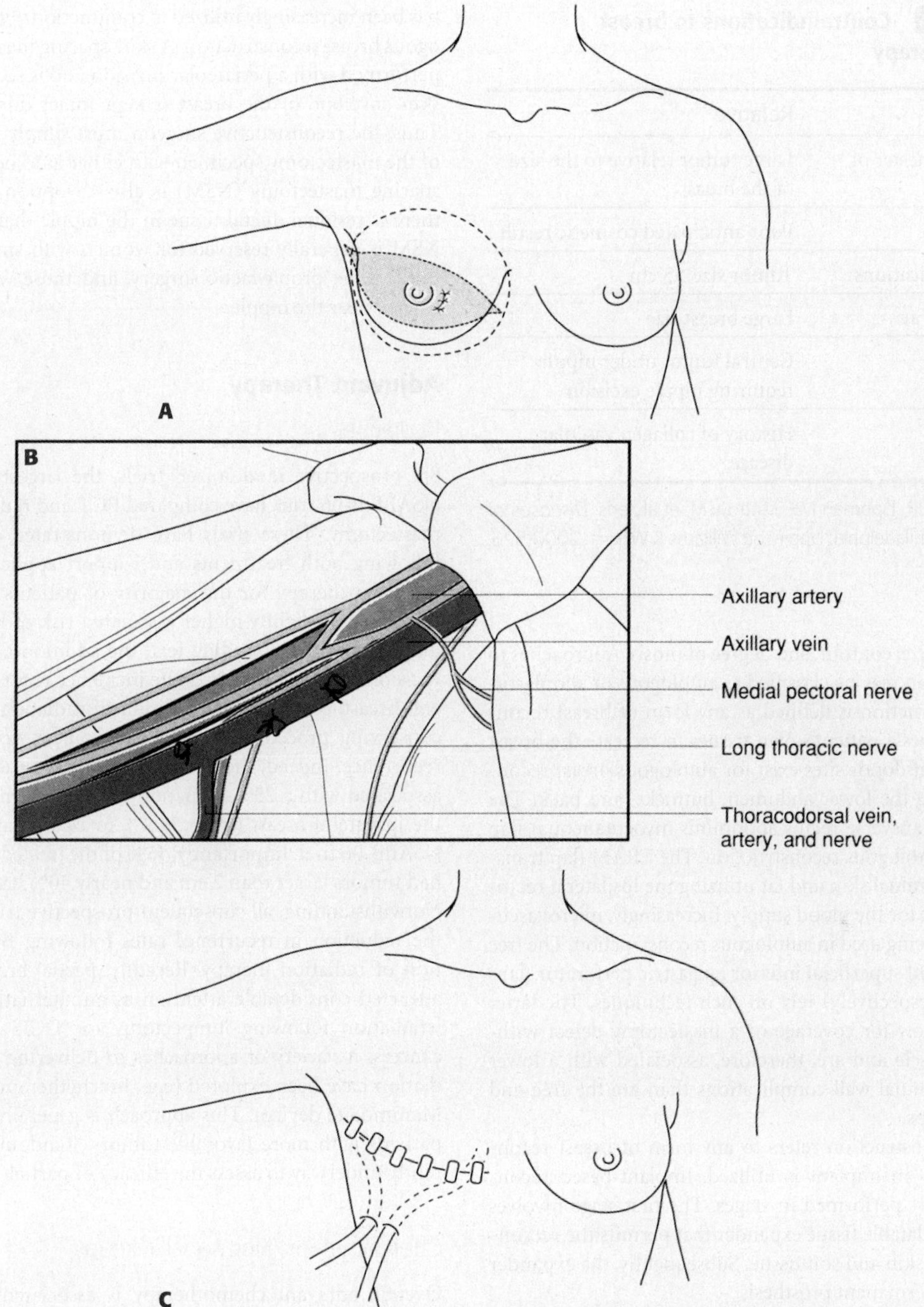

FIGURE 18.5 Technique of MRM. (From August DA, Sondak VK. Breast. In: Greenfield LJ, Mulholland M, Oldham KT, et al., eds. *Surgery: Scientific Principles and Practice*. 2nd ed. Philadelphia: Lippincott–Raven; 1997:1393, with permission.)

augmented by immunohistochemical staining. Contraindications to SLNB include clinically positive nodes, tumor size greater than 5 cm, locally advanced cancer, and prior axillary surgery.

Historically, patients found to have metastases in the sentinel node or nodes (i.e., a positive sentinel node biopsy [SLN]) undergo completion lymphadenectomy, or ALND. However, studies such as the ACOSOG Z0011 trial have dramatically changed current axillary management. This trial included patients with T1-2 tumors without clinical lymphadenopathy who underwent breast-conserving surgery including whole-breast irradiation, and who had no more than one to two positive sentinel lymph nodes. Patients were randomized to ALND versus no additional surgery; there were no differences between the two groups regarding locoregional recurrence or mortality after 6 years of follow-up. Currently, many women are spared the additional morbidity of an ALND with the changing paradigm of axillary management.

Breast Reconstruction

Breast reconstruction has become an essential component of the care of women with breast cancer. The goals of breast reconstruction are to recreate a natural-appearing breast mound that matches the

TABLE 18.7 Contraindications to breast conservation therapy

Absolute	Relative
First or second trimester of pregnancy	Large tumor relative to the size of the breast
Multicentric disease	Poor anticipated cosmetic result
Diffuse microcalcifications	Tumor size >5 cm
History of prior x-ray	Large breast size
Therapy	Central tumor under nipple requiring nipple excision
	History of collagen vascular disease

Source: From Harris JR, Lippman ME, Morrow M, et al., eds. *Diseases of the Breast*. 2nd ed. Philadelphia: Lippincott Williams & Wilkins; 2000:526, with permission.

opposite breast in size, contour, and degree of ptosis. Approaches to breast reconstruction may be classified as autologous or alloplastic. *Autologous* reconstruction is defined as any form of breast reconstruction that utilizes a patient's own tissues to recreate the breast mound. A variety of donor sites exist for autologous breast reconstruction, including the lower abdomen, buttocks, and back. The pedicled *TRAM* (transverse rectus abdominis myocutaneous) flap is often used for autologous reconstruction. The TRAM flap transfers the lower abdominal skin and fat utilizing the ipsilateral rectus muscle as a conduit for the blood supply. Increasingly, microvascular techniques are being used in autologous reconstruction. The free TRAM and deep and superficial inferior epigastric perforator flaps (*DIEP* and *SIEP*, respectively) rely on such techniques. The latter two approaches allow for coverage of a mastectomy defect without harvest of muscle and are, therefore, associated with a lower incidence of abdominal wall complications than are the free and pedicled TRAM flaps.

Alloplastic reconstruction refers to any form of breast reconstruction in which an implant is utilized. Implant-based reconstruction is typically performed in stages. The first stage involves placement of an inflatable tissue expander that permits the recruitment of additional skin and soft tissue. Subsequently, the expander is replaced with a permanent prosthesis.

The timing of, and approach to, reconstruction should take into account patient preference, age, comorbidity, requirement for adjuvant therapies, and body habitus. A history of RT or planned postmastectomy RT, in particular, influences the timing and choice of a reconstruction approach. Implant-based techniques are contraindicated in patients who are likely to receive radiation. *Delayed breast reconstruction*, defined as reconstruction that occurs after a patient has undergone a mastectomy, is most commonly performed for patients who require postoperative RT. While immediate reconstruction has traditionally been avoided in such patients, women requiring radiation therapy are now being offered immediate autologous reconstruction with increasing frequency, as evidence suggesting acceptable outcomes with this approach has grown.

Mastectomy techniques have a significant impact on the outcome of autologous breast reconstruction. Skin-sparing mastectomy has been increasingly utilized in conjunction with immediate autologous breast reconstruction. A skin-sparing mastectomy is typically performed with a periareolar incision and is so named because the skin envelope of the breast is kept intact during the procedure. Thus, the reconstructive surgeon must simply replace the volume of the mastectomy specimen with either autologous tissue. Nipple-sparing mastectomy (NSM) is also an option, with the risk that there is residual ductal tissue in the nipple that must be screened. NSM is generally reserved for women with smaller breasts, those undergoing prophylactic surgery, and those without evidence of disease near the nipple.

Adjuvant Therapy

Radiation

Six prospective randomized trials, the largest of which was the NSABP B-06 trial, have compared BCT and radiation therapy with mastectomy. These trials have demonstrated equivalent survival following both treatments and support application of BCT with radiation therapy for the majority of patients with invasive cancer despite a slightly higher associated risk of local recurrence. As discussed in the preceding text, the addition of radiation to wide excision for DCIS decreases the incidence recurrence in the ipsilateral breast. Similarly, the addition of radiation therapy to breast-conserving procedures for invasive cancer decreases the risk of recurrence. Indeed, the addition of radiation therapy to BCT was associated with a 25% reduction in the incidence of recurrence in the ipsilateral breast (from 39.2% to 14.3%) after 20 years in the NSAPB-06 trial. Importantly, 45% of the treated women in this trial had tumors larger than 2 cm and nearly 40% had nodal metastases. Notwithstanding, all subsequent prospective trials have confirmed the reduction in recurrence rates following BCT with the addition of radiation therapy. Recently, partial-breast irradiation has attracted considerable attention as an alternative to whole-breast irradiation following lumpectomy for DCIS and early invasive cancers. A variety of approaches to delivering partial-breast irradiation have been explored (e.g., brachytherapy delivery using the MammoSite device). This approach is generally reserved for older patients with more favorable tumors. Randomized trials are currently underway to assess the efficacy of partial-breast irradiation.

Chemotherapy/Hormonal Therapy

Overall, adjuvant chemotherapy is associated with an approximately 33% risk reduction. Established regimens for the treatment of breast cancer include CMF (cyclophosphamide, methotrexate, and 5-fluorouracil) and AC (anthracycline and cytoxan). Newer agents utilized in the treatment of advanced breast carcinoma include taxanes (e.g., paclitaxel and docetaxel) and vinca alkaloids (e.g., vinorelbine). Newer combinations of agents (e.g., taxol and cytoxan) may be more effective than traditional regimens. Additionally, humanized antibodies against the growth factor receptor HER-2/neu, such as trastuzumab and pertuzumab, are often used to treat patients with HER-2/neu overexpressing invasive cancers. Trastuzumab may be particularly effective when used with docetaxel and carboplatin. Historically, all patients with breast cancers larger than 1 cm and those with lymph node metastases were candidates for adjuvant chemotherapy (Table 18.8). Currently, genetic analysis of the tumor may be used to assess the benefit of

TABLE 18.8 Recommendations for use of adjuvant therapy in breast cancer

Patient Subset	Recommended Treatment
−Nodes, low risk	Physician judgment; no treatment; tamoxifen if ER+
−Nodes, higher risk	
ER+	Tamoxifen ± chemotherapy
ER−	Chemotherapy
+Nodes	
ER+	Chemotherapy + tamoxifen; or tamoxifen alone
ER−	Chemotherapy

[a]Low risk defined as negative ANs and tumor ≤1 cm, nuclear grade 1; or 1–2 cm ER+ tumor with low proliferation index.

Source: From Harris JR, Lippman ME, Morrow M, et al., eds. *Diseases of the Breast*. 2nd ed. Philadelphia: Lippincott Williams & Wilkins; 2000:627, with permission.

chemotherapy in selected patients. Oncotype Dx is a diagnostic test that quantifies the likelihood of disease recurrence and the response to chemotherapy when the patient receives 5 years of antiestrogen therapy (Tamoxifen); a Recurrence Score is given in categories of low, intermediate, and high risk. It may be used in premenopausal, ER-positive, node-negative patients with T1-2 tumors as well as postmenopausal, ER-positive, SLN-positive patients with T1-2 tumors.

Tamoxifen is a selective estrogen agonist–antagonist; the agonist activity explains its favorable effect on blood lipid profiles and bone mineral density. A role for tamoxifen in the treatment of ER-positive breast cancers, particularly in older patients, has emerged following several randomized trials and meta-analyses. Most notably, the NSABP trial B-14 evaluated the role of tamoxifen in node-negative patients. Patients who had ER-positive cancer and received tamoxifen had fewer recurrences, fewer contralateral breast cancers, and a lower mortality rate than did patients who received placebo. In a large meta-analysis, tamoxifen given to patients with ER-positive tumors resulted in an approximately 50% reduction in the annual risk of recurrence and 26% reduction in the annual risk of death. Selective aromatase inhibitors such as anastrozole, letrozole, and exemestane block the production of estradiol and estrone sulfate. These agents appear to improve event-free survival with fewer side effects in postmenopausal women following surgery for breast cancer when compared to tamoxifen or placebo and are typically incorporated into the treatment of such patients.

Chemoprevention with Tamoxifen

The aim of the 1993 NSABP P-1 Prevention Trial was to assess the efficacy of tamoxifen for the prevention of breast cancer. Inclusion criteria for the study included age greater than 60 years and a history of LCIS or a 5-year Gail risk of developing breast cancer greater than 1.66%. Tamoxifen therapy for a duration of 5 years was associated with a 49% reduction in the risk of invasive breast carcinoma overall. For women who had LCIS, the risk was reduced by 56%, and for women with ADH, it was reduced by 86%. In this study, tamoxifen was associated with an increased incidence of endometrial cancer and thromboembolic events, such as deep vein thrombosis and pulmonary embolus. Other side effects of therapy included hot flashes and vaginal discharge. Recently, it has been shown that the benefit continues when tamoxifen is taken for 10 years, and currently, this is the recommendation for women taking this medication. It remains to be determined if the selective aromatase inhibitors have similar improved efficacy past 5 years.

SPECIAL CONSIDERATIONS

Inflammatory Breast Cancer

Inflammatory breast carcinoma is characterized by erythema and induration of the skin. *Peau d'orange*, the characteristic orange peel appearance of the skin, results from dermal lymphatic congestions with tumor cells. Patients frequently present with axillary metastases, and remote metastases should be excluded. Chemotherapy is the initial treatment modality, often followed by mastectomy and radiation therapy.

Male Breast Cancer

Male breast cancer accounts for approximately 1% of all breast cancers, with an estimated 1,300 cases in 2003. The strongest risk factor for the development of male breast cancer is Klinefelter syndrome. Other risk factors include a family history of breast or ovarian cancer, a *BRCA2* mutation, a history of undescended testes, and chronic liver disorders such as cirrhosis. Male breast cancer usually presents as a painless, firm, subareolar mass, or as a mass in the upper outer quadrant. MRM is the treatment of choice. Frequently tamoxifen and occasionally adjuvant chemotherapy are recommended.

Paget Disease

Paget disease of the breast is a condition characterized by erythema, scaling, and ulceration of the nipple and the presence of Paget cells on histology, which are large, pale-staining cells with prominent nuclei interspersed among the normal keratinocytes of the nipple epidermis. Paget disease is associated with an underlying breast carcinoma (either *in situ* or infiltrating) in 97% of patients. Following evaluation with mammography and, more recently, MRI to identify an underlying malignancy or multicentric disease, patients may undergo either partial mastectomy, including excision of the nipple–areolar complex, or total mastectomy with or without axillary lymphadenectomy.

OTHER MALIGNANT TUMORS

Phyllodes Tumor (Cystosarcoma Phyllodes)

Phyllodes tumor is a nonepithelial tumor that occurs exclusively in the female breast. Phyllodes tumors represent a spectrum of diseases including *benign* (60%), *borderline* (15%), and *malignant* (25%) variants. These distinctions are made on the basis of microscopic features and are of limited value in predicting the clinical behavior of a given tumor; metastases occur in approximately 20% of malignant cases but 5% of benign cases as well. Phyllodes tumors are typically smooth mobile lesions and are often bulky. The mean age at the time of presentation is 45. Benign lesions are excised with 1-cm margins or with total mastectomy without axillary dissection if breast conservation is not feasible (e.g., for large tumors).

Metastatic lesions typically spread hematogenously to the lung, bone, or abdominal viscera. Such metastases are associated with a grave prognosis.

Angiosarcoma

Angiosarcomas of the breast are uniformly aggressive malignancies originating from either lymphatic or capillary endothelium. They may be classified as primary or secondary, the latter following a previous diagnosis of adenocarcinoma of the breast. The interval between the initial breast cancer and subsequent secondary angiosarcoma is typically 5 to 10 years and may affect a lymphedematous upper extremity after MRM or radiation therapy (Stewart–Treves syndrome), the chest wall after mastectomy, or the breast after partial mastectomy and radiation. Angiosarcomas typically present with a bluish nodule. Disease progression is characterized by the emergence of multiple nodules and soft tissue edema. Hematogenous spread to the lung and bone is common. In the absence of metastatic disease, *angiosarcoma* is treated with wide resection to achieve negative margins, most often requiring mastectomy. Unlike adenocarcinoma of the breast, which spreads hematogenously and through the lymphatics, malignant phyllodes tumors and angiosarcomas spread only via the hematogenous route.

Lymphoma

Lymphomas account for less than 0.5% of all breast malignancies. They most often present as a painless palpable mass, and ipsilateral axillary lymphadenopathy is seen in up to 50% of cases. Bilateral breast involvement is seen in 5% to 25% of cases. Breast lymphomas may be primary (i.e., limited to the breast) or secondary. The diagnosis of the latter is facilitated by the presence of widespread disease. Generally, excisional biopsy is required to establish or confirm the diagnosis. Additional therapy consists of radiation and/or chemotherapy. Radical surgery provides no advantage over limited excision.

ACKNOWLEDGMENTS

The authors would like to thank Dr. Robert Roses for his contribution to the prior edition of this book.

Suggested Readings

Boughey JC, Gonzalez RJ, Bonner E, et al. Current treatment and clinical trial developments for ductal carcinoma in situ of the breast. *Oncologist.* 2007;12:1276–1287.

Fisher B, Constantino JP, Wickerham L, et al. Tamoxifen for prevention of breast cancer: report of the National Surgical Adjuvant Breast and Bowel Project P-1 Study. *J Natl Cancer Inst.* 1998;90(18):1371–1388.

Giuliano AE, Hunt KK, Ballman KV, et al. Axillary dissection vs. no axillary dissection in women with invasive breast cancer and sentinel node metastasis: a randomized clinical trial. *JAMA.* 2011;305(6):569–575.

Iglehart JD, Kaelin CM. Diseases of the breast. In: Sabiston DC, ed. *Textbook of Surgery: The Biological Basis of Modern Surgical Practice.* 17th ed. Philadelphia: WB Saunders; 2004:867–927.

Paik S, Shak S, Tang G, et al. A multigene assay to predict recurrence of tamoxifen-treated, node-negative breast cancer. *NEJM.* 2004;351(27):2817.

Perou CM, Sørlie T, Eisen MB, et al. Molecular portraits of human breast tumours. *Nature.* 2000;406(6797):747–752.

Roses DF, Giuliano AE. Surgery for breast cancer. In: Roses DF, ed. *Breast Cancer.* 2nd ed. Philadelphia: Churchill Livingstone; 2005:401–459.

SECTION

IV

Cardiovascular and Respiratory Systems

CHAPTER 19

Cardiovascular Disease and Cardiac Surgery

ANN C. GAFFEY AND PAVAN ATLURI

KEY POINTS

- Upon taking initial breaths, the neonatal pulmonary vascular resistance drops, pressure in the left atria exceeds that in the right atria, and spontaneous closure of the foramen ovale occurs.
- The anterior leaflet of the mitral valve is in close proximity to the aortic valve.
- The coronary arteries are the first branches of the aorta.
- Eighty-five percent of the population has a right-sided dominate circulation with the posterior descending artery arising from the right coronary artery.
- Cardiac cells can maintain prolonged action potentials, conduct from cell to cell via gap junctions, and self-generate.
- Coronary perfusion occurs during diastole.
- The major resistance to blood flow occurs at the level of penetrating arteries.
- Myocardial oxygen demand is dependent on myocardial oxygen tension.
- VSD is the most common congenital heart defect, but ASD is the most common congenital condition encountered in adulthood.
- New-onset murmur following a myocardial infarction may signify either a postinfarction VSD or papillary muscle rupture.
- Rheumatic heart disease is the most common cause of mitral stenosis.
- Type A dissections require emergent operation, while type B dissections are managed conservatively.

Proper function of the cardiovascular system is essential to normal homeostasis. Alterations in the cardiovascular system's ability to supply oxygen and nutrient-rich blood result in multiple organ dysfunction. The heart is a complex pump with many intricate components. A thorough understanding of normal cardiovascular physiology allows for an intricate understanding of cardiovascular disease processes. Normal cardiovascular physiology as well as disease processes will be discussed in detail.

CARDIOVASCULAR PHYSIOLOGY

Fetal Circulation

Oxygenated blood from the placenta is brought to the fetus via the umbilical vein. Roughly half of the blood from the placenta passes through hepatic sinusoids, while the remainder bypasses hepatic circulation flowing directly into the inferior vena cava via the *ductus venosus*. In the inferior vena cava, oxygenated placental blood mixes with deoxygenated venous blood from the lower extremities before entering the right atrium. Once in the right atrium, the majority of blood passes directly to the left atrium via the foramen ovale, thereby bypassing the pulmonary circulation. Left atrial blood mixes with the small amount of deoxygenated blood in the fetal pulmonary circulation before entering the left ventricle and ultimately the ascending aorta.

A small portion of right atrial blood mixes with superior vena caval blood from the head and upper extremities as well as coronary sinus blood and passes into the right ventricle (5% to 10% of total cardiac output). From the right ventricle, the blood enters the pulmonary artery; however, due to the very high pulmonary vascular resistance (PVR) in the fetus, the majority of blood is shunted to the descending aorta via a patent ductus arteriosus (PDA). Roughly half of the descending aortic blood passes into paired umbilical arteries and is returned to the placenta. It is these two fetal shunts, a patent foramen ovale (PFO) and PDA, that allow many neonates born with cyanotic congenital heart disease to survive. Figure 19.1 illustrates the fetal circulation.

At birth, as the placental circulation is no longer present and the neonatal lungs expand, the PVR is greatly reduced. This reduction allows increased pulmonary blood flow. With increased pulmonary blood flow, left atrial pressure is greater than right atrial pressure. This allows closure of the foramen ovale by the septum primum pressed against the septum secundum. During the first days of life, this closure is reversible. When an infant cries, an increase in pulmonary pressure with a right-to-left shunt through the foramen ovale may be present. This is manifested as cyanosis in newborns.

Closure of the ductus arteriosus results from the release of bradykinin from the lung that mediates contraction of the muscular ductus wall. Functional closure of the ductus typically occurs within the first 15 hours after birth, and anatomic closure occurs by day 12 of parturition. Prior to birth, locally produced prostaglandins maintain patency of the ductus. The fibrotic, atrophied remnant of the ductus arteriosus is referred to as the ligamentum arteriosum.

Anatomy

The human cardiovascular system is composed of the systemic circulatory system and the pulmonary circulation, with the heart at the center of the circulatory system. The heart is situated

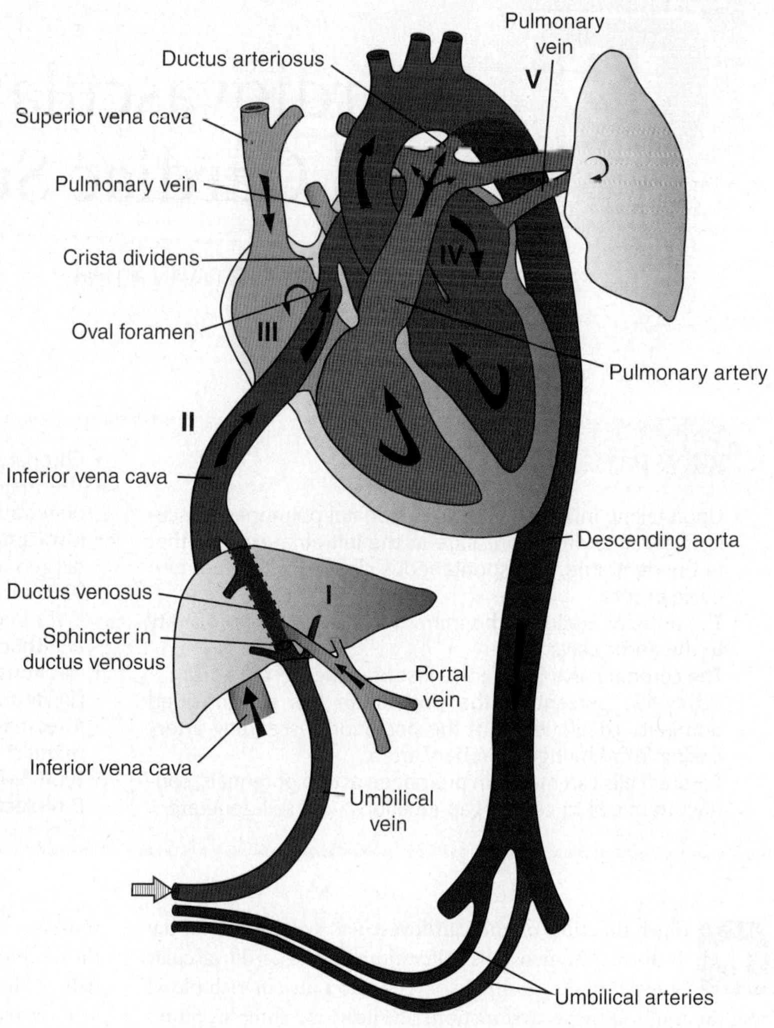

FIGURE 19.1 Diagram of the human circulation before birth. *Arrows* indicate the direction of blood flow. Note where oxygenated blood mixed with deoxygenated blood: in the liver (*I*), in the inferior vena cava (*II*), in the right atrium (*III*), in the left atrium (*IV*), and at the entrance of the ductus arteriosus into the descending aorta (*V*). (From Sadler TW. *Langman's Medical Embryology*. 13th ed. Philadelphia: Wolters Kluwer; 2015.)

obliquely within the pericardial sac, with one third of the heart situated to the right of the median plane and two thirds to the left. The right ventricle abuts the sternocostal surface and forms the anterior surface of the heart. The right side of the heart receives deoxygenated systemic blood via the superior and inferior vena cava as well as deoxygenated blood from the coronary circulation via the coronary sinus. The right heart then pumps this blood through the low-pressure, high-flow pulmonary arteries. Once the blood has circulated through the pulmonary circulation, it is returned to the left atrium via four posteriorly situated pulmonary veins (two superior and two inferior pulmonary veins). Blood from the left heart is ejected from the left ventricle into the systemic circulation via the aorta.

Valvular Anatomy

The mammalian heart is composed of four one-way valves. Two atrioventricular valves (mitral and tricuspid) provide unidirectional diastolic flow from the atria to the ventricles and allow a systolic pressure gradient between the atria and ventricles. The semilunar valves (aortic and pulmonary) allow systolic flow and maintain a diastolic pressure gradient between the ventricles and outflow circulations.

The tricuspid and mitral valves are fibrous endocardium–lined valves. The tricuspid valve separates the right atrium from the right ventricle and consists of a large anterior leaflet attached to the anterior wall of the heart, a posterior leaflet at the right margin, and a septal leaflet attached to the septum. Three chordae tendineae are attached to the free surface of the leaflets and to the papillary muscles at the right ventricular base. This apparatus prevents prolapse of the tricuspid valve leaflets into the right atrium during systole. The mitral valve, located at the orifice of the left ventricle, consists of a large anterior leaflet in continuity with the posterior wall of the aorta and a smaller posterior leaflet. The anterior leaflet of the mitral valve is anatomically in close proximity to the aortic valve. Chordae tendineae (Fig. 19.2) secure the leaflets to the anterior and posterior papillary muscles and ensure coaptation of the valve leaflets during systole.

The aortic and pulmonic valves are situated at the outflow of the left and right ventricles, respectively. The aortic valve is a trileaflet valve. These leaflets are named according to the origin of the coronary arteries, namely, the right coronary, left coronary, and noncoronary leaflets (Fig. 19.3). Similarly, the pulmonic valve is a trileaflet valve with a right, left, and noncoronary leaflet.

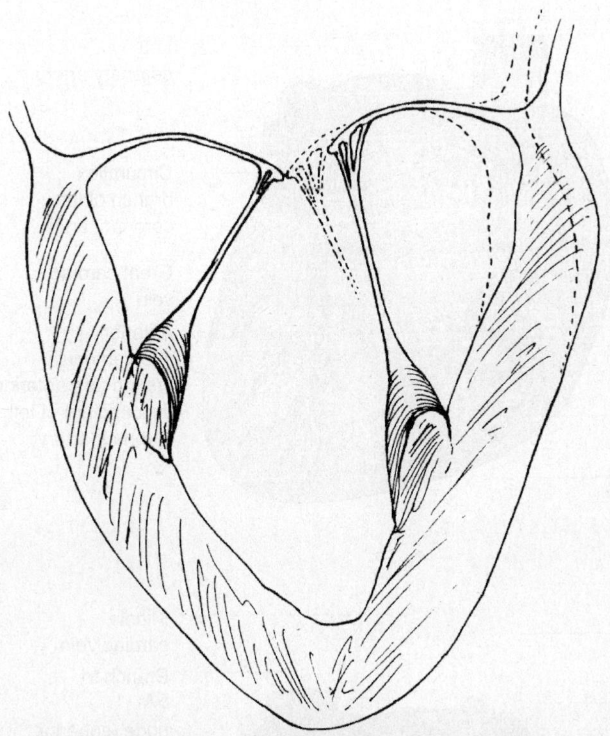

FIGURE 19.2 Chordae tendineae tether the leaflets of the mitral and tricuspid valves, allowing precise coaptation during systole. (From Chitwood WR Jr. Mitral valve repair: ischemic. In: Kaiser LR, Kron IL, Spray TL, eds. *Mastery of Cardiothoracic Surgery*. Philadelphia: Lippincott-Raven Publishers; 1998.)

Coronary Anatomy

The coronary circulation (Fig. 19.4) supplies oxygen-rich blood to the myocardium and epicardium. The endocardium is in continuous contact with intracardiac blood and does not require additional blood flow. The right and left coronary arteries of the heart arise just superior to the aortic valve in the coronary sinuses and are the first branches of the aorta.

The *right coronary artery* arises from the anterior (right) *sinus of Valsalva* in the aorta and runs along the atrioventricular (AV; coronary) groove. In about 60% of the population, the right coronary artery gives off a sinoatrial (SA) branch near its origin to supply the SA node. It traverses posteriorly toward the apex of the heart and gives off a *right marginal artery,* which supplies the right ventricle. After giving off this branch, it continues in the posterior interventricular groove. In roughly 85% of patients, the *posterior descending artery* arises from the right coronary artery and defines a right-sided dominant circulation. In approximately 5% of patients, a balanced pattern exists in which the right coronary and circumflex coronary arteries supply the posterior descending artery, branches to the septum, and AV node (Fig. 19.5).

The *left coronary artery* arises from the left *sinus of Valsalva* and passes between the left auricle (atrial appendage) and pulmonary trunk toward the anterior AV groove. In 40% of the patients, the SA branch arises from the left coronary artery. The left coronary artery divides at the AV groove to give off the *left anterior descending artery* (LAD) and *circumflex coronary artery* (Fig. 19.5). The LAD passes anteriorly along the interventricular groove to the apex and provides septal branches that supply the anterior two thirds of the interventricular septum and diagonals that supply the anterolateral wall of the left ventricle. The circumflex coronary artery follows the AV groove around the left border of the heart to the posterior surface of the heart and provides marginal branches (i.e., obtuse marginal) that supply the posterior left ventricle. In 10% of the population, the circumflex coronary artery ends in the posterior descending artery, providing blood flow to the posterior one third of the interventricular septum and AV node, defining a left-sided dominant circulation.

The venous drainage of the heart is via veins that drain into the coronary sinus as well as into smaller venae cordis minimae and anterior cardiac veins that drain into the right atrium. The coronary sinus is a large vein that receives coronary venous blood from the left (great cardiac, left marginal, and left posterior ventricular veins) and right (middle and small cardiac veins) side veins. It runs in the posterior AV groove.

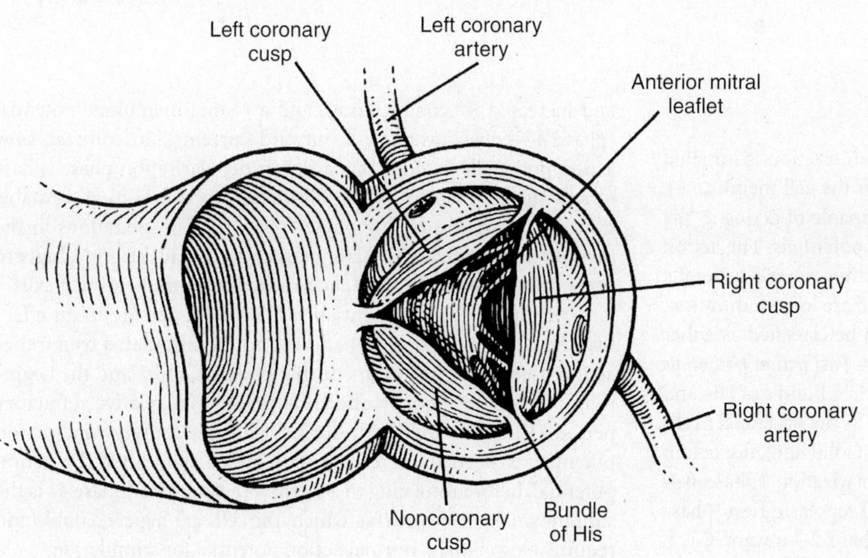

FIGURE 19.3 Normal aortic valve from a surgeon's point of view. (From Damiano RJ. Aortic valve replacement: prosthesis. In: Kaiser LR, Kron IL, Spray TL, eds. *Mastery of Cardiothoracic Surgery*. Philadelphia: Lippincott-Raven Publishers; 1998.)

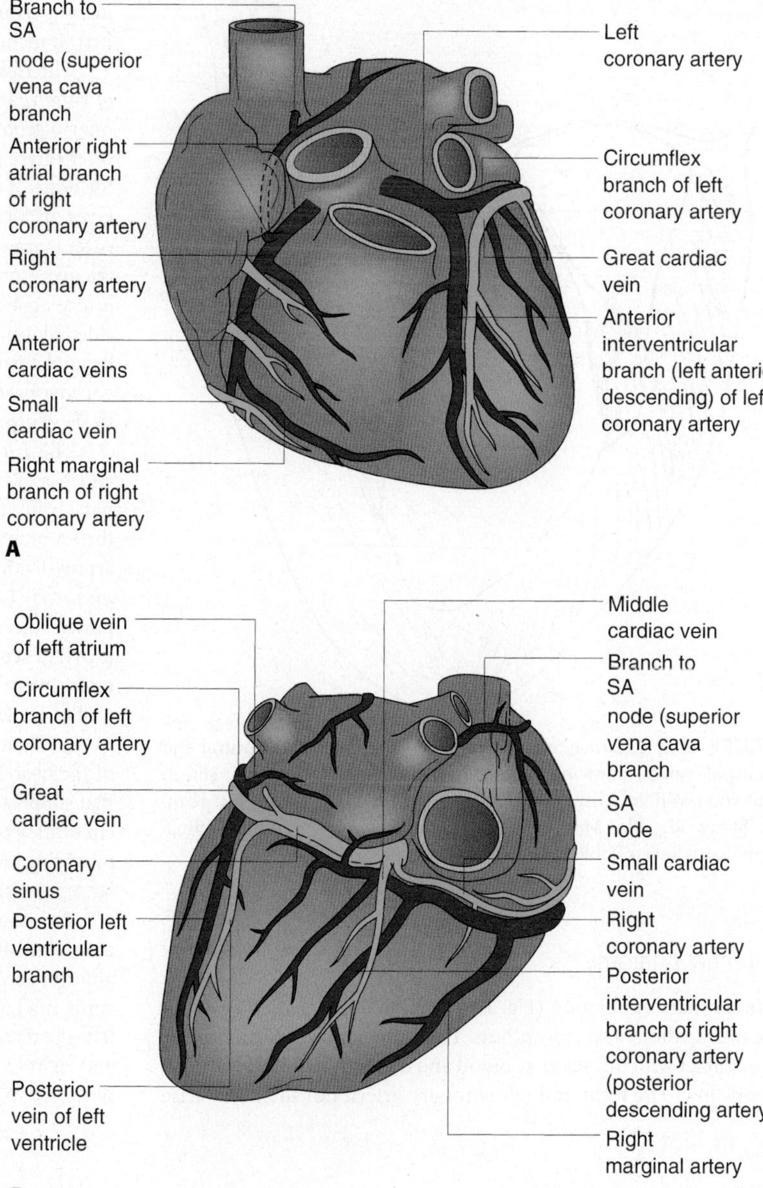

FIGURE 19.4 Anatomy of the coronary arteries and cardiac veins. **A.** Anterior view. The origin of the left main coronary artery is left lateral and somewhat posterior with respect to the aorta; it courses behind the pulmonary artery and then divides into the left anterior descending and circumflex coronary arteries. The origin of the right coronary artery is almost directly anterior, and it runs in the AV groove. **B.** Posterior view. The great, middle, and small cardiac veins come together at the level of the coronary sinus, which lies in the left inferior AV groove and empties into the right atrium. (From Mulholland MW. *Greenfield's Surgery: Scientific Principles and Practice*. 5th ed. Philadelphia: Lippincott Williams & Wilkins; 2011.)

Electrophysiology

As with any striated muscle, cardiac muscle contraction is initiated by action potentials (rapid voltage changes of the cell membrane). Certain cells within the cardiac muscle are capable of acting as the pacemaker and spontaneously initiate action potentials. The action potentials of cardiac muscle are special in that they can self-generate, conduct from cell to cell via gap junctions, and are long in duration.

Action potentials of the myocardium can be classified as either fast action potentials or slow action potentials. *Fast action potentials* occur in normal myocardium of the atria, ventricle, bundle of His, and Purkinje fibers. *Slow action potentials* are seen in the pacemaker cells of the SA and AV nodes. As seen in Figure 19.6 (solid line), fast action potentials are characterized by a rapid depolarization (phase 0—transient increase in Na^+ conductance), partial repolarization (phase 1—outward movement of K^+), a plateau (phase 2—inward Ca^{2+}), membrane repolarization (phase 3—decreased Ca^{2+} conductance and increased K^+ conductance), and a resting membrane potential (phase 4—equal inward and outward currents). In contrast, slow action potentials demonstrate a slower depolarization phase (phase 0) and shorter plateau and repolarization (phase 3) to an unstable slow depolarization resting phase (phase 4). The alterations in the membrane potential are a factor of a cell membrane's permeability to particular ions (Na^+, K^+, Ca^{2+}) and the resulting gradients that exist.

During an action potential, cardiac myocytes are in an effective refractory period (ERP) and cannot be stimulated by another action potential. This occurs during phases 1 and 2 and the beginning of phase 3. Shortly after this period is a relative refractory period (RRP, late phase 3), during which, a supranormal action potential is needed for excitation. Immediately after the action potential, before returning to a normal resting state (phase 4) is the supranormal period, during which, the cells are hyperexcitable and require a lower-than-normal action potential for stimulation.

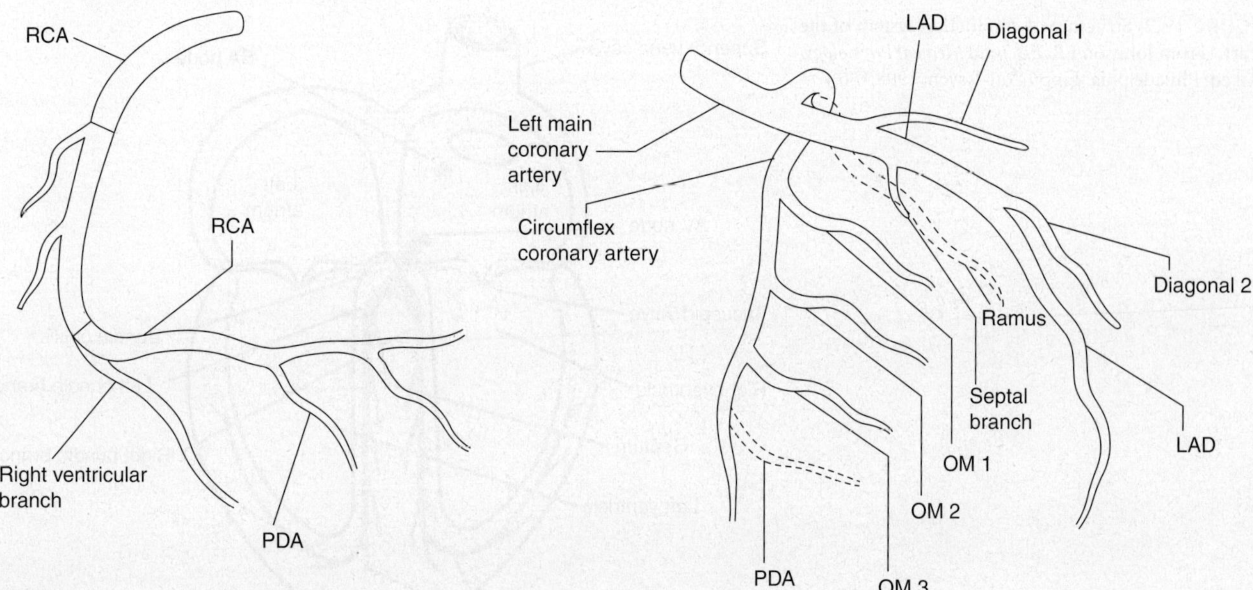

FIGURE 19.5 Coronary anatomy. RCA, right coronary artery; PDA, posterior descending artery; LAD, left anterior descending artery; OM, obtuse marginal artery.

Once an action potential arises, it is conducted across the cell membrane to adjacent cells via gap junctions. The speed of transmission of the action potential is determined by a combination of cell size and rate of depolarization. The smaller cells of the pacemaker cells demonstrate a slower conduction velocity than the larger Purkinje cells. Similarly, the slow response of the pacemaker cells mediates a slower conduction velocity when compared to the fast response of ventricular myocardial cells.

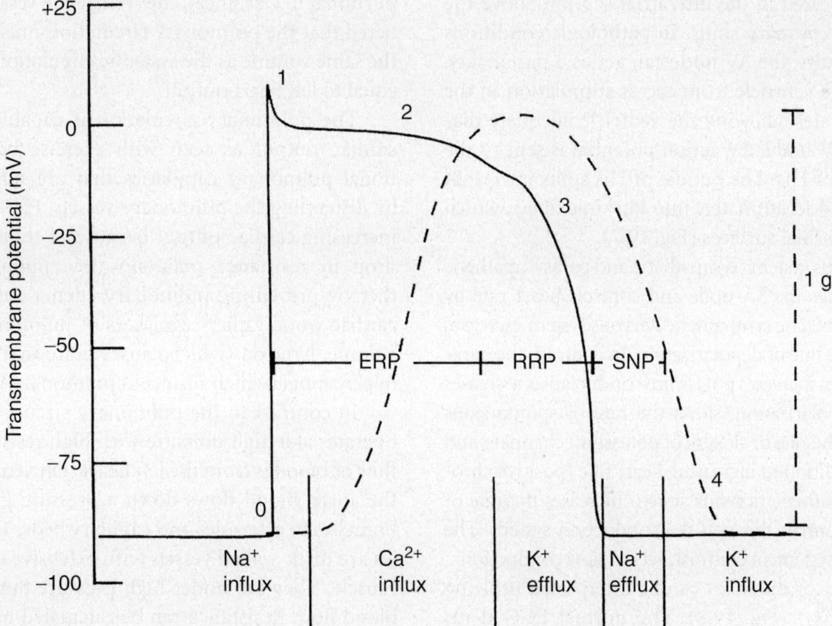

FIGURE 19.6 Schematic fast action potential of human ventricular myocardium (*solid*) with electrolyte movements, refractory periods (see text), and force generated (*dashed line*). The five phases of fast cardiac action potential are indicated as numbers. *Phase 4*: the resting membrane potential. Potassium conductance is high and sodium conductance is low. *Phase 0*: Upstroke of the action potential due to membrane depolarization. An increase in sodium conductance due to the opening of voltage-dependent fast sodium channels causes depolarization. There is a simultaneous decrease in potassium conductance. *Phase 1*: Period of partial repolarization due to a dramatic decrease in sodium conductance and a brief increase in chloride conductance. *Phase 2*: Plateau phase during which changes in potassium efflux (conductance decrease and then plateaus) is matched by calcium influx (conductance increases and then plateaus). *Phase 3*: Membrane repolarization phase due to an increase in potassium efflux (increase potassium conductance) and a decrease in calcium influx (decreased calcium conductance).

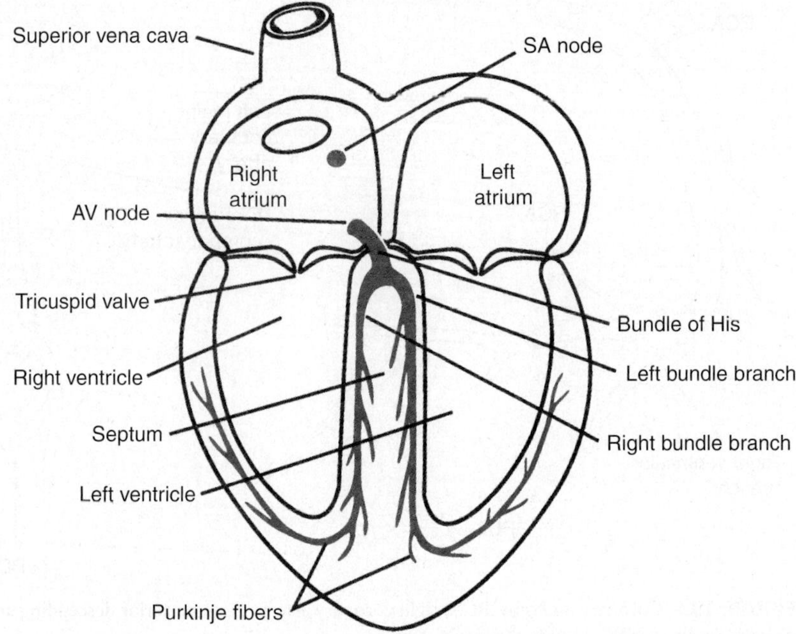

FIGURE 19.7 Structure of conduction system of the heart. (From Johnson LR. *Essential Medical Physiology*. 2nd ed. Philadelphia: Lippincott-Raven; 1998:166.)

SA nodal cells demonstrate the most rapid spontaneous depolarization and hence act as the pacemaker under routine conditions. This tissue lies within the wall of the right atrium at the junction of the right atrium and superior vena cava. Once the action potential is initiated in the SA node, it is propagated via the atria to the AV node. The AV node is located in the interatrial septum above the tricuspid valve near the coronary sinus. In pathologic conditions with SA nodal discontinuity, the AV node can act as a pacemaker. The AV node protects the ventricle from excess stimulation in the case of increased atrial rates, allowing the ventricle adequate diastolic filling. From the AV node, the action potential is sent to the ventricle via the bundle of His. The bundle of His splits into right and left bundle branches and ultimately into Purkinje fibers, which conduct to the subendocardial surfaces (Fig. 19.7).

The autonomic nervous system (sympathetic and parasympathetic nervous systems) innervates the SA node and controls heart rate by modifying SA nodal activity. The sympathetic nervous system increases heart rate by increasing the rate of depolarization. In contrast, the parasympathetic nervous system increases potassium conductance, increases the magnitude of hyperpolarization, slows the rate of spontaneous depolarization, decreases the rate of closure of potassium channels, and slows the heart rate. In addition to increasing heart rate (positive chronotropic effect), the sympathetic nervous system increases the rate of conduction of action potentials through the conduction system. The parasympathetic nervous system, in contrast, acts to slow conduction.

The electrical activity of the heart can be interpreted utilizing an *electrocardiogram* (ECG) (Fig. 19.8). The normal ECG demonstrates *P* waves and *QRS* complexes, which represent atrial and ventricular depolarization, respectively. Ventricular repolarization is demonstrated by the *T* wave.

Circulatory Physiology

As previously stated, the cardiovascular system is composed of the pulmonary circulation to provide perfusion to the lung parenchyma and the systemic circulation to provide systemic perfusion (and a very small degree of pulmonary circulation via the bronchial vessels). The pulmonary circuit is a low-pressure (mean PA pressure of 15 mm Hg), high-flow system. As compared to the systemic circulation, the pulmonary vessels contain very little smooth muscle and are much shorter. This results in highly compliant [compliance (mL/mm Hg) = volume (mL)/pressure (mm Hg); inversely proportional to elastance], low-resistance vessels. It should be remembered that the pulmonary circulation must be capable of handling the same volume as the systemic circulation, as right heart output is equal to left heart output.

The pulmonary circulation is capable of handling increased cardiac output as seen with exercise both by recruiting additional pulmonary capillaries that are not normally utilized and by distending the pulmonary vessels. PVR is able to decrease with increasing cardiac output because of these two mechanisms. This drop in resistance maintains low pulmonary artery pressures, thereby preventing pulmonary edema and decreasing right heart cardiac work. Other regulators of pulmonary blood flow are lung volume, hypoxia (which causes pulmonary vasoconstriction), and hypercapnia (which results in pulmonary vasodilation).

In contrast to the pulmonary circuit, the systemic circulation operates at a high pressure with high resistance to blood flow. The flow of blood is from the left heart (left ventricle) to the aorta. From the aorta, blood flows down a pressure gradient through various branches to arterioles and capillary beds. The large and small arteries are thick-walled vessels with extensive elastic tissue and smooth muscle. They are under high pressure but offer little resistance to blood flow. Resistance can be calculated using the following equation derived from the work of Jean Leonard Marie Poiseuille on flow mechanics:

$$\text{Resistance} = \frac{8(\text{viscosity of blood})(\text{length of vessel})}{\Pi(\text{radius of blood vessel})^4}$$

Aortic and arterial elasticity maintains perfusion during the diastolic/filling phase of left ventricular (LV) cycling. *Arterioles*, the short, terminal braches of the arteries, are the principal resistance vessels of the systemic circulation. They are comprised of a large percentage of vascular smooth muscle innervated by the autonomic nervous system

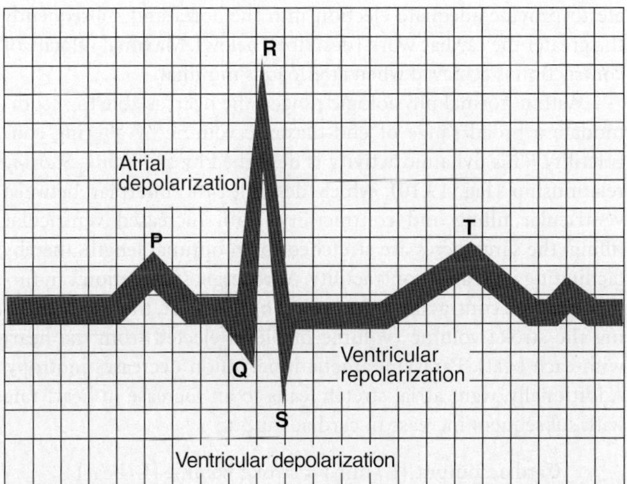

FIGURE 19.8 Normal ECG strip, which consists of components that indicate electrical events during one heartbeat. P wave indicates atrial contraction. QRS complex represents ventricular depolarization and contraction. T wave represents ventricular repolarization.

TABLE 19.3 Normal hemodynamic parameters

Cardiac output	4.0–8.0 L/min
Cardiac index	2.5–4.5 L/min/m^2
Stroke volume	60–130 mL
Systemic blood pressure	100–130/60–90 mm Hg
Mean arterial pressure (MAP)	70–105 mm Hg
Right atria/central venous pressure	2–10 mm Hg
Right ventricular pressure	15–30/0–18 mm Hg
Pulmonary artery pressure	15–30/6–12 mm Hg
Pulmonary capillary wedge pressure	5–12 mm Hg
SVR	700–1600 dynes/s/cm^2
Pulmonary vascular resistance	20–130 dynes/s/cm^2

mm Hg, millimeters of mercury; L/min, L/min; m, meter, cm, centimeter, s, second.

within the vessel wall that can constrict and impede the flow of blood. Arterioles provide the largest pressure drop in the circulation.

As arterial structures progressively branch from the aorta ultimately to the capillary bed, the cross-sectional area of the vascular bed continues to increase. On the outflow side of the capillary bed, the cross-sectional area decreases as capillaries drain into venules that merge into small veins, large veins, and ultimately the vena cava. The velocity of blood flow is directly proportional to volume of blood flow and inversely proportional to cross-sectional area:

$$\text{Velocity of blood flow}\,(\text{cm/s}) = \text{flow}\,(\text{cm}^3/\text{s})/\text{cross-sectional area}\,(\text{cm}^2)$$

As illustrated in Figure 19.9, there is a decrease in the velocity of blood flow as the cross-sectional area of the vascular bed increases. This is ideal at the capillary level (high surface area, low velocity), where a high contact surface area and low velocity provide for optimal exchange of metabolic products at a cellular level.

Cardiac Mechanics

The heart is a biomechanical pump. The mechanical force generated by the heart is utilized to eject blood from the heart to either the pulmonary or systemic circulations providing perfusion to end organs. There must be synchrony of the cardiac myocytes, valves, and four chambers of the heart for maximum efficiency. The heart is in a constant state of flux to ensure that adequate end-organ perfusion is achieved. The primary variables that alter cardiac function are preload, afterload, and autonomic nervous system stimulation. A proper understanding of these forces is a prerequisite to an adequate understanding of cardiac mechanics. The normal hemodynamic parameters are shown in Table 19.3.

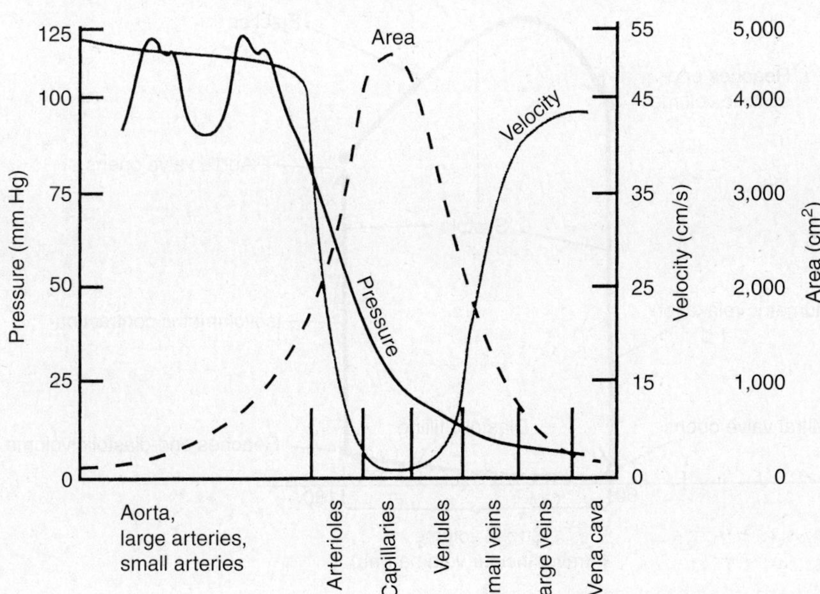

FIGURE 19.9 Pressure, area, and velocity relationship across the systemic circulation.

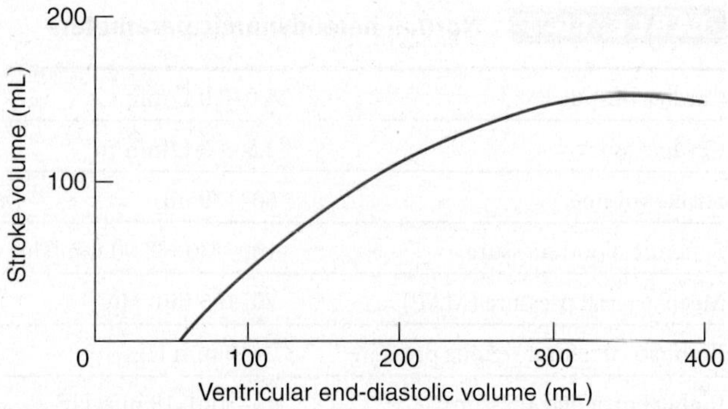

FIGURE 19.10 Frank–Starling law refers to the length–tension relationship of the cardiac muscle where length is determined by the end-diastolic volume and tension. As the ventricles become over filled, the heart is inefficient resulting in the stoke volume leveling off and eventually declining.

The left and right ventricles function in a cyclical manner. Contraction and ejection of blood occurs during *systole*. Myocardial perfusion as well as filling of the ventricles occurs during the relaxation phase known as *diastole*. To simplify the discussion, all references to ventricular function will focus on LV mechanics.

The LV intracavitary volume and pressure at end diastole (immediately prior to contraction) determines the *preload* of the heart. There are several factors that affect preload. Increasing venous return increases preload. Fibrotic, hypertrophied, and aging hearts become increasingly stiff and thus limit LV filling and preload. As described earlier, relaxation is an energy-dependent process (calcium ATPase), which is augmented by adrenergic stimulation, but is impaired in ischemia, hypothyroidism, and congestive heart failure (CHF)—all conditions that limit preload.

The afterload of a muscle is the pressure against which it must contract. For the left ventricle, this is equivalent to the aortic pressure against which it must eject blood during systole. Afterload for the right ventricle is equal to the pulmonary artery pressure. The greater the afterload, the greater the potential energy the heart must generate to provide adequate ejection into the aorta and subsequently the greater the cardiac work (described below). Maximal velocity of contraction is achieved when afterload is minimal.

Within normal physiologic ranges, the heart is able to accommodate a broad range of end-diastolic volume by altering contractility. This dynamic activity is described by the *Frank–Starling* relationship (Fig. 19.10), which describes the interplay between ventricular filling and contractility. With increased ventricular filling, the sarcomeres are stretched to an optimal length, thereby facilitating increased contractility. Adrenergic stimulation can further increase contractility (inotropy) of the heart, thereby increasing the stroke volume (volume of blood ejected from the heart with each beat). Parasympathetic innervation decreases inotropy. Additionally, right atrial stretch leads to an increase in heart rate with subsequent increase in cardiac output:

$$\text{Cardiac output } (\text{L/min}) = \text{stroke volume } (\text{L/beat}) \times \text{heart rate } (\text{beats/min})$$

The cardiac cycle, as well as the interplay between preload and afterload on stroke volume, can best be described using pressure–volume loops (Fig. 19.11). These pressure–volume loops are constructed by combining systolic and diastolic pressure curves. The diastolic component (dotted line) is determined by diastolic filling (preload). The shape of the loop is determined by both contractility and the afterload against which the ventricle must contract. The cardiac cycle begins at end diastole when the left ventricle is filled with left atrial blood and the cardiac muscle is relaxed. Upon excitation, the muscle begins to contract and generate force against closed valves (isovolumetric contraction). Once the pressure in the left ventricle exceeds aortic pressure, the blood is ejected into circulation during systole. This volume ejected is the stroke volume (depicted by the width of the pressure–volume loop). The remaining volume at the end of contraction is the end-systolic volume. At the end of contraction, the ventricle begins to relax (isovolumetric relaxation) and the aortic valve closes as the pressure in the aorta exceeds that of the left ventricle. With a drop in LV pressure, the mitral valve opens and

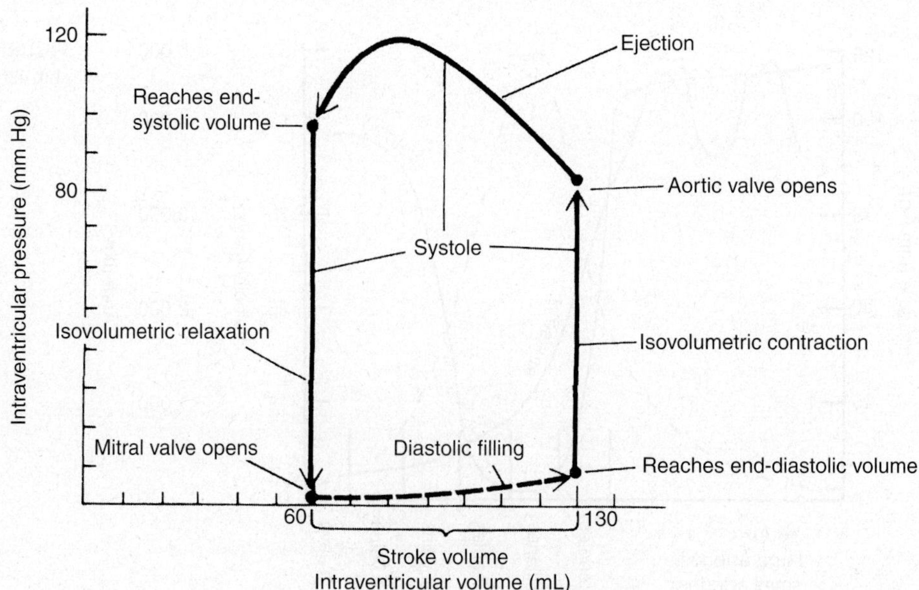

FIGURE 19.11 Pressure–volume loop of one cardiac cycle. (From Mohrman DE, Heller LJ. *Cardiovascular Physiology*. 3rd ed. New York: McGraw Hill; 1991:54.)

left atrial blood begins to fill the left ventricle during diastole. It should be noted that in the ideal system following passive flow of atrial blood, atrial contraction near the end of diastole optimizes filling of the left ventricle (*atrial kick*), thereby optimizing the Frank–Starling relationship. Loss of this end-diastolic atrial contraction as in atrial fibrillation in a heart with ventricular hypertrophy can have adverse systemic hemodynamic consequences.

There are several factors that affect the pressure–volume loops. Increased preload increases end-diastolic volume and stroke volume. Increased afterload increases pressure that is required to be generated during isovolumetric contraction to eject blood and decreases the stroke volume. Increased contractility, as with adrenergic stimulation, increases stroke volume and decreases end-systolic volume. The ability of a hypertrophic heart to increase stroke volume is severely limited by its decreased diastolic compliance, limiting preload.

Oxygen utilization by the heart is twofold. A small amount of oxygen is utilized for cellular homeostasis, and a large amount is utilized during contraction. Changes in myocardial oxygen consumption are directly related to the work of the heart and changes in contractility. Cardiac work can be quantified as *stroke work*, or work which the heart performs with each beat (stroke work = aortic pressure × stroke volume). The *minute work* of the heart is equal to the product of heart rate times the stroke volume multiplied by the aortic pressure (or cardiac output × aortic pressure), so an increase in any of these three variables will increase cardiac work and ultimately increase myocardial oxygen consumption and demand.

The major determinant of oxygen demand is *myocardial wall tension*. Tension in the wall of the ventricle is determined by both the pressure in the ventricle and the geometry of the ventricle. The normal left ventricle is a pressurized irregularly shaped chamber. If we were to consider the ventricle as a cylinder, then the *law of LaPlace* states that wall tension is proportional to internal pressure times the radius. Increasing the wall thickness decreases the wall tension by distributing the internal pressure over a greater number of muscle fibers. In other words, wall tension equals pressure times radius divided by wall thickness. Altering the geometrical configuration of the ventricle (as with cardiomyopathy), increasing the radius, decreasing the wall thickness, and increasing ventricular pressure all increase wall tension and myocardial oxygen demand. Changing the geometry of the ventricle requires extra energy consumption to realign the myocytes prior to each systolic contraction.

As stated previously, cardiac output is equal to the product of stroke volume multiplied by the heart rate. A clinically feasible means of calculating cardiac output is to utilize the Fick equation:

$$\text{Cardiac output} = \frac{\text{total body oxygen consumption}}{[O_2]\text{ arterial blood} - [O_2]\text{ venous blood}}.$$

Dye dilution and thermal dilution of heat are other clinically utilized methods of calculating cardiac output (described later in chapter). Given the varying sizes of patients (varying body surface area), simply calculating a cardiac output may not provide enough information regarding cardiac function and adequate systemic perfusion. The calculated parameter of *cardiac index* factors in patient size and expresses cardiac output per square meter of surface area, thereby eliminating the variable of patient size (cardiac index = cardiac output/body surface area). A cardiac index greater than 2 L/min/m^2 is accepted as adequate. Figure 19.12 demonstrates the mechanical and electrical events during the various phases of the cardiac cycle.

Coronary Physiology

Coronary blood flow follows the major vessels into smaller penetrating arteries, which provide the majority of the resistance to blood flow. There is a dense capillary network by which the extensive metabolic demands of the heart can be provided. At rest, coronary blood flow is approximately 1 mL/g of myocardium, but with demand, this flow is capable of increasing nearly fourfold. The increase in blood flow is accomplished with a combination of local vasodilatation of the penetrating arteries as well as recruitment of vessels that are collapsed at rest. Since nearly 70% of the oxygen is derived from delivered coronary blood, there exists a very tight regulatory system to ensure adequate perfusion of the myocardium. The myocardial tissue functions most optimally under aerobic conditions and is capable of sustaining only a few minutes of anaerobic activity.

Coronary perfusion is accomplished during the relaxing diastolic phase. During systole, the compressive forces within the myocardial wall are powerful enough to collapse the penetrating vessels and prevent myocardial perfusion. Therefore, increasing heart rate will not only increase myocardial oxygen demand but will also decrease myocardial perfusion. Regulation of coronary blood flow is accomplished by a combination of the autonomic nervous system, metabolic vascular mediators, and vascular endothelium–mediated vasodilatation. There is a combination of α- and β-receptors on the conductance vessels, which regulate nervous system–mediated vasoconstriction and vasodilatation, respectively. *Adenosine* is produced by cardiac myocytes in response to ischemia and is the primary metabolic vascular mediator. It acts locally on vascular smooth muscle to cause vasodilatation. The vascular endothelium is capable of releasing both vasodilatory and vasoconstricting mediators.

CARDIOVASCULAR PATHOPHYSIOLOGY

Congenital Heart Disease

Atrial Septal Defect

Atrial septal defects (ASDs) account for 10% to 15% of cardiac anomalies. Additionally, these are the most common congenital conditions encountered in adults. ASDs may occur in association with other complex congenital heart and genetic defects including Down, Turner, Marfan's, and Ehlers–Danlos syndromes.

A defect in formation of the septum primum results in ostium secundum–type ASD (Fig. 19.13). Ostium primum–type ASDs are a result of malformation of the AV canal.

Other less common types of ASDs include sinus venosus type (defect at the level of the superior and inferior vena cava) and coronary sinus ASD (defect in the wall between coronary sinus and left atrium). Roughly 20% of adults have a PFO, which is clinically inconsequential as it remains closed due to higher left atrial pressure compared to right atrial pressures. But, with high right-sided pressures, the foramen ovale may become patent causing right-to-left shunting of blood.

Often, patients remain asymptomatic. Symptomatic patients present with signs of heart failure, exercise intolerance, or arrhythmias. Echocardiography is usually diagnostic. Many small ASDs in children will close spontaneously and should be monitored. All symptomatic and large/significant ASDs should be closed either by percutaneous or surgical means. Prior to closure, it is critical to measure PVR by cardiac catheterization. Elevated PVR (>8 woods units) is a contraindication to closure.

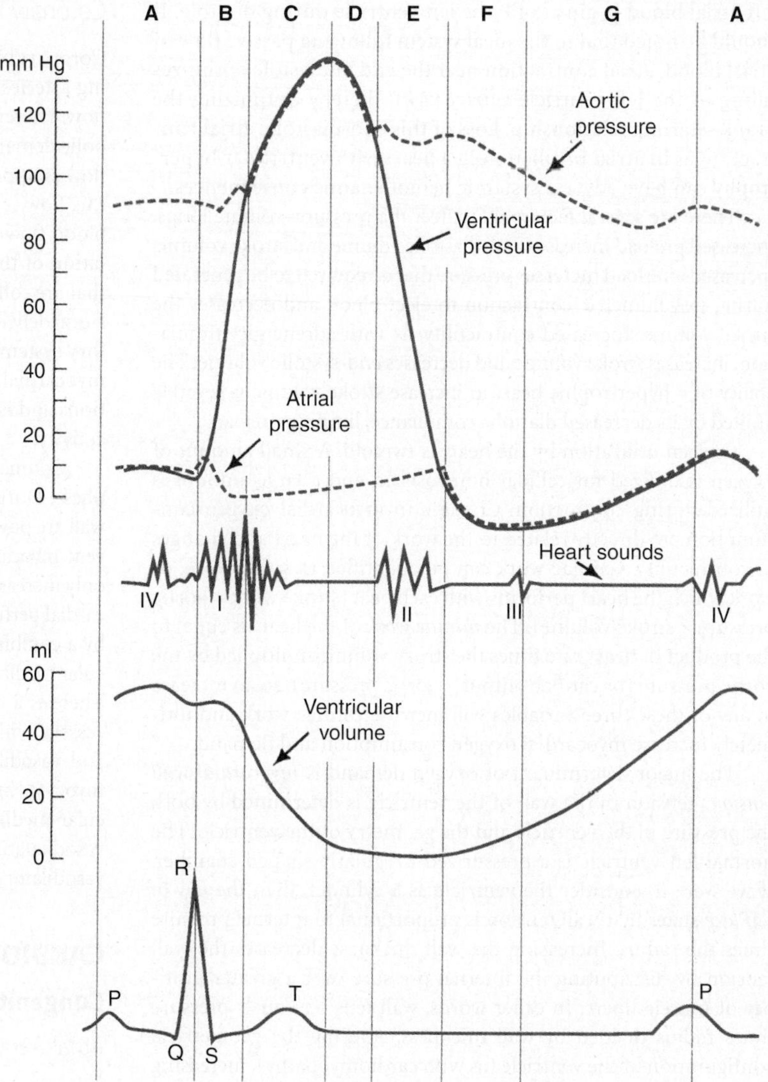

FIGURE 19.12 Mechanical and electrical events during a single cardiac cycle. The seven phases are denoted by letters as follows: (*A*) atrial systole, (*B*) isovolumetric ventricular contraction, (*C*) rapid ventricular ejection, (*D*) reduced ventricular ejection, (*E*) isovolumetric ventricular relaxation, (*F*) rapid ventricular filling, and (*G*) reduced ventricular filling. (From Johnson LR. *Essential Medical Physiology*. 2nd ed. Philadelphia: Lippincott-Raven; 1998:190.)

Ventricular Septal Defect

Ventricular septal defects (VSDs) account for roughly 25% of congenital heart defects. VSDs can either occur singly or multiply. One half of patients with VSDs will also have another cardiac anomaly and should therefore undergo thorough evaluation. VSDs are defined based upon their location in the ventricular septum, that is, outlet, septal, conoventricular, anterior muscular, midmuscular, apical muscular, and inlet septal (Fig. 19.14). Hemodynamically, VSDs result in left-to-right shunting of blood, thereby resulting in elevated PVR and left atrial and ventricular overload. With

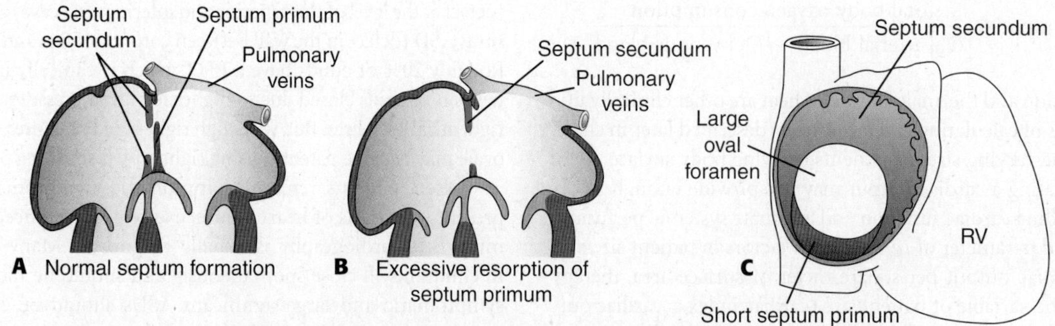

FIGURE 19.13 Normal atrial septum formation **(A)** and ostium secundum–type atrial septal defect caused by excessive resorption of the septum primum **(B** and **C)**. (From Sadler TW. *Langman's Medical Embryology*. 13th ed. Philadelphia: Wolters Kluwer; 2015.)

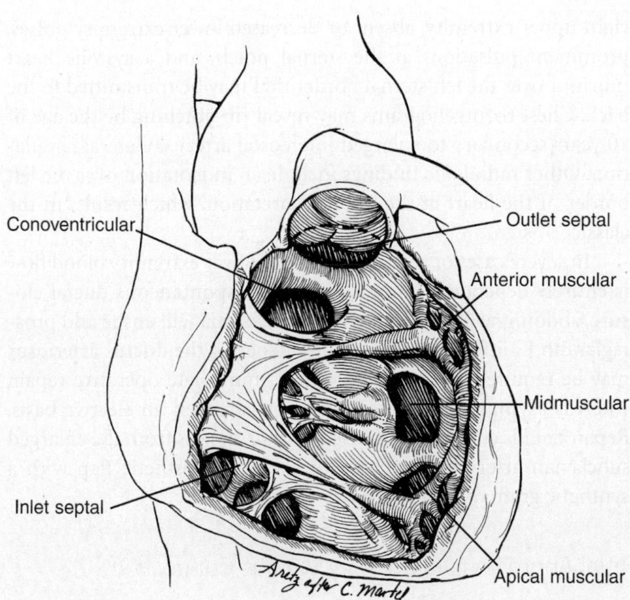

FIGURE 19.14 Major types of VSDs categorized by anatomic location. (From Kaiser LR, Kron IL, Spray TL, eds. *Mastery of Cardiothoracic Surgery*. Philadelphia: Lippincott-Raven Publishers; 1998.)

long-standing left-to-right shunting, there is medial hypertrophy of the pulmonary vasculature and an increase in pulmonary artery pressures. Over time, as the PVR increases, volume overload on the left heart decreases, and eventually, there is a reversal of flow through the VSD. With right-to-left shunting, there is a worsening cyanosis that ensues, referred to as Eisenmenger's syndrome. Once a diagnosis of Eisenmenger's syndrome has been made, operative repair is contraindicated given the high risk of right heart failure. With an intracardiac defect, a functioning right ventricle, and failing lungs secondary to elevated PVR, bilateral lung transplantation and intracardiac repair may be the only option. In the presence of a failing right ventricle, the only option would be a heart–lung transplant, of which few currently are done because of the scarcity of donors.

VSDs can be diagnosed by echocardiography. Early surgical repair is indicated for children with large VSDs with a pulmonary blood flow (Q_p):systemic blood flow (Q_s) ratio greater than 2. Moderate-sized defects are often monitored until childhood.

Patent Ductus Arteriosus

PDA results from failure of closure of the ductus arteriosus, which results in blood being shunted from the proximal descending thoracic aorta to the pulmonary artery bifurcation. PDAs take up to 3 months after birth to close and are therefore not considered pathologic until after this age. The male to female ratio is 1:2. Failure of closure after 3 months is thought to be secondary to immaturity of the medial muscular layer.

As with VSDs, left-to-right shunting of the blood occurs, resulting in increased pulmonary blood flow and left atrial and ventricular overload. On auscultation, a classic "machine-like" murmur is heard. Closure of the PDA can be attempted by pharmacologic means in newborns with inhibition of prostaglandins utilizing agents such as indomethacin. PDAs that fail to close may be

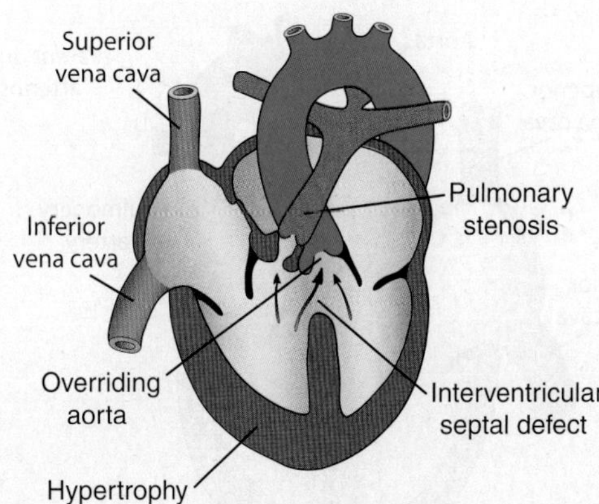

FIGURE 19.15 Tetralogy of fallot: schematic drawing. (From Sadler TW. *Langman's Medical Embryology*. 13th ed. Philadelphia: Wolters Kluwer; 2015.)

amenable to percutaneous embolization utilizing coils. In infants, if operative closure is required, these defects can often be approached thoracoscopically or via a small left thoracotomy.

Tetralogy of Fallot

Tetralogy of Fallot (TOF) results from an anterior misalignment of the infundibular septum. Classically, this malformation results in a VSD, overriding aorta, right ventricular outflow obstruction, and resultant right ventricular hypertrophy (Fig. 19.15). With the addition of an ASD, the condition is referred to as pentalogy of Fallot. Twenty-five percent of TOF patients have a right-sided aorta, and in addition, anomalies in the coronary circulation may also exist.

The extent of the cyanosis depends on the severity of the tetralogy. In severe cases, increased cyanosis can occur with agitation or crying. Older children often learn to squat to relieve cyanotic spells. Physical examination reveals a systolic murmur over the left heart border and an accentuated second aortic heart sound. Chest roentgenogram often demonstrates a boot-shaped heart. Conservative therapy includes a knee-to-chest position, supplemental oxygen, volume expansion, and sedation. Symptomatic infants should undergo immediate repair with elective repair done at 1 year of age for asymptomatic patients.

Tricuspid Atresia

Tricuspid atresia results from a lack of communication between the right atrium and ventricle. Associated anomalies include an ASD, enlarged mitral valve and left ventricle, and right ventricular hypoplasia. As with other congenital cardiac anomalies, echocardiography secures the diagnosis and nicely demonstrates the anatomic abnormalities. These patients require surgical correction in order to increase systemic oxygen saturation and avoid the development of heart failure. Surgical repair requires a Fontan procedure, an operation that results in the systemic venous return being connected directly to the pulmonary artery resulting in increased pulmonary blood flow, a decreased right-to-left shunt, and decreased volume overload of the left heart.

Transposition of the Great Vessels

Transposition of the great vessels (TGA) occurs when the aorta arises from the anatomic right ventricle and the pulmonary artery

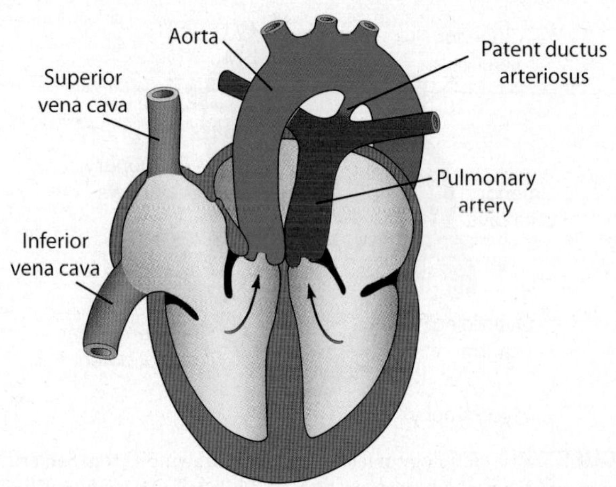

FIGURE 19.16 Transposition of the great vessels: schematic drawing. (From Sadler TW. *Langman's Medical Embryology*. 13th ed. Philadelphia: Wolters Kluwer; 2015.)

arises from the anatomic left ventricle (Fig. 19.16). TGA accounts for 8% to 10% of all congenital heart defects. Associated cardiac anomalies can include ASD, VSD, PDA, LV outflow obstruction, abnormal coronary branching, or PFO. Normal physiologic closure of the ductus arteriosus can result in profound cyanosis. In the case of complete TGA, survival depends upon early recognition and the presence of a right-to-left shunt in the form of a PDA or ASD. A closing ductus arteriosus can be maintained patent with infusion of prostaglandin E_1 to enhance the requisite left-to-right shunting, thereby providing temporary palliation. Alternatively, an ASD can be created percutaneously with a balloon septoplasty.

Diagnosis is confirmed by echocardiography. On physical examination, a systolic murmur and loud single heart sound can be appreciated. Chest roentgenogram reveals an oval or egg-shaped heart, narrow superior mediastinum, and increased pulmonary vascular markings. An arterial switch procedure in which the great vessels are transposed to their appropriate anatomic positions is the definitive operation for this anomaly.

Coarctation of the Aorta

Coarctation of the aorta is characterized by a focal narrowing of the thoracic aorta, most frequently just distal to the origin of the left subclavian artery usually near the ductus arteriosus. Coarctation accounts for 5% to 8% of all congenital heart defects. Associated anomalies include PDA, VSD, bicuspid aortic valve, subaortic obstruction, and mitral valve anomalies.

Coarctation has historically been categorized as either infantile or adult. In infantile coarctation, the aortic obstruction is most often preductal and leads to separation of the LV flow directed to the head and arms from the pulmonary artery flow directed to the lower body. This type of coarctation results in early LV failure and death if not surgically corrected. The more common adult type of coarctation is postductal and leads to proximal hypertension and eventual CHF over time, although patients may remain asymptomatic and appear healthy well into adulthood.

Physical findings of absent femoral pulses with poor distal perfusion should warrant a workup for coarctation of the aorta. Findings on physical examination include upper extremity systolic hypertension and a pressure differential between the left and right upper extremity, absent or decreased lower extremity pulses, prominent pulsations at the sternal notch, and a systolic heart murmur over the left sternal border that may be transmitted to the back. Chest roentgenograms may reveal rib notching by the age of 10 years secondary to enlarged intercostal artery collateral circulation. Other radiologic findings include an indentation over the left border of the heart at the site of coarctation, which results in the classic "3" sign.

In severe cases of aortic coarctation, lower extremity blood flow is entirely dependent upon a PDA. With spontaneous ductal closure, abdominal and lower extremity ischemia will ensue and prostaglandin E_1 infusion to maintain patency of the ductus arteriosus may be required. Severe cases require immediate operative repair, whereas asymptomatic cases can be repaired on an elective basis. Repair entails either an end-to-end repair, bypass from the enlarged subclavian artery to the descending aorta, prosthetic flap with a synthetic graft, or subclavian flap aortoplasty.

Total Anomalous Pulmonary Venous Connection

Total anomalous pulmonary venous connection (TAPVC) is a condition in which there is abnormal drainage of the pulmonary veins into the right atrium. The presence of either a PFO or ASD is required to maintain blood flow to the left heart and thus the systemic circulation. Severity of symptoms depends on whether there is obstructed or nonobstructed TAPVC. With obstructed TAPVC, the obstruction causes pulmonary hypertension, decreased venous return, low cardiac output, venous congestion, and acidosis. Obstructed TAPVC is a surgical emergency. Unobstructed cases present similar to that of an ASD. Operative repair is recommended for unobstructed TAPVC once diagnosed to prevent pulmonary hypertension and minimize mortality. Up to 80% of infants with TAPVC will die by 1 year of age if the condition is not surgically repaired.

Hypoplastic Left Heart Disease

Hypoplastic left heart syndrome (HLHS) accounts for 7% of congenital cardiac anomalies and accounts for 25% of deaths within the first week of life. HLHS is a complex anomaly with aortic and aortic valve hypoplasia, mitral valve stenosis, and a hypoplastic left ventricle. A PDA is essential for survival of the neonate and mandates infusion of prostaglandin E_1. Systemic blood flow is dependent on the parallel circulation that exists from the right ventricle to the systemic circulation via the PDA. Once the lungs expand and the PVR drops, blood flow preferentially flows to the pulmonary circulation. In order to balance pulmonary and systemic circulations, PVR should be controlled by adjusting ventilation, hematocrit should be increased, and SVR should be altered pharmacologically.

Newborns typically present within the first 48 hours of life with tachypnea and cyanosis. Echocardiography is almost universally diagnostic. Initial management includes prostaglandin E_1 infusion and pharmacologic balancing of the systemic and pulmonary circulations. Operative repair is carried out in three stages. The first operation, the Norwood procedure, involves connection of the diminutive aorta to the proximal pulmonary artery, at the same time a graft is placed between the innominate artery and pulmonary trunk. At the second stage, performed at 3 to 10 months of age, a hemi-Fontan procedure is performed whereby SVC blood is directed exclusively into the pulmonary artery. The final stage,

TABLE 19.1 Canadian Cardiovascular Society functional classification

Class I	Ordinary physical activity does not cause angina. Angina may occur with strenuous or prolonged exertion.
Class II	Slight limitation of ordinary activity. Angina may occur with walking or climbing stairs rapidly; walking uphill; walking or stair climbing after meals or in the cold, in the wind, or under emotional stress; or walking more than two blocks on the level or climbing more than one flight of stairs under normal conditions at a normal pace.
Class III	Marked limitation of ordinary physical activity. Angina may occur after walking one or two blocks on level ground or climbing one flight of stairs under normal conditions at a normal place.
Class IV	Inability to carry out any physical activity without anginal discomfort; angina may be present at rest.

From Braunwald E. The history. In: Braunwald E, ed. *Heart Disease: A Textbook of Cardiovascular Medicine.* 5th ed. Philadelphia: WB Saunders; 1997:1–14, with permission.

performed at 18 to 24 months, involves redirection of the IVC and SVC blood flow into the pulmonary circulation, the Fontan procedure. Some centers prefer to immediately list these neonates for heart transplantations and reserve the 3-stage procedure if a donor cannot be found.

Acquired Heart Disease

Cardiovascular disease is the number one killer of Americans, accounting for 37.3% of all deaths in the United States. The 2015 American Heart Association Heart Disease and Stroke Update estimates that there are 84 million people suffering from some form of cardiovascular disease, 15 million Americans suffering from coronary heart disease, and 5 million suffering from heart failure. Heart disease is the number one cause of death in the United States, killing over 375,000 people per year, which is more than all the cancers combined. With an increasing prevalence of diabetes, obesity, and a sedentary lifestyle, the incidence of cardiovascular disease is expected to increase dramatically with an increasing incidence in children and young adults.

Coronary Artery Disease

Coronary artery disease (CAD) is the leading cause of mortality in the United States. Similar to peripheral vascular disease, CAD is due to luminal narrowing with resultant decrease in blood flow secondary to progressive atherosclerotic disease. Risk factors for atherosclerotic disease include hypertension, diabetes, hypercholesterolemia, smoking, sedentary lifestyle, and family history. Men are at higher risk than women for developing premature coronary artery, but after menopause, the risk is equivalent. Patients with CAD can present with a spectrum of signs and symptoms ranging from asymptomatic to chronic severe angina, depending on the extent of disease and degree of luminal narrowing. Diabetic patients often have no symptoms until a major cardiovascular event ensues. The Canadian Cardiovascular Society Functional Classification has been developed to classify anginal symptoms related to CAD (Table 19.1). A second similar grading system for heart failure is the New York Heart Association Heart Failure Functional Classification, which is a subjective classification system (Table 19.2). Asymptomatic patients may present with myocardial

TABLE 19.2 New York Heart Association heart failure functional classification

Class I	Patients with cardiac disease but without resulting limitation of physical activity
Class II	Patients with cardiac disease resulting in slight limitation of physical activity. Ordinary physical activity causes fatigue, palpitations, dyspnea, or angina. No symptoms at rest
Class III	Patients with cardiac disease resulting in marked limitation of physical activity. Less than ordinary physical activity results in fatigue, palpitations, dyspnea, or angina. No symptoms at rest
Class IV	Patients with cardiac disease who are unable to carry on any physical activity without discomfort. Symptoms of cardiac insufficiency or angina may be present even at rest. Any physical activity increases discomfort.

From Braunwald E. The history. In: Braunwald E, ed. *Heart Disease: A Textbook of Cardiovascular Medicine.* 5th ed. Philadelphia: WB Saunders; 1997:1–14, with permission.

infarction (MI) or even sudden death related to malignant arrhythmias. Roughly one half of all fatal heart attacks occur in previously asymptomatic individuals.

Over 10% of patients undergoing noncardiac surgical procedures in the United States are estimated to be at risk for CAD. More than 15% of these patients suffer from cardiovascular complications in the postoperative period. This risk is even greater in patients with peripheral vascular disease. It is critical to appropriately identify patients at risk for CAD and evaluate them for critical disease. Diagnostic studies traditionally utilized to identify patients at risk for CAD have included stress echocardiography, stress electrocardiography and thallium tests, and intravenous (IV) dipyridamole thallium 201 or technetium 99m scintigraphy (DTS). Newer modalities including high-resolution cardiac computed tomography and magnetic resonance imaging become more prevalent for diagnosis. DTS is the best initial preoperative noninvasive screening test. As compared to exercise stress tests, DTS can be performed on patients who are unable to perform the exercise portion of the study. In DTS, a finding of reversible defects following infusion of the radiotracer at stress when compared to resting images reflects viable myocardium, where as a nonreversible defect signifies scar that not amenable nor responsive to revascularization. Results obtained by either thallium or technetium scintigraphy are 90% sensitive and 75% specific. The findings of CAD on DTS warrant a coronary angiogram to define any coronary lesions and appropriate therapy either in the form of coronary artery bypass grafting (CABG) or a percutaneous coronary intervention (PCI) to enhance myocardial perfusion. Coronary revascularization is generally performed to alleviate increasing anginal symptoms, preserve at-risk myocardium, and prevent MI and damage. Noncritical coronary lesions can often be managed medically until progression of disease ensues.

Based upon the large body of literature comparing medical therapy, PCI, and CABG, the American College of Cardiology and the American Heart Association have established guidelines for surgical revascularization. These in-depth criteria are beyond the scope of this chapter. The general guidelines include left main stenosis, disease in three or more vessels, proximal LAD stenosis, and failure of PCI. Diabetic patients have been shown to fare better with CABG as compared to PCI. In general, CABG is not performed on vessels with lesions less than 70% due to decreased patency rates related to outflow obstruction from competitive flow in the native circulation.

The long-term benefits of CABG are primarily related to patency of the conduit. Vein grafts develop intimal hyperplasia that limits long-term patency to 50% to 60% at 10 years. In contrast, the internal mammary artery (IMA) has been reported to have patency rates upward of 95% as far out as 20 years following operation. Statistically significant improvements in patient survival have been demonstrated in patients receiving an IMA to LAD bypass (Fig. 19.17).

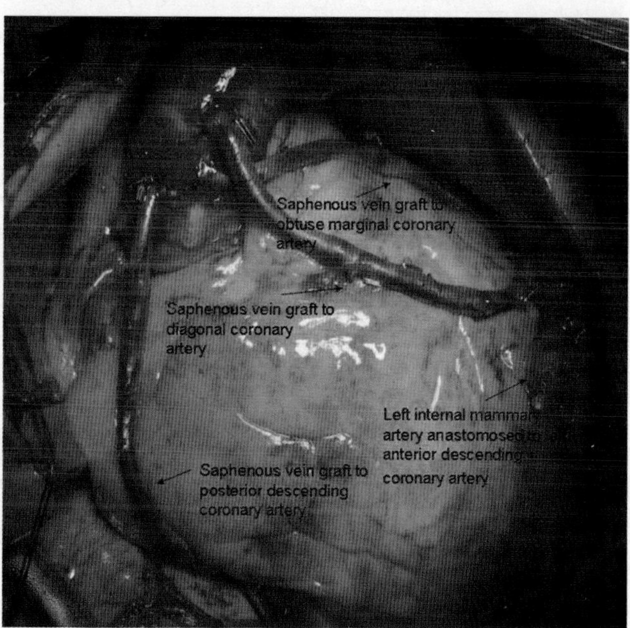

FIGURE 19.17 Coronary artery bypass grafting performed for atherosclerotic coronary artery disease.

Alternatives to Traditional Coronary Artery Bypass Grafting

CABG accounted for 300,000 operative procedures in 2014. CABG has traditionally been performed with the assistance of the cardiopulmonary bypass (CPB) circuit with an arrested heart. This allows for a still operative field and optimal circulatory management. The CPB circuit is utilized to isolate the cardiopulmonary system and thereby provide optimal, blood-free operative exposure for cardiovascular surgery. The CPB circuit must perform the functions of the cardiovascular system. It must oxygenate blood, remove carbon dioxide, and provide adequate perfusion to end organs. The cardiovascular surgeon can utilize either total or partial CPB. During total CPB, the venous return of the heart is circulated through the CPB circuit in its entirety, whereas during partial CPB, a fraction of the blood is allowed to circulate to the right ventricle and pulmonary circulation.

The basic components of the CPB circuit include the venous reservoir, oxygenator, heat exchanger, and pump. The venous reservoir stores systemic venous return. The oxygenator both adds oxygen and removes carbon dioxide from the blood. Thermoregulation of blood is controlled by the heat exchanger. Blood is returned to the systemic circulation via the ascending aorta or femoral artery by the pump. The pump can either be a kinetic centrifugal pump or the more common electric motor-driven, load-independent roller pump. It is important to note, however, that CPB activates the complement cascade, triggers the release of proinflammatory cytokines, up-regulates inflammatory mediators (IL-1, TNF-α, IL-6, IL-8, IL-10), initiates the systemic inflammatory response syndrome (SIRS), stimulates oxygen-free radical generation, and increases oxidative stress. In order to minimize these systemic manifestations, a renewed interest in beating heart surgery has arisen.

Off-pump coronary artery bypass (OPCAB) grafting is performed on a beating heart with the use of stabilization devices to minimize motion at the site of anastomoses. Blood flow to the affected myocardium can be sustained with the use of an intraluminal shunt, which minimizes blood in the operative field. Alternatively, Silastic tapes can be utilized as a tourniquet for proximal and/or distal control. The most critical vessels that supply the greatest amount of myocardium at risk are traditionally grafted first, that is, LAD, to maximize perfusion to the heart throughout the case. Randomized controlled trials have demonstrated significantly lower transfusion requirements, decreased systemic inflammation, shorter hospital stay, and decreased cost. Trends toward lower renal complications are also observed. Circulatory management is much more difficult in OPCAB and requires very close communication between the surgeon and anesthesiologist. OPCAB is associated with a significant learning curve and is therefore performed at the discretion of the surgeon based upon experience. Heart failure, hemodynamic instability, severe LV dysfunction, cardiomyopathy, frequent arrhythmias, and emergent operations were once absolute contraindications for OPCAB, but are now relative contraindications based upon surgeon experience and preference.

The rapid development of minimally invasive techniques in gynecologic, urologic, and general surgery has stimulated an interest in revascularizing myocardium utilizing smaller incisions. Initially, this consisted of performing beating heart revascularization through small partial sternotomies or anterolateral thoracotomies, depending on the target vessels of interest. This approach was originally termed minimally invasive direct coronary artery bypass (MIDCAB). Often, these incisions can be limited to between 8 and 10 cm and yield excellent cosmetic results. MIDCAB is amenable to single as well as multivessel coronary disease. However, it is most ideally suited for an isolated LIMA to LAD anastomosis. Clinical trials have demonstrated excellent patency and rapid recovery following MIDCAB.

Robotic Cardiac Surgery

The development of robotic technology has further advanced minimally invasive techniques in cardiac surgery. The progressively advancing technology has facilitated sternal sparing minimally invasive access to the heart. Robotic systems are comprised of miniaturized surgical instruments mounted on long thin shafts with multiple degrees of range of motion improving mobility and elimination surgeon tremor, coupled with a dual camera endoscope providing three-dimensional high-magnification visualization (Fig. 19.18). Most recently, excellent outcomes have been observed in large series including the ability to conduct coronary revascularization, mitral valve repair, ASD closure, LV pacing lead implantation, and aortic valve surgery.

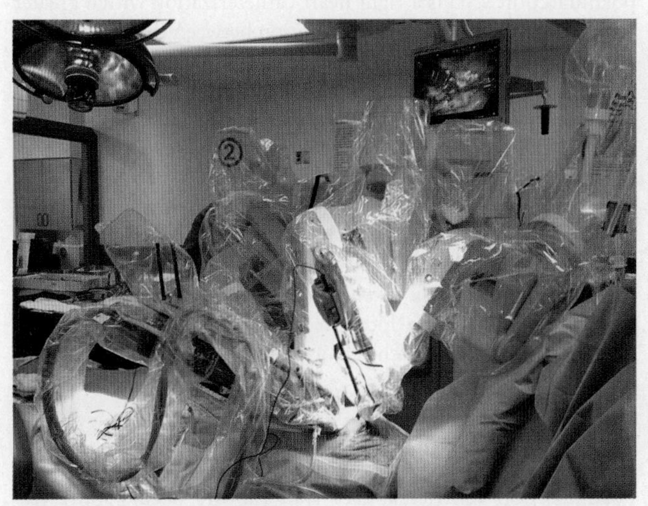
A

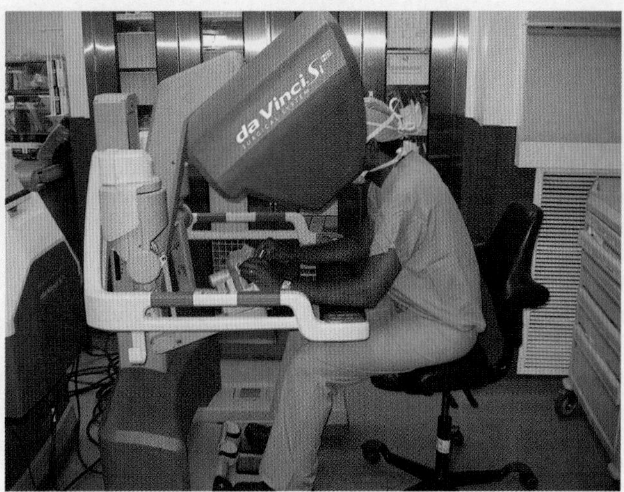

B

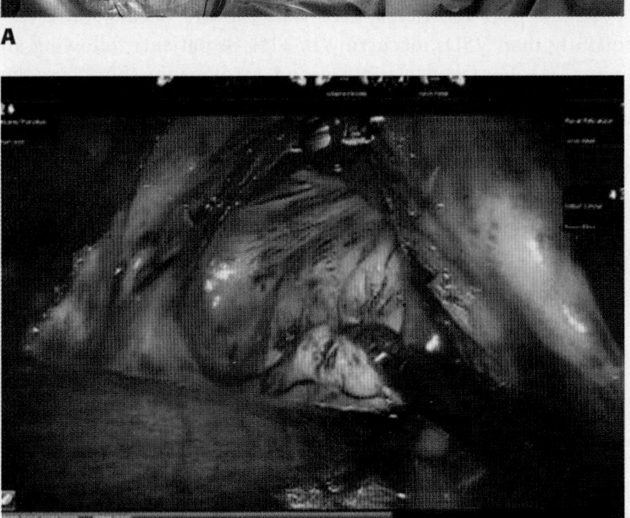
C

FIGURE 19.18 The da Vinci robotic telemanipulation system. **A.** The robotic endoscope and instruments inserted into the patient. **B.** Surgeon instrument control console. **C.** Surgeon optics during a robotic mitral valve repair.

Randomized clinical trials of robotically assisted totally endoscopic coronary artery bypass grafting (TECAB) performed using CPB with peripheral cannulation have demonstrated TECAB to be a safe procedure with angiographic patency, mortality, and morbidity equivalent to standard CABG procedures. Further advances in technology, surgical expertise, and reduced cost will be required before TECAB can become widespread.

The advantages of the robotic system over "traditional open" surgery are being investigated but primarily stem from the less invasive nature of the access to the heart resulting in less tissue trauma and less bleeding. Overall, studies have noted less pain, improved cosmesis, shorter hospital stay, faster recovery, and greater patient satisfaction.

Myocardial Infarction

The American Heart Association and the Centers for Disease Control and Prevention estimate that 735,000 Americans will have a heart attack, 525,000 will have a first heart attack, and 210,000 will have recurrent heart attacks. Furthermore, nearly 175,000 will have a silent heart attack. About 38% of patients suffering an MI will die in the ensuing year. Roughly, a heart attack is occurring every 20 seconds in an American with a death occurring every 60 seconds. Advances in medical management and interventions for MI have reduced the mortality from acute MI by 24% since 1989. The goal of therapy is to rapidly salvage as much myocardium as is feasible. Loss of more than 40% of functional LV mass often results in cardiogenic shock. Reperfusion of myocardium 40 minutes after onset of acute ischemia results in salvage of 60% to 70% of affected myocardium, while as little as 3 hours following ischemia, only 10% of myocardium can be salvaged.

Medical management of MI necessitates rapid intervention. Treatment should include decreasing myocardial oxygen demand, increasing arterial oxygen delivery, maintaining perfusion, and protecting the threatened myocardium. Early reperfusion should be the goal. Depending on the expertise of a given medical facility, thrombolytics or angioplasty can be utilized. Thrombolytic therapy is easy to perform in most community settings by trained health care professionals. Since time to reperfusion is essential, this is often the strategy utilized in facilities lacking cardiac catheterization laboratories. If feasible, the preferred approach to myocardial salvage is rapid evaluation and transfer to a cardiac catheterization lab for PCI with the potential for emergent CABG in the event of left main CAD or if the lesions are not revascularizable by PCI.

Vasopressors and inotropic agents are the first-line therapy for cardiogenic shock. Maintenance of optimal filling pressures is essential and may require insertion of a pulmonary artery catheter to optimize management. Ventilatory support and/or diuresis may be necessary to maintain proper oxygenation in the setting of acute cardiogenic pulmonary edema. While medical management is essential, early revascularization with either PCI or CABG is critical and has been shown to significantly improve long-term survival.

Complications of Myocardial Infarction

A number of structural sequelae may ensue in the early or late postinfarction period that require prompt surgical intervention. These complications include the following: VSD, ventricular free wall rupture, LV aneurysm, and ischemic mitral regurgitation (MR). Early recognition and treatment of these issues is critical to maximizing survival. Overall, these postinfarction complications are responsible for 20% of deaths following MI.

Ventricular Septal Defect

Postinfarction VSDs complicate 1% to 2% of MIs, accounting for 5% of deaths following an MI. Roughly 60% of postinfarction VSDs occur in the anteroapical septum as a result of a full-thickness anterior wall MI secondary to an LAD occlusion with limited collateral vessel formation. The remainder of patients have posterior septal VSDs resulting from occlusion of either a dominant right or circumflex coronary artery. Postinfarction VSDs occur most frequently 2 to 4 days following an acute MI, but can occur between a few hours to a few weeks following infarction. The VSD may be a simple rupture or may develop a serpiginous dissection tract.

Typically, patients present with a new-onset harsh holosystolic murmur that radiates to the axilla and is often associated with chest pain and a thrill. The gold standard for diagnosis of a postinfarction VSD is a right heart catheterization with a greater than 9% "step-up" in oxygen saturation between the right atrium and pulmonary artery. Color flow Doppler echocardiography is also a good diagnostic modality for VSD. Once diagnosed, immediate placement of an intra-aortic balloon pump (IABP) and early surgical intervention are necessary. Preoperative management centers on reducing systemic vascular resistance (SVR) while maintaining cardiac output and systemic perfusion. Without an operation, this condition is almost universally fatal, with 7% survival at 1 year if left untreated. Patients in cardiogenic shock should be immediately taken to the operating room. Operative repair depends on the location of the defect, but in general involves endocardial patch repair with possible exclusion of the infracted myocardium.

Ventricular Free Wall Rupture

Postinfarction ventricular free wall rupture occurs more frequently than VSDs, occurring in 11% of patients following an acute MI. Ventricular rupture and cardiogenic shock are the leading causes of mortality following an MI. Postinfarction ventricular free wall rupture is more common in elderly women suffering their first MI. In the present era, ruptures occur most frequently in hypertensive patients within 5 days of infarction. Rupture can affect the anterior, lateral, and posterior walls. LV ruptures are divided into three categories: acute, subacute, and chronic. Acute ruptures result in sudden chest pain, profound shock, electromechanical dissociation, and rapid death. Subacute rupture is characterized by a smaller defect that may be sealed by clot or fibrinous pericardial adhesions. They usually present with signs of tamponade and cardiogenic shock and may remain stable for several hours or days prior to intervention. A chronic rupture presents as a false aneurysm of the left ventricle with adhesions containing the aneurysm. Diagnosis of rupture is best made with echocardiography. Operative repair involves mattress closure of the defect buttressed with Teflon felt or a Dacron patch.

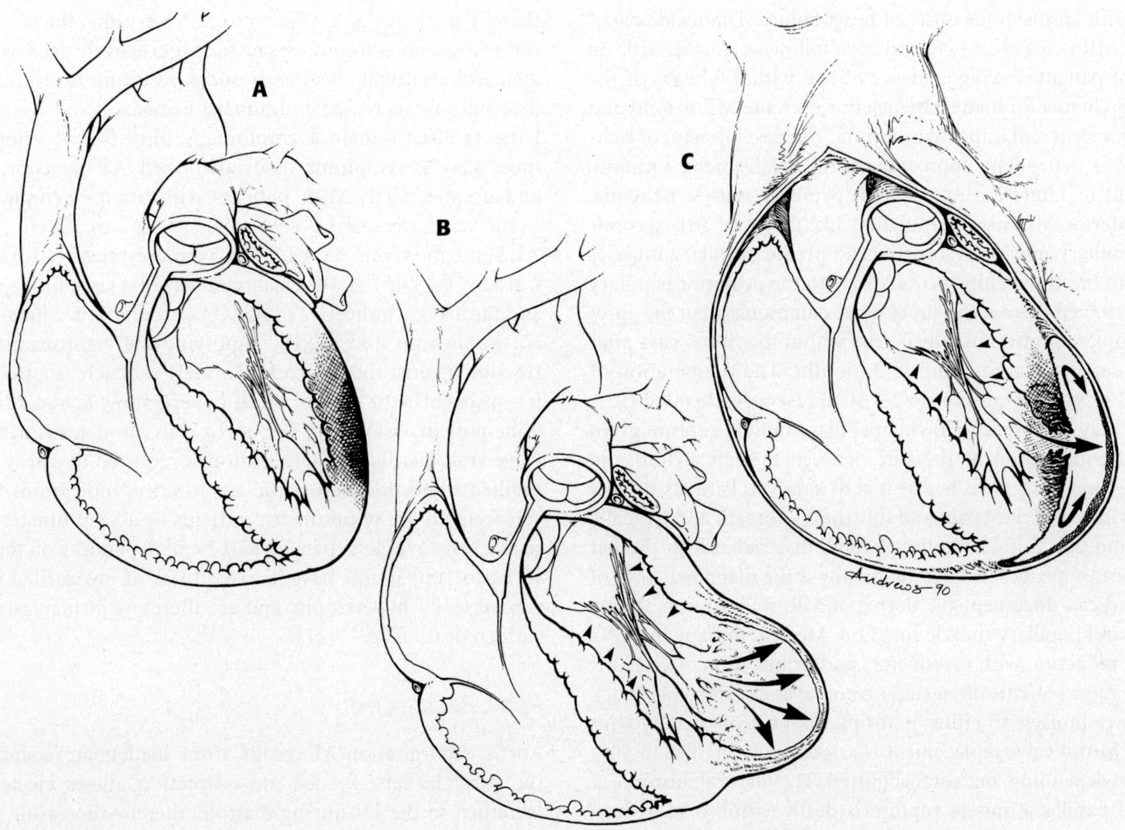

FIGURE 19.19 The pathophysiology of LV aneurysm formation. **A.** Area of infarction. **B.** True aneurysm. **C.** False aneurysm. (From Kaiser LR, Kron IL, Spray TL, eds. *Mastery of Cardiothoracic Surgery*. Philadelphia: Lippincott-Raven Publishers; 1998.)

Left Ventricular Aneurysm

LV aneurysms affect between 10% and 35% of patients following an MI (Fig. 19.19). Aneurysm formation occurs in 50% of patients by 48 hours following an MI. Aneurysm formation is thought to occur as a result of early infarct expansion and late remodeling of the aneurysmal wall with scar. Asymptomatic patients have an excellent prognosis following aneurysm formation with a 90% 10-year survival. Symptomatic patients have a much poorer prognosis. Angina related to underlying CAD and dyspnea are the most common presenting symptoms. Diagnosis can be made using multiple diagnostic modalities. ECGs frequently demonstrate Q waves with persistent ST elevation. Chest radiographs may demonstrate LV enlargement (Fig. 19.20). Echocardiography can often detect a paradoxical bulge during systole of the aneurysm. The gold standard for diagnosis remains left ventriculography. There are no absolute indications for operative repair. Symptomatic patients with angina, CHF, or arrhythmias appear to do better following repair. Surgical intervention involves either simple plication of the aneurysm, linear closure, or closure with a Dacron patch. In the absence of thrombus, there is a low thromboembolic risk, 0.35% per patient-year, and therefore, anticoagulation is not required. In the setting of large LV thrombus or diminished LV function, long-term anticoagulation is recommended.

Ischemic Mitral Regurgitation

MI or papillary muscle ischemia results in ischemic mitral regurgitation (MR). By definition, the leaflets and subvalvular apparatus are normal in ischemic MR. The disease is a manifestation of postischemic myocardial remodeling. The presentation may be acute and immediately life threatening or may present in a chronic

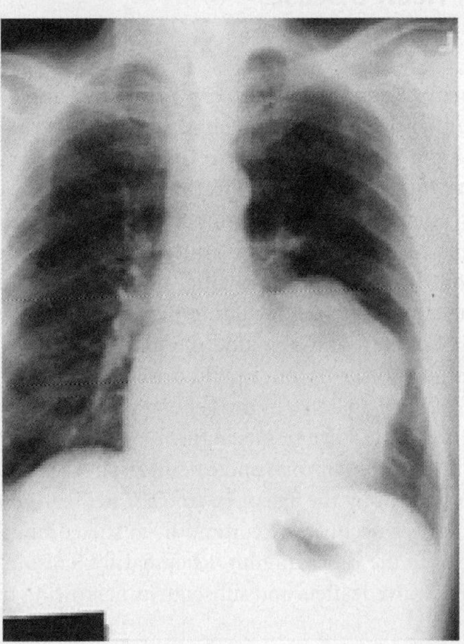

FIGURE 19.20 Chest radiograph demonstrating large ventricular aneurysm. (From Kaiser LR, Kron IL, Spray TL, eds. *Mastery of Cardiothoracic Surgery*. Philadelphia: Lippincott-Raven Publishers; 1998.)

fashion with an insidious onset of heart failure. The incidence of ischemic MR is between 17% and 55% following an MI, with up to 18% of patients having evidence of MR within 6 hours of the onset of ischemia. In many patients, however, the MR is mild and may be transient and improve over time. The development of ischemic MR is dependent upon transmural involvement, location, and extent of infarction or resultant papillary muscle ischemia. Posteroinferior MIs have the highest likelihood of MR secondary to papillary muscle dysfunction. Ruptured papillary muscles can lead to life-threatening acute MR, with the posterior papillary muscle involved three to six times more commonly than the anterior. Complete rupture usually occurs within the first 7 days after MI but may be delayed by up to 3 months. The presentation of acute MR represents only 1% to 2% of all cases of ischemic MR. A murmur may be absent following papillary muscle rupture given the rapid equalization of pressure between the left atrium and ventricle. Rapid diagnosis is essential to survival. Patients usually present with acute chest pain and shortness of breath and typically have a loud apical holosystolic murmur that radiates to the left axilla. Transesophageal echocardiography is the diagnostic tool of choice and can document the degree of MR, wall motion abnormalities, and papillary muscle function. Medical therapy includes afterload reduction with vasodilators and/or insertion of an IABP, although these patients often suffer from severe cardiogenic shock that is unresponsive to either inotropic support or therapy with an IABP. Mitral valve replacement is associated with 10% to 40% mortality depending on comorbidities. The natural history of untreated papillary muscle rupture is death within 3 to 4 days, although patients with partial rupture may survive for weeks. For patients with chronic ischemic MR, indications for operation include symptomatic coronary disease, severe MR (3+ or 4+), or significant LV dysfunction secondary to MR. Surgical intervention consists of either valve replacement or repair with potential CABG for severe CAD.

Valvular Heart Disease

Aortic Stenosis

The majority of aortic stenosis (AS) within the United States is a result of either degenerative or congenital AS, with rheumatic AS representing a small subset. Age-related degenerative AS is secondary to protein and lipid infiltration of the aortic valve leaflet with subsequent cellular infiltration and ultimately calcification. This results in increased valve stiffness and increasing valvular obstruction. Risk factors for calcific AS are the traditional risk factors for atherosclerosis including hypertension, hypercholesterolemia, diabetes, and smoking. Calcified bicuspid AS is the most common form of congenital aortic valve disease, with an incidence of 0.9% to 2.0% of the general population. The bicuspid structure of the valve results in turbulent flow, which disrupts the valve resulting in fibrosis and calcification. Clinically evident stenosis is present by the age of 50 to 60. Calcifications of bicuspid aortic valves occur more commonly at the commissures and often extend to the valve annulus. Rheumatic AS results in fusion of the aortic valve leaflets and subsequent narrowing of the outflow tract.

Physiologically, as the valve area narrows, the left ventricle hypertrophies (with resultant decreasing diastolic compliance) in order to generate increased pressures for ventricular ejection, thereby maintaining cardiac output. Over time, the left ventricle is no longer able to compensate for progressively decreasing valve area and eventually begins to dilate, resulting in decreased cardiac output, increased pulmonary pressures, and heart failure. Patients often remain asymptomatic until they develop one or more classic symptoms associated with AS: syncope, angina, and dyspnea/CHF. Most patients will become symptomatic at aortic valve areas of 1.0 cm^2 (normal = 2.5 to 3.5 cm^2, mild AS >1.5 cm^2, moderate AS = 1.0 to 1.5 cm^2, severe AS < 1.0 cm^2, critical AS < 0.7 cm^2). A weak arterial pulse that rises slowly ("parvus and tardus") is indicative of AS. On auscultation, a harsh systolic aortic murmur and loud S_4 signifying the vigorous atrial contraction against the noncompliant left ventricle is audible. ECG is consistent with LV and atrial hypertrophy. Echocardiography is helpful in visualizing the aortic valve and measuring aortic valve area. Cardiac catheterization is required to assess pressure gradients and flow across the aortic valve. Indications for valve replacement are symptomatic patients or asymptomatic patients with a valve area less than 1.0 to 0.7 cm^2 depending on the clinical scenario. AS patients have increased risk of myocardial ischemia related to LV hypertrophy and are therefore at increased risk of sudden death (Fig. 19.21).

Aortic Regurgitation

Aortic regurgitation/AI results from inadequate coaptation of the valve leaflets. Inadequate coaptation allows ejected blood to return to the LV during diastole, thereby increasing diastolic stress and resulting in concentric LV hypertrophy. Etiology of AI includes rheumatic heart disease, dilatation of the aortic root, aortic dissection, infective endocarditis, myxomatous degeneration, bicuspid aortic valve, rheumatoid arthritis, and systemic lupus erythematosus. With acute AI, the LV is unable to dilate to accommodate the large regurgitant flows producing a low cardiac output state with elevated heart rate and diastolic ventricular pressures.

Physical findings with AI vary depending on the duration of symptoms. For example, in acute AI, the pulse pressure is not widened, resulting in a lack of clinical symptoms. A classic "water hammer pulse" is present with chronic AI. Auscultation reveals a prominent S_3 and other symptoms of heart failure, including rales. Most patients with chronic AI remain asymptomatic for

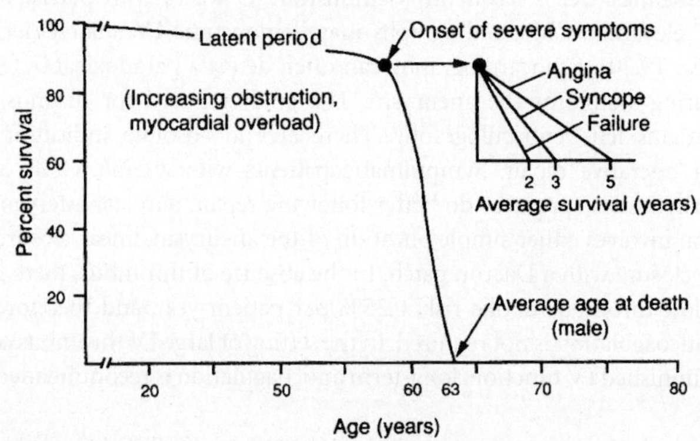

FIGURE 19.21 The natural history of medically treated AS. (From Kaiser LR, Kron IL, Spray TL, eds. *Mastery of cardiothoracic surgery*. 2nd ed. Philadelphia: Lippincott-Raven Publishers; 2007.)

years until there is an increase in the size of the regurgitant orifice leading to the onset of symptoms and heart failure. The onset of symptoms is associated with nearly 60% to 70% of regurgitant stroke volume to the left ventricle. Echocardiography is the most helpful diagnostic modality since it allows for measurement of the regurgitant jet and LV geometry and function. Asymptomatic patients may be followed with close observation and serial echocardiograms until they experience symptoms or noninvasive modalities demonstrate LV dilatation. Patients with acute AI and those with chronic disease and symptoms should undergo valve replacement.

Idiopathic Hypertrophic Subaortic Stenosis

Idiopathic hypertrophic subaortic stenosis (IHSS) is an asymmetrical, obstructive hypertrophic cardiomyopathy in which there is anatomic and physiologic obstruction of the LV outflow tract. Pathologically, IHSS results in marked thickening of the middle and upper ventricular septum. Histologic examination reveals an atypical whorled configuration of myocytes and connective tissue elements described as myocardial disarray.

LV outflow obstruction is dynamic, increasing with decreased ventricular volume and the use of inotropes. Patients with IHSS can be asymptomatic or present with symptoms of LV outflow tract obstruction (dyspnea, angina) or even sudden death. On physical examination, a systolic murmur can be heard over the left sternal border. ECG and chest radiographs demonstrate LV hypertrophy. Echocardiograms display various patterns of hypertrophy and mitral valve function. Cardiac catheterization provides pullback gradient measurements across the outflow tract as well as coronary arteriograms.

Usually, symptomatic patients can be treated nonsurgically with beta blockers and calcium channel blockers. Operation is reserved for patients with severe symptoms and resting or provocative gradients despite maximal medical therapy. Operative intervention is also indicated in patients who have survived sudden death episodes and have significant resting or provocative gradients. Surgical treatment of IHSS may involve LV myotomy and myomectomy or, in certain cases, elimination of systolic anterior motion of the mitral valve by mitral valve replacement or Alfieri repair of the mitral valve. Modern innovations also include alcohol ablation of the hypertrophic septum by injection into the first septal perforator using percutaneous techniques and synchronized AV pacing to reduce dynamic outflow obstruction.

Mitral Stenosis

Rheumatic heart disease is the most common cause of mitral stenosis (MS). In the United States and other developed countries, the incidence of MS has decreased dramatically. Pathologic changes include commissural fusion, leaflet fibrosis, and chordal fusion and shortening. With progression of disease and narrowing of the valve area, chronic pulmonary venous obstruction ensues with elevations of left atrial pressures, pulmonary hypertension, right ventricular enlargement, and CHF. Classically, patients present with dyspnea (initially on exertion but eventually even at rest), orthopnea, paroxysmal nocturnal dyspnea, and fatigue. Systemic thromboembolism may be the presenting symptom and occurs in up to 20% of patients. Auscultatory findings include a presystolic murmur, opening snap, and diastolic rumble. Chest radiography often reveals left

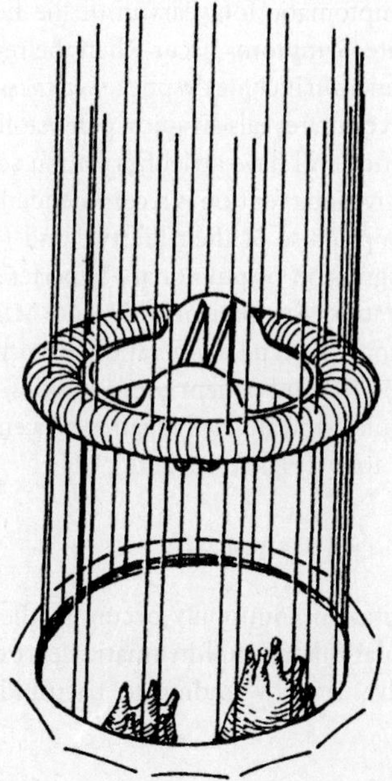

FIGURE 19.22 Conventional mitral valve replacement with complete excision of the leaflets and the entire subvalvular apparatus. The mitral prosthesis is implanted using a series of horizontal mattress sutures. (From Kaiser LR, Kron IL, Spray TL, eds. *Mastery of cardiothoracic surgery*. 2nd ed. Philadelphia: Lippincott-Raven Publishers; 2007.)

atrial enlargement and pulmonary congestion. Echocardiography is the primary means for assessing mitral valve anatomy and flow dynamics. Symptomatic patients often have mitral valve areas of 1.5 to 2.0 cm^2 (normal = 4.0 to 6.0 cm^2), whereas valve areas of 1.0 cm^2 or less are associated with severe symptoms. Surgery is indicated for patients with hemodynamically significant valve obstruction and NYHA class III to IV symptoms, onset of atrial fibrillation regardless of symptoms, increasing pulmonary hypertension, episodes of systemic embolization, or infective endocarditis. Operative intervention consists of mitral valve replacement (Fig. 19.22). The choice of a mechanical or tissue valve depends on the age of the patient, the probability of long-term survival, and risks/desire of anticoagulation. Mechanical valves have good long-term durability but require lifelong anticoagulation. Tissue valves often last between 10 and 14 years and require redocardiac surgery and valve replacement at that point.

Mitral Regurgitation

Mitral valve competence depends on the coordinated function of the annulus, leaflets, chordae tendineae, papillary muscles, left atrium, and left ventricle. Dysfunction of any of these components can result in MR. The most common etiology of MR is myxomatous degeneration. Other causes include ischemic heart disease, dilated cardiomyopathy, rheumatic heart disease, mitral annular calcification (MAC), endocarditis, chordal rupture, and collagen vascular disorders.

Clinically, left atrial pressures are elevated secondary to regurgitant blood flow. Progressive disease results in pulmonary venous obstruction, pulmonary hypertension, and right heart failure. Additionally, the left ventricle is chronically subjected to volume overload resulting in LV dilatation and left heart failure. Patients may remain asymptomatic for years until the heart is no longer able to compensate. Symptoms occur when the regurgitant volume approaches 50% and can include dyspnea, weakness, fatigue, and palpitations. Physical exam reveals an apical pansystolic murmur and S_3 gallop. Patients often will have atrial fibrillation secondary to atrial dilatation. Operative intervention is recommended for symptomatic patients with compromise of their lifestyle and for asymptomatic patients with progression of pulmonary hypertension, atrial fibrillation, or LV dilatation. Any patient with acute MR should undergo an urgent operation. The type of operation performed is dependent upon surgical expertise and patient comorbidities. Operative strategies include complex mitral valve repair, replacement, and in rare cases commissurotomy (Figs. 19.23 and 19.24).

Tricuspid and Pulmonic Valves

Tricuspid regurgitation commonly occurs in the setting of heart failure with annular dilatation. Rheumatic heart disease can affect the tricuspid valve, thereby leading to tricuspid stenosis and/or regurgitation. Acquired pulmonary valve disease is rare, although rheumatic involvement can occur. Valve fibrosis secondary to carcinoid syndrome most commonly affects right-sided valves.

Infective Endocarditis

Infection of the heart most commonly affects the valves. Predisposing factors for development of infective endocarditis include previous congenital or acquired cardiac lesions, immunocompromised status, IV catheters, and IV drug abuse. Gram-positive organisms are the most common cause of bacterial endocarditis (i.e., *Streptococcus viridans*, *Staphylococcus aureus*, and *Staphylococcus epidermis*), though gram-negative bacteria, fungus, and virus can also result in endocarditis. Classic presenting symptoms of endocarditis include fever, weakness, night sweats, and anorexia. Physical examination commonly reveals a cardiac murmur; splinter hemorrhages, Osler nodes, Janeway lesions, and Roth spots. Persistent bacteremia results in positive blood cultures in 85% to 95%. Echocardiography, either transthoracic or

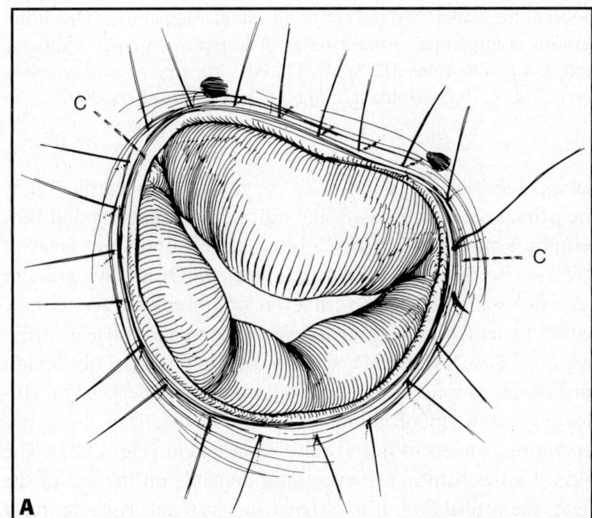

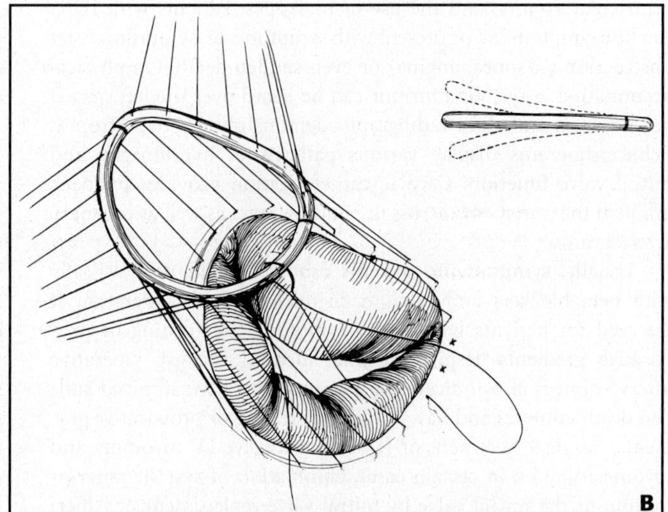

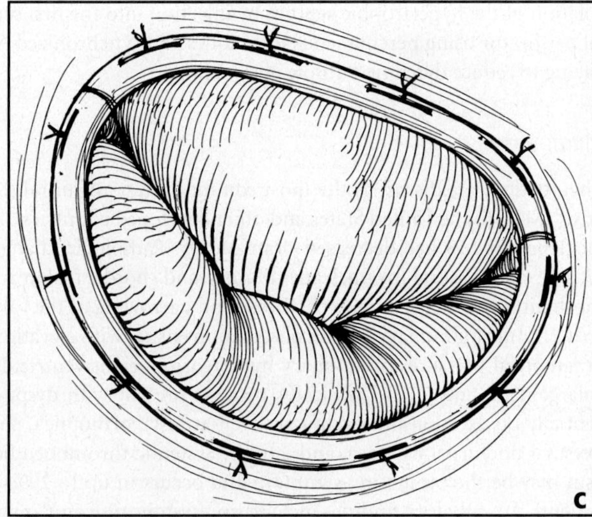

FIGURE 19.23 Technique of mitral ring annuloplasty. **A.** Placement of annular sutures. **B.** Placement of sutures on the annular ring prosthesis. **C.** Completed ring annuloplasty. (From Kaiser LR, Kron IL, Spray TL, eds. *Mastery of Cardiothoracic Surgery*. Philadelphia: Lippincott-Raven Publishers; 1998.)

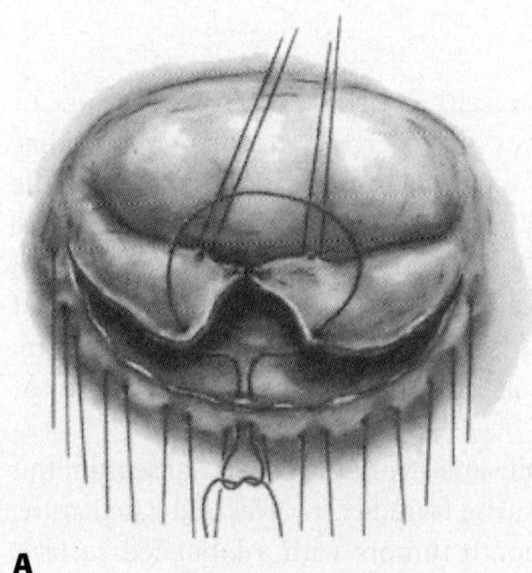

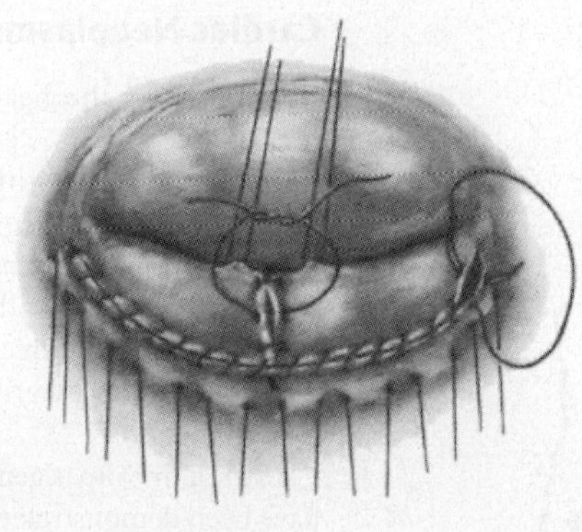

FIGURE 19.24 Quadrangular resection of the posterior mitral valve leaflet and mitral valve annuloplasty for mitral valve prolapse. The free edges of the resected margin are reapproximated in the midline, and the posterior valve is sutured to the annulus. (From Kaiser LR, Kron IL, Spray TL, eds. *Mastery of Cardiothoracic Surgery*. Philadelphia: Lippincott-Raven Publishers; 1998.)

transesophageal, can provide visualization of resultant valvular vegetations. Medical management with appropriate IV antibiotics is the treatment of choice and is often successful in clearing the bacteremia and vegetation. Valve replacement is reserved for prosthetic valve endocarditis, failure of medical management, life-threatening emboli, severe valvular insufficiency or obstruction, and CHF. Localized mitral valve endocarditis can occasionally be treated with partial leaflet resection and valve repair.

Heart Failure

Heart failure is a major global health concern. It is estimated that there are 5 million cases of CHF in the United States alone, with 550,000 new cases diagnosed each year. The major cause of heart failure is ischemic in etiology, with idiopathic dilated cardiomyopathy being the second leading cause. The majority of these patients are medically managed with angiotensin-converting enzyme (ACE) inhibitors, β-blockers, and diuresis to optimize preload, afterload, and contractility. Medical management has been shown to have beneficial effects on ventricular remodeling. Percutaneous and surgical interventions allow optimization of myocardial function by revascularization, mitral valve repair, and resynchronization therapy with biventricular pacemakers, myocardial reconstruction, and passive ventricular restraint devices. Mechanical ventricular restraints and surgical resections have attempted to restore myocardial efficiency and function by restoring ventricular geometry and preventing the progression of adverse ventricular remodeling. Surgical resections, such as the Dor procedure, have attempted to restore ventricular geometry and resect nonviable myocardium that hinders normal, efficient myocardial contractility. Multiple studies have reported variable success from improvements in LV function and geometry following these reconstructive procedures.

Orthotopic heart transplant remains the gold standard and definitive therapy for end-stage heart failure. Unfortunately, access to heart transplantation is limited by the shortage of available donor hearts, with only about 2,400 heart donors annually. Therefore, careful selection criteria and rational allocation of the organs have been developed. Traditionally, heart transplants were performed in a biatrial fashion with anastomoses performed between left and right atria, aorta, and pulmonary artery (Fig. 19.25). Newer techniques utilize bicaval anastomosis (superior and inferior vena caval, left atrium, aortic, and pulmonary artery anastomosis) in an attempt to diminish the need for pacemakers and diminish tricuspid regurgitation (Fig. 19.26). Long-term survival is institution specific, but can approach 90% at 1 year and 85% at 5 years. Long-term graft failure is most often secondary to accelerated coronary artery atherosclerotic disease.

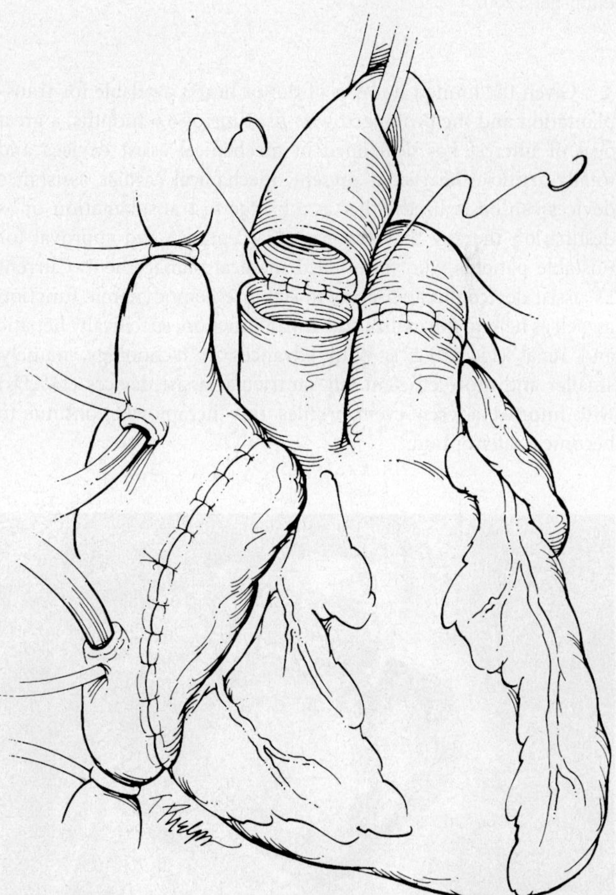

FIGURE 19.25 Orthotopic implantation of a cardiac allograft. The aortic anastomosis is being completed. (From Kaiser LR, Kron IL, Spray TL, eds. *Mastery of Cardiothoracic Surgery*. Philadelphia: Lippincott-Raven Publishers; 1998, with permission.)

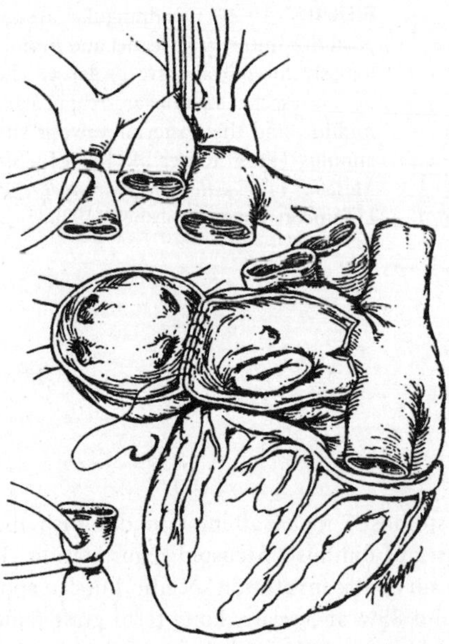

FIGURE 19.26 Bicaval orthotopic heart transplant starts with the left atrial anastomosis. (From Kaiser LR, Kron IL, Spray TL, eds. *Mastery of cardiothoracic surgery*. 2nd ed. Philadelphia: Lippincott-Raven Publishers; 2007.)

Given the limited number of donor hearts available for transplantation and the prolonged wait-list time of 6.6 months, a great deal of interest has developed in mechanical assist devices and totally artificial hearts. At present, mechanical cardiac assistance devices can be utilized either as a bridge to transplantation or as destination therapy that has gained acceptance and approval for unstable patients who have failed medical management. Current LV assist device therapy serves to stabilize hemodynamic function as well as help to normalize end-organ function, specifically hepatic and renal (Fig. 19.27). With advances in technology, namely, smaller and more efficient left ventricular assist devices (LVADs) with improve adverse event profiles, this therapy will continue to become a safer option.

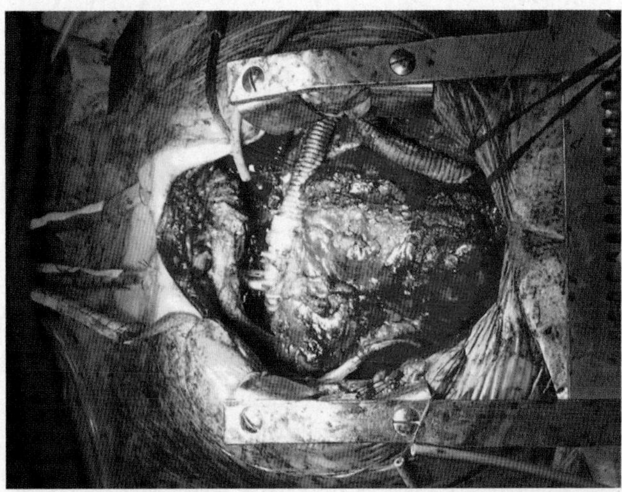

FIGURE 19.27 Left Ventricular assist device placement for ischemic cardiomyopathy.

Cardiac Neoplasms

Neoplasms of the heart are either primary cardiac tumors or metastatic tumors. Seventy-five percent of primary cardiac tumors are benign with the half of these being myxomas, while 75% of malignant primary cardiac tumors are sarcomas. Cardiac myxomas occur roughly twice as frequently in women than in men, with a peak incidence between the 3rd and 6th decades of life. Seventy-five percent of myxomas occur in the left atrium, with 5% demonstrating an autosomal dominant pattern of inheritance.

Atrial myxomas generally arise from the interatrial septum but have been demonstrated to arise from heart valves and vasculature. They appear as round, smooth tumors with a lobulated surface. Most of these lesions are asymptomatic and are incidentally discovered by echocardiography or computed tomography. Symptoms can include malaise, valve orifice obstruction, or embolism. Myxomas should be resected once discovered (Fig. 19.28). Newer minimally invasive approaches have allowed for resection with small incisions and rapid recovery.

Primary malignant tumors of the heart include angiosarcoma, malignant fibrous histiocytoma, and rhabdomyosarcoma. These aggressive tumors grow rapidly and invade surrounding structures. Metastatic lesions are present in 80% of all cases. The long-term prognosis is poor with median survival less than 1 year following resection. Primary malignancies that can metastasize to the heart include bronchogenic carcinoma, melanoma, leukemia, lymphoma, and carcinoma of the breast.

Thoracic Aortic Disease

Aortic Dissection

Aortic dissection occurs three times as frequently as rupture of the abdominal aorta. Up to 40% of patients suffering from an acute aortic dissection die immediately. Fifty percent of patients with an acute type A dissection will die within 48 hours. There are roughly 2,000 new cases of aortic dissection diagnosed in

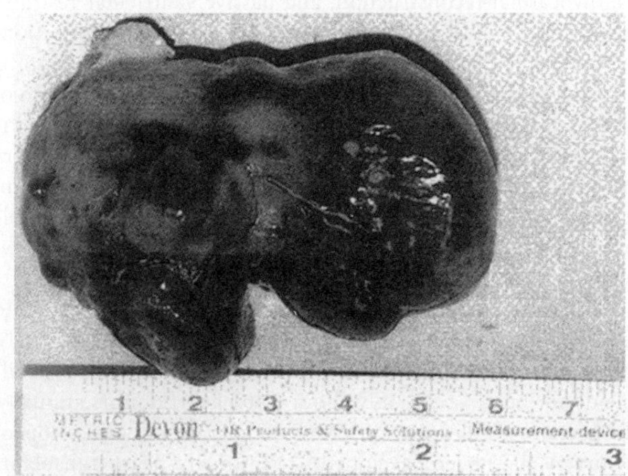

FIGURE 19.28 Gross pathologic appearance of this myxoma, which consists of large, mottled-tan hemorrhagic tissue, somewhat gelatinous and myxoid, measuring 6 cm in maximal dimension. (From Kaiser LR, Kron IL, Spray TL, eds. *Mastery of cardiothoracic surgery*. 2nd ed. Philadelphia: Lippincott-Raven Publishers; 2007.)

the United States annually. Aortic dissections arise from an intimal disruption that permits blood to form a plane of separation within the media of the aortic wall creating a false lumen. Patients with connective tissue disorders, that is, Marfan's disease, undergo cystic medial necrosis related to a tissue factor defect as the inciting event for dissection. Iatrogenic causes, that is, catheterization and cannulation, are also potential causes of aortic dissection. Dissection of the aorta has been linked to bicuspid aortic valve, hypertension, and AS. Dissections are classified as either acute (<2 weeks) or chronic (>2 weeks). By the Stanford classification system, type A dissections involve the ascending aorta and classically propagate to the arch and descending aorta, whereas type B dissections involve only the descending aorta (Fig. 19.29). Type A dissections are usually located in the right anterior aspect of the aorta from which they extend to involve the ascending aorta, arch, and descending aorta. Retrograde propagation can also occur whereby the coronary ostia are involved, resulting in myocardial ischemia and infarction. Type B dissections begin distal to the left subclavian artery origin and involve the descending thoracic and abdominal aorta.

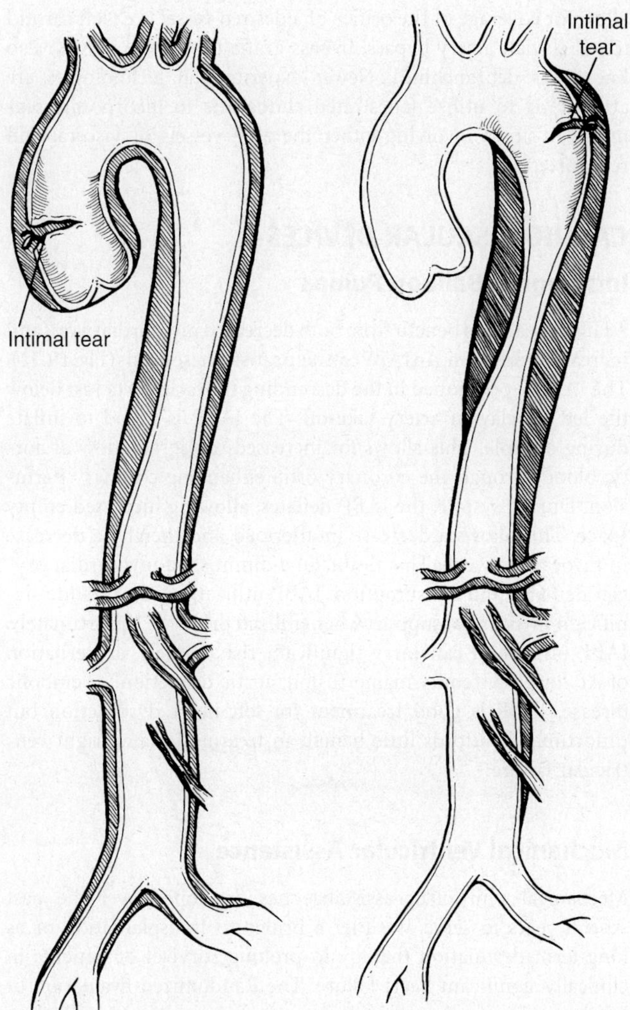

FIGURE 19.29 The Stanford classification of aortic dissections. (From Kaiser LR, Kron IL, Spray TL, eds. *Mastery of Cardiothoracic Surgery*. Philadelphia: Lippincott-Raven Publishers; 1998.)

Aortic dissection should always be considered in patients with severe, unrelenting chest or back pain that is described as ripping or tearing. Pain is usually midsternal for ascending dissections and midback for descending dissections. Findings may also include signs of malperfusion to the brain, viscera, limbs, or heart. Perfusion to end organs will be maintained as long as flow to the major vasculature remains patent either through a true (native) or false (new, artificial) lumen. Malperfusion will occur with occlusion of aortic branches secondary to dissection. Hypotension and tachycardia can be signs of free rupture, pericardial tamponade, acute aortic insufficiency (AI), or myocardial ischemia and should be immediately investigated.

ECG findings consistent with acute ischemia will be present if the dissection involves the coronary ostia with resultant limitation of coronary perfusion. The classic finding of a widened mediastinum by chest X-ray should prompt further investigation, but this finding is not necessarily always present. Diagnosis is established by either high-resolution computed tomography or transesophageal echocardiography. Magnetic resonance imaging, intravascular ultrasound, and aortography are second-line modalities for diagnosis. Initial management involves tight blood pressure control with the goal of minimizing the change in pressure over the change in time ($\Delta P/\Delta t$), thereby reducing aortic wall stress. Acute type A dissections mandate immediate operative treatment given the high rate of mortality. Acute type B dissections are initially treated medically with control of hypertension unless there is evidence of aortic rupture into the left chest or severe major organ or limb ischemia from aortic branch obstruction.

The indications for surgical repair of chronic dissections differ. Type A dissections that are not recognized acutely are repaired to prevent late development of AI and CHF or aneurysmal dilation of the ascending aorta exceeding 5 cm. Chronic type B dissections are repaired for aneurysmal dilation of the descending aorta greater than 6 cm or end-organ malperfusion.

The goal of surgical repair is to replace the segment of aorta containing the intimal tear with a prosthetic graft while maintaining or restoring perfusion of the heart, carotid and subclavian arteries, abdominal organs, spine, and lower body. In acute type A dissections, aortic replacement is limited to the ascending aorta and proximal aortic arch, even when the dissection extends distally. This procedure effectively eliminates the causes of death related to type A dissection without exposing the patient to the morbidity of replacement of the entire aorta. Lifetime follow-up with serial cross-sectional imaging is necessary to identify and follow the development of aneurysmal dilation of the remaining dissected aorta.

Thoracic Aortic Aneurysm

Aneurysm is defined as dilatation of a vessel by 50% or more of the normal diameter. Patients with connective tissue disorders and inherent vascular wall abnormalities have a greatly increased predisposition to aneurysm formation. The incidence of thoracic aortic aneurysms is estimated to be roughly 5.9 per 100,000 person-years. Risk of rupture is directly proportional to the size of the aneurysm. For the scope of this discussion, thoracic aneurysms will be classified as ascending aortic aneurysms, aortic arch aneurysms, or descending thoracic and thoracoabdominal aneurysms.

Ascending aortic aneurysms are most often asymptomatic but occasionally can present with chest pain. These aneurysms are often found incidentally. On physical exam, a clinician may detect a diastolic murmur or widened pulse pressure that indicates AI secondary to dilatation of the aortic root. A chest X-ray may reveal a widened mediastinum, thereby raising concern for an ascending aortic aneurysm or dissection. Concern of an aneurysm warrants further diagnostic workup. Currently, diagnostic modality consists of high-resolution helical CT with contrast, MRI, or transesophageal echocardiography. CT is the imaging study of choice given its ability to evaluate the entire aorta, dissections, and mural thrombus. Unfortunately, CT is contraindicated in patients with renal insufficiency. Emergent repair is indicated with rupture, impending rupture, or concomitant dissection. Symptomatic aneurysms, valvular dysfunction, an aortic diameter greater than 5 cm, and growth greater than 1 cm per year warrant elective repair. There are many choices for repair including simple tube graft replacement, composite valve graft conduit, or valve sparing operations with or without aortic root replacement. Smaller aneurysms should be closely monitored for progression of disease.

Aortic arch aneurysms have a similar pathophysiology to isolated ascending aortic aneurysms. However, involvement of the aortic arch branch vessels carries an increasingly greater risk with operative repair. Therefore, elective repair for arch aneurysms is reserved for patients with aortic diameters greater than 6 cm, secular aneurysms, or asymmetric aneurysms. Repair of arch aneurysms requires a period of deep hypothermic circulatory arrest, in which the core body temperature is cooled to 10°C and circulatory flow is temporarily arrested to allow repair. The procedure involves resection of the aneurismal aorta, leaving behind a patch(es) containing the arch vessels, and replacement of the diseased vessel with a synthetic graft to which the arch vessels are incorporated. Cerebral protection is achieved either by isolated hypothermia alone or by antegrade and/or retrograde perfusion of cold blood.

Thoracoabdominal aneurysms are traditionally classified according to the Crawford classification system. By this system, type I aneurysms are isolated to the thoracic aorta, and types II–IV involve varying portions of the thoracic and abdominal aorta (Fig. 19.30). As compared to ascending aortic aneurysms, roughly 50% of patients are symptomatic at the time of diagnosis of thoracoabdominal aneurysms. Diagnosis can be made with CT, MRI, or rarely aortogram. Repair of thoracoabdominal aneurysms carries a high morbidity, and for this reason, surgical intervention is reserved for aneurysms greater than 6 cm. All symptomatic aneurysms should be repaired, regardless of size. Thoracoabdominal aneurysms are traditionally repaired utilizing a prosthetic tube graft. Circulatory management consists of partial CPB (left atrium to femoral artery) or a shunt to provide blood flow to the viscera and lower extremities during cross clamping and repair. The major morbidity associated with this procedure is spinal cord ischemia resulting in paralysis. In addition, pulmonary insufficiency also commonly is seen following this procedure. The clamp and sew technique, the original repair strategy, was associated with a high rate of spinal cord ischemia. In order to minimize spinal cord ischemia, all large intercostal arteries should be preserved to maximize perfusion to the spinal cord. Intraoperative management includes utilization of a lumbar drain to maximize perfusion pressure to the spinal cord. Postoperatively, perfusion pressure should be maintained by increasing mean arterial pressure (MAP) and decreasing spinal cord pressure.

Endovascular Repair of Aortic Aneurysms

Endovascular repair of thoracic aortic aneurysms is a direct development of endovascular technology for repairing infrarenal AAA. Thus far, endovascular stent grafts are utilized for repair of thoracic aortic aneurysms that are distal to the left subclavian artery and proximal to the visceral segment (Fig. 19.31). As with open repair, there is a high incidence of spinal cord ischemia and paralysis, which mandates close postoperative monitoring with or without a spinal drain. In the high-risk patients, morbidity and mortality are markedly improved following endovascular thoracic aortic repair as compared to traditional open repair. Additionally, endovascular stent grafts have been used in the setting of isolated type B dissections and in combination with type A dissections to stent the descending thoracic aorta. Thus far, this modality is limited to segments of aorta without critical branches. Strategies to overcome this shortcoming have involved performing bypass procedures to allow for coverage of the orifice of a desired vessel (i.e., left carotid to subclavian artery bypass; bypass grafts to visceral vessels, also known as debranching). Newer experimental technologies are attempting to utilize fenestrated endografts to incorporate segments of aorta involving either the arch vessels or visceral and renal arteries.

CARDIOVASCULAR DEVICES

Intra-aortic Balloon Pumps

A failing heart can benefit from both decreased myocardial work and increased perfusion. An IABP can help satisfy these needs (Fig. 19.32). The IABP is positioned in the descending thoracic aorta just below the left subclavian artery take-off. The IABP is timed to inflate during diastole. This allows for increased retrograde flow of aortic blood through the coronary ostia enhancing coronary perfusion. During systole, the IABP deflates, allowing increased empty space. This allows a decrease in afterload and thereby a decrease in myocardial work. This results in a diminished myocardial oxygen demand and consumption. IABP utilization can provide significant myocardial support when utilized properly. Unfortunately, IABP utilization can carry significant risk, namely, exacerbation of AI, lower extremity malperfusion, aortic dissection, or embolic disease. IABP is good treatment for left heart dysfunction but unfortunately affords little benefit in treating isolated right ventricular failure.

Mechanical Ventricular Assistance

Mechanical ventricular assistance has developed over the past several years to serve as either a bridge to transplantation or as long-term destination therapy to prolong survival of patients in clinically significant heart failure. The Randomized Evaluation of Mechanical Assistance of the Treatment of Congestive Heart Failure (REMATCH) study demonstrated a significant improvement in

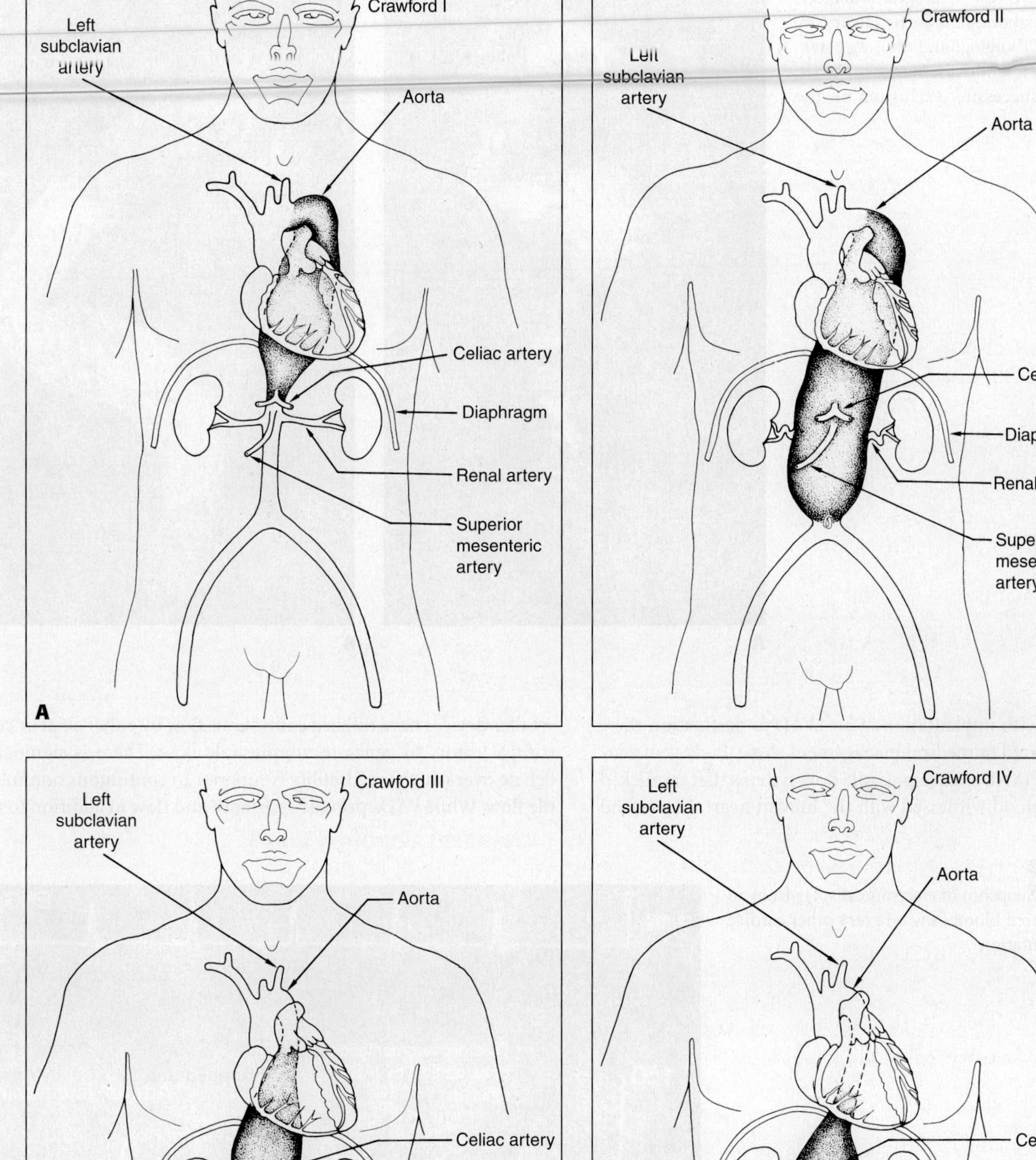

FIGURE 19.30 Crawford classification of thoracoabdominal aneurysms. (From Kaiser LR, Kron IL, Spray TL, eds. *Mastery of Cardiothoracic Surgery*. Philadelphia: Lippincott-Raven Publishers; 1998.)

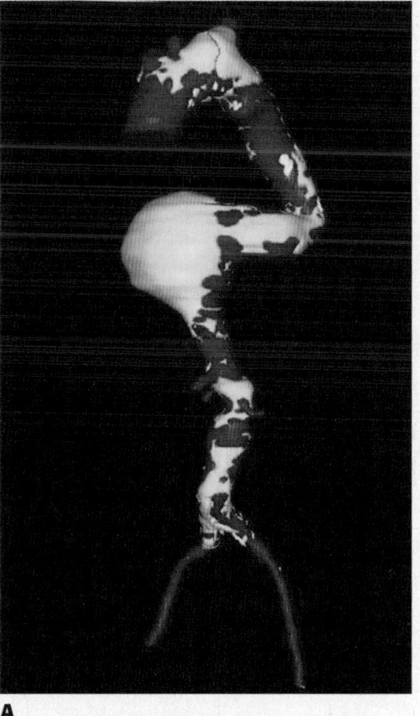

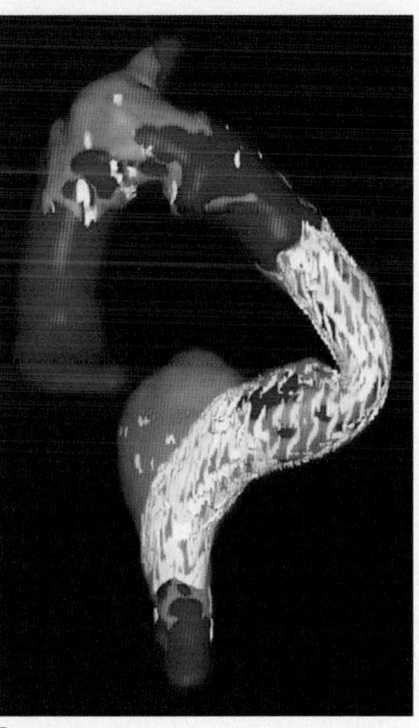

FIGURE 19.31 A. CT angiogram demonstrating a thoracoabdominal aortic aneurysm, preoperative. B. CT angiogram following placement of a thoracic endovascular stent graft, demonstrating successful exclusion of the aneurysm.

2-year survival with implantation of an LVAD as destination therapy when compared to medical management alone. Early ventricular assist devices (VADs) were pulsatile flow systems that mimicked the ejection of blood witnessed with the human heart. Newer and smaller devices have utilized continuous flow by either axial or centrifugal rotors to generate nonpulsatile flow. There is significant debate over whether pulsatility is superior to continuous nonpulsatile flow. While VADs provide assistance and flow in addition to the

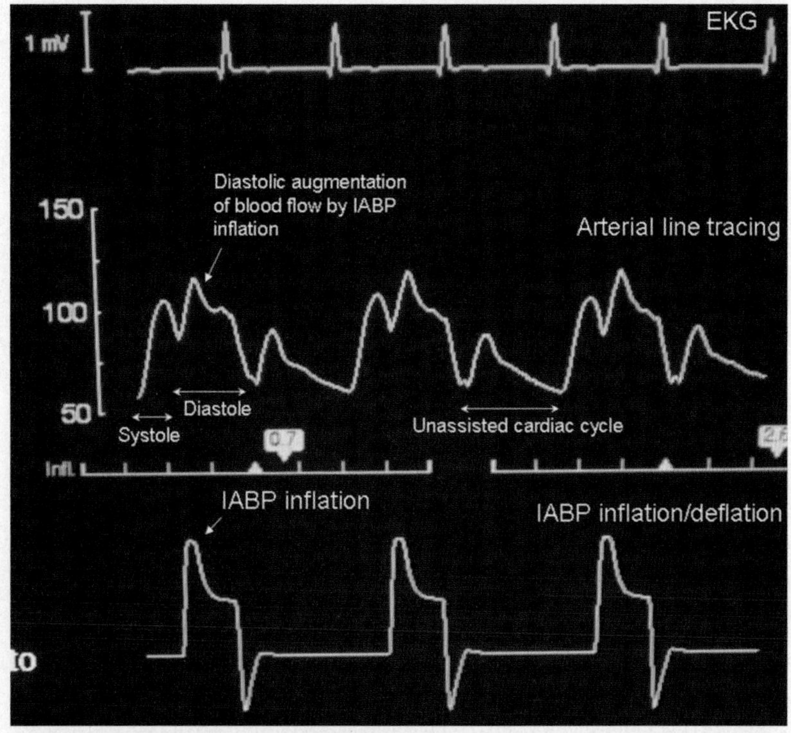

FIGURE 19.32 Snapshot of electronic display from an IABP set to augment blood flow on every other cardiac cycle (1:2 augmentation).

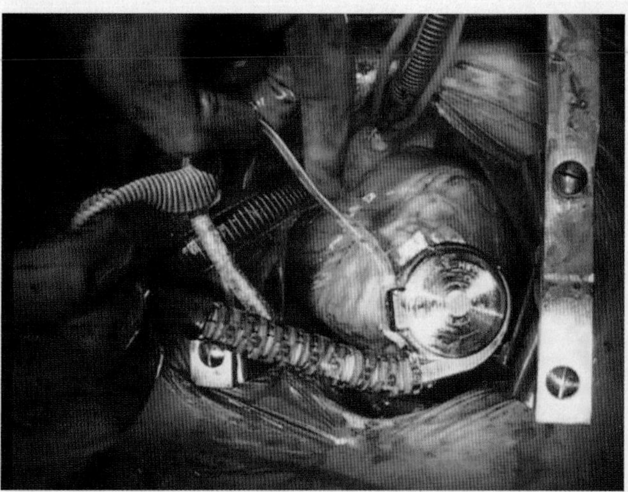

FIGURE 19.33 Intraoperative picture following placement of HeartWare VAD in the left apex.

mechanical activity of the heart, implantable total artificial hearts replace an existing heart with a mechanical device, which provides the entirety of inotropic activity (Fig. 19.33).

Extracorporeal Membrane Oxygenation

Extracorporeal membrane oxygenation (ECMO) is a form of partial CPB used for intermediate support (average of 7 days) of respiratory and cardiac dysfunction. The complexity of ECMO functions and applications are beyond the scope of this chapter. A brief description of the two varieties will be discussed: venoarterial (VA) and venovenous (VV). VA ECMO takes deoxygenated blood from a central vein or the right atrium, pumps it past an oxygenator, and then returns the oxygenated blood to the arterial circulation, commonly the aorta. VA ECMO supports both the respiratory system and normal cardiac output. VV ECMO is used for respiratory dysfunction, such as acute respiratory distress syndrome.

CHAPTER

20

Vascular Disease and Vascular Surgery

ERIC K. SHANG, J. RAYMOND FITZPATRICK III, AND BENJAMIN M. JACKSON

KEY POINTS

- Atherosclerosis is responsible for the vast majority of vascular diseases. The four major modifiable risk factors are hyperlipidemia, hypertension, diabetes mellitus, and smoking.
- Stroke resulting from cerebrovascular disease is the third leading cause of death in the United States. Diagnosis of carotid artery disease is best accomplished with a combination of duplex ultrasonography and axial imaging (CTA or MRA). Carotid endarterectomy is of proven benefit in patients with symptomatic carotid stenosis and select patients with asymptomatic stenosis. Endovascular therapy with angioplasty and stenting is an alternative in high-risk patients.
- Arterial occlusive disease can affect any portion of the arterial vascular tree but is most common in the aortoiliac, femoropopliteal, and tibioperoneal circulations. Initial treatment is conservative, though revascularization is indicated for patients with crippling claudication or critical limb ischemia. Bypass grafting is the traditional option, though endovascular angioplasty with or without stenting is rapidly emerging as a viable alternative.
- Aneurysms of the aorta, iliac arteries, visceral arteries, and peripheral arteries remain a major cause of morbidity and mortality. The majority of these aneurysms are caused by atherosclerosis. The main risks are bleeding and death due to rupture or acute ischemia due to embolization or thrombosis. The diagnosis and treatment of aneurysms in each of these locations is unique. Endovascular aneurysm repair is rapidly changing the practice of vascular surgery.
- TOS can cause neurologic, arterial, or venous symptoms by compression of the brachial plexus, subclavian artery, or subclavian vein. Neurologic TOS should be approached cautiously, as symptoms may not improve after surgery. Arterial and venous symptoms from TOS should prompt surgical resection of the compressing structure (either a cervical rib or a hypertrophied scalene muscle).
- Diagnosis of acute or chronic mesenteric ischemia requires a high degree of suspicion, and early intervention can be lifesaving. Surgical treatment involves resection of nonviable bowel and revascularization of the remaining intestine.
- DVT is common in surgical patients but can usually be avoided by appropriate prophylactic measures (sequential compression devices, subcutaneous heparin). Treatment involves anticoagulation and close monitoring for complications. When anticoagulation fails or is contraindicated, insertion of an inferior vena cava filter dramatically decreases the incidence of pulmonary embolism. Venous insufficiency may result from severe DVTs or inadequate anticoagulation.

Vascular diseases are epidemic in the Western world and account for more morbidity and mortality than does any other category of human disease. The most common cause of vascular disease is atherosclerosis, although many other vascular disorders cause significant morbidity. This chapter discusses vascular anatomy, the pathogenesis of atherosclerosis, atherosclerotic vascular diseases and their management, and other vascular pathology relevant to surgical practice.

ARTERIAL WALL ANATOMY

Arteries and veins are formed from endothelium, smooth muscle, and extracellular matrix synthesized by cells in the vessel wall. A common structure and composition recapitulates itself throughout the vascular system, with cells and matrix fibers arranging themselves into three layers: the tunica intima, tunica media, and tunica adventitia (Fig. 20.1).

The tunica intima lines the luminal surface of the vessel wall and is composed of a thin continuous layer of polygonal endothelial cells overlying subendothelial connective tissue. Through the release of vasoactive mediators, anti-inflammatory cytokines, and antithrombotic agents, endothelial cells modulate vascular tone, hemostasis, vessel permeability, and cell proliferation. Endothelial cells are covered by a glycocalyx, which is responsible for the antithrombogenic properties of the surface. In inflammatory conditions, portions of the glycocalyx coat are lost, leading to the trafficking of leukocytes, which has been theorized as one of the initiating factors in the development of atherosclerotic lesions.

The basal lamina borders endothelial cells on their abluminal surface and forms a boundary separating the endothelium from the underlying intimal structures. This layer is formed by glycoproteins, adhesion molecules such as fibronectin and laminin, various proteoglycans, and microfibrils of types IV and V collagen. The basal lamina not only serves to strengthen the vascular wall through polymer networks of type IV collagen and laminin chains but also regulates numerous functions such as endothelial cell regeneration and vessel permeability.

The internal elastic lamina is a layer of elastic fibers dividing the subendothelial intima from the tunica media. The elastin present in this layer is organized into cylindrical lamellae that are separated by smooth muscle cells. It has been suggested that the elastic lamellae function as barriers to macromolecule accumulation in the vessel wall, as defects have been associated with intimal thickening and atherosclerotic plaque development.

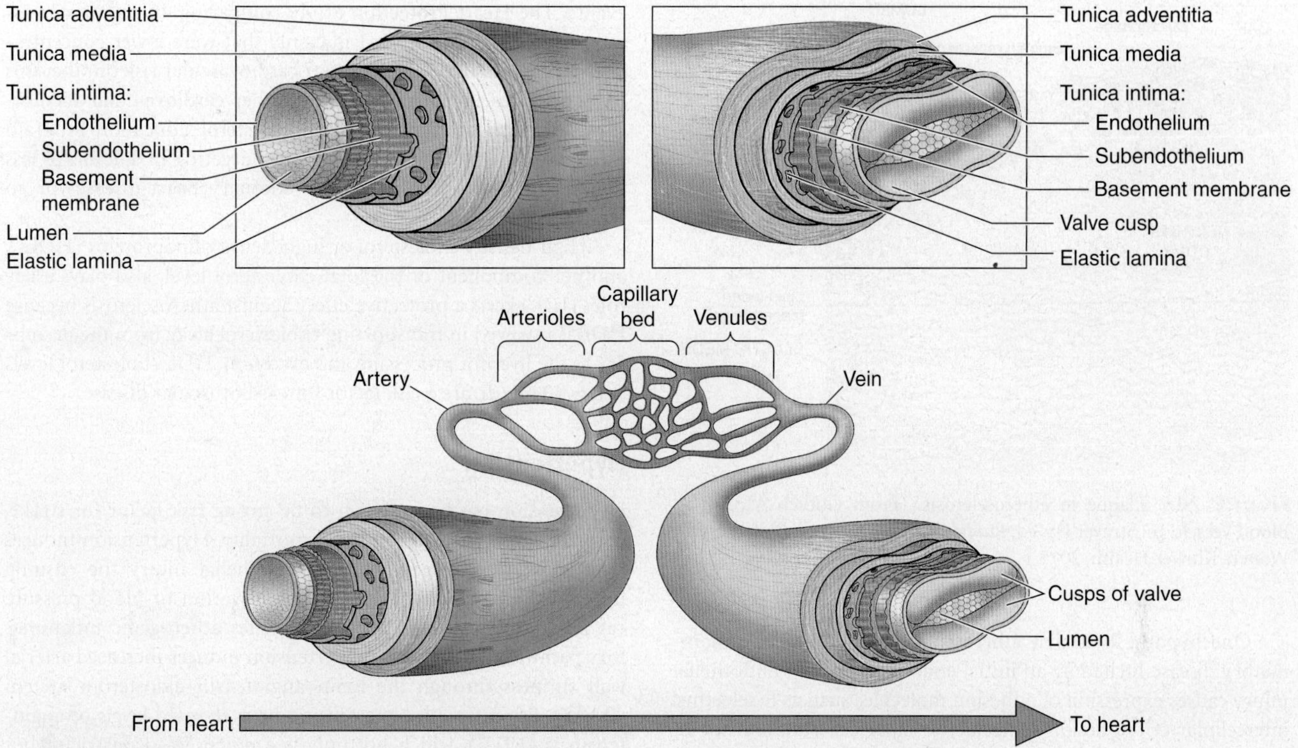

FIGURE 20.1 Structure of the vascular wall. (From Moore KL, Dalley AF, Agur AMR. *Clinically Oriented Anatomy*. 6th ed. Baltimore: Lippincott Williams & Wilkins; 2010.)

The tunica media layer is the muscular layer of the vessel wall comprising vascular smooth muscle cells, elastic, and collagen separating the internal elastic lamina from the adventitia. The components of the media are arranged in a highly organized manner, with closely packed layers of smooth muscle cells, elastin and collagen fibers surrounded by a basement membrane of laminin, type IV collagen, and fibronectins. At physiologic pressures, the media is the chief load-bearing portion of the arterial wall, and as such is the main determinant of arterial elastic wall properties.

The tunica adventitia is a collection of adipose and other supportive connective tissue that extends from the media to the perivascular connective tissue. The vasa vasorum, a collection of feeding vessels only present in large vessels, is contained in the adventitia and functions as the blood supply of the vessel wall. They arise from the parent vessel at branch points and arborize in the adventitial layer. Also present in the adventitia are vasomotor nerve fibers that mediate vasoconstriction and vasodilation via adrenergic α- and β-receptors, respectively.

Arteries are classified as elastic, distributing, or small. Elastic arteries are the largest and consist of the aorta and its largest branches, such as the brachiocephalic, common carotid, and common iliac arteries. Distributing arteries are the second largest and are exemplified by the coronary, renal, and hepatic arteries. The small arteries are contained within the substance of organs and tissues. Arterioles are the smallest arteries, and their primary function is to control tissue blood flow and systemic arterial pressure. Capillaries are the smallest vessels, typically about the diameter of a single red blood cell. In tissues, they are the primary site for exchange of oxygen, nutrients, and waste.

Lymphatics are small, thin-walled structures with an endothelial lining. These channels function as conduits, which carry extracellular fluids centrally away from tissues for processing in the lymph nodes and eventual return to the vascular system.

PATHOGENESIS OF ATHEROSCLEROSIS

Atherosclerosis is a disease whose hallmark is the deposition and accumulation of smooth muscle cells and lipids within the arterial intima. The lesions characteristic of late atherosclerosis are the fibrous and complicated plaques. Fibrous plaques consist of a necrotic core, containing foam cells (lipid filled smooth muscle cells or macrophages) and extracellular lipids, covered by a fibrous cap of smooth muscle cells, lymphocytes, and connective tissue (Fig. 20.2). The plaque is situated in the intima and may enlarge and ultimately intrude upon the vessel lumen.

Features of complicated plaques include calcification, ulceration, plaque rupture with subsequent hemorrhage, and thrombosis. Complicated plaques are the source of thromboembolic phenomenon through plaque rupture and thus are associated with clinically significant disease. The process by which a fibrous plaque evolves into a complicated one is currently poorly understood but is thought to be accelerated by extrinsic risk factors such as hypertension and cigarette smoking.

Numerous theories exist regarding the initial formation and the evolution of atherosclerotic lesions, but inflammation appears to be a common factor. Also common to all these theories is the overarching concept that arterial structures are not simply conduits for blood flow but rather modulators of complex and dynamic interactions between the vascular wall cells and the blood.

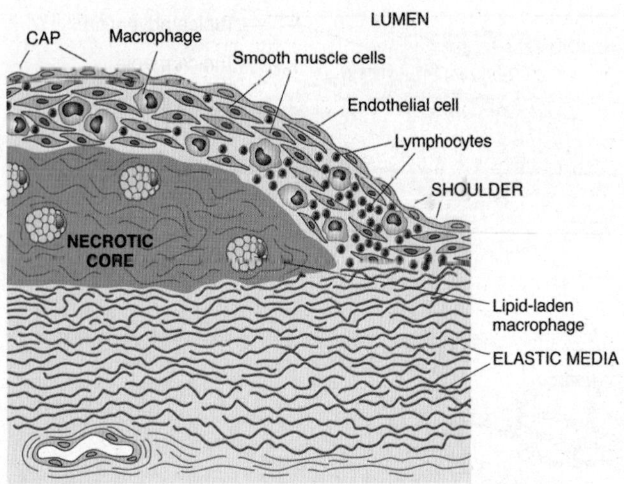

FIGURE 20.2 Plaque in atherosclerosis. (From Gotlieb AI, Liu A. Blood Vessels. In: Strayer DS, ed. *Rubin's Pathology*. 7th ed. Philadelphia: Wolters Kluwer Health; 2015.)

One hypothesis is that atherosclerosis is a complex inflammatory disease incited by an initial endothelial injury. Endothelial injury causes expression of adhesion molecules such as E-selectins, intercellular cell adhesion molecule, vascular cell adhesion molecule, and platelet endothelial cell adhesion molecule. These mediate binding, activation, and diapedesis of circulating platelets and leukocytes. Inflammatory cytokines and chemokines produced by activated cells then attract and activate monocytes to the site of injury. Differentiation of monocytes into macrophages allows these cells to engulf lipids, thus forming the foam cells characteristic of atherosclerotic lesions. Lymphocytes promote the migration and proliferation of smooth muscle cells in the lesion, creating an atheromatous plaque.

An alternative, but not mutually exclusive, hypothesis is one that emphasizes the roles of immune and inflammatory mediators such as cytokines and growth factors like TGF-α, gamma-interferon, and IL-2. The activation of the complement system by cholesterol particles has been shown to be an important step in the deposition of immune complexes in vascular tissues, producing proinflammatory molecules and the membrane attack complex, which has been identified in atherosclerotic lesions. Furthermore, plaque stability has been tied to the balance between matrix metalloproteinases (MMPs) and tissue inhibitors of metalloproteinases (TIMPs) produced by macrophages, which can be regulated by inflammatory cytokines such as IL-1 and TNF.

RISK FACTORS FOR ATHEROSCLEROSIS

Hyperlipidemia

Hypercholesterolemia is a major risk factor for atherosclerosis. Of particular importance is the level of low-density cholesterol, or low-density lipoproteins (LDLs). LDLs undergo oxidative modification in the bloodstream. The oxidized end products then function as inflammatory mediators, inducing adhesion molecule expression by endothelial cells. Furthermore, these end products are potent macrophage chemokines, promoting their migration into the tunica intima.

There exists a linear relationship between the absolute reduction of LDL and the reduction of coronary and other vascular events. The Heart Protection Study comparing 40 mg of simvastatin versus placebo showed not only that were lower concentrations of LDL associated with lower cardiovascular risk but that this reduction was independent of any other cardiovascular medications being taken. The National Cholesterol Education Program Adult Treatment Plan III recommends targeting LDL levels of less than 100 mg/dL in patients with coronary heart disease (or an equivalent).

High-density cholesterol or high-density lipoproteins (HDLs), another component of the total cholesterol level, also plays a key role. HDL exerts a protective effect against atherosclerosis because HDL is involved in transporting cholesterol away from the periphery to the liver for processing and excretion. HDL cholesterol levels below 40 mg/dL are a risk factor for cardiovascular disease.

Hypertension

Hypertension has been shown to be strong risk factor for stroke, coronary heart disease, and total mortality. Hypertension induces atherosclerotic changes through endothelial injury the ensuing inflammatory response. The chronic elevation of blood pressure causes endothelial damage, which incites atherogenic inflammatory pathways. In addition, hypertension induces increased arterial wall stiffness through the renin–angiotensin–aldosterone system (RAAS). Patients with hypertension have elevated levels of angiotensin II (AT II), which not only is a potent vasoconstrictor but also triggers matrix remodeling and decreases elastin and NO synthesis. Additionally, AT II induces the secretion of proinflammatory cytokines such as IL-6 from smooth muscle cells. Furthermore, aldosterone has been shown to promote vascular stiffness and hypertension by stimulating vascular smooth muscle cell hypertrophy and fibrosis.

Diabetes Mellitus

Diabetes is associated with a 2-fold increase in myocardial infarction and an 8- to 15-fold increase in gangrene of the lower extremities. Diabetic patients have impaired vasodilation due to dysfunction of endothelial nitric oxide synthase and increased production of endothelin 1, a potent vasoconstrictor. Platelet hyperactivity due to an increased number of glycoprotein IIb–IIIa receptors also contributes to decreased microvascular blood flow. Additionally, hyperglycemia results in the formation of reactive oxygen species and advanced glycation end products, which promote inflammatory pathways.

Clinical trials have shown that tight glycemic control decreases the incidence and progression of microvascular complications such as retinopathy, nephropathy, and neuropathy. However, in type II diabetics (90% to 95% of patients), large multicenter randomized controlled studies comparing standard versus intensive glucose control failed to show any reduction in macrovascular complications.

Tobacco

Cigarette smoking is a well-established risk factor for the development of atherosclerosis and has been linked to a threefold increase in risk for the development of symptomatic peripheral arterial disease (PAD). Cigarette smoke has been shown to alter endothelium-mediated vasoreactivity in both the peripheral and coronary circulations by decreasing the availability of nitric oxide.

In addition, cigarette smoke increases circulating proinflammatory markers, such as CRP and IL-6, as well as increases platelet aggregation.

Age

All forms of cardiovascular disease are more prevalent in the elderly. The risk for PAD increased 1.5- to 2.0-fold for every 10-year increase in age. The death rates from coronary artery disease (CAD) increase with each decade of life up to age 85, from 10 per 100,000 by the ages of 25 to 34 to nearly 1,000 per 100,000 by ages 55 to 64.

Gender

The epidemiology, manifestation, and progression of cardiovascular disease differ between men and women. Women appear to develop cardiovascular disease 10 years later than do men and typically after menopause. Premenopausal women have comparatively lower.

Family History

Familial predisposition to atherosclerosis has been determined to be multifactorial and can be related to the clustering of risk factors (hypertension, diabetes, etc.) or to atherosclerosis itself. So far, approximately 40 to 50 quantitative trait loci for atherosclerotic disease have been found through linkage analysis. As our understanding of the interplay between genetic and environmental factors increases, the continued identification of genetic markers through projects like the Human Genome Project will likely change the practice of cardiovascular medicine.

CEREBROVASCULAR DISEASE

Stroke is the third leading cause of death in the United States behind heart disease and cancer. Approximately 87% of strokes are ischemic, and 13% are hemorrhagic. Of ischemic strokes, recent studies estimate that approximately 15% are related to atherosclerotic disease. The remainder are lacunar (20%), cardioembolic (20%), or cryptogenic (45%) in etiology. Significant carotid stenosis (>50%) is seen in 12% to 20% of all anterior circulation ischemic strokes. In larger population-based studies, the overall prevalence of cerebrovascular disease was noted to be 2.5%. In subjects 60 to 79 years old, 10.5% of men and 5.5% of women had atherosclerotic disease on duplex examination.

Pathophysiology

Carotid artery disease, except that related to trauma, almost always occurs as a result of atherosclerosis. Cerebral ischemia occurs most commonly due to embolization from plaque rupture rather than thrombosis. The most common source of emboli is the internal carotid artery, followed by cardiac emboli. Ischemia can also occur as a result of a low-flow state through a severely stenotic lesion.

Risk Factors

Previously described risk factors for atherosclerosis, such as hyperlipidemia, smoking, diabetes, and hypertension, also contribute to the development of carotid stenosis. A history of atrial fibrillation significantly increases a patient's stroke risk. Transient ischemic attacks (TIAs) are a major risk factor for stroke. The 90-day risk for stroke has been reported to range from 3% to 17%, with greatest risk occurring in the first 30 days. This high risk for stroke in the immediate period following TIAs mandates aggressive evaluation of these patients. Other often-cited risk factors include a sedentary lifestyle, excessive alcohol consumption, and obesity.

Natural History

Carotid artery atherosclerosis predisposes patients to TIA and stroke, with risk being proportional to the severity of carotid stenosis. In a study of 500 patients with cervical bruits, the incidence of stroke in patients with 0% to 29% stenosis was 2.1%. This increased to 5.7% in patients with 30% to 74% stenosis, and 19.5% in patients with 75% to 100% stenosis. In the Veteran Administration Cooperative Trial, medical management of asymptomatic (≥50%) carotid stenosis resulted in 20.6% incidence of ipsilateral TIA or stroke over 4 years. The Asymptomatic Carotid Atherosclerosis Study (ACAS) reported a 11% risk of ipsilateral stroke risk for lesions greater than or equal to 60%.

Diagnosis

Typical carotid territory ischemic symptoms include contralateral weakness or sensory deficit of the face, arm, or leg, or transient ipsilateral blindness (amaurosis fugax). Left hemispheric symptoms include aphasia, alexia, and anomia. If the right hemisphere is involved, neglect, visual or sensory extinction, anosognosia, or asomatognosia may be present. Neurologic symptoms unlikely to be attributable to the carotid territory include vertigo, ataxia, diplopia, or syncope.

A carotid bruit may be detectable on physical examination. The North American Symptomatic Carotid Endarterectomy Trial (NASCET) found that carotid bruit is only 63% sensitive and 61% specific for high-grade carotid stenosis. The presence of Hollenhorst plaques on fundoscopic examination is also correlated with significant carotid bifurcation disease.

The initial study in many patients is carotid artery duplex ultrasonography (DUS), as it is both noninvasive and reliable. DUS estimates the degree of stenosis on the basis of flow velocity. A peak systolic velocity of greater than or equal to 230 cm/s has a sensitivity of 99% and specificity of 86% for lesions of greater than or equal to 70% stenosis. Despite its accuracy, there are several important limitations to DUS. It cannot reliably distinguish very high-grade stenoses from occlusions, and it cannot evaluate intracranial portions of the carotid artery system. Finally, performance of the test is highly dependent on technique, so testing should be performed in an accredited vascular laboratory.

Magnetic resonance angiography (MRA) is seeing increasing use in the diagnosis of carotid stenosis. It has the ability to assess the intrathoracic and intracranial portions of the carotid artery and does not require ionizing radiation. MRA has been shown to have a tendency to overestimate the degree of stenosis, making it difficult to differentiate moderate (50% to 69%) stenosis from severe stenosis. Additionally, MRA cannot be used in patients with metallic implants and is not advisable in critically ill or claustrophobic patients.

Computed tomography angiography (CTA) is less susceptible to overestimating the degree of carotid stenosis. Image acquisition is more rapid than MRA and offers superior (often submillimeter) spatial resolution. In addition, it has the ability to detect the calcium burden of atherosclerotic lesions and can visualize additional soft tissue structures surrounding the vessel. CTA has been shown by meta-analysis to be approximately 85% sensitivity and 93% specificity in detection of 70% to 99% stenosis, as compared to digital subtraction angiography (DSA). It is also 97% sensitive and 99% specific for detecting carotid occlusion. Limitations of CTA include contrast exposure, the use of ionizing radiation, and difficulties interpreting studies in patients with significant calcium burden.

Catheter-based DSA is the criterion standard test for carotid stenosis. It allows for visualization of the entire carotid artery circulation as well as the vertebrobasilar circulations. This invasive test historically carries a 4% risk of neurologic complications and a 1% risk of major stroke or death, and as such is an inappropriate screening tool. Use of contrast dye also limits the use of this modality in patients with renal insufficiency and/or severe iodine allergy. DSA is most useful when less invasive studies offer differing results.

We recommend CDUS as a screening test and CTA or MRA as a confirmatory adjunct to evaluate patients for carotid artery stenosis. Unless a percutaneous intervention is planned, angiography should be reserved for cases of complex or equivocal findings.

Medical Therapy

Medical management is an important component to the treatment of patients with carotid disease, regardless of the degree of stenosis or plan for intervention. These therapies not only lower the risk of stroke but also lower the incidence of overall cardiovascular events. Lowering blood pressure to a target less than 140/90 mm Hg with antihypertensive medications is recommended in patients who have hypertension with asymptomatic carotid stenosis. The Framingham Heart Study showed that each 10 mm Hg reduction in blood pressure reduces the risk for stroke by 33%. Despite studies showing tight glycemic control (ADVANCE, ACCORD) did not reduce risk of stroke in diabetics, glucose control to nearly normoglycemic levels (hemoglobin A1C < 7%) is recommended to reduce microvascular complications. Smoking has shown to nearly double to risk of stroke, and patients with carotid stenosis should be counseled to quit.

Patients with known atherosclerosis have reduced stroke risk when treated with lipid-lowering therapies such as statins. Specifically, 10% reductions in levels of serum LDL have been associated to reduce stroke risk by 15%. The Stroke Prevention by Aggressive Reduction in Cholesterol trial demonstrated that atorvastatin given to patients with recent stroke or TIA reduced the 5-year stroke rate by 16%.

The U.S. Preventative Service Task Force recommends daily aspirin as cardiovascular prophylaxis in patients with anticipated cardiac morbidity of greater than 3% for men more than 45 years old and women more than 55 years old. While there is evidence supporting antithrombotic treatment for secondary prevention of recurrent stroke in patients with symptomatic carotid artery atherosclerosis, the choice of antiplatelet therapy is not clear. The American Academy of Neurology guidelines on CEA suggest that a low dose of 81 to 325 mg daily be used prior to and after carotid endarterectomy (CEA).

Indications for Intervention

For symptomatic patients, stenosis greater than 50% should prompt consideration of CEA. Symptomatic patients with stenoses from 50% to 69% have an approximately 5% annual risk reduction with CEA. Because their risk is less than that of those with higher-grade stenoses, these patients should be considered for CEA if they are low-risk surgical candidates.

For asymptomatic patients, the ACAS demonstrated that patients with greater than 60% stenosis should be considered for CEA as long as their surgical mortality was not greater than 3%. In these conditions, CEA was superior to antiplatelet therapy alone in the reduction of long-term stroke risk.

Urgent/emergent CEA (within 2 weeks) should be performed for patients with severe stenosis and recent or crescendo symptoms. The traditional recommendation was to wait 4 to 6 weeks after a completed stroke to perform CEA; however, this recommendation is not supported by high-level evidence.

Carotid Endarterectomy

Surgical exposure to the carotid artery can be achieved through an incision along the medial border of the sternocleidomastoid muscle or an oblique transverse incision in the neck. After the administration of systemic heparin, the carotid is clamped and an arteriotomy is made from the common carotid artery to the distal extension of the atherosclerotic plaque in the internal carotid. The atherosclerotic plaque, which resides in the intima and inner media, is then removed from the vessel. Typically, patch angioplasty is then performed to close the arteriotomy with either Dacron or bovine pericardium. The ACAS study has demonstrated decreased restenosis rates with the use of a patch, as compared to primary closure. Other techniques exist, including eversion CEA where the internal carotid is divided at the bifurcation and the plaque is removed by everting the adventitia and media cranially.

CEA can be performed under local anesthesia with frequent neurologic checks or under general anesthesia using continuous electroencephalographic (EEG) monitoring. If the neurologic examination or EEG changes after clamping of the artery, a temporary shunt should be used to provide continuous ipsilateral blood flow while the artery is clamped. If general anesthesia is used without EEG monitoring, a shunt should be used if the internal carotid artery stump pressure is less than 50 mm Hg.

Complications

The most dreaded complication of CEA is stroke, occurring at a rate from 2% to 4%. This can be avoided with meticulous intraoperative technique and prompt reexploration if the patient develops an acute postoperative neurologic deficit. Myocardial infarction is the most common source of morbidity and mortality after CEA, due to the clustering of atherosclerotic diseases in this population.

Postoperative hypertension is due to manipulation of the carotid body and occurs in 20% of patients. Hypertension puts this population of patients at particularly high risk of intracranial hemorrhage due to vasoplegia induced by a long-standing low-flow state preoperatively. Therefore, postoperative hypertension and/or headache should be aggressively treated with an intravenous infusion of a vasodilator such as nicardipine or nitroprusside.

The vagus nerve (CN X) is the nerve most commonly traumatized during CEA. This injury is due to inadvertent clamping or stretching of the nerve and results in hoarseness and increased risk of postoperative aspiration. Injury to the hypoglossal nerve (CN XII) results in tongue deviation to the side of the injury, as well as speech and mastication difficulties. This often occurs due to retraction and is temporary.

Carotid Stenting

Percutaneous angioplasty with stenting has become an option in the treatment algorithm for carotid stenosis. The role for carotid artery stenting (CAS) versus CEA is the subject of considerable controversy. The Carotid Revascularization Endarterectomy versus Stenting Trial (CREST) demonstrated that both CEA and CAS can be performed with low complication rates in asymptomatic patients. In symptomatic patients, the International Carotid Stenting Sturdy Trial (ICST) showed an increased risk for stroke after CAS (7.7%) versus CEA (4.1%). Meta-analyses of all published trials comparing CEA and CAS have shown that CAS was associated with lower MI risk and significantly increased periprocedural stroke risk.

Carotid stenting is the currently preferred over CEA in patients with previous ipsilateral neck surgery or external beam radiotherapy, as obliteration of tissue planes in these cases leads to a more difficult operation with increased perioperative complications. Similarly, CAS is preferred in medically infirm patients with extremely high perioperative risk, such as those with severe and uncorrectable CAD, CHF, or COPD.

ARTERIAL OCCLUSIVE DISEASE

Arterial occlusive disease affects roughly 5% of the population 55 to 74 years of age. It affects all aspects of the vascular system, including the upper extremity, the aortoiliac circulation, the viscera, and the lower extremity. Occlusive arterial disease in these areas is primarily related to atherosclerosis. This section discusses occlusive disease related to the lower extremities, including aortoiliac occlusive disease. Upper extremity and visceral occlusive diseases are discussed elsewhere in this chapter.

PAD can be further classified into acute ischemia and chronic ischemia, with differing principles of management. The main tenet of ischemic diseases, however, applies to both acute and chronic ischemia: the highest likelihood of limb salvage is achieved by maximizing proximal inflow and distal outflow.

Acute Lower Extremity Ischemia

The etiology of acute lower extremity ischemia is either embolism of a clot or plaque from a proximal source or local development of thrombus, both of which occlude blood flow to the distal portion of the extremity. The Thrombolysis or Peripheral Artery Surgery (TOPAS) trial established that local thrombus is causative in 85% of cases. Patient outcome is directly related to the degree of ischemia and the time to revascularization. Without treatment, the natural history of acute arterial occlusive disease is that of progressive limb loss and potentially death. The amputation rate is clearly linked to the time between onset of acute limb ischemia and intervention, so timely diagnosis and intervention is paramount.

Diagnosis

Patients with acute ischemia will manifest the "six P's," which include pain, pallor, paresthesias, pulselessness, poikilothermia, and paralysis, in some variation. The most common presenting symptom is pain. Paralysis is a late finding and is indicative of advanced ischemia. Systemic effects of tissue necrosis include acidosis, hyperkalemia, myoglobinuria, renal failure, sepsis, and death. Diagnostic tests such as arterial DUS or noninvasive angiography (CTA vs. MRA) may be helpful, but these tests take valuable time to obtain. Once a clinical diagnosis has been made, it is more advantageous to proceed directly to arteriography and definitive management to maximize the likelihood of limb salvage.

Management

Systemic anticoagulation with heparin should be instituted immediately when a diagnosis of acute ischemia is made. This prevents clot propagation to the distal circulation and decreases morbidity and mortality. The first step in diagnosis and intervention is arteriography. Figure 20.3 outlines the treatment algorithm for acute limb ischemia.

Complications

The development of most complications is related to the duration of ischemia. Compartment syndrome arises in approximately 2% of patients and is due to reperfusion injury following revascularization. This syndrome is characterized by pain with passive stretch of the muscles and increased compartment pressures (>20 to 30 mm Hg). Diagnosis is made by history, physical examination, and a high index of suspicion. Four-compartment fasciotomy of the leg should be performed if there is any concern of compartment syndrome. It is worth noting that the extent of reperfusion injury is less when flow is gradually restored to the extremity, as in catheter-directed thrombolysis.

Other complications are those associated with thrombolysis and include minor catheter-related bleeding (10% to 15%), bleeding requiring transfusion (5%), and hemorrhagic stroke (1%).

Chronic Lower Extremity Ischemia

Chronic ischemia of the lower extremity most commonly results from occlusive atherosclerotic lesions of the aortoiliac, femoropopliteal, or infrapopliteal vascular systems. Most patients are asymptomatic despite having physical signs of chronic ischemia. The most common symptoms are intermittent claudication, rest pain, ischemic ulcers, and frank gangrene. In general, claudication alone is rarely limb threatening. In contrast, rest pain and ischemic ulcers usually lead to limb loss if left untreated.

Diagnosis

History and Physical Examination

A careful history and a detailed physical examination will often raise the level of suspicion and indicate the need for diagnostic testing or treatment. Many patients will report underlying medical disease including heart disease, diabetes, kidney disease, and hypertension. Advanced age, male gender, and family history may also be noted. Physical examination may reveal diminished peripheral pulses, hair loss, skin atrophy, nail hypertrophy, elevation pallor, and dependent rubor.

Intermittent claudication is typically the initial symptom. Claudication is defined as extremity discomfort, pain, or weakness consistently produced by exercise and promptly relieved by rest. Symptoms generally occur one level below the area of disease. Buttock claudication can likely be attributed to an aortic or common iliac lesion, while mid-thigh claudication is commonly associated with an external iliac lesion. Likewise, calf pain is most likely

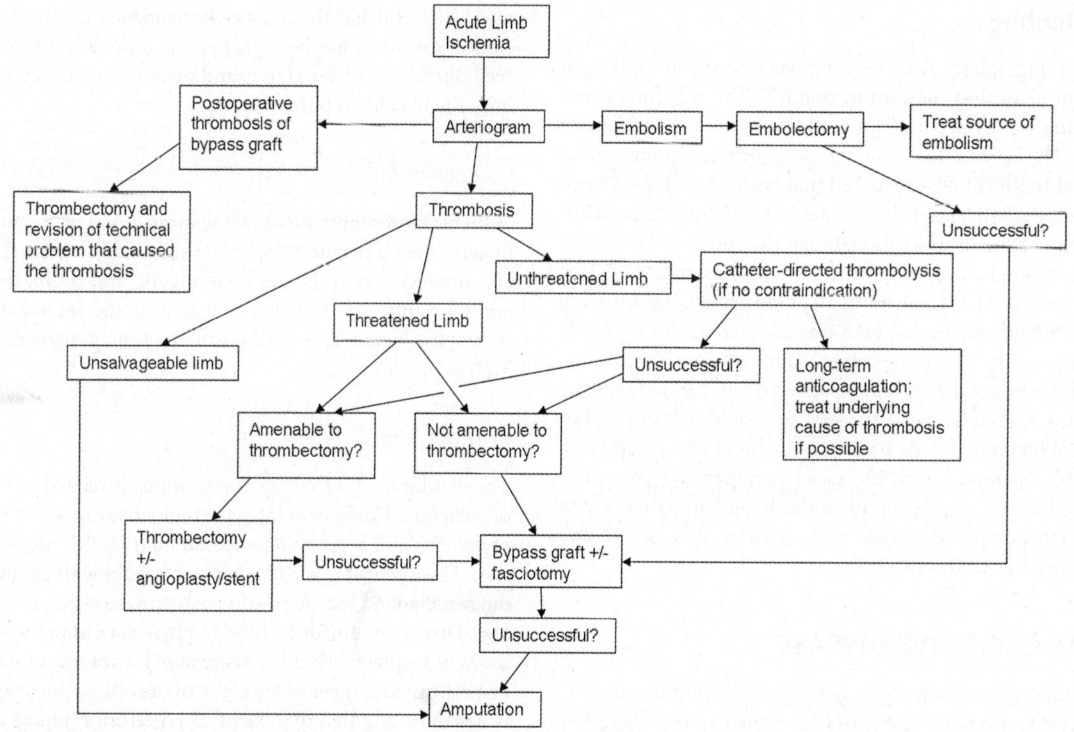

FIGURE 20.3 Treatment algorithm for acute limb ischemia.

due to a common femoral or superficial femoral artery (SFA) occlusion. Finally, an occlusion in the distal SFA or popliteal artery often results in foot claudication.

Claudication can be caused by nonvascular conditions, and alternative diagnoses should be considered. Neurogenic leg pain caused by spinal stenosis, nerve compression, and diabetic neuropathy are the most common conflicting diagnoses. It is worth noting that vascular and nonvascular diseases can coexist, which mandates that the vascular surgeon identify and treat vascular claudication, even in the presence of another condition.

The presence of ischemic rest pain, the presence of tissue loss, or gangrene secondary to arterial insufficiency is known as critical limb ischemia (CLI). Ischemic rest pain indicates that the arterial blood supply is insufficient to meet the metabolic demands of the resting tissue. It usually affects the forefoot and toes, but when pain is felt more proximally, distal areas are usually not spared. The pain is aggravated by elevation of the extremity and diminished or relieved by dependency. Therefore, pain commonly occurs while the patient is reclining or sleeping.

Ischemic ulcers usually result from minor traumatic injuries, which fail to heal because of lack of adequate blood supply. They are most common in areas of focal pressure on the foot and are usually dry and punctate. Conversely, the ulcers of venous insufficiency are usually located superior to the medial malleolus and are often moist, superficial, and diffuse. Venous ulcers are also associated with hemosiderin skin pigmentation and venous varicosities.

Gangrene is characterized by cyanotic, anesthetic tissue associated with necrosis due to inability of the arterial blood supply to meet minimal metabolic requirements. Gangrene can be classified as dry or wet. Dry gangrene is more common in patients with atherosclerotic disease and frequently results from embolization to the toes or forefoot. Elective amputation is required, although autoamputation of lower extremity digits commonly occurs. Wet gangrene is more common in diabetic patients who sustain unrecognized trauma to the foot. The severe infection present in wet gangrene makes it a true surgical emergency that mandates either complete debridement of infected, nonviable tissue or guillotine amputation. Guillotine amputation may be revised to a formal amputation once the infection has been controlled.

The blue toe syndrome refers to the sudden development of cool, painful, cyanotic toe(s) or forefoot. This develops as a result of embolic occlusion of digital arteries with atherothrombotic material from a proximal source. The affected digit(s) may require amputation, and because these episodes tend to increase in frequency and severity, localizing and eradicating the embolic source is indicated.

Diagnostic Testing

Patients with suspected arterial occlusive disease should undergo noninvasive testing to establish the diagnosis, quantify the severity of the disease, and localize the level of occlusion(s). Three simple tests include the measurement of segmental systolic blood pressures, the ankle–brachial index (ABI), and pulse volume recordings (PVRs) (Fig. 20.4). Normally, Doppler segmental pressures increase

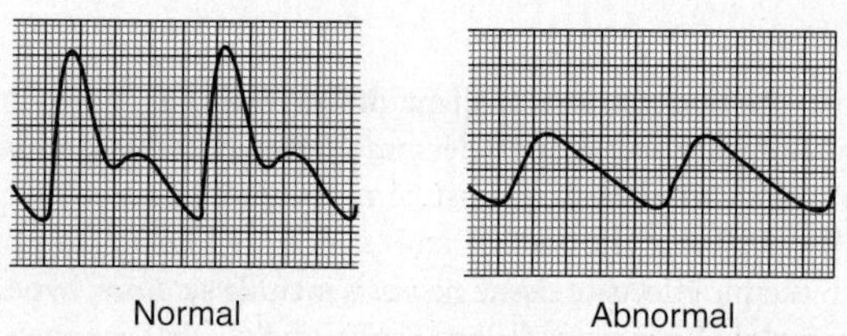

FIGURE 20.4 Normal and abnormal PVRs at ankle level.

20 mm Hg from the brachial artery to the proximal femoral artery. Any change less than a 20-mm Hg increase indicates significant aortoiliac disease. Pressures are then measured segmentally at the proximal and distal thighs and at the proximal and distal calves. A pressure drop of more than 30 mm Hg signifies a significant obstruction between two levels.

The ABI is the ratio of the ankle blood pressure to the brachial blood pressure. An ABI greater than 1.0 is considered normal. An ABI from 0.5 to 0.84 is usually accompanied by claudication, while an ABI less than 0.5 is often associated with CLI. In cases where the arteries are significantly calcified and therefore noncompressible, the pressure measurements may be artificially elevated. In this case, plethysmographic waveforms derived from calibrated cuffs placed at the proximal and distal thigh, calf, ankle, metatarsals, and toes can be useful to locate flow-limiting lesions. The cuffs measure the pressure waveform of each pulse; analysis of the quality of the waveform and the volume (proportional to the area under the curve) can yield important information about flow between each segment.

Duplex imaging can be a useful tool in determining the location and severity of arterial obstruction. However, the time, equipment, and experience required to perform a complete screening of the lower extremity vessels make its use impractical. Therefore, its use is primarily limited to the analysis of specific arterial segments and bypass grafts.

Axial imaging such as MRA and CTA are increasingly used to image significant occlusions identified by the previously mentioned tests. One notable limitation of CTA is that in small vessels with an abundance of calcific disease, differentiation of the flow lumen from calcification can be difficult. In addition, these modalities suffer the same limitations as with evaluation of carotid disease, most notably due to their use of nephrotoxic contrast agents. There are protocols such as time-of-flight (TOF) MRA that do not require contrast that can yield image sequences analogous to conventional angiography. However, TOF MRA has difficulty resolving areas of slow flow, or flow in a vessel parallel to the scan plan.

Contrast angiography remains the gold standard for the evaluation of lower extremity ischemia. A complete study of the abdominal aorta, iliac, femoral, popliteal, and runoff vessels is performed bilaterally since atherosclerotic disease commonly occurs at any of these sites. Angiography is reserved for patients who are expected to undergo intervention or revascularization.

Management

Patients with claudication and those with CLI are managed differently due to major differences in their natural histories. Patients with claudication have amputation rates of 1% to 7% at 5 years. In contrast, 25% of CLI patients progress to major limb amputation in 1 year, and 25% die of cardiovascular complications in that time period. Surprisingly, history studies of patients with intermittent claudication suggest that only a small fraction of these patients (<5%) progress to CLI.

All patients with PAD warrant medical therapy. Given the relatively benign natural history of intermittent claudication, surgical intervention is not necessarily warranted. In contrast, the natural history of untreated CLI is much more grim. Information from placebo arms of pharmacologic trials of patients with unrevascularizable disease suggests up to 40% limb loss rates at 6 months. Therefore, revascularization is indicated for all functional patients.

Initial management is medical and consists of antiplatelet therapy and risk factor modification, including smoking cessation, antihypertensive medication, weight loss, and statin therapy for hypercholesterolemia. Data from numerous trials have confirmed that exercise therapy is the best initial treatment of intermittent claudication. Exercise regimens promote the development of a robust collateral circulation, which supplies blood to the areas distal to significant stenoses. More importantly, they halt the downward spiral of cardiovascular deconditioning. The American Heart Association recommends that exercise training in the form of walking, performed for 30 to 45 minutes three to four times per week for a period not less than 12 weeks. Trials have shown those patients who underwent implementation of structured exercise resulted in a 5-year cardiovascular survival rate of 80%, compared to 56% in untreated matched controls.

Aortoiliac Occlusive Disease

Endovascular therapy provides excellent long-term patency with very low mortality in aortoiliac occlusive disease. For single stenoses of the common iliac artery (CIA) or external iliac artery (EIA), shorter than 3 cm, endovascular therapy is the preferred modality. It is also reasonable to employ endovascular therapy for (a) a single stenosis in the CIA between 3 and 10 cm in length, (b) two isolated stenoses in the CIA/EIA less than 5 cm, or (c) a single CIA occlusion. Angioplasty alone often produces an adequate result, and stenting can be used in cases of residual stenosis, dissection, or lesions with high embolic risk.

Surgical revascularization is the method of choice for more complex lesions. Aortobifemoral bypass grafting with a Dacron graft has 88% patency at 5 years, but the morbidity and mortality of aortic surgery are significant. In patients with a hostile abdomen or high surgical risk, who cannot be revascularized with an endovascular approach, axillobifemoral bypass grafting (or its equivalent) is the approach of choice. Unfortunately, due to the length of the synthetic conduit, the patency of these grafts is less than is that of the aortobifemoral graft. For patients with unilateral iliac disease not amenable to endovascular therapy, unilateral aortofemoral grafting yields the best results. In elderly or medically infirm patients unable to tolerate a midline laparotomy for aortic access, a femoral–femoral crossover graft is an option.

Femoropopliteal Disease

Endovascular therapy for infrainguinal disease as compared to aortoiliac disease has the following characteristics: (a) the patency rates are lower, though acceptable; (b) no more than two focal stenoses less than 3 cm in length should be treated; and (c) the role of primary stenting is unclear, though angioplasty remains well accepted. Bypass grafting is indicated when endovascular therapy is inappropriate or inadequate. When grafting to a target above the knee, vein grafts have only slightly higher patency than do polytetrafluoroethylene (PTFE) or other prosthetic grafts. However, vein grafts are far superior to PTFE for below-knee targets. Recently, percutaneous stent grafting to the suprageniculate popliteal has demonstrated highly favorable results.

Tibial–Peroneal Disease

The role of angioplasty and stenting for infrapopliteal disease remains controversial and is reserved for patients in whom revascularization is otherwise not possible. Bypasses to the distal circulation are typically performed only for limb salvage due to poorer success rates with these grafts. A femoral–distal bypass is the option of choice because it provides the best inflow. Autologous vein has an approximately 50% patency rate at 4 years, while PTFE has only 12% patency.

Postoperative Graft Surveillance

Bypass grafts fail at three common time point: early (<30 days), intermediate (30 days to 2 years), and late (>2 years). Early failure must be assumed related to a technical or judgment error, though infection and hypercoagulability are also possible. Intermediate failure is most often caused by neointimal hyperplasia within a vein graft or at anastomotic sites. Late failure is caused by natural progression of atherosclerotic disease. Meticulous postoperative surveillance of bypass grafts can significantly increase long-term success. A typical surveillance protocol includes DUS of the graft as well as ABI measurements. Examinations should be performed perioperatively, at 6 weeks, and then at 3-month intervals for 2 years and every 6 months thereafter.

Complications

Morbidity and mortality of intervention for chronic lower extremity ischemia fits into two categories: those related to concomitant systemic illnesses and those related to surgery. Myocardial infarction and renal failure are common examples of the first category. Surgical complications include pseudoaneurysm resulting from arterial puncture, compartment syndrome, and graft infection. All of these must be treated promptly and aggressively.

ANEURYSMAL VASCULAR DISEASE

Aneurysms of the aorta, iliac arteries, visceral arteries, and peripheral arteries remain a major cause of morbidity and mortality. Atherosclerosis is the major cause of aneurysmal disease in all locations except for the ascending aorta, where cystic medial necrosis accounts for the majority of aneurysms. Less common causes of aneurysms include dissection, connective tissue disorders (e.g., Takayasu arteritis, Marfan's disease), infection, and syphilis.

Abdominal Aortic Aneurysms

The Aneurysm Detection and Management Veterans Affairs Cooperative Study Group (ADAM) trial determined numerous risk factors for abdominal aortic aneurysm (AAA): advanced age, CAD, atherosclerosis, hypertension, and a smoking history. Men outnumber women by a ratio of approximately 5 to 1. Having a first-degree family member with history of aneurysm repair increases the relative risk of developing an AAA by a factor of 2. The risk for developing an AAA is lower in women, African Americans, and diabetics.

By far, the greatest risk of an untreated AAA is death due to rupture. Risk of rupture increases significantly with the size of the aneurysm because of the exponential increase in wall stress with increased radius. In addition to aneurysm size, the United Kingdom Small Aneurysm Trial (UKSAT) found that female gender, current smoking, and hypertension were independent risk factors for rupture.

Diagnosis

AAAs are usually asymptomatic. The presence of symptoms such as abdominal or back pain signifies impending or active rupture and should lead to urgent intervention. The presence of peripheral embolization of intraluminal thrombus is also reported with aortic aneurysms. Rupture of an AAA presents as severe abdominal or back pain with associated hypotension, tachycardia, and shock. Finally, AAAs may rupture into the third or fourth portion of the duodenum, producing exsanguinating gastrointestinal (GI) hemorrhage.

Physical examination may reveal a pulsatile abdominal mass, but only 30% to 40% of aneurysms are noted on physical examination. Detection is correlated with aneurysm size; aneurysms greater than 5 cm in diameter are detected in 76% of patients, but those 3 to 3.9 cm are detected only in 29%.

AAAs are often diagnosed accidentally by ultrasonography or abdominal CT scan ordered for an unrelated reason. Ultrasonography is reproducible, noninvasive, and cheap. While sensitivity and specificity approach 100%, in approximately 1% to 3% of patients the aorta is unable to visualized secondary to obesity of overlying bowel gas. While it is ideal of screening and surveillance of small aneurysms, it is imprecise in measuring aneurysm diameter, which is a key component of the decision to proceed with operative intervention.

CTA is more reproducible than is ultrasound and is the primary modality for operative planning. CT scanning can determine the extent and morphology aneurysm, in particular its involvement and proximity to key vessels such as the celiac, superior mesenteric, and renal arteries (Fig. 20.5). Software packages are now commonly available that enable multiplanar analysis and 3-D reconstruction, both of which are helpful in planning endovascular stent graft repair.

Patient Selection

Symptomatic patients presenting with AAA and abdominal or back pain are at an increased risk of rupture, and urgent intervention is recommended. Aneurysm rupture is associated with 50% prehospital mortality; those that reach intervention have a 40% to 70% perioperative mortality.

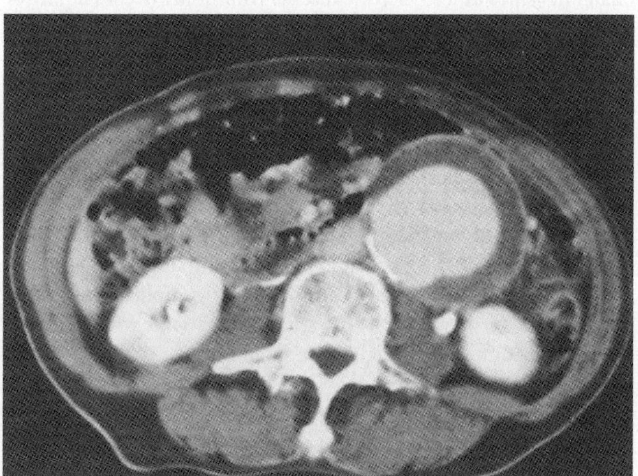

FIGURE 20.5 Abdominal computerized tomographic scan demonstrating AAA with mural thrombus. (From Goldstone J. Abdominal aortic aneurysms. In: Greenfield LJ, Mulholland MW, Oldham KT, et al., eds. *Surgery: Scientific Principles and Practice*. 1st ed. Philadelphia: J.B. Lippincott; 1993:1715, with permission.)

For patients with asymptomatic AAA, the decision for operative intervention is largely driven by diameter criterion. There is strong evidence that aneurysms greater than or equal to 5.5 cm should be electively repaired. Large randomized prospective trials in both the United Kingdom and United States indicate that there is no survival advantage to operating on AAAs up to 4.5 cm in diameter. Once the aneurysm has reached a size of 4.5 to 5.5 cm, operative repair should be strongly considered. The decision to operate involves many variables including size, recent expansion, operative risk, medical comorbidities, age, life expectancy, and family history of rupture.

Open Surgical Repair

Conventional AAA repair consists of a retroperitoneal approach through the left flank or a transabdominal, transperitoneal approach via a midline incision. No strong data exist favoring one exposure to the other in terms of perioperative or long-term outcomes. In current practice, the juxtarenal (aneurysms involving the takeoff of the renal arteries) and suprarenal aneurysms are best approached through the left retroperitoneal space and opening the left diaphragmatic crura.

Upon clamping of the aorta proximally, the aneurysm sac is entered, and bleeding lumbar arteries are ligated. A prosthetic graft is sewn proximally and distally to normal aorta. In the presence of significant iliac artery disease, a bifurcated graft can be sewn to either the iliac arteries or the common femoral arteries. The aneurysm sac is closed over the graft in an attempt to lessen the risk of aortoenteric fistulization from erosion of the duodenum or other viscera by friction from the prosthetic graft.

In the presence of a ruptured or inflammatory aneurysm, the aorta must be controlled at the supraceliac level before the infrarenal aorta is exposed. Once control of the aneurysmal segment of the aorta is established, the supraceliac clamp should be moved as caudally as possible ideally to an infrarenal location.

Some special anatomic considerations apply to AAA repair. Prior to aortic cross clamping, the left renal vein must be identified and protected to avoid injury. With regard to pelvic outflow, if the inferior mesenteric artery (IMA) is to be sacrificed, then at least one hypogastric (internal iliac) artery must have good flow to prevent colon ischemia and vasculogenic impotence. If both hypogastric arteries are sacrificed secondary to aneurysmal disease, the patent IMA should be reimplanted into the aorta.

Endovascular Repair

Endovascular aortic aneurysm repair (EVAR) was introduced by Parodi in 1991, and two stent graft devices obtained U.S. FDA approval in 2000 (Fig. 20.6). Stent grafting was initially reserved for patients who presented a prohibitive risk for open repair. As the technology has gained acceptance and long-term durability of the devices has been established, stent grafts are being offered to standard risk patients. Since its introduction, there has been a rapid increase in its adoption; EVAR now accounts for more than half of all AAA repairs. Multiple studies have shown that EVAR can be accomplished with shorter hospital stay and decreased morbidity compared with open repair, both in the elective and the ruptured setting.

The key anatomic factors, which determine eligibility for EVAR, are the size and location of the aneurysm neck (especially its proximity to the renal arteries), the degree of tortuosity of the aorta, and the size and shape of the access vessels (the femoral or iliac arteries). An adequate neck length (usually 15 mm) is necessary to ensure proper fixation of the device without compromising flow to the renal arteries.

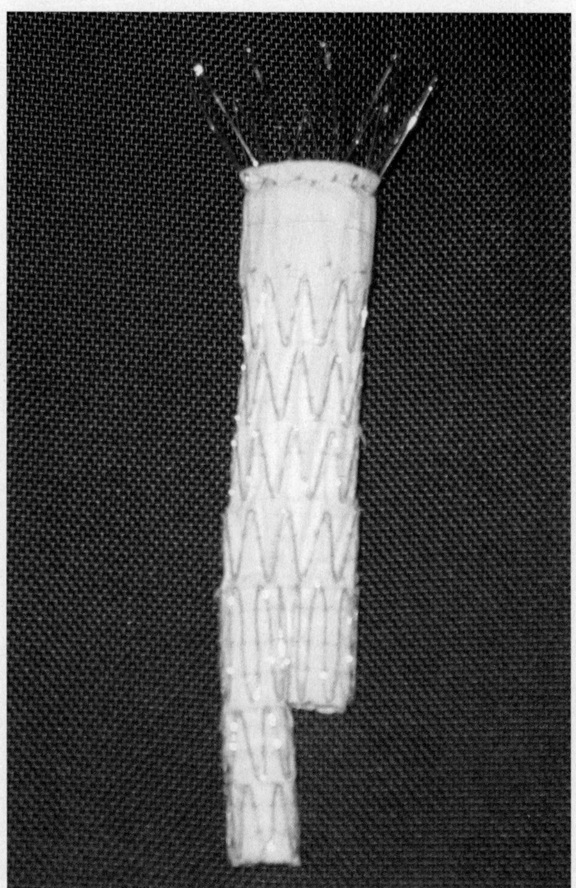

FIGURE 20.6 Zenith stent graft for treatment of endovascular repair of AAAs. Note the barbs for suprarenal aorta fixation.

Complications

The most common early complications following conventional open AAA repair are paralytic ileus, coronary ischemia, cardiac arrhythmias, renal dysfunction, and pneumonia. Less common early complications include ischemic colitis, impotence, paralysis, graft infection, and pseudoaneurysm. Late complications include incisional hernia, pseudoaneurysm development, atherosclerotic graft occlusion, graft thrombosis, and aortoenteric fistula. It should be noted that the complication rate following repair of ruptured aneurysms is significantly higher in all categories.

Endovascular aneurysm repair, despite having a lower rate of overall morbidity, has its own set of unique complications. Device-related complications include kinking, occlusion, thrombosis, and endoleak. Most concerning of these is the development of an endoleak, because this implies that the aneurysm sac is still filling with blood at arterial pressure, and therefore, the risk of rupture has not been eliminated. Figure 20.7 details the types of endoleaks. Non–device-related complications include dissection or thrombosis of the access vessels, contrast-induced nephropathy, and wound complications.

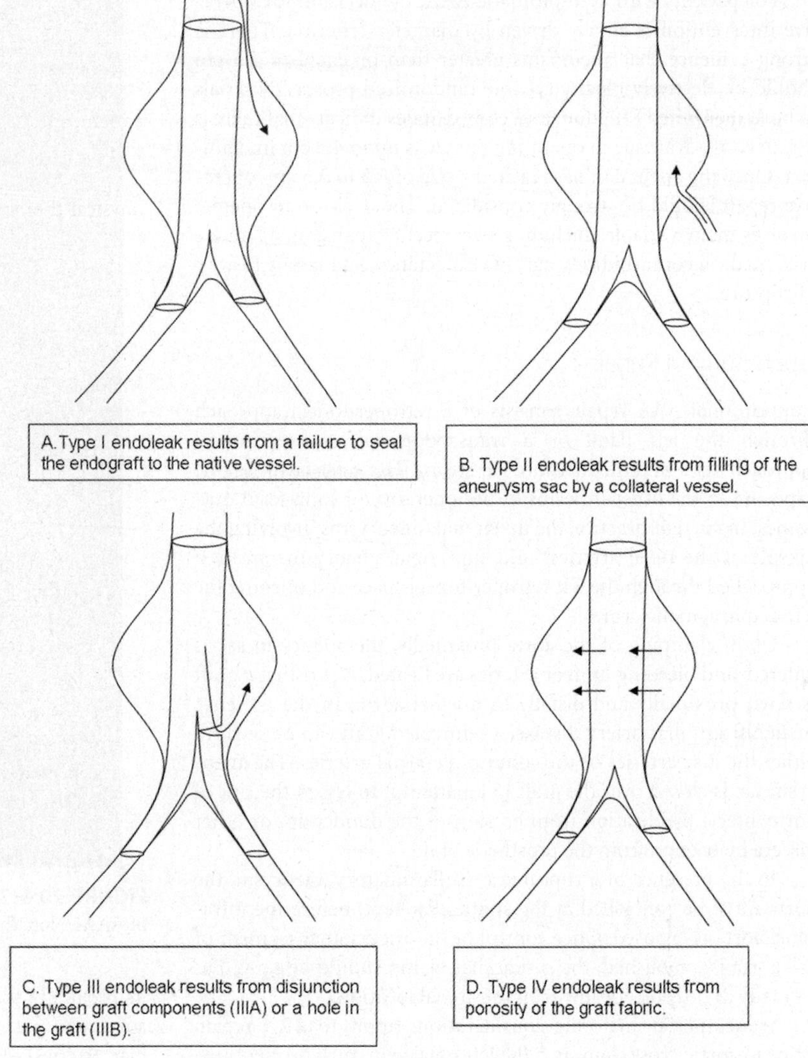

FIGURE 20.7 Graphic representation of the four types of endoleaks. **A.** Type I endoleaks result from an inadequate seal between the graft and the landing zones. These can be divided into IA (proximal) and IB (distal). **B.** Type II endoleaks result from collateral flow into the aneurysm sac. **C.** Type III endoleaks occur when graft components are inadequately sealed to each other (IIIA) or when a hole in the graft develops (IIIB). **D.** Type IV endoleaks result from porosity of the graft fabric and are usually self-limited.

Visceral Aneurysms

Aneurysmal disease also occurs in the renal, hepatic, and splenic arteries; however, these aneurysms are usually not of atherosclerotic etiology and tend to occur in younger patients. Renal and hepatic aneurysms should be repaired when discovered because of their high risk of rupture. Splenic artery aneurysms have a lesser risk of rupture and can be closely monitored, although there are exceptions to this rule. Splenic aneurysms in pregnant women (or women who may become pregnant) and those larger than 2 cm in diameter have a higher risk of rupture and should be repaired.

Renal, hepatic, and splenic aneurysms are typically treated with exclusion and bypass grafting. Proximal aneurysms of the hepatic and splenic arteries, however, can be simply excluded because of the rich collateral blood supply around these vessels. Endovascular coil embolization is useful in the treatment of saccular aneurysms, and covered stent grafts may also be utilized to repair fusiform aneurysms of these vessels.

Peripheral Aneurysms

Aneurysms of the iliac, femoral, and popliteal arteries are common in patients with atherosclerotic diseases. The primary risk of an iliac aneurysm is rupture, while femoral and popliteal aneurysms have a tendency to thrombose or embolize. Each of these aneurysms is strongly correlated with the presence of significant aneurysmal disease in other arteries. An abdominal aneurysm may be present in up to 85% of patients with femoral artery aneurysms and up to 62% of patients with popliteal aneurysms.

Iliac artery aneurysms should be repaired if they are symptomatic, larger than 3 cm, or mycotic. Repair is accomplished with either endovascularly with a covered stent or through open surgical bypass graft with exclusion of the aneurysm. Femoral artery aneurysms should be repaired if they are symptomatic, larger than 2.5 cm, or mycotic. Repair is carried out with exclusion of the aneurysm and bypass graft. Popliteal artery aneurysms are repaired if they are symptomatic, larger than 2 cm, or mycotic. Treatment is with exclusion and bypass with saphenous vein graft, although recently stent grafting has gained support, especially in high-risk patients.

Pseudoaneurysms

Pseudoaneurysms occur when arterial blood fills a cavity that is not enclosed by all three layers of the vessel wall. This most commonly occurs in the femoral artery after puncture for a percutaneous procedure but can also occur at vascular suture lines. Small pseudoaneurysms associated with puncture of the vessel can resolve spontaneously, but larger pseudoaneurysms and those present at surgical suture lines require intervention to avoid rupture. For pseudoaneurysms resulting from percutaneous puncture, treatment consists of either duplex-guided compression or thrombin injection. Operation is necessary for pseudoaneurysms associated with bypass grafts, as there is often a defect in the graft at the suture line.

UPPER EXTREMITY VASCULAR DISEASE

Clinically evident upper extremity arterial occlusive disease is relatively uncommon. Most lesions are proximal and have adequate collateralization, leaving the majority of patients asymptomatic. The most commonly affected vessel is the subclavian artery. Subclavian steal syndrome occurs in the presence of a proximal stenosis or occlusion of the subclavian artery. The delivery of arterial blood to the ipsilateral extremity thus depends on reversed flow through the ipsilateral vertebral artery via the circle of Willis. Thus, strenuous activity of the affected upper extremity may result in ischemic pain in the extremity or neurologic symptoms of vertebrobasilar insufficiency as blood is increasingly shunted away from the posterior cerebral circulation. Revascularization is indicated for symptomatic stenoses and is accomplished with either percutaneous transluminal angioplasty and stenting or carotid to subclavian artery bypass.

Thoracic Outlet Syndrome

Thoracic outlet syndrome (TOS) describes a constellation of vascular and/or neurologic symptoms, often without any physical findings and most commonly without an anatomic correlate. It usually occurs in younger patients and is caused by compression of the subclavian artery, vein, or branches of the brachial plexus. Patients complain of weakness, numbness, paresthesias, pain, and swelling of the extremity.

Anatomic Cause

The brachial plexus and subclavian artery pass through the narrow triangle formed by the anterior scalene muscle, the middle scalene muscle, and the first rib (the scalene triangle). The subclavian vein also passes over the first rib but lies anterior to the anterior scalene muscle. Presence of an anomalous cervical rib or hypertrophy of the anterior scalene muscle can cause compression of the brachial plexus, subclavian artery, and/or subclavian vein.

Neurologic Symptoms

The symptoms and signs caused by irritation and seemingly compression of the brachial plexus are far more common than are symptoms attributable to the subclavian artery or vein. Complaints include weakness, numbness, paresthesias, and pain; however, there may be no objective findings on neurologic examination. Pain is described in the subscapular, scapular, and cervical regions, while paresthesias and numbness typically occur in the hand and medial forearm (ulnar distribution). Elevation of the arm will often exacerbate symptoms. Physical findings are uncommon but may include weakness and atrophy of the triceps muscle, the intrinsic muscles of the hand, and the wrist flexors.

Diagnosis is difficult due to a lack of objective findings and is often based on history, physical examination, and exclusion of other conditions. Chest and cervical spine x-rays can demonstrate the presence of a cervical rib, but this is found only in the occasional patient, and EMG may be helpful in diagnosing a subtle neurologic defect.

The mainstay of treatment is conservative, with exercise and physical therapy providing symptomatic relief. Surgical treatment of neurologic TOS should be reserved for refractory cases because major neurovascular complications are not uncommon. It is critical that this operation be performed by a surgeon experienced in the management of TOS as outcomes are markedly improved. First rib resection may be performed via a transaxillary approach, or a supraclavicular approach can be used to perform anterior and middle scalenectomies with or without first rib resection.

Vascular Symptoms

Subclavian artery compression usually results from hypertrophy of the anterior scalene muscle in athletes but may also be caused by the presence of a cervical rib. Ischemic symptoms may be exacerbated by maximal abduction of the arm. Surgical intervention is indicated for arterial compressive symptoms resulting from TOS and involves release of the scalene muscles and resection of bony abnormalities. In the presence of acute ischemia, immediate anticoagulation should be followed with thrombectomy, and definitive repair can be accomplished at a later time.

Compression of the subclavian vein in TOS usually presents as effort-induced thrombosis (Paget–von Schrötter disease). Common in young men with a history of strenuous upper extremity activity, it presents as painful swelling of the affected arm. Diagnosis is made with venous duplex studies and venography. Initial treatment is directed at recanalizing the subclavian vein and consists of thrombolytics and anticoagulation. If the subclavian vein is reopened with medical therapy, surgical intervention such as first rib resection to relieve venous compression should follow. If the thrombosis does not respond to medical therapy alone, decompression should be performed earlier, and angioplasty may be required as an adjunct.

MESENTERIC ISCHEMIA

Acute embolic occlusion, responsible for 50% of acute mesenteric ischemia, usually affects the superior mesenteric artery (SMA), and the embolus is typically from a cardiac source. The most common site for an embolus to lodge is at the origin of the middle colic artery, distal to the first jejunal branches. Thus, the most proximal small bowel is typically spared. Rapid diagnosis and intervention are paramount, as patients who progress to the point of peritonitis usually have irreversible damage that is associated with a high incidence of mortality.

Early diagnosis depends greatly on a high degree of suspicion, as the classic finding is "pain out of proportion to physical examination." Common symptoms include sudden onset of periumbilical pain, diarrhea, vomiting, and GI bleeding. If the diagnosis is suspected before the onset of peritoneal signs, mesenteric angiography is the diagnostic procedure of choice. If an embolism is present, laparotomy should be performed immediately, with embolectomy of the SMA and resection of nonviable bowel.

Acute thrombotic occlusion is the cause of acute mesenteric ischemia in about 25% of cases. These events occur in the setting of preexisting atherosclerotic disease of the mesenteric vessels. The presenting symptoms are similar to those of embolic occlusion. In contrast to embolic events, angiography is likely to show an occlusion at or near the ostium of the SMA without sparing the jejunal vessels. Once the diagnosis is made, laparotomy is performed immediately to resect infarcted bowel and revascularize the remaining intestine.

Nonocclusive mesenteric ischemia accounts for 20% of acute mesenteric ischemia. This occurs almost exclusively in critically ill patients with severely diminished cardiac output and corresponding splanchnic vasospasm. The primary symptom is vague abdominal pain, though tube feeding intolerance, distension, leukocytosis, and metabolic acidosis may also be present. Angiography shows a patent vascular tree with nonvisualized mesenteric arcades ("pruning"). Treatment includes directed injection of vasodilators such as papaverine into the mesenteric vessels in conjunction with aggressive treatment of the underlying disorder.

Mesenteric venous thrombosis accounts for the remaining 5% of acute mesenteric ischemia. It primarily affects younger patients, most of whom will have an underlying hypercoagulability disorder. Thrombosis usually develops initially in distal vessels and then propagates to the larger veins. The most common complaint is diffuse abdominal pain, but some patients have vomiting, diarrhea, and GI bleeding as well. Peritonitis is rare. CT scan reveals marked bowel wall edema, mesenteric thickening, ascites, and an enlarged superior mesenteric vein with a central lucency suggestive of thrombus. The patient should be followed closely for peritonitis, as medical therapy with fluid resuscitation, bowel rest, antibiotics, and anticoagulation is usually curative.

Chronic mesenteric ischemia occurs primarily because of atherosclerotic disease at the ostia of the visceral vessels. Because of the rich collateral supply of the intestine, symptomatic chronic mesenteric ischemia usually does not occur until multiple vessels are severely stenosed. The classic symptom is postprandial pain, which is severe enough to deter the patient from eating, resulting in significant weight loss. Diagnosis is made with angiography. Revascularization should occur promptly, as this population is at high risk for acute thrombosis. Revascularization is accomplished with either PTA with or without stenting, bypass, or endarterectomy.

NONATHEROSCLEROTIC VASCULAR DISEASE

Fibromuscular dysplasia, previously mentioned in the setting of renal vascular hypertension, encompasses multiple subtypes, the most common of which is called medial fibrodysplasia (80% to 90%). In this type, degeneration of the media causes fibrous constrictions alternating with aneurysmal dilatation creating a "string of beads" appearance on angiography. Fibromuscular dysplasia is seen most commonly in young women and affects the renal arteries most often, followed by the carotid and iliac arteries.

Buerger disease (*thromboangiitis obliterans*) is a severe, progressive, nonatherosclerotic arterial occlusive disease. The typical patient is a young male smoker of Eastern European, Mediterranean, or Asian descent. Symptoms begin with lower extremity claudication and rapidly progress to rest pain and ischemic ulceration. Occasionally, the upper extremity is also affected by Raynaud phenomenon, with cyanosis or gangrene of the digits. Angiography shows (a) absence of atherosclerotic disease, (b) severe occlusive disease of small vessels, and (c) "corkscrew" collaterals along the course of the occluded vessels. Absolute cessation of smoking results in disease remission in most patients, and exercise therapy to develop collaterals is essential. Other therapies used with some success include vasodilators, antiplatelet agents, and even sympathectomy (loss of vascular tone produces vasodilation).

Autoimmune vasculitides: Takayasu arteritis and *temporal arteritis*, both classified as forms of giant cell arteritis, deserve mention in that they occasionally require intervention by a vascular surgeon. *Takayasu disease* causes stenotic or occlusive lesions, and occasionally aneurysms, of the aorta and its major branches. It occurs primarily in women younger than 35 years. The mainstay of treatment is immunosuppression with glucocorticoids; chemotherapy is used when recurrences present during steroid therapy. One quarter of patients are unresponsive to medical therapy. Those who require surgical intervention respond best to open vascular bypass, though angioplasty and stenting may have a role in renal artery lesions.

Temporal arteritis affects women more commonly than men and usually occurs in patients older than 50 years. The most commonly affected vessels are the temporal, occipital, subclavian, and axillary arteries. Besides constitutional symptoms, many patients present with visual deficits. Diagnosis is established by temporal artery biopsy. Corticosteroids are the treatment of choice.

Popliteal entrapment syndrome is a rare disease, which typically affects young adults. In this disorder, the popliteal artery deviates around the medial head of the gastrocnemius muscle. Most patients present with mild claudication; physical examination may reveal loss of distal pulses with plantar flexion of the foot. Treatment involves surgical resection of the medial head of the gastrocnemius muscle, though arterial reconstruction may be necessary.

VENOUS DISEASES

Deep venous thrombosis (DVT) is a common problem in surgical patients and can cause serious short- and long-term morbidity and mortality. Risk factors for DVT include age greater than 40 years, obesity, malignancy, prolonged immobilization, surgery, trauma, pregnancy, and hypercoagulability. DVT prophylaxis is a controversial and evolving topic; however, it is known that pneumatic compression stockings, subcutaneous doses of either unfractionated or low molecular weight heparin, and early mobility decrease the rate of DVT when applied both pre- and postoperatively.

The most feared acute complication of DVT is pulmonary embolism. Seventy percent of pulmonary emboli arise from DVTs in the pelvic and deep veins of the lower extremities. The upper extremity, the calf, and the superficial venous system are rare sources of pulmonary emboli.

The most common presentation of DVT is unilateral swelling of an extremity, though clinical diagnosis is difficult. Occasionally, in the case of iliofemoral venous thrombosis, massive swelling, pain, and cyanosis develop. This is referred to as *phlegmasia cerulea dolens* (swollen, blue, painful). If this condition progresses and arterial supply to the extremity is compromised because of swelling, *phlegmasia alba dolens* (swollen, white, painful) develops. In severe cases, gangrene can develop. Surgical thrombectomy or catheter-directed thrombolysis are indicated in these conditions.

Venography is the gold standard for diagnosis of venous thrombosis, but it is rarely as it is invasive and requires intravenous contrast. DUS has excellent sensitivity and specificity and is inexpensive and easy to obtain.

The mainstay of treatment for DVT is anticoagulation with heparin, followed by warfarin. Low molecular weight heparin, given subcutaneously twice daily, is now an accepted alternative to intravenous heparin. For a first occurrence of DVT, anticoagulation should continue for 6 months. For a second DVT, treatment is extended to 1 year. For patients who develop pulmonary embolism or a third DVT, lifelong anticoagulation is recommended. Placement of an inferior vena cava (IVC) filter should be considered for patients who have a contraindication to anticoagulation or develop pulmonary embolism or recurrent DVT despite therapeutic anticoagulation.

Increasing attention has been turned to the long-term sequelae of DVTs. Manifestations of postthrombotic syndrome arise from a combination of valvular damage and incompetence, and residual venous obstruction. This can lead to fluid translocation into the soft tissue resulting in persistent edema and venous stasis ulcers. Clinically significant postthrombotic syndrome can occur in up to 30% of patients. Predictors of disease severity include involvement of the common femoral or iliac veins, previous DVT, higher BMI, and advanced age.

The growing recognition of postthrombotic syndrome has lead to an increased interest in techniques for thrombus removal. Current techniques include surgical thrombectomy and catheter-directed thrombolysis. Recommendations are currently still in evolution, but early thrombus removal should be considered in severely symptomatic patients with acute iliofemoral DVTs, and who have no contraindication to thrombolytics.

ARTERIOVENOUS ACCESS

With the number of patients affected by end-stage renal disease (ESRD) increasing, surgeons must be familiar with the various options for hemodialysis access. AV access options can be classified as temporary or permanent.

Percutaneous catheters, usually considered a temporary solution, are typically used in patients who need urgent dialysis or who have exhausted all options for permanent surgical access. These large, double-lumen catheters are usually placed in the internal jugular, subclavian, or femoral veins. Catheters should be removed from the femoral veins as soon as possible due to the high risk of infection. If more than a brief period of dialysis is anticipated, a percutaneous cuffed, tunneled catheter should be placed as this significantly decreases the risk of infection. Catheter placement in the subclavian vein results in a high rate of vein thrombosis and stenosis, making the internal jugular vein the ideal target vessel.

The basic tenets of permanent AV access are as follows: (a) native fistulas are preferable to prosthetic grafts; (b) distal sites should be used before proximal sites; (c) the nondominant extremity should be used whenever possible; and (d) an access site should not be abandoned until reasonable efforts at revision have been exhausted. ·

In order of preference, AV fistula options include the radiocephalic fistula (Brescia–Cimino), brachiocephalic fistula, and basilic vein transposition. AV graft options include looped forearm grafts, upper arm grafts, and lower extremity or chest wall grafts.

ACKNOWLEDGMENTS

Special thanks to previous edition authors David G. Neschis, MD; Michael A. Golden, MD; Mireille A. Moise, MD; and Ronald M Fairman, MD.

SUGGESTED READINGS

Cameron JL, ed. *Current Surgical Therapy*. 8th ed. St. Louis: Mosby; 2004.

Moore WS, ed. *Vascular and Endovascular Surgery: A Comprehensive Review*. 7th ed. Philadelphia: WB Saunders; 2005.

Rutherford RB, ed. *Vascular Surgery*. 7th ed. Philadelphia: WB Saunders; 2005.

CHAPTER

21

Pulmonary Physiology and Thoracic Disease

JEFFREY E. COHEN AND SUNIL SINGHAL

KEY POINTS

- Definitions of pulmonary function tests
  - TV (Tidal volume): The amount of air inspired or expired during normal respiration
  - FRC: The amount of air contained in the lungs after normal expiration
  - VC: The amount of air exhaled following maximal inspiration and forced expiration
  - RV: The amount of air remaining in the lungs after maximal expiration
  - FEV1: The volume of air exhaled in 1 second with a maximum expiratory effort
- Criteria for operative risk for pulmonary resection
  - Preoperative FEV1:
    - Greater than 40% predicted: little increased risk
    - 30% to 40% predicted: increased risk of pulmonary complications
    - Less than 30% predicted: prohibitive risk
- Etiologies of hypoxemia
  - Hypoventilation
  - Diffusion gradient
  - *V/Q* mismatch
- Presence of a new solitary nodule in a patient with smoking history must be assumed to be a lung cancer until proven otherwise.
- Lung cancer is the most common cause of cancer-related death in men and women.
- 80% of lung cancer is NSCLC.
  - 20% are resectable
  - 70% 5-year survival of those resected
- Surgical resection is the cornerstone of therapy for stage I and II disease.
- Adjuvant therapy has demonstrated a clear benefit in stage II and III disease.
- Stage IIIB patients are generally considered not to be operative candidates, particularly with contralateral positive nodes.
- Signs of inoperability in lung cancer are bloody pleural effusion, Horner syndrome, SVC syndrome, and distant metastases.
- Myasthenia gravis is present in 30% of patients with thymoma.

RESPIRATORY PHYSIOLOGY

The central purpose of respiration is to deliver oxygen to erythrocytes and clear carbon dioxide. This enables the body's cells to undergo aerobic metabolism to efficiently produce ATP and thereby fuel the countless number of processes necessary for organ function. Additionally, the removal of carbon dioxide is a critical component of the body's acid–base homeostasis. This exchange of gases consists of *ventilation*, the process by which atmospheric air travels to the alveoli; the *blood–gas interface*, which is the site of gas exchange; and *perfusion*, whereby blood passes through this interface.

Air Movement

Atmospheric oxygen can enter the bloodstream only if it is delivered to the alveoli. Air must enter through the oropharynx or nasopharynx and then travel past the larynx, into the trachea, through the conducting airways of the tracheobronchial tree, and then into the alveoli. The pressure gradient required for air movement is generated by the primary and accessory respiratory muscles. These are regulated by components of the central nervous system.

Airways

The upper airway is composed of the mouth, pharynx, and larynx. The conducting zone of the lung is composed of the trachea and the first 16 generations of the airways. This zone is the anatomical dead space because there is an absence of alveoli, and thus, gas exchange is not possible while air dwells within them. The 17th to 19th generations consist of the respiratory bronchioles from which the first alveoli emerge. This region is termed the "transitional zone" of the lung. Generations 20 through 23 are lined with alveolar ducts and sacs and are known collectively as the respiratory zone. The segmental anatomy of the tracheobronchial tree is illustrated in Figure 21.1.

The conducting airways distal to the pharynx have cartilaginous walls with minimal smooth muscle. They are lined with ciliated epithelium interspersed with mucus-secreting goblet cells. The cilia and mucus are involved in the clearance of inhaled or aspirated particles. The mucociliary escalator carries particles in the tracheobronchial tree to the pharynx where they are either swallowed or expectorated. The cilia beat synchronously at 1,000 to 1,500 cycles per minute and can move particles 2 to 10 μm in diameter at a rate

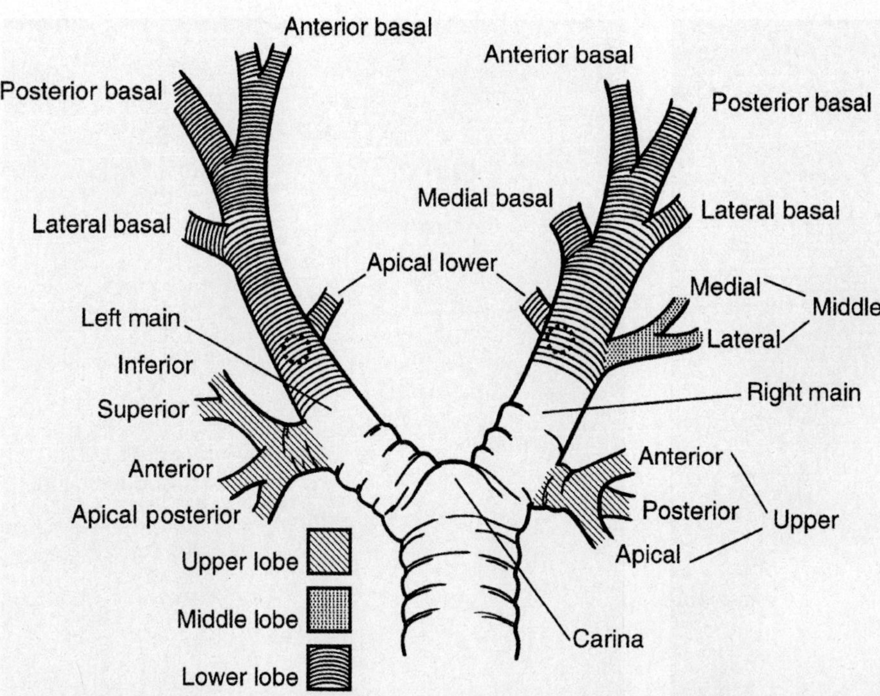

FIGURE 21.1 Schematic representation of airway branching in the human lung.

of 16 nm/minute. Smokers demonstrate abnormalities in both mucous production and ciliary motility that contribute to their difficulties with secretion clearance. Bronchiectasis is a condition in which the bronchi are dilated and a loss of ciliary action occurs. Secretions pool and can become chronically infected, a situation that may be associated with hemoptysis.

The transition zone is composed of membranous and terminal bronchioles. They do not contain cartilage and are innervated by the autonomic nervous system. Bronchoconstriction occurs due to cholinergic stimulation of muscarinic receptors in this zone, while adrenergic receptors cause bronchodilation. Several other chemokines including leukotrienes, thromboxane, and prostacyclins act on the bronchial lumen in this region.

The histologic morphology of the respiratory zone differs markedly from the conducting and transitional zones. There are 300 million alveoli with a total surface area of all the alveoli around 7 mm^2. The critical component of the alveoli that is integral for movement is the elastin that is embedded within the basal lamina in the alveolar septal interstitium. Elastin provides elastic recoil properties that prevent hyperextension of lung tissue. There are two major types of alveolar epithelial cells. Type I cells, the major lining cells, are large, flat, squamous cells with cytoplasmic extensions and are primarily responsible for gas exchange. Type II granular pneumocytes are thicker and are responsible for producing surfactant. Surfactant, a dipalmitoyl phosphatidylcholine, reduces alveolar surface tension, a force that decreases alveolar size and results in alveolar collapse. By Laplace's law, the distending pressure (P) to overcome the surface tension (T) is inversely proportional to the radius (r), $P = 2\ T/r$. Therefore, as the alveolus gets smaller, the surfactant becomes more concentrated, and its effect on lowering the surface tension becomes more essential to keep the alveolus open. This decrease in surface tension also helps equalize pressures within alveoli of differing sizes that would otherwise result in emptying of smaller alveoli into larger ones and subsequent collapse of smaller alveoli. Surfactant also counterbalances the hydrostatic pressure of blood. Without surfactant, unopposed surface tension would result in a 20-mm Hg hydrostatic force pushing fluid from the blood into the alveolus. Surfactant levels are increased by thyroid hormone and glucocorticoids. They are decreased in respiratory distress syndrome, acute pancreatitis, and smokers and at high oxygen tensions. The alveoli also contain pulmonary alveolar macrophages that pass through lung capillaries into the pulmonary interstitium. These cells can phagocytose particles less than 2 μm.

Mechanics of Ventilation

Ventilation is achieved by air movement to and from the alveoli. This is accomplished by a decrease in intrathoracic pressure relative to the atmosphere when the diaphragm contracts and the thoracic cavity expands. The force generated by the diaphragm generates peak force at approximately 130% of its resting length. The decline in force generated with decreasing muscle length, which corresponds to an increase in resting lung volume, assumes clinical importance. For example, in COPD, hyperinflation of the lung produces flattening of the diaphragm. The flattened diaphragm has a shorter length and produces less force. When large volumes of air are required, the external intercostal muscles contract, which further expands the thoracic cavity. This is important to recognize in patients with increased work of breathing. Expiration is a passive process by which the elasticity of the diaphragm, rib cage, and lung returns the thoracic cavity to its baseline dimension. During normal exhalation, the muscles of inspiration relax and the elastic recoil of the lung results in a passive decrease in alveolar volume, which produces a positive alveolar pressure. There is a pressure gradient for air to move out of the lungs until the functional residual capacity (FRC) of the lung is reached. At this point, the alveolar and atmospheric pressures are equal; thus, there is no gradient for air movement. Forced expiration can be achieved with contraction of the internal intercostal muscles and abdominal muscles. It is important to note that the forces involving inspiration and

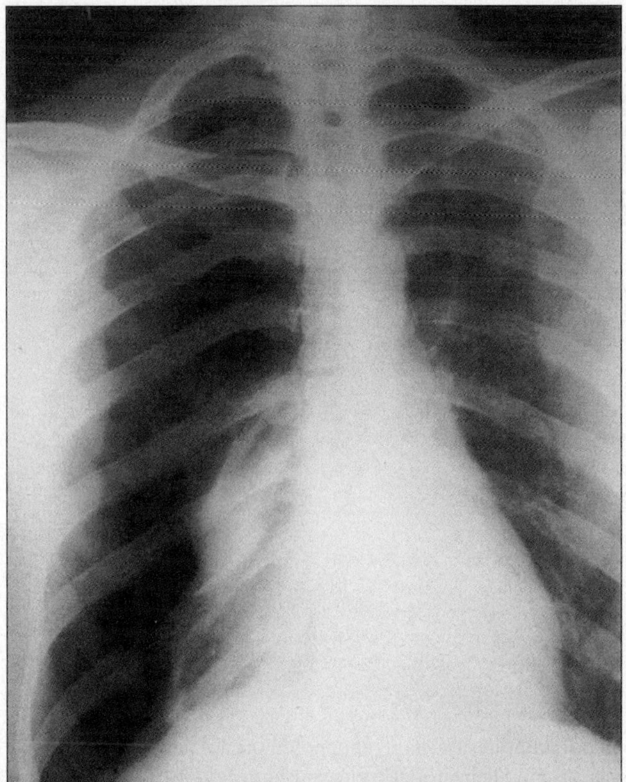

FIGURE 21.2 A chest radiograph of a right pneumothorax. (From Fidan F, Esme H, Unlu M, et al. Welder's lung associated with pneumothorax. *J Thorac Imaging.* 2005;20(2):120–122, with permission.)

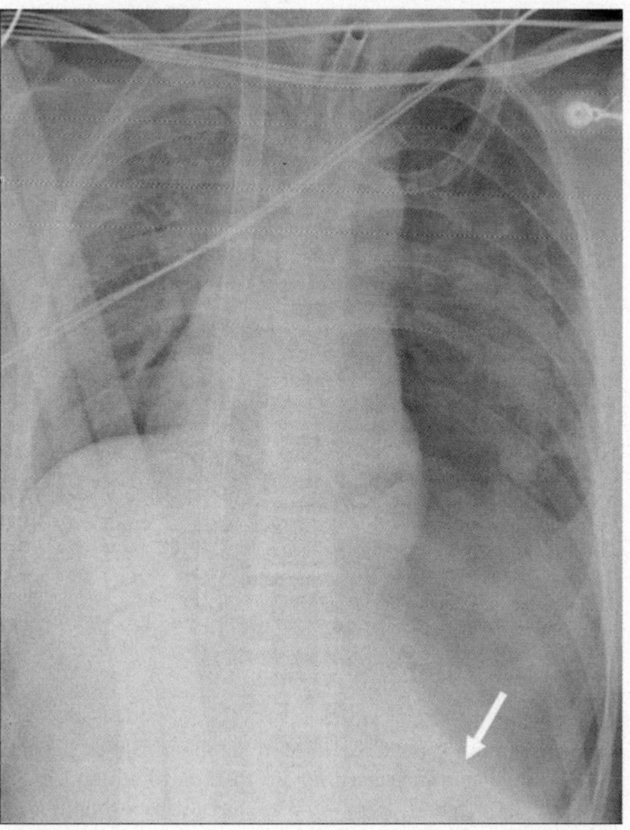

FIGURE 21.3 A left tension pneumothorax with depression of the left hemidiaphragm. (From Sur BW, Wandtke, JC, Hobbs SK, et al. Pneumothorax: how to recognize subtle signs and avoid pitfalls. *Contemp Diagn Radiol.* 2015;38(4):1–7.)

expiration are inherently coupled by the apposition of the visceral and parietal pleura. If this coupling is disrupted, as in the event of a pneumothorax (Fig. 21.2), this can lead to outward expansion of the chest wall, collapse of the lung, and eventual respiratory distress. In extreme cases, an ongoing air leak from the lung parenchyma can lead to a pressurized pleural space, creating a tension pneumothorax (Fig. 21.3), with resultant mediastinal shift, decreased venous return to the right atrium, and eventual circulatory collapse.

Ventilation is assessed by the measurement of the partial pressure of arterial carbon dioxide (PCO_2). Alveolar ventilation (V_A) is dependent on the depth of inspiration (tidal volume, V_T), the volume of the conducting airways (dead space, V_{DS}), and the rate of respiration (R). Mathematically, *alveolar ventilation* can be defined as:

$$V_A = (V_T - V_{DS}) \times R$$

The driving pressure for airflow through the entire system (from alveoli to atmosphere) is the difference between the alveolar pressure and pressure at the airway opening (atmospheric pressure). Alveolar pressure consists of two components, the elastic recoil pressure and the pleural pressure. Furthermore, elastic recoil pressure is determined by the intrinsic elastic properties of the alveoli and the degree of stretch imposed on the lung. The pleural pressure is generated by the elastic recoils of the lung and chest wall. At FRC, pleural pressure is approximately −5 cm H_2O. It becomes more negative with deeper inspiration and more positive with forced expiration. The pressure generated within the alveoli is dissipated in overcoming the resistance to airflow, including frictional resistance.

During the respiratory cycle, alveolar forces are balanced between the elastin, which allows recoil and prevents alveolar hyperextension, and surfactant, which reduces alveolar surface tension that would cause alveolar collapse. The compliance of the lung is a measure of the resistance of the lungs to expansion. Therefore, lungs with decreased compliance require greater work to allow alveolar expansion. This means that a larger pressure gradient is required to achieve a certain tidal volume. Figure 21.4 demonstrates how a disease state such as pulmonary fibrosis results in reduced compliance and decreased tidal volumes for a set pressure gradient. Conversely, patients with emphysema demonstrate increased lung compliance and augmented tidal volumes for a set pressure gradient. These patients have increased work of breathing because of increased expiratory resistance.

Control of Ventilation

Normal ventilation is involuntary and mediated by the respiratory center in the medulla, primarily in a dorsal nucleus and in a ventral group of nuclei. No definite pacemaker cells have yet been identified to explain the rhythmic nature of normal ventilation. Rather one major theory suggests within major clusters of respiratory neurons is a collection of cells whose pooled firing patterns produce inspiration and expiration—an oscillating respiratory network. Voluntary ventilation is mediated by the cerebral cortex via the corticospinal tracts. The efferent neurons from the pons and medulla

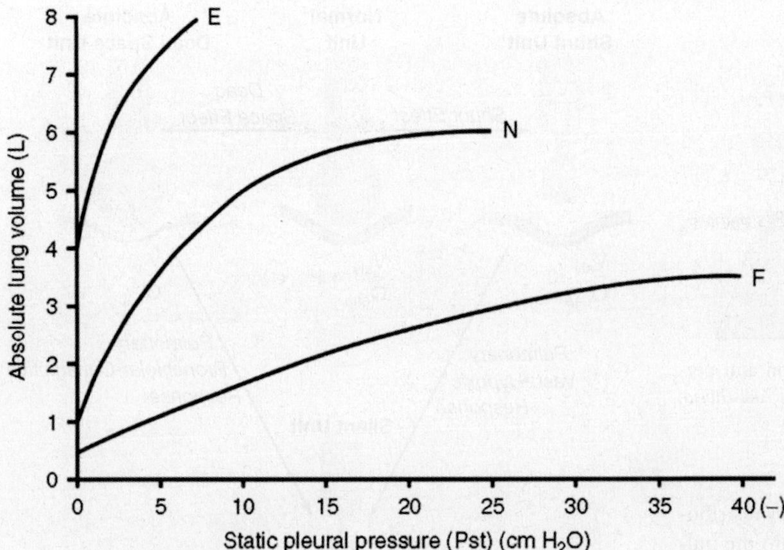

FIGURE 21.4 Demonstration of pulmonary compliance curves for normal and diseased lungs. (From Hyatt RE, Scanlon PD, Nakamura M, eds. *Interpretation of Pulmonary Function Tests: A Practical Guide.* 3rd ed. Philadelphia: Lippincott Williams & Wilkins; 2008.)

are in the white matter of the spinal cord between the lateral and ventral corticospinal tracts. All of the nerves concerned with inspiration join in the ventral horns of C3 through C5, in the phrenic motor neurons, or in the external intercostal motor neurons, which can be found in the ventral horns throughout the thoracic spinal cord. Dysfunction of any of these neural pathways, by either local inflammation, trauma, tumor, or systemic disease, can impair the ability to create an effective negative inspiratory effort.

Inspiratory and expiratory muscles are alternately inhibited and stimulated. Inspiratory neurons are located primarily in the dorsal nuclei group of the medulla. Expiratory neurons are at either end of the ventral group of nuclei, with additional inspiratory neurons in its midposition. Both are influenced by receptor afferents from the airways and the carotid and aortic bodies. Chemoreceptors located bilaterally in the carotid bodies and in the aortic bodies near the aortic arch are composed of type I and type II glomus cells. These cells contain several neurotransmitters, including large quantities of dopamine and other catecholamines, serotonin, acetylcholine, and several neuropeptides. Glomus cells are considered the actual chemosensing cells. Receptors in the ventrolateral medulla are stimulated to increase ventilation by increased CO_2 or a decrease in pH. The carotid body cells are affected primarily by hypoxemia. In general, the respiratory minute volume is proportional to the metabolic rate. The effective stimuli are mediated by CO_2. Elevated CO_2 levels stimulate an increased rate and depth of inspiration, with a resultant rise in minute volume, whereas low CO_2 levels decrease the respiratory drive. In addition, there are medullary chemoreceptors that respond to cerebral spinal fluid pH, which is primarily related to the amount of dissolved CO_2 in the serum. This pH change could reflect CO_2 changes of respiratory or metabolic origin.

The inherent rhythm of breathing is the result of complex interactions in the dorsal and ventral respiratory groups of the medulla that mediate the depth and the rate of breathing in response to a number of different stimuli. The pneumotaxic center in the pons is responsible for alternating between inspiration and expiration. There are stretch receptors within the lung that produce feedback signals to shut off inspiration (the Hering–Breuer reflex). These same stretch receptors indicate the degree of deflation and signal the respiratory center to initiate inspiration. Chemoreceptors also exist in the carotid and aortic bodies that respond primarily to changes in oxygen and carbon dioxide tensions. Other chemoreceptors in the ventral lateral medulla are pH sensitive and can initiate a ventilatory effort in response to altered CO_2 levels.

Perfusion

The lung has a dual blood supply. The pulmonary circulation receives the entire cardiac output from the right ventricle under low pressure and is composed of mixed venous blood with an approximate oxygen saturation of 68% to 76% in normal individuals. This blood consists of the systemic venous return mixed with cardiac venous return that enters the right heart via the thebesian veins and the coronary sinus. The bronchial circulation arises from the aorta and receives only 1% of the left ventricular cardiac output and has an oxygen saturation near 100%. The pulmonary arterial vessels are thin-walled vessels, containing much less vascular smooth muscle than the systemic vessels. This results in a vasculature that is under normal conditions, more distensible and thereby maintains relatively low pressure and low resistance within the pulmonary circulation. Normal pulmonary arterial pressures are one fifth of the systemic circulation.

The main pulmonary artery branches into the left and right pulmonary arteries, which subdivides into the lobar, segmental, and subsegmental branches that are intimately related to the airways with one or more branches of the pulmonary artery supplying each bronchopulmonary segment. These large elastic arteries give rise to the morphologically distinct arterioles that constitute the precapillary pulmonary vessels. The arterioles, capillaries, and venules constitute the microcirculation of the lung and establish the blood–air interface required for gas exchange. Other cellular components are important in the pulmonary microcirculation. Pericytes are found in the alveolar capillaries and are thought to be phagocytic and control vascular contraction. Mast cells are found in the connective tissue of the pulmonary vessels, which provide the vasoactive substances mediating pulmonary hypoxic vasoconstriction.

Blood returns to the pulmonary capillary network, pulmonary veins, and left atrium. These veins lack valves and drain into distinct superior and inferior pulmonary veins in either side. They do not

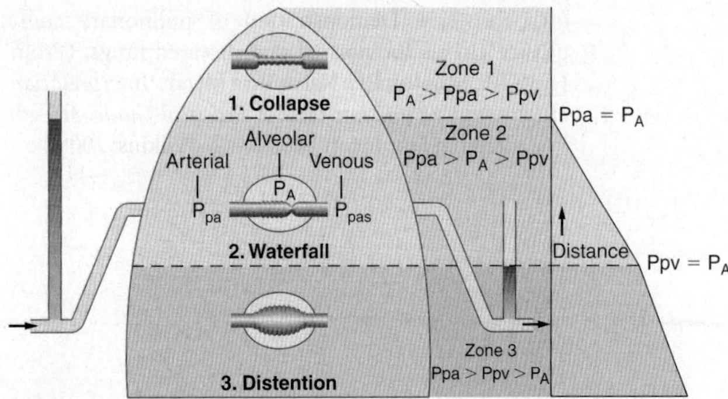

FIGURE 21.5 Representation of differences in ventilation and perfusion of the upright lung. (From Barash PG, ed. *Clinical Anesthesia*. 6th ed. Philadelphia: Lippincott Williams & Wilkins; 2009.)

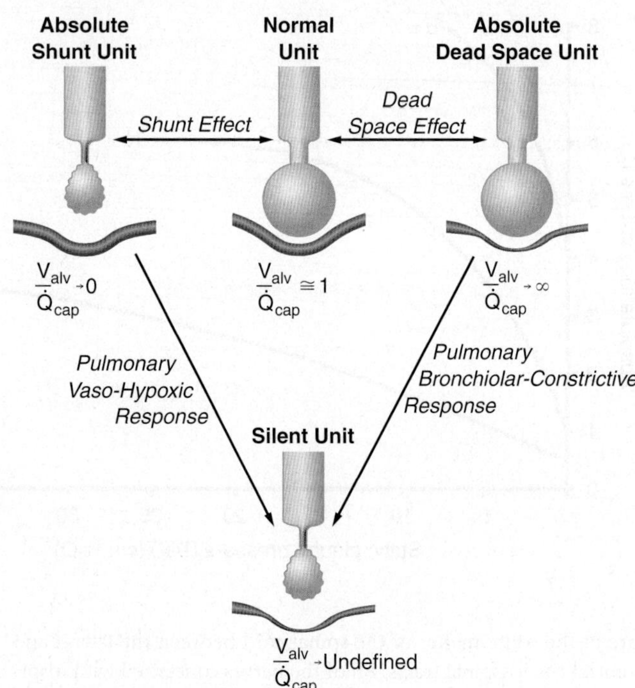

FIGURE 21.6 A schematic of normal and pathologic ventilation–perfusion ratios. (From Barash PG, ed. *Clinical Anesthesia*. 6th ed. Philadelphia: Lippincott Williams & Wilkins; 2009.)

follow the bronchial anatomy as closely as the pulmonary distribution. Of note, some bronchial arteries drain directly into the pulmonary venous system without entering the capillary network and contribute to physiologic shunting. The lungs may contain up to 20% of the total body volume, although only 10% of that volume is in the capillaries. The velocity of flow through the capillary bed depends on cardiac output; however, a red cell passes through the alveolar–capillary gas exchange area in 0.3 to 0.8 seconds.

The distribution of the blood flow to the lung is not uniform. Gravity and alveolar pressures influence regional lung perfusion (Fig. 21.5). Ventilation (V) and perfusion (Q) increase from the top to the bottom of the lung; however, Q increases more rapidly. Classic descriptions of the lung describe three zones based on the interrelationship between alveolar pressure (P_A), pulmonary arterial pressure (P_a), and pulmonary venous pressure (P_V). Zone 1 conditions ($P_A > P_a > P_V$) are those at the apex of the lung where pulmonary arterial pressure falls below alveolar pressure (normally close to atmospheric pressure). If this occurs, the capillaries are flattened, and no flow is possible. This zone does not occur under normal conditions because the pulmonary arterial pressure is just sufficient to raise blood to the top of the lung but may be present if the arterial pressure is reduced (e.g., following severe hemorrhage) or if alveolar pressure is raised (during positive pressure ventilation). This ventilated but unperfused lung is useless for gas exchange and is called alveolar dead space.

Further down the lung (zone 2), pulmonary arterial pressure increases because the hydrostatic effect exceeds alveolar pressure ($P_a > P_A > P_V$). However, venous pressure is still very low and is less than alveolar pressure, and this leads to remarkable pressure–flow characteristics. Under these conditions, blood flow is determined by the difference between arterial and alveolar pressures (not the usual arterial–venous pressure difference). Indeed, venous pressure has no influence on flow unless it exceeds alveolar pressure. Since arterial pressure is increasing down the zone but alveolar pressure is the same throughout the lung, the pressure difference responsible for flow increases. In addition, increasing recruitment of capillaries occurs down this zone.

In zone 3, ($P_a > P_V > P_A$) venous pressure exceeds alveolar pressure, and flow is determined in the usual way by the arterial–venous pressure difference. The increase in blood flow down this region of the lung is apparently caused by distension of the capillaries. The pressure within them (lying between arterial and venous) increases down the zone, while the pressure outside (alveolar) remains constant. Thus, their transmural pressure rises, and, indeed, measurements show that their mean width increases. Recruitment of previously closed vessels may also play some part in the increase in blood flow down this zone.

The thin-walled arteries contain smooth muscle that dilates in response to pain sympathetic stimulation with acetylcholine, β-sympathetic receptor stimulation (epinephrine and norepinephrine), bradykinin, prostaglandin E_1 (PGE_1), and prostacyclin. They constrict with α-receptor stimulation, histamine, serotonin, thromboxane A_2, and prostaglandin F and E and hypoxemia. Pulmonary arteries produce endothelial-derived relaxing factor (EDRF) or nitric oxide (NO), which have important implications toward ventilation and selective pulmonary venodilation.

When comprehending respiratory function as an interaction between ventilation and perfusion, it becomes more transparent how V/Q mismatch forms the basis of much of pulmonary pathology. For instance, in the case of alveolar obstruction, normal gas exchange cannot occur, and blood flows through the capillary bed without attaining oxygen or clearing carbon dioxide (Fig. 21.6). Conversely, in the case of no perfusion such as a pulmonary embolism, the affected alveoli become dead space where no gas exchange occurs.

Physiology of Blood–Gas Exchange

The lungs fundamental place of gas exchange is the acinus, which composes the terminal airway and its surrounding alveoli. There are around 300 million alveoli in an adult lung; each one is 0.25 mm in diameter. The total available surface area available for gas exchange is around 70 to 100 m^2. The alveoli are interdigitated with a capillary network. The alveolar–capillary border is anywhere from 0.2 to 0.3 mm thick, permitting the rapid exchange of gaseous compounds.

Gas exchange occurs at the alveolar level at the interface of the alveolar epithelium and the capillary endothelium. The alveoli are outpouchings of the respiratory bronchioles, alveolar ducts, and alveolar sacs. The alveolar septa are made up of a continuous flattened epithelium constituted of type I and type II alveolar epithelial cells covering a thin layer of interstitial tissue. Type I alveolar cells cover approximately 95% of the alveolar surface and functionally are involved in resorbing pathologic alveolar fluid or ingesting intra-alveolar particulate material. The type II epithelial cells are the source of alveolar surfactant and are also involved in the renewal of the alveolar surface by differentiation into type I cells. A continuous basal lamina underlies both type I and type II cells and is in apposition to the underlying endothelial cell. The alveolar septal interstitium is also composed of connective tissue made of a proteoglycan matrix embedded with elastin and collagen. Alveolar macrophages are important in clearance of intra-alveolar material, production of inflammatory mediators, and antigen presentation.

After delivery of oxygen to the alveoli, it diffuses through the alveolar–capillary interface. At the blood–air interface, there are approximately 300 million alveoli with a combined surface area of 70 to 100 m^2; thus, 120 L of air will come into contact with 25 L of blood per minute. For oxygen to be delivered to the blood, it must first dissolve into the layer of pulmonary surfactant, thus moving from the gas phase to the liquid phase. Oxygen then diffuses through the alveolar epithelium, interstitium, and capillary endothelium and into the plasma. Once in the plasma, some oxygen will remain dissolved. However, the majority of oxygen enters the erythrocyte where it becomes bound to hemoglobin.

The relationship between ventilation and perfusion determines alveolar and thus arterial PO_2 and PCO_2. Ideally, alveolar ventilation and perfusion should allow for complete hemoglobin saturation and removal of sufficient carbon dioxide to result in a normal pH level. This does not occur uniformly as described by the different zones of the lung. The extremes of these ratios are pure shunts (low V/Q) or pure dead space (high V/Q). Under normal conditions, alveolar PO_2 is 100 mm Hg and PCO_2 is 40 mm Hg. The mixed venous blood in the pulmonary arterial system has a PCO_2 of about 40 mm Hg and a PCO_2 of 45 mm Hg. The resulting gradients favor diffusion of oxygen into the blood and carbon dioxide into the alveolar space.

The amount of air inhaled does not equal the amount of gas seen by alveoli due to the inherent dead space in the conducting airways. On inspiration, the amount of gas reaching the alveoli (V_A) is less than the tidal volume (V_T) and is dependent on the volume of the dead space (V_{DS}):

$$V_A = V_T - V_{DS}$$

In each breath, the vast majority of gas is not exchanged. Each breath increases the alveolar P_AO_2 and decreases the alveolar P_ACO_2 by only 5% to 10%. The small changes are due to the buffer effect of the gas remaining in the lungs at the end of a normal breath (the FRC). Normal V_A is 300 mL, and the normal FRC is 3 L.

The pulmonary arterial blood enters the lung with a mixed venous oxygen tension and a mixed venous carbon dioxide tension, which is determined by the cardiac output and the metabolic rate of tissues. In blood, oxygen is carried in both dissolved form and on hemoglobin. Hemoglobin is composed of globin folded around heme, an iron-containing O_2 carrier. Each gram of hemoglobin can bind up to 1.39 mL/O_2. The strength with which O_2 binds the heme molecule decreases with each of four binding sites in a nonlinear fashion called the oxyhemoglobin dissociation curve (Fig. 21.1). The dissolved oxygen constitutes only a small amount of oxygen carried in the blood. The oxygen content of the blood can be described by:

$$O_2 \text{ content (mL/dL blood)} = (\text{HgB content in grams}) \times (1.39) \times (O_2 \text{ saturation}) + 0.003 \times PO_2$$

Many factors influence the relation between the partial pressure of oxygen and the blood content. Factors that are involved in increased O_2 use (increased PCO_2 and higher temperature and reduced pH) decrease the affinity of the hemoglobin for O_2, causing a rightward shift of the curve and facilitate the release of O_2 to tissues. The leftward shift causes increased loading of O_2 by hemoglobin. Factors such as increased production of 2,3-diphosphoglycerate move the curve to right. Carbon monoxide competes with O_2 for hemoglobin-binding sites and shifts the curve to the left. Temperature and acidosis similarly affect curve movement. Increased ATP concentrations, cortisol levels, and aldosterone levels move the curve to the right.

After oxygenation within the lungs, arterial blood is distributed to the body where oxygen is released and diffuses into tissues. Oxygen delivery to peripheral tissues and oxygen and consumption by organs can be calculated based on oxygen content:

$$O_2 \text{ delivery (mL/dL blood)} = \text{cardiac output} \times O_2 \text{ content (mL/dL blood)}$$

$$O_2 \text{ consumption (mL/dL blood)} = \text{cardiac output} \times (\text{arterial } O_2 \text{ content} - \text{venous } O_2 \text{ content})$$

In situations where arterial oxygen content remains constant, a fall in the mixed venous saturation indicates a fall in cardiac output. Clinically, a mixed venous specimen for oxygen saturation can be used as a surrogate measure of cardiac output.

Carbon dioxide is transported through the blood in three forms: 90% as bicarbonate, 5% is carried by hemoglobin, and 5% dissolved in plasma. In contrast to the frequent problems with oxygen, problems with CO_2 gas exchange becomes clinically important only with advanced pulmonary disease. CO_2 is 20 times more soluble in blood as oxygen and rapidly forms carbonic acid.

The rate at which oxygen and carbon dioxide can transfer between the alveoli and pulmonary arterial blood depends on:

1. Inspired gas concentration
2. The mixed venous oxygen tension and mixed venous carbon dioxide tension
3. Diffusion capacity of alveolar–capillary interface
4. Ratio of ventilation to perfusion (V/Q) in each acinus

The rate of diffusion of a gas, governed by the Fick law of diffusion, is proportional to the area available for diffusion, the diffusion coefficient of a particular gas, and the partial pressure gradient across the barrier and is inversely proportional to the thickness of the barrier. The area available for diffusion is relatively constant; however, during exercise, additional capillaries can be recruited, thus increasing diffusion. In hypovolemia, the reverse may be true. The diffusion coefficient is proportional to the solubility of a given gas and inversely proportional to its molecular weight. When comparing oxygen and carbon dioxide, although carbon dioxide is larger than oxygen, it is about 25 times more soluble in the liquid phase and thus diffuses more rapidly through the air–blood barrier. The diffusing capacity for oxygen is difficult to measure; therefore, the diffusing capacity of carbon monoxide (D_LCO) is measured.

Pathophysiology

Hypoxemia

Hypoxemia is clinically manifested as low oxygen tension in the arterial blood. This process typically results from four distinct processes: hypoventilation, diffusion gradients, shunt, and ventilation–perfusion mismatch.

1. Hypoventilation can be caused by drugs (opiates, barbiturates), mechanical impairments of the chest wall (painful incisions and binders), and paralysis of the respiratory muscles (muscular dystrophy, polio virus, and neuromuscular blockade). Since the level of alveolar PO_2 is a function of the balance between oxygen supply and oxygen consumed, any process that causes hypoventilation will cause the alveolar PO_2 to drop. As a result of hypoventilation, there is a subsequent rise in alveolar PCO_2. This relationship can be described by the alveolar gas equation:

$$P_AO_2 = P_{INSP}O_2 - P_ACO_2/(0.8)$$

Hypoventilation is always accompanied by hypercarbia and is secondary to a low minute ventilation, either on the basis of low tidal volume or rate. The addition of supplemental oxygen to the inspired gas of a hypoventilating patient will readily overcome the hypoxia of hypoventilation.

2. Increased diffusion gradients cause failures of equilibration between the hemoglobin in the red cell and the gas in the alveoli. Under normal conditions, the red cell has fully equilibrated with alveolar oxygen within one third of its passage through the alveolar capillary. However, any interstitial lung process such as collagen vascular disease, sarcoidosis, and idiopathic interstitial fibrosis can cause arterial hypoxemia.
3. Shunt, another cause of hypoxemia, is the fraction of blood that enters the systemic arterial system without passing through a ventilated portion of the lung. Shunts occur due to intracardiac communications such as in congenital heart disease, arteriovenous malformations of the lung, lung consolidation (i.e., pneumonia), and vasodilators such as nitroprusside. Of the four causes of hypoxemia, shunt is the only one that cannot be corrected by oxygen therapy because the shunted blood is never exposed to the airway. Also unlike the other three causes, P_aCO_2 is typically low to normal. An approximation of the shunt can be described by:

$$\text{Shunt flow/total flow} = Q_S/Q_T = (F_iO_2/2) - (P_aO_2/10)$$

A calculated shunt of less than 10% is compatible with normal lungs, 10% to 20% is rarely of clinical importance, 20% to 30% indicates significant pulmonary disease, and greater than 30% is life threatening.

4. Finally, ventilation–perfusion mismatch (i.e., "partial shunting") is the most common etiology of hypoxemia. Conditions such as oversedation, COPD, and the inability to take a deep breath that describe perfusion exceeding ventilation (shunts) or ventilation exceeding perfusion (dead space) create a mismatch. In patients with pulmonary disease, the lung will have alveoli with varying *V*/*Q* ratios. The hyperventilatory response to hypoxia, which results from chemoreceptors at the carotid bifurcation and below the aortic arch, is more effective in correcting hypercarbia than hypoxia. Thus, the net result of *V*/*Q* mismatch is hypoxemia and hyperventilation. Ventilation–perfusion is diagnosed primarily by exclusion of the other three causes of hypoxia.

Pulmonary blood flow can be actively redistributed to optimize the *V*/*Q* relationship by a process called "hypoxic pulmonary vasoconstriction." Alveolar hypoxia ($PO_2 < 70$ mm Hg), hypercarbia, or collapse result in local pulmonary arteriolar vasoconstriction. The exact mechanism for this response remains unclear but may involve local release of vasoactive mediators. This vasoconstriction will divert blood from areas that will undergo little gas exchange (low *V*/*Q*), thus lowering PO_2 and increasing PCO_2 to areas that are better ventilated (high *V*/*Q*).

Hypercapnia

An increase in P_aCO_2 is often associated as a compensation factor for an underlying metabolic alkalosis. However, if this is not the case, other primary respiratory causes need to be considered. The carbon dioxide level in arterial blood is directly proportional to the rate of CO_2 production by oxidative metabolism (VCO_2) and inversely proportional to the rate of CO_2 elimination by alveolar ventilation (V_A). Alveolar ventilation is the fraction of the total expired ventilation (V_E) that is not dead space ventilation (V_d/V_E). Therefore,

$$P_aCO_2 \text{ is proportional to } (VCO_2/V_A) = (VCO_2)/[(V_E)(1 - V_d/V_E)]$$

From this equation, it can deduced that there are three major sources of hypercapnia:

1. Increased CO_2 production (VCO_2)
2. Hypoventilation
3. Increased dead space ventilation (V_d/V_E)

1. Increased CO_2 production (VCO_2): Increased CO_2 production (i.e., hypermetabolism) is normally accompanied by an increase in minute ventilation. The ventilatory response tends to eliminate excess CO_2 and maintain a constant arterial P_aCO_2. Therefore, excess CO_2 production does not normally cause hypercapnia. However, when CO_2 exertion is prevented by an increase in dead space ventilation, an increase in CO_2 production can result in an increase in the arterial PCO_2. Therefore, increased CO_2 production is relevant in causing hypercapnia in patients with underlying lung disease. The rate of CO_2 production can be measured at the bedside by metabolic carts that assess body nutritional status. They measure total CO_2 excreted per minute. The normal VCO_2 is 90 to 130 L/min/m^2, which is roughly 80% of the VO_2. An increase in VCO_2 is evidence for one of the following abnormalities: generalized hypermetabolism, overfeeding, or organic acidoses.
2. Hypoventilation: Increased alveolar hypoventilation can occur due to either a primary neurologic defect or a muscular process. Oversedation with narcotics, obesity, shock, myasthenia gravis, or other neuromuscular diseases may result in a decreased respiratory drive. Opiates and benzodiazepines are the most common culprits for hypoventilation. Muscular weakness can also cause alveolar hypoventilation. The standard measure for evaluating respiratory muscle strength is the maximum inspiratory pressure (MIP) and maximal voluntary ventilation (MVV). Most healthy adults have an MIP above 80 cm water. Carbon dioxide retention develops when the MIP falls to less than 40% of the normal value.

3. Increased dead space ventilation (V_d/V_E): Dead space ventilation increases when the alveolar–capillary interface is compromised (i.e., emphysema), when blood flow is reduced (i.e., heart failure, pulmonary embolus) or when alveoli are overdistended by positive pressure ventilation.

End-tidal carbon dioxide can be measured from the ventilator circuit. This value is a close approximation of the arterial P_aCO_2. Typically, end-tidal CO_2 is 5 mm Hg higher than arterial carbon dioxide levels. An increasing gradient between end-tidal carbon dioxide and arterial carbon dioxide suggests increased dead space ventilation. A proportionate increase in end-tidal carbon dioxide and arterial carbon dioxide indicates the patient is either hypoventilating or increasing metabolic activity.

THORACIC DISEASE

A multitude of pathologies are manifested in the chest. As with most surgical cases, pathologies that alter the structure and function of the lung are most amenable to surgical intervention. The essential concepts for the surgeon in the management of thoracic disease entail restoration of pleural apposition, treatment of malignant disease, and understanding a patient's tolerance to lung resection.

Infectious Lung Disease

While the advancement of antimicrobial therapy and critical care over the last 60 years has lessened the thoracic surgeon's role in managing infectious lung disease, the rise of multidrug-resistant (MDR) bacteria and immunosuppressed patients presents a continued challenge and space for the surgeon in treating pulmonary infection.

Pneumonia refers to an infection of the lower respiratory tract, and community-acquired pneumonia (CAP) refers to a pneumonia acquired outside of the hospital. The most common organisms involved are *Streptococcus pneumoniae* and *Haemophilus influenzae.* In up to half of cases, a causative organism is not identified. These patients can typically be managed medically. Hospital-acquired pneumonia is the second most common nosocomial infection and has the highest mortality. Importantly, ventilator-associated pneumonia appears to have a higher incidence in surgical ICUs compared to medical. Aspiration refers to inhalation of oropharyngeal or gastric contents. This results initially in a pneumonitis from damage to the alveolar and capillary cells sometimes followed by a pneumonia if the gastric contents are infected. If aspiration is witnessed, bronchoscopy is recommended to clear residual fluid from the airway. Of note, antibiotic therapy is indicated only in patients where gastric colonization is suspected or when there is no improvement after 48 hours of supportive care. At this point, broad-spectrum coverage is warranted for treatment of pneumonia and prevention of complications such as lung abscess that can require surgical intervention. No clinical benefit of steroids has been found.

Bronchiectasis refers to the permanent dilation of the bronchi as a result of recurrent infection and inflammation. This condition is usually found in the more distal bronchial tree, usually presenting is subsegmental bronchi after a severe pneumonia, and may lead to decreased clearance of airway secretions. It has also been associated with multiple congenital disorders such as Kartagener syndrome, α1-antitrypsin deficiency, and cystic fibrosis. Autoimmune diseases like SLE and rheumatoid arthritis have been implicated as well. The most common presentation consists of a persistent productive cough, hemoptysis, and a history of recurrent pulmonary infections.

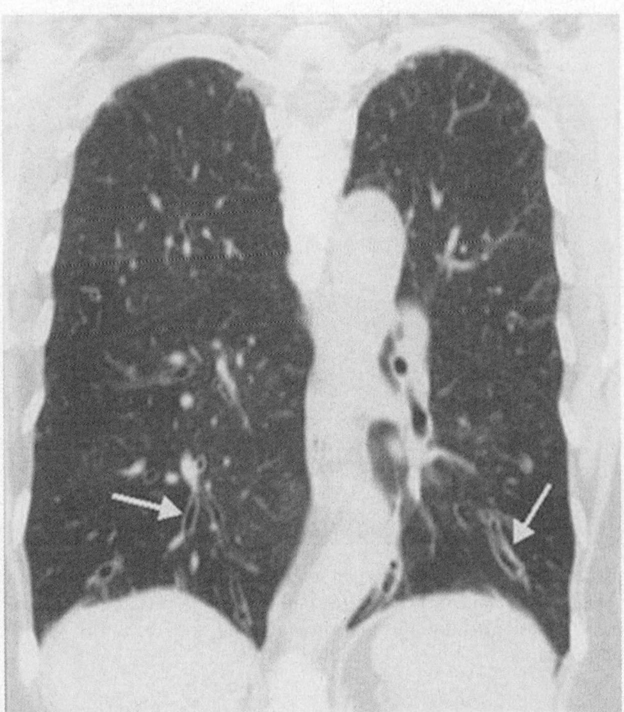

FIGURE 21.7 A CT scan demonstrating bronchiectasis (*arrows*). (From Collins J, Stern EJ, eds. *Chest Radiology: The Essentials.* 2nd ed. Philadelphia: Lippincott Williams & Wilkins; 2008.)

Of note, patients should also be evaluated for an obstructing lesion. Chest x-ray (CXR) usually demonstrates nonspecific findings encompassing atelectasis and increased lung markings, while CT scan can show more specific findings of bronchial dilation within the lung parenchyma (Fig. 21.7). While the pathology surrounding bronchiectasis can typically be managed medically, there is a role for surgical intervention (Table 21.1).

TABLE 21.1 Important pulmonary physiology equations

Alveolar gas equation[a]	$P_{AO_2} = P_{IO_2} - P_{aCO_2}/0.8 + F$
A–a gradient (NrI 15–20 mm Hg)[b]	$P(A-a)O_2 = P_{AO_2} - P_{aO_2}$
Shunt equation[c]	$Q_s/Q_T = C_{CO_2} - C_{aO_2}/C_{CO_2} - C_{vO_2}$
Pulmonary vascular resistance[d]	$PVR = PA_m - LA_m/CO$
Fick law of diffusion[e]	$V_{gas} = A \times D \times (P_1 - P_2)/T$

[a]P_{AO_2}, alveolar partial pressure of oxygen; P_{IO_2}, partial pressure of oxygen in inspired air; P_{ACO_2}, alveolar CO_2, arterial CO_2; F, correction factor (ignored).

[b]P_{AO_2}, alveolar partial pressure of oxygen; P_{aO_2}, arterial partial pressure of oxygen.

[c]Q_s/Q_T, shunt; C_{CO_2}, content of capillary oxygen; C_{aO_2}, content of arterial oxygen; C_{VO_2}, content of venous oxygen.

[d]PA_M, mean pulmonary artery pressure; LA_M, mean left atrial pressure; CO, cardiac output.

[e]A, area available for diffusion; D, diffusion coefficient; P_1–P_2, pressure gradient of the gas across the diffusion barrier; T, thickness of the barrier.

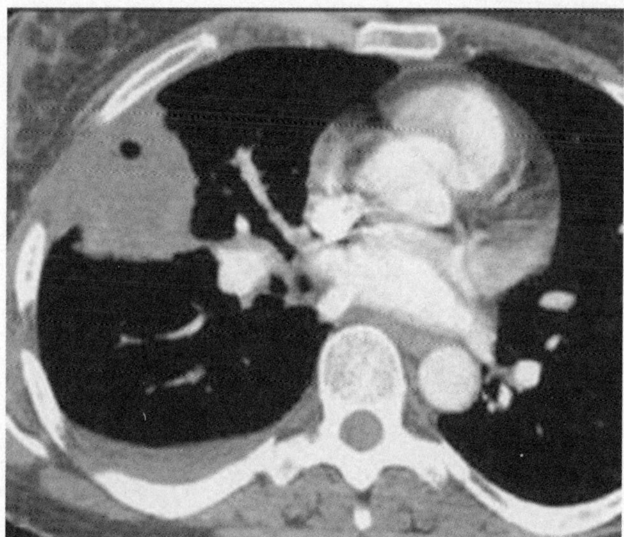

FIGURE 21.8 CT scan of a right lung abscess with a relatively smooth wall. (From Betancourt Cuellar, Sonia L, Palacio D. Imaging of pulmonary aspiration syndrome. *Contemp Diagn Radiol.* 2015;38(9):1–7, with permission.)

A lung abscess is an area of lung parenchyma filled with purulent material and air. Etiologies include aspiration resulting in an infection distal to the occluded bronchus and septic emboli. As with any infection, it is critical to identify the source for successful treatment. CT scan is very helpful in identifying a lung abscess (Fig. 21.8) since it can easily be mistaken for cavitation from a tumor. Importantly, an abscess typically demonstrates thin, smooth walls compared to the thick, irregular walls of a tumor. Treatment consists of prolonged antibiotics and successful drainage, which can usually be accomplished internally with postural techniques. Percutaneous drainage, if needed, has a very good response though it can infect the pleural space and/or result in a bronchopleural fistula. Generally, therapy lasts 6 to 8 weeks with resolution on imaging in 4 to 5 months. Approximately 90% of lung abscesses are managed medically. Surgical intervention is indicated in cases of empyema, bronchopleural fistula, suspected malignancy, significant hemoptysis, and inadequate abscess drainage. Importantly, it is critical to protect the contralateral lung during this procedure.

Pulmonary tuberculosis (TB) includes infection with *Mycobacterium tuberculosis* along with multidrug-resistant TB (MDR-TB) and extensively drug-resistant TB (XDR-TB). There are 16,000 new cases of TB in the United States annually compared to 7 to 8 million around the world. Drug-sensitive TB can almost always be cured with antimicrobial therapy, isoniazid and rifampin, over a 6- to 9-month course. Patients undergo surgery only for complications including airway stenosis, massive hemoptysis, bronchopleural fistula, suspicion of a malignant lesion, and decortication of a trapped lung. Patients with MDR-TB and XDR-TB are operated on, in addition to the scenarios stated above, for persistent cavitary disease, destroyed lobe, or a destroyed lung irrespective of sputum culture.

Fungal infections are also an important consideration when discussing infectious lung disease, particularly in immunosuppressed patients. The most common are histoplasmosis, coccidioidomycosis, blastomycosis, and aspergillosis. Surgical intervention is typically reserved for complications arising from residual cavitary lesions and assistance with diagnosis. In cases of aspergillosis, an individual with a preformed cavity from previous pathology can develop an aspergilloma (Fig. 21.9). These are typically noninvasive and asymptomatic. The most common symptom is hemoptysis followed by cough and weight loss. Surgical intervention is reserved only for uncontrolled hemoptysis or additional significant symptoms due to the aspergilloma.

Benign Lung Lesions

Benign lung masses can arise from epithelial, mesenchymal, or endothelial tissue and account for less than 1% of lung masses. The most common is a hamartoma, which is of mesenchymal origin, and 90% are asymptomatic. They are usually an incidental finding on CXR or CT and seen as discrete rounded nodules, often with "popcorn calcifications" (Fig. 21.10). When they do cause symptoms, they are typically due to obstruction or erosion into a bronchus. As with any mass demonstrated on imaging, hamartomas demonstrate a diagnostic dilemma as they must be differentiated from malignant tumors. The presence of a fat density within the nodule on CT supports the diagnosis of a hamartoma; however, it is not conclusive. Since needle biopsies do not provide sufficient positive or negative predictive value, surgical resection may be necessary for a diagnosis. Additional rare, but worthy of mention, masses include adenoma, cystadenoma, chondroma, fibroma, leiomyoma,

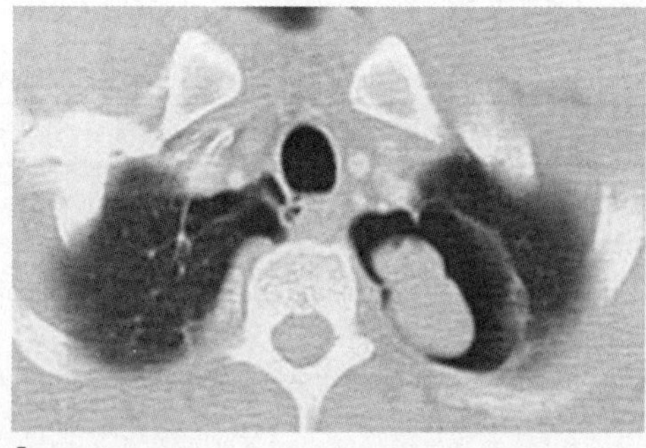

A

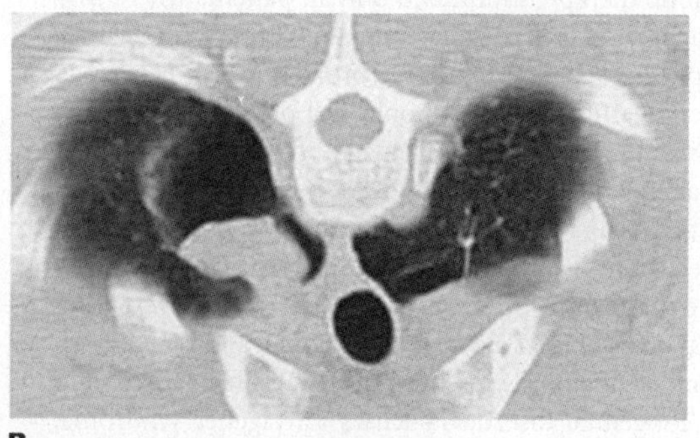

B

FIGURE 21.9 CT scan (**A** and **B**) of an aspergilloma. Movement of a fungus ball with change in patient position is typical of a noninvasive aspergilloma. (From Collins J, Stern EJ, eds. *Chest Radiology: The Essentials.* 2nd ed. Philadelphia: Lippincott Williams & Wilkins; 2008.)

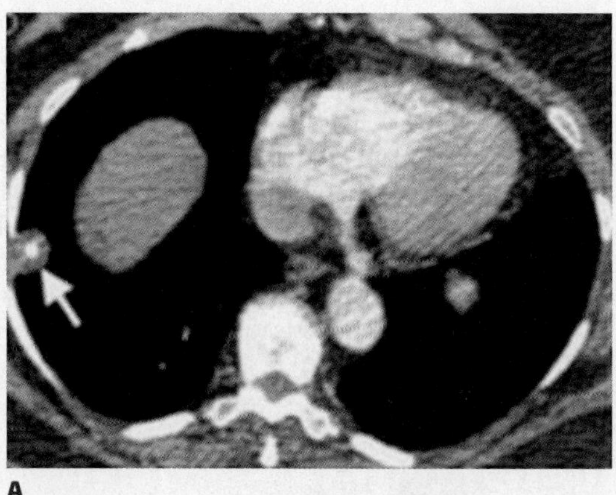

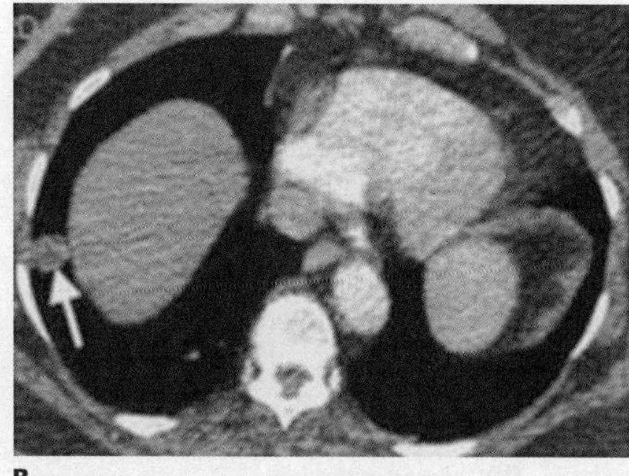

FIGURE 21.10 CT of a benign hamartoma (*arrow*) with **(A)** and without **(B)** calcification. (From Collins J, Stern EJ, eds. *Chest Radiology: The Essentials*. 2nd ed. Philadelphia: Lippincott Williams & Wilkins; 2008.)

lipoma, nodular amyloidosis, granular cell tumor, clear cell tumor, and a pulmonary paraganglioma.

Overall, benign tumors of the lung are rare and typically a diagnosis of exclusion. It is important for the surgeon to be aware of these, as he/she can be helpful in providing a diagnosis or intervening for symptomatic patients.

Lung Cancer

Lung cancer is the most common cause of cancer-related deaths in both males and females in the United States. While the mechanism behind the development of lung cancer is multifaceted, smoking is the most clearly defined risk factor and reversible cause. African Americans have a higher incidence of lung cancer compared to Caucasians (81.2 vs. 63.2 per 100,000). People exposed to radon, asbestos, polycyclic aromatic hydrocarbons, and chromate have been noted to have an increased risk of lung cancer. Multiple genetic mutations have also been associated with lung cancer development including p53, *p*16cyclin D1, *ras*, and *myc*. Bronchogenic carcinoma is divided into two subgroups: small cell lung cancer (SCLC) and non–small cell lung cancer (NSCLC). NSCLC includes adenocarcinoma (most common histologic subtype overall), squamous cell carcinoma, and large cell carcinoma. A correct tissue diagnosis is critical because SCLC has a high initial response rate to chemotherapy and radiation and is rarely treated by surgery alone. Conversely, NSCLC can be cured by surgery in certain stages and is not curable by chemotherapy alone. The overall 5-year survival rate for lung cancer remains 15%. With the increased utilization of CT scans in emergency departments, trauma bays, and surveillance for other medical problem, the identification of incidental pulmonary nodules has risen sharply over the last several years. General recommendations for solid nodules less than 5 mm and nonsolid nodules less than 8 mm entail a repeat CT scan in 6 months to 1 year. For nodules between 5 mm and 15 mm, a repeat CT scan should be performed in 3 months. An additional option in these patients is to initiate a 7- to 10-day course of antibiotics and repeat the scan in 1 month. If following repeat scan in any of these scenarios, a suspicion of lung cancer exists, a tissue diagnosis is critical. This can be accomplished via fine needle aspiration (FNA), which yields outcomes of malignant, specific benign, nonspecific benign, and nondiagnostic. More aggressive methods of obtaining a tissue diagnosis include bronchoscopic biopsy with or without ultrasound and video-assisted thoracoscopic surgical (VATS) biopsy.

Non–Small Cell Lung Cancer

Approximately 80% of lung cancers are NSCLC. Of these, about 80% involve disseminated disease that is not surgically resectable. Of the remaining 20% that are surgical candidates, these patients demonstrate a 70% 5-year survival rate. The most common type of NSCLC is adenocarcinoma, followed by squamous cell, and then large cell carcinomas. NSCLC is staged according to tumor, node, and metastasis (TNM) criteria. Table 21.2 illustrates the 2009 7th edition of TNM criteria for NSCLC.

The workup for a patient with suspected NSCLC begins as always with a thorough history and physical. This should also include evaluation for potential pulmonary resection. Before considering a patient for surgical resection of a bronchogenic carcinoma, it must be determined that adequate pulmonary reserve exists. Simple spirometry and an arterial blood–gas measurement are routinely required. Patients with a forced expiratory volume in 1 second (FEV_1) of greater than 60% predicted or more than 2.0 L likely will tolerate a pneumonectomy. When pulmonary function does not appear to be evenly distributed between right and left lungs, quantitative perfusion scanning, which correlates well with regional pulmonary function, may help estimate postoperative pulmonary function. Hypercarbia, unless solely on the basis of a low respiratory drive, is a predictor of poor postoperative outcome, but hypoxemia is not a strong indicator of poor outcome. In addition, the D_LCO has been shown to be a strong predictor of 30-day postoperative morbidity and mortality, and it is becoming increasingly used in the preoperative assessment of a candidate for pulmonary resection.

Once this initial evaluation is complete, CXR should always be performed followed by a high-resolution CT. Positron emission tomography (PET)-CT is valuable in assessing mediastinal

TABLE 21.2 Causes of hypoxia

Ventilation–perfusion mismatch
Shunt
Decreased alveolar P_{AO_2}
Hypoventilation
Increased diffusion gradient

nodal involvement. A standardized uptake value (SUV) over 2.5 or greater than the background of the mediastinum is consistent with an abnormal PET-CT. It is important to note that nonmalignant processes such as inflammation and infection can lead to an abnormal PET-CT. MRI has not been found to be any more effective than CT in identifying mediastinal metastases; however, it can be useful in assessing tumor invasion to the spinal canal. After noninvasive imaging, flexible bronchoscopy can be employed to obtain endobronchial biopsies and brushings. Additionally, transbronchial needle aspiration can be performed for diagnosis. For mediastinal lymph node biopsy, endobronchial ultrasound (EBUS) has become an effective tool and significantly less invasive than mediastinoscopy. Percutaneous transthoracic needle biopsy can be performed typically with CT guidance. The major complication is pneumothorax, with COPD being the greatest risk factor. Although slightly more invasive, cervical mediastinoscopy is the most accurate method of detecting mediastinal lymph node involvement. It has a sensitivity of approximately 80% and specificity of 100%. It is typically performed in the operating room just prior to formal resection. Figure 21.11 illustrates the Mountain–Dresler lymph

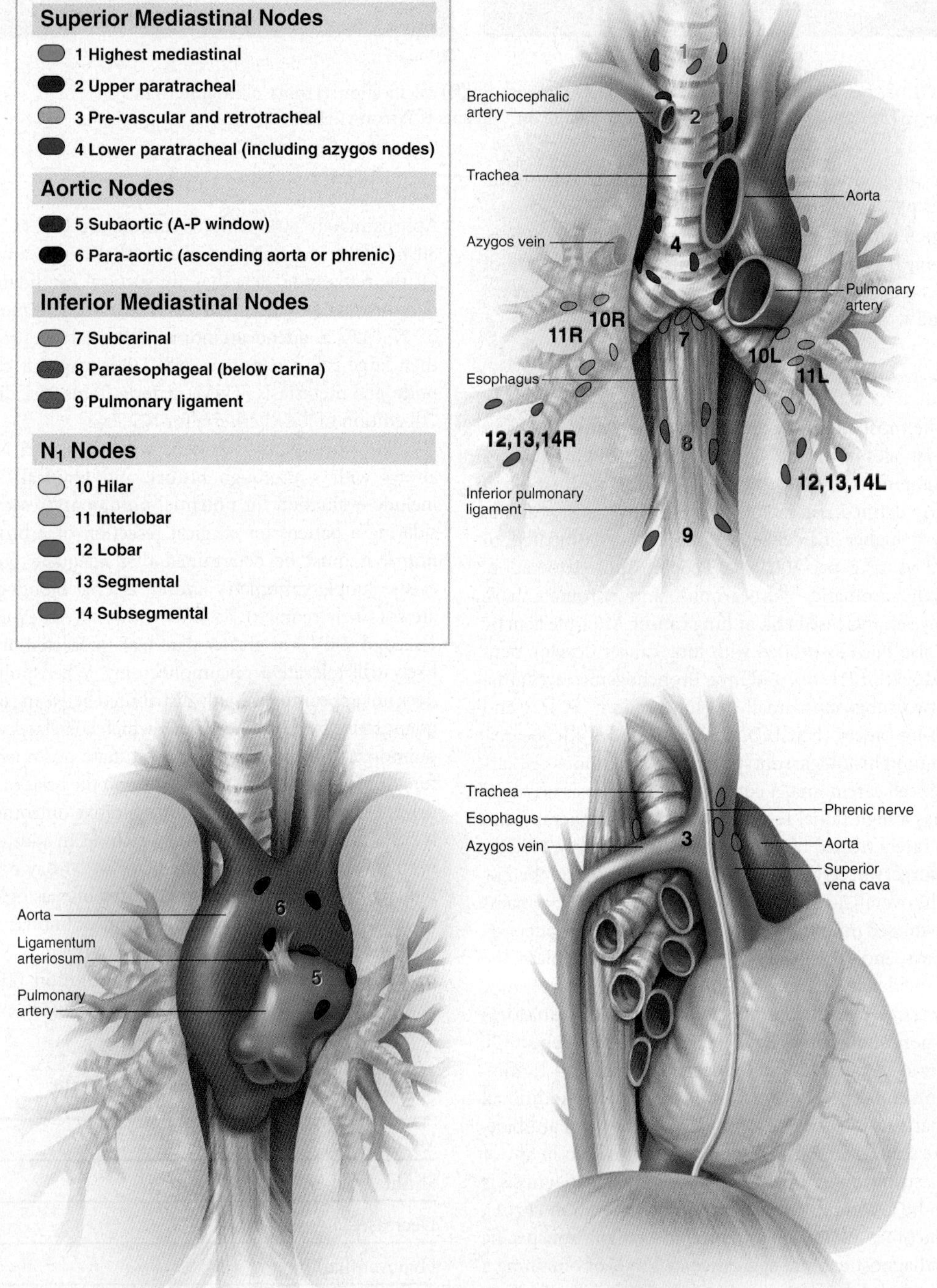

FIGURE 21.11 The Mountain–Dresler modification of the pulmonary lymph node map.

node stations. While debatable, indications for mediastinoscopy include a lymph node greater than 1 cm on CT, increased uptake on PET-CT, and consideration for neoadjuvant therapy. Importantly, the morbidity and complication rate are very low. If lymph nodes in the aortic–pulmonary window must be sampled, a left anterior mediastinoscopy, the Chamberlain procedure, can be performed via a small transverse incision over the second rib. Finally, VATS can be performed for mediastinal lymph node biopsy that is otherwise inaccessible from a standard cervical approach. The sensitivity and specificity approach 100% for diagnosis and staging with VATS. Finally, it is important to identify patients at risk for distant metastases. Findings on history, physical, and basic laboratory tests in including chemistry, LFTs, and CBC that suggest potential extrathoracic spread require further imaging. The most common sites of metastases are the brain, bone, and adrenal glands. In these cases, whole-body PET-CT, MRI of the brain, and CT of the abdomen should be performed prior to consideration of resection.

Adenocarcinoma is the most common histologic type and accounts for approximately 45% of all lung cancers. The increasing prevalence of this tumor is due to more frequent occurrence in women and changing environmental exposure. Most of these tumors (75%) are peripherally located. Adenocarcinomas tend to metastasize earlier than squamous cell carcinomas. Because of the frequent peripheral origin of this type of carcinoma, sputum cytology is seldom positive even when the disease is detected early by chest radiography. Histologically, adenocarcinoma comes from mucus-producing bronchial epithelial cells. These cuboidal to columnar cells have abundant vacuolated cytoplasm with evidence of gland formation. Half of adenocarcinomas exhibit markers for type II or Clara cells, such as mRNA for the surfactant proteins A, B, and C. The hallmark of adenocarcinomas is the tendency to form glands. Special stains demonstrate that the tumor cells contain mucins.

Squamous cell carcinoma accounts for a third of all lung cancers. Until recently, this was the most common lung cancer cell type, but in most centers, squamous cell subtypes have diminished and adenocarcinoma has become the most prevalent cell type. Squamous cell carcinoma tends to originate in the central airways. Squamous cell carcinoma arises from areas of chronically damaged bronchial epithelium in a progressive fashion from metaplasia to dysplasia and to neoplasia. The origin of squamous cell carcinoma from damaged bronchial epithelium explains the occasional occurrence of positive sputum cytology in the absence of chest radiographic abnormalities. Squamous cell carcinoma is the cell type most prone to cavitation. Histologically, squamous cell carcinomas are characterized by keratinization with "pearl" formation (i.e., flattened cells surrounding central cores of keratin). Squamous carcinomas are also characterized by predominant desmosomes that can be visualized on histologic sections as intercellular bridges.

Large cell carcinoma, often referred to as large cell undifferentiated carcinoma, accounts for 15% to 20% of tumors, but this diagnosis may be overestimated since tumors without clear differentiation are often placed in this category. Large cell carcinoma is a group of carcinomas undifferentiated at the light microscopic level. They exhibit neuroendocrine or glandular differentiation markers when studied by immunohistochemistry or electron microscopy. The location and behavior of large cell carcinoma tend to be similar to adenocarcinoma, although certain large cell variants such as giant cell tumors may be extremely aggressive. Most of these tumors are large peripheral lesions unrelated to bronchi except for contiguous growth. Two rare subtypes of large cell carcinomas are the giant cell carcinomas, associated with peripheral leukocytosis, and clear cell carcinomas, which resemble renal cell carcinomas.

The treatment for NSCLC, including the use of adjuvant and neoadjuvant therapy, is complex and dependent on many factors including patient condition and staging. The stage groupings based on TNM are illustrated in Table 21.3. Surgical resection is the cornerstone of therapy for stage I and stage II disease. Most patients should undergo a lobectomy or pneumonectomy to achieve negative margins. A segmentectomy or wedge resection may be appropriate in patients with marginal lung reserve such that the risk of not tolerating the proper oncologic operation outweighs the benefits. In these cases, segmentectomy seems to be superior to wedge resection with regard to local recurrence. An additional group of patients that can benefit from segmentectomy are those with T1N0 peripherally located tumors. There does not seem to be a negative impact on clinical outcome for this group of patients undergoing sublobar resection. For stage IIIA disease, resection is performed with the objective of removing all pulmonary and lymph node disease. Five-year survival is approximately 25% following resection with a 15% local recurrence rate. For patients with stage IIIA N2 disease, several clinical trials have supported the use of neoadjuvant therapy with resection. Of note, care must be taken to evaluate the risk–benefit calculation regarding resection following chemotherapy. For instance, high-risk patients may benefit from definitive radiotherapy rather than surgical resection in this situation. Currently, stage IIIB patients are generally not surgical candidates. This is especially true for N3 patients with involved contralateral nodes. Additionally, T4N2 patients generally do not benefit from surgical resection.

Regarding adjuvant therapy, the Lung Adjuvant Cisplatin Evaluation (LACE) demonstrated a clear survival benefit for patients with resected stage II and III disease; however, there was not a clear benefit for stage IB patients. More recently, patients with stage IB disease and tumors greater than 5 cm have been qualifying for postoperative chemotherapy. For adjuvant radiation therapy (XRT), there is no evidence to support its implementation in stage I and II patients unless there are positive surgical margins. The data is ambiguous at best for stage III patients. In terms of neoadjuvant therapy, recent studies suggest that it does confer some survival benefit in early-stage (I and II) patients; however, more data is needed to fully elucidate the indications for neoadjuvant therapy in specific patient populations.

Patients with lung cancer die because of disseminated disease that is sometimes, but not typically, associated with local recurrence. As mentioned previously, the most common sites of recurrences are the brain, bones, and adrenal glands.

The best predictor of survival is the patient's lymph node status. Overall 5-year survival is 67% for stage IA, 57% for stage IB, 55% for stage IIA, 39% for stage IIB, and 25% for stage IIIA. It is unfortunately 5% for stage IIIB and IV tumors.

Small Cell Lung Cancer

SCLC represents 15% of primary lung malignancies. Approximately 80% of small cell tumors originate centrally and are found in airway submucosa. This tumor spreads rapidly to regional hilar and mediastinal lymph nodes without involving the respiratory tract directly. They also expand against the bronchus, causing extrinsic compression. These tumors tend to undergo central necrosis and cavitation. The disease is characterized by a very aggressive tendency to metastasize. It spreads very early to mediastinal lymph nodes and distant sites, especially the bone marrow and brain.

TABLE 21.3 Classification of lung cancer

Stage	TNM Classification
IA	T1 N0 M0
IB	T2 N0 M0
IIA	T1 N1 M0
IIB	T2 N1 M0, T3 N0 M0
IIIA	T1 N2 M0, T2 N2 M0, T3 N1 M0, T3 N2 M0
IIIB	Any T N3 M0, T4, any N M0
IV	Any T any N M1
Primary tumor	
T1	Tumor ≤ 3 cm No bronchoscopic evidence of invasion into main bronchus
T2	Tumor > 3 cm Involvement of main bronchus ≥2 cm from the carina Invasion of visceral pleura Associated atelectasis or obstructive pneumonitis extending into the hilar region but not the entire lung
T3	Any size tumor invading chest wall (includes superior sulcus tumors), diaphragm, mediastinal pleura, parietal pericardium Tumor ≥2 cm from the carina, without carinal involvement Atelectasis or pneumonitis of the entire lung
T4	Any size tumor invading mediastinum, heart, great vessels, trachea, esophagus, vertebral body, or carina Separate tumor nodules in the same lobe Malignant pleural effusion
Regional lymph nodes	
N0	No lymph node metastases
N1	Ipsilateral peribronchial or hilar metastases Ipsilateral intrapulmonary nodes involved by direct extension
N2	Ipsilateral mediastinal and/or subcarinal lymph node metastases
N3	Contralateral mediastinal or hilar lymph node metastases Ipsilateral or contralateral scalene or supraclavicular lymph node metastases
Nodal levels	
N	Level/nodes
N2	1/highest mediastinal 2/upper paratracheal 3/pretracheal and retrotracheal 4/lower paratracheal, including azygous nodes
Aortic	5/subaortic (aortopulmonary window) 6/para-aortic (ascending aortic or phrenic) Inferior 7/subcarinal 8/paraesophageal (below carina) 9/inferior pulmonary ligament
N1	10/hilar 11/interlobar 12/segmental 13/subsegmental
Distant metastases	
M0	No distant metastases
M1	Distant metastases, including synchronous nodules in a different lobe

SCLC is assumed to be a systemic disease at the time of presentation. Thus, systemic chemotherapy is the treatment modality most commonly employed in these patients. At staging, about one third of patients will have "limited" disease (confined to the chest) and two thirds will have "extensive" disease. Management of limited disease typically consists of chemotherapy and XRT with a 5-year survival of approximately 15%. Extensive disease confers a median survival of about 12 months. While there have been case reports suggesting benefit of surgical intervention in limited SCLC, no trial has proven any benefit from surgical resection in these cases. As a result, surgery is typically not offered for these patients.

Carcinoid Tumors

Carcinoid tumors belong to a spectrum of neuroendocrine tumors that arise from the bronchial epithelial cells and are technically carcinomas, although they rarely metastasize. They make up 2% of all lung carcinomas. While usually associated with serotonin production, these tumors can produce and secrete various other neuroendocrine peptides such as bradykinin, glucagon, insulin, vasopressin, and calcitonin. The majority, however, do not actively secrete peptides. While typical carcinoids rarely metastasize, atypical carcinoids are associated with lymph node metastases in up to 50% of patients. The usual presentation involves hemoptysis, dyspnea, or recurrent pulmonary infections. Only 2% of patients present with carcinoid syndrome, which is usually associated with metastatic disease. The treatment consists of complete tumor resection, and survival is 90% for typical carcinoids compared to 60% for atypical.

Adenoid Cystic Carcinomas

Adenoid cystic carcinomas arise from the submucosal glands in the bronchi and trachea. They are slow growing and invade the submucosal plane along perineural lymphatics. As a result, they typically extend well past their gross margins. The mainstay of therapy is resection of the tumor and involved airway followed by XRT. When lesions are truly unresectable, palliation can be obtained with endobronchial laser therapy. The slow growth allows for long-term survival even in unresectable cases.

Mucoepidermoid carcinomas

Mucoepidermoid carcinomas are extremely rare and account for less than 5% of bronchial adenomas. They vary in degree of malignancy from low to high grade. The treatment is resection, and high-grade lesions can be treated as bronchogenic carcinomas with respect to resection and survival.

Metastases in the Lung

The lungs are a common site for metastases from a variety of tumors. The first pulmonary metastasectomy was described by Davis in 1927. Most patients with pulmonary metastases present with asymptomatic lesions on follow-up chest imaging. Guidelines for resection involve control of the primary cancer, absence of extrathoracic metastases, and sufficient physiologic reserve to tolerate lung resection. A 2011 study based on 10 years of a single-center experience with pulmonary metastasectomy demonstrated a significant survival benefit in patients undergoing complete resection relative to incomplete (Fig. 21.12). Additionally, one of the largest series of patients to undergo pulmonary metastasectomy was collected by the International Registry of Lung Metastases, which reported on over 4,000 resected cases of metastatic disease to the lung. It illustrated actuarial survival rates of 36%, 26%, and 22% at 5, 10, and 15 years, respectively. This was compared to 13% and 7% at 5 and ten years for incompletely resected tumors. As a result, there appears to be significant evidence supporting a role for pulmonary metastasectomy.

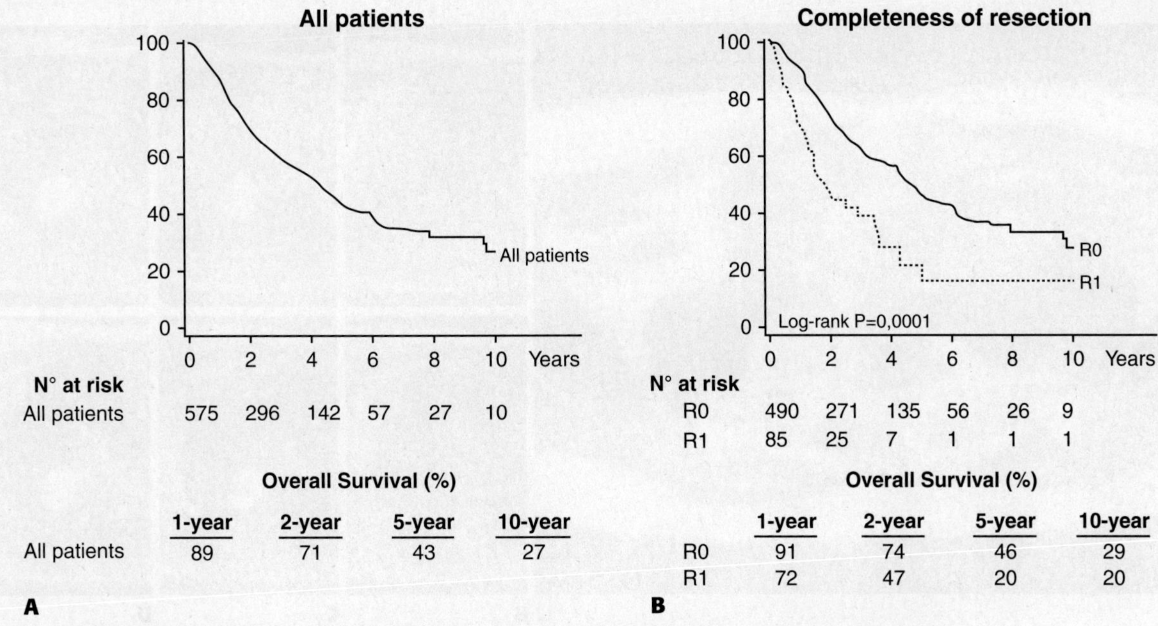

FIGURE 21.12 Overall survival for all patients **(A)** and according to completeness of pulmonary resection **(B)** after a mean follow-up of 34 months. (From Casiraghi M, De Pas T, Maisonneuve P, et al. A 10-year single-center experience on 708 lung metastasectomies: the evidence of the "international registry of lung metastases." *J Thorac Oncol.* 2011;6(8):1373–1378.)

TABLE 21.4 **Mediastinal structures**

Anterior	Middle	Posterior
Thymus	Heart	Esophagus
Aorta/great vessels	Pericardium	Vagus nerves
Lymphatics	Phrenic nerves	Sympathetic nerve plexus
Fatty areolar tissue	Carina	Thoracic duct
Upper trachea	Main bronchi	Descending aorta
Upper esophagus	Pulmonary hilum	Azygous vein
—	Lymph nodes	Hemiazygous vein
—	—	Paravertebral lymphatics
—	—	Fatty areolar tissue

Chest Wall Tumors

Primary tumors of the chest wall, of which between 50% and 80% are malignant, are relatively uncommon lesions that encompass both bone and soft tissue pathology. Table 21.4 lists the more common benign and malignant types of chest wall tumors. They represent less than 5% of thoracic neoplasms. The typical presentation is an insidious process with a slow-growing tumor that eventually becomes painful and apparent. Workup is initiated with CXR, which can identify the mass and demonstrate any clear pulmonary metastases. Cross-sectional imaging is then employed, with MRI being the preferred modality in that is able to more clearly delineate the tumor's relationship to the spine and thoracic inlet (Fig. 21.13). PET-CT is then useful to evaluate for primary versus metastatic disease. Excisional biopsy rather than incisional should be performed for tissue diagnosis in a manner that will not disrupt future treatment. If malignancy is diagnosed, then wide resection must be performed. A resection margin of 4.0 cm is recommended for a primary malignant chest wall neoplasm. A 2.0 cm margin is considered *inadequate* for these situations. Additionally, high-grade neoplasms should have the entire bone removed. Following appropriate resection, the other critical component of treatment is reconstruction of the chest wall that will support respiration and protect the thoracic organs. This may involve the use of polypropylene mesh (Fig. 21.14), polytetrafluoroethylene (PTFE), or methyl methacrylate sandwiched between polypropylene mesh. The overall 5-year survival rate for chest wall tumors is 60% with a recurrence rate of approximately 50%. Of the recurrences, the 5-year survival is 17%.

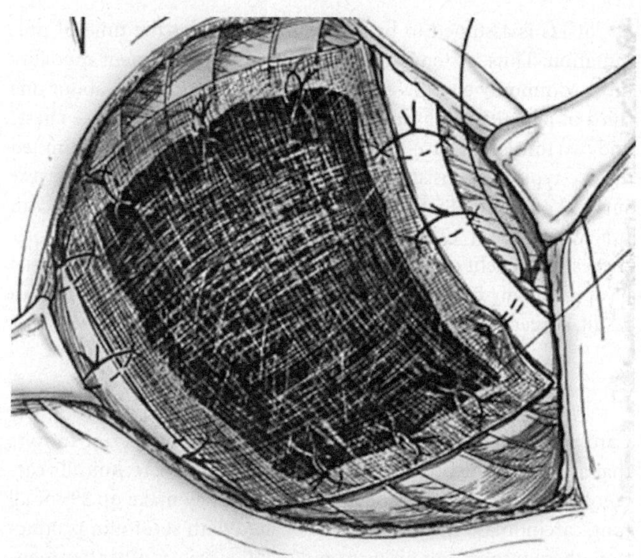

FIGURE 21.14 Chest wall prosthesis inset. (From Kaiser LR, Kron IL, Spray TL, eds. *Mastery of Cardiothoracic Surgery*. 3rd ed. Philadelphia: Wolters Kluwer Health; 2014.)

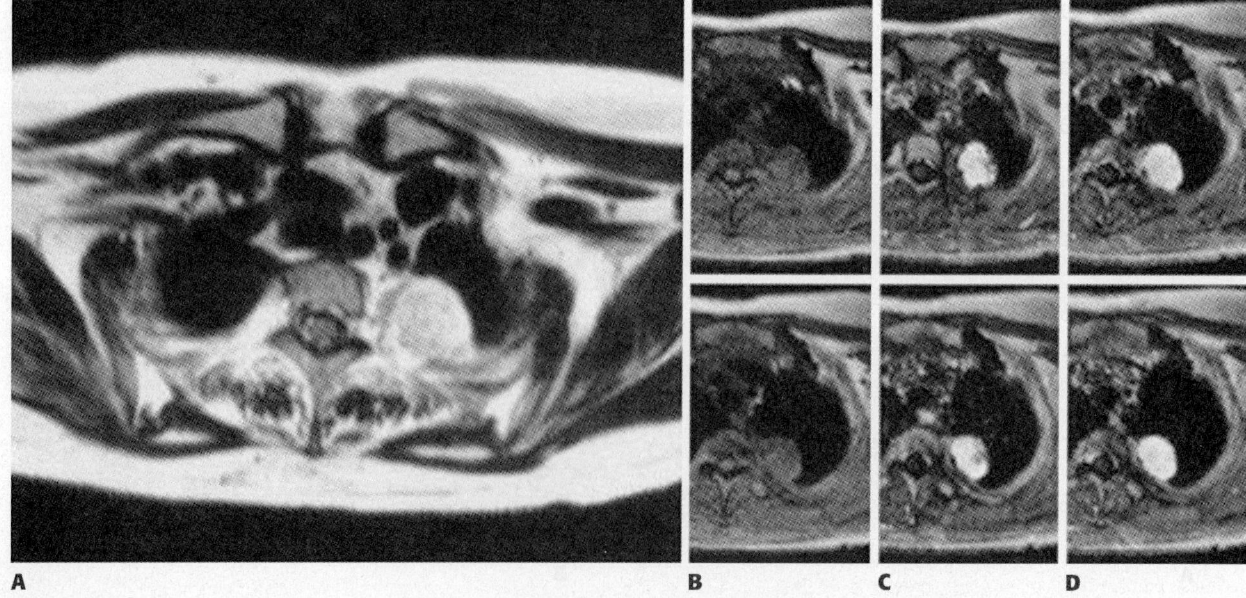

FIGURE 21.13 MRI demonstrating chest wall tumor's relationship to the great vessels **(A)**. Unenhanced **(B)**, early phase (C), and delayed phase (D) images are included. (From Yuan Y, Matsumoto T, Miura G, et al. Imaging findings of an intercostal hemangioma. *J Thorac Imaging*. 2002;17(1):92–95.)

Diseases of the Pleura and the Pleural Space

The pleural surface is a mesothelial layer that envelopes all of the structures of the thoracic cavity. It is further defined as parietal if it covers the chest wall, diaphragm, and mediastinum or visceral if it covers the lung. The pleura and its components are subject to the same benign and malignant processes that affect epithelial tissues throughout the body.

Pleural Space Disease

A pleural effusion can be a manifestation of a localized or systemic process. Effusions are classically divided into exudates and transudates. Exudative effusions are associated with pleural or lymphatic diseases, while transudative effusions are secondary to either increased production or decreased absorption of pleural fluid. Differentiation is crucial as their etiologies are extremely different. Almost 50% of exudates are due to a neoplastic process, while transudates are typically secondary to congestive heart failure (CHF). The diagnosis can easily be made by thoracentesis and laboratory evaluation of the pleural fluid. Exudative effusions are defined as follows: (1) ratio of pleural fluid to serum total protein, greater than 0.5; (2) ratio of pleural fluid to serum LDH, greater than 0.6; and (3) value of LDH in pleural fluid, greater than 200 U/L. Additionally, low glucose and pH are common in malignant effusions. Effusions are easily identified on CXR since as little as 125 to 250 mL of fluid is visible. CT of the chest can be helpful in determining if an effusion is loculated and whether an underlying disease is present. Ultrasound is an effective imaging aid to thoracentesis by identifying a safe path of entry into the thorax.

If the underlying cause of an effusion cannot be effectively contained, drainage is necessary in symptomatic patients. This is unfortunately a frequent occurrence with malignant effusions. In these cases, placement of a small silicone catheter with a valve that allows only drainage is an effective treatment. It enables the patient to leave the hospital and intermittently drain pleural fluid to relieve dyspnea. Additionally, patients with malignant effusions are frequently unable to maintain an expanded lung following drainage. To address this, a sclerosing agent such as talc or bleomycin can be delivered into the pleural space to accelerate pleurodesis by inciting an intense inflammatory response that results in strong adhesion development in the pleural envelope.

Another common condition requiring surgical intervention is spontaneous pneumothorax (SP). Primary SP usually occurs in young patients with blebs and otherwise normal lungs. Secondary SP is seen in patients with significant structural lung disease, which contributes to the SP. The incidence is between 8 and 18 cases per 100,000 in men and 1 and 6 cases per 100,000 in women. The typical patient is between 10 and 30 years old, tall, and thin. The most significant risk factor is smoking, which can raise the risk by as high as 20. Secondary SP is most frequently due to COPD with an incidence of about 6 per 100,000 among men and peaking at 60 to 65 years of age.

The etiology of primary SP is related to the rupture of a subpleural bleb. After the first episode of SP, the recurrence is approximately 30% and usually occurs 6 to 24 months following the initial episode. After the second episode, the recurrence rate approaches 80% and therefore warrants intervention. Patients typically present with pleuritic chest pain and dyspnea. With regard to management for the initial episode, small SPs in an asymptomatic patient can be managed with observation. A CXR should be repeated within 6 hours to monitor for any expansion. An enlarging SP is an indication for intervention. A large or symptomatic SP should be treated with chest tube placement, which is effective in 90% of patients for the first occurrence. In patients with recurrence, failure of the lung to re-expand, bilateral pneumothoraces, high-risk occupations (pilots, divers), and large pulmonary bullae, surgery is recommended. The procedure of choice is VATS blebectomy with pleurodesis.

For patients with secondary SP, the underlying cause is most commonly COPD with bleb rupture. Their clinical presentation is generally more severe because of baseline lung disease, and more aggressive chest tube placement is warranted. Since these patients are overall much higher operative risks than those with primary SP, it is argued that Heimlich valves are a low morbidity approach for managing persistent air leaks. A rare but notable form of pneumothorax is a catamenial pneumothorax. These usually occur within 72 hours of menstruation in young to middle-aged women. A variety of strategies, in addition to chest tube placement, are implemented to address this phenomenon including inspection of the diaphragm for fenestrations that could potentially allow endometrial implants on the visceral pleura.

A hemothorax refers to a collection of blood in the pleural space. Small hemothoraces are usually not even recognized and usually resolve without intervention. Larger collections can be successfully treated with chest tube placement if drained early. Complications of an undrained hemothorax include empyema and fibrothorax with entrapped lung. Empyema requires definitive drainage, often surgical, and is discussed later in the chapter. Fibrothorax and trapped lung result from an organized fibrous peel that encases the lung and leads to a functional reduction in volume. The treatment is to remove the peel from the chest wall and lung, referred to as decortication. This can be performed via thoracotomy or VATS.

A chylothorax refers to a collection of chyle in the pleural space following an injury to the thoracic duct or a branch. It can be confirmed by a cholesterol/triglyceride ratio of less than 1 and a triglyceride level of greater than 110 mg/dL. Of note, in a minority of cases, chylothorax can exist without meeting these criteria. In these cases, detection of chylomicrons in the pleural fluid can confirm the diagnosis. Typically, in a postoperative patient, the chest tube output will turn a milky-white color once the patient initiates a diet. The treatment can be conservative or interventional. Conservative treatment involves TPN and a medium-chain fatty acid diet. There is debate over determining when conservative management has failed; however, there is consensus that a leak of over 1 L/day should not be allowed to persist for greater than 7 days. There are a variety of interventional strategies with the common goal of stopping the leak and obliterating the space involved. Additionally, some centers have become increasingly comfortable with embolization of the duct during lymphangiography.

An empyema is defined as the accumulation of infected fluid in the pleural space. A sampling of the fluid typically demonstrates a pH < 7.0, glucose less than 40 mg/dL, LDH greater than 1,000 IU/L, and a positive Gram stain. Additional findings include a WBC greater than 15,000 cells/mL, protein greater than 3 g/dL, and a specific gravity greater than 1.016. Most empyemas occur secondary to a pneumonic infiltrate, with *Staphylococcus aureus* and enteric gram-negative bacilli being the most common organisms. Treating the empyema involves eradicating the primary infection, evacuating infected fluid, and re-expanding the lung to completely obliterate residual space. Some patients are not able to be adequately drained by chest tube alone and require more extensive procedures such as VATS drainage, decortication, or rib resection in conjunction with placement of an empyema tube. An empyema tube is a thoracostomy tube that is gradually backed

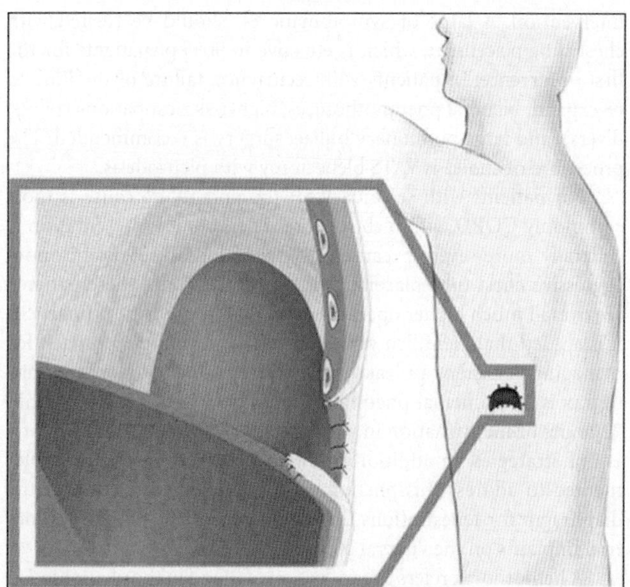

FIGURE 21.15 Illustration of the modified Eloesser flap. (From Althubaiti G, Butler C. Abdominal wall and chest wall reconstruction. *Plastic Reconstr Surg.* 2014;133(5):688e–701e.)

out of the infected space over a 3- to 4-week period such that the cavity closes around the tube. Of note, the use of thrombolytic agents, streptokinase and urokinase, has regained some popularity in managing empyema. This is because fibrin strands form between the visceral and parietal pleura during empyema development. The thrombolytic agents break these bands and enhance drainage. Randomized prospective studies have found significantly improved empyema drainage with thrombolytic therapy; however, this treatment has not been fully adopted. In patients that have failed to drain with chronic empyema, a more long-term solution is creation of the modified Eloesser flap (Fig. 21.15). This enables drainage over a long period of time, and the open thoracostomy window can be easily irrigated and dressed. There are multiple options for closing at a later date.

Pleural Cancer

Pleural malignancies most commonly present as metastases from lung, breast, stomach, and pancreas neoplasms. Primary malignant tumors of the pleura, the most common being malignant mesothelioma, are far less common than metastatic lesions. Exposure to asbestos is the biggest risk factor for developing mesothelioma; however, there exists a latency period of 20 to 50 years with a lifetime risk of 4.5% to 10% of developing the disease. Patients typically present with nonpleuritic chest pain, dyspnea, cough, fever, and weight loss. Chest radiographs may show classical pleural plaques or pleural thickening, and most patients either present with or will develop a pleural effusion some time during the course of their disease. Because mesothelioma may be difficult to distinguish from adenocarcinoma that has metastasized to the pleural cavity, a definitive diagnosis can only be achieved by obtaining a sample of the tumor. The prognosis without treatment carries a median survival of 4 to 12 months. Unfortunately, there is no evidence-based guideline regarding mesothelioma treatment. This is partly because there have been no randomized controlled trials examining different treatment strategies. XRT has demonstrated benefit in reducing local recurrence following VATS biopsy; however, no randomized study has demonstrated a clear benefit of XRT as an adjunct to extrapleural pneumonectomy (EPP). Evolution of chemotherapy strategies have led to combination therapy, which has demonstrated enhanced response rates. Currently, the combination of pemetrexed and cisplatin is the accepted chemotherapeutic regimen for mesothelioma. This approach is supported by a randomized phase III trial. Surgical treatment involves pleurectomy and decortication versus EPP. As expected, EPP carries a higher operative morbidity and mortality and, therefore, has stricter criteria for eligibility. Mortality rates are reported between 3.5% and 10% in high volume centers, while morbidity has been reported as at 25%. Currently, multimodality therapy involving surgery and chemoradiation seem to portend somewhat of a survival benefit compared to historical controls. Studies are ongoing to better quantify this benefit. Additional innovative therapies for mesothelioma include intracavitary lavage with hyperthermic chemotherapy, photodynamic therapy, gene therapy, and immunogenic modulators.

Mediastinal Disease

The mediastinum can be deconstructed into three compartments: the anterior/superior, middle, and posterior. This is based on the relation to the pericardium. The anterior mediastinum contains all structures anterior to the pericardium and great vessels. The middle mediastinum is bounded by the anterior and posterior pericardial reflections, while the posterior mediastinum contains everything posterior to the posterior pericardial reflections.

Mediastinitis

Bacterial contamination of the mediastinum, referred to as mediastinitis, can rapidly lead to sepsis and clinical deterioration. Early recognition is critical. It can be secondary to an esophageal perforation, contamination after a surgical procedure, or descend from an infectious process in the posterior pharynx. Patients present with the typical signs of infection and sepsis. They may have subcutaneous emphysema if there is an esophageal, tracheal, or bronchial perforation. If a pharyngeal abscess is the source, then patients may present with Ludwig's angina, pain over the anterior neck and chest. A standard CXR may demonstrate an air–fluid level in the mediastinum. A CT of the chest is critical in acquiring more information regarding a possible source. Bronchoscopy, esophagoscopy, and water-soluble contrast studies are the most useful diagnostic tools in confirming airway or esophageal perforation. Successful treatment consists of rapid identification, repair of the source, adequate drainage, and broad-spectrum antibiotics. Gross contamination from an esophageal perforation requires wide debridement and typically repair of the esophagus. If the esophagus cannot be repaired initially, it can be divided with a stapler, and a cervical esophagostomy can be created for temporary control. A patient in this scenario will require enteral access for nutrition until future repair. A postoperative sternal infection with mediastinitis, following cardiac surgery, for instance, will typically require sternal debridement with a pectoralis or omental flap.

Mediastinal Masses

Approximately half of mediastinal lesions are asymptomatic and are detected on chest radiographs taken for unrelated reasons. As a rough guideline, the absence of symptoms suggests that a lesion is benign, whereas the presence of symptoms suggests malignancy. The percentage of patients with symptoms from mediastinal masses precisely parallels, or equals, the percentage of malignant lesions. In adults, 50% to 60% of lesions are symptomatic, whereas the percentage of symptomatic lesions is higher in children—60% to 80%. Since the incidence of symptoms parallels the incidence of malignancy, a child with a mediastinal mass is considerably more likely to have a malignancy than is an adult with a mediastinal mass. The most common symptoms are cardiorespiratory, specifically chest pain and cough. Other manifestations are heaviness in the chest, dysphagia, dyspnea, hemoptysis, signs of superior vena caval obstruction with facial swelling, and cyanosis. Recurrent respiratory infections are a common complaint. As discussed below, several mediastinal lesions are associated with other clinical syndromes: thymoma with myasthenia gravis, red cell aplasia, hypogammaglobulinemia, and nonthymic cancers; Hodgkin's disease with recurrent fevers; and von Recklinghausen's disease with neurofibromas.

The masses are almost always initially identified on CXR. This should be followed up with a CT of the chest, which is excellent in evaluating mediastinal masses (Fig. 21.16). It can also be used to guide biopsy and potential surgical approach. MRI can be helpful and is superior to CT when evaluating a tumor's invasion to neuronal or vascular structures. Radionucleotide scanning can also be employed to help identify substernal thyroid masses, parathyroid, and paraganglioma. The decision to biopsy mediastinal masses is a complex one. The nuances are beyond the scope of this chapter, but an important concept is that biopsy carries significant benefit when there is a reasonable suspicion (i.e., elevated AFP or βhHC) that a mass will be managed by systemic chemotherapy rather than surgical resection. A germ cell tumor is an example of this where surgery is reserved for residual disease following chemotherapy.

Thymoma

Thymomas are the most common tumors found in the anterior mediastinum. They appear benign histologically even when they are invasive. They derive from either cortical or medullary epithelial cells. They are the most common of the thymic malignancies. Patients commonly present with local symptoms accompanied by paraneoplastic syndromes such as myasthenia gravis, Cushing syndrome, SLE, or rheumatoid arthritis. Five histologic grades have been described, based on lymphocytic infiltration: lymphocytic, lymphoepithelial (mixed), epithelial, spindle cell, and unclassified. Thus, a lymphocytic thymoma consists of 65% to 80% lymphocytes. Tumor stage at the time of treatment indicates prognosis better than tumor grade. Table 21.5 illustrates thymoma staging. Stage I lesions (encapsulated) are generally considered benign. Tumor–node–metastasis (TNM) staging has not been widely adopted. A peculiar characteristic of the benign histologic appearance of many of these lesions is that invasion of adjacent structures, and thus the stage of the tumor, can usually be more easily determined by the surgeon at the time of operation than by the pathologist at the time of microscopy. Thymomas most commonly are differentiated as being either "encapsulated" or "invasive" opposed to "benign" or "malignant."

The mainstay of therapy, even for extensive lesions, is surgical resection. Most surgeons, even those experienced in thoracoscopy, recommend median sternotomy for the procedure. Transcervical resection is also performed. Most recurrences are local, either in the pleural space or in the mediastinum. Distant recurrences, when they do develop, are most often in bone. Recurrences are potentially curable, requiring several therapeutic methods, including repeated surgical exploration. All patients in whom an invasive thymoma has been resected should receive postoperative radiotherapy, which is

A

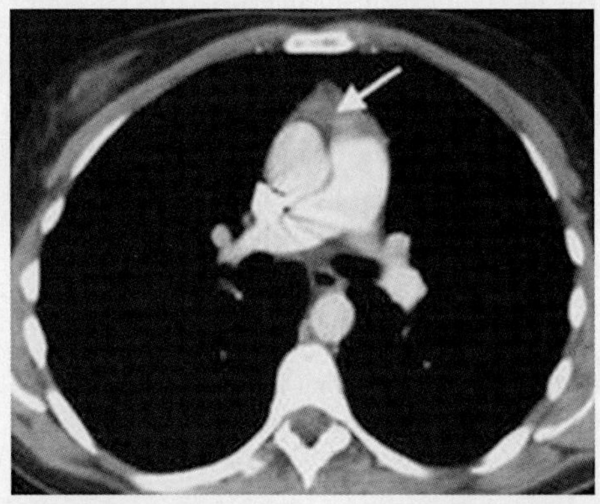

B

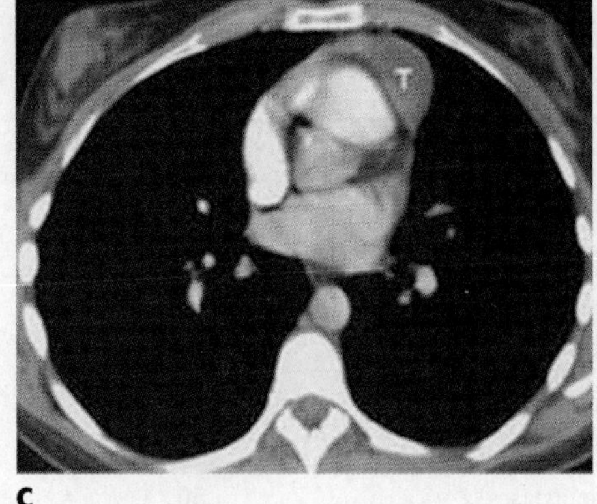

C

FIGURE 21.16 A PA CXR with an abnormal left mediastinum **(A)**. A CT showing soft tissue anterior to the ascending aorta **(B)**, and CT more inferior **(C)** demonstrating enlarged thymic tissue on the left. (From Collins J, Stern EJ, eds. *Chest Radiology: The Essentials*. 2nd ed. Philadelphia: Lippincott Williams & Wilkins; 2008.)

TABLE 21.5 Mediastinal masses

Anterior	Middle	Posterior
Thymoma (31%)	Cysts (61%)	Neurogenic (52%)
Lymphoma (23%)	Lymphoma (20%)	Cysts (32%)
Germ cell tumors (17%)	Mesenchymal (8%)	Mesenchymal (10%)
Carcinoma (13%)	Carcinoma (6%)	Endocrine (2%)
Germ cell tumors (17%)	Other (5%)	Other (4%)
Cysts (6%)	—	—
Other (10%)[a]	—	—

[a]Includes teratoma, lipoma, lymphangioma, hemangioma, parathyroid adenoma/carcinoma, thyroid adenoma/carcinoma/goiter.

strongly recommended for all but stage I patients. Surgery alone yields a recurrence rate of approximately 30%, whereas radiation and surgery together yield a recurrence rate of approximately 5%. Whether noninvasive encapsulated thymomas respond to irradiation is debatable. Patients with thymomas, even when the disease is unresectable, recurrent, or metastatic, often respond to treatment with cisplatin, doxorubicin, and cyclophosphamide (Table 21.6).

Myasthenia gravis is the most common thymoma-associated systemic syndrome. Patients with myasthenia gravis present with muscle weakness that intensifies with repetitive activity. The pathophysiology of myasthenia graves entails the autoimmune-mediated binding of antibodies to the acetylcholine receptor, followed by their lysis by complement-mediated factors. Striking clinical improvement may occur after thymectomy without any change in measurable immune parameters, including the absence of change in the serum levels of autoantibodies. Myasthenia gravis is present in approximately one third of patients with thymomas. This disorder may either precede or follow the development of thymoma by many years. Any type of thymic tumor may occur in patients with myasthenia gravis. Among patients with myasthenia gravis without thymomas, remission can be expected in up to one half: in about 20%, remissions are completely drug free; in up to 30%, remission is maintained by drugs, that is, a combined remission rate of 50%. Improvement can be expected in one third to one half of patients; no change is evident in 10%, and a rare patient gets worse after surgery.

TABLE 21.6 Staging and 5-year survival rates for malignant thymomas

Stage	Five-Year Survival (%)
I (encapsulated, no evidence of gross or microscopic capsular invasion)	85–100
II (pericapsular invasion into mediastinal fat, pleura, or pericardium)	60–80
III (invasion into adjacent organs or intrathoracic metastases)	40–70
IV (extrathoracic metastases)	50

Lymphoma

Lymphoma commonly presents in the mediastinum. Patients with Hodgkin's and non-Hodgkin's lymphomas can present with dyspnea, hoarseness, chest pain, SVC syndrome, fever, chills, and weight loss. A CXR can provide initial visualization, but CT and MRI are necessary for further information. A definitive diagnosis typically requires surgical biopsy as FNA is unreliable. Treatment is with chemotherapy.

Neurogenic Tumors

Neurogenic tumors commonly arise from neural crest cells and are located in the posterior mediastinum. They have the ability to secrete various hormones but are typically inactive. Most tumors found in adults are benign, while most in children are malignant. Intercostal nerve tumors include neurofibroma, neurilemoma (schwannoma), neurofibrosarcoma, and neurosarcoma. Sympathetic ganglia tumors include ganglioma, ganglioneuroblastoma, and neuroblastoma. A pheochromocytoma is a paraganglia tumor. Neurofibromas are poorly encapsulated, associated with neurofibromatosis type 1, and tend to form in the paravertebral gutters. Schwannomas are the most common neurogenic tumor. Both of these can be associated with von Recklinghausen's disease and can develop into neurosarcomas if not addressed.

Patients can present because of an incidental finding on CXR, respiratory symptoms, or neurologic symptoms. Further imaging with CT and MRI (Fig. 21.17) is necessary to first identify a potential neurogenic tumor and then to establish its relationship to the spinal canal. Tumors that extend into the canal through the intervertebral foramen are considered *dumbbell* tumors. This is critical for surgical planning. Percutaneous FNA can be performed for tissue diagnosis; however, surgical intervention is the standard of care for neurogenic tumors. As always, biopsy should be performed only if it will potentially affect further management. The traditional approach for posterior mediastinal tumor resection was a posterolateral thoracotomy; however, minimally invasive resection with VATS has gained significant popularity. The general prognosis for neurogenic tumors is variable and tied to the histopathology.

Congenital Chest Wall Deformities

The most common congenital abnormality of the chest wall is pectus excavatum that presents as a concave depression of the lower sternum. It is thought to be due to an overgrowth of costal cartilages during chest wall development. If a deformity is significant, it is apparent by 3 years of age. It occurs more frequently in males than females with a 4:1 ratio. It is well tolerated in infancy and childhood; however, teenagers tend to report pain and limited exercise ability. Palpitations have also been reported. There has been debate over the years regarding the significance of pectus excavatum on pulmonary function. A recent large analysis demonstrated that the median FVC and FEV_1 were 13% below predicted, and FEF was 20% below predicted. Indications for surgical repair include exercise intolerance, abnormal PFTs, abnormal echocardiogram, exercise-induced asthma, cosmetic reasons, and Haller index greater than 3.0 (transverse diameter of the thorax divided by the anteroposterior dimension on CT). Multiple open surgical strategies for pectus excavatum have been described including the established modified Ravitch repair. The minimally invasive Nuss repair, introduced in 1998, has gained significant popularity as well and is illustrated in Figure 21.18. Outcomes have been excellent in the

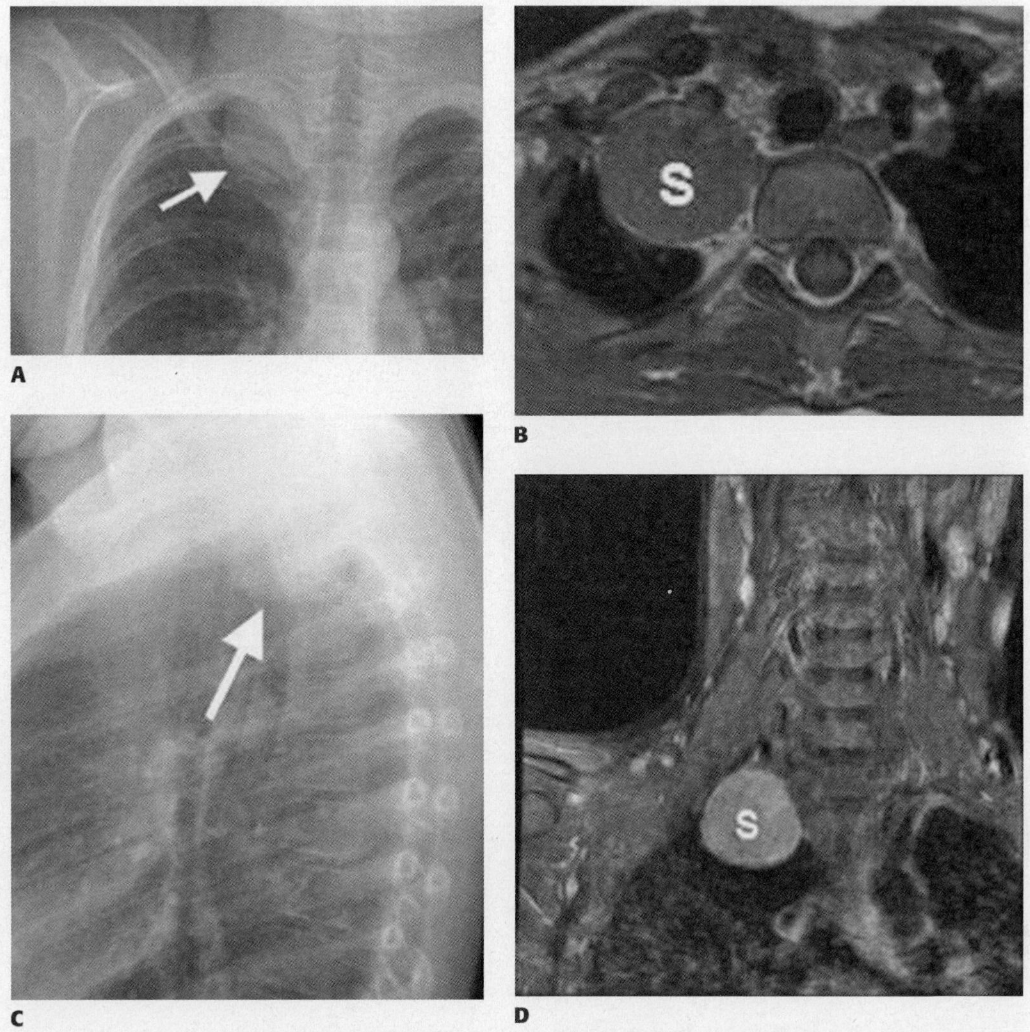

FIGURE 21.17 Benign schwannoma. PA **(A)** and lateral **(B)** CXR of a 9-year-old girl illustrate a right apical circumscribed mass. Axial MRI **(C)** demonstrates that the mass is paraspinal with no continuity with the spinal cord. Contrast **(D)** shows high signal intensity. (From Collins J, Stern EJ, eds. *Chest Radiology: The Essentials*. 2nd ed. Philadelphia: Lippincott Williams & Wilkins; 2008.)

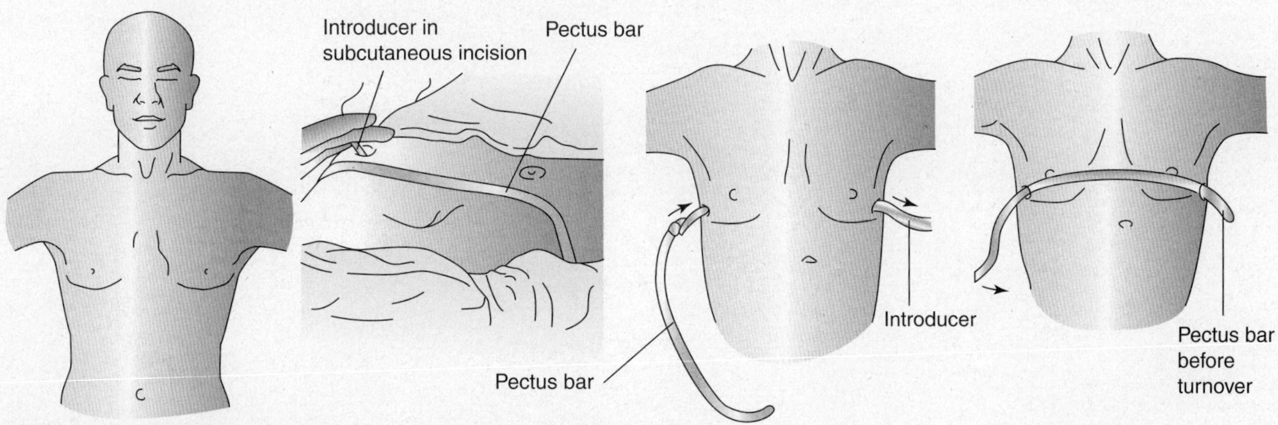

FIGURE 21.18 Illustration of the Nuss repair of pectus excavatum. (From Kaiser LR, Kron IL, Spray TL, eds. *Mastery of Cardiothoracic Surgery*. 3rd ed. Philadelphia: Wolters Kluwer Health; 2014.)

pediatric population, and it has even been applied to patients who have failed a modified Ravitch repair.

Pectus carinatum is an anterior displacement of the chest wall caused by an overgrowth of costal cartilage. It is not nearly as common as excavatum, and patients tend to present at an older age. Typically, patients are treated with a brace to reduce the carinatum. Indications for operation include body image, pain, respiratory symptoms, and ease of injury. Surgical intervention should be deferred until after puberty to avoid recurrence. If managed properly, recurrence is less than 1%.

Suggested Readings

Collins J. *Chest Radiology: The Essentials*. 2nd ed. Philadelphia: Lippincott Williams & Wilkins; 2008.

Grippi MA, Elias JA, Fishman JA, et al. *Fishman's Pulmonary Diseases and Disorders*. 5th ed. New York: McGraw-Hill; 2015.

Levitzky MG. *Pulmonary Physiology*. 8th ed. New York: McGraw-Hill; 2013.

Nason KS, Maddaus MA, Luketich JD. Chest wall, lung, mediastinum, and pleura. In: Brunicardi F, Andersen DK, Billiar TR, et al. eds. *Schwartz's Principles of Surgery*. 10th ed. New York: McGraw-Hill; 2014.

Selke FW, del Nido, PJ, Swanson, SJ. *Sabiston and Spencer's Surgery of the Chest*. 8th ed. Philadelphia: Elsevier; 2010.

SECTION

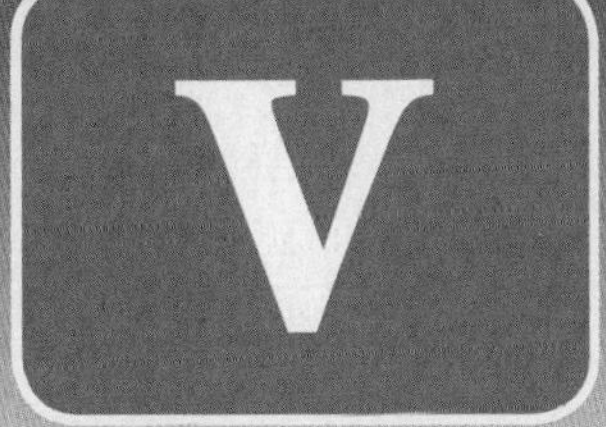

Trauma

CHAPTER

22

Trauma Evaluation, Resuscitation, and Surgical Critical Care

IAN W. FOLKERT AND BENJAMIN M. BRASLOW

KEY POINTS

- The primary survey of an injured patient is performed in an order that prioritizes and identifies the most acute life-threatening issues, which might cause the patient to expire next. Interventions should occur as these issues are identified.
- The safest place for an unstable trauma patient is in the operating room where hemorrhage control and resuscitation can occur simultaneously.
- Often, a neurologic assessment is imperative to obtain before pharmacologically sedating and paralyzing a patient. A rapid head CT obtained on the way to the operating room or an intra-op ICP monitor in an unstable blunt trauma patient may be necessary to identify life-threatening closed head injury that needs simultaneous intervention.
- Volume resuscitation in an exsanguinating patient is best achieved with blood component therapy in a 1:1:1 ratio of packed red blood cells, fresh frozen plasma, and platelets to prevent the deleterious effects of a high-volume crystalloid resuscitation.
- Critical care is a concept, not a location!
- Physiologic goal-directed therapy for resuscitation of the patient in shock from exsanguination, neurologic injury, sepsis, or cardiogenic etiologies should be initiated early and monitored invasively to maximize survival benefit.

EVALUATION AND RESUSCITATION OF THE TRAUMA PATIENT

Background

Trauma, including intentional and unintentional injury, is an enormous global health burden and is the leading cause of potential, unrealized loss of life. In the United States and worldwide, injury is the leading cause of death through age 45 years. Trauma is responsible for nearly 190,000 deaths and over 3 million hospitalizations annually in the United States. The economic and social impact of these injuries is staggering—with costs over $250 billion per year and countless potential life years lost.

Death from injury occurs in a trimodal distribution: immediate deaths (50%), early deaths (30%), and late deaths (20%). *Immediate deaths* happen seconds to minutes after injury and are usually secondary to severe brain or spinal cord injury (SCI) or from rupture of the heart, aorta, or other major blood vessel. These injuries are essentially untreatable, except by prevention, and patients rarely survive long enough to present to a hospital or trauma center. *Early deaths* occur within minutes to several hours following an injury and are often due to subdural or epidural hematoma or exsanguination from hemopneumothorax, ruptured spleen, lacerations of the liver, and/or pelvic fractures. Development of the U.S. trauma and Emergency medical staff/technicians (EMS) systems has resulted in expeditious management of patients with such injuries and reductions in mortality for patients in the critical "golden hour" after injury. *Late deaths* usually occur in the intensive care unit (ICU) several days to weeks after the injury, most often in the setting of sepsis and/or multiple organ system failure (MOSF).

A step-wise approach to the management of trauma patients (those suffering from life-threatening injury) was conceived in the development of the advanced trauma life support (ATLS) program. This program, adopted by the American College of Surgeons Committee on Trauma (ACSCT) in 1979, standardizes concepts and protocols in the management of trauma patients.

Preparation and Triage

Trauma patients are first evaluated and resuscitated at the scene of injury (Table 22.1). EMS in the prehospital phase provide rapid basic life support (BLS), whereas paramedics and flight nurses can perform ATLS, that is, more advanced interventions with the backing of a medical command physician. The goals of prehospital care are airway maintenance, control of external hemorrhage, early shock management, immobilization of the axial spine and injured limbs, and immediate transport to the closest appropriate trauma-receiving facility. At the hospital, the trauma team is assembled, and the needed ancillary services are mobilized. The composition of the trauma team can vary, but key components always include the trauma surgeon, trauma-trained nurses, an airway team (either an emergency medicine physician or anesthesia representative), and a respiratory therapist. The necessary ancillary services often include availability of a computerized tomographic (CT) scanner, blood

TABLE 22.1 Initial assessment and management

Phase	Action
Prehospital/inhospital	Preparation
Prehospital/inhospital	Triage
Prehospital/inhospital	Primary survey (ABCDEs)
Prehospital/inhospital	Resuscitation
Prehospital/inhospital	Adjuncts to primary survey and resuscitation
Prehospital/inhospital	Secondary survey (head-to-toe evaluation and history)
Prehospital/inhospital	Adjuncts to secondary survey
Inhospital/ICU/OR	Continued postresuscitation monitoring and reevaluation
Inhospital/ICU/OR	Definitive care

ABCDE, *A*irway establishment or maintenance with cervical spine protection, *B*reathing/ensuring adequate ventilation, *C*irculation/hemorrhage control and maintenance of adequate perfusion pressure, *D*isability/neurologic status, *E*xposure/environmental control/injury identification.

bank, interventional radiology, operating room (OR) staff, and a clinical perfusion team capable of operating autologous transfusion and cardiopulmonary bypass devices.

Triage involves the sorting of trauma patients according to their need for treatment within the context of available resources. The most severely injured are treated first when the number of patients and the severity of their injuries do not exceed the resources of the trauma facility. However, in mass casualties, when the number of patients and injury severity *do* exceed the capability of the trauma facility, a different protocol is followed. In that setting, those patients with the greatest chance for survival at the least expense are treated first. Physiologic parameters (i.e., vital signs) and injury assessment scoring protocols help medical control and prehospital personnel identify which trauma patients should be transferred to a trauma center (Fig. 22.1). If geographically and physically possible, the trauma patient should be transferred to a level I facility (Regional Resource Trauma Center), which by definition will have 24-hour in house surgical coverage, readily available ancillary services and medical subspecialties, a surgical residency, an active trauma research program, and act as a resource for other communities and institutions in the region. If a level I facility is more than 30 minutes away, transfer to a level II facility (Regional Trauma Center) may be preferable.

The trauma bay or resuscitation area should be readied prior to the arrival of the patient, with the necessary equipment based on the EMS prehospital report. Airway boxes, ALS Lifepak monitor/defibrillator, ultrasound machines, warmed intravenous (IV) fluids, blankets, and various surgical procedure kits (i.e., tracheostomy or thoracotomy trays) are just some examples of the standard equipment that should be readily available if needed. The importance of universal or standard precautions (wearing fluid impervious gowns and leggings, facemask, caps, eye protection, and gloves) cannot be overemphasized. All trauma team personnel who have contact with bodily fluids are required to follow standard precautions under Occupational Safety and Health Administration (OSHA) regulations.

Primary Survey: Assessment and Resuscitation

The "golden hour" when deaths are preventable requires accurate, decisive interventions. The tenet of initial evaluation and resuscitation is to establish and maintain sufficient perfusion of oxygenated blood to the vital organs. The most critical concept of ATLS is to *treat the greatest threat to life first.* Therefore, primary survey and resuscitation follows the mnemonic ABCDE: *A*irway establishment or maintenance with cervical spine protection, *B*reathing/ensuring adequate ventilation, *C*irculation/hemorrhage control and maintenance of adequate perfusion pressure, *D*isability/neurologic status, and *E*xposure/environmental control/injury identification. ATLS characterizes these steps as a guide to assessment and stresses that resuscitation is typically performed simultaneously under a "horizontal" team approach. Sound medical judgment is necessary to identify the patients who require an intervention to survive. The primary survey should be performed as quickly as circumstances permit. For instance, a primary survey is completed within a few seconds when the conscious, speaking patient is demonstrating equal breath sounds and palpable peripheral pulses, has been exposed, and is given appropriate cover. The findings of the primary survey are conveyed to the trauma team and the record keeper as it is performed, for example, "airway intact, breath sounds clear bilaterally, femoral pulses palpable bilaterally." Problems are identified and treated as they are sequentially encountered during the ABCDEs of the primary survey.

Airway and Cervical Spine Protection

An airway is required for gas exchange and adequate delivery of oxygen to tissues. However, when attempting airway control, cervical spine injury must be presumed in any trauma patient who sustains injury from a blunt trauma mechanism, displays an altered level of consciousness (LOC), or suffers a multiple system trauma. Hence, a patent airway is best established while upholding cervical spine immobilization. Proper inline immobilization techniques and stabilization equipment are maintained until cervical spine injury is excluded. The trauma patient's ability to maintain a patent airway can be rapidly assessed by asking a simple question such as "How are you?" A patient speaking in sentences with a clear voice suggests an intact airway. However, if the patient is hoarse, stridorous, cannot speak, has garbled speech, or does not follow commands, a patent airway needs to be established and maintained. Airway secretions or foreign bodies should be suctioned or removed.

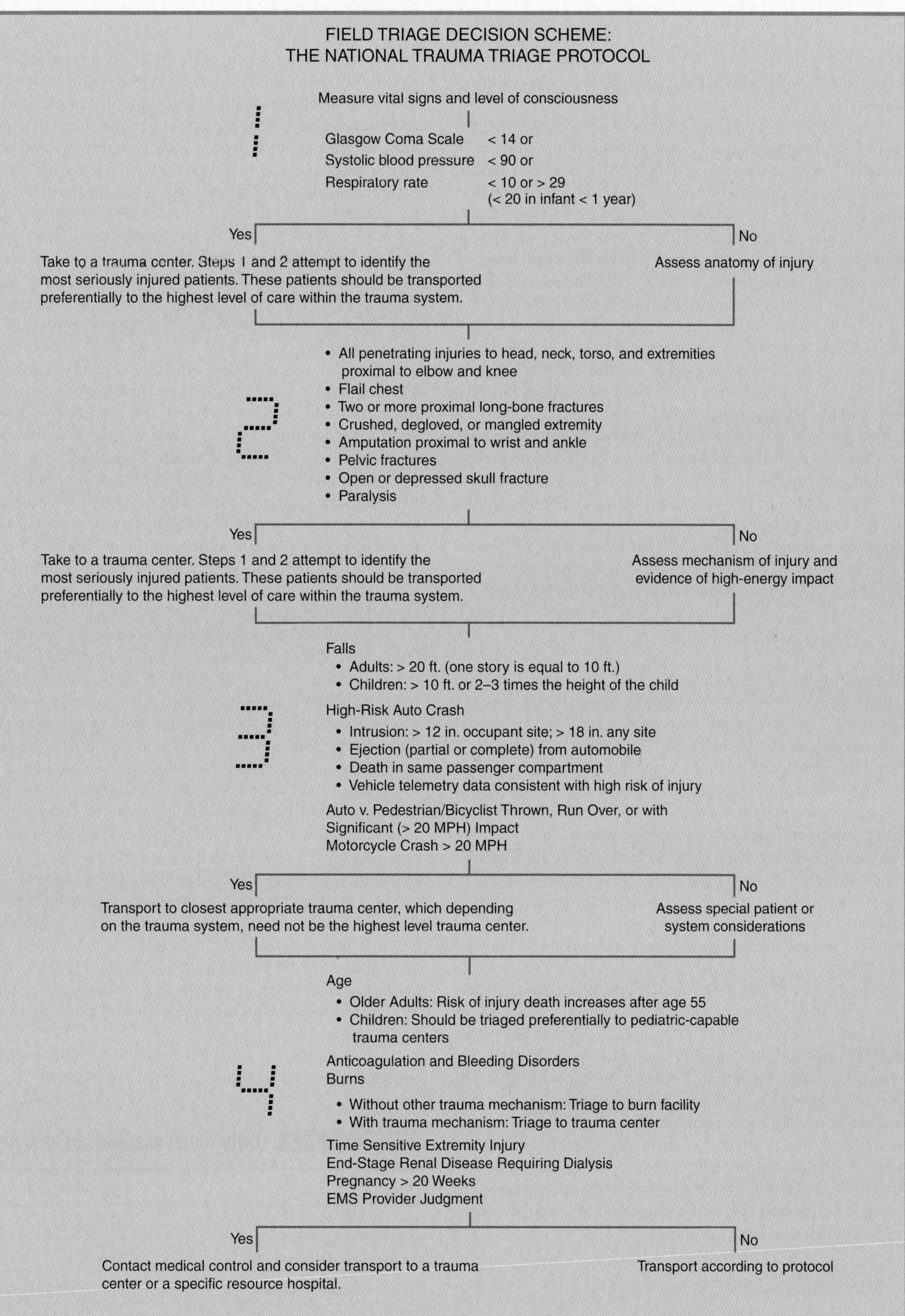

FIGURE 22.1 Field triage algorithm: The national trauma triage protocol. (From Mulholland MW, Lillemoe KD, Doherty GM, et al. *Greenfield's Surgery: Scientific Principles and Practice*. 5th ed. Philadelphia: Lippincott Williams & Wilkins; 2011:318, with permission.)

Fractures of the upper airway (facial bones, mandible, larynx, and trachea) should be identified. Pulse oximetry is a helpful adjunct and should be utilized.

In the obtunded trauma patient, jaw-thrust, chin-lift maneuvers, or naso/oropharyngeal airways alleviate obstruction from pharyngeal tissues or the tongue. Supplemental oxygen is applied up to 6 L via nasal cannula or up to 12 L via nonrebreathing oxygen mask, depending on the patient's oxygen requirement. A patent airway does not ensure sufficient oxygenation or ventilation. Arterial blood gas measurement may provide useful information early in resuscitation; however, it should not delay airway management. If there is any doubt about the patient's ability to maintain a patent airway and/or ventilate (see in subsequent text), or if their Glasgow Coma Scale (GCS) is 8 or less, a definitive airway should be obtained. Orotracheal placement of a cuffed endotracheal tube (ETT) is a standard procedure. In the conscious patient, this procedure requires pharmacologic sedation and paralysis. Other less common approaches are nasotracheal intubation, cricothyroidotomy (Chapter 23), and tracheostomy. Trauma patients who present with emergently placed rescue airway devices, such as a laryngeal mask airway (LMA) or an esophageal tracheal combitube, should have them exchanged for an ETT as soon as possible. An early cricothyroidotomy should be performed if the airway is not obtainable via above-mentioned approaches, such as in trauma patients with severe obesity, severe maxillofacial bleeding, or facial fractures.

Breathing/Ventilation

After the airway is secured, the function of the chest wall, diaphragm, and lungs must be investigated. Ventilation is determined clinically by gas exchange at the nose and mouth, chest excursion, palpation, percussion, auscultated breath sounds, capnometry, arterial blood gas, and the patient's GCS. In the unintubated patient, bag-mask ventilation will temporarily permit gas exchange. However, this technique is not a definitive airway—it will insufflate air into the stomach, raising the risk of aspiration, and is often uncomfortable for the semiconscious patient. To detect gas exchange upon intubation, an end-tidal carbon dioxide ($ETCO_2$) colorimeter or digital capnometer should be used. False-positive readings can occur if the patient recently ingested a carbon dioxide–containing beverage like soda or recently received positive pressure ventilation via a bag-valve mask.

A chest x-ray (CXR) (anteroposterior [AP], supine) should be promptly obtained after endotracheal intubation to confirm appropriate ETT position within the thoracic inlet, at least 2 cm above the carina, and also to identify chest pathology. This film may also reveal life-threatening injuries requiring immediate therapy or further diagnostic study, such as pneumothorax, hemothorax, or a widened mediastinum suggestive of aortic rupture. A tension pneumothorax may be present in an unstable patient with unilateral breath sounds, contralateral tracheal deviation, and a significant drop in $ETCO_2$. Immediate needle decompression relieves the hemodynamic compromise, and a large-bore tube thoracostomy provides definitive therapy (Chapter 23).

Circulation/Hemorrhage Control/Shock

Once the airway is secure and gas exchange is confirmed, the trauma patient's circulatory system must be interrogated. Hemorrhage is the most common cause of preventable postinjury death and may be suspected in the patient with shock-like symptoms, including altered LOC, skin pallor, and a rapid, thready pulse. External hemorrhage is immediately identified and controlled during the primary survey using direct manual pressure. Compression of the proximal palpable pulse either digitally or with a tourniquet may be necessary to temporarily control external hemorrhage. The presence of occult hemorrhage should be suspected in the chest and abdominal cavities, in the soft tissues surrounding a long bone fracture, or in the retroperitoneum of the hypotensive trauma patient. A minimum of two large-bore IV catheters should be established, and warm lactated Ringer's should be administered rapidly. Aggressive blood product and crystalloid resuscitation is adjunctive rather than definitive treatment. Manual or operative control of hemorrhage is essential.

Sufficient cardiac filling pressures are maintained in the bleeding trauma patient with appropriate volume resuscitation. Initial IV fluid administration is accomplished with isotonic electrolyte solutions. Normal saline has the potential to cause hyperchloremic acidosis, especially in patients with impaired renal function. Solutions containing glucose are not used in initial resuscitative efforts: most patients have high serum concentrations of epinephrine and cortisol, and the resulting excessive serum glucose levels can induce an osmotic diuresis. Early conversion to resuscitation with blood product components is recommended to avoid the morbidity associated with large-volume crystalloid resuscitations.

Pulses should be assessed early upon arrival to the resuscitation area. Prehospital pulseless electrical activity (PEA) in the trauma patient carries a dismal prognosis (Table 22.2). Trauma patients in PEA undergoing CPR require prompt evaluation to determine whether resuscitative thoracotomy might be of value. Blunt trauma patients are poor candidates because the causes of cardiopulmonary collapse following this mechanism of injury (e.g., massive brain and SCI or exsanguination from multiple injuries) are difficult to reverse (Table 22.3). However, penetrating trauma resulting in cardiac tamponade in the prehospital patient requiring CPR may be treated effectively by a left anterior thoracotomy (Fig. 22.2). In this approach, pericardial blood under pressure may be evacuated, intrathoracic exsanguination may be controlled, open cardiac massage performed as volume resuscitation is underway, and the descending aorta is cross-clamped to minimize caudal hemorrhage and increase brain and cardiac perfusion. Blood drained via tube thoracostomy can be reinfused by autotransfusion filter devices capable of collecting blood in a sterile manner.

Pulses should be evaluated centrally (carotid or femoral), peripherally (radial and dorsalis pedis), and bilaterally for quality,

TABLE 22.2 Differential diagnosis of PEA, 6Ts, 6Hs

Trauma	Hypovolemia
Tension pneumothorax	Hypothermia
Tamponade, cardiac	Hypoxia
Toxins (drug overdose)	Hyper/hypokalemia
Thrombosis, coronary	Hydrogen ion (acidosis)
Thrombosis, pulmonary (embolism)	Hypo/hyperglycemia

TABLE 22.3 Criteria for declaring patients dead on arrival

• Blunt trauma: prehospital CPR > 5 min, age > 12 y, no pulse on arrival
• Penetrating trauma: abdomen, head, neck, groin: prehospital CPR > 5 min, age > 12 y, no pulse on arrival
• Penetrating trauma: chest: prehospital CPR > 15 min, age > 12 y, no pulse on arrival
• Child with any of the above who has inhospital CPR > 15 min (open or closed) without pulse

Source: From Pasquale MD, Rhodes M, Cipolle MD, et al. Defining "dead on arrival": impact on a level I trauma center. *J Trauma.* 1996;41(4):726–730. Table 1: Lehigh Valley Hospital criteria for DOA in normothermic trauma patients: report of the ad hoc committee; April 1990, with permission.

rate, and regularity. Patients with full, slow, regular pulses are usually normovolemic, unless they are medicated with β-adrenergic blockade. Palpable pulses from the radial, femoral, and carotid arteries correspond to a systolic blood pressure (SBP) of at least 80, 70, and 60 mm Hg, respectively. Continuous intermittent noninvasive blood pressure monitoring and continuous electrocardiographic (ECG) monitoring should be established. Cardiac dysrhythmias such as sinus tachycardia, atrial fibrillation, premature ventricular beats, and ST segment elevations are all suggestive of blunt cardiac injury. Pulseless ventricular tachycardia or ventricular fibrillation requires prompt cardioversion as per advanced cardiovascular life support (ACLS) guidelines.

Shock, by definition, is the state of inadequate perfusion of oxygen to end organs and tissues and is subdivided into four classes by the severity of physiologic derangement and vital sign abnormalities (Table 22.4). Evidence of shock is often masked, especially in younger patients with excellent cardiovascular compensation capability, and clinically significant hemorrhage may occur before findings such as hypotension, tachycardia, and decreased urine output are noted.

If shock persists despite initial volume replacement with 2 L of crystalloid fluid, blood product administration should be started to augment the resuscitation effort. O-negative packed red blood cells (RBCs) are initially used until type-specific blood is available. New data from the U.S. military experience in the Iraqi conflict support the use of fresh frozen plasma and platelets as well in a 1:1:1 volume ratio with packed RBCs. Most high-volume trauma centers will have

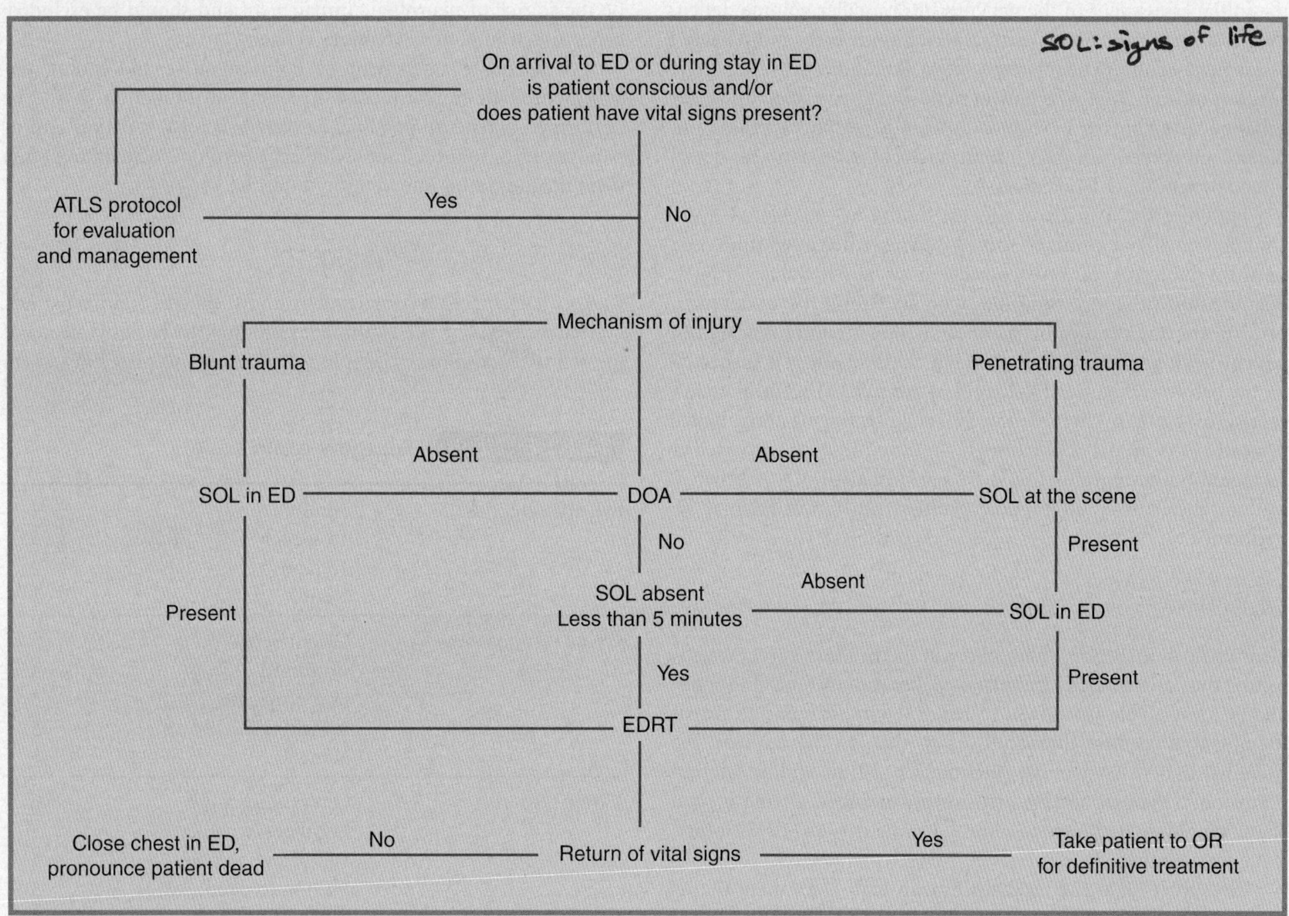

FIGURE 22.2 Algorithm for performing ED thoracotomy for penetrating trauma. (From Mulholland MW, Lillemoe KD, Doherty GM, et al. *Greenfield's Surgery: Scientific Principles and Practice.* 5th ed. Philadelphia: Lippincott Williams & Wilkins; 2011:333, with permission.)

TABLE 22.4 Classification of hemorrhagic shock based on initial presentation

	Class I	Class II	Class III	Class IV
Blood loss (mL)	≤750	750–1,500	1,500–2,000	>2,000
Blood loss (% blood volume)	≤15	15–30	30–40	>40
Heart rate	<100	>100	>120	>140
Blood pressure	Normal	Normal	Decreased	Decreased
Pulse pressure	Normal	Decreased	Decreased	Decreased
Respiratory rate	14–20	20–30	30–40	>35
Urine output (mL/h)	>30	20–30	5–15	Negligible
Mental status	Slightly anxious	Mildly anxious	Anxious, confused	Confused, lethargic
Replacement fluid	Crystalloid	Crystalloid	Crystalloid and blood	Crystalloid and blood

Source: From the Committee on Trauma of the American College of Surgeons. *Advanced Trauma Life Support for Doctors–Student Course Manual.* 9th ed. Chicago: American College of Surgeons; 2012, with permission.

a massive exsanguination protocol designed by the trauma team and the blood bank to ensure that large volumes of blood products are rapidly available for the exsanguinating patient. Regardless of the initial assessment of the patient's intravascular volume deficit, the most important measure in resuscitation is early and repeated assessment of the patient's response to fluid administration. The surgeon must evaluate the patient's end-organ perfusion and oxygenation, assessing the LOC, blood pressure, peripheral pulses and tissue capillary refill, urinary output, and acid–base status (as determined by repeated blood gases).

Placement of a urinary catheter should be considered upon completion of the primary survey, because urinary output is a sensitive indicator of renal perfusion or genitourinary injury. Examination of the rectum and genitalia should be undertaken prior to transurethral catheterization, which is contraindicated in patients with suspected urethral injury. Urethral injury is suspected on the basis of (i) blood at the urethral meatus, (ii) perineal ecchymosis, (iii) blood in the scrotum, (iv) a high-riding or nonpalpable prostate, or (v) a pelvic fracture. If urethral injury is suspected, a retrograde urethrogram should be performed prior to catheterization; alternatively, suprapubic bladder catheterization may be performed.

Disability/Neurologic Status

Neurologic evaluation should follow in the primary survey, establishing the patient's LOC, pupillary size/reaction, lateralizing signs, and SCI level. This assessment provides the opportunity to revisit the potential need for intubation, as an altered LOC can alert the examiner to deficiency in oxygenation, ventilation, and/or cerebral perfusion. If hypoxia and hypotension are excluded, altered mental status should be attributed to central nervous system (CNS) injury, until proven otherwise.

The GCS (Table 22.5) is a quick neurologic assessment that is predictive of the need for intervention (e.g., GCS ≤ 8 suggests a need for airway protection by intubation) and predictive of patient outcome (especially the best motor response). The GCS only assesses the brain and was not designed to assess for SCI. Patients should therefore also be asked to move all of their extremities (e.g., bilateral grip assessment and foot dorsiflexion and plantar flexion) to rule out SCI. Hypoglycemia, alcohol, narcotics, and/or other drugs may be the source of neurologic impairment and should be excluded; otherwise, traumatic CNS injury is likely.

An adequate assessment of both cognitive and motor/sensory neurologic function prior to emergent intubation should be performed whenever possible, as pharmacologic sedation and/or paralysis prior to intubation will mask neurologic deficits and often delay diagnosis and intervention if needed.

Exposure/Environmental Control

The primary survey is completed by undressing the trauma patient, cutting away his or her clothing, examining the back by means of log roll while keeping axial spine alignment, and providing warm

TABLE 22.5 Glasgow coma scale

Eye opening	Spontaneously	4
	To speech	3
	To pain	2
	None	1
Verbal response	Orientated	5
	Confused	4
	Inappropriate	3
	Incomprehensible	2
	None	1
Motor response	Obeys commands	6
	Localizes to pain	5
	Withdraws to pain	4
	Flexion to pain	3
	Extension to pain	2
	None	1
Maximum score	—	15

blankets or a warming convection device to prevent hypothermia. Temperature is a key physiologic determinant, and any hypothermia calls for rapid treatment. Exposure is necessary to accomplish the full head-to-toe physical examination comprising the secondary survey. However, all means should be used to warm the hypothermic patient and are necessary to prevent acidosis, arrhythmias, and coagulopathy. All IV crystalloid should be warmed to approximately 39°C via incubator, high-flow fluid warmer, or even microwave oven prior to infusion.

Additional Adjuncts to the Primary Survey

An oro- or nasogastric tube should be placed following endotracheal intubation of a trauma patient especially if a bag-valve-mask device was utilized to preoxygenate. Decompression of the stomach reduces the risk of aspiration. However, if fracture of the anterior skull, skull base, or midfacial bones is suspected, the gastric tube must be inserted orally to prevent passage of the catheter intracranially. In the unintubated patient, clear indications are necessary, as insertion of a nasogastric tube may induce emesis, increasing the risk of aspiration and chemical pneumonitis.

Cervical spine assessment is integral to developing an airway management plan and in evaluating for potential SCI. The majority of significant SCIs in adults arriving to the emergency department (ED) are at the C5–C7 levels; in children, the most frequent location of SCI is in the region between the occiput and C3. A good-quality cross-table lateral cervical spine film will reveal only approximately 80% of *unstable* fractures in the adult; three-view plain films (cross-table lateral, AP, and open-mouth odontoid) will reveal approximately 90%. Fine-cut CT scan of the entire cervical spine has emerged as the standard evaluation technique because of its accuracy and lack of dependence on body habitus to obtain adequate views. A lateral cervical spine film may be helpful in assessing a source of hypotension in a patient where it is not possible to do a definitive examination. The presence of hypotension may indicate a significant vertebral body alignment abnormality that could account for a high spinal cord disruption with a loss of sympathetic tone. This is one of the only times when vasoactive pressors must be utilized early in a trauma patient's resuscitation.

An AP pelvic film may assist in evaluating the trauma patient by identifying a pelvic fracture associated with pelvic hemorrhage (e.g., open-book type or vertical shear) that would need immediate stabilization, identifying or confirming a hip dislocation, or visualizing a retained foreign body (bullet). In general, stable, awake patients without symptoms suggestive of pelvic or hip injury do not need a pelvic x-ray, especially if they are going to have an abdominal–pelvic CT scan as part of their radiographic workup anyway.

Abdominal ultrasonography or focused assessment sonography in trauma (FAST) can be performed rapidly in a noninvasive manner to assess for intraperitoneal hemorrhage and to identify pericardial tamponade as well as pneumothorax. Four anatomic windows are generally examined: the pericardium (subxiphoid), the hepatorenal fossa, the splenorenal fossa, and the pelvis. A positive FAST in the unstable patient represents hemorrhage and mandates operative exploration. In the stable patient, contrast-enhanced abdominal and pelvic CT scan is obtained following a positive FAST (Fig. 22.3). Many centers have expanded the FAST to include bilateral thoracic windows to assess for "pleural sliding" and determine the presence of pneumothorax.

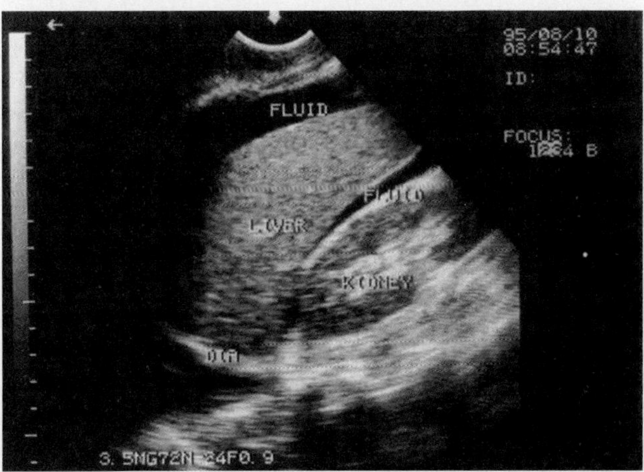

FIGURE 22.3 Sagittal ultrasound of the liver, kidney, and diaphragm demonstrating hemoperitoneum. DIA, diaphragm. (From Rozycki GS, Ochsner MG, Feliciano DV, et al. Early detection of hemoperitoneum by ultrasound examination of the right upper quadrant: a multicenter study. *J Trauma.* 1998;45(5):878–883, with permission.)

If ultrasound technology is not available, diagnostic peritoneal lavage (DPL) can be utilized to assess for intra-abdominal injury. This diagnostic procedure can be performed in either a percutaneous or an open fashion. Aspiration of gross blood or succus entericus on placement of the catheter constitutes a positive result and mandates surgical exploration. Otherwise, warmed crystalloid at 10 mL/kg of body weight is instilled into the peritoneum and allowed to remain for 5 to 10 minutes. It is then drained by gravity; either an RBC concentration greater than $10^5/mm^3$ ($10^4/mm^3$ for penetrating trauma) or a white blood cell count greater than $500/mm^3$ indicates the need for surgical exploration. DPL has largely fallen out of favor given the ready availability and noninvasive nature of bedside ultrasound. However, it remains a useful adjunct in the unstable patient with multicavity injury and can occasionally direct initial operative management (e.g., an unstable patient with a positive DPL in the OR may be best served by a laparotomy prior to a thoracotomy).

Initial Assessment and Management: Trauma Patient in Shock

Shock is classified according to its etiology: hypovolemic, cardiogenic, neurogenic, and septic or vasogenic. *Hypovolemic shock* is the most common type of shock following injury and results most commonly from hemorrhage. During hypovolemic shock, cardiac preload is insufficient and cardiac output falls (CO = HR × SV, where CO is cardiac output, HR is heart rate, and SV is stroke volume). Other causes for hypovolemic shock in injured patients include excessive third-space plasma losses, as might occur from severe burns or heat exhaustion.

Cardiogenic shock is the result of extrinsic and/or intrinsic pump failure. Extrinsic *compressive* (or obstructive) cardiogenic shock results from increased extracardiac forces, which limit blood return to the heart. Tension pneumothorax, pericardial tamponade, and extreme levels of positive end-expiratory pressure (PEEP) are examples of forces that may limit venous return to the heart and result in shock. A positive pericardial view on FAST and Beck's triad (hypotension, bilateral distended jugular veins, and muffled heart sounds) characterize pericardial tamponade. If the patient progresses to cardiac arrest, resuscitative thoracotomy is performed. Otherwise, pericardiocentesis can be attempted to temporize cardiac function until median sternotomy can be performed. Intrinsic cardiogenic shock may result from primary myocardial dysfunction such as myocardial contusion, myocardial ischemia or infarction, cardiac arrhythmia, valvular insufficiency or stenosis, papillary muscle rupture, or myocarditis. Right-sided heart failure may present after a large pulmonary embolus that results in an acute increase in right ventricular pressure. Neurogenic and vasogenic (or septic) shock are discussed in the section "Surgical Critical Care."

Secondary Survey

Once the primary survey is completed, resuscitation is underway, and the trauma patient demonstrates a normalization of vital signs, the secondary survey is started. A complete medical history and a head-to-toe physical examination, including a reassessment of the mnemonic ABCDEs, are performed. If a life- or limb-threatening injury is found at the time of secondary survey, then temporizing measures (i.e., splinting displaced fractures, suturing a bleeding scalp laceration) should be performed prior to continuing on with the survey. The mnemonic AMPLE—allergies, medications, past illnesses and surgeries, last meal, and events related to the injury—guides the initial medical history from the trauma patient, family, or prehospital personnel. Understanding the mechanism of injury can provide insight into patient injury patterns and resultant physiologic abnormalities (Table 22.6).

Each anatomic area is examined by inspection, palpation, and, if necessary, auscultation and percussion. This examination should systematically proceed from the scalp to toes in a routine pattern so as not to skip even areas of low suspicion for injury. The *head* and *eyes* are examined for direct trauma and foreign bodies. Basilar skull fracture is suggested by ecchymosis behind the ears (Battle's sign) or around the eyes (raccoon eyes), hemotympanum, and drainage of cerebrospinal fluid (CSF) from the nose or ears. Visual acuity, when possible, as well as pupillary size and reactions should be assessed. A brief cranial nerve examination is important when intracranial injury is suspected.

The *neck* is examined after removal of the anterior segment of the cervical collar, with in-line stabilization maintained. The cervical spine can be cleared clinically only in those patients without tenderness through a full range of motion who are awake, alert, and without evidence of intoxication or distracting injuries. In a patient who does not meet these criteria, a CT scan of the entire cervical spine is the diagnostic imaging modality of choice to rule out bony cervical spine injury. Moreover, in those patients where clinical examination is not possible, MRI evaluation of the cervical spine is often needed in addition to CT scan in order to rule out ligamentous injury prior to C-spine clearance and collar removal. Classically, wounds to zone II of the neck are managed by operative exploration or assessed with a combination of angiography, esophagoscopy, and bronchoscopy (Fig. 22.4). Wounds to zones I and III are managed initially by endoscopy, angiography (with possible embolization), and bronchoscopy, with selective operative exploration. In these zones, it is difficult to obtain both proximal and distal vascular control at the time of operation. For penetrating injuries of the neck, CT has been shown to accurately portray trajectory, and CT angiography is emerging as an appropriate single modality for injury screening.

The *chest* examination is repeated, and a portable AP chest radiograph should be obtained if not already performed. Patients who sustain blunt trauma, especially if subjected to high-speed deceleration injury, and are found to have any findings suspicious of an injury to a great vessel (e.g., a widened mediastinum, a pleural cap, a leftward tracheal deviation, an elevation of the left mainstem bronchus, or a left-sided hemothorax) should be evaluated for aortic transection. In addition, up to 30% of patients with aortic

TABLE 22.6 Mechanisms of blunt injury and suspected injuries

Frontal impact: bent steering wheel, knee-imprinted dashboard, bull's eye fracture, windshield	Cervical spine fracture, anterior flail chest, myocardial contusion, pneumothorax, traumatic aortic disruption, fractured spleen or liver, posterior fracture/dislocation at the hip, knee
Side impact	Contralateral neck sprain; cervical spine fracture; lateral flail chest; pneumothorax; traumatic aortic disruption; diaphragmatic rupture; fractured ipsilateral kidney, spleen, or liver; fractured pelvis or acetabulum
Rear impact	Cervical spine injury, neck soft tissue injuries
Ejection from vehicle	Greater risk for all injuries, precludes prediction of injury pattern
Pedestrian vs. motor vehicle	Head injury, traumatic aortic disruption, abdominal visceral injuries, fractured lower extremities/pelvis

Source: From the Committee on Trauma of the American College of Surgeons. *Advanced Trauma Life Support for Doctors—Student Course Manual*. 9th ed. Chicago: American College of Surgeons; 2012, with permission.

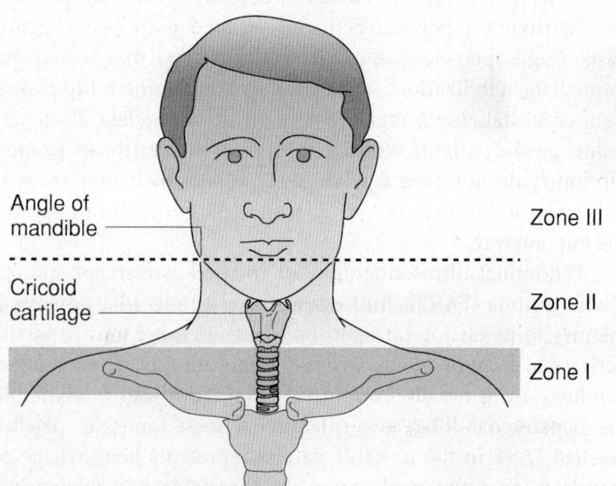

FIGURE 22.4 Zones of the neck in the trauma patient. (From Mulholland MW, Lillemoe KD, Doherty GM, et al. *Greenfield's Surgery: Scientific Principles and Practice*. 5th ed. Philadelphia: Lippincott Williams & Wilkins; 2011:333, with permission.)

injury have a normal chest radiograph; therefore, if the history and mechanism of injury are suggestive of possible aortic injury, investigation should continue. Contrast chest CT scan is the study most often used to evaluate for traumatic aortic injury. Transesophageal echocardiogram (TEE) is an excellent alternative to screen for aortic injury in an unstable patient, in the patient with impaired renal function, or in one who is already in the OR. Contrast aortography remains the criterion standard for detection of thoracic aortic injury and should be performed in the case of an equivocal CT or TEE.

The *abdomen* and *back* are examined, with special attention to penetrating wounds. In the unstable patient with a penetrating abdominal wound, emergent exploratory laparotomy is indicated. In the stable patient with a stab wound to the anterior abdominal wall, local wound exploration is performed; if the anterior fascia is violated, exploration in the OR is mandated. For stable patients who have a stab wound to the back or flank, contrast-enhanced CT scan is used to identify retroperitoneal and intraperitoneal injuries. In any patient with localized tenderness over the thoracic or lumbar spines, CT of the thoracic and/or lumbar spine with image reformatting is the best imaging modality, especially if a spiral CT evaluation of the chest, abdomen, and pelvis has already been performed on the patient. AP and lateral radiographs are very nonsensitive and nonspecific, especially in the frequently obese trauma patient.

The stability of the *pelvic ring* and *pelvis* is assessed by medial and AP compression or, if questionable, by AP pelvic radiograph. Unstable fractures (e.g., "open book" or vertical shear) need to be immediately stabilized by some form of circumferential compression to close down pelvic volume and help tamponade venous bleeding. This can be accomplished via a commercially available corset-like device (e.g., the trauma pelvic orthotic device ["TPOD"]) or more inexpensively by a tied bedsheet. Rectal tone is assessed to evaluate for gross bleeding, SCI, and the position of the prostate in males. In females with a pelvic fracture, the vagina should be inspected to rule out vaginal wall disruption and bleeding.

All *extremities* should be examined for deformity, bruising, lacerations, penetrating injuries, soft tissue injury, peripheral pulses, and neurologic function (including sensory/motor function or any spinal cord level deficit). External bleeding must be addressed if not adequately treated during the primary survey and resuscitation. A patient with obvious "hard signs" of vascular injury—pulsatile bleeding, expanding hematoma, palpable thrill, audible bruit, regional ischemia, and diminished or absent pulses (ankle–brachial index of <0.9)—should undergo operative exploration and repair without delay for further diagnostic studies. Less definitive "soft signs" of vascular injury—history of active bleeding, stable nonpulsatile hematoma, neurologic deficit due to primary nerve injury, or proximity of wound to major vascular structures—warrant further workup such as angiography or duplex ultrasonography to exclude vascular injury. Extremity compartment syndrome must be recognized early; causes include severe soft tissue injury, hematomas, fractures, arterial injuries, and massive fluid resuscitation. Femur fractures with significant bone displacement can be associated with significant internal bleeding as the thigh configuration becomes more spherical and less cylindrical. This requires prompt application of a traction splint for immobilization and reestablishment of normal thigh architecture. Consequences of compartment syndrome include muscle necrosis, myoglobinuria, renal failure, vascular compromise, and limb loss. Signs and symptoms of increased interstitial tissue pressure and decreased tissue perfusion include pain (especially with passive motion), paresthesias, a swollen tense extremity, paresis or paralysis, and loss of peripheral pulses (late finding). Compartment pressures can be measured using a needle catheter or handheld Stryker monitor inserted into the compartment in question; a pressure greater than 25 mm Hg associated with clinical suspicion of decreased tissue perfusion should prompt emergent fasciotomy.

Patient Transfer

At the completion of the primary survey, the attending physician often has sufficient information to determine whether it is necessary to transfer the patient to a specialty center (e.g., level I trauma center, burn unit, or SCI center) for definitive care. Once the need for transfer is identified, transfer should not be delayed for any further diagnostic study that will not change the immediate plan of care. All records and imaging studies should be sent with the patient to the receiving facility after a physician-to-physician report has occurred.

SURGICAL CRITICAL CARE

Continued Postresuscitation Monitoring and Definitive Care

The severely injured trauma patient will ultimately require care within a highly monitored setting whether that is after resuscitation in the trauma bay, in the interventional radiology suite, or in the OR. In this section, the aspects of critical care that are vital to the survival of the trauma/general surgical patient are discussed. Critical care begins with a verbal handoff from the surgical team to the critical care team (nurses and physicians) that will be assuming care of the patient. Pertinent patient information is shared, and the operative/resuscitative details are delineated. A total body assessment of the traumatically injured or critically ill surgical patient is then performed. An organ system approach is helpful in the evaluation and treatment of such patients.

Neurologic Critical Care

The critical care team of physicians and nurses should reevaluate the trauma patient for any unrecognized neurologic deficit consistent with SCI, progression of cerebral edema, or stroke. A patient presenting with altered LOC from a blunt mechanism of injury and incomplete radiographic evaluation for cervical spine injury necessitates cervical spine immobilization in a semi-rigid cervical collar. Neurosurgical staff should evaluate all traumatic CNS injuries. Use of corticosteroids in patients with nonpenetrating SCI has recently come under intense scrutiny. Recent reports including The National Acute Spinal Cord Injury Studies (NASCIS) II and III, a *Cochrane Database of Systematic Reviews* article of all randomized clinical trials, and other published reports all verified significant improvement in motor function and sensation in patients with complete or incomplete SCIs who were treated with high doses of methylprednisolone within 8 hours of injury. It was recommended that a bolus of 30 mg/kg be administered, and if started within 3 hours of the injury, a continuous infusion of 5.4 mg/kg/h be given for 24 hours. A 48-hour infusion was recommended if the injury was recognized within 3 to 8 hours of injury. Upon more intense scrutiny over the validity of the data, however, updated guidelines issued in 2013 by the CNS and the American Association of Neurological Surgeons (AANS) recommend against the early use of steroids after an acute SCI. The guidelines recommend that methylprednisolone not be used for the treatment of acute SCI within the first 24 to 48 hours following injury. The previous recommendation was revised because of a lack of medical evidence supporting the benefits of steroids in clinical settings and evidence that high-dose steroids are associated with harmful adverse effects including an increased incidence of infection and avascular necrosis. If steroid therapy is utilized, however, appropriate peptic ulceration prophylaxis should be initiated and maintained during the patient's hospitalization.

Sympathetic denervation from SCI, spinal anesthesia, or severe head injury often produces generalized arteriolar vasodilation and venodilation resulting in *neurogenic shock*. Traumatic SCIs generally must occur above the level of T6 to cause this level of disruption of the sympathetic outflow tract. Relative hypovolemia results when the normal blood volume is suddenly insufficient to fill the acutely increased intravascular space. These patients present with the characteristic findings of warm extremities and normal to decreased heart rate despite hypotension. The initial therapy is directed at restoring sympathetic tone by volume repletion and vasopressors. Dopamine is typically the agent that is initially selected, especially in the setting of bradycardia. Norepinephrine or neosynephrine can also be used. This is perhaps the only indication for early use of vasopressors in the hypotensive trauma patient where bleeding is the usual cause of hemodynamic instability.

Elevated *intracranial pressure* (ICP) should be suspected clinically in cases of head trauma when patients have diminished LOC, headache, nausea, vomiting, cranial nerve palsies, or the late, ominous finding, *Cushing triad* (hypertension, bradycardia, and respiratory depression). Normal ICP in adults is 15 mm Hg or less, whereas pathologic intracranial hypertension usually occurs at 20 mm Hg or greater. The fundamental goal in ICU management of the patient with severe traumatic brain injury (TBI) after recognition and/or evacuation of intracranial mass lesions is to prevent secondary brain injury from hypoperfusion. As little as 5 minutes of hypoperfusion can double the risk of death from TBI. Cerebral perfusion pressure (CPP) is equal to the mean arterial pressure (MAP) minus the ICP. For patients with elevated ICP, the CPP should be kept above 60 mm Hg. This value can be calculated by directly measuring arterial pressure via a peripheral transducer catheter and utilizing an ICP transducer (ICP bolt or ventriculostomy). Direct brain parenchyma oximetry (Licox Integra Neurosciences, Plainsboro, NJ) or monitoring for jugular venous oxygen desaturation (jugular bulb oximetry) will detect ischemic cerebral conditions often during elevated ICP. Elevated ICP can be treated by head elevation, osmotic diuresis with mannitol infusion if MAP will tolerate, hypertonic saline (3% to 7% NaCl) therapy, and/or removal of CSF (e.g., ventriculostomy). High-dose barbiturate therapy (barbiturate coma) and decompressive craniotomy are reserved for refractory intracranial hypertension.

Pain control and appropriate, judicious sedation are essential in the management of the critically ill surgery patient. Please refer to Chapter 7 for a description.

Patients with severe TBI often succumb to brain death despite maximal therapeutic intervention. This diagnosis cannot be made in the presence of severe hypothermia (≤30°C), barbiturate intoxication, metabolic derangements (e.g., uremia), and marked hypovolemia because these conditions are reversible. Criteria for brain death are the *absence* of the following: response to painful stimuli, seizure activity, pupillary light reflex, corneal reflex, gag reflex, oculocephalogyric (doll's head) reflex, vestibuloocular (caloric) reflex, and respiratory effort during an apnea test. In the apnea test, the patient is sufficiently preoxygenated before the ventilator is stopped and hypercarbia is permitted. The $Paco_2$ should rise at least 20 mm Hg or exceed 60 mm Hg before the absence of respiratory effort is considered confirmatory. Additional positive findings of brain death are 30 minutes of electrical silence on EEG and absence of cerebral blood flow on cerebral angiography (old criterion standard) or nuclear medicine scan. Brain death determination protocols are hospital specific and vary from institution to institution. Usually two brain death examinations performed by a neurologist, neurointensivist, or neurosurgeon, 6 to 12 hours apart, are required before a patient may be declared brain dead. The critical care team should maintain full resuscitation efforts until an organ procurement representative has a chance to discuss potential organ donation with the patient's family or power of attorney.

Pulmonary Critical Care

Acute respiratory failure following severe injury is common. Principal causes of respiratory failure following injury include direct chest trauma (i.e., rib fractures or pulmonary contusion), fluid overload following large-volume resuscitation, aspiration pneumonitis, acute respiratory distress syndrome (ARDS) (secondary to a systemic inflammatory response to injury, fat emboli syndrome, transfusion-related lung injury, etc.), and high thoracic and/or cervical SCI. The normal mechanics of breathing in an individual with an intact respiratory effort occurs by *negative pressure ventilation*. The thorax expands as the diaphragm moves downward, resulting in an increase in the negative intrapleural pressure. The lungs actively fill with air as they expand to fill the vacuum. Normal expiration is a passive process initiated by the relaxation of the chest wall bony skeleton and musculature and the intrinsic recoil of the lung itself. Augmenting ventilation requires the initiation of *positive pressure ventilation* by either a face mask (noninvasive) or intubation of the trachea (invasive).

Noninvasive Assisted Ventilation

For patients who are awake and breathing spontaneously, but are hypoventilating, noninvasive positive pressure ventilation can often correct the hypercarbia and prevent the need for intubation. The patient must also be cooperative and possess an intact cough reflex and ability to clear secretions. *Continuous positive airway pressure (CPAP)* and *bilevel positive airway pressure (BiPAP)* are two modes of ventilation that can be delivered via a tightly fitting face mask that covers the nose and mouth. CPAP delivers oxygenated air with positive pressure to the airways continuously throughout the respiratory cycle. This ventilatory mode decreases the overall work of breathing (WOB) by recruiting previously unventilated, atelectatic alveoli; increasing functional residual capacity (FRC); and enhancing overall lung compliance. The use of CPAP is beneficial to patients suffering from restrictive and neuromuscular lung diseases, and it has been shown to reduce the need for intubation when compared with conventional therapy in patients with acute exacerbations of chronic obstructive pulmonary disease (COPD). CPAP is also commonly used in the treatment of obstructive sleep apnea, where positive pressure provides the necessary support to maintain airway patency against the compressive forces of the collapsing chest wall and pharynx. BiPAP delivers a set volume at positive pressure with inhalation while maintaining a separate amount of PEEP during exhalation. This mode is most beneficial to hypoventilating patients with hyperinflated lungs, as in emphysema. It is also used in obstructive sleep apnea when patients cannot tolerate CPAP. By preserving the natural airway and competence of the glottis, noninvasive ventilatory assistance preserves important physiologic functions such as cough, speech, and oral alimentation, all of which are lost once the trachea is intubated.

Invasive Assisted Ventilation

Although a number of criteria have been proposed as guidelines, it should be emphasized that indications for the institution of mechanical ventilation are subjective and require clinical judgment. Support may be indicated secondary to derangements in any component of the respiratory system: CNS, chest wall, airway, respiratory muscles, or alveoli. Patients with CNS depression secondary to narcotic overdose or closed head injury often require intubation for airway protection and respiratory support. Abnormalities of the chest wall such as a flail chest, open pneumothorax, or acute paralysis may require mechanical support. Multiple rib fractures and the associated underlying pulmonary contusions and pain with inspiration and forced expiration (cough) can also result in respiratory failure secondary to severe atelectasis and often pneumonia. Intubation is often required in patients with maxillofacial trauma, inhalation injury (heated gases or caustic chemicals), anaphylaxis, or atelectasis from endobronchial masses or foreign bodies. Respiratory failure as a result of alveolar dysfunction may be due to a variety of causes including chronic lung disease, cardiogenic or noncardiogenic pulmonary edema, and extensive pneumonia. Mechanical support may be indicated in the setting of hypercarbia ($Paco_2 > 45$ mm Hg) or life-threatening hypoxemia ($Pao_2 < 55$ mm Hg) despite maximal noninvasive oxygen therapy. Others have suggested a respiratory rate greater than 35 as a criterion indicating an increased WOB. However, the most common indication for intubation and mechanical ventilation is the decision by an experienced clinician that the patient's respiratory system is in jeopardy and requires support.

There are two main categories of ventilatory support: volume control and pressure control. Volume control ventilation delivers a preset volume of oxygenated air to the patient with each breath. The two most commonly used modes of volume control ventilation are *assist control* (*AC*) and *intermittent mandatory ventilation* (*IMV*). In the AC mode, the ventilator is triggered to deliver a preset volume of gas with each patient breath. As a safety against hypoventilation or apnea, a respiratory rate is also preset, ensuring that a sufficient minute volume is delivered to the patient. Tidal volume and flow determine inspiratory (I) and expiratory (E) time and hence the I:E ratio. AC is considered maximal ventilatory support, because ventilation is supported by a set volume with every breath. In IMV ventilation, the patient can breathe spontaneously without full assistance from the ventilator. In this mode, respiratory rate and tidal volume are set and delivered to the patient intermittently between spontaneous breaths. Spontaneous breaths may be supported with some pressure, but a fixed volume is not delivered. The main difference between the two modes is that in IMV, a patient-initiated breath does not automatically trigger the ventilator. *Synchronized intermittent mandatory ventilation* (*SIMV*) is a variation of IMV, which synchronizes the ventilator with the patient so that delivered breaths are initiated only after the patient exhales completely. IMV ventilation allows a wide range of levels of ventilatory support, as the preset number of breaths can be titrated to provide maximal or minimal ventilation support to the patient. Traditionally, SIMV has been used as a primary ventilator weaning mode.

The selection of ventilatory mode is often dependent upon the lung compliance (Δvolume/Δpressure). AC and IMV modes are very effective in supporting patients with compliant lungs. A drawback to volume-cycled ventilation, however, is that airway pressures may escalate to harmful levels—that is, barotrauma—in poorly compliant (stiff) lungs. In this scenario, the ventilator must generate high airway pressures to deliver the preset volume of oxygenated air. One acute danger of elevated airway pressures is barotrauma with resultant alveolar rupture and pneumothorax.

A more suitable ventilatory approach in these patients is the use of *pressure control* (*PC*) *ventilation*. In this mode, the peak inspiratory pressure (PIP) rather than volume is preset, and tidal volumes vary depending on lung compliance. Respiratory rate is also preset, and gas flow in this mode is either time cycled (preset inspiratory time) or flow cycled (gas flow stops when the flow rate drops below a preset % of the initial flow rate, usually 25%). *Pressure support ventilation* (*PSV*) is a variation of the PC mode that requires a spontaneously breathing patient. In this mode, every patient breath (negative inspiratory force) triggers the ventilator to deliver a preset amount of positive pressure. Tidal volumes again depend on lung compliance. PSV is a popular weaning mode, as the patient can control both their inspiration and expiration spontaneously. The disadvantage of this mode is that minute ventilation can be insufficient, and apneic periods can occur. PSV is often combined with IMV or CPAP when attempting to wean patients from ventilatory support. This type of *mixed-mode* ventilation strategy allows patients to spontaneously breathe with just enough positive pressure support to overcome the airway resistance caused by the breathing circuit.

The main function of *PEEP* is to prevent alveolar collapse at end expiration. The addition of PEEP to any mode of ventilation can help decrease V/Q mismatch by increasing FRC and subsequently allow for a reduction in inspired oxygen. Criteria for weaning from the ventilator include adequate oxygenation on less than 40% to 50% Fio_2, PEEP less than 5 to 8 cm H_2O, manageable secretions requiring little suctioning, awake/alert mental status, minute ventilation of less than 10 to 15 L/min, respiratory rate less than 30, tidal volume 5 mL/kg, and at least −20 cm H_2O inspiratory force.

Acute lung injury (ratio of Pao_2: Fio_2 of 200 to 300) occurs for several reasons following trauma and major surgery, including pulmonary contusion, pulmonary laceration, resuscitative fluid overload, and systemic inflammation. In prolonged shock or septic shock, damage to lung parenchyma may result in ARDS, a more severe form of acute intrinsic lung injury (ratio of Pao_2:$Fio_2 \leq 200$). Intrapulmonary shunting results in hypoxemia, as underventilated or collapsed lung segments are perfused. Decreased levels of surfactant and pulmonary edema lead to a decrease in lung compliance (increased "stiffness"). CXR findings may lag behind the clinical picture by as much as 24 hours and are of little value early in the course of ARDS. In early, established ARDS, alveolar–interstitial infiltrates are initially seen in the central lung fields and then later diffusely as bilateral fluffy infiltrates (Table 22.7).

Treatment for ARDS is primarily supportive, including the provision of sufficient nutritional support with appropriate prophylaxis against stress gastritis and venous thromboembolism. Maintaining adequate oxygenation and ventilation usually requires intubation and mechanical ventilation. A low tidal volume ventilation of 6 mL/kg, keeping airway plateau pressures or peak alveolar

TABLE 22.7 Criteria for the diagnosis of ARDS

• Acute onset
• Hypoxemia (PaO_2:FiO_2 < 200)
• Noncardiogenic pulmonary edema (PA wedge pressure <18 mm Hg)
• Bilateral pulmonary infiltrates on CXR

pressures (a distinct drop from PIP, as gas distributes from the upper to lower airways) less than 30 mm Hg, has been shown to reduce mortality. In the poorly compliant lungs of a patient with ARDS, high PEEP maintains alveolar recruitment, which attenuates atelectasis and hopefully improves oxygenation.

A number of options are available in patients who are difficult to wean from the ventilator. Permissive hypercapnia is a strategy utilized to minimize barotrauma and volume trauma to the lung. Inverse ratio ventilation increases the inspiratory time to greater than 50% of the respiratory cycle, increasing mean airway pressure and recruiting alveoli by auto-PEEP (must be used with caution in asthma and COPD patients, given their tendency for air trapping). Prone positioning has not been shown to impact survival, but it can improve oxygenation by increasing ventilation/flow matching. Using pharmacologic muscle paralysis can serve to minimize oxygen consumption and synchronize the ventilator with the patient's chest wall dynamics. Airway pressure release ventilation (APRV) is a relatively new mode of ventilation that has gained significant popularity in the treatment of ARDS. It is a time-triggered, pressure-limited, time-cycled mode of mechanical ventilation that can be conceptualized as high CPAP with regular, brief (as low as 0.6 seconds), intermittent releases of airway pressure, which allow for ventilation. Patients can spontaneously breathe at this high-PEEP setting, which enhances comfort and limits the need for sedation and/or paralysis, even though the I:E ratio is markedly inversed. Overall peak airway pressures are lowered, and V/Q mismatching is minimized. High-frequency ventilation and extracorporeal membrane oxygenation are other rescue techniques that may be necessary if all other forms of respiratory support fail in these patients, but established, recalcitrant ARDS carries a mortality that approaches 50%.

Cardiovascular Critical Care

Surgical and trauma patients admitted to the ICU often require resuscitation for hemorrhagic shock. The early recognition and treatment of shock is essential for maintaining adequate physiologic support. When tissues are hypoperfused and oxygen delivery becomes inadequate to meet the demands of cellular metabolism, shock ensues. This alteration in cellular metabolism leads to cellular dysfunction, expression of inflammatory mediators, and cellular injury. When oxygen supply to the cell is insufficient, there is an uncoupling of oxidative phosphorylation, the cell begins to metabolize glucose anaerobically, and lactic acidosis develops. The cell membrane loses its ability to maintain its sodium gradient via the active ionic pump, thereby leading to cellular swelling. If perfusion is quickly restored, cellular injury is limited and the progression of shock can be halted. However, if oxygen delivery remains inadequate, irreversible cellular injury occurs and end-organ damage can result. The posttrauma and postoperative setting are strikingly similar because in both it is critically important to suspect, recognize, and treat shock. This effort necessitates sufficient invasive and noninvasive monitoring, accurate recording of fluid inputs and outputs, and frequent clinical reassessment.

Timely restoration of perfusion is the core concept when treating shock, regardless of the etiology. Even when the cause of shock is not immediately apparent, treatment—including volume resuscitation—is initiated immediately to halt the progression of the shock physiology and prevent the onset of MSOF. When the shock state results in end-organ damage in multiple (three or more) physiologic systems, the likelihood of survival is very low.

Hemodynamic monitoring is a critical component to the evaluation and ongoing resuscitation of the trauma patient in shock (Table 22.8). The determinants of oxygen delivery to tissues are pump function of the heart, vascular tone of the vessels, and oxygen

TABLE 22.8 Measurements and criteria for placement of hemodynamic monitors

Monitor	Measurement	Criteria for Insertion
Arterial catheter	Systolic, diastolic, and mean arterial pressures (SBP, DBP, and MAP)	• Use of vasoactive or cardiotonic drugs • Continuous blood pressure monitoring • Frequent arterial blood gases
Central venous catheter	CVP tracing	• Venous access for parenteral nutrition, caustic medications, or chemotherapy; avoiding devastating peripheral extravasations or compartment syndrome • Access for adjunctive therapy: transvenous pacing, pulmonary artery catheter • Hemodialysis
PA catheter	CVP, cardiac output, mixed venous blood gases, PA pressures: systolic, diastolic, mean, wedge (PAS, PAD, PAM, PAWP)	• Persistent high CVP and low MAP, often necessitating inotropic support • Baseline intrinsic cardiac dysfunction in the setting of major trauma or surgery

DBP, diastolic blood pressure; PAS, pulmonary artery systolic; PAM, pulmonary artery mean.

content of arterial blood (calculated using concentration of hemoglobin, oxygen saturation, and partial pressure of oxygen in blood). Arterial catheters provide a stable continuous display of arterial blood pressure. However, variation between actual and detected blood pressures may exist depending on the catheter's distance from the heart, the vessel's stiffness/resistance, and the presence of excessive catheter movement (whip). Central venous catheters provide an assessment of right-sided heart function and overall volume status via a continuous tracing of central venous pressure (CVP). Cardiogenic shock is suggested by elevated CVP, but this finding is often confounded by positive pressure ventilation, which increases CVP during the inspiratory phase. The opposite is true in physiologic respiration where right-sided filling pressures decrease during inspiration. Independent of the ventilator status, the CVP is best measured at the end of expiration when pressures are relatively independent of respiration.

CVP is considered less reliable for predicting left-heart function in the mechanically ventilated, critically ill patient. Acidosis, metabolic depressants, and ischemia may predispose the postsurgical/trauma patient to cardiac pump dysfunction. In the resuscitated trauma patient with no structural cardiac injury, an elevated CVP, and a low MAP, the likelihood of cardiogenic shock is high. This scenario calls for accurate assessment of pump function to guide therapy. Transthoracic echocardiogram (TTE) is an excellent noninvasive, operator-dependent tool that provides a direct measure of myocardial contractility, filling pressures, CO, and valvular dysfunction. Bedside continuous, transesophageal echo devices (hTEE, ImaCor Inc., Garden City, NJ) are now available; however, in most institutions, *continuous* echocardiography is offered only in the OR. In the critical care setting, pulmonary artery (PA) catheterization can provide similar information via serial or continuous evaluation of the left ventricular end-diastolic volume (LVEDV or preload), the cardiac index (CI = CO/total body surface area), and the oxygen saturation of mixed venous blood $S\bar{v}O_2$. Modern PA catheters have incorporated a laser oximeter in the distal end of the catheter to permit continuous measurement of $S\bar{v}O_2$. Preload is detected by the pulmonary artery wedge pressure (PAWP) or approximated by the pulmonary filling pressures, such as the pulmonary artery diastolic (PAD) pressure. CO and CI are calculated by the Fick equation or electronically using thermodilution principles. Finally, systemic vascular resistance (SVR) reflecting vasomotor tone of the systemic circulation is calculated: $SVR = \frac{MAP - CAP}{CO}$. Extensive usage of PA catheters in the critical care setting is always a topic of debate as data support that they are actually associated with higher morbidity and mortality secondary to the invasive positioning and the subjective nature of interpreting the data. Central venous catheters with continuous SVO_2 monitoring capabilities (PreSep Catheter, Edwards Lifesciences Corp., Irvine, CA) are being utilized more to help guide resuscitation based on oxygen delivery parameters.

With selective, invasive, and noninvasive monitoring, intensivists can determine the cause of shock and formulate further resuscitation strategies (Tables 22.9 and 22.10). Therapy for *cardiogenic shock* depends on the etiology. During myocardial ischemia, supplemental oxygen and continuous ECG monitoring are imperative. Anticoagulation with aspirin and possibly IV heparin should be considered (unless contraindicated by recent surgery or injury with high likelihood of bleeding), as should implementation of pharmacologic β-blockade. Dopamine, dobutamine, or milrinone are inotropes frequently utilized to temporarily augment CO. However, in the case of ongoing myocardial ischemia, inotropes are relatively contraindicated, as myocardial oxygen demand can exceed supply. Diuresis may be effective in alleviating symptoms of pulmonary compromise from left-sided heart failure and pulmonary edema. In the patient with myocardial ischemia, efforts should be made to transfuse and maintain a hemoglobin concentration that will ensure adequate oxygen delivery. Transfusion to an absolute hemoglobin value is controversial, although it is felt that these patients mandate a lower threshold for transfusion in order to support their oxygen-carrying capability. Severe blunt myocardial injury management is similar to that of myocardial ischemia. Patients with ongoing myocardial ischemia or infarction necessitate coronary angiogram and possible endovascular intervention. Coronary artery bypass grafting or valvular replacement or repair may be indicated. Mechanical support of cardiac function should be considered in the patient in profound or recalcitrant cardiogenic shock; intra-aortic balloon counterpulsation can be lifesaving in these patients, especially in cases of clear coronary insufficiency, mitral insufficiency (frequently caused by myocardial ischemia), and a competent aortic valve. This device actively deflates in systole, increasing forward blood flow by reducing afterload through a vacuum effect. It actively inflates in diastole, increasing blood flow to the coronary arteries via retrograde flow. These actions continue to decrease myocardial oxygen demand and increase myocardial oxygen supply thus increasing overall cardiac efficiency. The cardiac surgery team can also consider ventricular assist devices that provide temporary "bridges" to either cardiac transplantation or cardiac recovery, especially in the case of infectious myocarditis.

Vasogenic or *septic shock* results from a sudden decrease in vascular tone and hence a relative hypovolemia. Endogenous and exogenous vasoactive mediators are responsible for this type of shock,

TABLE 22.9 Physiologic derangements and resuscitation response

Derangement	Therapy
High PAWP and high CI	Slow fluids, consider diuresis
Low PAWP and high CI	Fluid resuscitation
Low PAWP and low CI	Increase PAWP 3–5 mm Hg with crystalloid fluid resuscitation and reassess CI
High PAWP and low CI	Inotropic agent or, if possible, afterload-reducing agent

TABLE 22.10 Types of shock and their physiologic derangements.

Type of Shock	CVP and PAWP	Cardiac Output	Systemic Vascular Resistance	Mixed Venous O_2 Saturation
Hypovolemic	↓	↓	↑	↓
Cardiogenic	↑	↓	↑	↓
Septic	↓ or ↑	↓ or ↑	↓	↑
Neurogenic	↓	↓	↓	↓

and causative mechanisms include systemic inflammatory response syndrome (SIRS), infection or sepsis, anaphylaxis, acute hypoadrenal states, traumatic injury, or ischemia–reperfusion injury. In addition to the loss of vascular tone, patients in septic shock suffer a generalized injury to the endothelium resulting in leakage of plasma into the interstitium, compounding the effective hypovolemia. Patients in septic shock have intact sympathetic tone and are therefore tachycardic, in contrast to patients in neurogenic shock. Fluid resuscitation is the initial measure used to reestablish adequate intravascular volume. Early physiologic parameter goal-directed therapy is the pervading strategy to guide resuscitation. Vasoactive drugs or vasopressors may be necessary to maintain an adequate tissue perfusion; however, these agents should only be employed after CVP or PAWP has been raised to a euvolemic range. Use of inotropes without adequate preload may precipitate cardiogenic shock. Septic shock requires administration of broad-spectrum antibiotics and the treatment of the cause (i.e., debridement of necrotic or gangrenous tissue or drainage of purulent collections). Please see Chapter 3 for discussion of surgical infectious diseases.

Renal Critical Care

Acute renal failure (ARF) is classified as prerenal, renal, or postrenal, and in the surgical ICU (SICU), the most common cause is hypovolemia. Postrenal causes, such as bladder outlet obstruction, are alleviated with Foley catheter placement. Urine output should be monitored closely as a surrogate marker of response to resuscitation. In the shock state, the kidney preserves salt and water. A drop in blood flow to the kidney causes a reflex constriction of the renal afferent arteriole, which results in a decrease in the glomerular filtration rate (GFR). As GFR falls, antidiuretic hormone (ADH) and aldosterone levels increase, producing oliguria (<0.5 mL/kg/h). The result is *prerenal azotemia*, as the serum urea nitrogen levels rise out of proportion to the creatinine level (≥20:1), urine sodium levels are less than 20 mEq/L, and the fractional excretion of sodium (FENa) is less than 1%. FENa is calculated: ([urine Na × plasma Cr]/[plasma Na × urine Cr]) × 100%. Prerenal azotemia is reversible if adequate volume resuscitation is given. Prolonged decreases in renal blood flow may result in ischemia and acute tubular necrosis (ATN). Restoration of renal blood flow at this point results in a reperfusion injury. A loss of renal concentrating ability may develop, such that urine output is no longer an accurate measure of adequate perfusion (high-output ATN). Conversely, if the ischemic injury was profound, the renal tubules may clog with cellular debris. Hence, urine output remains low despite adequate resuscitation (oliguric or anuric ATN). Renal parenchymal causes of ARF are evidenced by urine sodium levels greater than 40 mEq/L and an FENa of at least 3%.

Most renal failures from ATN resolve over time, but permanent renal insufficiency or failure can occur, especially in those with preexisting renal disease. Nephrotoxic drugs and contrast dyes should be avoided in ARF, and all renal excreted medications should be dose adjusted accordingly. Patients with preexisting renal insufficiency who require contrast-enhanced radiographic studies should be pretreated with crystalloid volume infusions and sodium bicarbonate, which has been shown to assuage the nephrotoxicity possibly by a free radical scavenger mechanism (3 ampules of $NaHCO_3$ in 1 L D5W solution run at 3 mL/kg × 1 hour prior to study, followed by a drip of 1 mL/kg × 6 hours postprocedure). Renal replacement therapy is indicated for patients with severe electrolyte disorders (especially hyperkalemia), severe acid–base disturbance, symptomatic fluid overload, and uremia-induced pericarditis or encephalopathy. The most common type of renal replacement therapy in the trauma patient is continuous venovenous hemodialysis (CVVHD). Unlike traditional intermittent hemodialysis (iHD), CVVHD often requires some anticoagulation but is less of a hemodynamic burden in the critically ill patient as rapid volume changes are avoided. Despite a presumed physiologic advantage to continuous hemodialysis, which may more closely mimic natural renal function, no clear survival benefit has been shown in head-to-head comparison studies of CVVHD versus iHD.

Hematologic Critical Care

Multiple factors play a role in the delayed consumptive and dilutional coagulopathy seen after trauma or surgery. Hypothermia and acidosis contribute to platelet dysfunction and abnormal enzymatic coagulation cascade. Dilution of platelets and clotting factors in the process of massive resuscitation also perpetuates coagulopathy. Transfusion of platelets, fresh frozen plasma, and cryoprecipitate are guided by measurements of serum fibrinogen, partial thromboplastin time, prothrombin time, and platelet count. Patients who have sustained severe CNS injury are especially prone to coagulopathy because of the release of endogenous anticoagulants, such as tissue thromboplastin from neural tissues. Thromboelastography (*TEG*) is an old method of testing the efficiency of blood coagulation that is making a resurgence in modern resuscitative medicine. A small sample of blood is taken from the selected person and rotated gently to imitate sluggish venous flow and activate coagulation. A thin wire probe is used to measure, which the clot forms around. The speed and strength of clot formation are measured in various ways, typically by computer-generated graphic. The speed at which the sample coagulates depends on the activity of the plasma coagulation cascade, platelet function, fibrinolysis, and other factors, which can be affected by genetics, illness, environment, and medications. The elasticity and strength of the developing clot changes the rotation of the pin, which is converted into electrical signals that a computer uses to create graphical and numerical output. The graphic patterns of changes in strength and elasticity in the clot provide information about how well the blood can perform hemostasis and how well or poorly different factors are contributing to clot formation and can direct blood component resuscitation by identifying which components are lacking.

Trauma patients and any surgical patient in the ICU commonly have Virchow's triad of stasis, hypercoagulability, and endothelial injury. Therefore, prophylaxis against deep venous thrombosis (DVT) is required. Signs and symptoms of DVT include fever, extremity pain, rubor, and swelling. The physician fails to recognize many cases of DVT. The major complication of DVT, pulmonary embolism (PE), accounts for as many as 200,000 deaths annually. The paucity of signs and symptoms and the unreliability of physical examination underscore the importance of prophylaxis for DVT and ultimately PE. In the absence of prophylaxis, the incidence of DVT after major trauma is estimated to be as high as 65%. Regardless of injury pattern, use of DVT prophylaxis, or method of detection, 1 - 2% of patients who develop a DVT after trauma will suffer a PE.

If no contraindication exists, low molecular weight heparin via subcutaneous dosing has been shown to be most effective in DVT prophylaxis in patients at highest risk for DVT, including trauma and orthopedic patients. However, in routine nontrauma postsurgical patients, low molecular weight heparin did not prove to be any more efficacious over cheaper subcutaneous unfractionated heparin. Inferior vena cava filter placement may be considered in patients who have a contraindication to anticoagulation and who have recurrent DVT/PE on therapeutic anticoagulation. Duplex ultrasonography is highly sensitive and specific for detecting DVT. Weekly surveillance is recommended while the trauma patient is hospitalized and nonambulatory. The duration of risk for DVT in the trauma population is not clear, and the continuation of surveillance beyond 3 to 4 weeks is controversial. Therapy for upper and lower extremity DVT is at least 3 months of therapeutic anticoagulation, and thrombolytic therapy is used only in the uncommon scenario of limb-threatening thrombosis of the iliofemoral system. Patients who have a PE may demonstrate tachycardia, hypoxemia, mental status change, tachypnea, and hypotension. Anticoagulation is begun with bolus heparin administration when the presence of a PE is suspected while diagnostic testing is performed. The arterial blood gas may have a marked arterial–alveolar gradient, but this is not a consistent finding. If the suspicion for PE is high, a high-resolution CT angiogram of the chest should be obtained as the definitive diagnostic study. Large saddle PE may cause cardiac arrest or severe cardiopulmonary collapse, requiring urgent PA embolectomy.

Heparin-induced thrombocytopenia (HIT) is characterized by thrombocytopenia and thromboembolic findings following heparin therapy (acutely, type I, or approximately 5 to 8 days after administration, type II). If HIT is suspected, heparin should be immediately discontinued and the presence of heparin-associated antiplatelet antibodies should be assayed. If no antibodies are present, heparin may be restarted, otherwise anticoagulation with an alternative agent such as the direct thrombin inhibitors (i.e., lepirudin, argatroban, bivalirudin) should be started.

Gastrointestinal Critical Care

Trauma/postoperative patients are at risk for stress-related gastric mucosal lesions, especially if they have coagulopathy, severe burn(s), head injury, or prolonged ventilator dependence (>48 hours). Equal efficacy has been demonstrated between H2-blockers (e.g., cimetidine, ranitidine, and famotidine), sucralfate, and antacid therapy. Antacids are no longer recommended because of bulky administration and an increased risk of pulmonary aspiration. There are no current level I data to support the use of proton-pump inhibitors (PPIs) for prophylaxis. However, use of PPIs for prophylaxis is widespread, especially among patients who are taking this class of drug in the outpatient setting. Otherwise, it has been suggested that the least expensive regimen be employed when possible.

Injured patients who have sustained abdominal trauma carry significant risk for abdominal compartment syndrome (ACS). Risk for ACS increases if the patient has a coagulopathy, requires intra-abdominal packing, or receives a resuscitative volume in excess of 6 L over 6 hours. This syndrome is defined as increased intra-abdominal pressure (IAP > 25 mm Hg) that compromises organ system function (i.e., cardiac, pulmonary, and renal). The diagnosis and decision for operative decompression involves not only the relative IAP but also assessment for decreased CI, decreased pulmonary compliance, high airway pressures, and oliguria. Patients with bladder pressures of 15 to 24 mm Hg warrant close observation, whereas those with 25 to 35 mm Hg eventually require decompression and the ones with greater than 35 mm Hg require emergent decompression. Early definitive closure within 3 to 4 days avoids the risk of intestinal fistulas associated with prolonged vacuum dressing use or mesh closures. Trauma and postoperative patients should be provided with nutritional support (preferably enteral or parenteral if no enteral access available) in the presence of preexisting malnutrition, 5 to 7 days without nutrition, or if their illness is anticipated to last longer than 10 days. Please see Chapter 4 regarding nutritional support.

Endocrine Critical Care

Shock due to *adrenal insufficiency* is a rare form of vasogenic shock. The hypothalamic–pituitary–adrenal axis is stimulated by internal and external stressors to release corticotropin-releasing hormone, adrenocorticotropic hormone, and cortisol. Trauma patients who have recent or chronic glucocorticoid use, signs and symptoms of hypercortisolism/Cushing syndrome, or Addison disease could potentially have adrenal insufficiency. Other risk factors include even a single-dose exposure to IV etomidate (an induction agent frequently used in rapid sequence intubation procedures). Hypoglycemia, hyponatremia, hyperkalemia, and eosinophilia occur in association with adrenal insufficiency. If suspected, a random serum cortisol level should be checked. A random cortisol level less than 15 μg/dL in a "stressed patient" is consistent with adrenal insufficiency, whereas a level between 15 and 34 μg/dL is considered equivocal and warrants a cosyntropin stimulation test. Here, if the stimulated cortisol concentration exceeds the basal concentration by 9 μg/dL or more, adrenal insufficiency is unlikely. Adrenal insufficiency is a diagnosis of exclusion, and if treatment is in error, the patient is at increased risk of sepsis.

Postoperative and trauma patients are at risk for developing glycemic metabolic syndromes such as diabetic ketoacidosis (DKA), hyperosmolar nonketotic dehydration syndrome (HONK), and commonly, stress-related hyperglycemia. Both DKA and HONK require aggressive fluid resuscitation and serial electrolyte assessments. Free water deficit ($=0.6 \times \text{weight}\ [1 - (140/\text{serum Na})]$) can only be calculated after the serum sodium is corrected for hyperglycemia (add 1.6 mmol Na/L for each 100 mg/dL of glucose over 100). Intensive insulin therapy to maintain blood glucose between 80 and 110 mg/dL was found to improve survival of critically ill patients in one landmark study, but these results have not been confirmed in any of the subsequent trials, which revealed high rates of hypoglycemia and related morbidities. While prolonged hyperglycemia carries greater risk for postoperative infections and worse outcome after myocardial infarction, stroke, and head injury, the choice of intermediate insulin target therapy has recently become the recommended guideline. A blood glucose target below 150 mg/dl is presently recommended by the Surviving Sepsis Campaign.

Surgical–Trauma Wound Care

Trauma patients and postoperative surgical patients have unique wounds that necessitate frequent assessment. Furthermore, the risk for pressure ulcer formation is increased in the immobilized spinal cord–injured patient or in the patient transferred a great distance. After approximately 2 hours of immobilization on the long spine board, decubitus ulcers may be evident over the occiput, scapulae, sacrum, and heels. Also, rhabdomyolysis can occur rapidly in this same setting from muscle necrosis. Pressure points should be padded, and frequent repositioning should be routine.

SUGGESTED READINGS

Committee on Trauma of the American College of Surgeons. *Advanced Trauma Life Support for Doctors—Student Course Manual*. 9th ed. Chicago: American College of Surgeons; 2012.

Heron M. Deaths: leading causes for 2004. *National Vital Statistics Report*. Vol. 56, No. 5. Hyattsville, MD: Centers for Disease Control and Prevention, National Center for Health Statistics; 2007.

Mattox KL, Moore EE, Feliciano DV. *Trauma*. 7th ed. New York: McGraw-Hill. 2012.

Moore FA, Moore EE. Initial management of life-threatening trauma. In: Souba WW, Fink MP, Jurkovich GJ, et al., eds. *ACS Surgery: Principles and Practice*. New York: WebMD Inc.; 2005.

Mulholland MW, Lillemoe KD, Doherty GM, et al. *Greenfield's Surgery: Scientific Principles and Practice*. 5th ed. Philadelphia: Lippincott Williams & Wilkins; 2011.

Peitzman AB, Rhodes M, Schwab CW, et al. *The Trauma Manual: Trauma and Acute Care Surgery*. 4th ed. Philadelphia: Lippincott Williams & Wilkins; 2013.

Schrier RW, Wang W. Acute renal failure and sepsis. *N Engl J Med*. 2004;351:159–169.

Tobin MJ. Advances in mechanical ventilation. *N Engl J Med*. 2001;344(26):1986–1996.

Townsend CM, Beauchamp RD, Evers BM, et al. *Sabiston Textbook of Surgery*. 17th ed. Philadelphia: Elsevier Saunders; 2004.

www.CDC.gov/injury/wisqars/

CHAPTER

23

Management of Specific Traumatic Injuries

DANIELLE SPRAGAN AND CARRIE A. SIMS

KEY POINTS

- There is a trimodal distribution of times of deaths for trauma. Roughly half of trauma-related deaths occur within minutes of the injury and are secondary to cardiovascular or neurologic injuries.
- The initial management of trauma patients includes the primary survey, which attempts to assess and address immediately life-threatening injuries. This is followed by the secondary survey, which includes a more detailed examination in otherwise stable patients.
- In patients with traumatic brain injury, the primary injury cannot be undone; the goal is to prevent secondary brain injury by maintaining tissue oxygenation to uninjured but at-risk brain parenchyma.
- Stable patients with penetrating neck injuries require both vascular and aerodigestive tract evaluation. Zone I and III injuries are classically managed by angiography and endoscopy, whereas zone II injuries can be evaluated either operatively or nonoperatively. Unstable patients require exploration irrespective of the zone of injury.
- All blunt trauma patients require cervical spine evaluation. Physical examination may be sufficient in the hemodynamically stable and neurologically intact patient without distracting injury or intoxication.
- Patients with penetrating trauma to the abdomen frequently require an exploratory laparotomy. Rare exceptions require advanced decision making and extensive clinical experience.
- All patients with blunt abdominal trauma must have an objective evaluation to exclude intra-abdominal injury. Evaluation may range from serial abdominal examinations, serial abdominal ultrasounds, diagnostic peritoneal lavage (DPL), and/or CT imaging.
- DPL is an invasive objective test for excluding intra-abdominal injury. It is very sensitive but not specific and currently has a limited role. Ultrasound, or the FAST examination, is more commonly used and identifies free fluid in the dependent portions of the abdomen; it also lacks specificity, however.
- All patients with extremity trauma require special attention to the vascular examination. Signs of vascular injury require angiogram or operative exploration.
- Surgeons must learn to recognize "conditions, complexes, and critical factors" that place patients at risk for hypothermia, coagulopathy, and acidosis. Early termination of procedures after the control of life-threatening hemorrhage is termed "damage control" surgery and will prevent death in severely injured patients.
- Pregnant trauma patients are evaluated initially in the same manner as nonpregnant patients. Early obstetric consultation in pregnancies greater than 20 weeks of gestation is encouraged. Secondary testing should be utilized as needed, as missed maternal injuries are more detrimental to the fetus than the theoretical risk of moderate radiation exposure.

GENERAL CONSIDERATION

Trauma is the number one cause of death for people under 40 and the fourth leading cause of death overall in the United States. Roughly half of trauma-related deaths occur within seconds to minutes of the injury and are due to aortic, heart, brain stem, brain, or spinal cord injuries. Most of these patients will die regardless of care given. A second group of patient deaths occurs within hours of the injury and accounts for nearly 30% of the overall deaths. These deaths are a result of hemorrhage and central nervous system injuries. There has been a sharp decline in mortality during this period as the result of trauma education (e.g., Advanced Trauma Life Support [ATLS] Certification) and the development of specialized trauma centers. A third group of deaths occurs several days or weeks later as the result of infection and organ failure (Fig. 23.1). Remarkably, the incidence of death from posttraumatic organ failure has also declined abruptly within the last 15 years.

The initial management of trauma begins with the primary survey (see Chapter 22), a step that seeks to rapidly identify and treat life-threatening injuries. The primary survey can be recalled by the simple mnemonic "ABCDE" assessment:

A: *Airway*—is the airway patent? Can the patient protect his airway?

B: *Breathing*—is the patient breathing adequately? Are the breath sounds equal?

C: *Circulatory*—are pulses present and symmetric? Is there evidence of exsanguination that need to be addressed?

D: *Disability*—can the patient speak? Follow commands? Move all extremities equally?

E: *Exposure*—all clothes should be removed to fully evaluate evidence of trauma

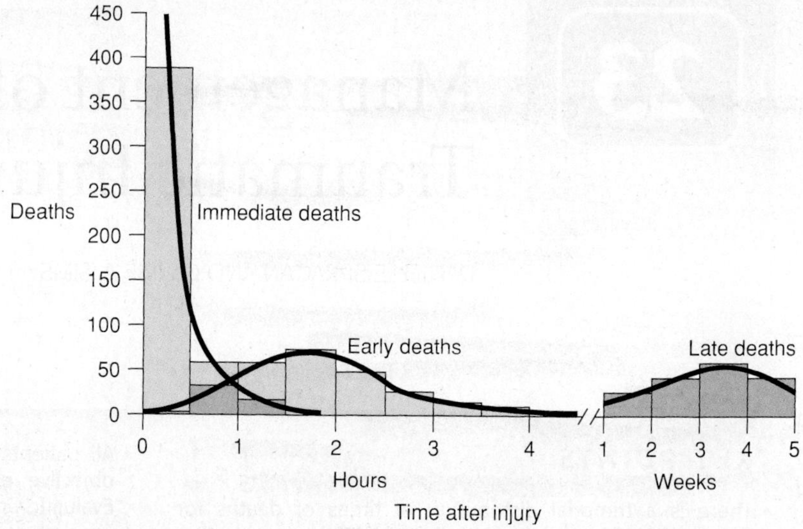

FIGURE 23.1 Three periods of peak mortality after injury. (From Mulholland MW, Lillemoe KD, Doherty GM et al., eds. *Greenfield's Surgery: Scientific Principles and Practices*, 5th ed. Philadelphia: Lippincott Williams & Wilkins, 2011, with permission.)

At each point of the assessment, life-threatening injuries should be identified and treated before moving on to the next part of the assessment. For example, if during the "Airway Assessment," the patient is found to be unable to protect the airway, intubation should be performed before moving to "B." If during the "Breathing Assessment," the patient is found to have decreased breath sounds consistent with a pneumothorax, a chest tube should be placed before moving on to "C," and so on. Identifying and attending injuries using the ABCDE platform not only ensures timely care, following this structured assessment can be lifesaving.

Once the primary survey is complete, a more thorough and detailed assessment, known as the secondary survey, can take place. The secondary survey is performed when the trauma patient is deemed stable and includes a detailed history, complete physical examination, and any necessary radiologic or diagnostic studies. Patients can thereafter be triaged based on degree of injury severity.

SPECIFIC INJURIES BY ANATOMIC REGION

Blunt Traumatic Brain Injury

Traumatic brain injury (TBI) is a common cause of death and long-term disability. TBI is classified both by the specific parenchymal lesion as well as the patient's neurologic function. Although the latter is more predictive of clinical outcome, effective treatment is based on both components. Therefore, irrespective of clinical findings at presentation, patients with suspected TBI should undergo head computerized tomographic (CT) scan as soon as possible after arrival to the trauma center.

The clinical classification of TBI is based on the Glasgow coma scale (GCS) (Table 23.1). The GCS is an easy, rapid assessment of consciousness that can help guide the immediate management of TBI. The GCS includes a ranked score for eye opening, verbal response, and motor response. Collectively, the score can be used to grade the initial injury severity. A GCS less than 8 indicates severe injury, whereas 8 to 12 indicates more moderate injury, and a score greater than 12 suggests mild injury. The GCS score guides initial management and can be tracked through the duration of a patient's hospitalization. For example, patients with a GCS less than 8 require early endotracheal intubation given their altered mental status and inability to protect their airway.

Although there are three components to the GCS, the motor score is the most important predictor of neurologic severity and recovery. For patients with mild TBI who have had a brief loss of consciousness but no focal neurologic deficit (GCS motor 6), the prognosis is excellent and mortality is rare. Patients with coma (GCS $\leq$ 8; motor $\leq$ 4), on the other hand, have a mortality that approaches 40%, and many survivors have a significant persistent neurologic deficit.

In addition to the clinical evaluation, TBI is frequently categorized anatomically based on CT scan findings. Even in the absence of CT findings, however, patients with a documented loss of consciousness in the setting of trauma are considered to have mild TBI or concussion. Although concussions rarely require surgical intervention or hospitalization, postconcussive symptoms are common and include headache, inattention, short-term memory loss, and mood swings. Unfortunately, these symptoms may persist for weeks to months postinjury. Patients and their families must be advised of these potential sequelae and provided resources for posttraumatic care. Patients

TABLE 23.1 Glasgow coma scale for head injury

Eye opening	
• Spontaneous	4
• To loud voice	3
• To pain	2
• None	1
Verbal response	
• Oriented	5
• Confused, disoriented	4
• Inappropriate words	3
• Incomprehensible sounds	2
• None	1
Best motor response	
• Obeys	6
• Localizes	5
• Withdraws	4
• Flexion posturing	3
• Extension posturing	2
• None	1

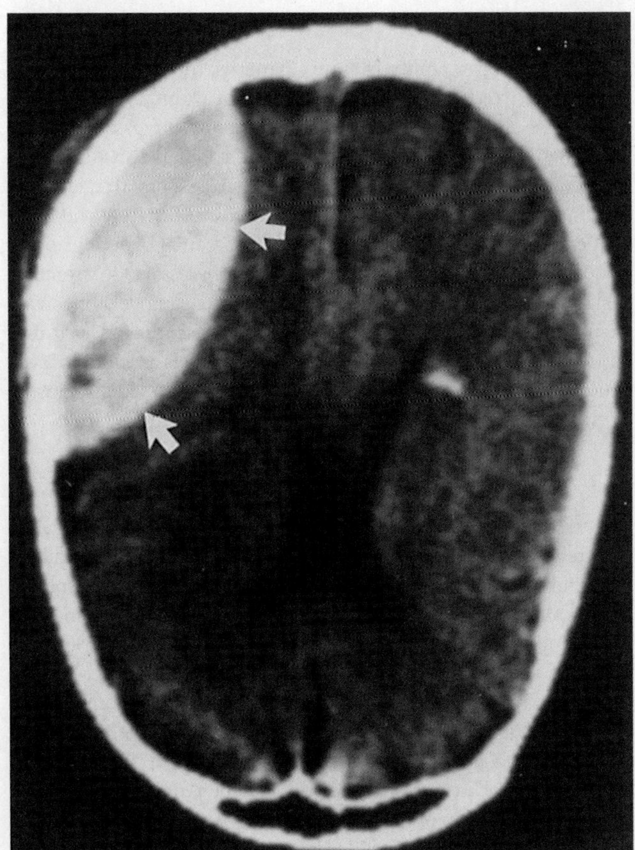

FIGURE 23.2 Typical computed tomography scan appearance of mixed-density, lens-shaped, acute epidural hematoma with mass effect. (From Mulholland MW, Lillemoe KD, Doherty GM et al., eds. *Greenfield's Surgery: Scientific Principles and Practices*, 5th ed. Philadelphia: Lippincott Williams & Wilkins, 2011, with permission.)

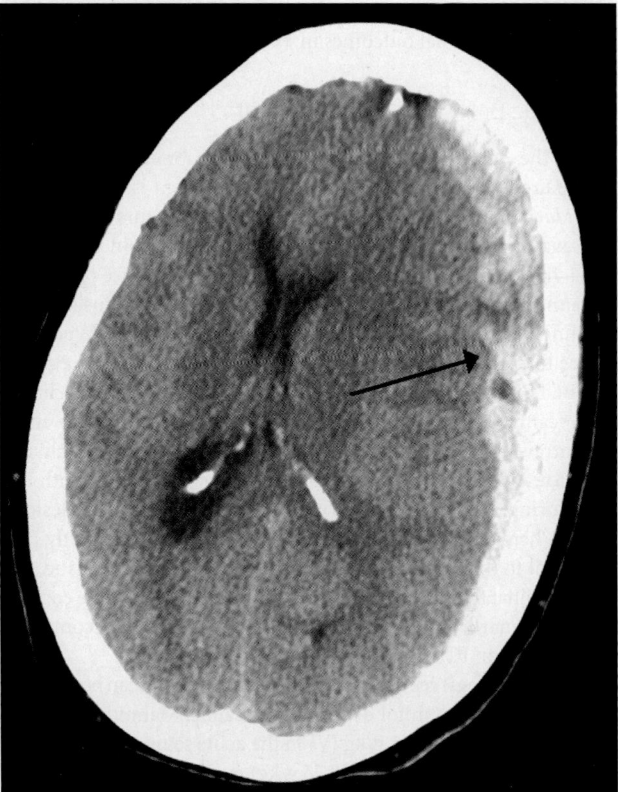

FIGURE 23.3 CT scan of crescent-shaped, high-density blood collection subdural hematoma. (From Mulholland MW, Lillemoe KD, Doherty GM et al., eds. *Greenfield's Surgery: Scientific Principles and Practices*, 5th ed. Philadelphia: Lippincott Williams & Wilkins, 2011, with permission.)

with concussion should avoid contact sports or other activities that may reinjure their brain for several weeks after they are symptom free.

TBI can be divided into parenchymal lesions and extra-axial collections. Parenchymal lesions include cerebral contusions and intraparenchymal hematomas. A cerebral contusion is essentially a "brain bruise" with localized intracerebral hemorrhage and edema adjacent to an area of impact. Depending on the degree of trauma sustained, these lesions can enlarge and coalesce into intraparenchymal hematomas. Parenchymal lesions may occasionally result in a mass effect leading to brain herniation and death.

In contrast, extra-axial hematomas are usually characterized by their relationship to the dural lining and include epidural, subdural lesions, and subarachnoid lesions. Epidural hematomas are most often seen after a direct lateral impact to the temporal region resulting in a skull fracture and laceration of the middle meningeal artery. Although blood subsequently accumulates between the skull and the dura, there may be little direct trauma to the underlying brain parenchyma (Fig. 23.2). Classically, patients with epidural hematomas experience a brief loss of consciousness and a subsequent lucid interval in which they may appear normal, sleepy, or even intoxicated. After a short interval, they lose consciousness again as the lesion expands and produces cerebral compression. On physical examination, ipsilateral pupillary dilation occurs as the result of direct compression of the third cranial nerve and reflects impending uncal herniation. Immediate surgical intervention is indicated in any patient with an altered mental status, a hematoma volume greater than 30 mL, or evidence of midline shift on CT scan. The prognosis following epidural evacuation is excellent and depends primarily on prompt surgical intervention and the degree of underlying cerebral trauma.

Subdural hematomas, on the other hand, accumulate between the dura and the brain itself (Fig. 23.3). The shearing or tearing of dural bridging veins is the most common underlying cause hemorrhage. In addition to the parenchymal compression secondary to the hematoma formation, significant direct brain injury and axonal shearing are frequently present. Therefore, patients with subdural hematomas have a worse prognosis and greater residual functional deficits than those with epidural hematoma. Similarly, subarachnoid hemorrhage often represents a shearing mechanism with local vascular disruption. Interestingly, subarachnoid lesions typically do not cause mass effect.

Occasionally, patients will have minimal findings on their initial CT scans but will present in coma (GCS ≤ 8). In these patients, diffuse axonal injury (DAI) must be suspected. DAI is an axonal shearing injury caused by rapid deceleration, often with little or no evidence of intracerebral trauma on CT scan. In these circumstances, magnetic resonance imaging (MRI) is much more sensitive in identifying scattered punctuate hemorrhages, loss of gray–white matter differentiation, and diffuse edema. Unfortunately, the prognosis for DAI is poor, with a high incidence of residual neurologic deficit.

Although these anatomic distinctions are helpful in terms of describing brain injuries, radiographically many patients present with a combination of intraparenchymal, extra-axial, and axonal injuries. Moreover, the initial CT findings do not necessarily predict long-term functional outcomes in TBI.

Traumatic Brain Injury Management

While the damage inflicted by the primary brain injury cannot be repaired, the basic tenant of TBI management is prevention of *secondary* injury. Secondary neurologic injury occurs when either hypoxia or impaired perfusion cause additional brain tissue ischemia. In addition to treatment strategies that emphasize preventing systemic hypoxia, therapies that maximize cerebral perfusion while minimizing intracerebral pressure (ICP) can mitigate hypoxia at the cellular level. In particular, targeting ICP has become a mainstay of TBI management. The ICP must be monitored if the clinical exam cannot be followed reliably and is accomplished with either an intraventricular (via ventriculostomy) or intraparenchymal monitor. A ventriculostomy has the advantage of allowing both ICP monitoring and treatment. With brain swelling or mass lesions, such as hematomas, the ICP rises. Because the ICP is directly proportional to the volume of intracranial blood, the brain tissue, and cerebrospinal fluid (CSF), therapies that target any of these components can markedly decrease ICP. Current guidelines recommend maintaining an ICP less than 20 mm Hg.

Pharmacologic reduction of intracranial swelling can be achieved transiently with mannitol or hypertonic saline. Mannitol is administered as a large bolus (1 g/kg IV) in the acute setting and is supplemented with smaller boluses (0.25 g/kg) every few hours as needed. Serum osmolarity must be monitored closely and maintained below 320 mOsm. Importantly, mannitol can cause a profound osmotic diuresis, and hypovolemia should be anticipated. In some centers, hypertonic saline is used, although there is currently no data to support its therapeutic superiority in adult trauma patients. Hypertonic saline is administered either as 30 mL boluses of 7.5% solution or as a continuous infusion of 3% solution with a goal of maintaining serum sodium levels between 155 and 160 mEq/L. Hypertonic saline has the advantage of maintaining intravascular volume and should be given when hypovolemia and hypotension are a concern.

Malperfusion can also contribute to tissue hypoxia and secondary brain injury. Because cerebral perfusion pressure (CPP) is defined as the difference between mean arterial pressure (MAP) and the ICP (CPP = MAP – ICP), therapies targeting either the systemic blood pressure or the ICP can directly influence brain perfusion. It is currently recommended that the CPP be maintained at greater than 60 mm Hg. In cases of intractably elevated ICP, adjunctive measures such as administration of vasopressor agents to increase MAP, neuromuscular blockade, and barbiturate coma to reduce cerebral metabolism are utilized. Finally, surgical removal of a large piece of skull via a decompressive craniectomy may have a role in the treatment of select patients with severe intracranial hypertension.

Lastly, conditions that cause increased cellular metabolism, such as fever or agitation, may lead to a relative hypoxia as oxygen demand surpasses supply. Although there is controversy regarding the benefit of therapeutic hypothermia, it is recommended that strict euthermia be maintained.

Because seizures can significantly increase cerebral metabolic demand, anticonvulsants such as phenytoin are often administered during the first week after TBI with intracranial hemorrhage. Corticosteroids, on the other hand, have no role in TBI management and have been shown to significantly increase both mortality and morbidity.

Penetrating TBI

Because of the variability in injury patterns, the optimal management of penetrating injuries (e.g., gun shot wounds) to the brain is less well established. Shock waves created by the passing missile cause significant cavitation and severe parenchymal disruption both in and away from the missile tract. As such, transcranial trajectories that injure both hemispheres are particularly devastating with subsequent hemorrhage, edema, and fatal intracranial hypertension.

While surgical intervention may be necessary to evacuate hematomas, debride devitalized tissues, and remove bone fragments, extensive debridement of the tract is discouraged, as it may cause further neurologic damage. Similarly, bullets are not retrieved unless they are infected or are very easily accessible. Lastly, closure of the dura should be attempted in order to prevent CSF leaks.

Spinal Cord Injury

The initial management of patients with spinal cord injury (SCI) is directed at stabilizing the injury while counteracting the vasodilatation and bradycardia that often occurs. All patients with suspected SCI should be maintained in cervical collar immobilization in order to minimize secondary trauma. Given the high (10% to 15%) incidence of synchronous fracture, the entire spine (thoracic, lumbar, and sacral) requires imaging, and absolute spinal precautions must be maintained until the radiographic evaluation is complete. Crystalloid resuscitation is initiated with the goal of euvolemia. If evidence of neurogenic shock exists, vasopressors may be required to maintain an MAP greater than or equal to 65 mm Hg. Although dopamine has been traditionally recommended given its inotropic, chronotropic, and vasoconstrictive effects, other vasopressors such as phenylephrine or epinephrine may also be used. Phenylephrine, however, may cause reflex bradycardia in an already sympatholytic patient.

The use of high-dose corticosteroids in SCI is still a common practice, although this practice is controversial and no longer supported by ATLS. Recently, the American Association of Neurological Surgeons and Congress of Neurological Surgeons have also concluded that the use of glucocorticoids in acute SCI is not recommended. While steroids theoretically reduce the inflammation and edema that occur postinjury, thus limiting additional loss of function, this benefit has not been universally demonstrated, and steroid use may increase the risk of pneumonia and sepsis. Neurologic deficits suggesting SCI, however, do require early neurosurgical consultation to expedite possible operative decompression.

Patients with SCI are susceptible to a variety of other medical issues, including pulmonary complications such as respiratory failure, pneumonia, thromboembolic events, pressure ulcers, gastrointestinal ulcers, and urinary retention. Thromboembolic prophylaxis in particular should be initiated early. Low molecular weight heparin is preferable to unfractionated heparin in the SCI population due to its longer half-life, lower risk of bleeding complications, and more predictable dose effect relative to unfractionated heparin. The routine use of inferior vena cava (IVC) filters is not recommended.

Neck Injury

The high density of vital structures in the neck makes injury to this region highly morbid and often fatal. Penetrating neck injuries are generally from stab or gunshot wounds but can also originate from penetrating debris. In contrast, blunt injury results from either direct impact to the neck or stretching of vital structures following a decelerating impact to the head or chest. The anatomic complexity of this region makes surgical intervention hazardous and requires a highly organized approach on the basis of the surgeon's experience and the patient's clinical condition.

Penetrating Neck Injury

Anatomic considerations are very important in evaluating penetrating neck injuries, and the trajectory of the knife or bullet will determine the anatomic injury. The platysma serves as an important superficial landmark, as patients without violation of this layer are unlikely to have significant injury to deeper structures. If the platysma has been violated or if violation cannot be excluded, further workup is needed. The anatomic "zone of injury" directs the diagnostic workup and is critical in terms of therapeutic options for vascular control. Zone I extends from the clavicles to the cricoid cartilage and includes the thoracic outlet, subclavian vessels, lung apices, thoracic duct, spinal cord, and esophagus. Injuries to zone I carry the highest mortality rate. Zone II includes all structures between the cricoid and the angle of mandible, including the carotid and vertebral arteries, the jugular veins, the trachea, and the esophagus. Zone III is the area between the angle of the mandible and the skull base and contains the distal internal carotid artery (Fig. 23.4). Not surprisingly, zones I and III require advanced operative techniques to obtain vascular control in the chest (sternotomy) or skull base (mandibular dislocation), respectively.

As with any injury, clinical presentation guides workup and therapy. Maintaining a patent airway is always the primary concern and is usually accomplished with endotracheal intubation. A surgical airway with emergent cricothyroidotomy, however, is sometimes required. Irrespective of the location of injury, immediate surgical exploration is required in patients who present with evidence of obvious vascular injury such as pulsatile hematoma, active bleeding, or hemorrhagic shock. Strong consideration should be given to angiographic embolization for zone III injuries, however, if this expertise is readily available given the difficulty of controlling vascular structures in this area. Bleeding is initially controlled with direct manual pressure; wounds should not be blindly probed nor should any attempt be made to blindly clamp bleeding vessels. With profuse

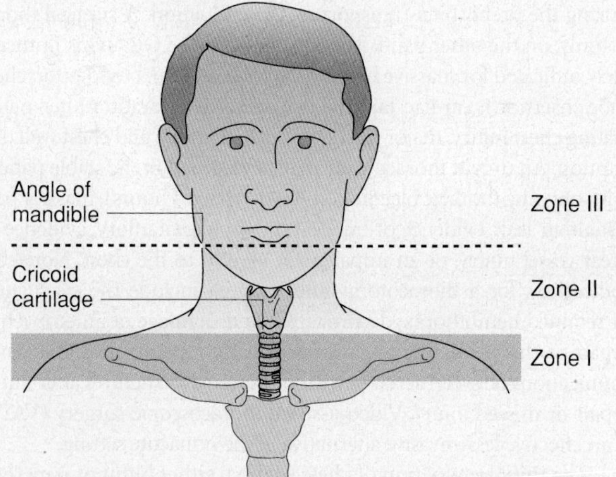

FIGURE 23.4 Zones of the neck. (From Mulholland MW, Lillemoe KD, Doherty GM et al., eds. *Greenfield's Surgery: Scientific Principles and Practices*, 5th ed. Philadelphia: Lippincott Williams & Wilkins, 2011, with permission.)

TABLE 23.2 Indications for immediate surgery after penetrating neck trauma

- Airway compromise
- Extensive subcutaneous emphysema
- Pulsatile hematoma
- Active bleeding
- Shock

bleeding, the compressing hand should be "prepped" into the operative field and removed only when formal surgical exploration begins.

In contrast, patients without an indication for immediate surgery (Table 23.2) are candidates for selective nonoperative management. Careful consideration must be given to identify and exclude injuries to the aerodigestive or vascular structures. In general, all neck injuries in stable patients can be initially triaged with an IV contrast-enhanced CT scan. If the trajectory is in doubt, patients with zone I penetration should subsequently undergo tracheobronchoscopy, and either barium swallow or esophagoscopy to rule out an aerodigestive injury. Positive findings are followed by appropriate surgical management. While the evaluation of zone II injuries has traditionally been operative, there is increasing support for a more selective nonoperative approach that includes CT angiography, esophagoscopy/barium swallow, and bronchoscopy. The presence of significant air on CT scan, however, suggests an aerodigestive injury that mandates operative exploration and drainage. Zone III injuries also require either traditional or CT angiograph as well as direct laryngoscopy/esophagoscopy.

Although a penetrating injury can cause SCI, this is rare. As such, a cervical collar should not be placed *unless* the patient demonstrates neurologic deficits. A cervical collar placed over a penetrating injury can hide on going hemorrhage or hematoma formation.

Blunt Cervical Injury

Blunt traumatic injury to the neck results from direct impact, crush injury, or stretch of vital structures caused by a rapid deceleration of the head. These injuries can be difficult to diagnose on clinical examination. A high index of suspicion is required to avoid missing injuries such as an unstable cervical spine, tracheal tears, and blunt cerebrovascular injury (BCI).

Until a systematic evaluation is complete, cervical spine immobilization should be maintained in all blunt trauma victims. The burden is on the trauma surgeon to prove that no injury exists before removing the cervical collar. Stable patients (<65 years of age) who meet appropriate clinical criteria, including no midline tenderness, normal mental status, no painful distracting injury, no clinical intoxication, and no neurologic deficits (transient or permanent), may have their cervical spine "cleared" without radiographic evaluation (Table 23.3). All other patients require complete cervical spine radiography from C1 to T1. Traditional three-view cervical radiographs include an open-mouth odontoid view, an anteroposterior view, and a lateral view. Inadequate visualization of the cervical spine must be supplemented by either a swimmer's view or, preferentially, a CT scan of the appropriate levels. Suspected areas of fracture should prompt imaging with CT scan. Because of the ease, efficiency, and sensitivity of modern CT technology, most centers

TABLE 23.3 Criteria for clinical cervical spine "clearance"

• Absence of midline tenderness
• Normal mental status
• Absence of intoxication
• Absence of significant distracting injury
• Absence of neurologic deficit

have abandoned the use of plain cervical radiographs in favor of complete cervical CT scan.

Patients who continue to have midline tenderness or pain with movement despite normal radiographs should undergo flexion–extension radiographs or MRI to help exclude ligamentous instability. Patients with a documented fracture on plain films or neurologic defects should undergo CT scanning of the entire spine. MRI should be performed in any patient with documented neurologic findings.

Blunt Cerebrovascular Injury

BCI is a rare but potentially devastating injury that occurs in approximately 1% of blunt trauma patients. Although the diagnosis of BCI should be entertained in patients whose neurologic deficits cannot be explained radiographically, this injury frequently occurs in the absence of neurologic findings but can rapidly progress to stroke. Thus, a high index of suspicion is required to make an early diagnosis. Patients with injuries that suggest either direct trauma (e.g., "seat belt sign" or bruising across the neck) or evidence of severe hyperextension, rotation, or flexion should undergo four-vessel cerebrovascular screening. Injuries associated with an increased risk of BCI include upper cervical spine (C1 to C3) fractures, cervical fractures that extend into the transverse foramina, basilar skull fractures through the petrous portion of the temporal bone, severe facial or mandibular trauma, or hanging/near hanging. Patients who have unexplained neurologic deficits also require urgent cerebrovascular screening. Although four-vessel angiogram is consider the gold standard, improved multislice CT scanning and magnetic resonance angiography (MRA) have emerged as acceptable noninvasive modalities. In most cases, treatment consists of early heparin anticoagulation or antiplatelet therapy with apparently equivalent results. If anticoagulation is selected, heparin can be transitioned to warfarin when clinically appropriate. Although minor luminal injuries can be managed medically, pseudoaneurysms (grade III injury) rarely resolve and should be managed either surgically or angiographically. In patients with complete thrombosis, operative or interventional repair should be undertaken if the patient is not moribund.

Thoracic Injury

Thoracic injury is extremely common after both blunt and penetrating trauma. Thoracic injuries are responsible for 25% of all trauma deaths. Immediate deaths usually involve cardiac or great vessel rupture. Deaths within the first few hours after injury are often caused by airway compromise, tension pneumothorax, or cardiac tamponade. Late complications are primarily due to pulmonary contusions and the development of pneumonia. All patients with thoracic complaints or injuries can initially be screened with

TABLE 23.4 Indications for thoracotomy after trauma

• Emergency department thoracotomy • Cardiac arrest after blunt trauma with loss of signs of life in the trauma bay • Cardiac arrest after penetrating trauma with loss of signs of life in the field or in the trauma bay
• Emergent (in OR) • Massive hemothorax 1,500 mL • Pericardial effusion after penetrating chest injury • Acute deterioration after penetrating chest injury • Major tracheobronchial injury • Chest wall disruption
• Urgent (in OR) • Ongoing thoracic bleeding 200 mL/h × 4 h • Ongoing massive parenchymal air leak • Radiographic evidence of vascular, tracheal, or esophageal injury after mediastinal traverse • Impalement
• Nonacute • Evacuation of retained hemothorax • Decortication/drainage of empyema • Repair chronic diaphragmatic hernia • Repair fistulous aerodigestive tract connection

a simple physical examination and a chest x-ray (CXR). Additional evaluation in selected patients may include arterial blood gas determination, CT scan, electrocardiogram (ECG), and echocardiogram.

The management of thoracic injuries is dictated by the clinical presentation. Despite the potential for significant injury, greater than 85% of all thoracic injuries can be managed nonoperatively with appropriate analgesia, aggressive pulmonary toilet, tube thoracostomy, and selective endotracheal intubation. An emergency department thoracotomy (EDT) is a potentially lifesaving procedure reserved for the patient *in extremis* (Table 23.4). These include patients who are profoundly hypotensive (SBP < 70 mm Hg) or who have lost vital signs during the prehospital transport or ED evaluation. A surgical thoracotomy, on the other hand, is usually done in the OR and is immediately indicated for massive hemothorax (>1,500 mL blood upon chest tube insertion), cardiac tamponade, acute deterioration after penetrating chest injury, major tracheobronchial injury, and chest wall disruption. An urgent thoracotomy may be required in the stable patient with ongoing thoracic bleeding (>200 mL/h for 4 hours), massive persistent air leak, evidence of tracheal or esophageal injury, evidence of great vessel injury, or an impalement wound to the chest. Nonacute indications for a thoracotomy after trauma include the evacuation of retained hemothorax, decortication and drainage of an empyema, repair of chronic diaphragmatic hernia, and repair of fistulous communications between aerodigestive and vascular structures after initial repair or missed injury. Video-assisted thoracoscopic surgery (VATS) is an effective less-invasive alternative in the nonacute setting.

The initial evaluation of chest trauma, either blunt or penetrating, proceeds according to ATLS guidelines with attention directed at identifying and treating the imminently lethal chest injuries such as tension pneumothorax, pericardial tamponade, open pneumothorax, massive hemothorax, and flail chest. Subsequent evaluation must identify or exclude other "hidden" causes of death in thoracic trauma such as aortic transection, tracheobronchial disruption, blunt cardiac injury, diaphragmatic tear, esophageal perforation, and pulmonary contusion. The index of suspicion for these injuries is formulated from pattern recognition on the basis of the mechanism of injury and the patient's clinical presentation.

Specific Conditions in Thoracic Trauma

Tension Pneumothorax

Tension pneumothorax can occur after both blunt and penetrating trauma and is caused by the injured lung parenchyma "leaking" air into the pleural space without a route of escape. Positive pressure subsequently builds in the pleural space leading to compression of the lung and an acute shift of the mediastinum. This mediastinal shift compresses the superior and IVC, thus significantly impairing venous return and progressively diminishing cardiac output. If unrelieved, cardiac arrest will eventually occur. Patients with tension pneumothorax classically present with unilaterally diminished breath sounds, jugular venous distension, severe respiratory distress, and hypotension. In severe cases, tracheal deviation away from the injured side may be present.

Treatment requires immediate decompression, which may be accomplished by inserting a 12- or 14-gauge intravenous catheter into the second or third intercostal space in the midclavicular line. A needle thoracostomy converts the tension pneumothorax into a simple pneumothorax. Although temporizing, needle decompression must always be followed immediately by definitive tube thoracostomy.

Massive Hemothorax

Massive hemothorax is rare following blunt trauma but is not uncommon following penetrating injuries. Etiologies include intercostal or internal mammary arterial bleeding, hilar vessel injury, great vessel injury, and cardiac injury. Clinically, patients are in hemorrhagic shock with absent breath sounds on the injured side. Neck veins may be flat secondary to hypovolemia or distended because of the mechanical effects of intrathoracic blood compressing the mediastinum. A chest radiograph will demonstrate a completely opacification of the hemithorax and occasionally mediastinal shift toward the contralateral side. Airway control, large-bore intravenous access, and volume infusion should be initiated immediately. A large chest tube (36 or 40 French) should be placed expeditiously and ideally should be attached to a collecting system with an autotransfusion reservoir. A thoracotomy is indicated if there is greater than 1,500 mL initial blood loss, ongoing bleeding of greater than 200 mL/h for more than 4 hours, or failure of a hemothorax to drain despite at least two functioning and well-positioned chest tubes. Importantly, a thoracotomy is also indicated if the patient remains hemodynamically unstable despite initial resuscitation attempts.

Pericardial Tamponade

Pericardial tamponade occurs most commonly after penetrating trauma to the heart, but it can also be seen following blunt chest trauma. Because the pericardial sac is not acutely distensible, as little as 75 to 100 mL of accumulated may produce tamponade in the adult. Classic signs such as distended neck veins, hypotension, and muffled heart tones (*Beck's triad*) are present in only a few patients with confirmed tamponade. *Pulsus paradoxus*, a decrease in systolic pressure of more than 10 mm Hg during inspiration, and *Kussmaul's sign*, a rise in venous pressure with inspiration, are rarely seen but classically described. Patients with tamponade are often extremely anxious with a sense of "impending doom." The diagnosis of pericardial tamponade considered in any patient who remains persistently hypotensive and acidotic despite adequate blood and fluid resuscitation. This is particularly true if the central venous pressure is found to be elevated despite systemic hypotension.

An ultrasonographic examination can quickly diagnose pericardial tamponade and can be easily performed at the bedside. A pericardial view demonstrating fluid or heterogeneous clot in the setting of hemodynamic instability is an indication for immediate operative exploration and decompression. An equivocal pericardial view with ultrasound in an unstable patient or a positive examination in a stable patient necessitates an operative pericardial window. Although a negative ultrasound in the unstable patient is usually satisfactory to exclude tamponade, cardiac tamponade cannot be excluded *in the presence of hemothorax*, as pericardial fluid can decompress into the pleural space.

If the patient is *in extremis*, an emergent left anterolateral thoracotomy can also be performed to relieve tamponade in the emergency room or trauma bay. In the unstable patient, urgent sternotomy or thoracotomy should be performed in the OR. Stable patients with pericardial fluid evident on focused assessment with sonography for trauma (FAST) should undergo a diagnostic subxiphoid pericardial window in the OR to confirm the diagnosis. A positive finding during pericardial window mandates extension to median sternotomy for evaluation and repair of cardiac injury. Although a pericardiocentesis can be used as a temporizing maneuver to relieve tamponade, it is generally not advisable because the pericardial blood is usually clotted, thereby making evacuation nearly impossible via this approach. Moreover, pericardiocentesis does not afford the opportunity to repair the underlying injury.

Open Pneumothorax

An open pneumothorax or "sucking chest wound" is most often caused by an impalement or destructive penetrating wound. A large open defect in the chest wall allows equilibration between intrathoracic and atmospheric pressure. When the defect is greater than two thirds of the tracheal diameter, air flows preferentially through the chest wall with each inspiration leading to profound hypoventilation and hypoxia. The chest wall defect should be temporarily occluded with the gloved hand and then closed with an occlusive dressing taped on three sides to act as a flutter valve. This maneuver allows the spontaneously breathing patient to preferentially breathe through the trachea but prevents the conversion to a tension pneumothorax. After temporary occlusion, a tube thoracostomy should be placed through clean tissue and away from the traumatic wound. The wound can then be completely occluded with a sterile dressing. Patients with large chest wounds should subsequently undergo formal operative thoracotomy to evacuate blood clot, debride devitalized tissue, and close the chest wall defect. Very large defects may require flap closure. Of note, any patient with respiratory distress or hemodynamic instability should undergo immediate positive pressure ventilation.

Chest Wall Injury

Direct injuries to the chest wall are very common in trauma victims. The chest wall comprised the rib cage, costal cartilage, and intercostal muscles. Specific clinical manifestations of chest wall trauma include pain with inspiration, tenderness, and chest wall instability. Significant chest wall instability, or "flail chest," can occur when two or more ribs are fractured in at least two more locations. Although paradoxical chest wall motion occurs during respiration, the major cause of respiratory compromise is the underlying *pulmonary contusion*. Initial care should occur in the intensive care unit (ICU) with monitoring to detect clinical deterioration, progressive hypoxia, or hypercapnia. Many patients with multiple rib fractures or flail segments will require endotracheal intubation and positive pressure ventilation.

Chest wall injuries are associated with significant morbidity because the presence of pulmonary contusions and "splinting" from pain significantly compromise pulmonary performance. As such, the major complication following chest wall trauma is pneumonia. Elderly patients are especially at risk for pulmonary complications following chest wall injuries; and patients over the age of 65 who sustain multiple rib fractures are five times more likely to die than younger patients with the same constellation of injuries. As such, adequate analgesia is paramount for all patients with chest wall trauma in order to facilitate aggressive pulmonary toilet and early mobilization. Optimal pain relief can be achieved with a *scheduled* multimodality regimen including nonsteroidal anti-inflammatory drugs (NSAIDs), acetaminophen and oral narcotics. Supplemental pain medication maybe necessary acutely and may include intermittent intravenous narcotics, patent controlled analgesia (PCA), epidural catheters, or paravertebral bupivacaine infusions. Although lidocaine patches are routinely used in some centers, randomized controlled trials suggest these devices are not superior to placebo and should not be routinely prescribed. Naturally, pain management should be tailored to the individual patient, their unique medical history, and their response to medical intervention. In particular, NSAIDs should be used cautiously in those over the age of 65.

Lung Injury

Pulmonary contusion not only occurs in 75% of patients with flail chest but may also occur in blunt trauma without fractured ribs. Pulmonary contusions are characterized by alveolar rupture with fluid transudation and extravasation of blood that result in localized airway obstruction and atelectasis. The diagnosis and subsequent treatment of pulmonary contusion is often delayed because both clinical and radiographic findings are often minor and nonspecific for 12 to 48 hours. Over time, clinical features may progress to copious blood-tinged secretions, chest pain, restlessness, labored respiration, and finally dyspnea and cyanosis. X-ray changes show patchy parenchymal opacification or diffuse linear peribronchial densities that progress to complete opacification within 12 to 48 hours after the injury. Treatment includes pain control, pulmonary toilet, supplemental oxygen, and occasionally mechanical ventilatory support.

Diaphragm Injury

Diaphragmatic laceration or rupture can result from bunt or penetrating trauma. Although diaphragmatic injury occurs in 5% of cases of severe blunt trauma, the incidence is significantly higher following penetrating trauma. In fact, nearly 40% of cases of penetrating trauma to the left chest will have a concomitant diaphragmatic laceration. The clinical presentation of diaphragm injuries, however, primarily depends on the associated injuries. Patients may complain of abdominal tenderness, dyspnea, or shoulder pain. Importantly, nearly 25% of patients with diaphragm injuries will present in shock as the result of concomitant thoracic or abdominal injuries.

As such, diagnosing diaphragm injuries can be exceptionally difficult. These injuries are rarely obvious using standard radiographic imaging, and concurrent injuries may take priority. Nonetheless, diaphragm wounds must not be overlooked as they rarely heal spontaneously. While injuries to the right diaphragm are usually well tolerated because the liver provides an element of protection, injuries to the left chest can result in herniation of abdominal viscera either immediately or years after the initial injury. While the chest radiograph is frequently used as a screening test, it may be entirely normal in 40% of cases. The most common finding on CXR is ipsilateral hemothorax, which is present in about 50% of patients. Occasionally, a distended, herniated stomach can be confused with a pneumothorax. Passage of a nasogastric tube before the chest radiograph will help to identify gastric herniation. CT scan or contrast x-rays may be used to establish the diagnosis in some cases. Alternatively, laparoscopy is useful, although invasive technique for detecting occult diaphragmatic injuries in patients who have no other indications for formal laparotomy.

Once the diagnosis is made, a transabdominal surgical approach should be used in cases of acute rupture to make sure that there are no other intra-abdominal injuries. Laparoscopic repair of the injury may be possible in selected cases. The diaphragm should be reapproximated and closed with interrupted nonabsorbable sutures. Figure of eight sutures are not recommended as these can cause tissue ischemia and lead to repair failure. Chronic herniation, on the other hand, should be approached via thoracotomy, with the addition of a separate laparotomy when indicated. Cases of chronic herniation can be quite challenging because the herniated abdominal viscera form adhesions to the adjacent thoracic structures.

Blunt Cardiac Injury

Blunt cardiac injury describes a spectrum of injury from myocardial muscle contusion to blunt rupture of the heart. Although blunt cardiac injury causing hemodynamic instability is rare, new-onset arrhythmia or cardiac failure in a patient after significant blunt trauma raises the suspicion of blunt myocardial injury. Sinus tachycardia is the most common arrhythmia seen with myocardial contusion followed by premature atrial contractions, atrial fibrillation, right bundle branch block, ST-segment elevation, and premature ventricular contractions.

The diagnosis of blunt cardiac injury requires a high index of suspicion based on mechanism of injury. A 12-lead ECG should be obtained; however, a completely normal ECG does not exclude blunt cardiac injury. Current recommendations now include sending troponin I levels. If both the ECG and troponin I level are normal, blunt cardiac injury can be safely excluded. If either test is abnormal, however, patients should be admitted for continued cardiac monitoring for 24 hours. An echocardiogram should be performed in patients with a new-onset murmur, hemodynamic instability, or new arrhythmia. Although a transthoracic echocardiogram (TTE) is convenient, noninvasive method of assessing anatomic function, transesophageal echocardiogram (TEE), may be necessary when the TTE is technically inadequate. Routine cardiac enzymes (creatine kinase [CK] with isoenzyme analysis) do *not* correlate with the severity of blunt myocardial injury nor do they predict complications. Myocardial enzyme levels, however, continue to be useful in diagnosing cardiac *ischemia* in trauma patients. Therefore, if a patient is suspected of a myocardial infarction before or after injury, cardiac enzymes should be sent.

Echocardiographic-proven cardiac contusion with either hypokinesis or abnormal wall movement mandates admission to the ICU. Invasive monitoring with a pulmonary artery catheter may be indicated to help guide therapy in patients who develop signs and symptoms of acute heart failure. Dobutamine or epinephrine may be useful in overcoming the impaired contractility experienced after blunt cardiac injury. Consultation with cardiology is warranted in patients with echo-proven myocardial injury.

Traumatic Aortic Injury

Traumatic rupture of the aorta (TRA) occurs after rapid deceleration injury, such as a fall from significant height or high-speed motor vehicle crash. The majority of individuals with this injury die at the scene. In survivors, there is typically a tear in the wall of the aorta that is contained by the adventitia and the parietal pleura. These patients are at risk for delayed free rupture into the mediastinum or pleural space with near-instant death. Because free rupture of the transected aorta is rapidly fatal, persistent or recurring nonlethal hypotension must be assumed to be from a cause than the aortic injury.

In 85% of patients, aortic laceration is located just distal to the ligamentum arteriosum, past the left subclavian artery. Less often, this injury occurs in the ascending aorta, at the diaphragm, or in the mid-descending thoracic aorta. Physical findings that increase suspicion of TRA include asymmetry of upper extremity blood pressures, chest wall contusion, intrascapular pain, and intrascapular murmur. Importantly, half of all patients with TRA have no external signs of blunt chest injury.

A chest radiograph can serve as a screening test; however, 30% of patients with known TRA will have a completely normal CXR. Radiographic signs suggesting TRA include a *widened mediastinum* (>8 cm), obliteration of the aortic knob, deviation of the trachea to right, presence of an apical pleural cap, depression of the left main stem bronchus, obliteration of the aortopulmonary window, and deviation of the esophagus (nasogastric tube) to the right (Table 23.5). No single sign on chest radiograph reliably confirms or excludes aortic injury, although mediastinal widening is the most consistent finding. Further, radiographic evidence of fractures of the first rib, sternum, and scapula are not specific for TRA but do imply a large force applied to the thorax. A high index of suspicion based on mechanism of injury and the presence of any of the previously noted findings should prompt further evaluation.

TABLE 23.5 Chest radiographic findings suggestive of traumatic rupture of the aorta

- Widened mediastinum (>8 cm)
- Obliteration of aortic knob
- Obliteration of aortopulmonary window
- Deviation of the trachea to right
- Presence of pleural cap
- Depression of the left main stem bronchus (4 cm)
- Deviation of the esophagus (nasogastric tube) to right

Although aortography has traditionally been the gold standard for diagnosis of TRA, chest CT has become the standard screening tool for TRA. Currently, in many centers, high-speed multidetector helical CT scan provides definitive diagnosis of aortic injury, allowing thoracic surgeons to proceed to repair without angiographic confirmation. Mediastinal screening with chest CT scan should be used liberally in patients whose mechanism or radiographic findings are suspicious for aortic injury.

Once the diagnosis of TRA has been made, the treatment goal is to decrease aortic wall stress by decreasing the heart rate and then the MAP. Typically, this is accomplished by the continuous infusion of short-acting β-blocker (e.g., esmolol). In the multiply injured patient, management may be complicated by competing interests such as maintaining cerebral perfusion or managing acute hemorrhage. Once the diagnosis of TRA has been made, a cardiothoracic surgeon should be consulted for possible repair via open thoracotomy or endovascular stent graft. However, in the presence of intra-abdominal bleeding, the abdominal injury should be dealt with prior to repair of a contained disruption of the thoracic aorta.

Transmediastinal Penetrating Injury

Missile injuries that traverse the mediastinum require special mention because of the complexity of their evaluation and the potential for devastating complications with any delay in diagnosis. One must remember that the heart, great vessels, tracheobronchial tree, and esophagus are all at risk when missiles traverse the mediastinum and an evaluation of *each* of these structures must be performed in *all* patients. Patients in *extremis* should undergo immediate median sternotomy or left anterolateral thoracotomy to control hemorrhage or relieve cardiac tamponade; if successful, further evaluation of the tracheobronchial structures and esophagus should continue in the OR. In the *unstable patient* with hypotension, a CXR should be obtained and chest tubes should be placed as needed to relieve pneumo- or hemothorax. A rapid ultrasound examination should be performed to exclude pericardial effusion. A thoracotomy can be performed in the trauma bay or OR as indicated based on the patient's hemodynamic status, the ultrasound results, and the volume of chest tube return. In the OR, after control of major hemorrhage, flexible esophagoscopy and bronchoscopy should be performed to diagnose aerodigestive tract injuries. If hemodynamic stability was achieved in the trauma bay but great vessel injury is suspected, formal *angiography*, embolization, and possibly endovascular stent placement can be performed followed by panendoscopy in the OR or ICU.

In the *stable patient*, evaluation must proceed in an organized and deliberate fashion to exclude injury to the heart, great vessels, esophagus, and tracheobronchial tree. Workup begins with a CXR and ultrasound examination. If ultrasonography is not available and there is concern for cardiac injury, one must proceed to the OR for a subxiphoid pericardial window. Angiography (or CT angiography) should be performed to rule out vascular injury. If injuries are found requiring operation, esophagoscopy and bronchoscopy can be performed in the OR or they can be completed in the ICU. A barium esophagogram can be used as a complement to esophagoscopy. When combined, these two tests have an overall sensitivity of 90%.

More recently, an alternative algorithm has arisen for the evaluation of mediastinal traversing injuries in highly selected *stable* patients and includes CT angiography as an imaging triage tool. If CT angiography is rapidly available, this modality can be used to determine missile trajectory and guide further workup. Angiography, bronchoscopy, and/or esophagoscopy are then performed selectively as needed on the basis of proximity of missile tract to individual structures. CT is best used to exclude injury on the basis of trajectory and proximity rather than to identify individual injuries.

Emergency Department Thoracotomy and Cardiac Injury

EDT can be lifesaving in properly selected trauma patients. The goals of EDT are to relieve pericardial tamponade, temporize bleeding, and improve perfusion to the coronaries and brain by temporarily occluding the descending aorta. The usefulness of EDT is determined by the presence (or absence) of signs of life and by the mechanism of injury. Accepted signs of life include a palpable pulse, spontaneous movement, pupillary response, spontaneous respirations, and an ECG-determined narrow complex electrical rhythm of greater than 40 bpm (Table 23.6). After blunt trauma, patients with cardiac arrest in the field or *en route* to the hospital are usually *not* candidates for EDT and should be declared dead on arrival. With blunt mechanism, thoracotomy should be performed *only* after the acute deterioration of signs of life *in the* ED. That being said, an EDT should not be performed in the setting of massive head trauma. The indications for EDT after penetrating trauma are slightly more liberal and reflect a greater potential for recovery. EDT should be *considered* if signs of life are lost on transport or during the ED evaluation. The treating surgeon must determine the amount of time without signs of life and assess if lethal injuries such as massive head injury would preclude EDT. The witnessed absence of signs of life by medical personnel precludes EDT regardless of mechanism.

The technique for EDT involves a left anterolateral thoracotomy below the nipple at the fourth intercostal space or in the inframammary crease in females (Table 23.7). A generous incision should be made from the right side of the sternum to the posterior axillary line. The initial incision should be through all subcutaneous tissues and onto the chest wall. The intercostal muscles are incised with scissors, and a large rib spreader is inserted with the crossbar down toward the stretcher. The pericardium is then incised longitudinally, anterior, and parallel to the phrenic nerve. The heart is delivered from the pericardial sac. The descending aorta should then be immediately crossed clamped in order to increase diastolic afterload and improve perfusion to both the coronary and cerebral circulation. Access to the descending aorta may require incising the inferior pulmonary ligament to retract the lung anteriorly and superiorly. In the exsanguinating patient, the thoracic aorta is flaccid and can be difficult to distinguish from the adjacent esophagus. Passing a nasogastric tube can help clarify the anatomy. Additionally, the aorta is covered with a dense parietal pleura that requires blunt dissection in order to effectively create enough space to apply an occlusive clamp.

TABLE 23.6 Signs of life

- Palpable pulse
- Spontaneous movement
- Pupillary response
- Spontaneous respirations
- Narrow complex electrical rhythm >40 bpm

TABLE 23.7 Steps in emergency department thoracotomy technique

1. Incise skin/subcutaneous tissue in the fourth intercostal space/inframammary crease from midline to posterior axillary line
2. Divide intercostal muscles and pleura with heavy scissors
3. Insert rib spreader (handle toward axilla)
4. Extend to right side if needed
5. Perform pericardiotomy with scissors
    - Incise anterior and parallel to phrenic nerve
    - Evacuate clots
6. Repair/control any cardiac injuries present
    - Digital pressure
    - Pledgeted mattress suture
7. Cardiac life support
    - Ventricular fibrillation: internal cardioversion
    - Asystole: epinephrine 1 mg and internal bimanual massage
8. If #7 is unsuccessful
    - Release left inferior pulmonary ligament
    - Gain digital control of aorta anterior to spine
    - Clamp with large vascular instrument to increase coronary perfusion
    - Repeat #7
9. Pulmonary hilar occlusion as needed for bleeding
    - Release affected inferior pulmonary ligament
    - Clamp hilum or perform 180-degree hilar twist
10. Cross-clamp aorta for intra-abdominal exsanguinations
    - Release left inferior pulmonary ligament
    - Gain digital control of the aorta anterior to the spine
    - Clamp with large vascular instrument
11. Proceed to operating room for definitive repairs/control
    - Ligate internal mammary arteries as needed

If the heart is lacerated, gentle wound compression with a finger usually controls bleeding until the patient can be transported to the OR for definitive repair. If manual compression of the injury is not possible, immediate closure is performed in the ED with a 2-0 pledgeted, monofilament, nonabsorbable suture. Balloon catheters should *not* be inserted into cardiac lacerations nor should attempts be made at clamping ventricular wounds. These maneuvers will not only fail to control bleeding, they will serve to only enlarge the hole in the myocardium. Atrial wounds may be controlled by vascular clamp occlusion followed by suture repair. Massive bleeding from the pulmonary parenchyma or hilum is controlled with a large hilar clamp or by finger occlusion. If the heart is not beating, internal massage is performed while resuscitation with fluids proceeds. If the heart is fibrillating, internal cardioversion is performed at 20 J initially, followed by 30 J. Unfortunately, in the absence of tamponade or easily controllable thoracic bleeding, survival after EDT for cardiac arrest is very poor.

On occasion, an EDT may be performed in profoundly a hypotensive or arresting patient who does not have obvious thoracic trauma. Temporarily occluding the descending aorta will slow all bleeding below the diaphragm and allow transport to the OR for laparotomy. Survival after EDT for penetrating *abdominal* or *extremity* injury, however, is very rare.

Abdominal Trauma

Blunt Abdominal Trauma: General Considerations

Physicians evaluating trauma victims must recall that the physical examination for abdominal trauma may be unreliable. In general, the reliability of the abdominal exam is increased in patients without distracting injuries or intoxication. Notable physical exam findings include abdominal distention, abdominal guarding, rebound tenderness, hypotension, and abdominal wall ecchymoses.

Blunt trauma patients who are hemodynamically unstable or who have considerable ongoing fluid requirements should be considered to have an uncontrolled source of hemorrhage. These patients are not candidates for CT scanning and should undergo immediate cavitary triage with CXR, pelvis x-ray, and either FAST or DPL (see Chapter 22). Immediate surgery is indicated in these unstable patients if the FAST exam is positive or the DPL is grossly bloody.

Blunt trauma patients who remain hemodynamically stable and in whom abdominal injury is suspected should have a contrast-enhanced abdominal–pelvic CT scan. A CT scan with IV contrast is both highly sensitive and specific for detecting solid organ injury after blunt trauma. Although a CT scan is less sensitive for hollow viscus injuries, a *completely normal* abdominopelvic CT scan reliably exclude both solid organ and hollow viscus injuries. Alternatively, serial FAST examinations by an experienced ultrasonographer in conjunction with a urinalysis and serial abdominal exams over 24 hours can also be used to exclude injury. A positive FAST, microscopic hematuria, or change in the clinical presentation mandate additional imaging. Deterioration of vital signs or a change in clinical status (e.g., fever, tachycardia, new or persistent abdominal pain tenderness, or leukocytosis) should prompt repeat CT scanning or exploratory laparotomy.

Penetrating Abdominal Trauma: General Considerations

Most patients with a penetrating injury to the abdomen will require a laparotomy. A laparotomy, however, can be avoided in select cases provided the patient is hemodynamically stable and nonperitonitic. For stab wounds, a plain film of the abdomen should be performed to confirm that the absence of a retained foreign body (e.g., knife blade). For gunshot wounds, a chest, abdominal, and pelvic x-ray should be performed in order to identify retained bullets and determine the trajectory. The number of gunshot wounds and bullets identified should always be an even number. An odd number suggests either a missing wound or an unaccounted bullet.

The diagnostic workup in hemodynamically stable patients is based on the anatomic location of the abdominal wound. For anterior abdominal wounds, a local wound exploration can be performed using sterile technique and local anesthesia. A laparotomy can be safely avoided if the anterior abdominal fascia can be directly visualized and is found to be intact. If the anterior fascia is violated, however, either an open laparotomy or diagnostic laparoscopy should be performed. If peritoneal violation is seen on laparoscopy, an open exploratory laparotomy is indicated.

In contrast, hemodynamically stable patients with penetrating wounds to the back or flanks should undergo a CT scan in order to identify trajectory and evaluate the potential for abdominal penetration and visceral injury. Laparotomy can be avoided in some patients whose trajectory is clearly away from all abdominal or retroperitoneal organs. In this setting, CT is not used to identify specific injuries but only to safely exclude them. Proximity to vital structures or questionable findings on CT scanning should prompt operative exploration and evaluation.

Trauma Laparotomy

Patients who require urgent laparotomy for trauma should have tetanus status updated and should receive preoperative broad-spectrum antibiotics that cover skin flora, enteric organisms, and anaerobes. In addition, a nasogastric tube, Foley catheter, and calf compression boots should be placed before commencing surgery. Skin preparation and towel draping should routinely be from the chin to knees and to both sides of the operating table irrespective of the area of injury. A consistently wide operative field allows the trauma surgeon to be prepared to explore any cavity or harvest a leg vein if necessary without reprepping or draping.

In general, a midline incision from xiphoid to pubis is used and affords the greatest exposure and flexibility. Consideration to possible stoma placement should be given when incising around the umbilicus. When immediate access to control hemorrhage is needed in patients with a previous laparotomy, a bilateral subcostal incision can be used as it will avoid midline adhesions and gives adequate exposure for immediate hemorrhage control. Once the abdomen in entered, the cavity should be systematically packed and the zones of the abdomen quickly explored (Fig. 23.5). Starting in the right upper quadrant, the liver should be compressed and packed lateral and medial of the falciform ligament. The spleen should then be protected with the nondominant hand to prevent secondary trauma, and several lap pads should be placed superiorly. Abdominal viscera should then be swept out of the left lateral gutter, and lap pads are placed along zone II. Lap pads are then placed in bilateral pelvic quadrants, and zone III is quickly evaluated. Abdominal viscera are then swept out of the right lateral gutter, and packing is placed in zone II. The upper portion of zone I is then quickly inspected by incising the gastrohepatic ligament followed incising the gastrocolic omentum and lifting the stomach cephalad. The lower portion of zone I is evaluated by lifting the transverse colon cephalad and inspecting the root of the small bowel mesentery. Active hemorrhage must be dealt with immediately. Enteric soilage can be initially contained with umbilical ties, GIA stapling devices, 2.0 silk sutures, or even Babcock clamps. Packs can then be sequentially removed in order to identify and treat injuries.

Hepatic Trauma

The liver is the most commonly injured organ in blunt injury. Patients with a history of right upper quadrant, right lower chest, or flank trauma should raise suspicion for hepatic injury. On exam, patients may complain of right upper quadrant pain or right shoulder pain secondary to diaphragmatic irritation. Hepatic lacerations,

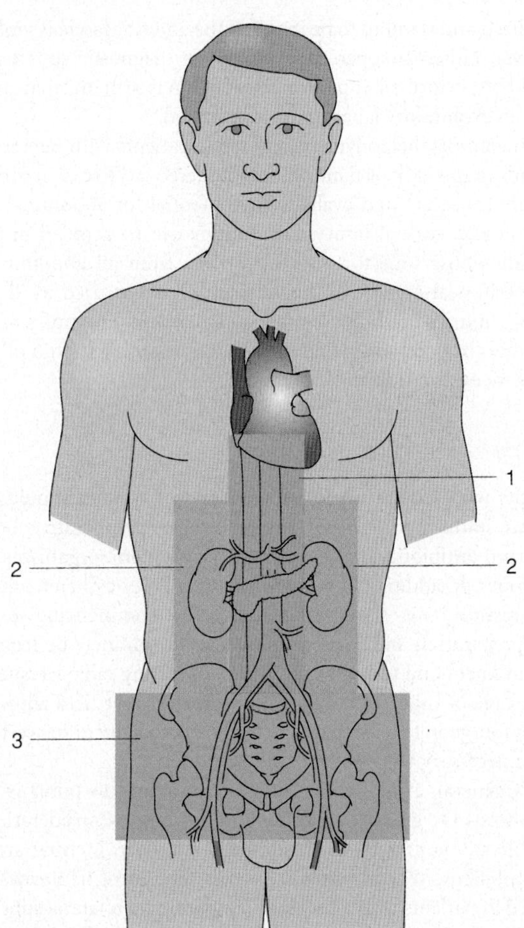

FIGURE 23.5 Zones of retroperitoneum. (From Mulholland MW, Lillemoe KD, Doherty GM et al., eds. *Greenfield's Surgery: Scientific Principles and Practices*, 5th ed. Philadelphia: Lippincott Williams & Wilkins, 2011, with permission.)

hematomas, or active bleeding are most easily demonstrated by abdominopelvic CT scanning with intravenous contrast. The majority of hepatic hemorrhage is venous in nature and is generally self-limited. Therefore, most isolated hepatic injuries can be managed nonoperatively regardless of injury grade provided the patient is hemodynamically stable. The presence of hepatic contrast extravasation ("blush") on initial CT scan suggests active hemorrhage and warrants angiography and possible embolization. Patients who are managed nonoperatively will require ICU admission, serial hemoglobin determination, and repeated abdominal exams. A falling hemoglobin concentration should prompt repeat abdominal CT scan to exclude ongoing hepatic hemorrhage with consideration of angiographic intervention at that time. Additionally, if signs of peritoneal irritation develop, laparotomy is required to explore for hollow visceral injury.

At laparotomy, most liver injuries can be controlled with suture ligation, cautery, or topical hemostatic agents. Finger fracture may be used to expose specific vessels in deeper parenchymal injuries. The elective ligation of injured vessels and bile ducts is preferable to mass ligation of liver tissue, which increases hepatic necrosis. If necessary, nonanatomic debridement and resection is preferable to formal anatomic resection.

With massive hemoperitoneum from hepatic hemorrhage, opening the peritoneum may release tamponade and precipitate profound hemodynamic instability. In this situation, the liver should be compressed manually until the anesthesia team can match blood losses with transfusion of red cells, plasma, and platelets. The use of autotransfusion and cell-saving devices is highly recommended. In severe liver trauma, occluding the portal triad at the hepatoduodenal ligament manually or with a Rumel tourniquet (a Pringle maneuver) will significantly reduce bleeding by occluding hepatic arterial and portal venous inflow. Ongoing hemorrhage after a Pringle maneuver suggests a retrohepatic vena caval injury or hepatic venous avulsion (Fig. 23.6). These complex injuries carry a very high mortality. If manual compression can control hemorrhage (in the absence of a Pringle maneuver), the liver should be firmly packed supra- and infrahepatically without dividing the hepatic suspensory ligaments. The upper midline fascia should be reapproximated in order to improve packing tension. If bleeding continues, however, despite tight packing, total hepatic vascular isolation with control of both the suprahepatic and infrahepatic venae cavae may be necessary. A sternotomy or thoracotomy may be required to gain access to the suprahepatic vena cava. Atriocaval (Schrock) shunting has been described, but despite its theoretical appeal, is rarely successful. Total hepatic isolation with venovenous bypass has also been described, although few hospitals have this capability readily available.

Massive hepatic trauma quickly leads to physiologic derangements including coagulopathy, hypothermia, or metabolic acidosis. As such, hemorrhage should promptly be controlled and the laparotomy abbreviated in favor of subsequent abdominal angioembolization and a second laparotomy when the patient is physiologically more stable. This "damage control" approach will prevent the development of irreversible physiologic deficits and subsequent death.

After definitive repair of hepatic injuries, the use of drains is controversial. If drains are placed, closed suction drainage is preferred and is associated with fewer infectious complications when compared to sump drains. Postprocedural complications include recurrent bleeding, intrahepatic or perihepatic abscess formation, biloma, and hemobilia. Recurrent bleeding or hemobilia may require reoperation or angioembolization. Abscess and biloma are generally treated by percutaneous drainage. The majority of biliary leaks are self-limited, but high-volume leaks may require endoscopic retrograde cholangiogram with sphincterotomy and/or stent placement.

Splenic Trauma

A history of trauma to the left upper quadrant, flank, or left chest wall should prompt a concern for splenic trauma. Patients with splenic injuries may complain of pain in the left upper quadrant, left shoulder pain, left chest wall discomfort, or abdominal tenderness. As with hepatic trauma, a contrast-enhanced CT scan is both sensitive and specific for splenic trauma.

In the hemodynamically stable patient, isolated blunt splenic injury can be managed nonoperatively. The success of nonoperative management, however, depends on the severity of splenic injury as determined by CT imaging (Table 23.8) and must be made in the context of concurrent injuries and the likelihood of patient compliance.

Patients with isolated low-grade splenic injuries (grades I–III) without evidence of a "blush" on CT scan can be managed initially

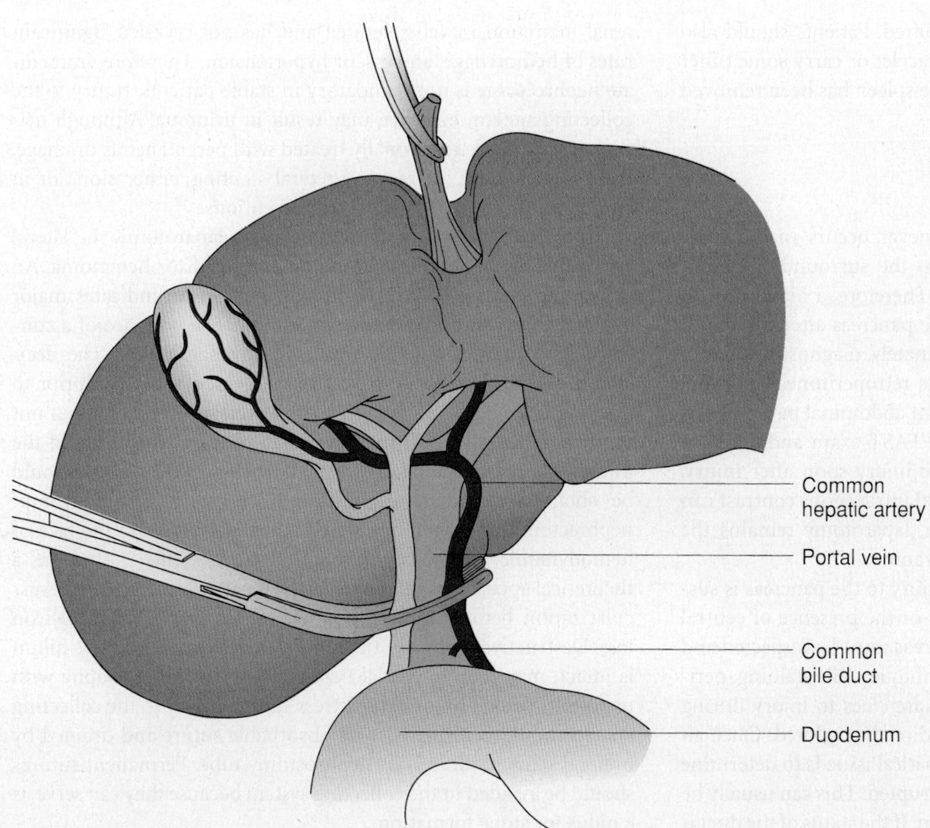

FIGURE 23.6 Pringle Maneuver compression of the portal triad structures with a noncrushing vascular clamp for hepatic inflow control. (From Mulholland MW, Lillemoe KD, Doherty GM et al., eds. *Greenfield's Surgery: Scientific Principles and Practices*, 5th ed. Philadelphia: Lippincott Williams & Wilkins, 2011, with permission.)

with bed rest, serial abdominal examination, close monitoring of vital signs, and serial hemoglobin evaluation. Angioembolization should be considered for all patients with more severe splenic injuries (greater than grade III) and in those with a contrast blush,

TABLE 23.8 The American Association for the Surgery of Trauma (AAST) Grading Scale for splenic injuries

Grade I	Hematoma: subcapsular, <10% of surface area Laceration: capsular tear <1 cm in depth into the parenchyma
Grade II	Hematoma: subcapsular, 10%–50% of surface area Laceration: capsular tear, 1–3 cm in depth, but not involving a trabecular vessel
Grade III	Hematoma: subcapsular, >50% of surface area OR expanding, ruptured subcapsular, or parenchymal hematoma OR intraparenchymal hematoma >5 cm or expanding Laceration: >3 cm in depth or involving a trabecular vessel
Grade IV	Laceration involving segmental or hilar vessels with major devascularization (i.e., >25% of the spleen)
Grade V	Hematoma: shattered spleen Laceration: hilar vascular injury that devascularizes the spleen

moderate hemoperitoneum, or evidence of ongoing bleeding. Although a number of algorithms have been suggested for the nonoperative management of hemodynamically stable splenic injuries, most recommend a period of inpatient observation and bed rest based on the degree of injury. For example, for every grade of injury (I–III), an 8-hour shift in the ICU and 24-hour shift of bed rest are frequently prescribed. Following nonoperative management, it is essential that patients be discharged with a limitation on physical activity especially contact sports. Again, the duration of limitation depends on the severity of injury. Conservatively, a rule of 1 month per grade is recommended. Splenic injuries are not typically followed by serial imaging unless a clinical need arises.

If necessary, the safest operative approach is splenectomy via midline laparotomy. This incision allows access to the spleen as well as inspection of other intra-abdominal structures. If a minor or nonbleeding splenic injury is discovered, splenic salvage may theoretically be considered. Historically, splenic salvage techniques have included splenorrhaphy and partial splenectomy. Splenorrhaphy may be performed using a Vicryl mesh to wrap the spleen. Partial splenic resection is performed with pledgeted mattress sutures. That being said, if there is any concern for hemodynamic compromise or ongoing hemorrhage, splenectomy is the safest option. Patients who undergo splenectomy, as well as those who have had a significant portion of their spleen embolized, should receive vaccinations to pneumococci, meningococci, and *Haemophilus influenza*. Postsplenectomy vaccinations limit but do not completely prevent overwhelming postsplenectomy sepsis (OPSS); a rare but grave complication of total splenectomy. Postsplenectomy vaccinations are frequently given just prior to discharge; however, current recommendations suggest that these vaccines be given at least 14 days postprocedure for maximal immunity. Additional "booster" vaccinations may also be required. Patients should also be encouraged to wear a Medic Alert bracelet or carry some other medical identification indicating that the spleen has been removed or embolized

Pancreatic Injury

Pancreatic injury is rare and almost never occurs in isolation. Moreover, hemorrhage from injuries to the surrounding vascular structures usually takes precedence. Therefore, a high index of suspicion is needed when evaluating the pancreas after trauma in order to avoid missing injuries. Unfortunately, diagnosing pancreatic injury can be challenging. Given its retroperitoneal location, patients frequently do not have significant abdominal pain or peritonitis. Noninvasive studies such as the FAST exam and CT scan are not reliable for detecting pancreatic injury soon after injury. Repeating the CT scan with both oral and intravenous contrast can improve diagnostic sensitivity; however, laparotomy remains the gold standard for excluding pancreatic trauma.

During the trauma laparotomy, if injury to the pancreas is suspected on the basis of missile trajectory or the presence of central hematoma, the entire length of the pancreas must be inspected and palpated utilizing wide mobilization techniques. Bile staining, peripancreatic or periduodenal hematomas are clues to injury during the time of laparotomy and should be directly explored. Once an injury to the pancreas is identified, the critical issue is to determine if the major pancreatic duct has been disrupted. This can usually be accomplished by inspection and palpation. If the status of the duct is unclear, an intraoperative cholangiopancreaticogram or Endoscopic retrograde cholangiopancreatography (ERCP) can be performed. Operative management is then based on the status of the duct itself. The operative principles of managing pancreatic injuries include hemorrhage control, debridement of devitalized tissue, wide closed-suction drainage, and either placement of a nasojejunal feeding tube or a feeding jejunostomy. Injuries involving the pancreatic duct typically require distal pancreatectomy at the point of ductal injury. Severe injuries to the pancreatic head and duodenum that involve the ampulla require a pancreaticoduodenectomy, which should be performed in a staged fashion according to the operative complexity. Pancreatic fistulae are common after pancreatic trauma and are usually managed successfully with nonoperative management.

Genitourinary Tract

Hematuria, either gross or microscopic, is the most common presenting sign of genitourinary tract trauma. That being said, the *absence* of hematuria does not necessarily exclude genitourinary tract trauma. Therefore, renal injury should be considered in any blunt trauma victim with impact to the back and flanks, especially in the presence of posterior rib fractures. Renal injuries after blunt trauma are most commonly diagnosed by CT scan, which may demonstrate renal laceration, contusion, perinephric hematoma, collecting system disruption, or devascularization. In the absence of active hemorrhage, nearly all renal injuries heal without intervention including those with urinary extravasation. Arteriography and selective embolization should be considered for those patients with a contrast "blush" on CT scan or those with persistent gross hematuria.

Traditionally, nephrectomy has been advocated for hemodynamically stable patients with severe grade V renal injury ("shattered kidney") or renal infarction. However, expectant management of renal infarction is well tolerated and has not revealed significant rates of hemorrhage, abscess, or hypertension. Therefore, immediate nephrectomy is not mandatory in stable patients. Injury to the collecting system, however, may result in urinoma. Although urinomas have been traditionally treated with percutaneous drainage, there is increasing interest in ureteral stenting, either alone or in combination with percutaneous interventions.

If a renal injury is suspected during a laparotomy, the lateral retroperitoneum (zone 2) should be examined for hematoma. An expanding hematoma irrespective of mechanism indicates major vascular injury and mandates exploration. The presence of a contralateral kidney should be confirmed by palpation. The decision of whether or not to gain proximal vascular control prior to opening Gerota's fascia is highly controversial but likely does not improve renal salvage. If the hematoma obscures the hilum of the injured kidney, proximal and distal aortic and IVC control should be obtained quickly. A significant hilar injury should prompt nephrectomy, as should any significant renal injury in the face of hemodynamic instability. Although renal revascularization has a theoretical appeal, it is rare to make the diagnosis and achieve revascularization before warm ischemia leads to irreversible nephron loss. Destructive lesions of the renal parenchyma, where the hilum is intact, may require partial nephrectomy and renorrhaphy with use of pledgeted horizontal mattress suture. Injury to the collecting system should be repaired with absorbable suture and drained by ureteral stent (double J) or nephrostomy tube. Permanent sutures should be avoided in the collecting system because they can serve as a nidus for stone formation.

Nonexpanding hematomas of the lateral retroperitoneum should not be routinely explored in blunt trauma patients. For victims of penetrating trauma, this remains controversial. Because injury to the collecting system cannot be excluded, the safest approach in penetrating trauma to zone II is to evaluate the kidney directly by exploring the organ.

Ureteral injury is rare in blunt injury but should be suspected in patients with microscopic hematuria and no other genitourinary tract injury. Following a penetrating injury to the flank, the ureter requires evaluation and even exploration based on trajectory. Ureteral injury should be repaired primarily with absorbable suture over a double J stent after debriding and spatulating the cut ends to avoid stricture. If primary ureteroureterostomy is not feasible because of tension, options include mobilizing both the kidney and bladder, creating a psoas bladder hitch, or constructing a Boari flap (bladder tube neoureter). Although transureteroureterostomy has been described, it places the noninjured kidney at risk and should not be performed.

Trauma to the urethra or bladder should be considered in all patients with severe pelvic trauma or straddle type injuries. Physical findings include blood at the urethral meatus, scrotal or labial hematoma, and/or abnormal position of the prostate on rectal examination. If any of these signs are present, retrograde urethrogram should be performed prior to placement of a Foley catheter in the male. If no urethral injury is identified, bladder catheterization can be safely performed. Return of gross hematuria on Foley placement should prompt a cystogram to rule out bladder injury. Classically, a plain film cystogram is utilized with two views of the contrast-filled bladder (AP and oblique) followed by a postvoid film. Recently, CT cystogram has emerged as an option.

The anatomic location of the bladder injury will dictate management. Extraperitoneal bladder injuries are typically managed by Foley catheter drainage alone, whereas intraperitoneal bladder injuries require formal operative repair followed by Foley catheter drainage. Bladder injuries are repaired in two or three layers with absorbable suture to create a watertight seal. Closed suction drains should be placed adjacent to the repair. A suprapubic catheter is almost never required as a supplement to Foley catheter drainage after bladder repair.

Hollow Viscus Injury

Hollow viscus injury following blunt trauma is difficult to diagnose in the acute setting. The physical examination may be unreliable because of altered mental status or distracting injuries. Moreover, it can take up to 6 hours before symptoms of peritoneal irritation develop. The presence of an abdominopelvic "seat belt sign" (hematomas or contusions) should alert the physician to possible intestinal and mesenteric injury caused by abrupt deceleration. With sudden deceleration, the intra-abdominal viscera can be avulsed from the mesentery, especially near relatively fixed areas such as the ileocecal valve. The presence of an anterior lumbar compression fracture (Chance fracture) suggests extreme hyperflexion, and injuries to the duodenum, proximal jejunum, and pancreas should be suspected.

CT scan can be used to evaluate hollow viscous injury but with certain key caveats; a *completely* normal abdominopelvic CT is sufficiently accurate to *rule out* hollow viscus injury with a negative predictive value of 99.6%. CT signs suggestive of hollow viscus injury include bowel wall thickening, free intra-abdominal fluid (in the absence of solid organ injury), mesenteric stranding, and extraluminal air seen. CT findings concerning for bowel injury warrant surgical exploration. Stable patients with any equivocal CT results should be admitted for observation including serial physical examination and serial labs (amylase and white blood cell count). Patients with fever, changes in vital signs, worsening physical examination findings, or new leukocytosis should undergo urgent operative exploration.

All victims of penetrating injury to the anterior abdomen with facial violation should be considered to have a bowel injury. Although various treatment algorithms have been proposed in recent literature, exploratory laparotomy should be the default management of penetrating abdominal trauma. FAST and DPL may be falsely negative immediately postinjury, and a CT scan is not indicated in this setting.

At laparotomy, the bowel should be examined in its entirety including both sides of the stomach, the entire small intestine, the colon, the visible rectum, and, if indicated by missile trajectory or by adjacent hematoma, the entire duodenum. Contamination by enteric contents should be rapidly controlled with figure-of-eight sutures, umbilical ties, or Babcock clamps until all injuries are identified. Definitive repair begins with debridement of nonviable edges. Primary repair may be considered if the resulting defect is less than 50% of the circumference of the bowel. Defects should be closed in two layers transversely to avoid luminal compromise. More extensive injury or concern on the part of the surgeon should prompt segmental resection with anastomosis. Serosal tears and bowel wall hematomas should imbricated with Lembert silk suture.

Colonic injuries are common after penetrating injuries but can also occur after blunt trauma. During exploration, the entire colon is inspected, and small injuries with minimal contamination can be debrided and repaired in two layers. More significant injuries require segmental or anatomic resection, with primary anastomosis. In the presence of shock, heavy contamination, or destructive injury, a colonic resection with colostomy may be indicated. Traditionally, the threshold for performing colostomy for left colon injuries is lower than for right colon injuries, although there appears to be no difference in anastomotic breakdown based on anatomic location. If there is doubt about primary repair or diverting colostomy, the surgeon is best advised to perform colostomy after resection. Colostomy is best done out of the zone of injury.

Intraperitoneal rectal injuries are managed as if they were colonic injuries. Minor injuries can be debrided and repaired primarily. Significant injuries require resection and creation of a Hartmann's pouch with end colostomy. Extraperitoneal rectal injuries, on the other hand, have traditionally been managed by the "three Ds": diversion, distal washout, and presacral drainage. Although diversion can be either loop or end colostomy, creating a loop colostomy is significantly less morbid and can be reversed several weeks later if barium enema confirms healing. Presacral drainage and distal rectal washout, however, are rarely performed since their efficacy in preventing pelvic sepsis has never been proven in civilian trauma

Retroperitoneal Hematoma

Penetrating injuries to the back and flank can injure both intra- and retroperitoneal structures. The management of retroperitoneal hematomas is based both on injury mechanism as well as anatomic zone (Fig. 23.5). Given the central location of zone 1, there is a high likelihood of major injury to the aorta, vena cave, porta hepatis, pancreas, and duodenum. Zone 1 hematomas are always explored regardless of mechanism or size of hematoma. Zone 2 is lateral to zone 1 and includes the renal pedicle as well as the kidney on either side. Zone 2 hematomas caused by penetrating injuries are explored, while those caused by blunt trauma are observed. Zone 3 is inferior to zone 1 and includes the iliac vessels and sacral venous plexus. Penetrating injuries to zone 3 should be explored, although controlling the iliac vessels and their branches can be difficult. Venous control with direct pressure usually stems the bleeding enough to allow dissection and placement of vessel loops above and below the injury. Occasionally, the right iliac artery may need to be divided in order to gain access to the right iliac vein. While the pelvic veins can be ligated in cases of exsanguinating hemorrhage, the iliac arteries must be repaired or shunted. In contrast, zone 3 hematomas associated with blunt trauma should be left alone. These hematomas are frequently associated with pelvic fractures. Incising the pelvic peritoneum and dissecting the hematoma can release tamponade and cause massive life-threatening bleeding. In these circumstances, the pelvis should be packed and the patient brought to interventional radiology for potential angioembolization.

Extremity Trauma

The extremities are commonly injured by both blunt and penetrating mechanisms. The vascular integrity and neurologic function of the injured extremity must be rapidly assessed. With simple physical examination, most vascular injuries can easily diagnosed by the presence of "hard" and "soft" signs. *Hard signs* mandate immediate intervention and include (i) absent or diminished pulses, (ii) pulsatile bleeding, (iii) expanding or pulsatile hematoma, (iv) palpable thrill or bruit, and (v) evidence of distal ischemia. *Soft signs* include proximity of the wound to a major artery, small nonpulsatile hematoma, neurologic deficit, and prehospital history of "pulsatile

TABLE 23.9 Hard/soft signs of vascular injury

- Hard signs
  - Pulsatile bleeding
  - Expanding or pulsatile hematoma
  - Absent distal pulse
  - Palpable thrill or audible bruit
  - Signs of distal ischemia (6 Ps)
    - Pain
    - Pallor
    - Pulselessness
    - Paresthesias
    - Poikilothermia (temperature change)
    - Paralysis
- Soft signs
  - Proximity to known vessel
  - History of pulsatile bleeding
  - Neurologic deficit
  - Small, nonpulsatile hematoma

bleeding." Although these signs do not require immediate intervention in the absence of a deficit, they should increase the surgeon's awareness of possible vascular injury and lead to further evaluation or serial examination (Table 23.9). Consideration should be given to the use of a tourniquet for major vascular injuries as a temporizing measure prior to operative repair. Vascular injuries associated with open fractures should also be treated with systemic antibiotics and tetanus prophylaxis.

In addition to palpating pulses, the initial vascular examination of the injured extremity includes an ankle–brachial index (ABI). This simple diagnostic maneuver compares the systolic pressure of the affected extremity to that of an uninjured extremity using a handheld Doppler and manual blood pressure cuff. A normal ABI is greater than or equal to 1.0 and usually requires no further workup. An ABI less than 0.9 indicates a high probability of a vascular injury requiring operative intervention. Interventional angiography is reserved for those patients with ABIs between 0.9 and 1.0. Angiography may also be indicated with soft signs of injury, multilevel injury (gunshot), or where clinical suspicion is high.

Vascular injury after blunt trauma is most often caused by long bone fracture or joint dislocation (e.g., knee) with arterial compromise. An absent pulse may return after a fracture is placed in alignment or a joint is relocated. Both a pulse exam and an ABI should be performed after reduction with subsequent workup as needed. The surgeon must be mindful that intimal injuries may be present and serial vascular exams must be performed. Given the high likelihood of a popliteal injury in the setting of a knee dislocation, either a traditional angiogram or screening CTA should be performed.

Penetrating extremity injuries require rapid determination of trajectory by examination of the wound locations and radiographic localization of any foreign bodies. Physical examination including ABI measurement guides the workup. Hard signs of vascular injury lead the surgeon directly to the OR. A tourniquet above the injury or direct pressure can be used to control external hemorrhage until operative control can be obtained.

An operative "on-table" angiogram can be performed by accessing the artery proximal to the injury. If available, digital subtraction angiography is recommended. A direct approach to the injured vessel with an incision over the area of injury can be used for immediate vascular exploration. Alternatively, if hemorrhage is controlled with direct pressure, a femoral or high brachial cut down can be used to provide proximal control before the area of injury is explored. After identifying the injury, proximal and distal vascular control allows bidirectional embolectomy, local heparinization, and subsequent repair. Proximal, large vessel injuries can be repaired with interpositions of either artificial material such as polytetrafluoroethylene (PTFE) or autogenous reversed saphenous vein with relatively equal outcomes provided the wound is clean and does not have extensive soft tissue damage. In contaminated or compromised wounds, an autogenous bypass is preferable. Distal vascular repairs and "bypasses" should also use autogenous saphenous vein given their higher long-term patency. A completion angiogram must be performed after every repair with the surgeon prepared to redo any unsatisfactory anastomosis. If necessary, wide debridement of damaged tissue is then carried out. Prophylactic four compartment fasciotomy should be consider in any patient with interruption of arterial flow greater than 6 hours, a history of hemodynamic instability or concomitant venous injury. Although not specifically studied in trauma patients, there is increasing enthusiasm for starting a statin and aspirin postoperatively.

Mangled Extremity/Crush Syndrome

The mangled extremity deserves special mention owing to the tremendous complexity of care and the great potential for associated complications. The mangled extremity is most frequently seen following farm machinery and industrial mishaps, high-speed motorcycle crashes, and combat explosions. These devastating injuries are accompanied by concomitant soft tissue, bony, vascular, and often nerve injury. Although most severely injured extremities can be salvaged with an aggressive multidisciplinary approach, the trauma surgeon, as the team leader, must keep the patient's overall condition as the central focus. The Mangled Extremity Severity Score (MESS) may be helpful in terms of predicting which patients may benefit from amputation rather than attempted salvage. The MESS takes into consideration the degree and contamination of the bone and soft tissue injury, evidence of limb ischemia, the degree of shock, and the patient's age (Table 23.10). While the MESS ranges from 2 to 14 (14 being most severe), a score greater than 7 suggests a poor prognosis for limb viability. Factors predictive of a poor outcome include prolonged ischemia (longer than 6 hours), age older than 50 years, crush injury, significant comorbidities (diabetes, smoking, and heart disease), and major neurologic injury to the extremity. Prolonged ischemia, however, is the only absolute contraindication to attempted limb salvage. In the presence of these factors, limb salvage may be more detrimental than early amputation. In general, named nerve disruption with an insensate foot, ischemia, and large soft tissue and bone defects predict very poor long-term outcome and the need for eventual amputation.

If the decision is made to proceed with limb salvage, early restoration of blood flow must be a priority, and preoperative discussions between the orthopedic, vascular, and trauma specialists are needed to plan the best approach. Depending on the clinical scenario, surgeons must decide between immediate revascularization versus temporary shunting and internal versus external fixation. The patient's clinical condition and the amount of contamination present guide these decisions. Typically, these injuries will require multiple surgeries and washout procedures with eventual muscle flap and skin graft closure of remaining wounds.

TABLE 23.10 The mangled extremity severity score

Limb ischemia	
1 pt	Reduced pulse but normal perfusion
2 pt	Pulseless, paresthesias, cold capillary refill
3 pt	Cool, paralysis, numb/insensate
Age	
0 pt	<30 y
1 pt	30–50 y
2 pt	≥50 y
Shock	
0 pt	SBP > 90 mm Hg consistently
1 pt	Hypotension transiently
2 pt	Persistent hypotension
Injury mechanism	
1 pt	Low energy (stab, gunshot, simple fracture)
2 pt	Medium energy (dislocation, open/multiple fractures)
3 pt	High energy (high-speed MVC (motor vehicle crash) or rifle shot)
4 pt	Very high energy (high-speed trauma with gross contamination)

Crush syndrome can occur with any severely injured extremity and refers to the metabolic derangements that occur after restoration of blood flow. It is caused by rhabdomyolysis with systemic manifestations of ischemia–reperfusion injury including shock, acidosis, hyperkalemia, myoglobinuria, and, at times, acute renal failure. In severe cases, multiorgan failure occurs with cardiac dysfunction, respiratory failure, and dialysis dependence.

The diagnosis of crush syndrome requires a high index of suspicion. The urine is usually dark tea colored. Although the diagnosis of myoglobinuria confirms the diagnosis, this is usually a send-out test that may take several days. A quicker study is to send the urine for routine analysis. The diagnosis is made if the urine is positive for hemoglobin in the absence of red blood cells. Patients suspected of developing crush syndrome should have serial labs (CK, electrolytes, and acid–base status). Worrisome trends should prompt preemptive intervention with aggressive crystalloid resuscitation and potentially forced diuresis with furosemide. Although mannitol diuresis and urine alkalinization with bicarbonate have been proposed in the past, they do not appear to be more beneficial than aggressive resuscitation. Early dialysis is indicated in the setting of persistent hyperkalemia, acidosis, or oliguria. Muscle beds should be examined for devitalized tissue requiring debridement, and in some cases, amputation will be lifesaving.

Compartment Syndrome and Fasciotomy

A compartment syndrome occurs when pressures within fascia-restricted compartments exceed the perfusion pressure therein causing tissue ischemia. Over time, the increased pressure causes muscle and nerve cell death that can result in a devastating loss of function with significant morbidity. In extremity trauma, swelling and bleeding are the most common factors causing elevated pressures with vascular injury, crush injury, and fractures being the usual culprits.

The keys to preventing compartment syndrome after extremity trauma include a high index of suspicion, pattern recognition, and the liberal use of fasciotomy in the appropriate clinical setting. In reality, the morbidity of fasciotomy is low compared to that of the compartment syndrome, and certain injury constellations should lead the surgeon to perform prophylactic fasciotomy at the time of the initial surgery. Injuries that benefit from prophylactic fasciotomy include (i) crush injuries, (ii) prolonged ischemia time (longer than 6 hours) prior to reestablishing perfusion, and (iii) combined arterial and venous injuries.

In patients with extremity trauma who have not undergone fasciotomy, recognition of compartment syndrome can be difficult. Typical symptoms and signs occur late after tissue death has occurred. Symptoms include pain out of proportion to examination and paresthesias. Signs include a cool and tense swollen extremity, pain on passive stretch, sensory nerve deficits, and progressive motor weakness. In the lower extremity, the first sign may be numbness in the first digital web space because of compression of the deep peroneal nerve in the anterior compartment. Pulselessness is a very late sign and indicates extremely high compartment pressure. Because tissue perfusion pressure is only 25 mm Hg, compartment pressures of only 30 mm Hg cause muscle ischemia while allowing a normal blood pressure to be transmitted to the distal extremity. Therefore, a palpable pulse does not exclude the compartment syndrome. If clinical suspicion suggests elevated compartment pressures, they should be quantified with a special monitoring device (Stryker needle) or with a modified arterial-line transducer setup. If compartment pressures exceed 25 to 30 mm Hg or if clinical suspicion is high, fasciotomies should be performed.

Compartment syndrome can occur in any part of any extremity, but the lower leg is by far the most common site. It has four compartments that are generally accessed by a two-incision fasciotomy. The anterior and lateral compartments are accessible through a lateral incision, whereas the superficial and deep posterior compartments can be released through a medial incision. Incisions should be generous to decompress the entire compartment, as inadequate fasciotomies may not prevent compartment syndrome. The muscle should be assessed at the time of fasciotomy, but only grossly necrotic tissue should be debrided. All other tissues can be reinspected at a later time to assess recovery and viability utilizing conservative debridement. Postoperatively, the extremity should be elevated and nonrestrictive circumferential bandage applied.

Fasciotomy incisions can often be closed within 5 to 10 days. The goal is to provide skin coverage of the muscle, and reapproximation of the fascia should not be attempted. Techniques include primary skin closure or split-thickness skin grafting. Vessel loops applied in a crisscross or "Roman sandal" to the skin edge can apply constant tension and improve the opportunity for skin closure. Often only one side can be closed primarily owing to excessive tension. In this setting, the lateral incision should be closed primarily for cosmetic purposes and to allow comfort when crossing one's legs. The medial side can then undergo skin grafting.

DAMAGE CONTROL

Damage control, or early termination of operative procedures, is recognized as one of the major advances in surgical care in recent history. This concept evolved from the realization that, during exsanguinating hemorrhage, patients die from a triad of coagulopathy, hypothermia, and metabolic acidosis. Once this metabolic

TABLE 23.11 Factors for pattern recognition leading to damage control application

Conditions
• High-energy blunt torso trauma
• Multiple torso penetrations
• Hemodynamic instability
• Coagulopathy or hypothermia at presentation
Complexes
• Combined major abdominal vascular injury and major visceral injury
• Multifocal or multicavitary bleeding with concomitant visceral injury
• Multiregional injury with competing priorities
Critical factors
• Severe metabolic acidosis (pH < 7.30)
• Hypothermia (temperature <35°C)
• Resuscitation and operative time >90 min
• Coagulopathy (nonmechanical bleeding)

TABLE 23.12 Phases of damage control from abdominal trauma

1. Operative control of hemorrhage and contamination
a. Control of active hemorrhage
b. Pack solid organ injuries
c. Resect injured bowel without anastomosis
d. Rapid temporary abdominal closure
2. Retreat to surgical intensive care unit (SICU)
a. Aggressive resuscitation with blood products
b. Active rewarming
c. Correction of coagulopathy
3. Reoperation
a. Complete reexploration
b. Remove packing
c. Complete vascular repairs
d. Restore gastrointestinal continuity
e. Facial closure (if possible)

failure has developed, it is often intractable and terminal. Victims of multiple trauma and other acute surgical emergencies are more likely to die from metabolic failure rather than from failure to achieve a technically complete operation. From this knowledge arose the theory that early operative termination, with retreat to the ICU for physiologic and metabolic recovery, could allow patients to regain metabolic stability and survive. Once stable, the patient could then be returned for staged operative repair of injuries.

The trauma surgeon must rely on pattern recognition to help identify, as rapidly as possible, those patients who require an abbreviated procedure in order to prevent metabolic failure. Pattern recognition incorporates certain "conditions, complexes, and critical factors" that serve to alert the surgeon that prolonged operative efforts to achieve technical completion of all repairs may be detrimental. Patients with high-energy mechanism or abnormal physiologic status on presentation, severe combined vascular and visceral injuries, multicavitary bleeding, or prolonged operative times should all be considered for "damage control" and subsequent staged procedures (Table 23.11).

The damage control approach to the severely injured patient is a three-stage procedure (Table 23.12). In the first stage of damage control, the priorities are *rapid and simple* control of hemorrhage and contamination. Once the decision is made to abbreviate the initial procedure, all efforts must concentrate on this goal. Simple techniques, such as "stapling off" injured bowel segments rather than restoring bowel continuity and ligating (or shunting) bleeding vessels rather than repairing them, help keep operative times short. Liberal packing of nonarterial bleeding and rapid temporary abdominal closure complete the initial procedure.

The second stage of damage control is a return to the ICU for aggressive rewarming, resuscitation, and restoration of normal physiology. Correction of metabolic acidosis and coagulopathy with biologically active colloid blood products is performed with frequent laboratory monitoring to assess progress. Failure of metabolic parameters to normalize may indicate ongoing surgical bleeding from inadequate hemorrhage control and should lead the surgeon back to the OR.

After correction of the metabolic derangement, which typically takes 24 to 48 hours, patients are ready to be returned to the OR. This third stage of damage control requires a careful and complete abdominal reexploration with removal of packing, definitive repair of injuries, restoration of intestinal continuity, and abdominal wall closure if possible provided that the patient's physiologic status remains normal. If there is evidence of recurrent metabolic failure, the surgeon must have the confidence to terminate the procedure and again retreat to the ICU. Occasionally, patients may require prolonged "open" abdominal management and eventually require abdominal closure with split-thickness skin grafting. In these cases, it is best to minimize the number of anastomosis and avoid placement of surgical feeding access. The open abdomen is a hostile environment in which sutures lines are at increased risk of failure and any hole in the viscera is likely to enlarge.

Lastly, it is important to note that although most commonly applied to abdominal trauma, the concept of damage control can be used in any traumatic or emergent surgical situation where metabolic failure occurs. Septic abdominal catastrophes from perforated viscus and ruptured aortic aneurysm are common examples where damage control can be lifesaving. The same tenets of pattern recognition and early decision making can achieve survival when operative persistence would lead to death. Interestingly, damage control techniques have also been described in orthopedic and neurologic surgery.

THE PREGNANT TRAUMA VICTIM

Trauma complicates an estimated 1 in 10 pregnancies and is the leading nonobstetric cause of maternal death. Although pregnant women can be injured in motor vehicle crashes and falls, domestic abuse and intimate partner violence account for most cases of death. While the initial evaluation and treatment priorities of the pregnant trauma patient do not differ from trauma management in general, there are a few important maternal–fetal issues that warrant special consideration. Additionally, patients may present to the trauma center unaware of their pregnancy or unable to convey their condition to the trauma team. Therefore, pregnancy should be considered as a possibility in all women of childbearing age (10 to 50 years) with routine use of pregnancy testing.

When evaluating and treating the injured pregnant patient, the surgeon must recognize that the priority is to save the mother, thereby saving the fetus as well. Although unnecessary interventions should be avoided in all patients, essential diagnostic or therapeutic procedures must not be withheld from the pregnant patient solely for fear of harming the fetus. The best possible outcome for both the patient and fetus is early, rapid, and efficient diagnosis and treatment of sustained injuries. In particular, the use of CT scans and other radiographic imaging should not be withheld if clinically indicated. Delays in diagnosis or missed injuries lead to significantly increased maternal–fetal morbidity and mortality. Moreover, the indications for operative intervention do not differ from non-pregnant trauma patients.

Anatomic and Physiologic Changes in Pregnancy

Normal physiologic changes during pregnancy can alter the physical findings and response to injury after trauma. Cardiovascular changes, in particular, can complicate the trauma assessment. Although there is a 15% increase in red blood cell mass with pregnancy, there is a concomitant 30% to 40% increase in plasma volume. This results in a dilutional "anemia," and the hemoglobin may be as low as 11 g/dL in an otherwise healthy pregnant patient. Additionally, pregnancy is associated with a 10 to 15 beat increase in pulse rate and hormone-mediated vasodilation results in relative hypotension (systolic blood pressure of approximately 105 mm Hg). This increased preload and decreased afterload creates a 25% increase in cardiac output. Importantly, late in pregnancy, the weight of the gravid uterus in the supine position may occlude the vena cava, thereby reducing venous return and dramatically limiting cardiac output.

Important pulmonary and airway changes in pregnancy may also complicate the trauma evaluation. With increasing gestational age, the uterus displaces the diaphragm and decreases pulmonary functional residual capacity (FRC). In addition, estrogen and progesterone significantly impair gastrointestinal motility leading to increased gastric distention and risk of aspiration with emergent intubation.

Assessment and Management

The initial evaluation and management of the pregnant patient are identical to that of other trauma victims. Airway, breathing, and circulation are assessed, and interventions are initiated quickly. Circulatory stability is improved by placing the patient in the left lateral decubitus position, thus relieving IVC compression by the gravid uterus. One must remember that with the expanded intravascular volume of the pregnant patient, significant blood loss may occur before signs of shock are present. Furthermore, during early shock, the maternal circulation will shunt blood away from the uterus depriving the fetal perfusion as a compensatory mechanism. As such, the fetus may be in distress, while the mother is relatively asymptomatic. Indeed, an increase in fetal heart rate may be the earliest sign of significant blood loss and hemodynamic instability.

The secondary survey in the pregnant patient includes a thorough prenatal history, obstetric examination, and fetal monitoring. A comprehensive prenatal history should include the last menstrual period, the expected delivery date, and a recent history of fetal movement. Additionally, any history of pregnancy-induced hypertension, gestational diabetes, or other complicating factors should be documented, and the patient's obstetrician should be notified. On physical examination, the uterine fundal height can be used to estimate fetal age: at 20 weeks, the uterus is at the level of the umbilicus and grows roughly 1 cm/week thereafter. The secondary examination should specifically evaluate the presence of vaginal bleeding, premature rupture of membranes, perineal bulging, uterine contractions, or an abnormal fetal heart rate or rhythm. The abnormal presence of amniotic fluid or blood on sterile vaginal examination and the degree of cervical effacement or dilation must also be noted.

Secondary diagnostic testing is essential when evaluating the gravid trauma patient. Ultrasonography is performed early to confirm or modify fetal age, to assess the fetal position, and to examine the placenta for evidence of abruption. In addition, beyond 20 to 24 weeks of gestation, cardiotocographic monitoring (CTM) is indicated to correlate any maternal contractions with changes in fetal heart rate. Both bradycardia (<110 bpm) and tachycardia (>160 bpm) are indicative of fetal distress. Patients with frequent contractions (>6 per hour), abdominal pain, vaginal bleeding, hypotension, or an altered cervical examination should have a minimum 24 hours of CTM.

Although radiation exposure is an important concern in the first 8 weeks of gestation (the period of organogenesis), it is much less important as the fetus enters the second and third trimesters. The accepted limit for direct fetal radiation exposure is less than 10 rads (0.10 Gy), and the risk to the fetus with direct exposure of less than 5 rads (0.05 Gy) is extremely small. Furthermore, with proper shielding of the abdomen and pelvis, actual direct fetal exposure with nonregional radiography is quite limited. Therefore, it must be stressed again that despite any concerns on the part of the mother or trauma team members about fetal radiation exposure, essential radiographic studies should not be withheld during the trauma evaluation. This includes abdominopelvic CT scans in patients in whom there is concern for intra-abdominal injury. Abdominopelvic CT results in a direct fetal radiation exposure that is estimated at only 0.5 rads (0.005 Gy).

In addition to routine trauma labs, all pregnant patients should have their Rh status and the presence of fetal hemoglobin determined. Fetal hemoglobin F (HbF) in the maternal circulations can be detected in a maternal sample by using commercial kits that rely on differential staining between HbF and adult hemoglobin A (HbA). This is a quantitative test that can be used to estimate the volume of fetomaternal transfusion. A positive test indicates the possibility of maternal sensitization to fetal blood in the Rh-negative mother and should prompt the administration of Rh immune globulin (RhoGAM) (300 μg per 30 mL of estimated fetomaternal transfusion) within 72 hours. The volume of fetomaternal transfusion also correlates with the risk of spontaneous miscarriage after trauma.

Because the likelihood of fetal viability is high after a gestational age greater than 20 to 24 weeks, early obstetric consultation is indicated in such patients. Furthermore, most patients in this group, irrespective of injury or mechanism, will be monitored for cardiotocographic changes for 24 hours on an obstetric ward and are typically released at the discretion of the evaluating obstetrician. Evidence of placental abruption in a gestationally viable pregnancy will typically prompt immediate operative delivery.

In cases of maternal arrest, a perimortem cesarean section should be considered if the fetus is greater than or equal to 24 weeks. Although it is recommended that cesarean be performed within 4 minutes of maternal arrest, this procedure can sometimes result in a viable delivery if performed within 20 minutes of maternal death. Fetal neurologic outcome, however, is directly related to the delivery time following maternal cardiac arrest. In contrast to elective procedures, a perimortem cesarean section is performed via generous midline laparotomy. Similarly, the uterus is entered with care to avoid injuring the fetus via midline vertical incision.

Suggested Readings

EAST Practice Management Guidelines: www.east.org

Feliciano DV, Moore EE, Mattox ML, eds. *Trauma*. 7th ed. New York: McGraw-Hill; 2012.

Peitzman AB, Schwab CW, Yealy DM, et al., eds. *The Trauma Manual: Trauma and Acute Care Surgery*. 4th ed. Philadelphia: Lippincott Williams & Wilkins; 2012.

Trauma and emergency care. In: Cameron J, ed. *Current Surgical Therapy*. 11th ed. Philadelphia: Elsevier Mosby; 2013:981–1143.

Surgical practice: Trauma. In: Mulholland MW, Lillemoe KD, Doherty GM, et al., eds. *Greenfield's Surgery: Scientific Principles and Practice*. 5th ed. Philadelphia: Lippincott Williams & Wilkins; 2010.

Western Trauma Association Algorithms: www.westerntrauma.org/algorithms/algorithms.html

CHAPTER

24

Burn Management

LINDSAY E. KUO AND PATRICK K. KIM

KEY POINTS

- Initial assessment of all burn victims must focus on airway, breathing, and circulation (the ABCs) to identify and treat any immediate life-threatening injuries.
- Burn shock is a result of hypovolemia due to fluid shifts. Most adults with burns greater than 15% of their TBSA require fluid resuscitation. The amount of fluid infused is initially calculated from the Parkland formula (4 mL lactated Ringer solution/kg/% TBSA, given over 24 hours) but should be adjusted on the basis of the patient's hemodynamic status and urine output.
- Inhalation injury should be suspected in all burn patients and can greatly increase fluid resuscitation needs. Upper airway injuries can be immediately life threatening, and caregivers must have a low threshold to intubate burn victims early for airway protection. Lower airway injuries are generally responsible for delayed mortality.
- Topical antibiotics are used to prevent local burn wound colonization from becoming burn wound infection. Systemic antibiotics are reserved for treating burn wound infection and systemic infections such as pneumonia but are not used to treat burn wounds prophylactically.
- Early excision and grafting of any wound that will not heal within 3 weeks (deep partial- and full-thickness burns) decrease mortality and improve functional and cosmetic outcomes. Autologous skin is the first choice for wound coverage.
- Burn victims require adequate nutrition to fuel the metabolic response to the burn. Enteral nutrition should be provided as soon as possible. High-protein and high-calorie enteral nutrition improves wound healing and anabolism, although it has had no proven direct effect on mortality.

INTRODUCTION

Significant burns account for approximately 450,000 hospital and clinic visits, 40,000 hospital admissions, and 3,400 deaths each year. Patient survival and quality of life have been greatly improved by advancements in fluid resuscitation and local wound care.

Injury is most commonly the result of thermal burns, and the pathophysiology and treatment is described in the next section. Electrical burns, chemical burns, and frostbite can also lead to significant morbidity and will subsequently be described as special cases.

THERMAL BURNS

Local Burn Wound Injury

Adult skin has a surface area of 1.5 to 2.0 m^2. Skin has an outer layer of epidermis consisting of a keratinized squamous epithelium that extends into underlying dermal appendages. The underlying dermis provides flexibility, support, and strength through its attachment to subcutaneous tissues (Fig. 24.1). Skin functions as a protective barrier that has thermoregulatory, neurosensory, immunologic, and metabolic functions.

Burns damage skin in several ways. The initial heat energy causes cell membrane damage, protein denaturation, and surface vessel thrombosis. After the initial heat-mediated injury, there is an inflammatory process that can cause local tissue destruction. This destruction manifests as three histologic zones of injury. The zone of coagulation is at the center of the burn injury and is the most severely damaged area of tissue because cells are necrotic and unsalvageable. In the surrounding zone of stasis, the cells are viable but vulnerable to further injury. The deeper and most peripheral zone of hyperemia is an area characterized by vasodilatation and minimal tissue damage.

Burn depth is assessed visually. These depths are classified as *superficial*, *partial-thickness*, or *full-thickness* burns (Table 24.1). Treatment protocol is dependent on the depth of the burn.

In addition to depth, the severity of burns is described by the percentage of the total body surface area (TBSA) that is covered by partial- and full-thickness burns. This percentage is estimated most commonly by the "rule of 9s," in which the body is divided into 11 parts, each making up 9% with the perineum making up 1% of TBSA (Fig. 24.2). However, the rule of 9s is inaccurate in young children, as their head and thighs represent a much greater percentage of the TBSA relative to adults. Formal burn diagrams, available in any emergency department, are more accurate and can help avoid miscalculations.

Burn wounds heal by a combination of contraction and reepithelialization from epidermal cells lining the periphery of the wound and dermal appendages. In general, burn depth is associated with scar formation;

Systemic Effects of Burn Wound Injury

Cardiovascular Effects

Burns not only cause local damage, but extensive burns can have several physiologic consequences. Burns greater than 35% to 40% TBSA usually result in a set of cardiovascular derangements known as burn shock: decreased cardiac output, decreased plasma volume, and oliguria. Following thermal injury, there is a significant

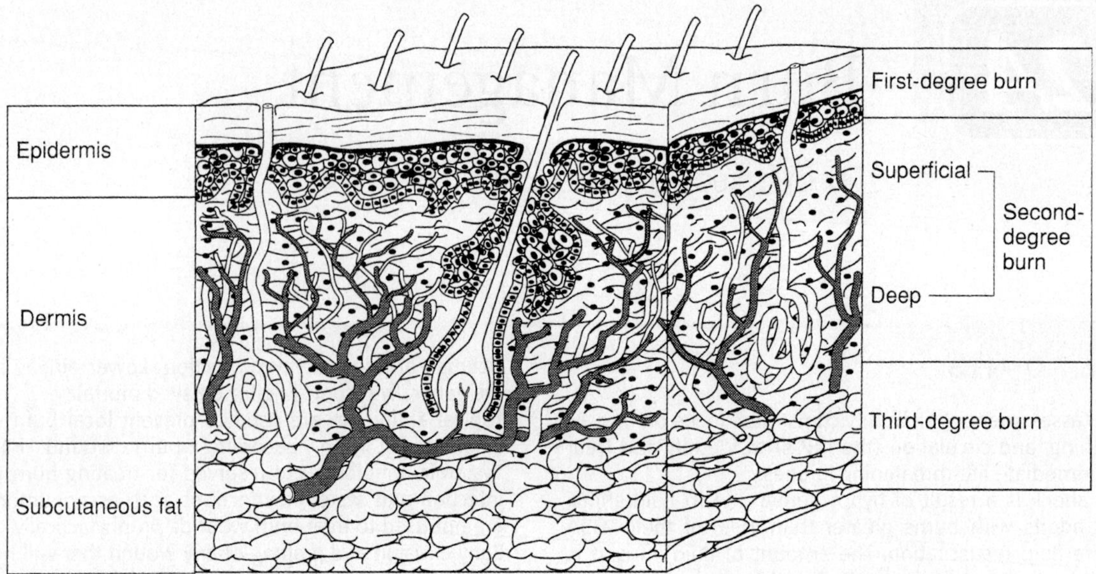

FIGURE 24.1 Depiction of skin. Degree of burn injury is classified based on depth of penetration. (From Sheridan RL, Tompkins RG. Burns. In: Greenfield LJ, Mulholand MW, Oldham KT, et al., eds. *Surgery: Scientific Principles and Practice*. 2nd ed. Philadelphia: Lippincott-Raven Publishers; 1997:423, with permission.)

inflammatory response causing a massive fluid shift from the intravascular to the interstitial space; simultaneously, there is direct extravasation of plasma into the burn site. These processes result in effective arterial hypovolemia that requires large amounts of resuscitative fluids to correct. In patients with burns greater than 20% to 30% TBSA, soft tissues that are not involved in the burn also become edematous. Cardiac output decreases within minutes after injury in proportion to burn size, although the heart is typically hyperdynamic. Following successful resuscitation, cardiac output normalizes within 24 to 72 hours and then increases to supernormal levels during the wound-healing phase.

Pulmonary Effects

The initial hypovolemic state usually results in fast, shallow breathing. A few days after a burn, adequately resuscitated patients are hypermetabolic and typically have hyperventilation with subsequent respiratory alkalosis. Resuscitated patients can also have mild hypoxemia secondary to pulmonary edema from significant fluid resuscitation.

Chest wall injury can cause further pulmonary dysfunction. Circumferential burns of the thorax can restrict chest wall excursion and impair ventilation, and an escharotomy may be needed if oxygenation and ventilation are impaired. Direct thermal injury to structures above and including the vocal cords leads to rapid upper airway edema that can cause obstruction. This edema typically increases progressively over the first 24 to 36 hours, after which it subsides.

Inhalation injury, which is a risk factor for mortality, is divided into upper airway and lower airway patterns. Upper airway injury can result in acute mortality. Lower respiratory injury tends to result in delayed morbidity and mortality. Toxic products of incomplete thermal combustion cause lower airway inhalation injury. Type I pneumocyte damage results in insufficient gas exchange, whereas type II pneumocyte damage leads to inefficient surfactant secretion and small airway collapse. This cellular damage causes intrapulmonary shunting, compromised endobronchial debris clearance, and progressive hypoxia with respiratory failure. Notably, chest x-rays are insensitive at diagnosing early inhalational injuries, and a normal film does not preclude a diagnosis of inhalational injury.

TABLE 24.1 Burn depth classification

Depth	Description	Healing
Superficial (first degree)	Red, sometimes painful No blister Sunburn	No scar Heals within 5 d
Partial thickness (second degree)	Red and painful Blisters Itching	Superficial heals with minimal scar <3 wk Deep heals with considerable scar
Full thickness (third degree)	Whitish, translucent, may be charred. Involves deep tissue Insensate due to nerve loss	Considerable scar

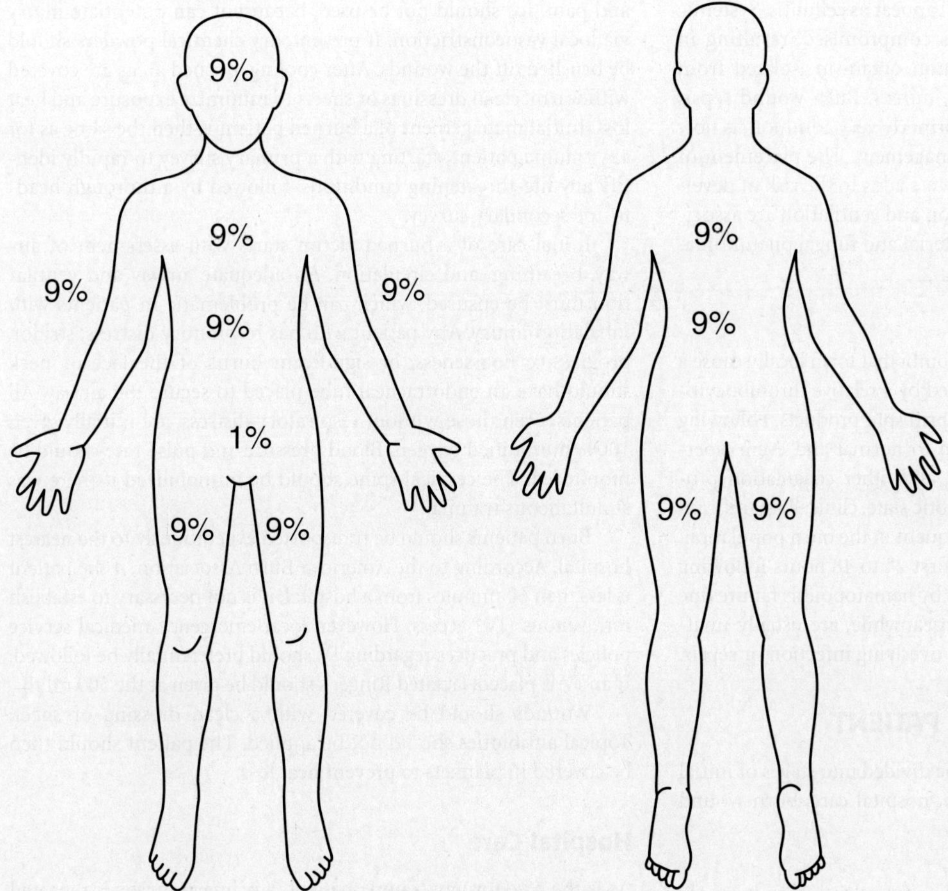

FIGURE 24.2 Burn estimate based on body surface area.

Pneumonia is the most common infectious complication in the burn patient, occuring in 40% of patients with inhalation injury and accounting for approximately 50% of burn fatalities. *Staphylococcus aureus* or gram-negative bacteria most commonly cause pneumonia in the burn patient. Additional significant complications of inhalational injury are carbon monoxide (CO) and cyanide (CN) toxicities, which should be considered in all patients with significant smoke exposure.

Metabolic Effects

The metabolic response to thermal injury is biphasic. The immediate, or ebb phase, is a 12- to 24-hour period of hypometabolism. After resuscitation, the patient enters the flow phase, in which the metabolic rate can be double that of resting values. This period can last for several weeks. Elevated oxygen consumption and increased body temperature to as high as 38.5°C are often seen. This process, driven mainly by catecholamines, cortisol, and glucagon stimulated by the needs of the burn wound, results in protein catabolism with muscle wasting, lipolysis, and profound weight loss if the patient does not receive adequate nutritional support. In turn, insufficient nutrition can result in respiratory failure, pneumonia, and other infections.

Gastrointestinal Effects

The initial decrease in cardiac output leads to decreased splanchnic blood flow, which weakens gastrointestinal mucosal defenses and can result in ulceration (Curling ulcer). Additionally, an ileus persisting for 3 to 5 days after the burn incident may occur in patients with larger burns.

Renal Effects

Acute renal failure is significantly associated with mortality in the burn patient. Changes in renal function after burns are often a result of the initial hypovolemic insult, although acute kidney injury can develop despite appropriate fluid resuscitation and normal urine output. However, patients with extensive muscle damage from high-voltage electrical injury or extensive thermal burns can have significant myoglobinemia, which can lead to renal dysfunction if a brisk diuresis is not achieved. Renal failure may also develop later in the postburn period, as a result of multiorgan dysfunction syndrome, sepsis, or nephrotoxic agents.

Immunologic Effects

A systematic inflammatory response syndrome (SIRS) can occur immediately after a burn injury is sustained. In the wake of this immunologic response, there is a period of immunosuppression, during which alterations in cellular and humoral immunity are seen. This immunosuppression combined with protective skin loss significantly increases susceptibility to infections. The depth and size of the burn are related to the risk of infection, and inhalation injury is a risk factor for pneumonia.

Burn wounds are initially sterile but quickly become colonized by endogenous bacteria within 72 hours of injury due to loss of the epithelial barrier. Gram-positive bacteria predominate initially, but by the 5th day after the burn, gram-negative organisms are more prevalent. Bacteria proliferate and penetrate the avascular zone of coagulation until reaching the nonviable/viable tissue interface.

Clinically, an infected burn wound will appear as cellulitis. Systemic invasion can occur if host defense is compromised, resulting in burn wound sepsis. The most common organism isolated from the blood of the burned patient is *S. aureus*. Burn wound sepsis caused by *Pseudomonas aeruginosa*, formerly very common, is now rare because of aggressive wound management. The placement of central venous and urinary tract catheters adds to the risk of developing an infection. Similarly, intubation and ventilation are associated with developing nosocomial bacterial and fungal pneumonia.

Hematologic Effects

Initially after burn injury, the microthrombi that form locally cause a consumptive coagulopathy characterized by a relative thrombocytopenia, low fibrinogen level, and high fibrin split products. Following resuscitation, there is a prompt return to normal and even supernormal levels of platelets, fibrinogen, and other coagulation proteins. Despite this apparent prothrombotic state, clinically significant thromboembolic phenomena are infrequent in the burn population.

A leukocytosis is expected in the first 24 to 48 hours following a burn, followed by leukopenia caused by hematopoiesis failure due to traumatic injury. Platelet counts, meanwhile, are usually unaffected by a burn injury, unless there is overlying infection or sepsis.

TREATMENT OF THE BURN PATIENT

Management of the burn patient can be divided into stages of initial assessment, initiation of resuscitation, hospital care, burn wound care, and wound coverage.

Initial Assessment

At the scene of the burn injury, the first treatment step is removing the patient from the heat source and stopping the burning process. All burning clothing and jewelry should be removed, but adherent clothing should not be peeled off. Warm tap water or saline is poured directly on the burned area to reduce the depth of the burn and pain. Ice should not be used, because it can potentiate injury via local vasoconstriction. If present, dry chemical powders should be brushed off the wounds. After cooling, burned areas are covered with warm, clean dressings or sheets to minimize exposure and heat loss. Initial management of a burned patient is then the same as for any trauma patient, starting with a primary survey to rapidly identify any life-threatening conditions, followed by a thorough head-to-toe secondary survey.

Initial care of a burned victim starts with assessment of airway, breathing, and circulation. An adequate airway and ventilation must be ensured, which can be problematic in patients with inhalation injury. Any patient who has respiratory distress, stridor, progressive hoarseness, or significant burns of the face or neck should have an endotracheal tube placed to secure the airway. All patients, even those without respiratory distress, are initially given 100% humidified oxygen. Blood pressure and pulse rate should be monitored. The cervical spine should be immobilized if there was simultaneous trauma.

Burn patients should be transported expeditiously to the nearest hospital. According to the American Burn Association, if the patient is less than 60 minutes from a hospital, it is not necessary to establish intravenous (IV) access. However, local emergency medical service policies and practices regarding IV should preferentially be followed. If an IV is placed, lactated Ringer's should be given at the 500 mL/h.

Wounds should be covered with a clean dressing or sheet. Topical antibiotics should not be applied. The patient should then be covered in blankets to prevent heat loss.

Hospital Care

As is the case for any trauma patient, a primary survey is repeated at the hospital, followed by a thorough secondary survey. There are a number of considerations for both the secondary assessment and subsequent hospital care that are unique in the burn patient. Indications for inpatient care depend on both the size of the burn as well as the circumstances surrounding the injury. Table 24.2 lists the criteria for transfer to a burn center.

TABLE 24.2 American Burn Association criteria for transfer to a burn center

Partial- and full-thickness burn involving TBSA > 10% in all patient age groups
Full-thickness burns of any size in all patient age groups
Burns that involve the face, hands, feet, eyes, ears, perineum, or overlying major joints
Significant chemical burns
High-voltage electrical injury, including lightning injury
Inhalation injury
Multiple trauma patients in whom the burn is thought to pose the greatest risk of morbidity and mortality
Burned children in hospitals that are not equipped or able to care for children
Patients with significant comorbidities that can potentially complicate treatment, prolong recovery, or affect mortality
Patients with burns who are expected to require extensive social, emotional, or rehabilitative support (e.g., substance abuse, child abuse)

TBSA, total body surface area.

Upon arrival to the hospital, the patient's respiratory status should be continually monitored and reassessed, particularly since patients with a lower airway inhalation injury may not manifest signs and symptoms until a few days after the initial injury. Evaluation for an inhalation injury is immediate and begins with a thorough oronasopharyngeal inspection. Singed eyebrows or facial hair suggest an inhalational injury. The supraglottic passages are examined for signs of upper airway injury, which include edema, erythema, or a carbonaceous coating; the presence of carbonaceous sputum is also suggestive. Patients who were in a confined burn environment and patients who experienced an explosion with a burn to the head or torso should also be assumed to have an inhalational injury. The treatment of inhalation injury is supportive: early intubation, mechanical ventilation, and transfer to a burn center. Patients with progressive hypoxia or respiratory distress may require mechanical ventilation. All patients requiring mechanical ventilation should receive 100% humidified oxygen. Those who do not require mechanical ventilation should be given supplemental oxygen, and other maneuvers including therapeutic coughing, chest physiotherapy, early ambulation, and tracheobronchial suctioning should be performed to assist airway clearance of debris and reduce, the incidence of pneumonia should be instituted. CO exposure should also be assumed in patients who were burned in an enclosed area and can be diagnosed with a carboxyhemoglobin (COHb) level. All patients with suspected CO exposure should receive high-flow oxygen through a nonrebreather mask.

Once the primary survey is complete, a secondary survey should be performed. This includes a thorough history-taking to better understand the events related to the burn. An understanding of the mechanism of the burn, the surrounding environment, related trauma, the possibility of chemical exposure, and smoke inhalation is critical. A head-to-toe physical exam should also be performed.

Every patient's chest must be exposed and assessed for adequate chest wall excursion with respiration, as the eschar of circumferential full-thickness burns can restrict chest movement. Escharotomy is needed if ventilation is impaired or if airway pressures are significantly elevated. This procedure can be performed at the bedside with minimal blood loss using electrocautery. The eschar is incised in the bilateral anterior axillary lines, extending from the clavicle to below the costal margin (Fig. 24.3). The incision should be made through the eschar but should not penetrate the subcutaneous tissues.

Extensive burns result in sequestration of fluid from the vascular space to the interstitial space, resulting in an intravascular hypovolemic state. Treatment of this hypovolemia with appropriate fluid resuscitation is critical for the survival of burn patients. Large-caliber IV lines should be placed and fluid resuscitation with crystalloid begun immediately for all patients with burns greater than 10% to 20%, inhalational injury or nonburn trauma. Large-bore peripheral catheters are preferred and should be placed through normal skin if possible, although placement through the burn wound is acceptable if it is the only option. Placement of the IV lines in the upper extremities is preferred over the lower extremities. Central access is obtained if no peripheral site is available or invasive hemodynamic monitoring is needed. Patients with smaller burns generally can be "orally resuscitated." For extensive burns, a Foley catheter should be placed to monitor hourly urine output to gauge the adequacy of resuscitation.

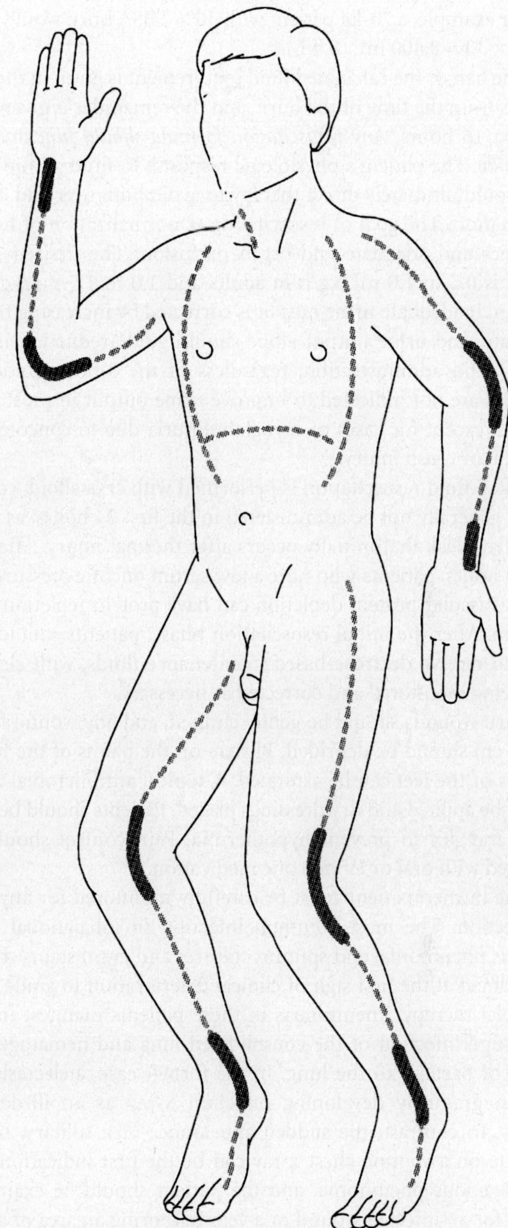

FIGURE 24.3 Preferred sites for escharotomy incisions. (From Moylan JA, Wellford, WJ, Pruitt BA. Circulatory changes following circumferential extremity burns evaluated by the ultrasonic flowmeter: an analysis of 60 thermally injured limbs. *J Trauma.* 1971;11:767, with permission.)

A careful evaluation of the burn wounds is performed in order to determine the extent of the burn. The extent of burn can be easily estimated by the rule of 9s (Fig. 24.2) and is a helpful guide in determining the amount of fluid resuscitation needed. The most commonly used formula to calculate fluid needs is the Parkland formula, which calculates the total fluid requirement as follows:

Parkland formula:

$$\text{Total fluid needed} = (4\text{ mL lactated Ringers}) \times (\text{body weight in kg}) \times (\%\text{ TBSA burned})$$

For example, a 70-kg patient with 30% TBSA burn would need $4 \times 70 \times 30 = 8{,}400$ mL (8.4 L).

One half of the calculated fluid requirement is given in the first 8 hours from the time of the burn, and the remainder is given over the next 16 hours. *Any resuscitation formula should function only as a guide.* The patient's physiologic response to fluid administration should ultimately direct therapy to avoid both over and under resuscitation. The goal of resuscitation is normalization of hemodynamics and adequate end-organ perfusion. The desired urine output is 0.5 to 1.0 mL/kg/h in adults and 1.0 to 1.5 mL/kg/h in children. Inadequate urine output is corrected by increasing the IV fluid rate, and urine output alone should guide reduction in the rate of fluid administration, regardless of the 8-hour guideline. Diuretics are not indicated to improve urine output in most burn patients, except for cases of myoglobulinuria due to concomitant electrical or crush injury.

Initial fluid resuscitation is performed with crystalloid; colloid should generally not be administered in the first 24 hours, as there is capillary leak that initially occurs after thermal injury. After the first 24 hours, patients who have a low serum oncotic pressure due to intravascular protein depletion can have protein repletion with albumin. After the initial resuscitation phase, patients should also begin to receive dextrose-based maintenance fluids, with electrolytes being monitored and corrected as necessary.

Burn wounds should be gently cleaned, and any wound larger than 2 cm should be debrided. Blisters on the palms of the hands or soles of the feet can be aspirated. A topical antimicrobial agent should be applied and dry dressings placed. Patients should be kept warm and dry to prevent hypothermia. Pain control should be managed with oral or IV narcotic medication.

The burned patient must be carefully monitored for any sign of infection. The most common infection in inhalational burn injury is pneumonia, and sputum cultures and gram stains should be obtained at the first sign of clinical deterioration to guide antimicrobial therapy. Pneumonias in these patients manifest in two ways: superinfection of the consolidated lung and hematogenous spread of bacteria to the lung. In the former case, atelectasis can be seen gradually developing on chest x-ray as an ill-defined process. In contrast, the sudden appearance of a solitary, round infiltrate on a routine chest x-ray can be the first indication of a hematogenous pneumonia, and the patient should be examined closely for an infected wound or a vein harboring an area of septic thrombophlebitis.

Assessment of extremity perfusion with a pulse examination must be performed both initially and during the 1st few days after the burn. Constricting circumferential eschar can compromise blood flow to the arms and legs. Escharotomy may be required if pulses are diminished or absent by Doppler examination or if the patient has any signs or symptoms of compartment syndrome. The five Ps of a compartment syndrome (pain, paresthesia, pallor, pulselessness, and poikilothermia) can be difficult to assess in a charred extremity; clinical suspicion is sufficient reason for an escharotomy (Fig. 24.3). Fasciotomy is rarely needed and performed only when escharotomies do not decompress the limb in patients with deep thermal or electrical burns.

Patients with large burns likely require stress ulcer prophylaxis and deep vein thrombosis (DVT) prophylaxis. Initial stress ulcer prophylaxis with sucralfate, H2-blockers, proton pump inhibitors, or antacids and early institution of total enteral nutrition has virtually eliminated the incidence of perforation of and bleeding from Curling ulcers, which had been the most life-threatening gastrointestinal complications seen after burn. Although burn patients have a lower-than-expected incidence of DVT after injury, patients with a prolonged hospital course need some form of prophylaxis, either with compression devices or with heparin.

Inhalation injuries often coincide with CO poisoning and, occasionally, CN poisoning. CO exposure should always be suspected, particularly for burns that occurred within an enclosed space or in any patient with neurologic signs or symptoms. Oxygen saturation measured by a pulse oximeter can give an erroneously normal saturation in the context of CO poisoning, so diagnosis must be made by direct measurement of the amount of COHb. CO binds hemoglobin 200 times stronger than oxygen. Treatment for CO poisoning is 100% oxygen in an attempt to displace the CO. Hyperbaric oxygen therapy should be considered in patients with neurologic signs or symptoms or COHb levels greater than 25% without major concomitant burns. The cumbersome resuscitation of the burned patient in an enclosed hyperbaric chamber, however, precludes its general use.

Treatment for CN poisoning should also be based on clinical suspicion. CN is a combustion product of nitrogen-containing polymers and is often present in closed space industrial fires. CN acts to inhibit oxidative phosphorylation in aerobic metabolism; as a result, these patient have a high lactic acid level. Standard CN level testing can take hours to perform, and the symptoms of CN poisoning are indistinguishable from that of CO poisoning; as a result, suspected patients should be given 100% oxygen along with IV sodium thiosulfate (125 to 250 mg/kg) and hydroxocobalamin (4 g).

All burn wounds are tetanus prone, and all patients should receive tetanus toxoid. Any patient whose immunization status is unknown or whose last booster was more than 10 years ago should also receive 250 IU of tetanus immunoglobulin concurrently in the contralateral arm.

Nutritional support in the postburn period is essential, during both the initial hypodynamic period and the subsequent hyperdynamic period, when the patient's resting energy expenditure is 1.5 to 2.5 times the basal level. Several indices are available to help estimate the burn patient's caloric requirements, although no one method is considered a gold standard. The burn patient's nutritional needs should be reassessed daily, as the requirements may increase or decrease over the hospital course and both overfeeding and underfeeding should be avoided. Enteral nutrition is the preferred source of nutritional supplementation. TPN can be used if gastrointestinal function is absent but is associated with a higher mortality rate. When possible, the transition should be made to oral intake. There are several enteral nutrition products available to provide nutrition to burn patients. Glucose is the primary source of calories in this population, while glutamine is essential for maintaining small bowel enterocytes.

Burns can be the result of child abuse or neglect. A high level of awareness is required to identify child or elder abuse. Whenever an odd mechanism, inconsistent history, sharply defined borders, or circumferential injury is involved in the burn of a dependent child or elderly person, abuse should be considered. Accidental burns should always manifest an unequal pattern of injury as one moves away from the heat. Any burn that conforms exactly to the shape of an object or is uniform in all directions because of prolonged contact may have been intentional. Cases suspicious for abuse or neglect should be admitted to the hospital and reported to the appropriate local agency for proper investigation.

Burn Wound Care

Initial care and assessment of the burn wound should include gentle cleaning with soap and water and removal of loose nonviable skin. The burn site can be cooled for up to 30 minutes. Evaluation of burn wound depth is very important in the first few days following successful resuscitation, as burn wound depth guides burn wound care, as described in subsequent text. Although numerous technical aids such as laser Doppler flowmeter, vital dyes, and staining have been devised to aid in this determination, clinical observation remains the standard for the assessment of burn wound depth.

Superficial burns, including sunburns, are erythematous and painful but do not require treatment. The dead epidermis is replaced by new skin within 3 to 4 days.

Shallow partial-thickness burns, characterized by blisters, will generally heal within 3 weeks and therefore are managed nonoperatively, requiring neither topical agents nor dressings. Management of these burns is daily wound care consisting of loose skin debridement, cleansing with soap and water, topical antimicrobials, and sterile dressing application. Intact blisters are left alone unless they limit extremity range of motion, as unroofing blisters exposes a painful underlying wound that is potentially more susceptible to infection. Deep partial-thickness classically present with mottled pink and white skin and take at least 3 weeks to heal. There are generally no blisters. Treatment is otherwise the same as for shallow partial-thickness burns. If the burn has not healed in 3 weeks, excision of the burn is required. Partial-thickness burns not requiring excision can be treated with application of a nonadherent dressing, which is changed daily. An alternative to daily dressing changes for the treatment of superficial partial-thickness burns is the immediate application of a biologic dressing, which is left in place until healing is complete. Examples of biologic dressings are TransCyte®, BGC Matrix®, Biobrane®, Acticoat®, porcine xenograft, and cadaveric cutaneous allograft. These dressings are fairly expensive and must be used with care as underlying infection can be masked.

Full-thickness burns extend into the subcutaneous tissues. Early excision of the burn, followed by skin grafting, is necessary. The advantages of early excision include increased survival, reduced pain, a shorter hospital stay, a shorter duration of the hypermetabolic period, earlier reversal of immunosuppression, decreased incidence of burn wound sepsis and other infectious complications, and less hypertrophic scarring.

The most common technique for burn wound excision is tangential excision, which involves removal of the eschar in thin layers down to a healthy bed characterized by brisk bleeding from patent vessels. Use of tourniquets and/or topical hemostatic agents such as thrombin or epinephrine decreases bleeding. These cases are limited to a few hours and excision of less than 20% of TBSA to minimize blood loss and morbidity of long cases. For full-thickness burns involving substantial subcutaneous tissue death, fascial excision is necessary. Fascial excision, in which both skin and subcutaneous tissues are resected, is associated with less blood loss than tangential excision, but inferior cosmetic results. Fascial excision may also be needed in cases of sepsis or invasive wound infection. Excision is performed within 7 days of injury to minimize conversion of colonized wound to infected wound. Delay is often necessary in patients with concomitant nonthermal trauma or multiorgan dysfunction. Patients are brought back to the operating room every few days until all nonviable tissue is removed. Wounds are closed with full- or split-thickness skin grafts (STSGs), depending on the depth of coverage needed (see below).

Wounds should be covered with nonadherent dressings. Dressings are removed on postoperative days 3 or 4 and thereafter should be changed at least once a day for inspection and cleansing of the wound and to allow early identification of infection and prevention of systemic complications. There is no role for prophylactic systemically administered antibiotics in uninfected local burn wound care, as therapeutic levels are not achieved in the burn wound. Topically applied agents, in contrast, are used to provide high drug concentrations at the wound surface to control the bacterial population. Three topical antimicrobial agents are currently used in routine burn wound care: silver sulfadiazine (Silvadene®), mafenide acetate (Sulfamylon®), and silver nitrate. Each agent is bacteriostatic and has specific advantages and side effects as described in Table 24.3.

TABLE 24.3 Topical antibiotics used in burn wound care

Agent	Advantages	Disadvantages
Silver sulfadiazine (Silvadene®)	Well tolerated Painless application	Poor eschar penetration *Transient leukopenia in 5%–15% of cases* Rash in 5% of cases Not for use with sulfa allergy Limited activity against *Pseudomonas* and *Enterobacter*
Mafenide acetate (Sulfamylon®)	Eschar penetration Broad spectrum of activity	Painful application (especially with cream) *Carbonic anhydrase inhibition can cause hyperchloremic metabolic acidosis* Not for use with sulfa allergy Rash in 5% of cases No fungal coverage
Silver nitrate	Painless application Broad spectrum of activity, including fungi	Poor eschar penetration Difficult to apply, stains everything black *Can cause electrolyte disturbances by leaching sodium, potassium, chloride, and calcium from the wound*

Noninvasive burn wound infections present as cellulitis and occasionally as an abscess. Treatment of a noninvasive burn wound involves cleaning the wound, application of topic antibiotics, and administration of systemic antibiotics. An invasive burn wound infection may develop. Signs of invasive burn wound infection are conversion of a partial-thickness to a full-thickness burn, early eschar separation or loss of the overlying skin graft, and discoloration of the burn wound. Rapid development of bullae and necrosis of previously health tissue may occur. The most accurate way to confirm the diagnosis of invasive infections is histologic examination of a sample of tissue from the burn wound. A portion of the sample is sent to the microbiology laboratory for identification of the organisms, and a portion is sent to pathology for frozen section analysis. Quantitative counts of greater than 10^5 organisms per gram of tissue indicate the presence of invasive infection, particularly if microorganisms are seen extending into viable uninjured tissue. Topical therapy should be switched to mafenide acetate for increased eschar penetration; systemic antibiotics are promptly administered, and prompt and aggressive excision of all necrotic tissue. Reoperation for removal of necrotic tissue may be required. Antimicrobial soaks, such as silver nitrate, are often used. Empiric antibiotics, including coverage of gram-positive, gram-negative, and fungal organisms, are first administered, with subsequent narrowing of coverage once microbial identification and sensitivities have been determined. Patients treated on an outpatient basis should be seen frequently in clinic. If the area remains free of infection, the patient is monitored as an outpatient until the wound heals. Any sign of wound infection mandates immediate hospitalization and the initiation of systemic antibiotics.

Burn Wound Coverage

The benefits of early excision of the burn injury are realized only if the wound is properly covered. Both biologic and synthetic dressings have been developed for this purpose and can be grouped as either permanent or temporary coverage. The advantages and disadvantages of each are listed in Table 24.4.

The most common and best coverage for extensive body burns is a split-thickness autograft to the affected area (STSG). The STSG comprises epidermis and part of dermis, which is excised from an unaffected donor site from the burn patient. The STSG is usually meshed to increase surface area of the graft. Small bridges of skin reepithelialize to fill in the gaps in the mesh. Adhesion to the underlying tissue is weak until about 7 days. Shear forces on the graft, underlying hematoma, seroma, or infection can cause graft failure. Grafts initially receive nutrients from the tissue below them by a process called imbibition until the growth of capillary buds from the recipient area occurs by days 2 to 3. Donor sites for STSG can be reharvested after the site has epithelialized in 2 to 3 weeks. While waiting for the donor site to regenerate, temporary coverings are

TABLE 24.4 Materials for burn wound coverage

Material	Advantages	Disadvantages
STSG	Donor sites close in 2–3 wk Harvest from anywhere Same donor site multiple times Can cover large sites	More contraction Poorer cosmetic result
Full-thickness skin graft	Reduced wound contraction Better cosmetic result	Less available tissue Limited coverage Fail more often than STSG
Integra™ (bovine collagen) AlloDerm® (cryopreserved human dermis) Dermagraft® (human neonate fibroblasts)	No need to harvest from donor site Can act as temporary or permanent cover	Cost Learning curve
Cultured epithelial autograft (Keratinocytes from patient skin biopsy)	Can provide large amounts of tissue Not rejected by host immune system	Cost Long time to grow skin culture Tissue is fragile Contracture is common
Cutaneous allograft (homograft) (cadaver skin)	No need to harvest from donor site	Immune-mediated rejection in 3–4 wk Possible disease transmission Limited supply
Cutaneous porcine xenograft	Extensive temporary skin cover No need to harvest from donor site Abundant supply	Will not vascularize
Amniotic tissue	Extensive temporary skin cover	Risk of disease transmission Frequent desiccation

STSG, Split-thickness skin graft.

used to prevent wound desiccation and infection. Full-thickness skin grafts have improved cosmesis, but may not "take" as well as split-thickness grafts because of the thicker depth, and the donor site must be closed or grafted. As a result, STSGs are preferred.

ELECTRICAL BURNS

Electrical injury is responsible for approximately 4% to 7% of burn center admissions annually. Injury results from the conversion of electrical energy to heat with the passage of current through tissue. The severity of electrical burns is determined by the voltage, the amount and type of current, the path of the current, and the duration of contact with the electrical source. Low-voltage burns are defined as less than 1,000 volts (V) and are often confined to the area directly surrounding the contact point, while high-voltage burns are defined as greater than 1,000 V and cause deep tissue damage. Nearly all domestic burns are low-voltage burns.

Initial treatment of an electrical burn patient follows the traditional pattern of airway, breathing, and circulation. All electrical injuries can produce dysrhythmias, and a 12-lead electrocardiogram should be obtained. Patients who experienced a loss of consciousness, required cardiopulmonary resuscitation, or with abnormal electrocardiographic (ECG) findings or a dysrhythmia should have continuous cardiac monitoring begun immediately and continued for at least 24 hours. Electrical injury greater than 380 V can cause paraspinal muscle tetany and warrants a complete spine series to rule out spinal compression fractures. Electrical injury may also result in local arterial and venous thrombosis.

High-voltage injury (>1,000 V) can cause significant muscle and soft tissue destruction. Because heat is lost at differing rates from superficial and deep tissues, significant deep tissue necrosis may be present despite unremarkable looking wounds. Rhabdomyolysis resulting myoglobinuria can cause acute renal failure and should be assumed and treated prior to laboratory diagnosis if dark urine is present. Urine output should be monitored with placement of an indwelling urinary catheter. Aggressive fluid administration should maintain a urine output of at least 100 mL/h in adults or 2 mL/kg/h in children. Mannitol may be required if aggressive fluid infusion does not maintain an adequate urinary output. High-voltage injuries to the extremities may result in compartment syndrome within 48 hours of the burn and necessitate fasciotomies.

Treatment of the wounds is staged. Mafenide acetate cream is initially applied to the contact points. Surgical excision and debridement of necrotic tissue is performed 2 to 3 days after the burn if compartment syndrome is not present. Second-look operations are performed 48 hours later until all necrotic tissue has been excised. Wounds are closed with skin grafts or flaps as appropriate.

Deep burns of the oral cavity and lips are the most common electrical burn in young children, often the result of chewing on an electrical cord. Significant bleeding can occur from the labial artery 10 to 14 days after injury, and families need to be carefully instructed to apply pressure to the bleeding point and return to the hospital immediately if bleeding occurs.

Neurologic changes can occur after an electrical injury. Immediate neuropathy results from electrical injury directly and usually resolves with time. Late manifestations are localized deficits, paralysis, and cataracts.

CHEMICAL BURNS

Chemical burns make up only 3% of all burns but are responsible for 30% of burn-related deaths. Chemical burns are associated with prolonged hospital stays and healing times.

Strong acids and bases destroy tissue by protein denaturation and thermal energy from chemical reactions. The severity of a chemical burn is affected by the concentration of the chemical, the amount of the chemical present, the duration of contact with the skin, and the mechanism of action of the chemical. As a result, rapid removal of the chemical is highly important. Alkali burns are generally more severe because exposure to an alkalotic agent results in liquefaction necrosis of the tissue, causing a deeper burn. Acidic burns result in coagulation necrosis.

Treatment consists of prompt removal of contaminated clothing and copious irrigation with cold water for at least 30 minutes and up to 2 hours. Neutralization with acid or base is avoided as the resultant exothermic reaction can cause further damage. Chemical burn patients should otherwise be managed in the same manner as thermal burn patients: attention to airway, breathing, and circulation, and fluid resuscitation and urine output monitoring. Wound care is similar to the care of thermal burn wounds.

FROSTBITE

Frostbite occurs when the tissue temperature falls below the freezing point of water (approximately −2°C or 28.4°F). Tissue damage in frostbite is due to intracellular ice crystal formation and subsequent distortion of cellular architecture. Skin is more resistant to freezing than deeper tissues, namely, nerves and blood vessels. Deep tissue microvasculature can be occluded by platelet aggregation at the site of vascular endothelial damage, resulting in ischemic damage.

Treatment consists of rewarming the injured area in a circulating water bath at 40°C until perfusion to the area returns and the skin is in pink color. Dry heat and massaging should be avoided. This is an extremely painful process, and analgesics are usually required. In contrast to thermal burns, demarcation can take several weeks to months, and earlier debridement is not necessary unless the affected area becomes infected. Local care focuses on preventing infection via cleansing and topical antimicrobials while the tissue demarcates. Systemic antibiotics should not be empirically administered.

SUGGESTED READINGS

American Burn Association. Available at: http://www.ameriburn.org. Accessed August 2014.

Endorf FW, Gzibran NS. Burns. In: Brunicardi F, Anderson D, Billiar T, et al., eds. *Schwartz's Principles of Surgery*. 9th ed. New York: McGraw-Hill; 2010.

Herndon D, ed. *Total burn care*. 4th ed. London: Saunders Elsevier; 2012.

Holmes JH. Burns/inhalation. In: Peitzman AB, Fabian TC, Rhodes M, et al., eds. *The Trauma Manual*. 4th ed. Philadelphia: Lippincott Williams & Wilkins; 2012.

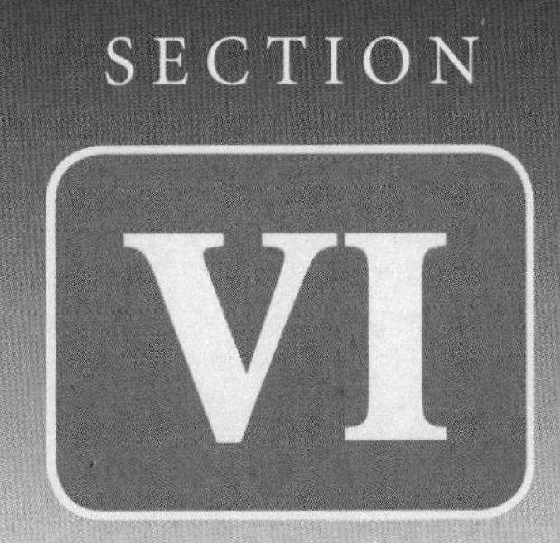

Surgical Subspecialties

CHAPTER

25

Neurosurgery

NIKHIL R. NAYAK, ERIC D. HUDGINS, AND JAMES M. SCHUSTER

KEY POINTS

- The development of the nervous system is a complex process. Errors at different points of this process cause numerous structural abnormalities requiring surgical intervention.
- The blood supply to the brain is from the internal carotid and vertebral arteries. Vascular pathology, such as intracranial aneurysms and arteriovenous malformations, may present with acute hemorrhage or be identified incidentally.
- Hydrocephalus afflicts children, adults, and the elderly due to a number of etiologies. Ventricular shunting procedures are extremely common in neurosurgical practice.
- While plain x-rays are still used, CT and MRI have become the mainstay for diagnosis and treatment planning in the modern neurosurgical practice.
- Successful management of TBI requires rapid assessment, diagnosis, and treatment of primary injuries and avoidance of secondary injuries from hypoxia, hypotension, elevated intracranial pressure, and seizures.
- Progressive obtundation, pupillary abnormalities, or other lateralizing neurologic findings in combination with intracranial lesions such as epidural hematoma, subdural hematoma, and intracranial hemorrhage causing pathologic brain shift are generally surgical emergencies.
- Patients with significant trauma are considered to have spinal injuries until proven otherwise. Clinical clearance may be performed in the awake and cooperative patient, and negative radiographs are required in symptomatic patients or those with altered mental status. Surgical stabilization is commonly performed if there is structural compromise.
- Degenerative disease of the spine leads to compression of the neural elements from disk herniations, bone spurs, ligamentous hypertrophy, malalignment, and possible instability.
- Metastases are the most common brain tumors in adults. Tumors that commonly metastasize to the brain include lung, breast, melanoma, and renal cell carcinoma. High-grade gliomas are the most common primary brain tumor in adults and have an overall poor prognosis.
- Common infections of the nervous system include meningitis, intracranial abscess, subdural empyema, spinal epidural abscess, osteomyelitis/discitis, and parasitic infections. Treatment varies from antibiotics alone to surgical debridement.

DEVELOPMENT

The development of the central nervous system (CNS) begins with the transformation of the inner cell mass into the bilaminar disc at approximately 14 days of gestation. The bilaminar disc is composed of the epiblast (primitive ectoderm) and hypoblast (primitive endoderm). By the 3rd week, gastrulation begins and the primitive streak develops at the posterior portion of the embryo, which gives rise to both endoderm and mesoderm. A collection of cells at the primitive streak, known as Henson's node, forms the notochord at approximately 16 days of gestation. The notochord is derived from mesoderm and induces the differentiation of overlying ectoderm cells to become specialized neural ectoderm, which then forms the neural plate. The edges of the neural plate thicken and fold in to create the basic tubular structure of the embryonic CNS, a structure called the neural tube. The anterior neuropore of the developing neural tube closes around 24 days of gestation and goes on to form the brain, while the posterior neuropore closes around day 26 and goes on to form the spinal cord. This process by which the neural tube develops is called primary neurulation. The neural tube is further subdivided into a basal plate, which gives rise to motor neurons, and an alar plate, which gives rise to sensory neurons. The notochord persists and lies deep in the developing neural tube to ultimately form the central portion of intervertebral discs, the nucleus pulposus. Cells at the periphery of the developing neural tube become neural crest cells. Derived from ectoderm, these cells form numerous structures including neurons and glia of the peripheral nervous system (PNS), pia and arachnoid, some skeletal elements, tendons and smooth muscle, chondrocytes, osteocytes, melanocytes, adrenal chromaffin cells, and hormone-producing cells in certain organs (Fig. 25.1).

By the 4th week of development, the cranial end of the neural tube expands to form three primary vesicles: the prosencephalon (forebrain), mesencephalon (midbrain), and rhombencephalon (hindbrain). The remaining caudal element of the neural tube will become the spinal cord. The five-vesicle stage closely follows the three-vesicle stage, as the prosencephalon divides to become the paired telencephalon and paired diencephalon. The mesencephalon does not divide, and the rhombencephalon divides to become the metencephalon and the myelencephalon. The telencephalon becomes the cerebral hemispheres and basal ganglia, the diencephalon becomes the thalamus, the mesencephalon becomes the midbrain, the metencephalon becomes the pons and cerebellum, and the myelencephalon becomes the medulla oblongata. The ventricular system develops later during embryogenesis, although its basic structure is formed during the five-vesicle stage, as the lateral ventricles are related to the formation of the telencephalic vesicles, the third ventricle to the diencephalic vesicle, and the fourth ventricle to the rhombencephalic roof.

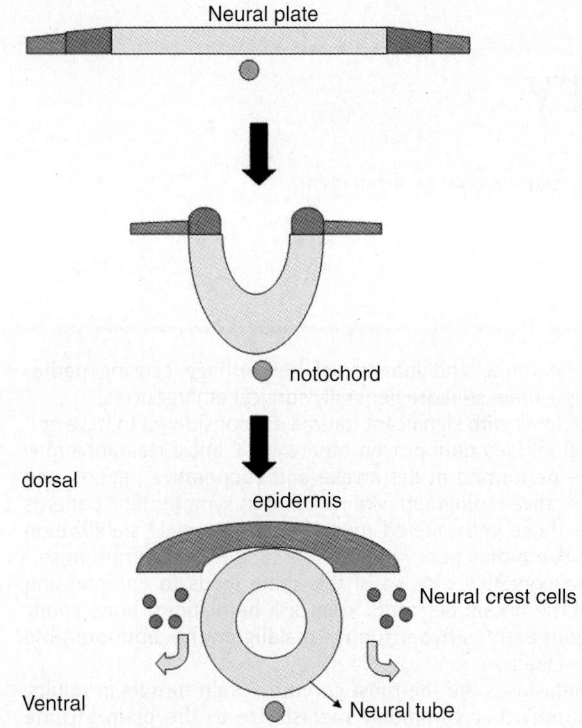

FIGURE 25.1 Early neuraxis development.

Errors during neuroembryogenesis result in a range of malformations of the fetus. Failure of fusion of the anterior neural tube leads to anencephaly, the most severe neural tube defect and one that is incompatible with life. While the orbits are generally well formed, the cranial vault is maldeveloped, hypoplastic, and contains a mass of immature blood vessels. Failure of the posterior end of the tube to close leads to a family of disorders categorized as spinal dysraphism. Spinal dysraphism is caused by incomplete formation of the dorsal midline structures during embryogenesis, resulting in abnormalities of the skin, vertebral arch, neural tissue, or a combination.

Spina bifida occulta, a failure of midline fusion of the bony structures without involvement of the meninges or neural tissue, is generally an incidental finding and asymptomatic, with a prevalence of 5% to 10% in the North American population. Spina bifida occulta is frequently accompanied by one or more cutaneous stigmata such as a hairy patch, subcutaneous lipoma, skin tag, sacral dimple, or port-wine stain. Spina bifida aperta includes meningocele and myelomeningocele and occurs when the bone and overlying skin fail to fuse in the midline, thereby allowing meninges and, sometimes, neural tissue to herniate through the defect. A meningocele is a defect in vertebral arches with cystic distension of meninges but no abnormality of neural tissue. One third, however, have some neurologic deficit. A myelomeningocele is a defect in the vertebral arch with cystic dilatation of meninges and structural or functional abnormality of the spinal cord or cauda equina. Almost all neonates with a myelomeningocele have a Chiari II malformation of the brain and associated hydrocephalus. A Chiari II malformation is characterized by caudal displacement of the cerebellar vermis, medulla, and fourth ventricle through the foramen magnum, a characteristic kink in the brain stem, and fusion of the tectum (dorsal region of the midbrain). A lipomyelomeningocele is a subcutaneous lipoma that passes through a midline defect through the fascia, neural arch, dura, and merges with an abnormally low tethered cord. The neural elements remain within the spinal canal.

A congenital dermal sinus tract is a dysraphic condition characterized by an opening in the skin overlying an epithelial-lined tract that can end outside the dura or extend through it. The opening at the skin is usually 1 to 2 mm in diameter and most commonly found in the lumbar region. Affected individuals often present with recurrent episodes of meningitis, sometimes with atypical organisms. Tethering of the spinal cord occurs when the cord itself or the nerve roots are attached to surrounding nonneural structures, such as the meninges. As the affected child grows, resultant stretching of the cord leads to neurologic deficits. Older children and adults present with pain, progressive neurologic dysfunction, urinary abnormalities, or lower extremity weakness; such symptoms often require surgical detethering.

Risk factors for spinal dysraphism include maternal relatives with affected children, siblings with dysraphism, and maternal perinatal folic acid deficiency. Since the neural tube closes at the end of the 3rd week of gestation, often before a woman is aware of her pregnancy, folate supplementation is recommended for all women of childbearing age at a dose of 400 μg daily.

ANATOMY

The scalp consists of five layers: the skin, underlying connective tissue, the galea aponeurotica, and the pericranium (periosteum of the skull). Blood vessels of the scalp are found in the connective tissue above the galea. The galea is continuous with the musculature of the face and neck. Subgaleal hematomas result from bleeding into the loose connective tissue deep to the galea and above the pericranium. These hematomas can attain substantial volume as the potential space between the galea and the pericranium is large. It is therefore imperative that the galea be reapproximated when repairing scalp lacerations.

The skull can be broadly divided into the cranial vault and the skull base. The cranial vault is composed of the frontal, parietal, squamous temporal, occipital, and sphenoid bones. The skull base is composed of the frontal, ethmoid, sphenoid, petrous temporal, and occipital bones. The skull base is further subdivided into the anterior, middle, and posterior fossae (compartments), which house the frontal lobes, temporal lobes, and brainstem/cerebellum, respectively. At birth, the skull contains unfused sutures, or fibrous joints, at the interfaces of the different bones that allow expansion and growth, which is driven primarily by brain growth. While there are several sutures, the most clinically useful ones at an introductory level include the metopic, coronal, sagittal, squamosal, and lambdoid sutures. The metopic and sagittal sutures are midline structures, while the coronal, squamosal, and lambdoid sutures are paired, bilateral structures.

The anterior fontanelle is the confluence of the frontal, bilateral coronal, and sagittal sutures and allows for deformation of the skull during birth and subsequent growth. It generally fuses by 2.5 years of age. The anterior fontanelle is clinically relevant in the assessment of an infant, as a sunken fontanelle may indicate dehydration and a bulging fontanelle, in the absence of distress, may indicate raised intracranial pressure (ICP). The posterior fontanelle is triangular in shape, found at the intersection of the sagittal and bilateral lambdoid sutures, and generally closes by 2.5 months of age. Other important skull surface landmarks include the bregma, which is the

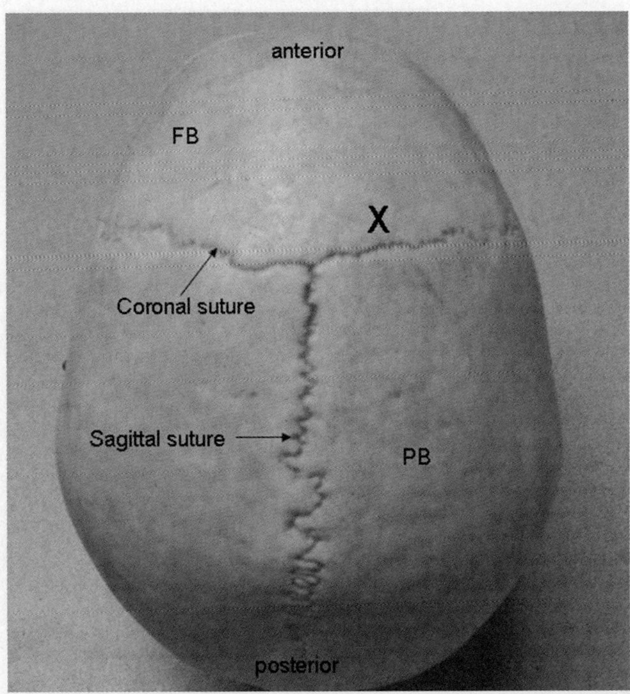

FIGURE 25.2 External skull anatomy and landmarks. X marks a common entrance point for a right frontal ventriculostomy. FB, frontal bone; PB, parietal bone.

intersection of the coronal and sagittal sutures; pterion, which is the region where the frontal, parietal, temporal, and sphenoid bones intersect; asterion, which is the confluence of the lambdoid, parietomastoid, and occipitomastoid sutures. These surface landmarks serve as important reference points for determining intracranial anatomy and surgical planning (Fig. 25.2).

The brain and spinal cord are covered by three meningeal layers. The most superficial layer is the dura mater, a tough, leathery membrane. The cranial dura has an outer periosteal layer and inner meningeal layer. These layers are tightly opposed except in areas that contain the venous sinuses, which accommodate the bulk of venous outflow from the brain and lay in between the two leaflets of dura. Spinal dura has a single meningeal layer. Deep to the dura mater is the arachnoid layer, a very thin, translucent layer composed of interdigitating loose connective tissue. The subarachnoid space contains cerebrospinal fluid (CSF) and traversing blood vessels that supply the brain and spinal cord. Finally, the deepest meningeal layer is the pia mater, which is tightly adherent to the surface of the brain and spinal cord and pierced by smaller blood vessels as they enter the neural parenchyma.

The supratentorial brain is divided into left and right hemispheres. The left hemisphere controls motor and sensory function for the right body; the right hemisphere controls the left body. Right-handed individuals almost all show left hemisphere dominance with regard to language function. Even in left-handed people, language localizes to the left hemisphere over 85% of the time. The cortical regions of each hemisphere are divided into four lobes: frontal, temporal, parietal, and occipital. The frontal lobes are the anterior-most aspect of the brain and extend back to the central sulcus of Rolando. They are separated inferiorly from the temporal lobes by the sylvian fissure. Posterior to the central sulcus are the parietal lobes, which, when viewing from the surface, do not have discrete separations from the temporal lobes inferiorly or the occipital lobes posteriorly. When viewing from a medial perspective, the parieto-occipital sulcus can be seen separating the parietal and occipital lobes. The left and right hemispheres are separated in the midline by the interhemispheric fissure, and a large, midline subcortical white matter structure called the corpus callosum connects the two hemispheres.

In general, the frontal lobes control executive function, personality, and motor function. In the dominant hemisphere, the inferolateral portion of the frontal lobe also controls speech production. The dominant temporoparietal region (known as Wernicke's area) is the site of language processing, and both temporal lobes perform basic processing of sound information. The parietal lobes process sensory information, and the occipital lobes are chiefly responsible for processing visual information. The infratentorial space houses the brain stem and cerebellum. The brain stem gives rise to the 12 pairs of cranial nerves and contains numerous nuclei and white matter tracts that control such basic functions as level of consciousness to modulating cerebral cortical activity. The cerebellum, which is also divided into hemispheres, is responsible for coordination of the smooth motor movements of the limbs, upright posture, and the motor fluency of speech. These functions are distributed to different locations in the cerebellum, but unlike the cerebral cortex, injury to one hemisphere of the cerebellum results in a deficit on the ipsilateral side of the body.

The cells of the CNS include neurons (nerve cells) and supporting cells, including oligodendrocytes, astrocytes, microglia, and ependymal cells. Neurons are the cells primarily responsible for signaling within the nervous system. Oligodendrocytes surround neuronal axons with their foot processes (myelination). Each oligodendrocyte myelinates several axons. Schwann cells, which are responsible for myelination of peripheral nerves, are only capable of myelinating a single axon. Microglia function as macrophages in the CNS, and ependymal cells line the internal CSF spaces of the CNS. Astrocytes play a role in myelination, help maintain the intracellular chemical environment of the neurons, and stimulate formation of the blood–brain barrier (BBB). The BBB has three components: tight junctions between endothelial cells of the CNS capillaries, the basal lamina, and astrocytic perivascular foot processes. The BBB is relatively permeable to lipid-soluble substances and small hydrophilic molecules but is relatively impermeable to large molecules and water-soluble components, which require specific transport mechanisms to enter the CNS from the bloodstream.

The vertebral column consists of 7 cervical, 12 thoracic, 5 lumbar, 5 fused sacral, and 4 fused coccygeal bones. The first and second cervical vertebrae are known as the atlas and axis, respectively, and are unique in their anatomy and function. C1 is essentially a ring of bone and lacks a true vertebral body. It articulates with both the base of the skull and with a peg-like extension of the C2 body called the dens (Fig. 25.3). The C1 ring rotates around the dens with head turning. The C1 ring also articulates bilaterally with the C2 body through facet joints, which help modulate head turning. While there is regional variability, the remaining vertebrae share a similar basic structure: a cylindrical vertebral body and paired arm-like structures (pedicles) that extend posteriorly to meet the lamina. The posterior vertebral body, pedicles, and lamina form a bony ring around the dura and neural elements. There is a spinous process that extends posteriorly from the midline of the lamina and bilateral transverse processes that extend laterally from the intersection

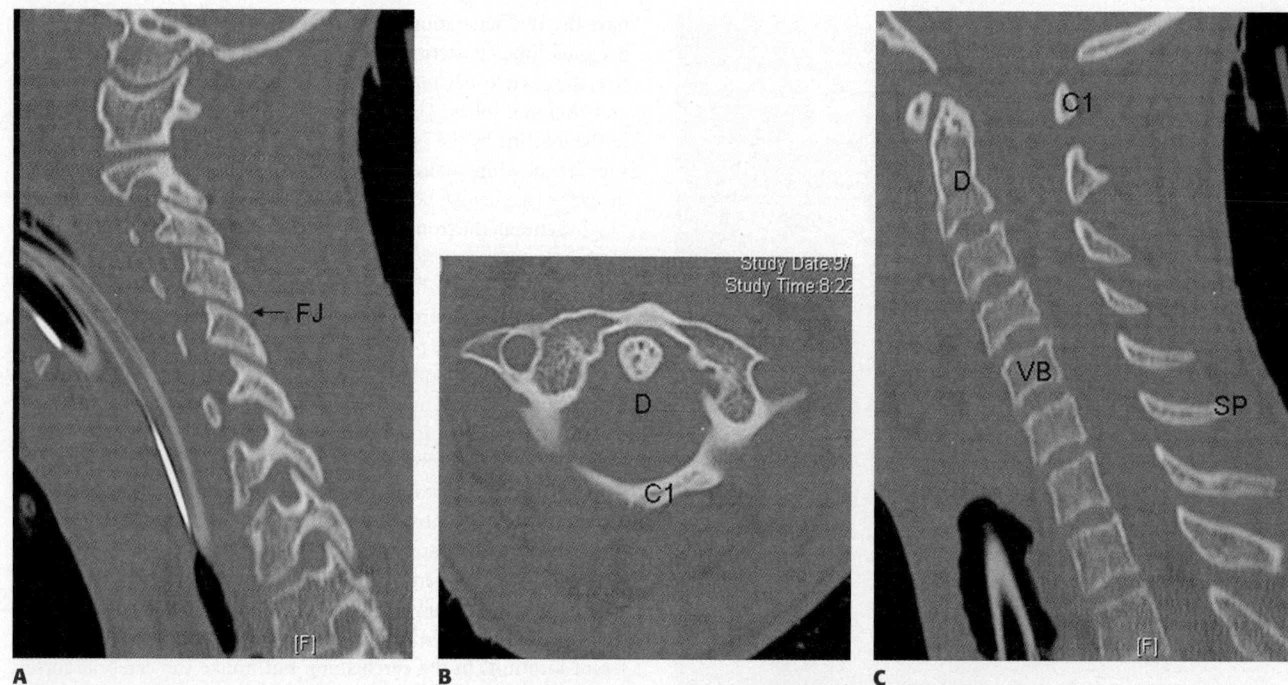

FIGURE 25.3 Bone anatomy of the cervical spine by **(A)** sagittal section through facet joints, **(B)** axial section through C1–C2, **(C)** midline sagittal section. FJ, facet joint; VB, vertebral body; D, dens of C2; C1, first cervical vertebral ring; SP, spinous process.

of the pedicles and the lamina (Fig. 25.4). From a sagittal view, there is a space between adjacent pedicles called the neural foramen, from which nerve roots exit the spinal canal. The subaxial vertebrae (below C2) articulate with each other through specialized joints. Additionally, the thoracic vertebrae articulate with the ribs, and the sacral bones articulate with the hip bones to form the pelvis.

There are multiple structures that hold the bones of the vertebral column together and allow them to move. Sandwiched between the vertebral bodies are the intervertebral discs. These consist of an outer, collagenous ring called the annulus fibrosus that surrounds the inner remnant of the notochord, the more gelatinous nucleus pulposus. Cartilaginous endplates attach the discs to the vertebral bodies. Posteriorly are the interspinous and supraspinous ligaments that connect adject spinous processes. These ligaments help limit flexion of the spinal column, and the supraspinous ligament serves as attachment point for some of the paraspinal muscles.

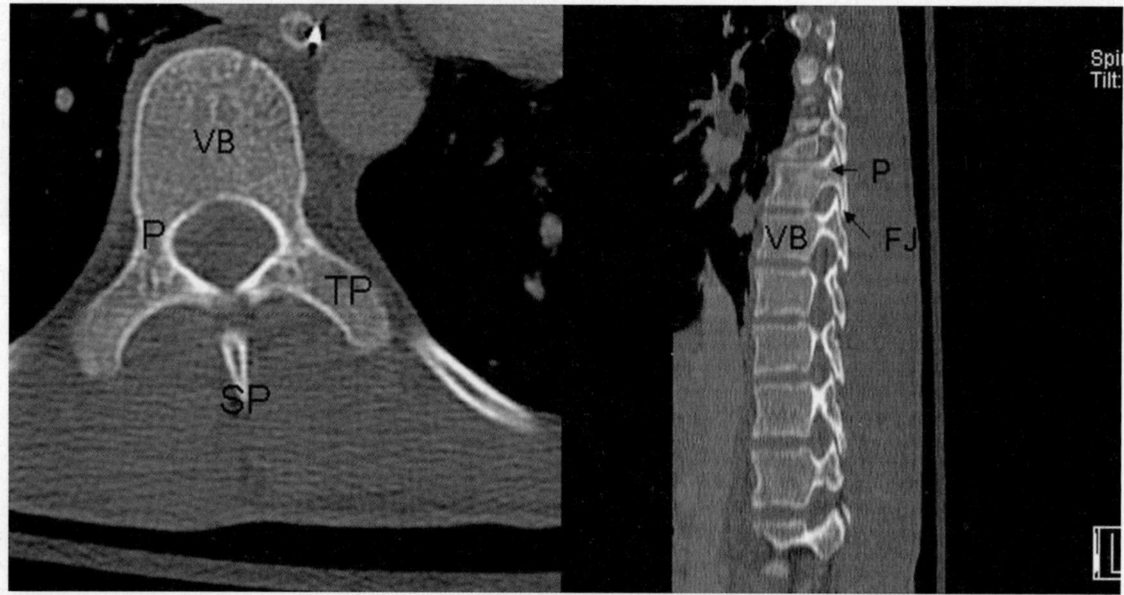

FIGURE 25.4 Axial and sagittal sections through the thoracic spine. VB, vertebral body; P, pedicle; SP, spinous process; TP, transverse process; FJ, facet joint.

The ligamentum flavum lies anterior to the lamina and connects adjacent lamina and limits flexion. The anterior longitudinal ligament runs along the anterior surface of the vertebral bodies and limits extension of the spine, while the posterior longitudinal ligament runs along the posterior aspect of the vertebral bodies and serves to limit flexion of the spine. Extending superiorly and inferiorly on both sides from the pedicle/laminar interface are synovial facet joints that modulate and constrain spinal movement and maintain alignment.

The joints of the spine (discs and facet joints), like all other joints in the body, are subject to degeneration with repetitive use. In the case of discs, this degeneration can lead to disc herniation (i.e., the nucleus pulposus extends out through the annulus fibrosis, leading to painful compression of an exiting nerve root) or desiccation and collapse potentially leading to malalignment and neural compression. Facet degeneration can lead to the formation of bone spurs and joint incompetence with malalignment and instability, potentially resulting in crowding of the spinal canal (stenosis) or neural foramen.

Nerve roots consist of both sensory and motor fibers and exit the spinal canal at the neural foramina. In the cervical spine, the nerve roots exit above the pedicle of the vertebrae with the same numbered level. The C8 nerve root does not have a corresponding vertebra and exits between C7 and T1. The nerve roots below the cervical spine exit beneath the pedicle of the vertebrae with the same number. The spinal cord ends at the approximate level of the first lumbar vertebral body (L1). The inferior-most tip of the cord is known as the conus medullaris. The cauda equina ("horse's tail") is the collection of lumbosacral nerve root fibers inside the dura beneath the level of the conus medullaris. The areas of the skin served by sensory fibers of specific nerve roots have a dermatomal distribution (Fig. 25.5).

In general, nerve roots are more resistant to compression than is the spinal cord; compression of the spinal cord produces myelopathy, whereas compression of a nerve root typically causes radiculopathy. Myelopathy occurs when the upper motor neurons malfunction, leading to symptoms such as hyperreflexia, pain, numbness, weakness, and sometimes bowel and bladder dysfunction. Patients with cervical myelopathy often present with a spastic gait and complaints of hand tingling, numbness, weakness, and loss of dexterity. In contrast, patients with a cervical radiculopathy complain of pain, which radiates down the arm in a pattern that matches the dermatomal distribution of the nerve being compressed. For example, a herniated disc between the C5 and C6 vertebral bodies causes pain in the C6 dermatome (traveling down the lateral aspect of the arm and into the thumb and forefinger). Concomitant weakness of muscles innervated by the C6 nerve root, such as the biceps and wrist extensors, as well as sensory loss in the C6 dermatome and a diminished biceps reflex are sometimes also present. In the lumbar spine, posterior–lateral herniation of a disc will generally cause a radiculopathy.

Cauda equina syndrome results from compression of the cauda equina by a herniated disc, tumor, hematoma, or other mass.

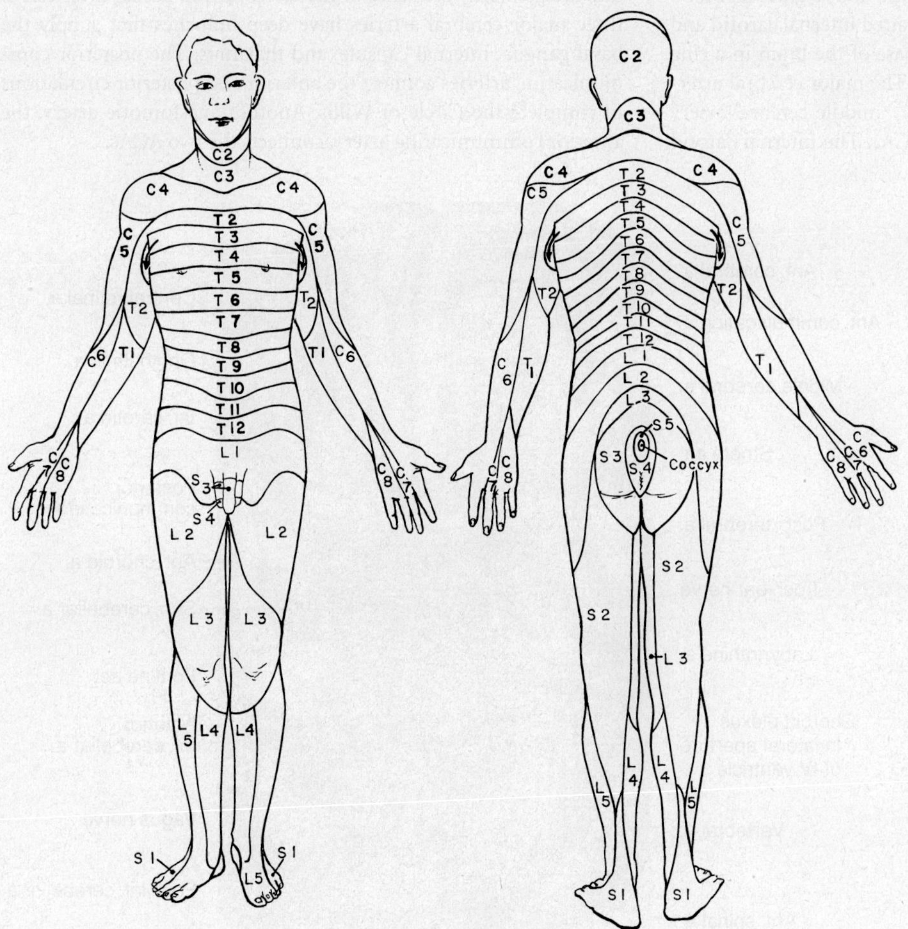

FIGURE 25.5 Dermatomes. The sensory innervation of the spinal roots. (From Barr ML, Kiernan JA. *The Human Nervous System*. Philadelphia: JB Lippincott Co; 1993, with permission.)

Compression of the roots typically leads to radicular pain and symptoms caused by dysfunction of the sacral nerve roots, specifically numbness in the perineum and groin, urinary retention, and occasionally bowel incontinence. Injury to the conus medullaris (terminal portion of the spinal cord) will result in similar bowel and bladder dysfunction, although pain is less prominent. Both are considered neurosurgical emergencies, requiring emergent magnetic resonance imaging (MRI) and sometimes surgical decompression if a structural cause is identified.

As stated previously, spinal stenosis is a degenerative condition of the spine characterized by accumulation of disc material, osteophytes, and thickening of the ligaments around the thecal sac and nerve roots leading to compression. Classically, spinal stenosis is associated with pain that is worsened by standing or walking (neurogenic claudication). It can be differentiated from vascular claudication with a thorough history. Neurogenic claudication causes pain that is often relieved by flexion at the waist or sitting and worsened by extension of the back or standing. In contrast, these maneuvers have no effect on symptoms of vascular claudication. The pain of neurogenic claudication is typically dermatomal in its distribution, although several dermatomes may be involved, and associated loss of sensation and tendon reflexes are sometimes present.

Vascular Anatomy

The brain receives roughly 15% of the heart's cardiac output but consumes an even greater proportion of the body's glucose. Blood reaches the brain via four arteries—the paired internal carotid and vertebral arteries, which coalesce at the base of the brain in a ring known as the Circle of Willis (Fig. 25.6). The major cerebral arteries are the anterior cerebral artery (ACA), middle cerebral artery (MCA), and posterior cerebral artery (PCA). The internal carotid arteries constitute the anterior circulation and give rise to the ACA and MCA, and the vertebral arteries join to form a single basilar artery, which constitutes the posterior circulation and gives rise to the PCA.

While variations exist, the right common carotid artery generally arises from the brachiocephalic trunk, the left common carotid arises directly from the aortic arch, and the vertebral arteries arise from their respective subclavian arteries. Both common carotid arteries bifurcate at approximately the level of the fourth cervical vertebral body forming the external and internal carotid arteries. The external carotid artery gives rise to several branches supplying the face, head, neck, and sinuses including the middle meningeal artery, which supplies the meninges and is a frequent culprit in the development of epidural hematomas. The internal carotid enters the skull through the carotid canal. It passes through the cavernous sinus and then bifurcates into the ACA and MCA at the base of the brain. The MCA provides blood to the lateral portion of the frontal lobe and the majority of the temporal and parietal lobes. The ACA provides blood to the medial portions of the frontal lobes and paramedian portions of the parietal lobes. Both vertebral arteries enter the bony transverse foramina of the cervical vertebrae at approximately the C6 level. They arch posteriorly around the C1 lamina and enter the foramen magnum after piercing the dura mater. The vertebral arteries join to form the basilar artery, which ascends anterior to the brain stem and finally bifurcates as the two PCAs. The PCA primarily supplies the occipital lobe and medial–inferior temporal lobe. The arteries supplying the brain stem and cerebellum are primarily branches of the vertebral and basilar arteries. All three major cerebral arteries have deep branches that supply the basal ganglia, internal capsule, and thalamus. The posterior communicating arteries connect the anterior and posterior circulations to complete the Circle of Willis. Another anastomotic artery, the anterior communicating artery, connects the two ACAs.

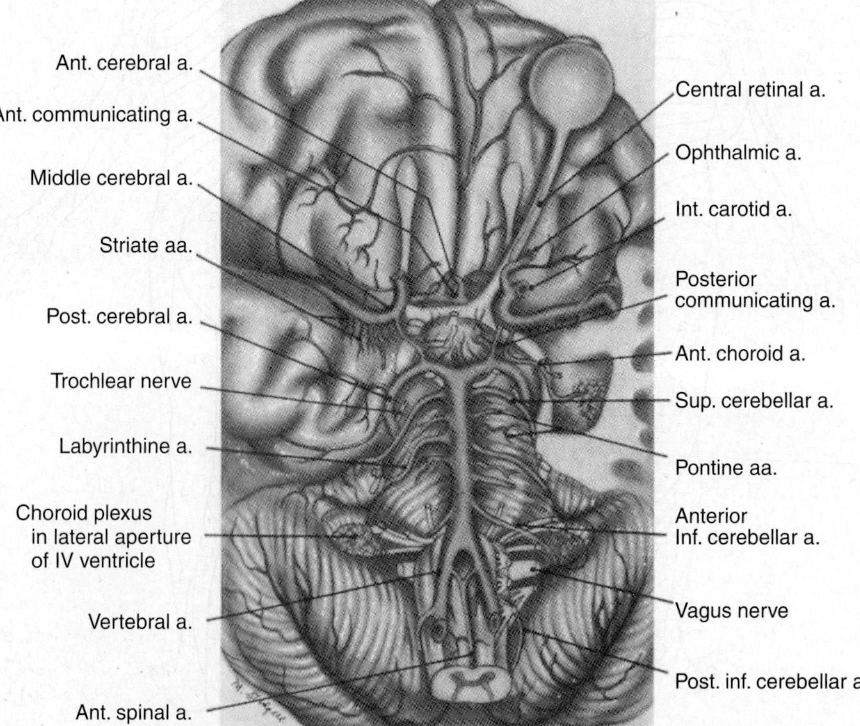

FIGURE 25.6 The ventral surface of the brain and the arterial anatomy. (From Carpenter MB. *Core Textbook of Neuroanatomy*. Baltimore: Williams and Wilkins; 1991, with permission.)

TABLE 25.1 Hunt and Hess classification system for aneurysm SAH

Grade	
0	Asymptomatic, unruptured
1	Asymptomatic, mild headache, or mild nuchal rigidity
1a	Fixed neurologic deficit (no headache or nuchal rigidity)
2	Cranial nerve palsy, moderate-to-severe headache, nuchal rigidity
3	Mild focal deficit, lethargy, or confusion
4	Stupor, moderate-to-severe hemiparesis, early decerebrate posturing
5	Deep coma, decerebrate posturing, moribund
	Add one grade for serious systemic disease or severe angiographic vasospasm

Cerebral aneurysms generally form at predictable branch points in the cerebral vasculature (e.g., the ACA origin, MCA bifurcation/trifurcation, origin of the posterior communicating artery, and the vertebrobasilar junction). Blood that flows from a ruptured aneurysm coats the surface of the gyri and sulci of the brain, usually in a pattern specific to the location of the ruptured aneurysm. This is termed subarachnoid hemorrhage (SAH). Ruptured aneurysms are the second most common cause of blood in the subarachnoid space after trauma, although the two entities have very different clinical behavior. Other causes of nontraumatic SAH include ruptured arteriovenous malformations (AVMs), hypertensive arteriopathy, and amyloid angiopathy.

Patients who present with aneurysmal SAH may complain of a slight headache or be completely comatose. The Hunt–Hess grading system (Table 25.1) is a useful prognostic tool. The initial diagnostic evaluation should include a computerized tomography (CT) scan and usually a four-vessel cerebral angiogram (the most sensitive and detailed study to evaluate cerebral arterial anatomy). Prompt treatment is generally undertaken to prevent ongoing hemorrhage and death or worsening neurologic outcomes. Therapeutic options include coil embolization of the aneurysm or open surgical clipping. Even after successful aneurysm occlusion, patients with SAH are at risk for secondary complications such as vasospasm (constriction of vessels possibly resulting in stroke); thus, aggressive monitoring is of paramount importance during the at-risk period, which lasts up to approximately 14 days from the initial bleed. Therapy is aimed at reducing vasospasm (calcium channel blockers) and maintaining intravascular volume and adequate blood pressure. Balloon angioplasty can be employed in refractory cases.

The primary vascular supply for the spinal cord is the anterior and posterior spinal arteries, which arise in the cervical region primarily from branches of the vertebral arteries. The single anterior spinal artery runs along the ventral surface of the cord, while the paired posterior spinal arteries run along the dorsal surface of the cord. The thoracic and lumbar regions of the cord are supplied by radicular arteries arising from the aorta. The largest of these is the artery of Adamkiewicz, which originates from the left side of the aorta between T10 and L2 in the majority of patients (Fig. 25.7).

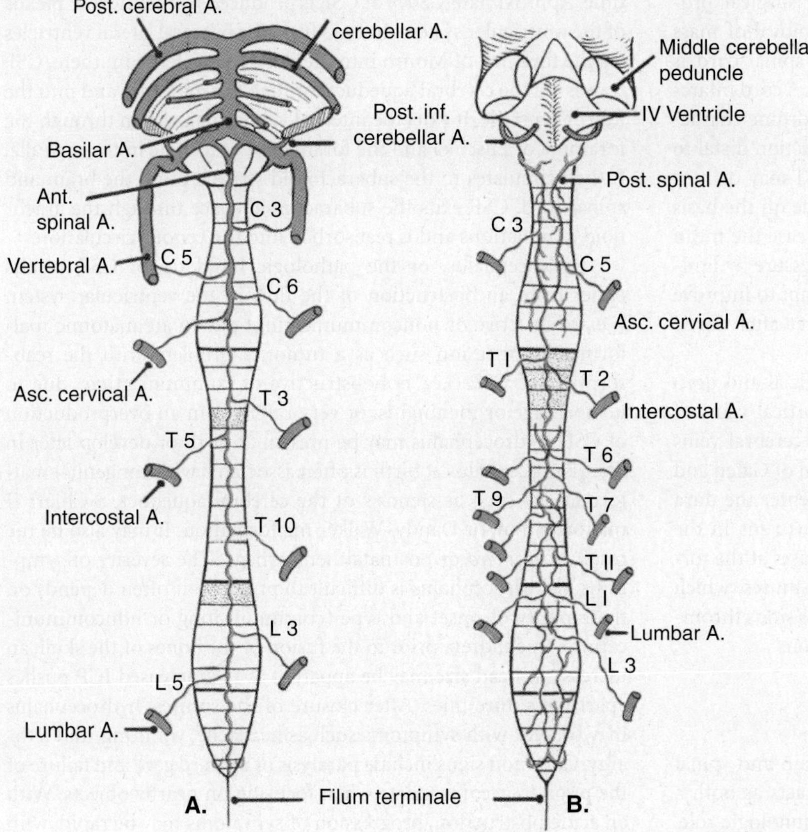

FIGURE 25.7 The arterial supply of the spinal cord. The watershed zones are stippled. **A.** Anterior view. **B.** Posterior view. (From Carpenter MB. *Core Textbook of Neuroanatomy*. Baltimore: Williams and Wilkins; 1991, with permission.)

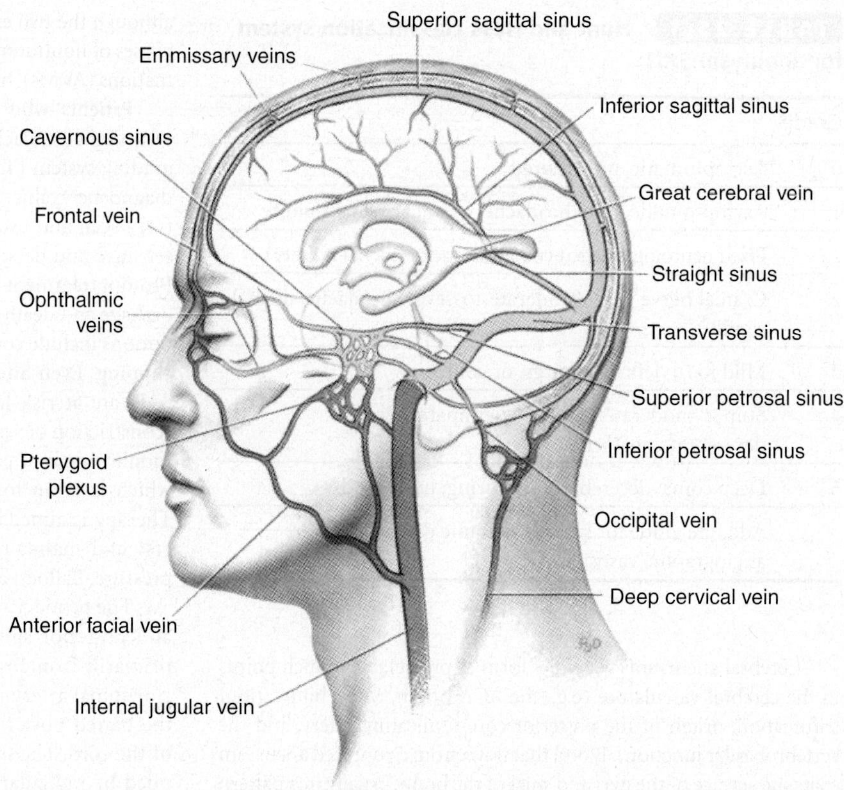

FIGURE 25.8 The venous drainage of the brain. (From Carpenter MB. *Core Textbook of Neuroanatomy*. Baltimore: Williams and Wilkins; 1991, with permission.)

The area of the thoracic spinal cord superior to the artery of Adamkiewicz is a watershed area with a relative paucity of blood flow, rendering it susceptible to infarction during surgical procedures such as repair of thoracic aneurysms or removal of mass lesions along the spine. The posterior half of the spinal cord is served by a more robust and redundant blood supply. A cord infarction will often result in an anterior spinal artery syndrome characterized by preserved sensation but lack of motor function distal to the lesion, and bowel and bladder dysfunction. MRI may or may not demonstrate a lesion; thus, the diagnosis is made on the basis of clinical findings. The chief intervention is to increase the mean arterial pressure (MAP). Reduction in intradural pressure by lumbar drain CSF diversion has been utilized in an attempt to improve spinal cord perfusion in cases of spinal cord infarct after aortic repair, but this technique is not universally practiced.

Venous drainage of the brain consists of superficial and deep systems (Fig. 25.8). Superficial veins include the cortical veins of Labbé and Trolard. Deep veins include the internal cerebral veins and basal veins of Rosenthal, which flow into the vein of Galen and subsequently into the straight sinus. Cortical veins enter the dura and drain into the venous sinuses. The sagittal sinus runs in the interhemispheric fissure and joins the transverse sinuses at the torcula. The transverse sinuses flow into the sigmoid sinuses, which become the jugular veins as they exit the skull. Venous sinus thrombosis can result in increased ICP and venous infarction.

CEREBROSPINAL FLUID

CSF is an ultrafiltrate of plasma that bathes the brain and spinal cord and resides within the subarachnoid space. It acts as both a mechanical cushion for the CNS and serves an immunologic role. CSF is produced at a rate of approximately 450 mL/day, although there is only approximately 150 mL of circulating CSF at any given time. Approximately 80% of CSF is produced by the choroid plexus of the ventricular system. It flows from the bilateral lateral ventricles via the foramen of Monro into the third ventricle. From there, CSF travels via the cerebral aqueduct through the midbrain and into the fourth ventricle. It exits the internal ventricular system through the foramina of Luschka and the foramen of Magendie in the medulla. It then circulates in the subarachnoid space around the brain and spinal cord. CSF exits the subarachnoid space through the arachnoid granulations and is reabsorbed into the venous circulation.

Hydrocephalus, or the pathologic build up of CSF, results either from an obstruction of the flow in the ventricular system (i.e., obstructive or noncommunicating) due to an anatomic malformation or lesion such as a tumor, a problem with the reabsorption of CSF (i.e., nonobstructive or communicating) due to hemorrhage or meningitis, or very rarely from an overproduction of CSF. Hydrocephalus may be present at birth or develop later in life. Hydrocephalus at birth is often associated with congenital malformations such as stenosis of the cerebral aqueduct, a Chiari II malformation, or Dandy–Walker malformation. It may also be the result of *in utero* or postnatal hemorrhage. The severity of symptoms of hydrocephalus is difficult to predict but often depends on the rapidity of onset and type (communicating or noncommunicating). In children, prior to the fusion of the bones of the skull, an increase in head size may be apparent as the increased ICP pushes apart the suture lines. After closure of the sutures, hydrocephalus may present with symptoms such as headache, vomiting, and lethargy. Common signs include paralysis of upward gaze and failure of the pupil to accommodate when focusing on nearby objects. With an acute obstruction, progression of symptoms may be rapid, with increasing somnolence and death due to herniation from elevated ICP. Chronic obstruction or communicating hydrocephalus has a more indolent course, with predominant symptoms such as behavior changes, lethargy, and headaches. Normal pressure hydrocephalus afflicts the elderly with a classic triad of symptoms including abnormal gait, cognitive slowing, and urinary incontinence. CT scan reveals dilated ventricles and no evidence of an obstructive lesion. Symptoms often improve following high-volume lumbar punctures or permanent CSF diversion.

Surgeons often find themselves evaluating patients with new-onset hydrocephalus as well those who have previously undergone CSF diversion procedures. Shunts function by diverting CSF from within the ventricular system to some other location, most commonly the peritoneal space, although other areas, such as the pleural space, a large central vein, or the atrium of the heart, are also used. Shunt systems are equipped with a valve to prevent backflow of contents into the brain and regulate the rate or pressure above which CSF is shunted out of the ventricles. This valve is then connected to distal tubing and tunneled subcutaneously to its site of termination. The most common causes of shunt failure are obstruction and infection. Treatment of an obstructed catheter consists of replacement of the defective or clotted portion. In the case of infection, the entire system must be removed with temporary external CSF drainage, treatment with antibiotics, and eventual reinternalization.

A CSF leak can occur following trauma, skull base or sinus surgery, lumbar surgery, chronic ear infections, or sinusitis or can be due to an invasive or destructive tumor. The presence of concomitant effluent from the nose or a surgical site can confound attempts to diagnose a CSF leak. CSF is thinner than mucus or blood, and, unlike mucus, it contains glucose. The most specific test for CSF is measurement of β-2 transferrin, a low molecular weight protein found only in the CSF.

NEURORADIOLOGY

Modern neuroimaging modalities, such as CT and MRI, serve a routine role in the diagnosis of neurosurgical disorders and are becoming increasingly utilized in treatment planning. Plain film x-rays are useful for the intraoperative and postoperative evaluation of hardware placement in the spine, and in select circumstances to evaluate abnormal spinal movement. Dynamic films such as flexion–extension views can be useful to assess spinal stability in a variety of clinical settings including degenerative, destructive, and traumatic conditions.

CT scans were developed from x-ray technology and measure the density of tissue. Thus, the terms hyperdense (brighter), isodense (similar in appearance), and hypodense (darker) are used to describe findings on CT scans relative to normal brain. CT can identify a variety of neurosurgical abnormalities including bony pathology, hemorrhage, infarction, tumors, vascular abnormalities, and foreign bodies. CT is the imaging modality of choice for most acute processes, such as acute hemorrhage or fractures (Fig. 25.9). CT is more sensitive than plain x-rays for visualizing fractures and is routinely used in evaluation of major spine trauma in many centers. The appearance of blood on CT scan depends on the age of the blood, with recent hemorrhage appearing hyperdense relative to brain and chronic blood appearing hypodense after 2 to 3 weeks. A caveat to the above generalization is that acute hemorrhage may appear relatively isodense in the anemic patient. Fresh, unclotted

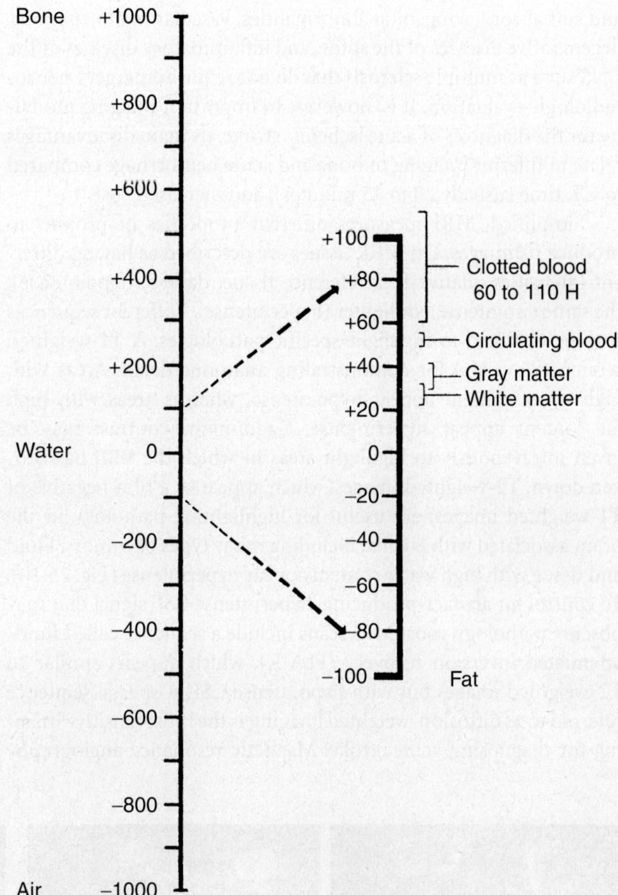

FIGURE 25.9 Hounsfield number scale with values of certain body tissues. This determines the appearance of the tissue CT scan. (From Taveras JM. *Neuroradiology*. Baltimore: Williams and Wilkins; 1996, with permission.)

blood appears isodense, as well. Mixed-density blood in an acute clot often reflects active hemorrhage, and in patients, with underlying iatrogenic or pathologic coagulopathies, blood may remain unclotted and isodense for extended periods. Infarction, on the other hand, is not readily visualized in the first 4 to 6 hours but then appears hypodense in the vascular territory of the infarct due to neuronal and glial cell death and subsequent cerebral edema. In addition, there may be mass effect associated with the edematous, infarcted tissue pushing against healthy structures. Over time, the infarcted tissue shrinks and remains relatively hypodense due to gliosis, or scarring, of the injured tissue. Tumors have a variable appearance depending on the pathology and may appear hypodense, isodense, or hyperdense. They may or may not have cystic components, areas of hemorrhage, or calcifications. The addition of intravenous contrast is routinely used when a neoplasm is suspected and highlights areas where the BBB has broken down. Not all tumors contrast enhance, thus the contrast pattern aids in formulating a differential diagnosis. Other enhancing processes include infections and abscesses. With correct timing, the cerebral vasculature may be imaged while contrast is passing through and 3-D reconstructions created, a technique called CT angiography.

MRI provides greater resolution and is useful in the evaluation of low-contrast or chronic processes, including tumors of the brain and spinal cord, congenital abnormalities, vascular malformations, degenerative diseases of the spine, and inflammatory diseases of the CNS such as multiple sclerosis that do not require emergent neuroradiologic evaluation. It is, however, an important imaging modality for the diagnosis of acute ischemic stroke. Its main disadvantages relate to inferior imaging of bone and acute hemorrhage compared to CT, time (usually 20 to 45 minutes), and increased cost.

Simplified, MRI measures different properties of protons to produce its images. On MRI, tissues are described as having different intensities relative to a reference tissue: darker (hypointense), the same (isointense), or lighter (hyperintense). Different sequences may be obtained to highlight specific pathologies. A T1-weighted sequence is useful for demonstrating anatomic detail. Areas with high water content appear hypointense, whereas areas with high fat content appear hyperintense. Gadolinium contrast may be given intravenously to highlight areas in which the BBB has broken down. T2-weighted images, which appear as a film negative of T1-weighted images, are useful for highlighting pathology in the brain associated with edema, including many types of tumors. Fluid and tissue with high water content appear hyperintense (Fig. 25.10). To control for artifact-producing, hyperintense CSF signal that may obscure pathology, most MRI scans include a sequence called fluid-attenuated inversion recovery (FLAIR), which appears similar to T2-weighted images but with hypointense CSF. A special sequence referred to as diffusion-weighted imaging is the most sensitive imaging for diagnosing acute stroke. Magnetic resonance angiography (MRA) is useful in evaluating the extracranial carotid arteries and the major intracranial arteries. Magnetic resonance venography (MRV) can be used to evaluate the venous sinuses.

More recently, specialized MRI techniques including magnetic resonance spectroscopy (MRS), diffusion tensor imaging (DTI), and functional MRI (fMRI) are being using for even further diagnostic evaluation of pathology. MRS delineates levels of biochemicals and neurotransmitters in the brain and can aid in such situations as differentiating a tumor from an abscess, MS plaque, or radiation-induced necrosis. DTI allows white matter tracts to be identified and is increasingly used intraoperatively to permit surgeons to approach or resect pathology while not disturbing critical tracts, such as those that transmit visual signals or connect language areas. Finally, fMRI may be used to localize the function of various areas of the brain, such as language and motor function, and has been used both clinically and in research.

Cerebral angiography is an invasive procedure used to diagnose and potentially treat vascular abnormalities of the CNS. It is associated with a risk of stroke of between 0.5% and 3%. Most commonly, it is used in the evaluation of a patient with SAH, carotid stenosis or dissection, traumatic arterial injury, AVM, or vasculitis. Therapeutic procedures may be performed with angiography including coiling of an aneurysm, embolization of a vessel that is bleeding, thrombolysis of a thrombus to treat acute ischemic stroke, and stenting of stenotic vessels.

Myelography is another invasive procedure in which contrast dye is instilled into the thecal sac via a lumbar puncture and allowed

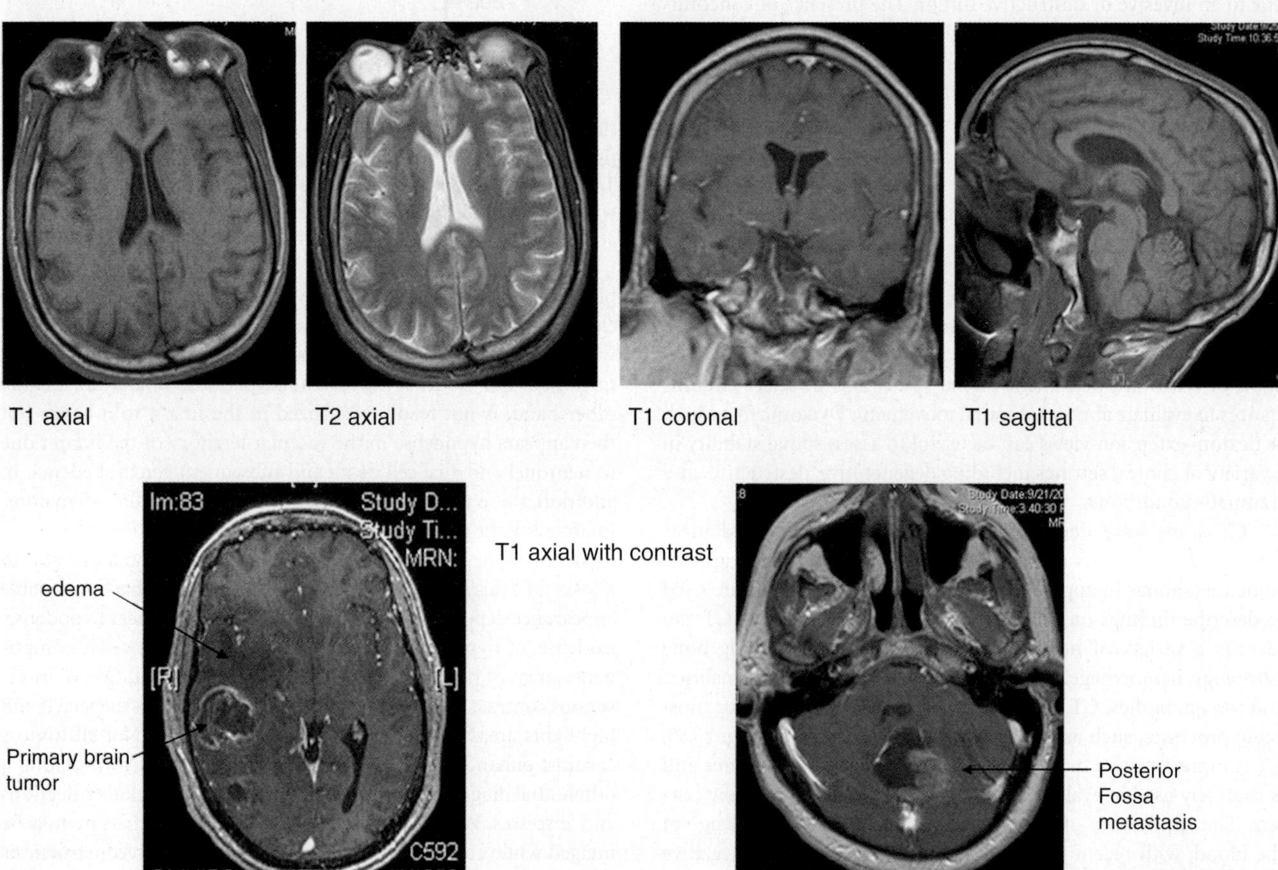

FIGURE 25.10 Composite brain MRI with representative sequences (T1, T2) and orientations for normal and pathologic conditions.

to diffuse. Previously, plain film x-rays were taken to localize any blockage of flow. CT has enhanced the utility of myelography by allowing axial images to be obtained. Myelography has largely been supplanted by MRI; however, it remains useful in situations in which MRI scanning is contraindicated or nondiagnostic.

CRANIAL TRAUMA

Evaluation of the trauma patient with a suspected head or spinal cord injury (SCI) begins with an assessment of airway, breathing, and circulation and initiation of advanced trauma life support (ATLS) protocols as indicated. Responders should determine the patient's Glasgow coma scale (GCS) score (Table 25.2). Coma is defined as a GCS of 8 or less. GCS can also be used to define the severity of the head injury. After initial resuscitation or hemodynamic stabilization, clinical and radiographic examinations are performed to rapidly identify life-threatening injuries that require immediate attention. Physical examination should include a search for external injuries that suggest a brain injury, such as a leakage of CSF from the nose or ears or bruising around the orbit or on the mastoid process, indicative of a basal skull fracture. Physical examination should always include a check for pupillary reactivity. Medications such as atropine may alter pupillary findings, although systemic paralytics used for rapid sequence intubation are unlikely to alter the pupillary light response. Lateralizing neurologic signs, such as hemiparesis, eye deviation, or facial asymmetry, should be assessed. The initial evaluation usually includes a CT scan of the cervical spine and a noncontrast CT scan of the head in addition to a more focused trauma evaluation. Patients with severe head injury commonly harbor an epidural, subdural, or intraparenchymal hematoma and may require emergent craniotomy for clot evacuation and hemostasis.

Head injuries may be subdivided into primary and secondary phases. Primary injury occurs at the time of the initial trauma and often results in irreversible damage to neurons. The goal of management of traumatic brain injury is to minimize secondary injury, which results from elevated ICP, ischemia, metabolic abnormalities, seizure, and hyperthermia. Primary injuries can be further subdivided into intracranial hemorrhages (e.g., epidural, subdural, subarachnoid, intraparenchymal) and cerebral contusions. Secondary injuries occur hours to days after the primary injury and include cerebral edema, excitotoxic damage, and impaired cerebral blood flow. Careful management of blood pressure (systolic blood pressure >90 mm Hg), cerebral perfusion, oxygenation (Pao_2 > 60 mm Hg), and control of elevated ICP can prevent secondary injuries.

Epidural hematomas most commonly occur with blunt trauma to the side of the head that results in fracture of the temporal bone with associated laceration of the middle meningeal artery. Less commonly, injury to a dural sinus may result in a hematoma. Both events result in bleeding into the epidural space, dissecting the dura mater away from the bone. A characteristic lentiform mass appears on CT scan respecting the suture lines, where the dura is adherent to the bone (Fig. 25.11). Patients with epidural hematomas do not often follow the classically described course of a lucid interval following an initial injury with subsequent deterioration. Focal neurologic deficits, such as hemiparesis, a third nerve palsy, or aphasia, are often associated with epidural hematomas.

Acute subdural hematomas result from injury to the bridging veins, classically as they enter the dura to drain into a dural sinus. The shifting of the brain inside the skull generates shear forces on the veins as the dura remains relatively fixed against the overlying skull. Blood accumulates into the subdural space, creating the characteristic crescent-shaped collection that crosses suture lines on CT scan (Fig. 25.11). Blood may also be seen collecting along the falx cerebri between cerebral hemispheres or along the tentorium above the cerebellum. Definitive treatment of acute subdural hematomas associated with mass effect on the brain, and depressed GCS is an urgent craniotomy for clot evacuation.

Chronic subdural hematomas are generally seen in older patients with less severe traumatic mechanisms. They are also caused by ruptured bridging veins that result in the accumulation of subdural blood. This can happen with trivial trauma in the elderly or coagulopathic patient. Patients are often initially asymptomatic. Eventually, membranes composed of dural border cells and extracellular substance form to wall off the blood and the coagulated blood liquefies. Such collections can expand over time, resulting in brain shift and focal symptoms (Fig. 25.11). Symptoms are often mistaken for a transient ischemic attack (TIA) or ischemic stroke. Because the collections are often liquid, they can be drained with burr holes rather than a larger craniotomy; however, loculated or recurrent collections sometimes require more extensive surgical intervention. Recurrent subdural collections with extensive membranes often require a craniotomy for subdural drainage and lysis of membranes to prevent recurrence.

Traumatic SAH often accompanies other forms of head injury. The rupture of small vessels in the subarachnoid space spills blood around the gyri of the brain (Fig. 25.11). The antiepileptic drug (AED) phenytoin is recommended in cases of traumatic SAH to prevent the occurrence of early seizures. No evidence suggests AEDs prevent late seizures, as such the drug is only recommended for 7 days following the traumatic injury. Increasing evidence suggests alternative AEDs, including levetiracetam, may be equally effective as phenytoin at preventing early seizures after TBI.

TABLE 25.2 Glasgow coma scale

Function	Score
Eye opening	
Spontaneous	4
To voice	3
To pain	2
None	1
Best verbal response	
Coherent speech	5
Confused speech	4
Words only, incoherent	3
Sounds only	2
None	1
Best motor response	
Obeys commands	6
Localizes to pain	5
Withdraws to pain	4
Flexor posturing to pain	3
Extensor posturing to pain	2
None	1

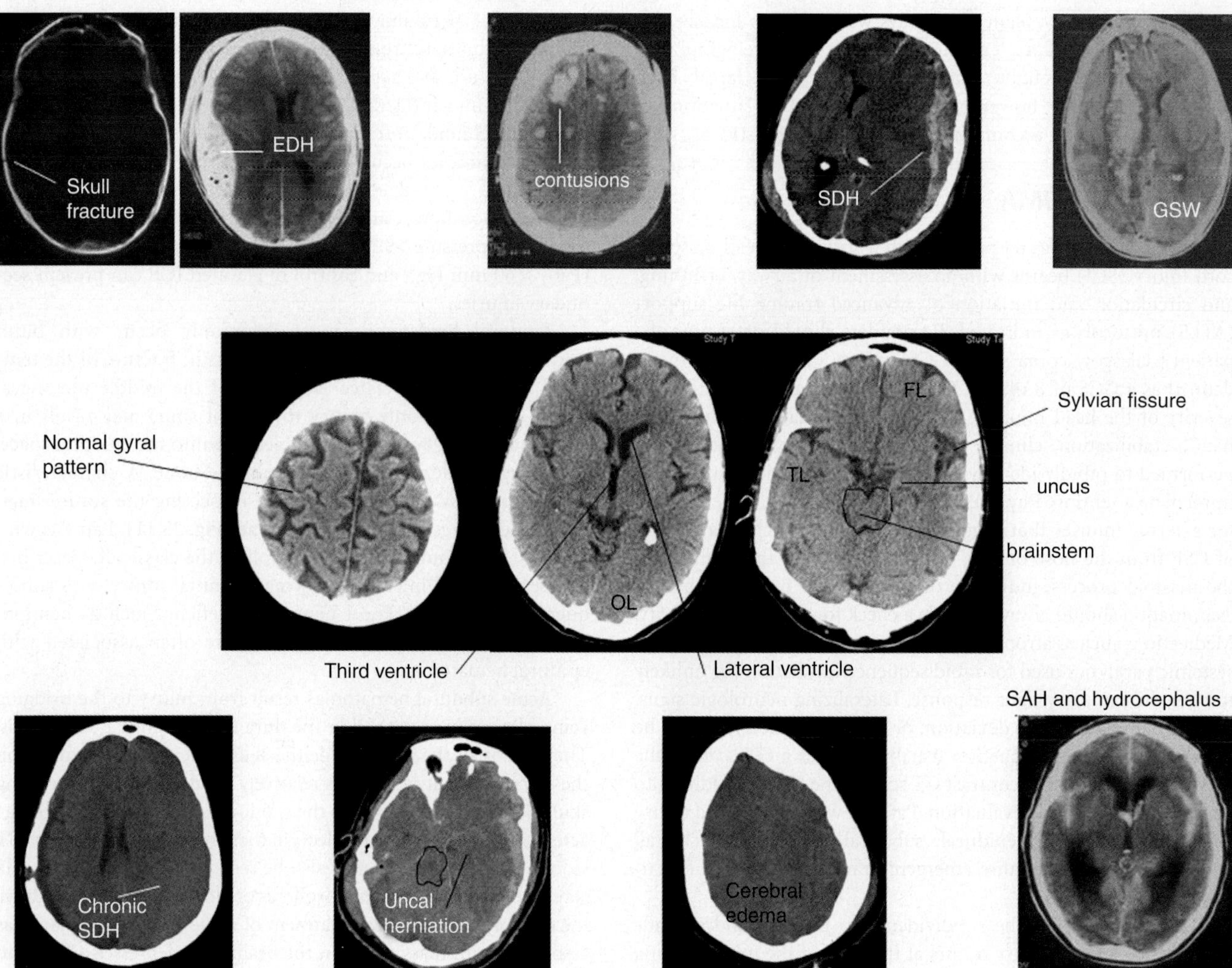

FIGURE 25.11 Composite head CT scans for normal and representative pathologic conditions.

Intraparenchymal hemorrhage may also occur following trauma or can result from hypertension, hemorrhagic conversion of an ischemic stroke, or in the setting of anticoagulation. Location, size, cause, neurologic status, and ICP are evaluated to determine the need for surgical evacuation. Smaller areas of hemorrhage inside the brain parenchyma are called contusions (Fig. 25.11). They result from deformation of the brain as it is subjected to shearing forces during blunt trauma. The inferior frontal and anterior temporal lobes are the most common sites of contusions. Coup injuries occur in the cortex directly beneath the cranial location of the impact, whereas contrecoup injuries occur at sites remote from the area of impact.

Mechanisms of injury that impart a large amount of force to the brain can induce diffuse axonal injury without a large focal contusion or hemorrhage. Microscopically, deformation in the shape of the brain puts strain on the relatively stiff axons of certain populations of neurons, leading to their disruption. Radiographically, small hemorrhages may be seen in white matter tracts, especially the corpus callosum, pons, or at the junction of gray matter and white matter in the cortex. Deficits are unpredictable, and prognosis bears little relation to the specific radiographic abnormalities identified.

Elevated ICP and/or lateralizing mass lesions can cause midline brain shift and brain stem compression termed herniation. The specific type of herniation depends on the area of the brain involved (central, uncal, subfalcine). The classic trauma herniation syndrome (uncal herniation) results from a lateralizing lesion such as a subdural or epidural hemorrhage. With expansion of the blood clot, the temporal lobe is displaced medially toward the brain stem. The most medial portion of the temporal lobe (uncus) pushes against the third cranial nerve, causing dysfunction of the parasympathetic fibers that control pupillary constriction. This results in unopposed sympathetic input to the pupil resulting in an ipsilateral, dilated, "blown pupil." With further displacement, the uncus pushes against cerebral peduncle of the brain stem, causing dysfunction in the as yet uncrossed cerebral spinal fibers, causing contralateral weakness, and, sometimes, abnormal posturing. As the brain herniates through the tentorium (the opening in the dura separating the cerebellum from the cerebral hemispheres), compression of the PCAs may lead to bilateral strokes. Central or transtentorial herniation can occur with more centralized swelling or mass lesion, resulting in progressive compression of the brain stem at the tentorium. Progressive lethargy, respiratory irregularity, and abnormal posturing and hyperreflexia generally precede pupillary dysfunction. Subfalcine herniation occurs when the structures of the medial frontal lobes herniated toward the contralateral side beneath the falx, sometimes leading to occlusion of the ACAs. The

Cushing triad of hypertension, bradycardia, and respiratory irregularity may reflect a near-terminal event with swelling in the posterior fossa, resulting in displacement of the cerebellar tonsils against the brain stem at the foramen magnum (tonsillar herniation).

Abnormal "posturing" results when higher cortical functions no longer suppress primitive brain stem and spinal reflexes. Patients with decorticate posturing present with arms flexed, or bent inward on the chest, hands clenched into fists, and legs extended. This generally corresponds to dysfunction above the level of the red nucleus in the midbrain. In decerebrate posturing, the head is arched back, the arms are extended by the sides (extended elbows), and the legs are extended. This corresponds to dysfunction below the level of the midbrain, as in late herniation or brain stem infarction.

The Brain Trauma Foundation recommendations for management of severe traumatic brain injury have undergone multiple revisions since their initial publication in 1995, commensurate with rapid advances in our understanding of optimal management for this condition. Table 25.3 outlines specific recommendations for a variety of clinical scenarios. The decision to place a monitor for ICP depends on the patient's neurologic examination (e.g., GCS < 8), the mechanism of injury, evidence of mass effect on CT imaging, and the likelihood of surgical intervention. For example, an epidural hematoma with mass effect is a surgical emergency; time should not be taken to place an ICP monitor. The type of monitor placed varies according to a surgeon's preference and institutional practice. Intraventricular catheters are often utilized because of their accuracy, low cost, and ability to help reduce ICP through the drainage of CSF. A host of fiberoptic and microstrain devices are also available; those placed in the brain parenchyma to monitor pressure are more accurate than subdural or subarachnoid monitors. An ICP monitor can guide hyperosmolar therapy (mannitol or hypertonic saline), although placement can cause hemorrhage necessitating surgical evacuation. If elevated ICP is refractory to medical therapy (including hyperosmolar agents and sedation), the first intervention available to the surgeon is CSF diversion via placement of a ventriculostomy catheter. Draining even a few milliliters of CSF per hour can have dramatic effects on pressure.

In cases of refractory increased ICP and poor brain oxygenation, decompressive craniectomy can be utilized. A portion of the skull is removed, the dura is opened, and the scalp is closed. The bone flap is stored either subcutaneously in the abdomen or sterilely in a freezer. When brain swelling resolves, the bone can be replaced. While this is a very effective method for reducing ICP, the ultimate clinical outcome is closely tied to the severity of the initial injury.

The management of penetrating injuries does not differ significantly from that of blunt injuries: medical support, ICP control, monitoring, and surgery are initiated using similar criteria. One caveat is that penetrating injuries, especially gunshot wounds, are associated with the development of pseudoaneurysms days to weeks after the initial traumatic event. Dedicated vascular imaging is recommended to aid in management.

Brain death inexorably follows the most severe brain injuries despite intervention. Guidelines for the determination of brain death are not universal; the most consistent features are the absence of brain stem reflexes, motor response to pain, and spontaneous respirations in the absence of pharmacologic paralysis or excessive sedation. Two neurologic examinations separated by 6 to 12 hours must consistently demonstrate the absence of these functions. Demonstration of the loss of respiratory drive in response to increased PCO_2 (apnea test) is also often required. Some institutions additionally require a confirmatory test such as an electroencephalogram (EEG) or a nuclear medicine perfusion scan showing a lack of blood flow or uptake of radioisotope into the brain. Guidelines are institution specific and should be strictly adhered to ensure consistency.

Spinal Trauma

Spinal column and spinal cord injuries are common in patients who have incurred significant trauma, and patients are assumed to harbor spinal injuries until proven otherwise. Thus, management begins in the prehospital setting. Trauma patients undergo immobilization of the entire spine with a rigid cervical collar and rigid backboard until injuries have been ruled out. The neck should be neutrally aligned; if the patient is awake and cooperative, they may move their neck into alignment, and if the patient is unconscious or uncooperative, the responder may passively move the neck into alignment. Any resistance to movement, pain, or neurologic deterioration makes further attempts contraindicated, and the neck should be braced in that position. Full spine precautions are also maintained to logroll a patient to allow inspection and palpation of the spine looking for bruising, swelling, tenderness, and step-offs. These assessments should be done in a timely fashion to reduce the amount of time the patient spends on a backboard and thus avoid skin breakdown. Of note, spinal immobilization should not be prioritized over the standard ATLS primary survey (airway, breathing, circulation) or other lifesaving interventions such as cardiopulmonary resuscitation. It is unclear whether all patients need to undergo immobilization, as many do not have spinal injuries, which is an area for further research and triage guidelines.

Cervical spine clearance generally requires negative radiographic imaging and/or lack of clinically significant tenderness to palpation in awake, cooperative patients. If a patient is alert, neurologically intact, and without head injury, distracting injury (e.g., leg fracture), and intoxication with drugs or alcohol, clinical clearance may be obtained if there is no bruising, deformity, pain at rest, pain with active palpation, and pain-free range of motion. Radiographs should be obtained in all other patients who do not meet the aforementioned criteria for clinical clearance. Difficulties arise in unresponsive patients, patients with altered mental status, or distracting injuries. Neurologic examinations need to be performed in a systematic and objective manner, including an assessment of intact motor/sensory levels, perianal sensation, rectal tone, and the presence or absence of normal and abnormal reflexes. Radiographs include both plain x-rays and CT scans. Patient with low-impact trauma may have spine radiographs performed as the first step. The standard cervical spine x-ray series include anterior–posterior, lateral, and open-mouth views. In high-impact trauma, CT scans have generally supplanted plain x-rays as the initial radiographic assessment. Helical scans of the cervical spine and often reconstructions of the thoracic and lumbar spines from the CT of the chest and abdomen are routinely performed to assess for injury at most centers. If a fracture is identified, a search for additional fractures should ensue as approximately 20% of patients will have a second spinal injury at a different level. In patients with normal radiographic studies and persistent symptoms, such as a neurologic deficit or persistent pain, MRI scan is pursued to evaluate the ligaments, soft tissue, spinal cord, and nerve roots. The trend for unconscious or severely brain-injured patients with suspected cervical spine

TABLE 25.3 Therapeutic recommendations in traumatic brain injury

Parameter	Recommendation	Clarifications and Qualifications
Blood pressure	Avoid SBP <90	
Oxygenation	Avoid hypoxia (Pao_2 < 60, saturation <90%)	
Mannitol	Used as needed, 0.25–1 g/kg	Avoid use of mannitol without ICP monitoring device, except as single dose emergently prior to surgical intervention
Hypertonic saline	Constant infusion, parameters in flux	Use governed by practice guidelines of individual institutions
Prophylactic hypothermia	Not universally recommended	May have benefit for specific subgroups
Infection prevention	Periprocedural antibiotics not universally recommended	Ventricular catheter changes or periprocedural antibiotics for ventricular catheters not recommended Early tracheostomy recommended
DVT prophylaxis	Intermittent compression devices are recommended	Pharmacologic prophylaxis is associated with risk of hemorrhage; no evidence to support its use
ICP monitoring	Recommended for TBI patients with GCS 3–8 and abnormal CT scan findings	May be fiberoptic bolt or intraventricular catheter
ICP monitoring devices	Ventricular catheters are the most accurate means	Parenchymal fiber optic or strain gauge monitors are acceptable; subarachnoid or subdural bolts are less accurate
ICP targets	Target ICP <20	Clinician must account for CT scan findings and comorbidities when deciding to treat elevated ICP
Cerebral perfusion pressure (CPP, where CPP = MAP–ICP)	Avoid aggressive attempts to keep CPP >70 out of concern for respiratory distress	Avoid CPP <50
Brain oxygen monitoring (with either jugular venous saturation monitor or intraparenchymal fiber optic monitor)	No strong consensus data exist to support targets for oxygen monitoring	Less robust data favor maintaining brain oxygen saturation >15 mm Hg and jugular venous saturation >50%
Anesthesia	Propofol is recommended for sedation Barbiturate coma is restricted to elevations in ICP refractory to other therapies	Propofol is associated with specific morbidities Hemodynamic instability with barbiturate coma should be avoided
Feeding	Patients should be fed by postinjury day 7	
Seizure prophylaxis	Anticonvulsants do not prevent late (>7 d after injury) posttraumatic seizures. They prevent early seizures. Valproate or phenytoin is recommended	Early seizures may not be associated with worsened outcome
Hyperventilation	Hyperventilation ($Paco_2$ < 25) is not recommended	Hyperventilation may be used as an emergency intervention to lower ICP before more definitive therapy is initiated
Steroids	Steroids should not be used	Strong evidence against the utility of steroids

injury is for early MRI scan, rather than prolonged immobilization until able to be clinically cleared or practitioner-assisted active flexion–extension fluoroscopy.

Considering the specific mechanisms and forces involved in a traumatic spine injury helps a clinician anticipate injuries and plan interventions. These forces can generally be classified as axial loading, distraction, rotation, flexion, extension, translational shear, or some combination thereof. It is also useful to separate the spine into the axial (occiput to C2) and subaxial segments (C3–C7) for purposes of classification. Distraction can lead to occipitocervical dissociation, an extremely dangerous injury in which the ligaments holding the skull to the spine are disrupted. Respiratory arrest may ensue as the brainstem is stretched. Compression injuries occur when an axial load is applied along the long axis of the spine. In the upper cervical spine, it can lead to a fracture of C1, called a Jefferson fracture, which was classically a four-point fracture of the ring of C1, but now is used to describe both two- and three-point fractures, as well. Nearly 40% of patients with a Jefferson fracture have a concomitant C2 fracture. C2 fractures include odontoid (dens) fractures and the hangman's fracture, which is fracture of the bilateral pars interarticularis components of C2, effectively disconnecting the lamina of C2 from the vertebral bodies. Odontoid fractures are most commonly flexion injuries, while hangman's fractures are typically extension injuries. Axial loading and flexion injuries are common in the cervical spine, leading to burst-type fractures and subluxation of the facet joints with resultant spinal cord compression. These injuries are often treated with cervical traction with progressive addition of weights to reduce fractures/subluxations (Fig. 25.12). These maneuvers are performed under light anesthesia to permit frequent neurologic examinations and require serial radiographic imaging as weight is added. After reduction, these injuries often require surgical stabilization.

The management of fractures of the thoracic and lumbar spine follows similar principles. Radiographs are indicated if there is pain, bruising, deformity, or neurologic deficit in the thoracolumbar region. Plain radiographs or a CT scan may be initially obtained to evaluate for fractures, although MRI is necessary if there is neurologic deficit without an obvious source, as well for evaluating the posterior ligamentous complex. Because of the significant energy transfer required to cause these injuries, concomitant chest and abdominal injuries are common. Burst-type injuries in the thoracolumbar spine are particularly common (Fig. 25.13). Decisions regarding the need for operation and/or external bracing are based on several factors including the extent of bony injury, the neurologic status of the patient, and the integrity of the posterior ligamentous complex.

SCI is a complication of spine trauma and may be associated with a fracture, a herniated intervertebral disc, ligamentous disruption, or penetrating injury. SCI may be classified as either "complete" or "incomplete" injuries and is graded by the American Spinal Injury Association (ASIA) classification (Fig. 25.14; Table 25.5). "Complete" injuries result in complete loss of motor and sensory function below the level of injury, and "incomplete" injuries range from mild findings to complete loss of motor with preserved sensation below the level of injury. Injuries are classified according to the lowest motor level at which function is retained (at least 3/5 motor strength) (Table 25.4). For instance, a patient with preserved biceps and wrist extension function but no triceps strength has a

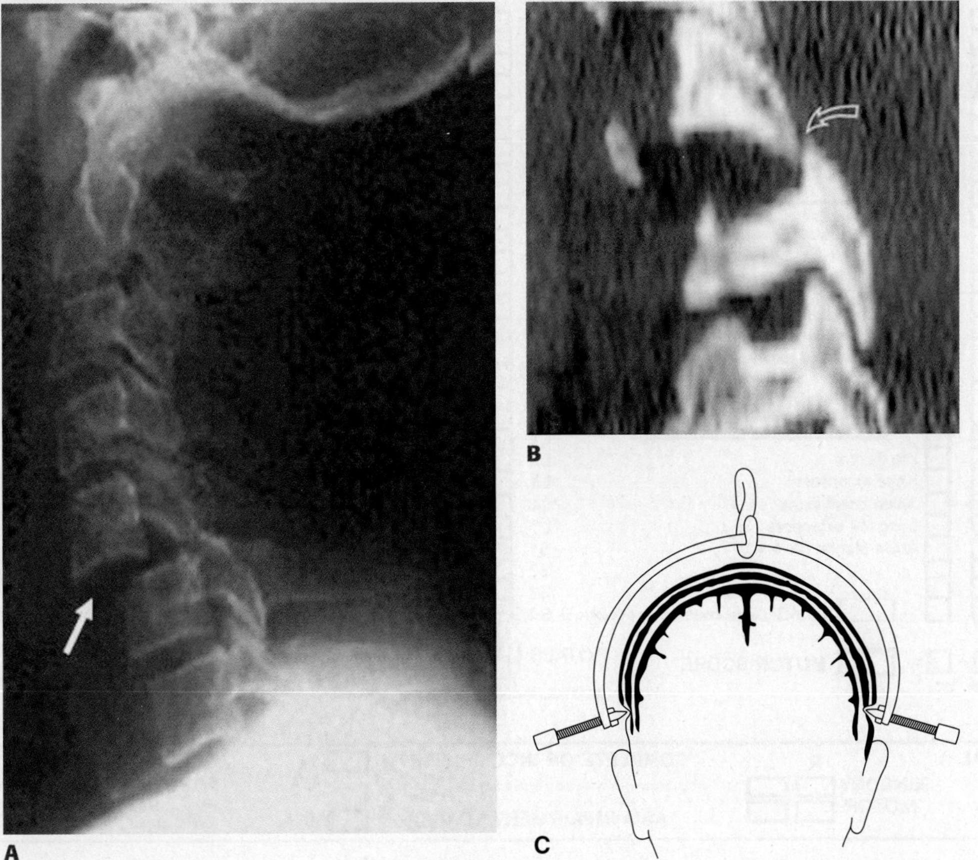

FIGURE 25.12 A. Lateral C-spine x-ray showing vertebral subluxation. **B.** Sagittal CT reconstruction showing subluxed facets. **C.** Drawing showing placement of Gardner–Wells tongs.

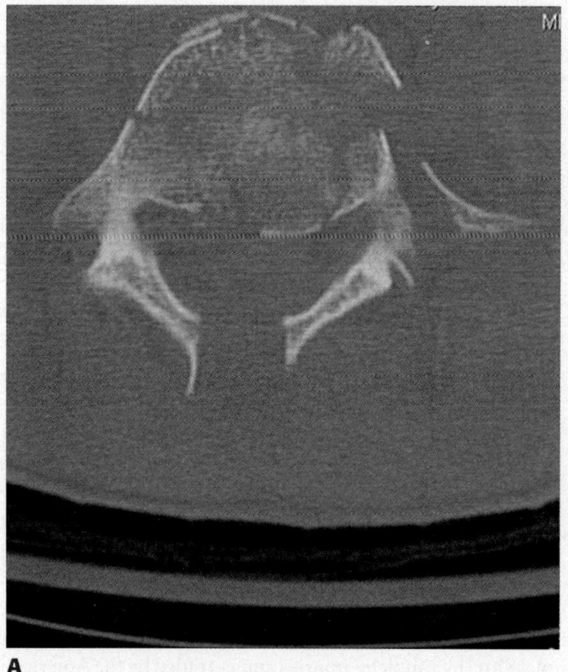

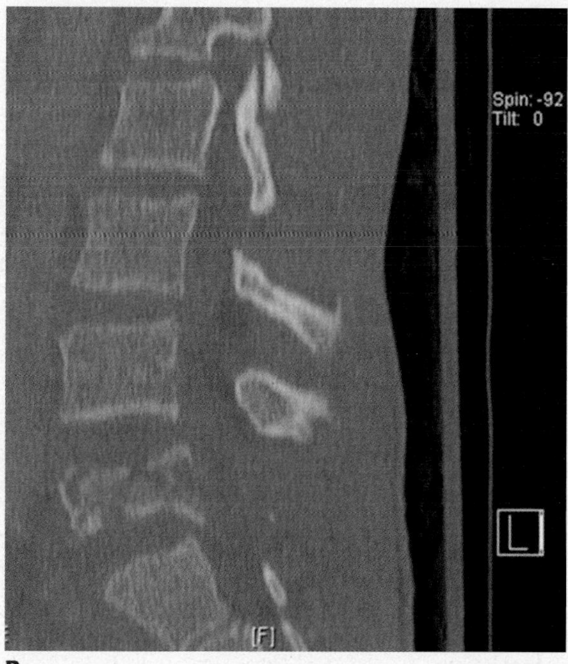

A **B**

FIGURE 25.13 Axial **(A)** and sagittal **(B)** images of an L5 burst fracture.

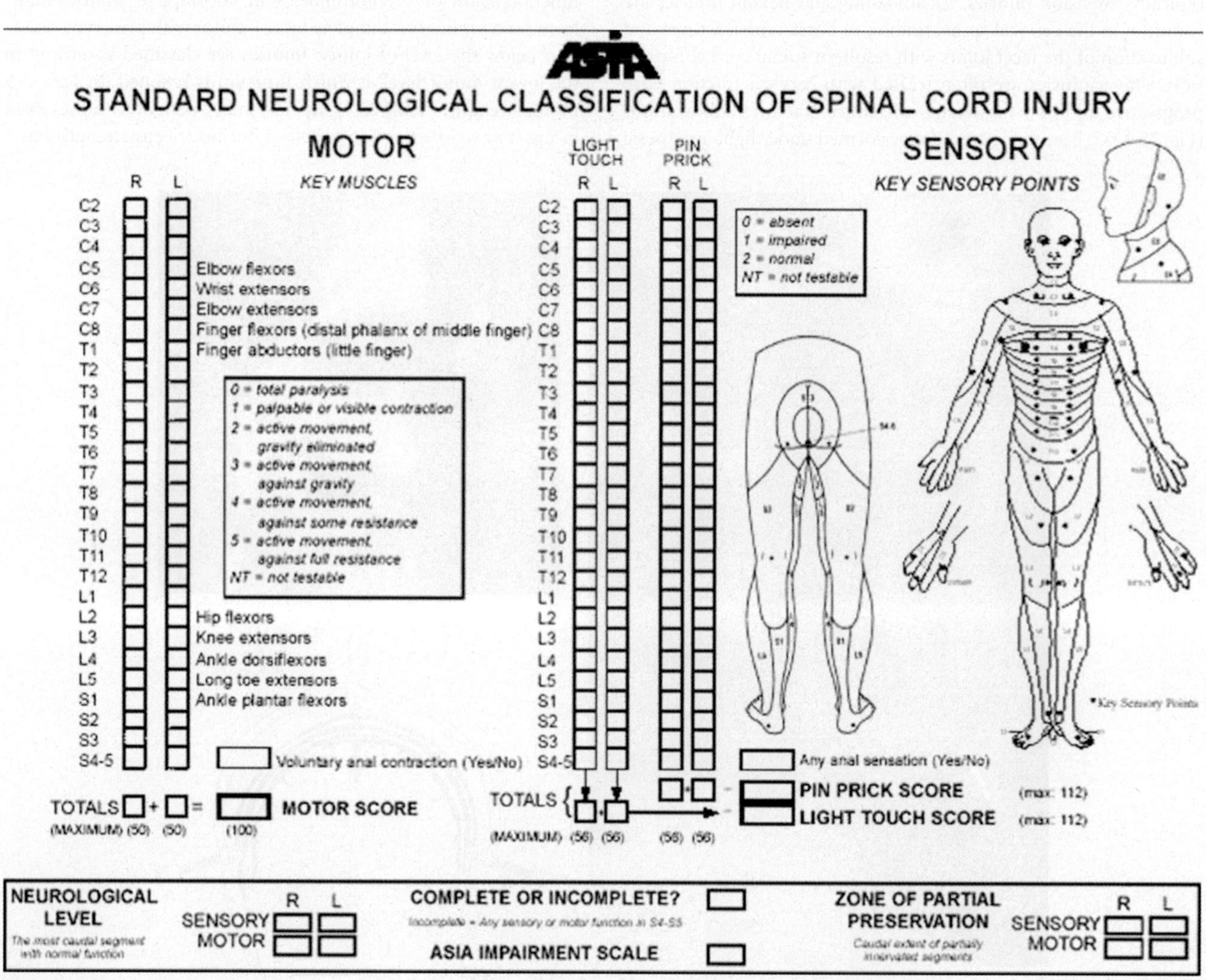

ASIA

STANDARD NEUROLOGICAL CLASSIFICATION OF SPINAL CORD INJURY

MOTOR

KEY MUSCLES

	R	L	Key muscles
C2			
C3			
C4			
C5			Elbow flexors
C6			Wrist extensors
C7			Elbow extensors
C8			Finger flexors (distal phalanx of middle finger)
T1			Finger abductors (little finger)
T2			
T3			
T4			
T5			
T6			
T7			
T8			
T9			
T10			
T11			
T12			
L1			
L2			Hip flexors
L3			Knee extensors
L4			Ankle dorsiflexors
L5			Long toe extensors
S1			Ankle plantar flexors
S2			
S3			
S4-5			Voluntary anal contraction (Yes/No)

0 = total paralysis
1 = palpable or visible contraction
2 = active movement, gravity eliminated
3 = active movement, against gravity
4 = active movement, against some resistance
5 = active movement, against full resistance
NT = not testable

TOTALS ☐ + ☐ = ☐ MOTOR SCORE
(MAXIMUM) (50) (50) (100)

SENSORY

KEY SENSORY POINTS

LIGHT TOUCH R L — PIN PRICK R L

C2, C3, C4, C5, C6, C7, C8, T1, T2, T3, T4, T5, T6, T7, T8, T9, T10, T11, T12, L1, L2, L3, L4, L5, S1, S2, S3, S4-5

0 = absent
1 = impaired
2 = normal
NT = not testable

Any anal sensation (Yes/No)

TOTALS ☐ + ☐ = PIN PRICK SCORE (max: 112)
LIGHT TOUCH SCORE (max: 112)
(MAXIMUM) (56) (56) (56) (56)

*Key Sensory Points

NEUROLOGICAL LEVEL — *The most caudal segment with normal function* — SENSORY R L; MOTOR R L

COMPLETE OR INCOMPLETE? ☐ — *Incomplete = Any sensory or motor function in S4-S5*

ASIA IMPAIRMENT SCALE ☐

ZONE OF PARTIAL PRESERVATION — *Caudal extent of partially innervated segments* — SENSORY R L; MOTOR R L

FIGURE 25.14 American Spinal Injury Association (ASIA) spinal cord injury classification system.

TABLE 25.4 Muscle strength grading scale

Grade	Strength
0	No contraction
1	Trace contraction
2	Active movement with gravity eliminated
3	Active movement against gravity
4	Active movement against resistance can be overcome
5	Normal strength

C6 level injury. Cord injury above the C3 level leads to respiratory compromise due to phrenic nerve dysfunction. Injuries above the upper thoracic spine may lead to neurogenic shock, a situation where the sympathetic output is disrupted and the patient suffers a precipitous drop in systemic vascular resistance. Heart rate remains low, and the skin is classically warm despite low blood pressure. Patients with complete SCI have a poor prognosis for good functional recovery.

Incomplete spinal cord injuries have a better prognosis than complete injuries. The central cord syndrome often follows a fall in an elderly patient with spinal canal narrowing from degenerative changes or in a younger patient with an acute disc herniation. Patients suffer loss of motor function worse in the upper than lower extremities (numb, clumsy hands with gait dysfunction), varying sensory loss, and bladder and bowel dysfunction. The Brown–Séquard syndrome most often follows penetrating spinal injury, in which half the spinal cord is injured. Patients suffer ipsilateral motor dysfunction, ipsilateral loss of touch and position sense, and contralateral loss of pain and temperature sensation. Anterior cord syndrome is due to infarction of the region supplied by the anterior spinal artery (roughly the anterior two thirds of the cord). Symptoms include paraplegia or quadriplegia and loss of pain and temperature below the injury. Generally, proprioception, vibration, and deep pressure are preserved.

TABLE 25.5 ASIA classification system

ASIA Score	Clinical Impairment
A Complete	No motor or sensor function preserved in sacral segments S4–S5 below level of injury
B Incomplete	Sensory but not motor function is preserved below the neurologic level including the sacral segments S4–S5
C Incomplete	Motor function is preserved below the neurologic level, and more than half of muscles below the level have a strength grade <3
D Incomplete	Motor function is preserved below the neurologic level and at least half have a muscle grade of 3 or more
E Normal	Motor and sensory functions are normal

After the initial assessment of spinal injuries, decisions regarding treatment are based on the level and extent of the injury, the patient's neurologic status, other underlying injuries, and general health. In general, patients with acute SCI are monitored in an ICU or similar setting, with hemodynamic and respiratory monitoring. Maintenance of MAP above 80 mm Hg for the first 7 days following SCI has been suggested as a treatment guideline to help maintain spinal cord perfusion. Ileus is common in this population, thus nasogastric suctioning is frequently employed to decompress the abdomen and prevent vomiting and aspiration. Additionally, Foley catheterization is frequently employed for accurate measurement of fluid balance and to prevent bladder overdistention injuries due to neurologic dysfunction. Because the patients are typically immobilized, they are at high risk for venous thromboembolic events (VTEs), thus VTE prophylaxis in paramount in this population. However, there has been ongoing debate as to the appropriate VTE prophylaxis among SCI patients, and institutions vary widely in their use of unfractionated heparin, low molecular weight heparin, therapeutic anticoagulation, mechanical prophylaxis, or combinations thereof. Early closed and/or open reduction and stabilization of spinal fractures may improve outcome, allow earlier mobilization, prevent pulmonary and other complications, and enhance rehabilitation potential.

The initiation of methylprednisolone therapy for SCI is also controversial as the evidence supporting its use is inconclusive. The National Acute Spinal Cord Injury Studies (NASCIS) 2 (in which steroids were administered within 8 hours of nonpenetrating SCI) and 3 (in which steroids were administered for 24 hours if initiated within 3 hours of injury and 48 hours if initiated between 3 to 8 hours of injury) trials concluded that use of steroids within 8 hours of injury were beneficial. However, subsequent critiques have commented on flaws in study design, statistical analysis, as well the meaningfulness of clinical improvement associated with the NASCIS trials. Furthermore, meta-analyses have failed to replicate the results of the original studies. Given these concerns, as well as the risks of prolonged steroid use such as immunosuppression and musculoskeletal compromise, the American Association of Neurological Surgeons and Congress of Neurological Surgeons advised against the use of methylprednisolone in SCI in 2013.

PERIPHERAL NERVE

The brachial plexus is a complex of nerves formed by the C5, C6, C7, C8, and T1 nerve roots that begins in the neck with extension to the axilla following a progressive reorganization from the nerve roots to form trunks (upper, middle, and lower), divisions (anterior and posterior) of the trunks to form cords (lateral, medial, and posterior), and subsequent terminal branches of the cords that supply the motor and sensory innervation of the upper extremities. While several nerves arise from different portions of the brachial plexus to supply the chest, back, and shoulder girdle, the five most clinically important terminal branches to the upper extremity are the axillary, musculocutaneous, radial, median, and ulnar nerves. The lumbosacral plexus is formed by the L1–L5 and S1–S4 nerve roots to provide the major sensory and motor innervation of the lower extremities. The most clinically important nerve branches of the lumbosacral plexus include the sciatic, femoral, obturator, peroneal, and tibial nerves. While details regarding the function and anatomic relationships of these nerves are beyond the scope of this chapter, it is imperative that any surgeon operating in the vicinity of a major peripheral nerve have a working knowledge of these relationships.

TABLE 25.6 Representative brachial plexus injuries

Injury	Mechanism	Clinical Findings
Erb upper plexus injury (C5–C6)	Forceful separation of humeral head from shoulder—birth injury, motorcycle fall	Paralysis of deltoid, bicep, brachioradialis, rhomboids, supra, and infraspinatus; hand unaffected "Bellhops tip position"—arm hangs at side with internal rotation and elbow extension
Klumpke lower plexus injury (C8, T1)	Tumor (pancoast) invasion, traction of the abducted arm in falls	Claw hand deformity with wasting of intrinsic hand muscles (also seen with ulnar neuropathy), can have Horner syndrome if T1 involved
Radial nerve injury	Pressure/injury to radial nerve at humerus level. "Saturday night palsy" from sleeping on arm or injury secondary to humerus fracture	Weakness of wrist extension (wrist drop) and finger extension. The triceps are spared (differentiates from higher lesion involving axillary nerve)

The brachial and lumbar plexuses and associated nerves are susceptible to various insults including neuropathy/plexopathy secondary to tumor invasion, vasculitis, diabetes, postradiation changes, and trauma. Traumatic causes of injury include entrapment, stretch, compression, crush, blast, and penetrating injuries. The most common entrapment neuropathies are carpal tunnel syndrome (compression of the median nerve at the wrist), followed by cubital tunnel syndrome (compression of the ulnar nerve at the elbow). Stretch injuries are frequently traumatic in nature. For example, an infant's neck may be stretched during delivery, or an outstretched limb is stretched beyond anatomic norms during bicycle and motorcycle accidents. In addition, certain nerves are at high risk for pressure injury, such as the common peroneal nerve at the lateral knee. Because some compression injuries are preventable, attention to detail with regard to positioning and protecting peripheral nerves during surgical procedures can avoid most of these problems. Hence, rigorous fixing of the shoulder inferiorly can stretch the brachial plexus and should be avoided, whereas a soft axillary role is commonly placed at the dependent axilla during the lateral decubitus position to help reduce pressure on the components of the brachial plexus (Table 25.6).

The diagnosis of a nerve injury is usually clinical and suggested by a motor and/or sensory deficit in the distribution of a peripheral nerve, along with a logical mechanism of injury. Differentiating a nerve injury from a radiculopathy can be challenging in a patient who suffers multiple injuries or when the mechanism of injury is associated with unpredictable forces such as a high-speed motor vehicle accident. Careful physical examination is the most useful tool in the acute and subacute setting. Supplemental diagnostic studies include electromyography (EMG), which generally requires 3 weeks from the injury to demonstrate findings, and nerve conduction studies. Often, MRI is necessary to exclude other anatomic causes for the deficit, such as a radiculopathy from a herniated disc or nerve root avulsion.

In the acute setting, attempted repair of peripheral nerve injuries is only appropriate when they result from sharp lacerating mechanisms, such as iatrogenic injuries during surgery. These should be explored, and an anastomosis should be attempted within 24 to 48 hours. Blast-type penetrating injuries, such as gunshot wounds or shrapnel, are generally not explored immediately. Crush injuries also do not warrant early exploration. In these instances, the patient is re-evaluated 3 months after the injury with electrodiagnostic studies, and a decision about possible surgical intervention is made at that time. After 24 months of denervation, however, most muscles cannot adequately recover useful function even with reinnervation procedures. Exceptions do exist, however, such as the muscles of the face and some large muscle groups. Entrapment neuropathies tend to have extremely good outcomes with adequate surgical decompression.

TUMORS

Brain tumors account for approximately 10% of all neoplasms. Primary tumors arise from neurons and glial cells, the meningeal layers covering the brain and spinal cord, the pituitary gland, and cranial nerves. Metastatic tumors can spread by local extension or through the blood, lymph, or CSF and are 10 times more common than primary tumors. The location of brain tumors varies with age. In adults, 70% of primary brain tumors are supratentorial. In children, 70% of brain tumors are located within the posterior fossa. The brain is the most common site for solid tumors in childhood.

Patients with brain tumors may present with signs and symptoms of increased ICP, focal deficits, or seizures. Increased ICP is a result of additional tumor mass within the skull, vasogenic edema, obstructive hydrocephalus, or tumor hemorrhage. Symptoms of elevated ICP include headache, nausea and vomiting, and progressive lethargy with slowed cognitive function. Signs of elevated ICP also include third and sixth cranial nerve palsies and papilledema. A third cranial nerve palsy results in down and outward deviation of the eye with impaired pupillary light response due to compression of peripherally located parasympathetic fibers. Sixth nerve palsy results from compression of the abducens nerve resulting in impaired lateral eye gaze. Depending on the location of the tumor, the patient may present with neurologic deficits such as hemiparesis, visual changes, aphasia, and cranial nerve palsies. In children with tumors in the posterior fossa, deficits include ataxia, nystagmus, cranial nerve palsies, and symptoms of elevated ICP from obstructive hydrocephalus.

When a brain mass is suspected, either a CT scan or MRI should be obtained to characterize the size and location of the lesion. Because CT scanning is quick, readily available, and relatively inexpensive, it is often the initial test of choice. MRI provides far greater soft tissue detail and will allow for better characterization of the intracranial mass.

Metastases are the most common brain tumors in adults, peaking between the fifth to seventh decades of life. Among metastatic lesions found in the brain, 50% arise from lung malignancies, 25% from breast cancer, 10% from melanoma, 10% from renal cell carcinoma, and 5% from colorectal cancer. On MRI or CT scan, metastatic lesions are often located at the junction between the gray and white matter, are associated with extensive surrounding edema, and are often multiple in number (Fig. 25.10). The preferred therapeutic approach is dictated by the size of the lesion, the severity of associated symptoms, and the number of additional lesions. Surgical resection, usually followed by whole brain or stereotactic radiation, is the preferred treatment for isolated and symptomatic metastatic lesions with the notable exception of small cell lung cancer, which is exquisitely sensitive to chemotherapy and radiotherapy. Stereotactic radiosurgery with or without whole-brain radiation may be effective for multiple and smaller metastatic lesions.

Primary brain tumors can be broadly categorized into those derived from cells normally present in the CNS and those derived from embryonic remnants. The latter group includes craniopharyngiomas, germinomas, teratomas, epidermoids, and dermoids. Tumors that arise from cells normally found in the CNS may be further divided into tumors that arise from neural tube derivatives (astrocytomas, glioblastomas, oligodendrogliomas, ependymomas, and choroids plexus papillomas), tumors that arise from neurons (medulloblastomas and gangliomas), tumors that arise from neural crest derivatives (meningiomas and acoustic neuromas), and tumors that arise from other cells present in the CNS (lymphomas, hemangioblastoma, glomus jugulare tumors, and pituitary adenomas). In adults, gliomas are the most common primary brain neoplasm followed by meningiomas, pituitary adenomas, and nerve sheath tumors. Astrocytomas are the most common primary brain neoplasm in the pediatric population, followed by ependymomas and medulloblastomas (primitive neuroectodermal tumor [PNET]).

Glioma is a general term for any tumor arising from a stromal cell of the CNS, including astrocytomas and oligodendrogliomas. The WHO grading system classifies these tumors into grades I through IV (Table 25.7). A grade I pilocytic astrocytoma is the most benign type of glioma. These tumors are more common in children and are often found in the cerebellum. The 10-year survival rate is greater than 90% following surgical resection with adjuvant therapy for a cerebellar pilocytic astrocytoma. Grade II gliomas include astrocytomas and oligodendrogliomas. These tumors often do not enhance with gadolinium on MRI, are slow growing, and demonstrate low cellularity compared with other tumors. A low-grade glioma may transform into a high-grade tumor over time. Grade III gliomas exhibit features of a more malignant tumor such as contrast enhancement on MRI, rapid growth rate, pleomorphic cells, and increased cellularity. These tumors often require surgical resection, radiation, and sometimes chemotherapy. Grade IV gliomas include glioblastoma multiforme (GBM) and gliosarcoma (Fig. 25.10). GBM is one of the most common primary intracranial tumors in adults. The diagnosis of a GBM is suggested by imaging characteristics of necrosis and enhancement; however, identification of pseudopalisading cells around necrotic areas and neovascularization on histology are required to confirm the diagnosis. Because of the diffuse, infiltrative nature of these tumors, complete surgical resection is challenging. Even with radiation and chemotherapy, 2-year survival rates are low and are inversely correlated to age and functional status.

Ependymomas are glial tumors derived from the ependymal cells that line the ventricular system. These tumors are more common in children and often grow from the floor of the fourth ventricle in the posterior fossa. In adults and children, ependymomas often cause obstructive hydrocephalus. In addition, they may seed the CSF and disseminate throughout the spinal cord. Choroid plexus papillomas are tumors that are derived from the cells that produce CSF. They often present with hydrocephalus.

Medulloblastomas originate from primitive bipotential cells of the cerebellum. These tumors are called PNETs, a broad term that also refers to other tumor subtypes, and commonly present as posterior fossa masses in children. They are generally midline lesions and cause obstructive hydrocephalus. Children present with signs of increased ICP and cerebellar dysfunction such as ataxia and nystagmus. These tumors are malignant, densely cellular, and may metastasize through the CSF. After detection of a lesion concerning for PNET, complete imaging of the brain and spinal cord is important to identify other lesions spread through the CSF.

Meningiomas account for nearly 20% of intracranial tumors. They are benign tumors that arise from arachnoid cap cells located within the meninges. These tumors are more common in women and may be located wherever there is dura. Meningiomas often

TABLE 25.7 WHO grading system for primary brain tumors

WHO Grade	Tumor Type	Imaging Features	Prognosis	Treatment
1	Pilocytic astrocytoma	Discrete, enhancing, often cystic with mural nodule	>80% survival in cerebellum	Surgery +/– chemotherapy
2	Astrocytoma or oligodendroglioma	Nonenhancing, associated with edema	>50% 5-y survival	Surgery Chemotherapy +/– radiation
3	Anaplastic astrocytoma	Enhancement, +/–necrosis	Average survival is 2 y	Surgery Chemotherapy Whole-brain radiation
4	Glioblastoma multiforme	Enhancement, necrosis, infiltrative, edema	Average survival is 1–2 y	Surgery Chemotherapy Whole-brain radiation

compress the brain but generally do not invade it; however, they may more commonly invade the adjacent bone. On MRI, they enhance brightly and homogeneously and may have a signature "dural tail." Treatment for large or symptomatic lesions is usually surgical resection, although small or asymptomatic meningiomas may be followed and/or treated with radiation, depending on the tumor and the surgical risk profile of the patient. Meningiomas are associated with good long-term prognosis and a low rate of recurrence.

Vestibular schwannomas, which arise from the vestibular portion of the eighth cranial nerve, arise from Schwann cells. They are frequently called "acoustic neuromas," although this term is a misnomer due to its relationship with the vestibular nerve. They typically present with hearing loss, vertigo or loss of balance, and sometimes with facial numbness from compression of the fifth cranial nerve. Vestibular schwannomas are benign lesions and depending on their size, treatment may involve either surgery and/or radiotherapy.

Neurofibromatosis (NF) is a heritable neurocutaneous disorder. NF type 1 (NF-1), also called von Recklinghausen disease, is more common than NF type 2 (NF-2) and accounts for more than 90% of cases. The gene responsible for NF-1 is found on chromosome 17q11.2 and has a simple autosomal dominant pattern of inheritance with variable expressivity but 100% penetrance after age 5. The clinical features of NF-1 include café au lait spots, neurofibromas on peripheral nerves, hyperpigmentation in the axillary or inguinal areas, optic gliomas, Lisch nodules (i.e., iris hamartomas), and thinning of the cranial bones. These patients are treated with resection of lesions that are symptomatic. The most important clinical feature of NF-2 is bilateral acoustic neuromas, which is pathognomonic for the diagnosis. Other clinical features include meningiomas, gliomas, schwannoma, seizures, and skin nodules. NF-2 also has as autosomal dominant inheritance pattern and is due to a mutation at chromosome 22q12.2. The treatment is also surgery or radiosurgery for symptomatic lesions. Eventual bilateral deafness is almost inevitable in patients with this condition.

The hypothalamic–pituitary axis regulates the diurnal endocrine oscillations of the body. The pituitary gland extends beneath the hypothalamus tucked into a cavity at the skull base known as the sella turcica, beneath the third ventricle and optic chiasm. The infundibulum connects the hypothalamus to the pituitary. The pituitary is divided into the anterior adenohypophysis and the posterior neurohypophysis. Axonal terminals of neurons that originate in the hypothalamus comprise the latter, which secretes antidiuretic hormone and oxytocin. The anterior hypophysis secretes six hormones under hypothalamic control: prolactin, growth hormone, follicle-stimulating hormone, luteinizing hormone, adrenocorticotropic hormone (ACTH), and thyroid-stimulating hormone.

Pituitary adenomas arise from the anterior lobe of the pituitary gland and are either detected because they overproduce a pituitary hormone (secretory) or because of local mass effect (nonsecretory). Tumors less than a centimeter are called microadenomas and lesions larger than 1 cm are called macroadenomas. Common presentations include amenorrhea and galactorrhea secondary to overproduction of prolactin or acromegaly from excess growth hormone production. Cushing disease results from overproduction of ACTH. Macroadenomas compress surrounding structures to cause symptoms. Bitemporal hemianopsia, or "tunnel vision," is caused by compression of the medial aspect of the optic chiasm by the tumor. Macroadenomas may also invade the nearby cavernous sinus and cause third, fourth, or sixth cranial nerve palsies. A macroadenoma may cause elevated prolactin levels by compressing the pituitary stalk, thereby interrupting the dopaminergic inhibition of prolactin release. Macroadenomas can also compress the normal pituitary, resulting in lower production of thyroid-stimulating and gonadal-stimulating hormones.

Cushing syndrome is the constellation of findings caused by hypercortisolism including weight gain, accumulation of fat on the upper back (i.e., "buffalo hump"), hypertension, purple striae, osteoporosis, muscle wasting, and hyperglycemia. Cushing syndrome may be due to one of several causes (Table 25.8). Cushing disease refers to endogenous hypercortisolism specifically due to oversecretion of ACTH by a pituitary adenoma. Because of cross-reactivity with a precursor of melanin-secreting hormone, these patients also often exhibit hyperpigmentation of the skin and mucous membranes. To test for Cushing syndrome, obtain a 24-hour urine-free cortisol level and perform a low-dose dexamethasone suppression test. Urine-free cortisol will be elevated, and upon administration of low-dose dexamethasone, cortisol levels will remain elevated in patients with Cushing syndrome. The high-dose dexamethasone test will help determine the etiology of the disorder. In Cushing disease, administration of high-dose dexamethasone will suppress cortisol production. Ectopic ACTH production from lung tumor or cortisol production by adrenal tumors will not exhibit lower cortisol levels after high-dose dexamethasone challenge.

The approach to the treatment of pituitary adenomas is influenced by several factors including the secretory status of the tumor, the hormonal deficits of the patient, and the presence of neurologic findings; specifically visual changes. Prolactinomas are the most common secretory adenomas and are usually initially treated with dopamine agonists such as bromocriptine or cabergoline. Other secretory lesions often require surgery. Likewise, large macroadenomas that compress the optic nerves and cause pituitary dysfunction most often require resection. The currently recommended surgical resection involves the transnasal approach through the sphenoid sinus, often in collaboration with otorhinolaryngology service for the endoscopic transnasal approach.

TABLE 25.8 Evaluation of increased cortisol production

Diagnosis	Overproduction	Frequency (%)	ACTH Level
Pituitary adenoma (Cushing disease)	ACTH	70	Elevated
Ectopic ACTH production (lung tumor)	ACTH	10	Markedly elevated
Adrenal tumor	Cortisol	15	Low

NERVOUS SYSTEM INFECTIONS

Infections of the CNS can have devastating consequences. Pyogenic infections can occur *de novo*, generally from hematogenous spread (systemic infection, endocarditis, or other cardiopulmonary abnormalities), or direct extension from head and neck infections such as sinusitis, mastoiditis, or tooth abscess. Infections can also occur as a result of previous craniospinal surgery, penetrating injuries, or other traumas. Infections include meningitis, subdural empyema, brain abscess, ventriculitis, spinal epidural abscess, and osteomyelitis/discitis.

The most common pathogens in cerebral abscess are *Streptococcus* species. Presentation can be nonspecific but are generally related to symptoms of elevated ICP, seizures, and local mass effect causing focal neurologic deficits. The most dreaded presentation of an intracranial abscess is rupture into the ventricular system causing ventriculitis, rapid neurologic deterioration, and frequently death. Radiographically, an early abscess may cause nonspecific cerebritis, which eventually evolves into a lesion with a well-defined capsule. Fever and leukocytosis may be present; however, often there are few signs of a systemic inflammatory response. Diffusion-weighted MRI can aid the diagnosis of intracranial lesions concerning for abscesses since these lesions characteristically diffusion restrict. Early cerebritis and smaller abscesses (i.e., those <3 cm) may be treated empirically with antibiotics alone. Surgery is generally indicated for larger lesions with mass effect, neurologic decline, location near the ventricles, or if the diagnosis is in doubt. Aspiration alone can be effective, but with recurrent lesions, excision may be required. Subsequently, patients are treated with pathogen-specific antibiotics. Subdural empyema is considered a neurosurgical emergency and requires prompt craniotomy for evacuation and subsequent antibiotic therapy. Untreated subdural empyema results in inflammatory thrombophlebitis of the vasculature and resultant infarction.

Herpes simplex encephalitis is one of the more common viral infections of the CNS. Patients present with progressive confusion and obtundation with associated seizures. Classically, there are hemorrhagic lesions in one or both temporal lobes. Diagnosis can be made from CSF studies and rarely brain biopsy, and treatment consists of acyclovir, an antiviral agent. Cysticercosis is a parasitic brain infection caused by the pork tapeworm *Taenia solium*, which is common in endemic areas. Patients often present with seizures and obstructive hydrocephalus. The diagnosis is made by radiographic studies and serology. Treatment consists of anthelmintic drugs, such as albendazole, and occasionally surgery.

Excluding infections related to previous surgical procedures or open trauma, the vast majority of cases of spinal epidural abscess and osteomyelitis/discitis are associated with intravenous drug abuse, immunocompromised states such as diabetes mellitus, dialysis-dependent renal failure, posttransplant, and systemic sources of bacteremia (e.g., bacterial endocarditis). Patients generally present with back pain, variable fever, and leukocytosis. Elevations in erythrocyte sedimentation rate and C-reactive protein levels are also characteristic, although nonspecific. Early infections can be treated with pathogen-specific antibiotics. CT-guided biopsies are frequently the ideal method of choice to safely obtain a tissue diagnosis and culture in cases of osteomyelitis with minimal risk as compared to open biopsy. Culture results from CT-guided biopsies can assist with narrowing antibiotic therapy. Surgery is often indicated in cases of progressive deformity, neurologic compromise, or failure of antibiotic therapy.

Suggested Readings

Bracken MB, Shepard MJ, Holford TR, et al. Administration of methylprednisolone for 24 or 48 hours or tirilazad mesylate for 48 hours in the treatment of acute spinal cord injury. Results of the third national acute spinal cord injury randomized controlled trial. National Acute Spinal Cord Injury Study. *JAMA.* 1997; 277(20):1597–1604.

Bullock R, Povlishock J, eds.; Brain Trauma Foundation; American Association of Neurological Surgeons; Congress of Neurological Surgeons. Guidelines for the management of severe traumatic brain injury. *J Neurotrauma.* 2007;24(Suppl 1):S1–S106.

Gunnarsson T, Fehlings MG. Acute neurosurgical management of traumatic brain injury and spinal cord injury. *Curr Opin Neurol.* 2003;16(6):717–723.

Louis DN, Ohgaki H, Wiestler OD, et al. The 2007 WHO classification of tumours of the central nervous system. *Acta Neuropathol.* 2007;114(2):97–109.

Patchell RA, Tibbs PA, Walsh JW, et al. A randomized trial of surgery in the treatment of single metastases to the brain. *N Engl J Med.* 1990;322(8):494–500.

Wiebers DO, Whisnant JP, Huston J III, et al.; International Study of Unruptured Intracranial Aneurysms Investigators. Unruptured intracranial aneurysms: natural history, clinical outcome, and risks of surgical and endovascular treatment. *Lancet.* 2003;362(9378):103–110.

Willinsky RA, Taylor SM, TerBrugge K, et al. Neurologic complications of cerebral angiography: prospective analysis of 2,899 procedures and review of the literature. *Radiology.* 2003;227(2): 522–528.

Winn HR, ed. *Youman's Neurological Surgery*. 6th ed. Philadelphia: WB Saunders; 2011.

CHAPTER 26

Pediatric Surgery

JESSE D. VRECENAK AND MICHAEL L. NANCE

KEY POINTS

- Malrotation and volvulus should be considered in the differential diagnosis of any child with bilious emesis; though most common among infants, volvulus can present at any age and is a surgical emergency. Malrotations discovered incidentally on imaging or at the time of another procedure in the pediatric population should be repaired to minimize this risk.
- Appendicitis is the most common cause of an acute abdomen among pediatric patients; though ultrasound is commonly performed to confirm the diagnosis, it is acceptable to perform an appendectomy based upon a clinical exam and CT scans should not be performed routinely.
- Necrotizing enterocolitis (NEC) is the most common surgical emergency among neonates, and a major cause of acquired gastointestinal-related morbidity and mortality. Though the mortality rate is significant (20-30%), pneumoperitoneum is the only absolute indication for surgery and most cases of uncomplicated NEC can be managed nonoperatively.
- Inguinal hernia is among the most common pediatric surgical problems, and occurs most often in males (4:1). Due to the risk of incarceration, these congenital hernias should be repaired when diagnosed and usually require only high ligation of the hernia sac without mesh or fascial repair.
- Injury is the most common cause of death among children older than 1 year, and providers should be aware of common signs of abuse or neglect. Children can compensate for hypovolemia until relatively late (>40% volume loss) and severely injured children may present with normal vital signs. Likewise, anatomic differences in the child (e.g. the greater elasticity of the pediatric rib cage, thinner abdominal wall musculature) increases the risk of injury.

ESOPHAGEAL ATRESIA AND TRACHEOESOPHAGEAL FISTULA

Esophageal atresia (EA) and tracheoesophageal fistula (TEF) form a spectrum of structural defects resulting from abnormal foregut development during the 4th week of gestation. Though poorly understood, the etiology is likely multifactorial; EA/TEF has been linked with exposure to agents such as methimazole, diethylstilbestrol, and endogenous sex hormones as well as maternal factors including alcohol or tobacco use, agricultural employment, first-trimester diabetes, and advanced maternal age. Heredity does not seem to play a major role, with low likelihood of a second child born with the same defect (approximately 1%) and low twin concordance (approximately 2% to 3%). Associated anomalies may be present in up to 25% of affected infants and often include the VACTERL spectrum (*v*ertebral, *a*norectal, *c*ardiac, *t*racheo*e*sophageal, *r*enal and *l*imb deformities). Genetic syndromes also associated with EA/TEF include Feingold syndrome (MYCN gene), CHARGE syndrome (CHD7 gene), and trisomy 18, among others.

There are five commonly recognized anatomic variants of EA/TEF (Fig. 26.1). Type C, a blind-ending upper esophageal pouch and distal TEF, is the most common, occurring in up to 85% of cases. Infants with pure EA (type A) are at highest risk for VACTERL anomalies.

Classically, EA/TEF is detected soon after birth with feeding difficulties and excessive oral secretions; the inability to pass a nasogastric tube is highly suggestive, and plain films will support the diagnosis. When a distal fistula is present, abdominal distention may result from passage of inspired air into the stomach, and reflux of gastric contents may lead to a chemical pneumonitis. Respiratory distress may be compounded by reduced diaphragmatic excursion in the setting of significant gastric dilation. H-type fistulas may be more difficult to diagnose and may present in delayed fashion with recurrent pneumonias or reactive airway disease. Though rarely required otherwise, in these cases, contrast imaging may help to confirm the diagnosis. Prenatally, affected infants may be identified based upon the presence of polyhydramnios with an absent or small stomach bubble and/or a dilated proximal esophageal pouch. However, the sensitivity and specificity of these findings remain relatively low despite advances in imaging techniques.

Initial management of the infant with EA/TEF should include upright positioning, aspiration precautions, acid suppression, and Replogle tube decompression of the proximal esophageal pouch. In those infants with a distal TEF, positive pressure ventilation should be avoided to prevent gastric distention and further respiratory compromise. Preoperatively, echocardiogram should be obtained to exclude major cardiac abnormalities and determine the location of the aortic arch, which will determine the laterality of the operative approach. In most cases (approximately 95%), a left-sided aortic arch will dictate repair through the right chest. Before proceeding to surgical repair, initial bronchoscopy is recommended to document the presence and location of the distal fistula and to assess for the presence of a proximal fistula.

The standard surgical approach involves a muscle-sparing posterolateral thoracotomy, with ligation of the TEF and primary esophagoesophagostomy. The distal fistula is usually located deep to the azygous vein, and mediastinal pleura may be used to buttress the tracheal suture line following division. In most cases, the

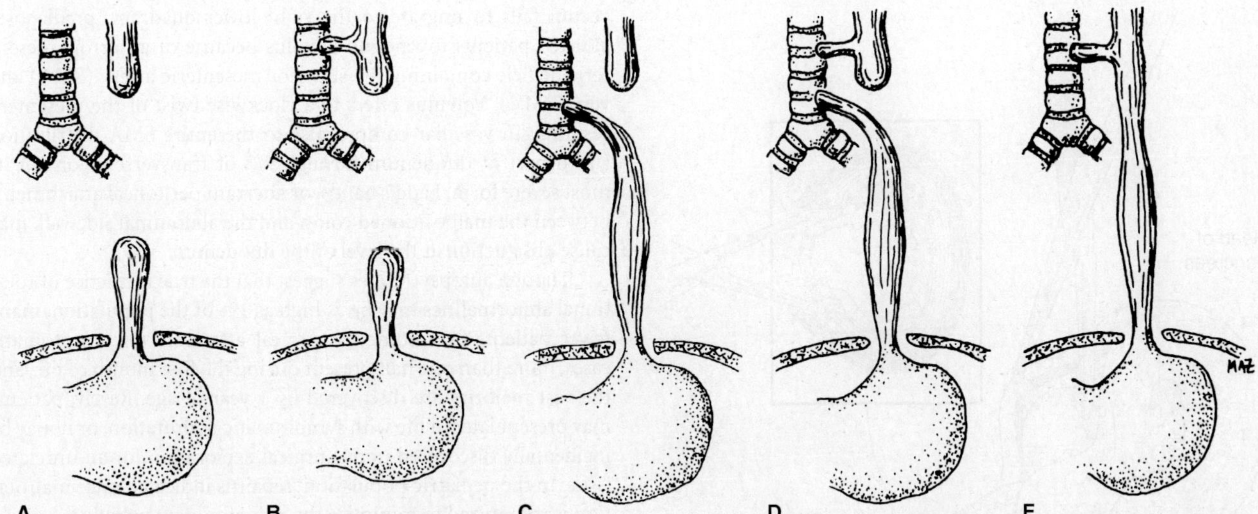

FIGURE 26.1 Variants of tracheoesophageal fistula. **A.** Atresia without fistula (8%). **B.** Atresia with proximal fistula (1%). **C.** Atresia with distal fistula (85%). **D.** Atresia with both proximal and distal fistulas (2%). **E.** Fistula without atresia (H type, 4%).(From Doherty GM, Lowney JK, Mason JE, et al. *The Washington Manual of Surgery*. 3rd ed. Philadelphia: Lippincott Williams & Wilkins; 2002:642, with permission.)

proximal and distal esophageal pouches can be mobilized to achieve a primary anastomosis without tension, and a proximal esophagomyotomy may be used to gain additional length; long-gap EAs may require placement of a gastrostomy tube and delayed primary repair with or without an esophageal lengthening procedure, or the use of an esophageal conduit (stomach, colon, jejunum). Thoracoscopic repair has increasingly been employed but requires appropriate technical expertise in suturing the esophageal anastomosis. In experienced hands, the rates of leak and stricture are comparable to open thoracotomy. Though postoperative pain and length of hospitalization may be slightly lower with the thoracoscopic approach, its main benefit lies in avoiding the potential for chest wall deformities with thoracotomy in neonates. Appropriate patient selection is critical to the success of this technique, which is best suited to short-gap atresias in relatively normal birth weight infants without multiple associated defects.

Postoperatively, an esophagram should be obtained 5 to 7 days postrepair to assess for leak, which may be seen in 15% to 25% of cases. Many patients with EA/TEF may have reflux symptoms postoperatively, but few ultimately require an antireflux procedure. Anastomotic strictures may also occur and can generally be managed with endoscopic- or fluoroscopic-guided dilation procedures. Overall, the survival of EA/TEF is generally related to the presence of other associated anomalies; survival rates for isolated EA/TEF approach 100%.

HYPERTROPHIC PYLORIC STENOSIS

Hypertrophic pyloric stenosis (HPS) is the most common cause of gastric outlet obstruction in infants, resulting from the progressive hypertrophy of pyloric smooth muscle with resultant luminal narrowing. Though the etiology has not been identified, the increased incidence in firstborn male children of affected individuals suggests a significant genetic component. In addition, environmental factors including method of feeding, blood type, erythromycin exposure, and seasonal variability have been associated with increased risk of HPS.

Affected infants classically present between 2 and 8 weeks of age with progressive nonbilious vomiting, often projectile and occurring within minutes of feeding. Peak onset is between 3 and 5 weeks of age, and the color of the emesis should closely resemble feeds. Though some infants may experience diarrhea due to nutritional deprivation, associated symptoms are rare, and most affected patients appear well and maintain a healthy appetite until late in the disease course.

Physical examination reveals a palpable "olive" in the epigastrium or right upper quadrant—the firm, hypertrophied pylorus that may be accompanied by visible gastric peristaltic waves. Though dependent upon the patient's cooperation and the skill of the examiner, these pathognomonic findings may allow the diagnosis to be made with an appropriate history and physical exam. Both ultrasonography and upper gastrointestinal series are sensitive and specific, though ultrasonography allows measurement of the pyloric channel. A pyloric length of 16 mm or greater or a wall thickness of 4 mm or greater is diagnostic for HPS.

Preoperative preparation is of critical importance in patients with pyloric stenosis, who often present with a significant hypokalemic and hypochloremic metabolic alkalosis. Prompt IV access should be obtained for correction of metabolic derangement, which generally requires a bolus of 20 mL/kg normal saline followed by 1.5 to 2 times maintenance fluids until adequate urine output is achieved. Pyloric stenosis is a medical emergency, not a surgical emergency, and operative repair should be deferred until the serum bicarbonate level is less than 30 and serum chloride reaches 100 or greater.

Pyloromyotomy is the surgical treatment for HPS (Fig. 26.2), and traditionally, a Fredet–Ramstedt procedure was performed after delivering the pylorus into a right upper quadrant incision. However, laparoscopic pyloromyotomy has been shown to be at least as safe as open pyloromyotomy, and several prospective trials have suggested that benefits may include a shorter recovery and fewer wound complications in addition to improved cosmesis. Many centers now perform laparoscopic pyloromyotomy as a standard of care. Regardless of the approach, adequate surgical treatment of pyloric stenosis relies upon complete division of the hypertrophied muscle from the

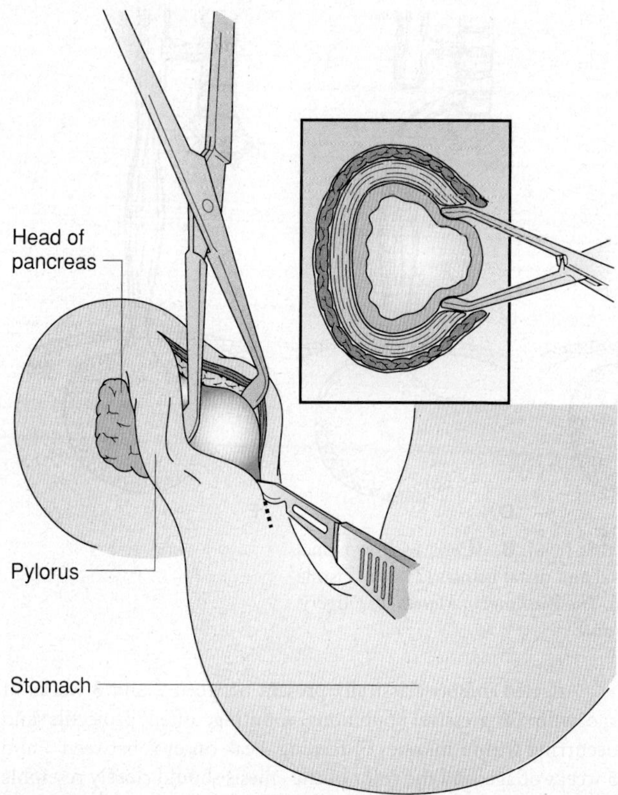

FIGURE 26.2 Ramstedt pyloromyotomy. Longitudinal division of the hypertrophied pyloric muscle allows the submucosa to herniate into the myotomy site. (From Mulholland MW. *Greenfield's Surgery: Scientific Principles and Practice*. 5th ed. Philadelphia: Lippincott Williams & Wilkins; 2011.)

prepyloric antrum to the pyloroduodenal junction using a single longitudinal incision. An adequate myotomy should allow visualization of the circular fibers of the stomach wall and independent movement of both halves of the pylorus. An incomplete myotomy is the most common cause of persistent symptoms (>5 days). Postoperative edema and antral or pyloric spasm may lead to some emesis initially despite an adequate myotomy, and parents should be counseled preoperatively regarding such symptoms. Apart from incomplete myotomy, mucosal perforation represents the most significant technical risk of the procedure and can be managed either by closing the longitudinal incision and performing a transverse myotomy or by mucosal closure and omental patch.

MALROTATION AND MIDGUT VOLVULUS

Normal midgut development in utero is characterized by herniation of the midgut loop into the umbilical cord during the 6th week of gestation, followed by a 270 degree rotation, reduction into the abdominal cavity during the 10th week of gestation, and fixation to the posterior body wall of the duodenojejunal junction at the ligament of Treitz and fixation of the ascending and descending colon. Rotation is complete by 12 weeks, and fixation continues through the second and third trimesters. Malrotation includes a broad spectrum of abnormalities, which are of varying clinical significance.

Classic malrotation, in which the ligament of Treitz is not appropriately fixated to the posterior abdominal wall and the cecum fails to migrate to the right lower quadrant, predisposes affected patients to midgut volvulus because of a narrow mesenteric pedicle containing the superior mesenteric artery (SMA) and vein (SMV). Volvulus refers to a clockwise twist of the mesentery resulting in vascular compromise to the entire SMA distribution (third part of duodenum through 2/3 of transverse colon) in its most severe form. Ladd's bands, or aberrant peritoneal attachments between the malpositioned colon and the abdominal sidewall, may cause obstruction at the level of the duodenum.

Though autopsy studies suggest that the true incidence of rotational abnormalities may be as high as 1% of the population, many fewer patients ever come to surgical attention. Of symptomatic cases, more than one half present during the first month of life, and the vast majority are discovered by 1 year of age. Rarely, patients may present later in life with symptomatic malrotation, or it may be incidentally discovered upon surgical exploration for an unrelated issue. In the pediatric population, repair is indicated once malrotation is recognized to minimize the risk of midgut volvulus.

In contrast to the nonbilious emesis seen with pyloric stenosis, hallmark of malrotation is bilious emesis due either to obstruction from extrinsic duodenal compression by Ladd's bands or midgut volvulus. Any neonate presenting with such symptoms should undergo urgent upper gastrointestinal series to rule out the diagnosis given the potential for significant vascular compromise to a majority of the intestine. An ultrasound can be useful to assess the orientation of the mesenteric vessels.

Surgical repair involves the Ladd procedure, comprised of four basic steps: (i) evisceration of the bowel and reduction of the volvulus (if present) via counterclockwise rotation, (ii) division of Ladd bands, (iii) broadening of the narrow mesenteric pedicle, and (iv) appendectomy (Fig. 26.3). Any necrotic bowel should be resected, taking care to preserve as much intestinal length as possible. Upon completion of the Ladd procedure, the small bowel should lie primarily in the right abdomen, and the cecum should be as far left as possible to maximally widen the mesenteric pedicle. The traditional approach to this procedure involves a supraumbilical right transverse incision through which the entire bowel can be eviscerated. Laparoscopic approaches are gaining favor, though no data can yet support a definitive recommendation. Regardless of approach, a nasogastric tube or catheter should be passed through the duodenum to exclude a proximal intestinal obstruction or web. The Ladd procedure minimizes risk, but does not completely prevent future volvulus. Notably, nonrotation is increasingly diagnosed incidentally on imaging studies and should be distinguished from malrotation by the existence of a "Ladd configuration," in which the cecum lies already in the left lower quadrant and the small bowel mesentery is wide. Though this group remains at some risk for midgut volvulus due to the lack of fixation, surgical intervention likely offers little benefit.

INTUSSUSCEPTION

Intussusception refers to the pathologic invagination of a proximal segment of intestine (*intussusceptum*) into adjacent distal bowel (*intussuscipiens*) and is the most common cause of small bowel obstruction in children under age 5. Ileocolic intussusception is most often pathologic, as incidentally discovered small bowel intussusception may simply represent normal peristalsis and rarely requires intervention. Intussusception in children is most often idiopathic; in 95% of cases, no pathologic lead point is identified.

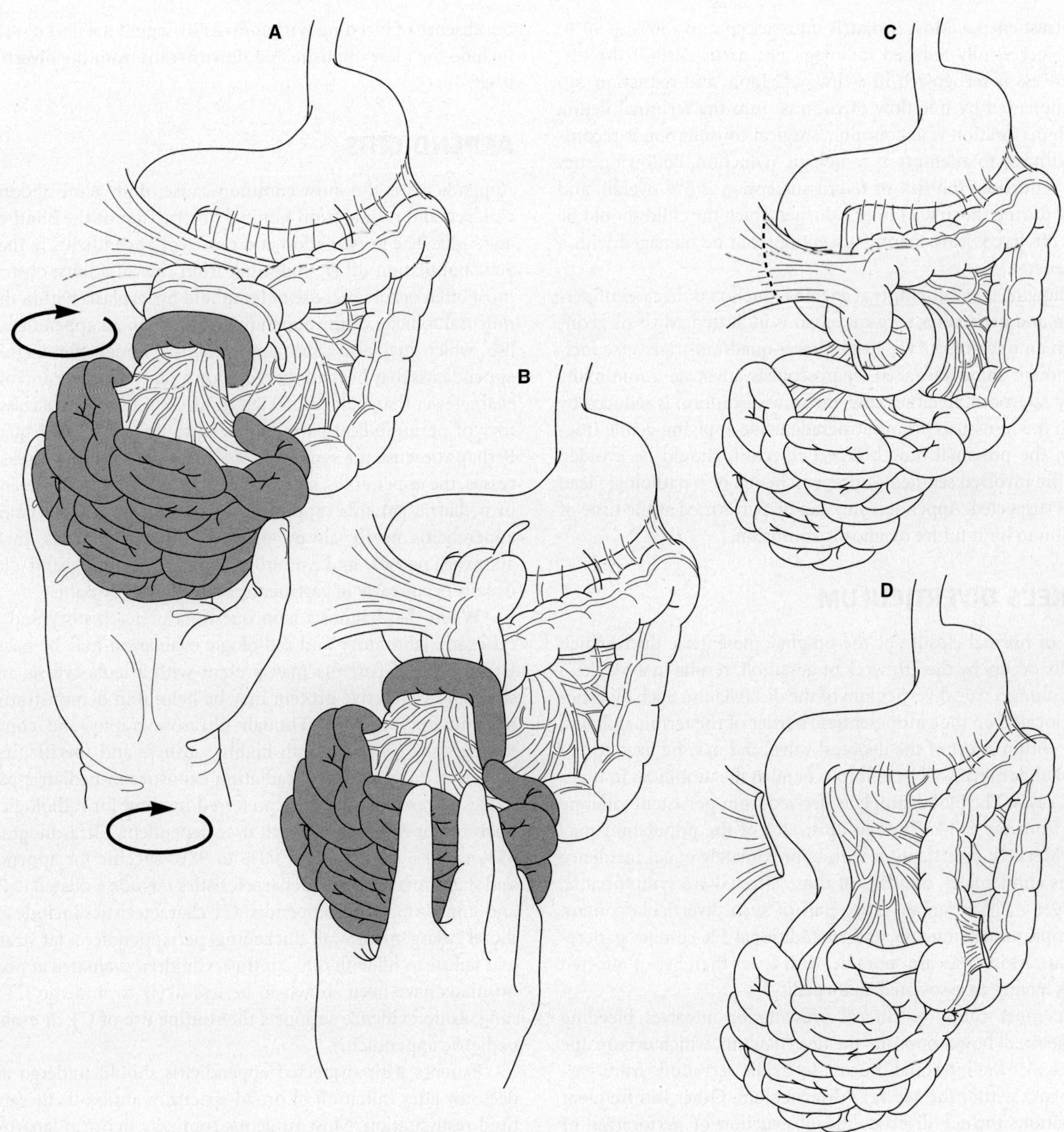

FIGURE 26.3 Ladd procedure. **A, B.** Counterclockwise detorsion of midgut volvulus. **C, D.** Division of peritoneal attachments (Ladd bands) of cecum to abdominal cavity. (From Greenfield L, Mulholland MW, Zelenock GB, et al. *Surgery: Scientific Principles and Practice*. 3rd ed. Philadelphia: Lippincott Williams & Wilkins; 2001:1998, with permission.)

Often, patients have experienced a recent viral illness (most commonly adenovirus), and hypertrophied Peyer's patches may predispose to intussusception. Peak incidence occurs between 3 months and 2 years of age, and older children have a higher risk of a pathologic lead point, which may include Meckel's diverticulum, polyps, or neoplasms. Cystic fibrosis and rotavirus vaccination may also increase the risk of intussusception.

Affected patients commonly present with colicky abdominal pain, characterized by intermittent crying and drawing up of the legs. Children are often asymptomatic between bouts of pain early in the disease process. "Currant jelly stools," the classic finding of pediatric intussusception, result from focal mucosal ischemia and are generally a late finding. The natural history of unreduced intussusception involves progression of ischemia, resulting in gangrene and perforation of the proximal intussusceptum. Bilious emesis and abdominal distention are late findings, and physical exam may reveal a palpable right lower quadrant mass.

Ultrasonography reliably demonstrates the presence of intussusception and is usually the initial diagnostic study of choice, revealing a "target" appearance in cross-section. Children suspected to have intussusception should undergo contrast enema (air, water soluble, or barium) for both diagnostic confirmation and therapeutic intent. The "coiled-spring sign," representing the ileum folded upon itself within the cecum is the classic finding of intussusception on contrast enema. Most pediatric intussusceptions (80% to 90%) can be successfully reduced radiologically, particularly if the disease process is recognized in a timely fashion, and reduction can be documented by free flow of contrast into the terminal ileum. Though perforation is uncommon, surgical consultation is recommended prior to attempts at radiologic reduction. Following successful reduction, the risk of reintussusception is 5% overall, and greatest during the first 24 hours, during which the child should be closely observed. Most reintussusceptions can be managed with a repeat enema.

Following failed attempts at enema reduction or in cases of perforation and peritonitis, surgical repair is indicated. Most surgeons perform an open repair via a right lower quadrant transverse incision, though some advanced laparoscopists advocate a minimally invasive approach. In either case, the intussusception is reduced by milking the intussusceptum retrograde while applying gentle traction on the proximal bowel. Bowel resection should be avoided unless the involved segments appear ischemic or a pathologic lead point is suspected. Appendectomy can be performed at the time of operation to limit future diagnostic confusion.

MECKEL'S DIVERTICULUM

Failure of normal closure of the omphalomesenteric duct, which normally occurs by the 7th week of gestation, results in a Meckel's diverticulum, a true diverticulum of the distal ileum. Such diverticula are located on the antimesenteric border of the terminal ileum, usually within 2 feet of the ileocecal valve, and may be fixed to the anterior abdominal wall by a fibrous band at the umbilicus in up to 25% of cases. The blood supply is derived from persistent vitelline vessels from the SMA. Though up to 2% of the population may have a Meckel's diverticulum with approximately equal incidence in males and females, only 2% of those affected are symptomatic, with a 2:1 male to female ratio. Half of such diverticula contain heterotopic gastric mucosa, and an additional 5% contain pancreatic tissue. Most cases are sporadic, with fewer than 5% of affected patients having an associated abnormality.

The most common clinical presentation involves bleeding from the small bowel opposite the diverticulum, which occurs due to erosion of the intestinal mucosa by acidic secretions from gastric mucosa within the Meckel's diverticulum. Other less frequent presentations include diverticulitis, obstruction or perforation of the diverticulum. Patients suspected to have a Meckel's diverticulum should be evaluated with a technetium 99m pertechnetate radionuclide study, or Meckel's scan, which demonstrates the presence of heterotopic gastric mucosa, allowing diagnosis of 60% to 80% of Meckel's diverticula. The relatively high false-negative rate dictates that a negative scan be repeated if the clinical suspicion remains high.

Other manifestations of Meckel's diverticula include inflammation causing right lower quadrant pain easily mistaken for appendicitis as well as small bowel obstruction related to either intussusception or volvulus around a diverticular attachment. Neoplasia is found in 0.5% to 4% of all Meckel's diverticula, and most such neoplasms are malignant. Of these, carcinoid is the most common, though leiomyosarcoma, adenocarcinoma, villous adenoma, and GIST have all been reported.

Though the data are mixed on resection of the asymptomatic Meckel's diverticulum, any symptomatic diverticulum should be resected either via wedge resection with transverse ileal closure in the absence of bleeding symptoms or by segmental ileal resection to include the ulcer opposite and downstream from the diverticulum itself.

APPENDICITIS

Appendicitis is the most common cause of an acute abdomen in children and results from luminal obstruction of the blind-ending appendix. The presentation and causes of appendicitis in the pediatric population differ somewhat from that of adults; obstruction most often occurs because of lymphoid hyperplasia within the submucosal follicles of the appendix, rather than an appendiceal fecalith, which may also cause appendicitis. Though the diagnosis of appendicitis may be made based upon a careful history and physical exam, fewer than half of affected children present with a classic history of periumbilical pain migrating to the right lower quadrant. Perhaps because the symptoms are mistaken for other disease processes, the appendix is more likely to be perforated at presentation in pediatric patients (approximately 50%). In general, pain from appendicitis nearly always precedes other symptoms, including anorexia, nausea, and vomiting, whereas vomiting and diarrhea usually occur early in gastroenteritis, followed by pain.

When the diagnosis is in question after a history and physical exam, laboratory and radiologic evaluation may be necessary. Up to 90% of patients may present with a leukocytosis and left shift, and C-reactive protein may be helpful in demonstrating the inflammatory process. Though ultrasonography and computed tomography (CT) are both highly sensitive and specific, increasing focus on minimizing radiation exposure in pediatric patients makes ultrasonography the preferred method for radiologic diagnosis of appendicitis. Though user dependent, ultrasonography is 85% to 90% sensitive and 90% to 98% specific for appendicitis, and the primary imaging characteristics include a dilated (>7 mm) and noncompressible appendix. CT characteristics include appendiceal enlargement, wall thickening, periappendiceal fat stranding, and failure to fill with oral contrast. Children evaluated at pediatric hospitals have been shown to be less likely to undergo CT scanning, as no evidence supports the routine use of CT in evaluating pediatric appendicitis.

Patients with suspected appendicitis should undergo appendectomy after initiation of broad-spectrum antibiotic therapy and fluid resuscitation. Most surgeons routinely perform laparoscopic appendectomy, which may be of particular utility in the adolescent female as it allows exclusion of gynecologic pathology from the differential diagnosis. Open appendectomy can be performed through a right lower quadrant incision, through which the appendix can be delivered into the wound. In either case, ligation of the appendiceal artery and base of appendix is performed.

Appendicitis can be broadly characterized into simple (nonperforated) and complicated (gangrenous, perforated) appendicitis, which may increase the risk of abscess from less than 5% to 20% or more. Antibiotic therapy is not necessary beyond the perioperative period in simple appendicitis. For complicated appendicitis, fever and leukocytosis may guide therapy duration, though there is no clear consensus on the duration or route of antibiotic therapy. In general, broad-spectrum oral antibiotics are preferred once a patient can tolerate a diet. Clinically stable patients known to have a perforation upon presentation may alternatively be managed nonoperatively with intravenous antibiotics, drain placement if necessary, and interval appendectomy in 6 to 12 weeks.

HIRSCHSPRUNG'S DISEASE

A functional large bowel obstruction of infancy, Hirschsprung's disease is characterized by the absence of ganglion cells in the myenteric (Auerbach) and submucosal (Meissner) plexus of the intestinal wall, likely related to a failure of neural crest cells to complete their migration to or proliferation within the distal bowel during the 13th week of gestation. Such aganglionic segments lack the parasympathetic innervations necessary for relaxation during peristalsis, creating obstructive physiology despite otherwise normal anatomy. Though most cases (85%) are limited to the rectum and sigmoid colon, aganglionosis begins at the rectum and may extend proximally as far as the distal small bowel (long-segment disease). Most cases are sporadic, but Hirschsprung's disease may be associated with various genetic syndromes, including Waardenburg syndrome and RET protooncogene mutations. The sporadic forms of the disease have a strong male predominance (4:1 male:female), while familial forms are associated with female gender and are more likely to involve long-segment disease.

Most affected infants fail to pass meconium within the first 24 hours of life, and many also present with abdominal distention and bilious emesis. In some cases, the presentation may be subacute, characterized by chronic constipation, abdominal distention, and failure to thrive. Delayed presentation may be more common in breast-fed infants, in whom weaning unmasks severe constipation. The first step in the evaluation of an infant suspected to have Hirschsprung's disease should be a water-soluble contrast enema, as this may be both diagnostic and therapeutic for other conditions with similar presentation, such as meconium ileus or meconium plug syndrome. A transition zone between small-caliber aganglionic bowel and dilated ganglionated bowel can often be visualized on contrast enema (Fig. 26.4), though this may be absent in younger infants or those with short-segment disease. Regardless of the timing, rectal biopsy should reveal aganglionosis in all intramural plexuses, increased staining for acetylcholinesterase, and the presence of hypertrophied nerve bundles. Suction rectal biopsy is the gold standard of diagnosis in the newborn period. Older children require operative biopsy to obtain tissue of adequate depth for interpretation.

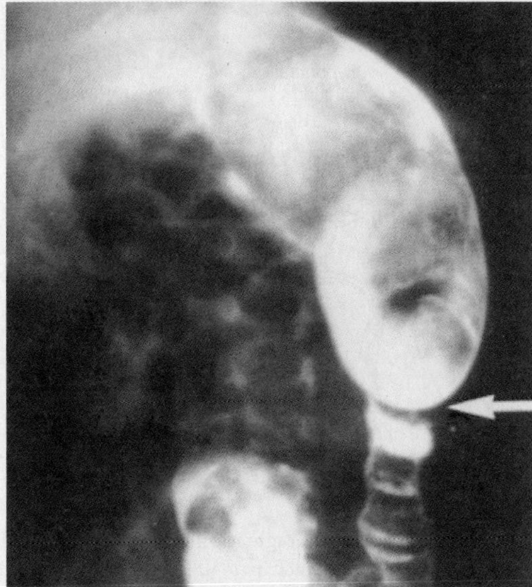

FIGURE 26.4 Hirschsprung's disease. Contrast enema demonstrating a classic rectosigmoid transition zone. (From Greenfield L, Mulholland MW, Zelenock GB, et al. *Surgery: Scientific Principles and Practice*. 3rd ed. Philadelphia: Lippincott Williams & Wilkins; 2001.)

Affected patients may also present with Hirschsprung-associated enterocolitis, which is associated with a poorer prognosis and may be life threatening, with progression to intestinal perforation and sepsis within 24 hours. Symptoms include fever, abdominal distention, and explosive diarrhea, and more severe cases may also involve anorexia, emesis, rectal bleeding, lethargy, or shock. Such patients require urgent decompression via rectal irrigation, aggressive fluid resuscitation, and intravenous antibiotics and the most severe cases may require diverting colostomy. The pathogenesis is not well understood, though partial obstruction leading to stasis and bacterial overgrowth may play a role, along with mucosal immunity defects, motility issues, and a dysfunctional mucosal barrier. Importantly, enterocolitis may present at any time either before or after surgical repair, suggesting that the disease process is not only related to obstructive physiology.

Surgical treatment of Hirschsprung's disease requires resection of the aganglionic segment of bowel with endorectal pull-through and anastomosis of ganglionated bowel to the anus. Though traditionally performed in three stages (leveling colostomy, pull-through at 6 to 9 months of age, stoma closure), many surgeons now choose a single-stage primary pull-through, avoiding a colostomy altogether. Prior to any pull-through, an intraoperative biopsy should be obtained to confirm the diagnosis and the level of the transition zone. Three approaches to the pull-through are commonly used with excellent long-term results, and the decision on which to employ relies primarily upon surgeon preference. The Swenson procedure was the original surgical approach to Hirschsprung's disease and consists of colon resection, extensive rectal dissection, and colorectal anastomosis above the anal sphincter. The Soave procedure was designed to avoid the risk of injury incurred by the deep pelvic dissection of the Swenson procedure, relying upon submucosal endorectal dissection to perform a coloanal anastomosis, which places the ganglionated bowel within a "cuff" of aganglionic muscle. The Duhamel–Martin procedure leaves the aganglionic rectal stump in situ, bringing the ganglionated bowel down through the plane between the rectum and sacrum, joining the two walls in a patulous anastomosis, sparing rectal dissection, and creating a "reservoir." Each of these procedures may also be performed laparoscopically with excellent short-term results, and laparoscopic mobilization allows the procedure to be performed using a transanal approach. Complications after surgical repair include constipation, obstruction, dysmotility, increased stool frequency, incontinency, or stricture in addition to local wound issues, infection, and intra-abdominal bleeding. Definitive repair will reduce (but not eliminate) the risk of future enterocolitis.

NECROTIZING ENTEROCOLITIS

Necrotizing enterocolitis (NEC) is a major cause of acquired gastrointestinal morbidity and mortality, particularly among low-birth-weight premature infants. Though the pathogenesis is poorly understood, NEC causes hypoxic–ischemic injury during the newborn period, usually within 2 to 3 weeks of birth. As the most common surgical emergency of neonates, the incidence is roughly 1 to 3/1,000 live births, though 1% to 2% of all neonatal ICU (NICU) patients and 7% to 10% of premature infants weighing less than 1,500 g may develop NEC at some point during their NICU stay.

The mortality associated with NEC is significant; 20% to 30% of affected infants do not survive. Much research has focused on the role of the intestinal microbiome and an inflammatory response, which may be of particular importance in very premature patients. Notably, 90% of NEC cases occur after the initiation of enteral feedings, suggesting that compromised barrier function may contribute, and though some studies have suggested that the prolonged use of trophic feedings may permit gut maturation and decrease the risk of NEC, randomized clinical trials have not detected a significant difference. Because of its immunologic and anti-inflammatory components, breast milk may be protective, and formula-fed infants are known to have a higher incidence of NEC. In addition to prematurity, known risk factors include hypoxia, hypotension, sepsis, umbilical vein catheterization, and maternal drug use. Most experts agree that NEC represents the final common pathway of intestinal damage related to decreased splanchnic perfusion, mucosal ischemic injury, and bacterial translocation in infants predisposed to such an insult because of an underdeveloped mucosal barrier, decreased motility, and an immature immune system.

The clinical presentation of NEC may be easily confused with neonatal sepsis, as early signs are nonspecific, including fever, lethargy, abdominal distention, increased gastric residuals, bilious emesis, and diarrhea. Twenty five to fifty percent of infants may have grossly bloody stools, and advanced disease is characterized by hemodynamic instability, erythema, edema or crepitus of the abdominal wall, a fixed abdominal mass, peritonitis, or discoloration of the scrotum, all of which suggest intestinal perforation. Laboratory findings may be similarly nonspecific, though neutropenia, thrombocytopenia, and metabolic acidosis are commonly observed. Radiographic evidence of advanced disease includes pneumatosis intestinalis, portal venous gas, or pneumoperitoneum. Serial abdominal radiographs should be obtained in suspected cases of NEC to detect pneumatosis or other evidence of disease progression.

The primary goal of clinical management is to distinguish between reversible mucosal injury and transmural necrosis, which requires urgent surgical intervention. Up to 90% of patients with NEC are managed nonoperatively ("medical NEC"), with nasogastric decompression, broad-spectrum antibiotics, and serial examination both clinically and radiographically. Enteral feedings should be avoided, and infants should be maintained on total parenteral nutrition (TPN) until the disease process is controlled.

Pneumoperitoneum is generally acknowledged to be the only absolute indication for operation, and most infants who require surgical management do so within 48 hours of diagnosis. The goal of operative management should be to preserve as much viable intestine as possible, and focal disease is defined as a single section of gangrenous bowel involving less than 25% of total intestinal length. As many as 55% of affected infants requiring operative management will have multisegmental disease, which involves several discontinuous segments representing a cumulative total of less than 50% of the bowel length. At laparotomy, all frankly gangrenous bowel should be resected and viable proximal and distal ends should be exteriorized, though some authors suggest the use of primary anastomosis for otherwise stable infants with multisegmental disease. In patients with diffuse disease, limited resection with planned second-look laparotomy can be of value. In infants weighing less than 1,000 g, the use of primary peritoneal drainage under local anesthesia has been associated with improved outcomes, though most of these infants require delayed laparotomy, and two randomized clinical trials comparing the use of peritoneal drainage and early laparotomy failed to show a significant difference between treatment groups with respect to mortality, TPN dependence, or length of stay.

In general, outcomes for infants with NEC are roughly equivalent to long-term outcomes for other premature infants, and overall survival exceeds 60%. Recurrent NEC occurs in 4% to 6% of patients. Important late complications include intestinal strictures, which develop in 9% to 36% of patients with NEC regardless of whether operative treatment was required, short bowel syndrome, and anastomotic ulcers, and some studies suggest that NEC may be an independent predictor of neurodevelopmental deficit. In patients managed with diversion, barium enema should be performed to evaluate for stricture prior to enterostomy closure.

THORACIC AND PULMONARY DISORDERS

Congenital Diaphragmatic Hernia

Incomplete development of the posterolateral portion of the diaphragm results in a hernia defect through the foramen of Bochdalek. In 80% to 90% of affected infants, the defect occurs on the left side, and the severest forms result in complete agenesis of the diaphragm. Herniation of abdominal contents through this defect creates a space-occupying process in the chest cavity, limiting normal lung development (Fig. 26.5). Anterior parasternal defects through the foramen of Morgagni occur far less commonly (<5%) and are less likely to cause physiologic derangement during the neonatal period. Congenital diaphragmatic hernia (CDH) can be diagnosed prenatally as early as 11 weeks, and the mean gestational age at diagnosis is 24 weeks. The specificity of prenatal diagnosis has been reported to range from 40% to 90%, and prenatal imaging can assist in predicting outcome through calculation of the lung-to-head ratio (LHR), which compares the area of the contralateral lung to the fetal head circumference. An LHR greater than 1.4 predicts nearly 100% survival, while LHR less than 1 portends poorer outcomes. Liver position remains the strongest prognostic sign, with liver herniation into the chest strongly

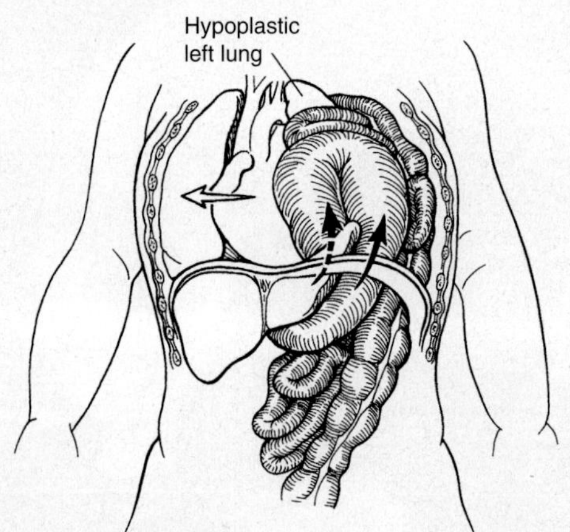

FIGURE 26.5 Congenital diaphragmatic hernia. Left-sided CDH with herniation of stomach (*solid black arrow*), liver (*dashed black arrow*), and intestine into the left hemithorax. The mediastinum is shifted right, and a hypoplastic left lung is seen at the apex of the left chest. CDH, congenital diaphragmatic hernia. (From Baker RJ, Fischer JE. *Mastery of Surgery*. 4th ed. Philadelphia: Lippincott Williams & Wilkins; 2001:699, with permission.)

associated with more severe disease. Because LHR changes with gestational age, many centers now utilize an observed-to-expected LHR (O/E-LHR), with severe disease marked by an O/E-LHR of less than 25%.

Despite prenatal diagnosis, the overall mortality of CDH ranges from 10% to 40%, as the mechanical compression of local structures leads to both pulmonary hypoplasia and pulmonary hypertension, which may result in right-to-left shunting. In severe cases, mediastinal shift may occur and both the ipsilateral and contralateral lungs may be affected. Histologic examination of lungs in affected neonates demonstrates decreased bronchial and pulmonary arterial branching as well as thickening of pulmonary arteriolar smooth muscle. Long-term outcomes are primarily determined by the degree of uncorrectable pulmonary hypoplasia and potentially reversible pulmonary hypertension, though loss of abdominal domain may complicate surgical repair.

At delivery, affected infants generally demonstrate a scaphoid abdomen and respiratory distress. Postnatal diagnosis is confirmed by the typical finding of intrathoracic intestine, absent diaphragmatic silhouette, and contralateral mediastinal shift. Up to half of all infants with CDH have other congenital anomalies, often cardiac, which may significantly decrease overall survival. Resuscitation should begin with placement of an orogastric tube for bowel decompression. Stabilization of cardiopulmonary function and resuscitation should be the primary initial goal, as more severely affected infants are often hypoxic, hypercarbic, and acidotic. Supplemental oxygen should be provided as needed, and early endotracheal intubation should be undertaken for any infant requiring mechanical ventilation. Bag–mask ventilation should be avoided due to the subsequent distention of the intrathoracic stomach and intestine. Ventilation strategies including permissive hypercapnia and spontaneous breathing have been shown to be successful in modifying pulmonary vascular tone. High-frequency oscillating ventilation and extracorporeal membrane oxygenation (ECMO) may be required in severe cases (10% to 20%). Controversy exists regarding the criteria for offering ECMO support, though this therapy should be reserved for those infants with potentially reversible disease rather than those with pulmonary hypoplasia incompatible with life.

No consensus exists regarding the optimal timing for surgical repair; approaches include early repair with or without ECMO, delayed repair once pulmonary function improves, or delayed repair once pulmonary hypertension has stabilized or resolved. Open repair of the defect is usually performed using an abdominal approach, though the repair can also be approached via thoracotomy or thoracoscopy. Regardless of technique, herniated abdominal viscera must be reduced and the diaphragmatic defect repaired. The defect should be closed primarily when possible, using nonabsorbable suture or, for larger defects, a prosthetic patch may be employed to bridge large defects with poorly defined tissue margins, anchored either to the diaphragmatic remnant or to the thoracic cage.

Survivors of CDH remain at risk for late complications, including recurrence, persistent pulmonary hypertension, and chronic neurologic, developmental, gastrointestinal, and nutritional disorders. Long-term pulmonary consequences may include bronchopulmonary dysplasia, reactive airway disease, and pneumonia; affected lungs never reach normal alveolar number and may be prone to emphysematous changes. CDH survivors have a unique constellation of lifelong management challenges, and multispecialty clinics play an increasing role in their care.

Congenital Pulmonary Cystic Diseases

Congenital lobar emphysema (CLE), congenital cystic adenomatoid malformation (CCAM), bronchopulmonary sequestration (BPS), and bronchogenic cysts are all part of a spectrum of congenital foregut abnormalities. Many of these lesions may be diagnosed prenatally, confirmed postnatally by plain radiography, and distinguished via CT angiogram. When diagnosed prenatally, the ratio of CCAM volume (length × height × width × 0.52) to head circumference, or CCAM volume ratio (CVR), predicts the risk of fetal hydrops; a CVR greater than 1.6 reflects an 80% risk of hydrops, and serial measurements to detect growth are necessary through 28 weeks, after which point, the lesion usually reaches a plateau. Any of these lesions may require resection for respiratory compromise, and the prognosis is related to the size of the lung mass and the secondary physiologic derangement related to mediastinal shift, lung hypoplasia, and cardiovascular compromise.

CLE is a rare condition characterized by hyperexpansion of one or more lobes of the lung due to the affected bronchus acting as a one-way valve to allow inspiration, but only limited expiration. The resultant air trapping leads to hyperexpansion, which causes compression of the adjacent normal lung and mediastinal shift. CLE may be distinguished from other cystic lesions prenatally by increased echogenicity relative to CCAM and the absence of systemic arterial supply. CLE occurs most frequently in the right upper or middle lobes, and preoperative management may require high-frequency ventilation or selective bronchial intubation to minimize air trapping with mechanical ventilation. CLE is effectively managed by thoracotomy and lobectomy except in infants with minimal air trapping whose mild symptoms do not progress; such patients may be safely observed.

CCAM lesions are cystic or hybrid solid/cystic lesions that communicate with the normal tracheobronchial tree and have a "swiss cheese" appearance on chest radiograph. Proliferation of the terminal airway yields cystic structures lined with respiratory epithelium capable of producing mucus. Microcystic CCAMs appear as a solid echogenic mass, while macrocystic lesions contain one or more cysts that are 5.0 mm or larger on prenatal ultrasonography. CCAM lesions are most commonly found in the lower lobes, and bilateral involvement is rare. Though many affected patients may be diagnosed prenatally, the most common postnatal presentation is with superinfection of the cystic lesion. CCAM lesions of any size require resection postnatally due to their rare incidence of malignant degeneration, or infection, either via thoracotomy or thoracoscopy.

BPS is characterized by anomalous lung parenchymal tissue, which does not communicate with the normal tracheobronchial tree, and generally takes its systemic blood supply from the abdominal aorta either above or below the diaphragm. Extralobar BPS drains systemically, usually via the azygous vein, while intralobar BPS drains via the pulmonary venous system. Prenatally diagnosed BPS lesions at risk of developing hydrops may often respond dramatically to maternal steroid administration. Small asymptomatic extralobar lesions rarely require surgical resection, though intralobar lesions may present with recurrent pneumonia requiring lobectomy. At resection, the systemic feeding vessel, which usually lies in the inferior pulmonary ligament, must be identified and divided.

Bronchogenic cysts reflect abnormal budding of the tracheal diverticulum and consist of immature bronchial tissue that neither communicates with the normal tracheobronchial tree nor possesses a unique blood supply. Two thirds of such cysts are located in the lungs, though they may be located at any level of the mediastinum or even below the diaphragm. Hilar and carinal bronchogenic cysts are thought to represent clusters of epithelial cells that become separated from the tracheobronchial tree and lung buds. Rather than undergo further differentiation as would a BPS, these lesions become extrapulmonary masses lined with ciliated columnar epithelium and surrounded by a fibrous tissue wall. Like CCAM lesions, malignant transformation has been reported, and all such lesions should be resected to avoid hemorrhage, expansion, superinfection, or malignancy.

BILIARY DISORDERS

Biliary Atresia

Biliary atresia is a progressive obliterative process affecting the extrahepatic biliary ducts; in the majority of patients, the entire extrahepatic biliary tract is obliterated, including the gallbladder. Though the inciting event for this process has not been identified, genetic, inflammatory, and infectious etiologies have been proposed. Animal models of perinatal viral infection seem to reproduce the clinical appearance of biliary atresia, but isolation of virus in clinical cases has been inconsistent at best. Furthermore, the relatively low incidence of biliary atresia suggests that, while perinatal infection may play a role, the disease process is likely multifactorial. Bile duct proliferation, cholestasis, and portal fibrosis may cause hepatic parenchymal dysfunction and cirrhosis if left untreated. Thus, a suspected diagnosis of biliary atresia should prompt thorough evaluation, as early intervention and establishment of biliary drainage are most important in preserving liver function long term.

Supporting an acquired etiology, affected neonates are most often anicteric full-term infants who develop progressive jaundice persisting beyond the first few weeks of life. Most infants become symptomatic by 1 month of age, with jaundice accompanied by acholic stools and dark urine, though many initially have normal-appearing meconium and initial stools. Physical exam may be significant for firm hepatomegaly; splenomegaly, ascites, failure to thrive, and malnutrition appear if untreated. Laboratory evaluation reveals elevations in both direct and indirect bilirubin, with a mild transaminitis and Gamma Glutamyltransferase (GGT) disturbance, though synthetic function generally remains intact. An abdominal ultrasound should be obtained to assess the biliary anatomy, with absence of extrahepatic biliary structures suggestive of biliary atresia. Technetium-labeled diisopropyl iminodiacetic cholestasis (DISIDA) scan reveals normal uptake with failure of excretion into the duodenum. To confirm the diagnosis, delayed images should be obtained at 24 hours. Liver biopsy, whether performed percutaneously or open, should demonstrate ductal proliferation and hepatic fibrosis and may further show bile stasis with plugging and giant cell transformation.

Prior to planned operative repair, the diagnosis should be confirmed using intraoperative cholangiogram; if the duodenum fills with contrast, the procedure should be aborted. The Kasai procedure, a Roux-en-Y hepaticoportoenterostomy performed through a right upper quadrant transverse incision, is the procedure of choice for operative repair. A laparoscopic approach has been reported, but several trials suggest decreased survival of the native liver versus the traditional open procedure. Evaluation of the hepatoduodenal ligament reveals a nonpatent fibrous cord replacing the common bile duct. Transsection of this cord distal to the cystic duct allows dissection to be carried up into the porta hepatis at the bifurcation of the portal vein, an important landmark of the procedure. The fibrous cone of extrahepatic biliary structures should be placed on traction and transected at the portal plate. Following dissection of the portal plate, the roux limb should be brought up in a retrocolic orientation to create a single-layer anastomosis between the jejunum and portal plate.

Postoperative outcomes not only depend on the technical adequacy of the procedure but also are inversely related to the age of the patient at operation. Jaundice will resolve postoperatively in 40% to 50% of affected infants, though surgical repair prior to 75 days has been associated with superior transplant-free survival. Because of this, some older infants (>120 days) may be listed for primary liver transplantation. Cholangitis may occur as a late complication in up to 50% of patients and requires early and aggressive resuscitation and intravenous antibiotics. Portal hypertension may be present in 35% to 75% of children following portoenterostomy and may occur despite excellent bile drainage. Lastly, some children may develop a malabsorptive syndrome related to the Roux-en-Y reconstruction, which requires treatment with medium-chain triglycerides.

Choledochal Cysts

Choledochal cysts are congenital malformations of the biliary tree involving cystic dilation of any portion of the intra- or extrahepatic bile duct. Though relatively rare in western countries, the incidence has been reported to be as high as 1 in 1,000 births in Japan. The "long common channel theory" postulates that choledochal cysts result from an anomalous proximal insertion of the pancreatic duct into the common bile duct (pancreatobiliary malformation), resulting in reflux of pancreatic enzymes and damage to the ductal wall. Distal obstruction at the duodenal insertion may further contribute to ductal damage and dilation, and this damage predisposes to carcinoma of the gallbladder and the involved portions of the biliary tree.

There are five main types of choledochal cysts (Fig. 26.6), of which type I, cystic/saccular of fusiform dilation of the common bile duct with minimal proximal disease, is most common (90% to 95% of cases). These cysts are generally large and may extend from the porta hepatis into the pelvis, displacing other abdominal viscera and predisposing to obstructive jaundice. Choledochal cysts may be diagnosed prenatally, and the differential diagnosis for a cyst seen in the porta hepatis includes hepatic cysts, mesenteric or omental cysts, intestinal duplication cysts, duodenal atresia, and ovarian cysts. In the absence of prenatal diagnosis, most patients will experience symptoms by 10 years of age, and most older children present with obstructive jaundice. The classic triad of symptoms includes jaundice, abdominal pain, and a palpable right upper quadrant mass, though this constellation of symptoms is present in no more than 50% of cases.

Radiographic evaluation of the suspected choledochal cyst should begin with abdominal ultrasound, followed by HIDA scan, which is highly sensitive for type I cysts, though somewhat decreased sensitivity for intrahepatic variants. In contrast to biliary atresia, contrast will enter the duodenum, though both filling and emptying of the cyst will be delayed. Percutaneous cholangiography, magnetic resonance cholangiopancreatography (MRCP), or endoscopic retrograde cholangiopancreatography (ERCP) may help in defining the anatomy of a cyst and planning the appropriate operative strategy.

Operative repair should begin with a cholangiogram performed via the gallbladder prior to cholecystectomy. Due to the risk of malignant transformation, the cystic portions of type I and IV choledochal cysts should be entirely excised and reconstructed with Roux-en-Y hepaticojejunostomy. With sparing of the common proximal to the bifurcation, choledochoduodenostomy is an option. Type II

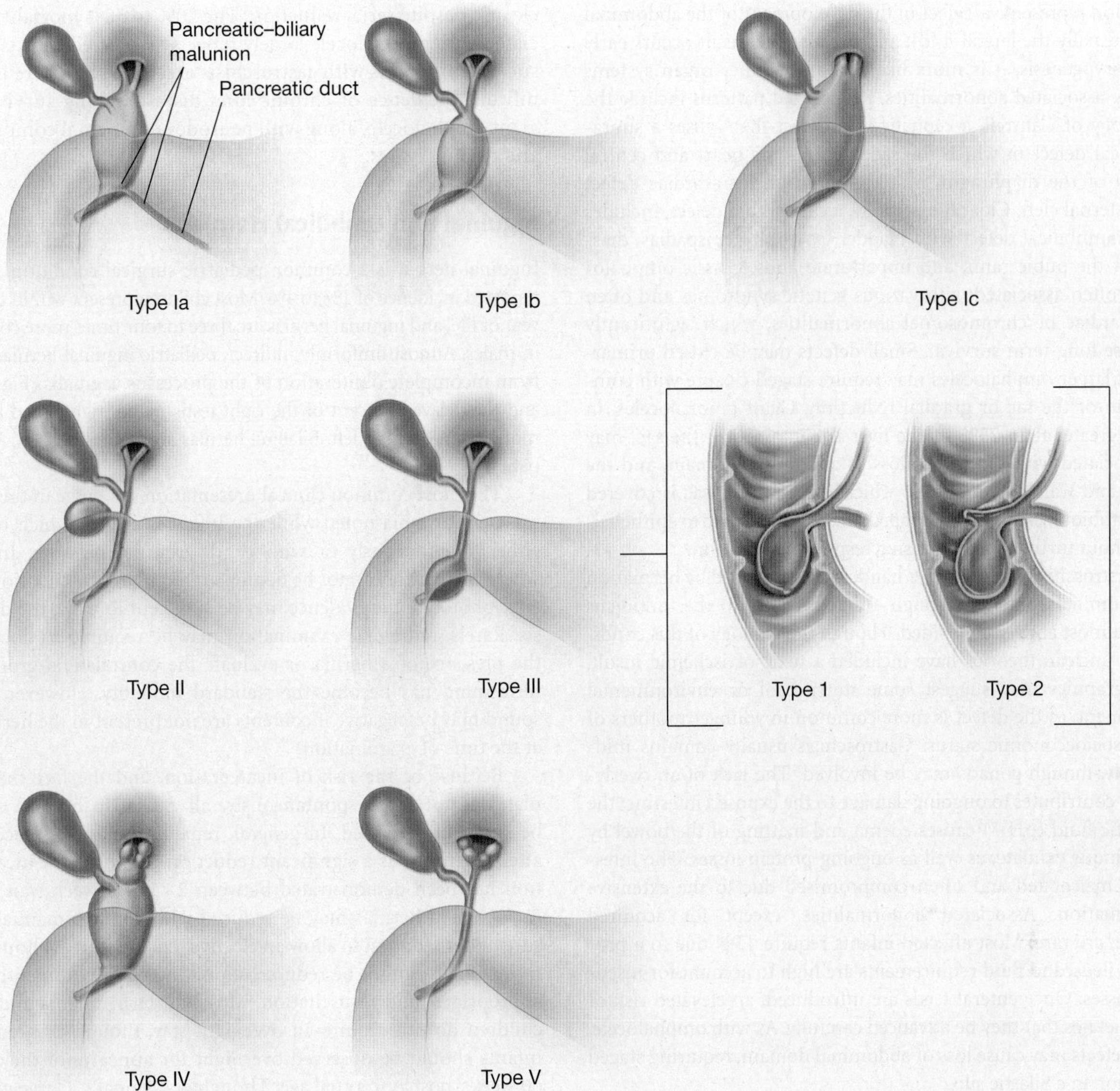

FIGURE 26.6 The five major classifications of choledochal cysts. (From Mulholland MW. *Operative Techniques in Surgery*. Philadelphia: Wolters Kluwer Health; 2015.)

choledochal cysts appear to have low malignant potential and may be managed with simple cystectomy, while type III cysts (choledochoceles) require marsupialization either endoscopically or via an open transduodenal approach. For these intraduodenal or intrapancreatic lesions, the risk of malignancy is unclear but is likely elevated. Surgical management of type V choledochal cysts, or Caroli disease, depends upon the intrahepatic extent; segmental resections may be performed if anatomically feasible, but for extensive disease, liver transplantation may be necessary. Long-term complications may include recurrent cholangitis, stricture or stone formation, and pancreatitis.

ABDOMINAL WALL DEFECTS

Omphalocele and Gastroschisis

Though both are developmental malformations of the anterior abdominal wall leading to herniation of abdominal contents, the anatomical differences between omphalocele and gastroschisis belie their distinct etiologies (Table 26.1). Omphalocele is a defect in the umbilical ring ranging from 2 to 10 cm or more, covered by amniotic membrane and resulting in herniation of midgut and possibly other abdominal organs including liver, spleen, and gonads. This

TABLE 26.1 Comparison of omphalocele and gastroschisis

	Omphalocele	Gastroschisis
Presence of sac	Yes	No
Location of defect	Midline	Lateral
Appearance of bowel	Normal	Inflamed
Associated anomalies	Yes	No
Mortality	30%	10%

condition represents a defect in the development of the abdominal folds (usually the lateral fold), and because the insult occurs early in embryogenesis, it is more likely to affect other organ systems causing associated abnormalities. Recognized patterns include the pentalogy of Cantrell, a cephalic fold defect that causes a supraumbilical defect in which the sac contains the heart and central tendon of the diaphragm, in addition to an intracardiac defect and a sternal cleft. Cloacal exstrophy, a caudal fold defect, includes an infraumbilical defect with bladder exstrophy, epispadias, diastasis of the pubic rami, and imperforate anus. Classic omphalocele is often associated with various genetic syndromes and often with cardiac or chromosomal abnormalities, which significantly decrease long-term survival. Small defects may be closed primarily, but larger omphaloceles may require staged closure with compression of the sac or gradual reduction. Giant omphaloceles, in which greater than 75% of the liver is contained in the sac, may be associated with significant loss of abdominal domain, and the "paint and wait" technique, in which the amniotic sac is covered with antibiotic cream and wrapped, may allow the sac to epithelialize without further compromising respiratory function.

Gastroschisis, on the other hand, is characterized by herniation of abdominal contents through a defect lateral to the umbilicus and is almost always right sided. Though the etiology of this condition is unclear, theories have included a toxic or ischemic insult. Demographics may suggest some nutritional or environmental component, as the defect is more common in younger mothers of lower socioeconomic status. Gastroschisis usually contains midgut only, though gonads may be involved. The lack of an overlying sac contributes to ongoing damage to the exposed intestine; the amniotic fluid (pH 7) causes edema and matting of the bowel by a gelatinous exudate, as well as ongoing protein losses. The intestine is malrotated and often compromised due to the extensive inflammation. Associated abnormalities, except for acquired atresias, are rare. Most affected infants require TPN due to a prolonged ileus, and fluid requirements are high to account for insensible losses. Once enteral feeds are introduced, an elevated risk of NEC dictates that they be advanced carefully. As with omphalocele, large defects may cause loss of abdominal domain, requiring staged reduction in a Silastic silo.

Both omphalocele and gastroschisis may be diagnosed prenatally by ultrasound, which allows visualization of a sac, if present. Cesarean section offers no benefit, though delivery should be carefully planned and coordinated to allow the pediatric surgical team to be prepared. When a fetus known to have either of these defects is born, the immediate priorities must be resuscitation and protection of the exposed bowel. Nasogastric decompression should be employed to decompress the bowel and prevent aspiration, and the herniated contents should be protected by wrapping with moist gauze and covering with a sterile plastic drape. Both fluid resuscitation and broad-spectrum antibiotics should be started while examining the infant for any other abnormalities. The presence of severe or life-threatening–associated anomalies may require that operative repair be deferred. Primary closure can be accomplished in 60% to 70% of all infants with abdominal wall defects, and mechanical ventilation may be required temporarily to accommodate the restriction of diaphragmatic excursion. In those that cannot be closed initially, serial bedside reductions generally allow delayed primary closure. Tissue expanders, skin grafting, and flap reconstruction may be options for repair of the rare defect too large for primary closure despite serial reduction. The 20% to 30% mortality associated with omphalocele largely reflects associated defects, while survival of infants with gastroschisis exceeds 90%. There is a significant incidence of chronic lung disease among survivors of giant omphalocele, along with neurodevelopmental compromise and feeding issues.

Inguinal and Umbilical Hernias

Inguinal hernia is a common pediatric surgical condition, with a reported incidence of 1% to 4%. Most children present within the first year of life, and inguinal hernias are three to four times more common in males. Almost uniformly indirect, pediatric inguinal hernias result from incomplete obliteration of the processus vaginalis (Fig. 26.7), and the delayed descent of the right testis makes right-sided hernias more common than left. Bilateral hernias are found in 5% to 10% of patients.

The most common clinical presentation is a bulge in the groin, scrotum, or labia noted while the infant is crying, which reduces either spontaneously or with gentle external pressure. In cases where the hernia cannot be demonstrated upon examination, parents' photographic evidence may be sufficient to make the diagnosis. Rarely, radiologic examination may be required to document the presence of a hernia or evaluate the contralateral groin, and ultrasound has become the standard modality. However, ultrasound may be negative if contents are not present in the hernia sac at the time of examination.

Because of the risk of incarceration, and the fact that hernias do not close spontaneously, all pediatric hernias should be surgically repaired. In general, repair should take place soon after diagnosis, as a significant reduction in the risk of incarceration has been demonstrated between 2- and 4-week wait times. Incarcerated hernias may be reduced with gentle bimanual pressure under sedation to allow an elective repair within 24 hours, and those which cannot be reduced should be repaired urgently after appropriate fluid resuscitation. Most full-term infants and older children do not require an overnight stay, though ex-premature infants should be observed overnight for apnea until they reach 60 weeks' postconceptual age. Though occasionally a large chronic hernia in a child or adolescent may require fascial repair, mesh is not generally used in the pediatric population; high ligation of the hernia sac at the internal inguinal ring is the procedure of choice. The hernia sac, located medially, and the cord structures, located laterally, can be delivered into a very small incision in a groin skin crease over the external inguinal ring. Great care must be taken to preserve all cord structures as well as the delicate testicular blood supply. The repair is competed by excising and tying off the sac at the level of the internal ring. Laparoscopic approaches may also be employed, in which the internal ring is obliterated by either a Z stitch or purse-string suture following reduction of the hernia contents. Laparoscopy may also be utilized to evaluate for the presence of a contralateral hernia.

A communicating hydrocele also results from a patent processus vaginalis, which permits intermittent accumulation of fluid within the tunica vaginalis. Because the anatomic defect is identical to that of indirect inguinal hernia, so too is the treatment. A noncommunicating hydrocele is an accumulation of fluid in the tunica vaginalis "trapped" by an obliterated processus vaginalis. Typically, a noncommunicating hydrocele does not require surgical treatment and resolves spontaneously by 1 year of age. Though the simple

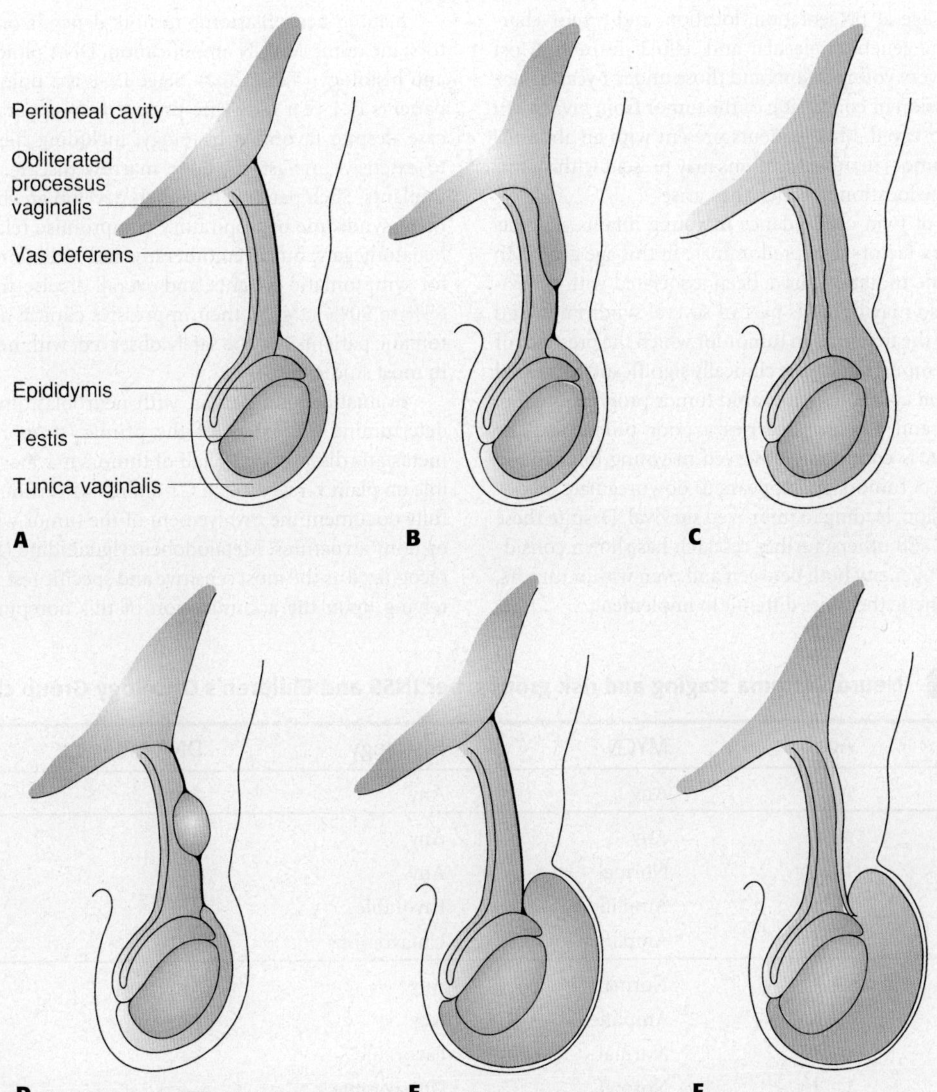

FIGURE 26.7 Variations in obliteration of the processus vaginalis. **A.** Normal, obliterated processus vaginalis. B. Proximal hernia sac, distal obliterated processus. **C.** Hernia sac extending into scrotum, no obliteration. **D.** Proximal and distal obliteration with hydrocele of the cord. **E.** Hydrocele of the scrotum, obliterated processus. **F.** Patent processus with communicating hydrocele. (From Mulholland MW. *Greenfield's Surgery: Scientific Principles and Practice*. 5th ed. Philadelphia: Lippincott Williams & Wilkins; 2011.)

fluid collection transilluminates, this technique does not reliably distinguish between hydrocele and hernia because fluid-filled bowel may transilluminate as well. A careful history is the most important diagnostic tool, and surgical approach should permit repair of an associated hernia if found.

Congenital umbilical defects may occur in 5% to 10% of Caucasian children and up to 25% to 50% of African-American children. Despite this being the most prevalent abdominal wall defect, most close spontaneously by 4 years of age. Prematurity is a significant risk factor, as these hernias result from incomplete closure of the umbilical ring. Incarceration is rare, and surgical repair should be deferred until the child is old enough to determine that the defect has failed to close. The repair may be performed through a small curvilinear infraumbilical incision with reconstruction of the umbilical appearance at the conclusion of the procedure.

NEOPLASTIC DISEASE

Neuroblastoma

Though pediatric malignancies are uncommon, cancer represents the second leading cause of death in children after traumatic injury. Neuroblastoma is one of the most common childhood cancers, representing 10% of all tumors and 15% of pediatric cancer deaths. Derived from primitive neural crest cells, neuroblastoma can arise anywhere along the migratory pathway along which the sympathetic ganglia descend. The adrenal medulla is the most common location (50%), though tumors may arise in cervical, posterior mediastinal, retroperitoneal, or pelvic sites, including the organ of Zuckerkandl. Neuroblastoma is typically a disease of early childhood, with 40% of cases diagnosed by age 1, 75% by age 7, and 98% by age 10; it is the most common malignancy diagnosed congenitally and within 1 year of birth. The behavior of the tumor is highly variable and depends upon the age at presentation, location, and tumor characteristics, including genetic molecular and cellular features. Most commonly seen in very young infants and those under 1 year of age, spontaneous regression or conversion of the tumor from invasive to benign has been observed. Most patients present with an abdominal mass, though tumors in other locations may present with symptoms referable to the location in which they arise.

A high degree of twin concordance in young infants suggests genetic or hereditary factors may predominate in this age group. In fact, multiple genetic mutations have been associated with neuroblastoma, which also may occur as part of several syndromes, and neuroblastoma was the first human tumor for which the presence of an oncogene was demonstrated to be clinically significant. Increased MYCN amplification correlates with rapid tumor progression and, along 1p deletion and 17q gain, carries a poor prognosis. The neurotrophin Trk-A is commonly observed in young infants and those with stage IV-S tumors and appears to downregulate angiogenic factor expression, leading to improved survival. Despite these promising findings and others, further research has shown considerable genetic heterogeneity both between and even within tumors, making targeted genetic therapies difficult to implement.

Staging neuroblastoma tumors depends on a number of factors, including MYCN amplification, DNA ploidy, age at diagnosis, and histology (Table 26.2). Stage IV-S is a unique group of young patients (<1 year old) who present with apparently advanced disease despite favorable histology, including hepatomegaly related to extensive metastasis, bone marrow disease, and subcutaneous implants. Such patients may even develop an abdominal compartment syndrome or respiratory compromise related to the massive hepatomegaly, but chemotherapy and radiation are only required for symptomatic patients, and overall disease-free survival exceeds 85% to 90%. Despite their impressive clinical appearance, asymptomatic patients may be safely observed, with nearly 100% survival in most studies.

Evaluation of a patient with neuroblastoma should focus on determining the extent of the primary tumor and assessing for metastatic disease. Up to half of tumors may have calcifications visible on plain x-ray, though CT and/or MRI should be performed to fully document the involvement of the tumor with adjacent organs or bony structures. Metaiodobenzylguanidine (MIBG) scanning is recognized as the most sensitive and specific test for neuroblastoma, relying upon the accumulation of this norepinephrine derivative

TABLE 26.2 Neuroblastoma staging and risk groups, per INSS and Children's Oncology Group classifications

INSS Stage	Age	MYCN	Histology	DNA Index	Risk Group
1	Any	Any	Any	Any	Low
2A/2B	<1 y	Any	Any	Any	Low
	1–21 y	Normal	Any	—	Low
	1–21 y	Amplified	Favorable	—	Low
	1–21 y	Amplified	Unfavorable	—	High
3	<1 y	Normal	Any	Any	Intermediate
	<1 y	Amplified	Any	Any	High
	1–21 y	Normal	Favorable	—	Intermediate
	1–21 y	Normal	Unfavorable	—	High
	1–21 y	Amplified	Any	—	High
4	<1 y	Normal	Any	Any	Intermediate
	<1 y	Amplified	Any	Any	High
	1–21 y	Any	Any	—	High
4S	<1 y	Normal	Favorable	>1	Low
	<1 y	Normal	Any	1	Intermediate
	<1 y	Normal	Unfavorable	Any	Intermediate
	<1 y	Amplified	Any	Any	High

INSS Stage 1	Localized tumor, complete gross resection, negative lymph nodes
INSS Stage 2A	Localized tumor, incomplete gross resection, negative lymph nodes
INSS Stage 2B	Unilateral tumor, complete or incomplete gross resection, positive ipsilateral lymph nodes, negative contralateral lymph nodes
INSS Stage 3	Tumor crosses midline, with or without regional lymph node involvement; unilateral tumor with positive contralateral lymph nodes; midline tumor with bilateral lymph node involvement
INSS Stage 4	Dissemination to distant lymph nodes, bone, bone marrow, liver, or other organs
INSS Stage 4S	Patient <1 y with localized tumor disseminated to skin, liver, or bone marrow with <10% tumor cells and negative MIBG scan in marrow

within the tumor to localize and follow response to treatment. Bone scintigraphy may be useful in detecting bony disease, and bone marrow biopsy should be performed to fully assess for marrow involvement, reflected by rosettes of tumor cells. Greater than 90% of affected children will have elevated levels of urinary catecholamines (HMA, VMA, vanillylglycolic acid, adrenaline, noradrenaline, dopamine, and metanephrine), and 24-hour urine collection should be conducted.

Low-risk patients often may be managed with surgery alone if the tumor can be completely resected with negative margins. Locally advanced tumors may rarely require en bloc resection of nearby structures, particularly the kidney, though this should be avoided whenever possible, and care should be taken to preserve the blood supply to other abdominal viscera. The tumor should be handled carefully, as catecholamine release may trigger dangerous hypertension, and rupture of the friable pseudocapsule can lead to tumor spillage and upstaging. Patients with more advanced disease, particularly those with stage III or IV tumor, should be initially managed by tumor sampling, bone marrow biopsy, and placement of a vascular access device for four to five rounds of chemotherapy with planned second-look surgery to decrease tumor burden. In these second-look procedures, the goal should be gross total resection of the primary tumor. External beam radiation may be useful for control of residual disease after surgical resection, or as treatment for bulky metastatic disease, though concerns remain about its potential toxicity. Proton beam therapy may represent a novel method to limit radiation dose to surrounding normal tissues, and a Children's Oncology Group trial is underway.

Wilms' Tumor

Like neuroblastoma, Wilms' tumor tends to present in young children, often between 1 and 5 years of age, and represents 6% of all pediatric tumors. Several conditions are known to be associated with Wilms' tumors, including WAGR syndrome (Wilms' tumor, aniridia, genitourinary malformation, and mental retardation), Beckwith–Wiedemann syndrome, and Denys–Drash syndrome. Most Wilms' tumors are focal and unilateral, though 7% of patients have multifocal unilateral disease and an additional 7% have bilateral tumors. Histologically, Wilms' tumors are embryonic renal tumors consisting of blastemal, stromal, and epithelial elements. Anaplastic histology is considered unfavorable.

Most Wilms' tumors present as an asymptomatic abdominal mass, though spontaneous tumor rupture can occur, causing pain. Hematuria, either gross or microscopic, may be present in a minority of affected patients, and still others experience coagulopathy or hypertension related to up-regulation of the renin–angiotensin–aldosterone pathway. Plain x-ray may identify a classic pattern of "eggshell" or linear calcification, but ultrasound is commonly the first radiologic evaluation of a suspected tumor, allowing definition of its size, origin, and any involved structures including intracaval extension of tumor or thrombus. Chest CT should be performed to assess for pulmonary metastasis, and advanced imaging with either abdominal CT or MRI allows detection of contralateral tumors and locoregional or lymphatic metastases and further defines vascular involvement.

Staging includes both the abdominal disease burden and distant metastasis, and nearly all patients undergo initial surgical resection (Table 26.3). Tumors are generally considered to be unresectable if

TABLE 26.3 Staging for Wilms' tumor

Stage	Description
I	Tumor limited to kidney, complete resection with intact capsule
II	Tumor extends beyond kidney or spillage during resection, but margins negative
III	Residual nonhematogenous tumor present in the abdomen (positive margins, positive lymph nodes in hilum or pelvis, peritoneal implants)
IV	Hematogenous metastases (brain, bone, liver, lung, etc.)
V	Bilateral renal involvement (each side staged individually)

the tumor thrombus extends above the hepatic veins, if the involvement of adjacent structures would require complete removal of vital organs, or if pulmonary metastases cause significant respiratory compromise. Tumors in a solitary kidney or bilateral tumors may be amenable to partial nephrectomy. In cases of bilateral Wilms' tumor, both sides may be considered to have a stage if neither has evidence of distant disease. For unresectable lesions, neoadjuvant chemotherapy may cause sufficient tumor shrinkage to allow delayed resection.

Surgical treatment provides necessary staging information and should include unilateral nephrectomy with lymph node dissection. Historically, routine exploration of the contralateral kidney was considered necessary, but the sensitivity of modern imaging protocols has improved sufficiently that palpation and examination of the contralateral kidney are not mandated unless a lesion is suspected on preoperative CT or MRI. The renal vein should be carefully palpated to exclude tumor thrombus, and the tumor should be handled carefully throughout to avoid rupture of the kidney capsule. Bloody ascites should raise suspicion for spontaneous tumor rupture. Final tumor staging depends upon the depth of invasion observed histologically and observations upon abdominal exploration. Certain young patients (<2 years) with very low-risk tumors and favorable histology may be treated with surgery alone, but the vast majority of patients with Wilms' tumors require postoperative chemotherapy, and those with advanced stage disease may receive external beam radiation to the primary tumor bed.

Outcomes for patients with Wilms' tumor are generally excellent, with greater than 90% survival for stage I, 85% to 90% survival for stages II and III, and greater than 60% survival even for stage IV disease. All patients should be monitored for disease recurrence, which occurs in 15% of those patients with favorable histology and up to 50% of those with anaplastic features. Though most recurrences occur within 2 years of the initial presentation, long-term follow-up is needed. In addition to the tumor bed, common sites of recurrence include the lung and liver.

PEDIATRIC TRAUMA

Trauma represents the leading cause of death in children between 1 and 18 years of age. Each year, approximately 20,000 children die from injuries, exceeding the total number of pediatric deaths from all other diseases combined. An additional 100,000 children sustain injuries causing permanent disabilities yearly. Pediatric trauma carries significant costs both financial and psychosocial, and care at pediatric-focused trauma centers has been shown to improve outcomes. Optimizing the care of the pediatric trauma patient requires understanding common patterns of injury and considering the unique physiologic and anatomic concerns inherent in the treatment of children.

The vast majority of pediatric traumatic injuries result from blunt trauma (greater than 80% to 90%), commonly associated with falls and motor vehicle crashes. Head injuries are more common after falls, while chest and abdominal injuries predominate in motor vehicle crashes. Child abuse, or nonaccidental trauma, represents a relatively unique category of injury and is among the most highly lethal mechanisms. Brain injury is common among the youngest victims of nonaccidental trauma, often related to shaking. Subdural hematoma is the most common intracranial finding in such cases, which may present with seizure activity or depressed level of consciousness at some interval from the injury. Motor vehicle crashes account for the highest number of pediatric trauma deaths, but case fatality rates are highest in cases of drowning, abuse, and penetrating wounds.

Pediatric trauma providers should be aware of common signs of child abuse or neglect, as patients are often unable or unwilling to provide an accurate history. Children whose weight or height is low for age, with oddly shaped injury patterns, burns of uncommon distribution or in areas normally protected ("glove," "stocking," thighs, upper arms, or stomach), retinal hemorrhage, or whose injuries are inconsistent with the mechanism provided should raise suspicion for abuse or neglect. Up to 80% of abuse cases are recognized radiographically, with multiple fractures in various stages of healing. Likewise, long bone fractures in a premobile infant are highly suspicious. Injuries to the genitals and the presence of sexually transmitted disease should prompt investigation of childhood sexual abuse. Most pediatric hospitals have teams dedicated to the evaluation of suspected abuse, and all providers are legally required to report any suspicion of abuse to the appropriate state agency.

Evaluation of the pediatric trauma patient, as with adults, begins with a primary survey including airway (A), breathing (B), and circulation (C). The cervical spine should be immobilized, and a variety of pediatric-specific collars exist to ensure appropriate sizing. The face should be moved anteriorly and superiorly ("sniffing position") to provide optimal airway protection due to the anterior position of the larynx in children. Surgical airways in children are rarely necessary; for children under 10 years of age, they should be accomplished via needle cricothyroidotomy with conversion to a formal tracheostomy in the operating room.

Assessment of circulation in children is complicated by their ability to compensate for hypovolemia until relatively late; tachycardia is the first indicator of hypovolemia, and many severely injured children may present with normal vital signs. Due to their ability to constrict small- and medium-sized arteries, hypotension may be absent until greater than 40% of the blood volume has been lost. Furthermore, the small blood volume in young children allows even what appears to be limited blood loss to have dramatic physiologic consequences. Venous access should be obtained rapidly, and if two attempts fail to obtain large-bore IV access in the extremities, an intraosseous (IO) line should be placed. Preferred sites for venous access include the cephalic vein at the antecubital fossa, the greater saphenous vein at the ankle, and the external jugular vein. An initial bolus of 20 mL/kg lactated Ringer solution should be given and repeated if the patient remains hypotensive. Hypotension that does not respond to 40 mL/kg of crystalloid should raise concern for surgical bleeding, and RBC transfusion should be initiated (10 mL/kg). Exposure is of particular concern in children, whose large surface area to volume ratio predisposes them to significant heat loss. Following a rapid secondary survey including a head-to toe exam, hypothermia should be aggressively corrected and body temperature maintained above 36°C.

Brain injury is the most common cause of trauma-related death among children, whose thin skull, weaker cervical spinal musculature, and relatively large heads predispose to head injury. Primary brain injury is a direct reflection of the structural damage sustained in the initial insult, and children are prone to white matter shear, diffuse axonal injury, punctuate hemorrhage, and linear, nondepressed skull fractures. Secondary brain injury, however, is related to the decreased cerebral perfusion following a head injury, and aggressive treatment of hypoxia, hypotension, and intracranial hypertension is critical in its prevention. Though excessive hyperventilation has been shown to worsen outcomes, careful management of pCO_2 around 35 and an alkalotic pH may help to limit intracranial pressure through cerebral vasoconstriction. Children may require placement of an intraventricular monitor to directly measure intracranial pressure. Fever and seizures may further injure the damaged brain, though the use of routine seizure prophylaxis is controversial.

Because the rib cage is more elastic in children than adults, thoracic organs are less well protected from blunt force trauma to the chest, and kinetic energy is more directly transmitted to underlying structures. Twenty-five to thirty percent of patients treated in level I pediatric trauma centers sustain injuries to the chest wall, lungs, or mediastinal structures, with an associated mortality rate as high as 25% in children under 5 years. The absence of rib fractures can mask major thoracic trauma, and suspicion for major thoracic injury should remain high even in their absence. If present, rib fractures suggest a particularly high-velocity mechanism. Because the mediastinal structures are particularly mobile in children, tension pneumothorax may present as severe hypotension with obstruction of venous return to the heart. Pneumothorax generally requires chest tube drainage, though small asymptomatic pneumothoraces (up to 15%) may be safely observed. In general, appropriate chest tube sizes are as follows: newborn—12 to 16 Fr, infant—14 to 18 Fr, child—18 to 24 Fr, and adolescent—20 to 32 Fr.

Though abdominal injuries occur in up to 25% of children after multisystem trauma, successful nonoperative management of solid organ injury in children has served as a template for widespread introduction of observation protocols in adult trauma. Though the focused abdominal sonography for trauma (FAST) exam is widely used in adult trauma protocols, its use in children has been associated with low sensitivity and inconsistent detection of abdominal injury, and CT remains the primary method of radiographic evaluation in the setting of high clinical suspicion. Dose reduction protocols should be employed to minimize radiation exposure–related CT scanning in the pediatric population. The liver and spleen are the most common organs injured and represent a combined total of nearly 75% of all pediatric abdominal injuries. Decades of experience have validated the safety and efficacy of serial observation and hematocrit determinations. Very few children require laparotomy for blunt injury to solid organs, though refractory hypotension and suspicion of perforated viscus require operative exploration.

Though injury prevention programs have increased the use of common child safety devices, education remains an important means of addressing this public health epidemic, as most pediatric trauma deaths are preventable.

Suggested Readings

Coran AG, Adzick NS, Krummel TM, et al., eds. *Pediatric Surgery*. 7th ed. Philadelphia: Elsevier; 2012.

Mattei P, ed. *Fundamentals of Pediatric Surgery*. New York: Springer; 2011.

Mulholland MW, Lillemoe KD, Doherty GM, et al., eds. *Surgery: Scientific Principles and Practice*. 5th ed. Philadelphia: Lippincott Williams & Wilkins; 2011.

Ziegler MM, Azizkhan RG, von Allmen D, et al., eds. *Operative Pediatric Surgery*. 2nd ed. New York: McGraw Hill'; 2014.

Urology

EUGENE J. PIETZAK III AND THOMAS J. GUZZO

KEY POINTS

- *Iatrogenic ureteral injury* most commonly occurs during complicated operations with distorted anatomy secondary to severe inflammatory changes or pelvic malignancy. Although preoperative prophylactic stent placement may help with intraoperative identification of a ureteral injury, they do not reduce the risk of injury.
- Prostate cancer is the most common cancer among males and is the second leading cause of cancer death in men. Risk factors include older age, family history of prostate cancer, and African American race. The management of prostate cancer depends on the grade and stage of the tumor, PSA level, comorbidities, and patient preference.
- It is estimated that approximately 80% of solid renal masses are malignant, with an incremental increase in malignancy risk as size increases. If localized, renal cell carcinoma surgery may be curative. However, the prognosis for metastatic renal cell carcinoma is poor.
- Patients with bladder cancer can broadly be divided into muscle-invasive and non–muscle-invasive disease depending on the involvement of the lamina propria (detrusor muscle). This distinction has significant implications for treatment.
- Benign prostatic hyperplasia (BPH) is a histologic diagnosis that can result in significant lower urinary tract symptoms from bladder outlet obstruction that results from enlarged static stromal tissue and increased dynamic smooth muscle tone.

SURGICAL ANATOMY OF THE GENITOURINARY SYSTEM

The Kidneys

The kidneys are paired, bean-shaped, retroperitoneal organs that are embryologically derived from the metanephric blastema. In adults, the kidney spans 10 to 12 cm in the craniocaudal direction. The renal pelvis and renal hilum are oriented medially with an approximately 30-degree anterior rotational access. The posterior aspect of the kidney is protected by the inferior rib cage (T11 and T12) and by the overlying musculature. The lung pleura usually attaches to the 11th rib and might be inadvertently entered with an open flank incision or with a nephrostomy tube placed in the renal upper pole. The right kidney is caudally displaced because the liver occupies the space below the right hemidiaphragm. The kidney is also protected by perirenal fat that is contained within the perirenal renal fascia (Gerota's fascia). Also contained within Gerota's fascia is the adrenal gland superiorly. Gerota's fascia serves as a barrier to spread of malignancy and can keep perinephric fluid collections (i.e., blood or urine) contained, but the anterior and posterior layers of Gerota's fascia are incompletely attached inferiorly.

The right kidney lies in proximity to the liver, right adrenal gland, ascending colon, psoas muscle, and duodenum. The left kidney lies in proximity to the spleen, left adrenal gland, tail of the pancreas, and descending colon (Fig. 27.1).

The arterial blood supply to each kidney is supplied by the renal artery, which branches directly from the aorta just inferior to the superior mesenteric artery. The renal vein usually courses anterior to the renal artery. The renal pelvis and proximal ureter lie posterior to the renal artery. The artery to the left renal unit is shorter in length than the right renal artery. The renal artery branches as it approaches the kidney. The divisions are as follows: renal segmental arteries (usually five divisions), lobar arteries, interlobar arteries, arcuate arteries, interlobular arteries, and finally afferent arterioles of the glomeruli. The incidence of renal vascular anatomic variation is common (i.e., as high as 30%). The most common variations are accessory renal arteries, a more common finding on the left than on the right. Renal arteries, including accessory arteries, are end-organ blood supply; therefore, ligation at any level of arterial supply will result in ischemic nephron loss.

The venous drainage of the kidney follows closely the arterial supply. However, the venous system, unlike the arterial segmental branches, is freely communicating, and occlusion of segmental venous vessels has little effect on overall venous outflow. The segmental veins drain into the main renal vein, which is shorter on the right side secondary to its proximity to the vena cava. Importantly, the left adrenal vein, the left gonadal vein, and the lumbar branches drain into the left renal vein, while all these vessels on the right side drain directly into the IVC. The lymphatic drainage of the kidney follows the blood vessels.

Adrenal Gland

The adrenal glands are found within Gerota's fascia superomedially to the kidney. The left adrenal is usually semicircular or crescent shaped, while the right adrenal is usually shaped like an inverted pyramid. The arterial supply is from branches of the aorta, inferior phrenic artery, and renal artery, but discrete adrenal arteries are often not identified during adrenalectomy. As previously mentioned, the left adrenal vein drains into the left renal vein, whereas the right adrenal vein drains directly into the IVC. The adrenal gland is of neuroendocrine origin, so in cases of renal ectopia (i.e., when

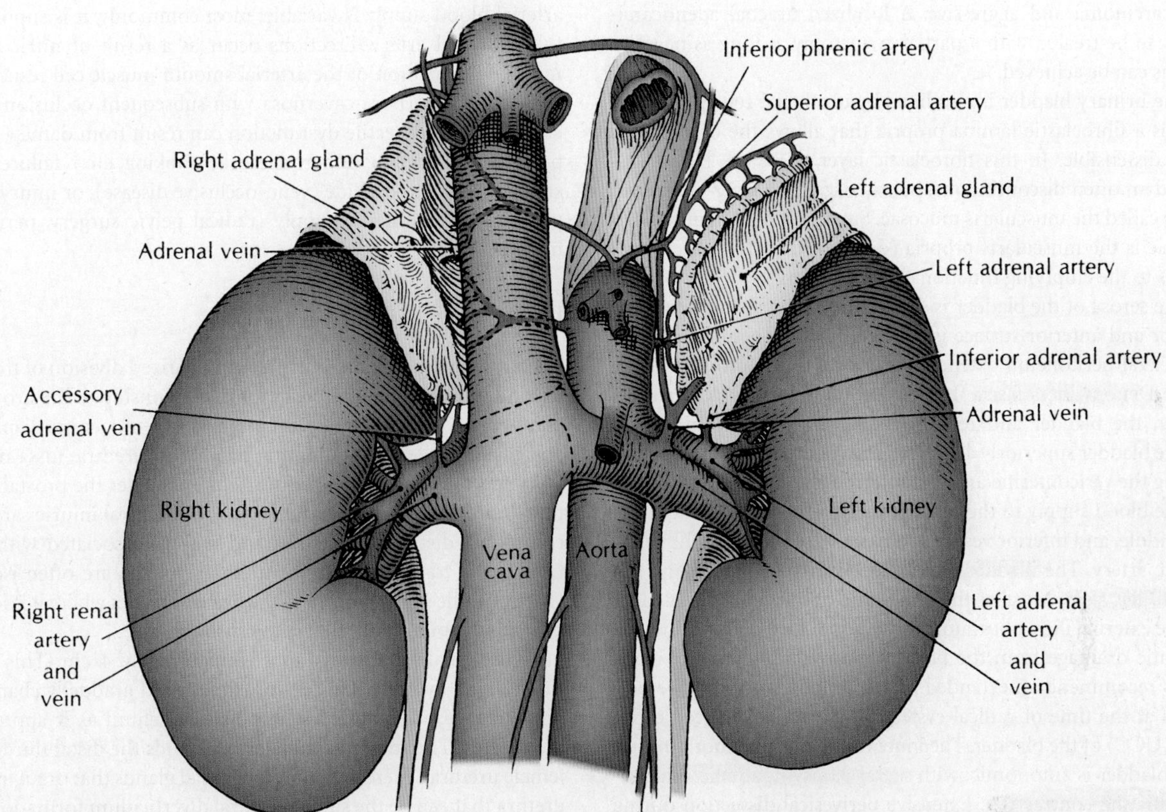

FIGURE 27.1 Relationship of kidneys to other retroperitoneal structures. (From Graham SD, Keane TE, eds. *Glenn's Urologic Surgery*. 7th ed. Philadelphia: Wolters Kluwer/Lippincott Williams & Wilkins Health; 2010, with permission.)

the kidney is not in its usual location), the adrenal gland remains in its typical location. Likewise, congenital absence of a kidney is not associated with absence of the adrenal gland.

Renal Collecting System

The kidney's major role is to filter the blood removing excess water, salts, and by-products of protein metabolism through the production of urine. After production in the microscopic working unit of the kidney, the nephron, urine passes through the collecting ducts (found in the renal medulla) and into the papillary ducts found at the tips of the renal papillae. The minor calyces surround the papillae. Each minor calyx narrows to form an infundibulum. Groupings of infundibulum join, giving rise to major calyceal branches (commonly called upper, middle, and lower pole calyces). These branches then coalesce to form the renal pelvis, which lies posterior to the renal artery and vein.

Ureter

The renal pelvis drains into the ureter at the ureteropelvic junction (UPJ). The ureter and collecting system (renal pelvis, calyces) are lined with urothelial cell epithelium. Beneath the urothelium lie the lamina propria and the muscularis propria. The ureter traverses the retroperitoneum inferiorly along the psoas muscle. It traverses the bony pelvis crossing over the iliac vessels near the common iliac bifurcation. The ureter passes posterior to the cecum and ascending colon on the right and the sigmoid and descending colon on the left. The ureter then enters the bladder posterolaterally at the ureteral vesicular junction (UVJ). There are three points of relative narrowing of the ureter from proximal to distal: the UPJ, the crossing of the iliac, and the UVJ. These are significant because ureteral calculi are more likely to get lodged at these locations. The blood supply to the ureter is derived from multiple arteries. The abdominal ureter is supplied from medial vessels (the renal artery, gonadal artery, and aorta), but the pelvic ureter receives blood supply from lateral vessels (internal iliac, superior vesical, uterine, middle rectal vaginal, and inferior vesical). There is a vast plexus surrounding the ureter that allows the ureter to be mobilized during surgery and retain adequate blood flow; however, it is imperative that the delicate periureteral adventitia be preserved.

Bladder

The urinary bladder serves two functions: (i) low-pressure *storage* of urine and (ii) emptying urine, ideally when socially appropriate. The adult bladder typically stores approximately 500 mL of fluid. In children, the normal bladder capacity can be as approximated in fluid ounces by adding 2 to age in years.

The bladder is derived from the urogenital sinus. During its early development, the bladder is attached to the umbilicus by the urachus. In normal development, the urachus becomes obliterated leaving a remnant, the median umbilical ligament. Rarely, a tumor within the urachal remnant may arise, which is typically adenocarcinoma and aggressive. A localized urachal adenocarcinoma can be treated with a partial cystectomy as long as negative margins can be achieved.

The urinary bladder is also lined by urothelial cell epithelium. There is a fibroelastic lamina propria that allows the organ to be highly distensible. In this fibroelastic layer, there are blood vessels and an often discontinuous, poorly organized layer of smooth muscle called the muscularis mucosae. Surrounding the muscularis mucosae is the muscularis propria (detrusor muscle), which contributes to the emptying function of the bladder.

The serosa of the bladder is surrounded by perivesical fat. The superior and anterior surface is covered by peritoneum. In males, the parietal peritoneum extends posteriorly to the prostate forming the Denonvilliers fascia. In women, the vagina and uterus lay between the bladder and rectum. Thus, the peritoneum drapes over the bladder superiorly and extends over the uterus and rectum forming the vesicouterine and rectouterine pouches, respectively.

The blood supply to the bladder is rich and includes the superior, middle, and inferior vesical arteries and branches of the internal iliac artery. The bladder drains via the vesical plexus into the internal iliac vein. Most of the lymphatic drainage of the bladder is to the external iliac, obturator, and internal iliac nodes. However, lymphatic drainage from the bladder is variable; therefore, many experts recommend an extended pelvic lymphadenectomy be performed at the time of radical cystectomy for urothelial cell carcinoma (UCC) of the bladder. The innervation of the smooth muscle of the bladder is autonomic, with sacral parasympathetic innervation initiating contraction. Extensive perivesical dissection during pelvic surgery (e.g., abdominoperineal resection [APR]) can lead to bladder acontractility and urinary retention.

Prostate

The prostate abuts the bladder at the bladder outlet and surrounds the prostatic urethra. Anteriorly, the puboprostatic ligaments fix the prostate to the bony pelvis. Posteriorly, the Denonvilliers fascia lies between the prostate and the rectum and envelops the seminal vesicles, which has clinical significance during radical prostatectomy. The verumontanum is the exit point of the ejaculatory duct. The lateral border of the prostate is formed by the pubococcygeus.

The internal architecture of the prostate can be divided into several zones: the transition zone, the central zone, the peripheral zone, and the anterior fibromuscular stroma. The transitional zone is the most common site of benign prostatic hypertrophy (BPH). The peripheral zone is the most frequent location of adenocarcinoma of the prostate.

The inferior vesical artery provides the major blood supply to the prostate. The pelvic plexus of Santorini (periprostatic plexus) provides the major venous drainage. The venous drainage of the penis, the deep dorsal venous complex (DVC), travels on the anterior surface of the prostate. Care must be taken during radical prostatectomy to ligate the DVC to reduce a significant amount of blood loss during the operation. The majority of the lymphatic drainage of the prostate is to the obturator and external iliac lymph nodes.

Penis

The penis is composed of paired erectile bodies, the corpora cavernosa, and the corpus spongiosum ventrally, which contains the male urethra and is continuous with the glans penis. The penile arterial blood supply is variable; most commonly, it is supplied by the pudendal artery. Erections occur as a result of nitric oxide–mediated relaxation of the arterial smooth muscle cell resulting in filling of the corpora cavernosa with subsequent occlusion of the emissary veins. Erectile dysfunction can result from damage to the penile arterial inflow (atherosclerosis, smoking, etc.), failure of the emissary veins to occlude (veno-occlusive disease), or injury to the parasympathetic nerve supply (radical pelvic surgery, peripheral neuropathy, etc.).

Urethra

The urologic trauma literature has popularized division of the male urethra into anterior and posterior in relationship to the urogenital diaphragm. The anterior urethra starts at the urogenital diaphragm and includes the bulbar urethra, pendulous urethra, fossa navicularis, and meatus. The posterior urethra includes the prostatic urethra and membranous urethra. Posterior urethral injuries are most commonly distraction injuries and may be associated with multiple pelvic fractures; anterior urethral injuries are often isolated. Classic saddle injuries occur at the bulbar urethra where it is located beneath the pubis and subject to crushing.

The female urethra is approximately only 4 cm. This structure is lined by urothelial cells proximally but gradually changes to non–keratinized-stratified squamous epithelium as it approaches the meatus. The striated sphincter surrounds the distal third of the female urethra. There are numerous small glands that drain into the urethra that can be the site of urethral diverticulum formation. The layers of the mucosa and submucosa are estrogen dependent and may atrophy at menopause.

Scrotum

The muscular dartos layer is continuous with Colles fascia in the perineum and Scarpa fascia in the abdominal wall. Fournier gangrene (necrotizing fasciitis) may track along these fascial planes, but the testicles are usually unaffected due to their different blood supply.

Testicles

The testicles are paired ovoid organs that are normally located in the scrotum. The functions of the testicle include sperm production and testosterone secretion. The organ is made up of tightly packed seminiferous tubules held together by dense fibrous connective tissue (the tunica albuginea). The seminiferous tubules contain Sertoli cells and germ cells and are the site of spermatogenesis. They connect to the epididymis via the rete testis. Sperm traverse these structures before traveling to the vas deferens. They are then expelled into the posterior urethra during emission. The parenchyma of the testicle also includes Leydig cells that are responsible for the production of testosterone under the control of gonadotropins released by the anterior pituitary gland.

The blood supply to the testicle is provided by the testicular artery, the cremasteric artery, and the vasal artery. The testicular arteries arise from the abdominal aorta near the origin of the renal arteries as the testicles develop *in utero* as abdominal organs and descend into the scrotum. Failure of one or both testicles to descend into the scrotum (cryptorchidism) is associated with an increased risk of infertility and testicular cancer.

IATROGENIC INJURIES TO THE GU SYSTEM

Ureteral iatrogenic injury occurs most commonly during operations for inflammatory bowel disease, diverticulitis, pelvic malignancy, abdominal hysterectomy vascular procedures, or ureteroscopy. Uncontrolled blood loss and inflammatory or neoplastic processes are obvious risk factors. Prophylactic stent placement does not reduce the risk of ureteral injury but may help with intraoperative identification.

When a ureteral injury is detected early, surgical repair should be attempted. If a clip is placed on the ureter and is immediately recognized, it may be removed and treated with only ureteral stenting. Excision of the affected segment and reanastomosis may be necessary if a crush injury is more severe. Upper and middle ureteral injuries can be managed with debridement and end-to-end anastomosis. Distal injuries should be managed with ureteral reimplantation with a psoas hitch or possibly a Boari flap (i.e., a distal neoureter is created using a flap of the bladder wall). All ureteral repairs should be coupled with urinary diversion with a ureteral stent or a percutaneous nephrostomy tube for approximately 4 to 6 weeks. Perforation or mucosal damage during ureteroscopy can usually be managed with ureteral stenting alone. A dreaded complication of ureteroscopy, ureteral avulsion, can occur from aggressive basketing of large stones. Surgical repair is required.

Treatment of recognized *iatrogenic injuries to the bladder* depends on the severity of injury as well as the presence of other injuries that may require exploration. Small cystotomies near the dome that occur intraoperatively can usually be primarily repaired without difficulty. If there is concern for an injury near the trigone, the bladder should be opened widely to inspect the entire mucosal surface and ureteral orifices. All devitalized tissue should be debrided. Most cystotomies can be closed watertight in one or two layers of absorbable suture. Around 250 to 300 mL of sterile water should be instilled to check for potential leaks. Continuous drainage with an indwelling Foley or a suprapubic tube ensures maximal drainage of the healing bladder, and a surgical drain should be maintained until healing is confirmed with a cystogram 1 to 2 weeks postoperatively. Between 1.5% and 5% of transurethral resections of bladder tumors (TURBT) are associated with a bladder perforation. The vast majority are extraperitoneal perforations, which can usually be managed with continuous Foley catheter drainage with or without antibiotic prophylaxis. Surgical exploration is required for most intraperitoneal perforations and for large symptomatic collections from an extraperitoneal perforation. The small intestine should be run to ensure no concomitant injury. The perforated bladder edges should be debrided and closed in two layers with continuous Foley catheter drainage and surgical drain placement for 1 to 2 weeks. A voiding cystogram is recommended prior to catheter removal.

Iatrogenic urethral trauma is reduced if duration of indwelling catheterization is limited and small caliber silicone catheters are used. The most common iatrogenic penile injury is a complication from circumcision. Older boys and adults are at higher risk than neonates, likely related to phimosis. Circumcision complication rates range from less than 1% up to 30%. Bleeding, infection, glans necrosis, and partial glans amputation are possible.

UROLOGIC NEOPLASMS

Prostate Cancer

Prostate cancer is the most common cancer among men and is second only to lung cancer as the most common cause of cancer death in men. There is estimated to be approximately 233,000 new cases of prostate cancer diagnosed in 2014 with approximately 29,480 prostate cancer specific deaths. The incidence of prostate cancer peaks in the 65- to 74-year-old age range, with less than 10% of cases occurring before age 55. Major risk factors include older age, family history of prostate cancer, and African American race.

Early-stage prostate cancer is usually asymptomatic. Screening for prostate cancer using a prostate-specific antigen (PSA) assay and digital rectal examination (DRE) is used widely. More prostate cancer is detected with the use of both of these tests than with either test alone. PSA has a sensitivity of 80% and a specificity of 35% to 50%. Other serologic markers are being investigated to improve the specificity. Although there is significant controversy surrounding the utility of widespread screening for prostate cancer, a baseline PSA around the age of 45 years can reasonably predict a man's subsequent risk of developing clinically significant prostate cancer. Those with an elevated baseline PSA or have risk factors for prostate cancer (African Americans and those with a family history of prostate cancer) are generally offered more frequent screening. A randomized control trial in the United States Prostate, Lung, Colorectal, and Ovarian screening trial (PLCO) failed to show annual PSA screening reduced the risk of prostate cancer mortality and potentially lead to overdiagnosis and overtreatment. There are several criticisms of this study including contamination with screening in the control arm and prior PSA testing in both arms resulting in a lower-risk cohort. The European Randomized Study of Screening for Prostate Cancer (ERSPC) showed a relative benefit from PSA every 2 to 4 years, but the absolute benefit was small. Ultimately, prostate cancer screening needs to be individualized and requires informed shared decision making.

Currently, patients with an abnormal serum PSA level or an abnormal DRE undergo transrectal ultrasound–guided biopsy of the prostate and undergo systematic sampling of the prostate with retrieval of approximately twelve core biopsy specimens. Despite prophylactic antibiotics, the risk of postbiopsy is sepsis and is approximately 1%, so limiting "unnecessary" biopsies is important. The use of endorectal coli magnetic resonance imaging (MRI) techniques has shown some promise in improving biopsy technique with better lesion-directed targeting and may one day be able to reduce the number of unnecessary biopsies.

Prostate cancer is graded using the Gleason scoring system (Fig. 27.2). The tumor growth pattern is graded from least dysplastic to most dysplastic, and a Gleason score between 6 and10 is assigned by adding the two most common patterns. The Gleason score is a reliable prognostic indicator.

The most common sites of metastasis of prostate cancer are bone and pelvic lymph nodes. The staging workup for prostate cancer is dependent on a patient's risk for metastatic disease taking into account pretreatment variables such as Gleason score, PSA, and digital rectal exam. For patients with low-risk prostate cancer, no further staging workup is recommended by the National Comprehensive Cancer Network. For patients at higher risk for metastasis, a radionuclide bone scan is commonly used to detect bony metastases. CT scan of the pelvis can detect obturator or iliac lymph node metastases in the pelvis. MRI with an endorectal coil can be useful, at the discretion of the physician, in the detection of extension of the tumor beyond the capsule of the prostate, a finding that significantly alters treatment recommendations.

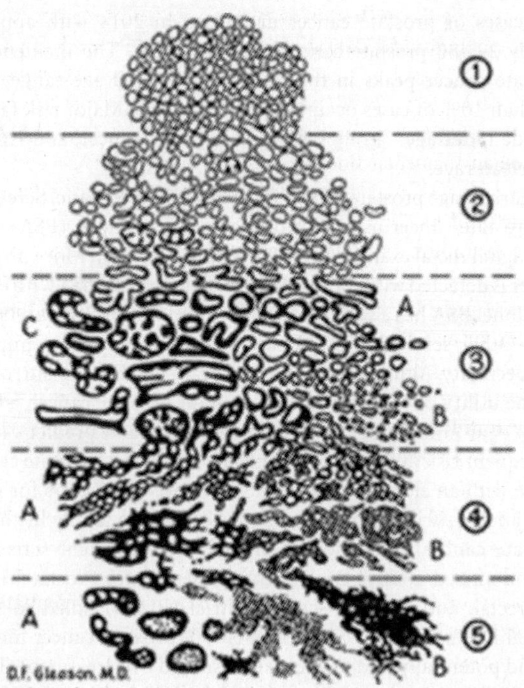

FIGURE 27.2 Gleason grading system. (From Amin MB, Grignon DJ, Humphrey PA, et al, eds. *Gleason Grading of Prostate Cancer: A Contemporary Approach*. Philadelphia: Lippincott Williams & Wilkins; 2004, Figure 1.2, with permission.)

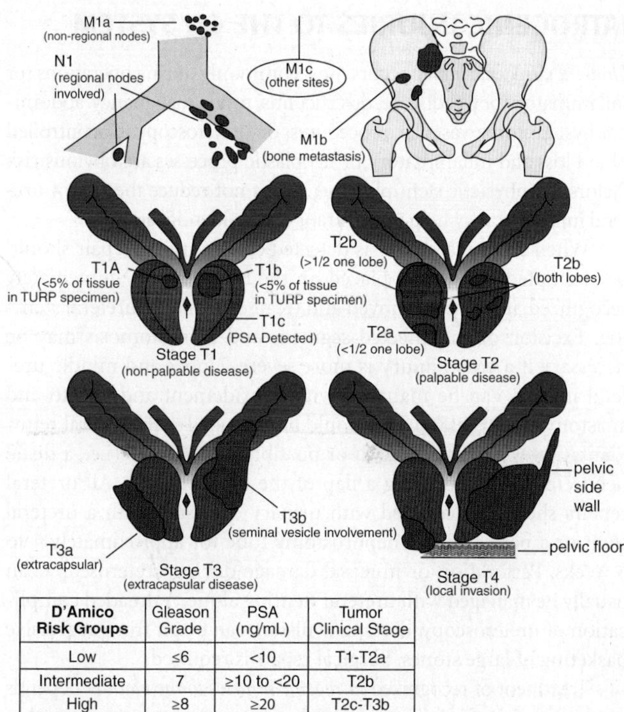

D'Amico Risk Groups	Gleason Grade	PSA (ng/mL)	Tumor Clinical Stage
Low	≤6	<10	T1-T2a
Intermediate	7	≥10 to <20	T2b
High	≥8	≥20	T2c-T3b

FIGURE 27.3 TNM staging for prostate cancer and D'Amico risk stratification groups for localized prostate cancer. (From Siroky MB, Oates RD, Babayan RK, eds. *Handbook of Urology: Diagnosis and Therapy*. 3rd ed. Philadelphia: Lippincott Williams & Wilkins; 2004, with permission. Revisions and annotations by Pietzak E and Guzzo T.)

The management of prostate cancer depends on the grade and stage of the tumor, PSA level, comorbidities, patient preference, and treatment availability (Fig. 27.3). The various treatment options include:

1. Radical prostatectomy: The definitive surgical treatment in men with a life expectancy of more than 10 years with organ-confined disease. It may be performed via an open approach (retropubic or perineal) or laparoscopic (pure or robotic assisted). Major complications include bleeding, rectal injury, bladder neck contracture, erectile dysfunction, and incontinence. The neurovascular bundles run just lateral to the prostatic fascia. Preservation of the neurovascular bundle at the time of surgery has been shown to improve erectile function rates; however, erectile function after surgery is dependent on other factors as well including comorbidity, age, and preoperative baseline function.
2. External beam radiation therapy (EBRT): This modality of therapy can be curative for organ-confined disease and is frequently used in combination with androgen deprivation therapy (ADT) for intermediate and high-risk disease. EBRT is associated with voiding and bowel symptoms, as well as erectile dysfunction. Adjuvant or salvage EBRT may be given after radical prostatectomy for suspected local recurrence or in some cases of adverse pathology or positive surgical margins. The safety profile of EBRT has improved with the introduction of advanced technology, such as intensity-modulated radiation therapy. This can be combined with image-guided or stereotactic techniques.
3. Brachytherapy: Is an alternative form of radiation provided with radioactive seeds composed of palladium or iodine implanted within the prostate for curative treatment of patients with low-grade, organ-confined disease. The advantage over external beam therapy is that it is a one-time treatment. Its side effects include irritable bowel and urinary symptoms.
4. Active surveillance: Active surveillance is a management strategy for the low-risk prostate cancer patient that involves monitoring with serial PSA levels, DREs, and interval prostate biopsies with the intent for curative therapy if disease progression occurs. With our improved understanding of the indolent nature of many PSA-detected, low-risk prostate cancers, active surveillance has become increasingly more popular over the last decade. This is a relatively new strategy that is still being developed but may avoid or delay the morbidity of localized treatment without compromising survival for selected men with low-risk disease.
5. Watchful waiting: This strategy differs from active surveillance as there is no attempt to monitor for disease progression or provide curative therapy. Watchful watching involves palliative treatment of metastatic lesions that become symptomatic or treatment of obstructive urinary symptoms. Periodic PSA levels can be checked to monitor for "impending" bone metastasis. Watchful watching is more appropriate in men with a poor life expectancy that are more likely to die from a competing risk than prostate cancer.
6. ADT: Prostate cancer is initially dependent upon testosterone for growth and survival. Historically, surgical castration with bilateral simple orchiectomy was used as a quick, effective,

and reliable way to reduce testosterone levels. Few patients are now treated with surgical castration, and ADT is typically provided with oral, implantable, or injectable therapies. Luteinizing hormone-releasing hormone (LHRH) agonists are widely used to achieve chemical castration in the United States. Side effects of antiandrogen therapy include impotence, decreased libido, hot flashes, and worsening of cardiovascular disease risk factors. ADT is usually reserved for combination therapy with EBRT for intermediate- and high-risk disease, localized treatment failures, and metastatic disease. ADT as a primary therapy for localized disease does not improve survival. Prostate cancer may eventually progress despite ADT to a state called castrate-resistant prostate cancer.

7. Cryoablation: This modality is offered as a salvage therapy for patients with local recurrence after radiation therapy or brachytherapy. This technique can lead to irritative symptoms and fistula formation. Nearly all patients develop erectile dysfunction. Cryoablation is approved as a primary therapy for organ-confined disease, though it is generally not the preferred approach.
8. Systemic therapies: Over the last few years, there has been an "embarrassment of riches" with regard to systemic therapy for castrate-resistant prostate cancer. Therapies including docetaxel, enzalutamide, and abiraterone are just a few of the growing list of therapy for patients with disease progression on ADT.

Follow-up for treated prostate cancer consists of serial PSA levels and DREs with repeated radiographic imaging performed as clinically indicated. Most patients with PSA recurrences following definitive treatment can initially be monitored with serial PSA measurements and the initiation of ADT if a rapid doubling of PSA or metastasis are identified.

Renal Masses and Renal Cell Carcinoma

Due to the widespread use of cross-sectional imaging, the incidence of renal masses has increased severalfold, and an incidental finding is one of the most common presentations for renal cell carcinoma (RCC).

Most renal masses are cysts, which exist on a spectrum from simple cysts with an imperceptible wall and without septations without a risk for malignancy to an increasing complexity from wall thickening, septations, calcifications, or enhancement. The most common cyst classification system is the Bosniak classification system, which ranges from relatively benign type I and II cysts that have such a low risk of malignancy that require no follow-up imaging to Bosniak type III and IV complex cysts, which should be surgical excised due to the associated risk of cystic RCC. Bosniak IIF cysts can be followed with interval surveillance imaging to better define their risk of malignancy and need for intervention. The Bosniak system has only been validated in CT scans, and controversy exists as to where the system can be applied to ultrasound or MRI.

It is estimated that approximately 80% of solid renal masses less than 4 cm are malignant, with an incremental increase in malignancy risk as size increases. Although the majority of solid renal masses are RCC, some commonly benign tumors are also encountered, including angiomyolipoma (AML) and oncocytoma. AML is a hamartoma of the kidney, the hallmark of which is the presence of macroscopic fat within the tumor. CT scans will show a well-circumscribed mass containing fat (< −20 HU). It may occur sporadically and is more common in women; 20% to 30% of AMLs are found in patients with tuberous sclerosis (TS) syndrome. TS in its most serious form is characterized by mental retardation; seizure disorder; hamartomas of the brain, lung, and kidney; and adenoma sebaceum. AMLs may be an incidental finding or found in the setting of an acute retroperitoneal bleed from the lesion (Wunderlich syndrome). Treatment of AML is based on the size and symptomatology of the lesion. Asymptomatic lesions may be observed, but lesions that are symptomatic, particularly those larger than 4 cm, should be treated with angioembolization or partial nephrectomy when possible. Excision or angioembolization of asymptomatic lesions that grow significantly during follow-up should be considered.

Oncocytoma is a benign tumor that may be difficult to distinguish from RCC by imaging alone. It is thought to be derived from distal tubular cells and tends to be asymptomatic and discovered incidentally. Grossly, oncocytomas may be large and have central scars that extend to the periphery in a stellate pattern. Histologically, oncocytomas are well differentiated and highly eosinophilic, with significant mitochondrial hyperplasia and rare mitoses. On cross-sectional imaging, there is no reliable way to differentiate this tumor from RCC, but angiography may show a typical "spoke-wheel" appearance caused by the stellate scar. Even with percutaneous renal biopsy, it is difficult to differentiate from chromophobe RCC as they are both oncocytic neoplasms. Although oncocytomas are benign, excision remains the standard of care because of the difficulty in making a definitive diagnosis. Like all small renal masses, partial nephrectomy is the preferred approach if feasible. Oncocytomas can also be found along with chromophobe RCC and hybrid tumors in the hereditary Birt–Hogg–Dube syndrome.

Despite the increasing incidence of small renal masses from cross-sectional imaging, the mortality rate for RCC remains the same, as RCC is the most lethal of the common GU cancers. In the United States, there are approximately 63,920 new cases of cancer within the kidney and renal pelvis reported each year, with more than 13,860 deaths. Of note, renal pelvic tumors are usually UCC, but Surveillance, Epidemiology, and End Results Program (SEER) does not differentiate these from the far more common RCC, which account for approximately 95% of renal cancers. RCCs are adenocarcinomas derived from the renal tubular epithelial cells. The tumors are usually sporadic, but up to 4% can be familial as seen in von Hippel–Lindau disease, hereditary papillary RCC, familial leiomyomatosis, and Birt–Hogg–Dube syndrome. Known risk factors for sporadic RCC include smoking (associated with a twofold increase in risk), hypertension, male sex, and acquired cystic kidney disease associated with hemodialysis in end-stage renal disease patients (associated with a 30-fold increased risk). Most patients are affected in the sixth and seventh decades of life.

Patients with RCC may be asymptomatic at the time of presentation or may present with one or more of the symptoms of the "classic triad" (i.e., flank pain, abdominal mass, and hematuria). Only 10% of patients will present with all three of these symptoms. Fever, weight loss, and hypertension may also be presenting features. Certain paraneoplastic syndromes have been associated with RCC. Hypercalcemia may be related to tumor production of PTH-related peptide. Stauffer syndrome, hepatic dysfunction not related to metastatic disease, is a transient elevation of liver enzymes that resolves following tumor excision. Reappearance of the abnormality may herald recurrence of tumor. Polycythemia may be related to inappropriate production of erythropoietin by the tumor.

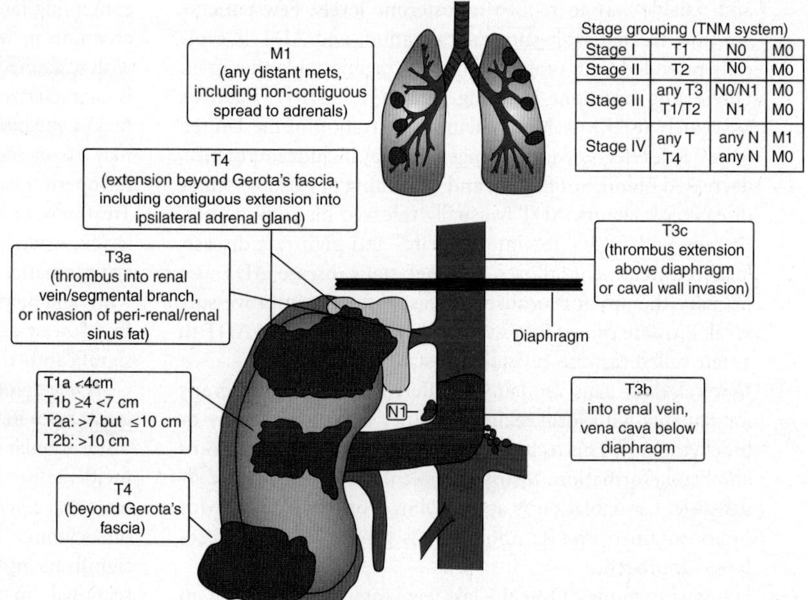

FIGURE 27.4 TNM staging for renal cell carcinoma. (From Siroky MB, Oates RD, Babayan RK, eds. *Handbook of Urology: Diagnosis and Therapy*. 3rd ed. Philadelphia: Lippincott Williams & Wilkins; 2004, with permission. Revisions and annotations by Pietzak E and Guzzo T.)

Physical examination is rarely helpful in the diagnosis, as most patients will have a normal physical examination until the tumor is locally advanced. Radiography is the mainstay of diagnosis. Renal ultrasonography will show a solid renal mass. CT scanning should be performed before and after intravenous contrast administration. A solid mass that enhances by more than 15 to 20 HU after administration of intravenous contrast is consistent with RCC. In patients who are unable to receive contrast or in those in whom CT is nondiagnostic, MRI with gadolinium may be helpful.

Staging of RCC uses the tumor, node, metastasis (TNM) staging system (Fig. 27.4). The most common sites of metastases are the lung, liver, and bone. Staging workup includes CT scan of the abdomen to evaluate local extent and distant metastases. RCC has an interesting predilection for venous thrombus formation. Chest x-ray (CXR) or noncontrast chest CT is used to rule out lung metastases. In patients with bone pain, elevated serum alkaline phosphate, or hypercalcemia, a radionucleotide bone scan should be obtained. Chemistry panel and liver function studies are performed as well, and patients with abnormal renal function may benefit from split-function renal scanning. Patients with metastatic disease and neurologic symptoms should have a brain MRI.

RCC is a surgical disease. Surgery alone can be curative for most cases of localized disease. Partial nephrectomy should be considered whenever feasible. Although the short-term complication rate is higher with partial nephrectomy (bleeding and urinoma), these risks are usually offset by the long-term benefits of renal preservation from nephron-sparing surgery. Tumors most amenable to partial nephrectomy are smaller (<4 cm) and more exophytic; however, larger and more endophytic tumors may also be amenable. Ablative therapies with radiofrequency ablation or cryotherapy are reasonable alternatives for some patients, but these modalities are less effective for tumors greater than 3 to 4 cm and usually reserved for patients with contraindications to surgery.

For larger tumors with adverse features, such as venous or perinephritic fat invasion, radical nephrectomy should be performed, which consists of removal of the entire kidney with the surrounding Gerota's fascia. The adrenal gland can safely be spared in most settings in which no evidence of radiographic or intraoperative involvement. Open and laparoscopic (pure, hand-assisted, and robotic-assisted) approaches have all been utilized for both radical and partial nephrectomy.

Since an important principle of a radical nephrectomy is that the renal artery should be ligated before the renal vein, some surgeons will obtain angiographic embolization of large tumors prior to surgery in hopes to reduce blood loss and facilitate arterial control. Angiographic embolization has never conclusively been shown to reduce blood loss or improve outcomes.

Patients with thrombus extending into the renal vein and as far as the right atrium may be treated with radical nephrectomy and removal of the tumor thrombus. This usually requires a multiteam approach with involvement of vascular or cardiothoracic surgeons, and sometimes, venovenous or cardiopulmonary bypass must be employed. Ten-year survival of up to 40% has been reported for select patients undergoing nephrectomy and tumor thrombectomy.

Approximately 30% of patients with RCC present with metastatic disease. For carefully selected patients, there is a role for primary tumor debulking with cytoreductive nephrectomy. Patients most likely to experience an improved survival from cytoreductive nephrectomy are patients with a good performance status without systemic symptoms or extrapulmonary metastasis. For patients previously treated with nephrectomy who develop subsequent distant metastatic disease, the time to disease recurrence is also an important prognostic factor. Selected patients might benefit from metastasectomy, particular if only a solitary pulmonary lesion is present.

Historically, the mainstay of medical therapy of RCC has been immunotherapy with IL-2 or INF-α. IL-2 is still offered at some experienced centers as it is the only therapy that can be potentially curative in approximately 8% of metastatic RCC patients; however, the substantial toxicity of the therapy requires intensive care monitoring and can result in mortality. In the current era of molecular-targeted therapies, small molecule tyrosine kinase inhibitors (sunitinib, sorafenib, pazopanib, etc.) that target vascular endothelial growth factor (VEGF) and similar pathways have gained FDA approval for use in metastatic RCC, though their effects are more tumorostatic with only a modest survival benefit.

Of note, the randomized controlled trials supporting cytoreductive nephrectomy utilized INF-α, but two large ongoing randomized trials, Clinical Trial to Assess the Importance of Nephrectomy (CARMINA) and European Organization for Research and Treatment of Cancer (EORTC), seek to investigate the role of cytoreductive nephrectomy in the molecular-targeted era.

Bladder Cancer and Upper Tract Urothelial Cell Carcinoma

Urothelial carcinoma can occur anywhere in the urinary tract, from the collecting system of the kidney to the proximal urethra; however, the bladder is the most common site. It is estimated that for 2014 in the United States, 74,690 new patients will be diagnosed with bladder cancer, with 15,580 patients expected to die from the disease. Bladder cancer is about three times more prevalent in men than in women. UCC is frequently multifocal, and there are two predominant hypotheses for UCC carcinogenesis with evidence to support both hypotheses. The first hypothesis to explain multifocal disease is monoclonal seeding from a primary tumor. The second hypothesis is that multifocal tumors arise from multiple epithelial mutations throughout the entire urothelium due to exposure to carcinogens within the urine ("field cancerization"). Known bladder carcinogens are nitrosamines and aromatic amines from cigarette smoke, aniline dyes and several aromatic amines from occupational exposure, and phenacetin. Cigarette smoking accounts for approximately 50% of bladder cancers in both men and women.

The most common presentation of bladder cancer is painless gross hematuria, occurring in around 70% of patients. Cystoscopy, urine culture, cytology, and upper tract imaging should be performed in all patients with gross hematuria.

Upper tract imaging historically was done with intravenous pyelography (IVP), but this has been replaced by CT urogram (three-phase CT with noncontrast phase, nephrographic contrast phase, and a delayed excretory phase) looking for upper urinary tract filling defects. Alternatively, the upper tracts can be evaluated with retrograde pyelograms at the time of cystoscopy. This approach may be performed in individuals with poor renal function, which precludes intravenous contrast; however, imaging of the renal parenchyma with noncontrast CT or ultrasound is still required. MR urography can also be used but lacks the sensitivity to reliably detect small (<5 mm) filling defects. Patients with upper tract lesions should have brush biopsy or ureteroscopic biopsy of the tumor.

Cystoscopy will identify most papillary lesions in the bladder or urethra but can miss carcinoma *in situ* (CIS). Newer imaging techniques using narrow band cystoscopy and so-called "blue light" cystoscopy using photosensitizing agents (hexyl aminolevulinate) may improve the detection of CIS over traditional "white light" cystoscopy. Urinary cytology is another useful adjuvant for detecting CIS as the sensitivity of urinary cytology increases as the grade of the lesion increases. Patients with bladder lesions should undergo complete transurethral resection (TUR) including removal of the underlying detrusor muscle so that the depth of invasion can be determined. An examination under anesthesia should ideally be performed before and after TURBT to provide information on tumor extent. Treatment of UCC depends on the grade, stage, and location of the lesion, as well as the overall health of the patient. Staging of bladder cancer uses the TNM staging system (Fig. 27.5), but patients can also be broadly divided into muscle-invasive and non–muscle-invasive disease depending on the involvement of the lamina propria (detrusor muscle).

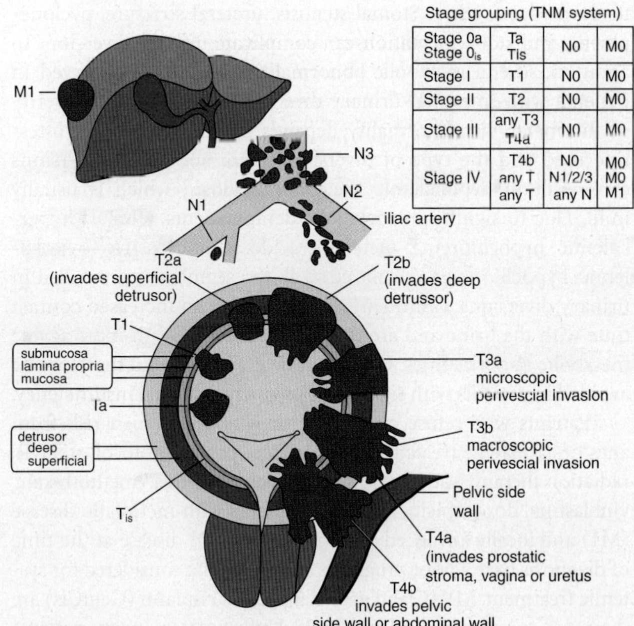

Stage	T	N	M
Stage 0a Stage 0_{is}	Ta Tis	N0	M0
Stage I	T1	N0	M0
Stage II	T2	N0	M0
Stage III	any T3 T4a	N0	M0
Stage IV	T4b any T any T	N0 N1/2/3 any N	M0 M0 M1

FIGURE 27.5 TNM staging for bladder cancer. (From Siroky MB, Oates RD, Babayan RK, eds. *Handbook of Urology: Diagnosis and Therapy*. 3rd ed. Philadelphia: Lippincott Williams & Wilkins; 2004, with permission. Revisions and annotations by Pietzak E and Guzzo T.)

Non–muscle-invasive disease accounts for approximately 75% to 80% of bladder tumors with the vast majority being low-grade tumors. Typically, papillary tumors (Ta and T1) are treated conservatively with TUR followed by surveillance cystoscopy every 3 to 6 months initially then annually for life. For many patients, an immediate post-TURBT instillation of intravesical mitomycin reduces the risk of tumor recurrence. Those at higher risk of disease progression or recurrence (high-grade tumors and multifocal tumors) may benefit from early restaging TURBT followed by additional treatment with intravesical therapy. Intravesical therapy may include bacille Calmette–Guérin (BCG) or mitomycin. Some urologists have advocated for early cystectomy for patients with recurrent or multifocal high-grade T1 lesions who have good performance status because of the high risk of progression to muscle invasion and death from bladder cancer.

Clinical staging for muscle-invasive bladder cancer is notoriously inaccurate, but involves cross-sectional imaging of abdomen and pelvis with CT scan or MRI, along with chest imaging. The mainstay of treatment for muscle-invasive disease without distant metastases is radical cystectomy with extended pelvic lymph node dissection and urinary diversion. Randomized trials and a subsequent meta-analysis support the use of neoadjuvant cisplatin-based chemotherapy, which provides a 5% overall survival benefit over radical surgery alone. Radical cystectomy is associated with significant perioperative morbidity, mainly from the required bowel resection to create the urinary diversion and the usually comorbid patient population. Following radical cystectomy, several either incontinent or continent urinary reconstructions can be created. Ileum is the most frequently used segment of bowel to create an incontinent cutaneous conduit, but colon can also be used if ileum is unavailable due to prior radiation or short-gut syndromes. Continent diversions can be achieved through creation of a catheterizable pouch or an orthotopic neobladder, which is connected to the native urethra. Stomal stenosis, ureteral stricture, pyelonephritis, and stone formation can complicate urinary diversion. In addition, several metabolic abnormalities have been observed in patients with intestinal urinary diversion. The type and severity of the metabolic abnormality depends on the segment of intestine used and the type of diversion. Ileum and colon diversions can result in hypokalemic metabolic acidosis, which is usually mild. Due to significant metabolic derangements, jejunal (hyperkalemic, hypochloremic metabolic acidosis) and gastric (hypokalemic, hypochloremic metabolic alkalosis) segments are avoided in urinary diversions. Continent reservoirs have an increased contact time with the urine and are therefore associated with more severe metabolic abnormalities. Continent diversions should therefore be avoided in patients with significant preoperative renal insufficiency.

Patients who refuse cystectomy or who are at high risk from anesthesia may be treated with a bladder-sparing protocol of TUR, radiation therapy, and chemotherapy such as MVAC (methotrexate, vinblastine, doxorubicin, cisplatin). Patients with metastatic disease (M1) and locally advanced (T4b and N2 or N3) disease at the time of diagnosis have a poor prognosis and should be considered for systemic treatment. MVAC and gemcitabine and cisplatin (GemCis) are the most commonly used protocols. Unfortunately, many patients with bladder cancer are unable to receive cisplatin due to renal insufficiency or poor performance status, and currently, second-line systemic therapy for bladder cancer is an unmet medical need.

Other bladder neoplasms include squamous cell carcinoma, which is associated with indwelling urinary catheters and *Schistosoma haematobium* infection. Small cell carcinoma and carcinosarcoma are rare and have a poor prognosis. Rhabdomyosarcoma is typically a pediatric disease and is usually treated with radiation and chemotherapy with good results.

Unlike UCC of the bladder, UCC of the upper urinary tract is a rare tumor, which represents only 5% of all urothelial tumors and about 5% of all renal tumors. For these reasons, much of the treatment and management of upper tract UCC (UTUCC) is extrapolated from bladder cancer. The clinical staging for UTUCC is even worse than bladder cancer as ureteroscopic biopsies and brush biopsies cannot provide details regarding the depth of invasion; extirpative surgery is therefore frequently warranted. The general principle guiding surgical management of UTUCC is that the tumor and all the ureter distal to the tumor should be removed as there is a significant risk of downstream recurrence. Therefore, UTUCC of the renal pelvis or proximal ureter is generally treated with nephroureterectomy (en bloc removal of the kidney, the entire ureter, and bladder cuff via a laparoscopic, open or combined approach), while UCC of the distal ureter can be managed with distal ureterectomy and ureteral reimplantation. Depending on the length of ureter excised, a psoas hitch, Boari flap, or ileal ureter may be necessary to bridge the gap from the kidney to the bladder. In cases of small volume, low-grade UCC, an initial approach with endoscopic or percutaneous ablation can be utilized, but there is a high recurrence rate mandating close surveillance. A conservative approach may also be favored in patients with lesions in solitary kidneys, chronic renal insufficiency, or high surgical risk.

Postoperative management of patients with UCC after extirpative surgery includes interval upper tract imaging, CXR, and urinary cytology. Approximately 3% to 4% of patients with UCC of the bladder will develop UTUCC, whereas between 25% to 40% of patients with UTUCC will eventually develop UCC of their bladder. Interval surveillance cystoscopies for patients with UTUCC are thus a necessary component of follow-up.

Testicular Cancer

Testicular cancer is a relatively rare and unique cancer. Although testis cancer is the most common solid malignancy in male between the ages of 15 to 35 years, it is only estimated to effect 8,820 individuals in the United States. Although testis tumors most often affect young men, prepubertal males and older men may also be affected. Because of the effectiveness of available treatments, testis cancer has emerged as the model for multidisciplinary cancer care success and is one of the most curable cancers. Only 380 Americans are estimated to die from the disease in 2014. Given the effectiveness of therapy and the young age of affected patients, much focus has been placed on reducing the morbidity of treatment and on survivorship issues.

The main risk factors for testis cancer are family history, infertility, and an undescended testicle (cryptorchidism). Although the risk of malignancy is not diminished by orchiopexy, the operation is recommended in part because it aids in future self-examination and identification of tumor. For patients with cryptorchidism treated with early orchiopexy, the risk of testicular cancer is still double that without cryptorchidism, but this risk increases to sixfold if orchiopexy is performed after 13 years of age. Orchiopexy around the age of one is considered a quality-of-care indicator as recommended by the American Academy of Pediatrics. Dysgenesis of testicular germ cells is a hypothesis, which links testicular cancer with infertility and cryptorchidism. Testicular dysgenesis syndrome may result from *in utero* exposure to environmental xenoestrogens, but this is only speculative at this time.

Approximately 95% of testis tumors are derived from germinal elements, referred to as germ cell tumors (GCT). GCT are further classified as pure seminoma or as nonseminomatous germ cell tumors (NSGCTs) for which treatment differs. NSGCTs are further characterized by their histologic components, embryonal carcinoma, yolk sac tumor, teratoma, or choriocarcinoma. NSGCT may include mixes of more than one cell type, including elements of seminoma with nonseminomatous components.

A testis tumor usually presents as a hard, painless scrotal mass in a young man. It is not uncommon for patients to delay presentation for several months. The differential diagnosis of a testis mass includes hydrocele, hernia, hematoma, orchitis, and spermatocele. Scrotal ultrasonography can differentiate among these diagnoses if the history and physical examination leave any doubt. In the case of a testis tumor, ultrasonography shows a hypoechoic, often hypervascular, mass in the testis.

Patients diagnosed with testis tumors should undergo radical orchiectomy via an inguinal incision as promptly as possible. Scrotal orchiectomy is not performed when testicular cancer is suspected because of the theoretical risk of contamination of scrotal lymphatics with tumor cells and the risk of inadvertently incising into the tumor. The inguinal portion of the spermatic cord is removed en bloc with the testis, and a nonabsorbable suture is left long on the distal end as a tag in case a subsequent retroperitoneal lymph node dissection (RPLND) is required, since the remainder of the spermatic cord is removed doing an RPLND.

Since the testis originates as an intra-abdominal organ, testis tumors metastasize most commonly to the retroperitoneum via lymphatics. The staging workup includes contrast CT scan with PO contrast of the abdomen and pelvis and imaging of the chest. Serum concentrations of lactate dehydrogenase (LDH), α-fetoprotein (AFP), and human chorionic gonadotropin (hCG) should also be

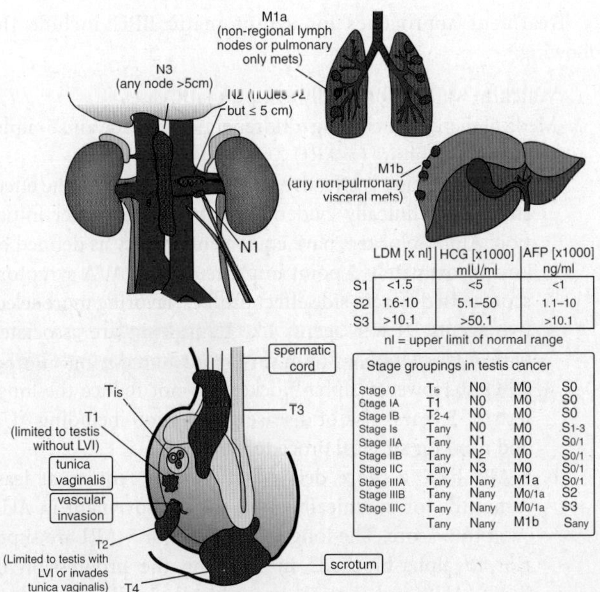

	LDM [x nl]	HCG [x1000] mIU/ml	AFP [x1000] ng/ml
S1	<1.5	<5	<1
S2	1.6-10	5.1–50	1.1–10
S3	>10.1	>50.1	>10.1

Stage groupings in testis cancer

Stage 0	T_{is}	N0	M0	S0
Stage IA	T1	N0	M0	S0
Stage IB	$T_{2\text{-}4}$	N0	M0	S0
Stage Is	T_{any}	N0	M0	$S_{1\text{-}3}$
Stage IIA	T_{any}	N1	M0	$S_{0/1}$
Stage IIB	T_{any}	N2	M0	$S_{0/1}$
Stage IIC	T_{any}	N3	M0	$S_{0/1}$
Stage IIIA	T_{any}	N_{any}	M1a	$S_{0/1}$
Stage IIIB	T_{any}	N_{any}	$M_{0/1a}$	S2
Stage IIIC	T_{any}	N_{any}	$M_{0/1a}$	S3
	T_{any}	N_{any}	M1b	S_{any}

FIGURE 27.6 TNM staging for testicular cancer. (From Siroky MB, Oates RD, Babayan RK, eds. *Handbook of Urology: Diagnosis and Therapy*. 3rd ed. Philadelphia: Lippincott Williams & Wilkins; 2004, with permission. Revisions and annotations by Pietzak E and Guzzo T.)

included in the initial workup. Staging is based on the histology of the primary specimen, imaging results, and serum markers (Fig. 27.6). Tumor markers can help in the determination of tumor type, prognosis, and response to treatment.

- AFP (half-life about 5 days) is produced by NSGCTs only; thus, the presence of AFP rules out a pure seminoma. Yolk sac tumors or yolk sac elements in mixed GCT are the main source of AFP. Embryonal carcinoma and teratoma can also produce AFP.
- hCG (half-life about 24 hours) is produced by syncytiotrophoblasts in choriocarcinoma. It may be present in NSGCTs and 10% to 15% of patients with pure seminoma can have an elevated hCG.
- LDH is a marker that is related to bulk of disease. It is also an independent prognostic indicator.

Patients with a negative metastatic workup and who have tumor markers that appropriately decline based upon their half-lives after orchiectomy are considered to have clinical stage I disease. Patients with NSGCT can elect for active surveillance (close follow-up, serial tumor markers, and serial CXR and CT imaging), primary RPLND, or primary chemotherapy (one to two cycles of bleomycin–etoposide–cisplatin [BEP]). Each option has unique risks and benefits, but in general, survival approaches 98% with any of these options. Currently, most patients who would be reliable with close follow-up are counseled towards surveillance to avoid morbidity from overtreatment; however, if disease recurs while on surveillance, a more intensive induction chemotherapy regimen would be required. The risk of occult retroperitoneal metastasis with surveillance is approximately 20% to 25% with clinical stage 1 NSGCT but can be as high as 40% for patients with lymphovascular invasion or predominant embryonal carcinoma. Most patients recur within the first 1 or 2 years; however, late recurrences are still possible.

NSGCT management is also complicated by the fact that teratoma elements are chemotherapy and radiotherapy resistant. Although teratoma is histologically benign, it can undergo malignant transformation or develop into a "growing teratoma syndrome." The absence of teratoma within the primary specimen cannot reliably exclude teratoma within the retroperitoneum. Patients without evidence of distant metastasis but have persistently elevated (or rising) tumor markers after orchiectomy are considered to have clinical stage 1-S disease and require induction chemotherapy as they have systemic disease that is not radiographically evident.

Patients with NSGCT and nonbulky retroperitoneal lymph node involvement can be treated with RPLND with 50% to 75% not requiring additional therapy, or alternatively, they can be treated with induction chemotherapy. Patients with bulky retroperitoneal disease or with metastasis outside the retroperitoneum require treatment with induction chemotherapy. Residual NSGCT masses after induction chemotherapy should be treated with RPLND if markers normalize or with salvage chemotherapy if tumor markers do not normalize. In patients undergoing postchemotherapy RPLND (PC-RPLND) after induction chemotherapy, approximately 40% will have teratoma and 10% to 15% will have viable GCT. The remainder will have necrosis and could be considered overtreated by PC-RPLND. Unfortunately, there are currently no reliable predictors of post-PC-RPLND pathology.

The treatment of seminoma differs from NSGCT in that seminoma is very radiosensitive and not associated with teratoma. Clinical stage 1 seminoma (no evidence of retroperitoneal or distant metastasis) can be managed with active surveillance, retroperitoneal radiation (20 Gy is current standard), or single cycle of carboplatin. Similar to NSGCT, active surveillance is usually advocated in the United States. The risk of occult retroperitoneal disease with seminoma is approximately 20% and associated with tumors greater than 4 cm and rete testis invasion in some studies. For retroperitoneal only metastasis, higher-dose radiation therapy to the retroperitoneum and ipsilateral iliac chain (so-called "dog-leg configuration") can be considered for nonbulky disease; otherwise, induction chemotherapy is given. "Poor-risk" metastatic disease does not exist in seminoma, as even in the setting of nonpulmonary visceral metastasis patient have an excellent survival rate.

Seminoma management further differs from NSGCT with regard to postchemotherapy masses. In seminoma, masses less than or equal to 3 cm can be observed, while for masses greater than 3 cm a CT/PET, scan is obtained 6 weeks after completion of therapy. If PET avid, masses greater than 3 cm have a high likelihood of viable seminoma being present, therefore, a PC-RPLND can be performed if technically feasible; otherwise, salvage chemotherapy is needed. Non-PET avid masses in seminoma can be safely observed as they likely represent only necrosis. Currently, CT/PET scan does not have a role in the management of postchemotherapy masses in NSGCT because teratoma is not PET avid.

RPLND is performed through a midline incision or thoracoabdominal incision. Nodal tissue surrounding the great vessels are dissected from the level of the renal vessels to the bifurcation of the iliac vessels, with the ureters representing the lateral borders of dissection. Beside the morbidity of the operation, the major long-term risks of the procedure are lack of emission or retrograde ejaculation from disruption of sympathetic nerve fibers. A nerve-sparing approach should be utilized using a "split-and-roll" technique. Alternatively, some advocate the use of modified dissection templates to reduce the risk of sympathetic nerve fiber injury; however, modified templates remain controversial. The use of laparoscopic- and robotic-assisted approaches to RPLND can be performed at select high-volume centers. Ultimately, if a testis cancer patient is going to under a significant surgical procedure, RPLND should be performed completely with curative intent to "control the retroperitoneum." Performing a "diagnostic" RPLND, even with minimal invasive approaches, should be discouraged. PC-RPLND can be very technically challenging due to the desmoplastic reaction, particularly in seminoma. PC-RPLND should only be performed at experienced centers, and many experts argue that primary RPLND should also only be performed at experienced testis cancer centers.

Benign Prostatic Hyperplasia/Low Urinary Tract Symptoms

Lower urinary tract symptoms (LUTS) are common in males, and nearly 90% of men between the ages of 45 and 80 years have some degree of urinary symptoms. Benign prostatic hyperplasia (BPH) is a histologic diagnosis from the proliferation of smooth muscle and epithelial cells within the prostatic transition zone resulting in adenomatous overgrowth. BPH can result in significant LUTS from direct bladder outlet obstruction (BOO) from enlarged stromal tissue (considered to be the static component) and increased smooth muscle tone and resistance (considered the dynamic component).

Most agree that hyperplasia is largely mediated by the action of DHT, and indeed, inhibitors of the production of DHT have been shown to decrease and even reverse BPH. Finasteride, a 5α-reductase inhibitor, inhibits the formation of DHT from testosterone and has been shown to significantly decrease the volume of the prostate in men with BPH. The smooth muscle in the prostate and bladder is rich in α-adrenergic receptors, and administration of α-adrenergic antagonists such as terazosin, doxazosin, and tamsulosin can result in significant improvement in LUTS.

Complications from BPH/BOO include renal insufficiency, urinary retention, recurrent infections, and bladder calculi. However, most patients with LUTS are unlikely to experience any adverse health effects in the future, and treatment is thus not indicated for all patients with BPH/LUTS. LUTS from BPH/BOO result from many factors, including detrusor hypertrophy, increased voiding pressures, and incomplete emptying. LUTS can be separated into obstructive voiding symptoms (e.g., hesitancy, straining, decreased stream, postvoid dribbling) and irritative storage symptoms (e.g., urgency, frequency, and nocturia). Detrusor overactivity can also contribute to storage symptoms from BPH/BOO.

The American Urologic Association (AUA) symptom index is an objective scoring system ranging from 0 to 35 that can be helpful in assessing the efficacy of treatment. Higher scores indicate more severe symptoms. Men with moderate to severe AUA symptom scores (≥8) are at risk for progression of symptoms and to acute urinary retention (AUR). An improvement in AUA symptom score greater than or equal to 3 is considered clinically significant.

Treatment approaches for symptomatic BPH include the following:

1. Watchful waiting for mildly symptomatic cases
2. Medical therapy, including α-adrenergic blockade and 5-alpha reductase inhibitors (5-ARI)
   a. Alpha-blockade is effective within a few days and the effect should be clinically evident by 2 to 4 weeks after initiation. Alpha-blockers have equivalent efficacy as defined by an approximately 3-point improvement in AUA symptom score with different side effect profiles, favoring more selective agents. Newer agents like tamsulosin are associated with intraoperative floppy iris syndrome during cataract surgery. However alpha-blockers do not reduce the long-term (>5 years) risk of disease progression including AUR and need for surgical procedures.
   b. 5-ARI have a more delayed effect and require at least 3 months for a clinically apparent improvement in AUA symptom score. The long-term effects of 5-ARI are superior to alpha-blockade in reducing the progression of BOO (AUR and surgical procedures). 5-ARI also reduce prostatic bleeding. However, because 5-ARI work by reducing prostatic size, they are reserved for individuals with prostatic enlargement usually with prostate volumes over 30 cc.
   c. Combination therapy with alpha-blockade and 5-ARI. Two randomized control trials, the Medical Therapy of Prostate Symptoms (MTOPS) trial and the CombAT trial, have demonstrated that combination therapy with alpha-blockade and 5-ARI was superior to either agent as a monotherapy in reducing the long-term risk of AUR and need for surgical procedures. This is primarily important for individuals with large prostates greater than 30 to 40 mL based on volume assessment, PSA level as proxy for volume, and/or enlargement on DRE,
   d. Anticholinergic therapy can be used for select men with predominantly irritative symptoms without an elevated postvoid residual volume (PVR). Clinical trials have excluded men with PVR greater than 250 to 300 mL, but in clinical practice, volumes are usually even lower than this.
3. Clean intermittent catheterization can be used for patients who have failed or refused medical and surgical therapies, with elevated postvoid residuals complicated by infection or significant symptoms. This may be the only viable option for some patients with detrusor failure from long-standing obstruction.
4. Transurethral resection of the prostate (TURP). TURP is a highly effective treatment reserved for patients who have failed medical therapy or who present with significant complications including upper tract deterioration, gross hematuria, AUR, and/or bladder stones. This operation typical requires a 1- to 2-day hospital stay and is associated with complications including bleeding, infection, and retrograde ejaculation. The VA cooperative study found the risk of incontinence to be less than 1% after TURP. A post-TURP syndrome (hyponatremia, fluid overload, and mental status) might develop after prolonged monopolar TURP from significant absorption of hypotonic irrigant required for the procedure. Newer technology utilizing bipolar electrocautery allows normal saline to be used as the irrigant, which eliminates the risk of post-TURP

syndrome. Alternative techniques to debulk the surgical outlet have been developed more recently and may be considered less invasive. These include microwave therapy, thermotherapy, laser ablation, and transurethral incision of the prostate.

5. Simple prostatectomy. The indications for open prostatectomy are similar to those for TURP, but open surgery is performed in those with very sizable glands (usually >80 g). The operation is performed either via a suprapubic approach by opening the bladder or via a retropubic approach by incising the capsule of the prostate. This operation causes the greatest improvement in symptoms of all the possible treatments but also requires a 2-day hospital stay and may result in significant complications.

Urinary Retention

Many patients, particularly men, will experience urinary retention following nonurologic procedures. This retention may result from several factors, including underlying BPH, anticholinergic effects of certain medications, and detrusor hypocontractility secondary to the effects of anesthesia. Furthermore, certain radical pelvic surgeries, most notably APR, may interrupt autonomic pathways mediating normal voiding function. The treatment of postoperative urinary retention consists of assisted bladder drainage (Foley catheter or preferably clean intermittent catheterization) with or without adjuvant alpha-blockade therapy until emptying function has returned. In rare instances, normal voiding does not resume, and surgical therapy or prolonged catheter drainage is required. Pressure flow urodynamics are beneficial to determining if the urinary retention is from BOO or detrusor hypoactivity.

RENAL PHYSIOLOGY

The kidney plays an integral role in the regulation of intravascular volume, salt and water balance, acid–base balance, blood pressure, red blood cell production, calcium, and potassium regulation. The kidneys receive about 20% of the resting cardiac output, approximately 1,440 L of blood per day (higher in men than women). Approximately 20% of this plasma is filtered at the glomeruli to create a glomerular filtrate (GFR) of about 170 L/day. Unfiltered plasma (80%) leaves the glomerulus via the efferent arteriole and postglomerular capillaries. Approximately 99% of the filtrate is reabsorbed by passive and active forces along the length of the nephron, ultimately creating 1 to 2 L of urine/day.

Renal blood flow (RBF) travels through the renal artery into the interlobar, arcuate, interlobular, and afferent arterioles before entering the glomerulus, where the plasma is filtered. The filtration fraction (renal plasma flow [RPF]/GFR) is dependent on the oncotic and hydrostatic forces acting in the glomerulus (g) and Bowman space (bs), which determine the ultrafiltration pressure (P_{uf}). Increased hydrostatic forces (P) within the glomerulus increase P_{uf} and increased P within the Bowman space decreases P_{uf}. Because the glomerulus is located between the afferent and efferent arterioles, changes in the arteriolar resistances can have a significant impact on the filtration fraction. The glomerular basement membrane is impermeable to most proteins; therefore, oncotic forces play a role in filtration. Increased oncotic pressure (π) within the glomerulus decreases P_{uf}, whereas increased π within Bowman space increases P_{uf}. In general, $P_{uf} = ([P_g - P_{bs}] - [\pi_g - \pi_{bs}])$. Because the act of filtration changes the P and π along the glomerulus, the fraction of the plasma filtered per unit length decreases.

The GFR is the volume of plasma that is filtered into Bowman space per unit time. Given a substance that is freely filtered at the glomerulus and neither secreted nor absorbed, the GFR is equal to the clearance of that solute, defined as the volume of plasma that is cleared of that substance per unit time. Creatinine is a plasma solute that is for practical purposes neither secreted nor absorbed, and thus, creatinine clearance (urine$_{cr}$ × volume/plasma$_{cr}$) is a proxy for GFR. However, as true GFR declines with worsening renal insufficiency, the amount of creatinine that is secreted increases significantly. A mathematical formula (the Cockcroft–Gault) was developed to better estimate GFR on the basis of plasma$_{Cr}$, accounting for the influences of patient age and weight (in kg): CrCl = ([140 − age] × [ideal body weight in kg])/(72 × P_{cr}) (×0.85 for women). The Cockcroft–Gault formula was originally calculated using normal healthy individuals, and therefore, it is less accurate in individuals with impaired renal function. Attempts to improve upon the Cockcroft–Gault formula include the Modification of Diet in Renal Disease (MDRD) formula and Chronic Kidney Disease Epidemiology Collaboration (CKD-EPI) formula, which give an estimated GFR from serum creatinine, age, gender, and race.

Glomerular filtration flows through the various segments of the nephron, where all but a fraction of 1% of the filtrate is reabsorbed. In the proximal convoluted tubule (PCT), almost three fourths of the GFR is reabsorbed by passive diffusion. In the loop of Henle, energy is consumed to reabsorb salt in greater proportion than water to make relatively dilute, hypo-osmotic urine and to create the hyperosmotic medullary gradient necessary for countercurrent exchange and urine concentration. The active transport of sodium is mediated by the sodium-potassium-2-chloride cotransporter (NaK2Cl). This transporter is inhibited by "loop" diuretics, such as furosemide. In the distal convoluted tubule (DCT), the fine-tuning of salt and water reabsorption occurs via the apical sodium chloride cotransporter, which is inhibited by thiazide diuretics. The final urine may be as dilute as one third or as concentrated as fourfold the osmolality of plasma.

The kidney's role in maintaining blood pressure, RBF, and electrolyte balance involves a complex system of hormones, neural stimuli, and vasoactive substances. The *renin–angiotensin–aldosterone* axis is initiated with the production of renin by the juxtaglomerular apparatus (a specialized group of cells located at the afferent arteriole of each nephron). Renin production is stimulated by decreased intravascular volume as manifested by (i) decreased hydrostatic pressure in the afferent arteriole, (ii) decreased salt delivery to the macula densa of the distal tubule, and (iii) increased sympathetic tone. Renin cleaves angiotensinogen to form angiotensin I. This peptide is further cleaved to form angiotensin II in the lung by angiotensin-converting enzyme (ACE). Angiotensin II is a powerful peripheral vasoconstrictor. In the kidney, its effect is mainly on the efferent arteriole. It reduces renal sodium excretion by increasing its reabsorption by proximal tubules. Angiotensin II also acts on the zona glomerulosa of the adrenal gland to stimulate secretion of aldosterone, a potent mineralocorticoid that increases sodium reabsorption and potassium secretion in the collecting duct. The net effect is an increase in intravascular volume.

Increased *sympathetic tone* causes afferent arteriolar vasoconstriction, leading to decreased RBF and GFR, and promotes renin secretion and proximal tubular reabsorption of sodium. These changes cause decreased delivery of salt and water to the distal nephron.

Atrial natriuretic peptide (ANP) is a polypeptide secreted by the atrium in response to stretch and increased sodium concentration. It causes a salt and water diuresis as well as a significant peripheral vasodilation and inhibits renin secretion and antidiuretic hormone (ADH) action. ANP is able to increase GFR in the setting of a constant RBF.

ADH is released by the posterior pituitary gland (neurohypophysis), mainly in response to osmotic stimuli on the hypothalamus, although some volume stimuli are a secondary influence. ADH makes the collecting duct more permeable to water, which is reabsorbed into the medulla because of the high concentration of medullary solutes. Without the medullary concentration gradient, ADH cannot function and the concentrating ability of the kidney is hampered. The syndrome of inappropriate ADH secretion causes inappropriately concentrated urine in the face of plasma hyposmolality. In contrast, diabetes insipidus, or a lack of ADH action, leads to polyuria.

Sodium Balance

The aforementioned factors act in concert with several others to regulate electrolyte homeostasis. The balance of *sodium* is largely regulated by factors affected by intravascular volume. An increase in intravascular volume is sensed by baroreceptors and receptors in the juxtaglomerular apparatus, leading to the following changes, which increase the excretion of sodium:

1. Increased RBF, RPF, and glomerular hydrostatic pressure, all of which lead to an increased GFR
2. Decreased renin and aldosterone levels, which cause decreased reabsorption of sodium in the PCT and collecting duct, respectively
3. Increased ANP level, which leads to increased sodium excretion by increasing delivery of salt to the distal tubule and by inhibiting ADH action
4. Decreased sympathetic tone, which leads to increased GFR, decreased PCT sodium reabsorption, and increased delivery of sodium to the distal nephron

Water Balance

Water balance is responsible for the sodium concentration and osmolality of the plasma and is regulated by osmoreceptors in the hypothalamus. The osmolality of the plasma is a function of the concentration of solutes that do not freely cross the cell membrane. The main determinants of the osmolality of plasma are sodium and glucose. Plasma osmolality can be estimated using the formula: $(2 \times [Na^+]) + ([glucose]/18) + ([urea]/2.8)$.

Increased osmolality triggers the osmoreceptors, leading to increased thirst for free water, as well as the release of ADH from the anterior pituitary. ADH acts to make the collecting duct permeable to water, thereby allowing the urine to equilibrate with the medullary concentration gradient. This causes reabsorption of free water and concentration of the urine.

Potassium

Potassium is mainly an intracellular ion. Plasma potassium concentration in the short term is mainly dependent on shifts of the extracellular store of potassium into and out of the intracellular store. Factors that cause a shift of potassium into cells, thus decreasing the plasma potassium level, include:

1. Alkalosis, by driving protons out of the cell. This increases the positive charge gradient allowing potassium to move into the cell.
2. Insulin level, by increasing the active cotransport of glucose and potassium into cells

Factors that may cause a shift of potassium out of the intracellular space, thereby increasing plasma potassium, include:

1. Acidosis, by driving protons into the cell. This decreases the positive charge gradient allowing potassium to move into the cell.
2. Cell lysis, by rapidly releasing intracellular potassium. This may occur during certain pathologic states such as transfusion reaction and rhabdomyolysis.

The total body store of potassium is dependent on intake and excretion. The excretion of potassium by the kidney occurs primarily in the distal tubule and collecting duct. It is almost solely dependent on the following two factors:

1. Aldosterone level. Aldosterone makes the collecting duct permeable to potassium, leading to passage of potassium from the cells of the collecting duct into the urine.
2. Urine flow rate in the collecting duct. The increased flow of urine leads to a washout of the potassium gradient in the collecting duct, causing an increase in the secretion of potassium.

Acid–Base Metabolism

By-products of normal metabolism constitute a significant *acid load*, which must be excreted each day. This is accomplished by the secretion of hydrogen ions, the reabsorption of bicarbonate, and the buffering of the urine with ammonium in the distal tubule. In response to acid loads, the body maintains *acid–base homeostasis* in several ways. The pH level of the plasma is dependent on the concentration of bicarbonate and carbon dioxide. In response to an acid load, the body has a short-term and a long-term response. In the short term, the acid load is buffered by the bicarbonate buffer system. Furthermore, increased ventilation causes a decrease in plasma carbon dioxide concentration. In the long term, acid loads are neutralized by increased bicarbonate reabsorption in the kidney, a process that is dependent on a sodium–proton exchange and on carbonic anhydrase.

Distal renal tubule acidosis (RTA), also known as type I RTA, is the most common and most clinically significant RTA to urologists. Distal RTA is a failure to excrete the protons in the distal tubules leading to a nonanion gap metabolic acidosis with relatively alkaline urine. Hypokalemia will often also occur. Patients with distal RTA frequently have nephrocalcinosis and recurrent calcium phosphate urolithiasis because of increase calcium load from the bone buffering of the acidosis combined with the alkaline urine of calcium in the urine. Distal RTA can be treated with oral potassium citrate, which reduces the acidosis, replaces potassium losses, and inhibit stone formation.

Calcium Balance

The kidney plays an important role in the regulation of calcium balance. It metabolizes 25-hydroxy vitamin D to its highly active form, 1,25-dihydroxy vitamin D. Furthermore, under the regulation of parathyroid hormone (PTH), it excretes most of the daily calcium load. PTH increases renal tubular reabsorption of calcium within the DCT. Thiazide diuretics promote reabsorption of calcium in DCT and can be used as a medical treatment for recurrent calcium stone formers.

Red Blood Cell Regulation

Erythropoietin is secreted by the kidney in response to decreased oxygen delivery to the renal cortex. This hormone acts on the bone marrow to increase the production of erythrocytes. Patients with chronic renal failure may develop anemia responsive to exogenous erythropoietin because of their decreased viable renal parenchyma. Erythropoietin secretion by some RCCs may cause a paraneoplastic polycythemia.

ACUTE RENAL FAILURE

Acute renal failure is a precipitous deterioration in renal function that results in the retention of nitrogenous wastes and/or a failure to regulate the extracellular fluid volume/composition. Renal failure may be classified according to its various causes as prerenal, intrarenal, or postrenal.

Prerenal failure (prerenal azotemia) is caused by a decreased blood flow to the kidneys. This may be secondary to decreased intravascular volume, decreased cardiac output, or relative vasodilatation of the peripheral vasculature. Decreased RBF leads to the conservation of salt via an increased sympathetic tone and increased renin/angiotensin II/aldosterone activity by decreasing the amount of glomerular filtration but increases the filtration fraction and thus the reabsorption in the PCT. The increase in resorption by the PCT (which passively resorbs blood urea nitrogen [BUN] but not creatinine) is greater than the decrease in GFR; therefore, the BUN level rises faster than the creatinine level. A BUN–creatinine ratio of greater than 20:1 is typical in prerenal azotemia.

Intrarenal failure is caused by reversible or irreversible insults to the kidneys. Common medical etiologies include acute glomerulonephritides, acute vasculitides, or acute interstitial nephritides. The vast majority of hospital-acquired intrarenal failure is caused by acute tubular necrosis. Etiologies include hypoxia, drug toxicity, myoglobinuria, profound hypotension, and sepsis. Intrarenal failure may cause oliguria but rarely results in complete anuria.

Postrenal failure is caused by urinary tract obstruction. This obstruction may occur at any level of the collecting system, ureter, or bladder outlet. Causes of obstruction include stones, tumors, extrinsic compression by tumor or retroperitoneal fibrosis, and BOO from BPH, urethral stricture, or detrusor overactivity. The cause and completeness of the obstruction, the rapidity of onset, and the duration of obstruction are important determinants of reversibility. Complete acute obstruction of one ureter usually leads to a temporary increase of the serum creatinine level followed by a gradual return to the baseline caused by contralateral renal compensation. True anuria in a patient with two normal kidneys suggests BOO or bilateral ureteral obstruction, which is rare. In cases of suspected postrenal failure, the passage of a Foley catheter should confirm or exclude the possibility of BOO. Renal ultrasonography can suggest upper tract obstruction by showing hydronephrosis and hydroureter. Obstruction can be confirmed by diuretic renogram, intravenous urogram, or antegrade/retrograde pyelography. Upper tract obstruction may be relieved percutaneously or by retrograde placement of ureteral stents. BOO may be relieved by placement of a Foley or suprapubic catheter. Prompt relief of acute obstruction usually leads to a return to normal renal function, although it may sometimes require several weeks for the serum creatinine concentration to reach its nadir.

Relief of bilateral upper tract obstruction may lead to a brisk postobstructive diuresis. A temporary concentrating defect in the kidney leads to derangements in serum electrolytes and volume status. Most patients who are alert and have relatively short-term obstruction may be followed as outpatients, as their thirst and hunger mechanisms will compensate for renal losses of sodium, potassium, and water. Obtunded, elderly, or demented patients, as well as those with long-term obstruction, require intravenous fluids and close monitoring of electrolytes.

Suggested Readings

Hanno PM, Guzzo TJ, Malkowicz B, et al. *Penn Clinical Manual of Urology*. 2nd ed. Philadelphia: Saunders Elsevier; 2014.

Graham SD Jr, Keane TE, Glenn JF. *Glenn's Urologic Surgery*. 7th ed. Philadelphia: Lippincott Williams & Wilkins; 2009.

Guzzo TJ, Drach GW, Wein AJ. *Primer of Geriatric Urology*. 1st ed. New York: Springer; 2012.

McAninch JW, Lue TF. *Smith and Tanagho's General Urology*. 18th ed. New York: McGraw-Hill; 2012.

Wein AJ, Kavoussi LR, Novick AC, et al., eds. *Campbell-Walsh Urology*. 10th ed. Philadelphia: Saunders Elsevier; 2011.

CHAPTER

28 Gynecology

STEPHANIE JEAN, EVELYN B. MARSH, AND CHRISTINA S. CHU

KEY POINTS

- The embryologic development of the female genital tract involves fusion of the müllerian ducts. The most common congenital anomalies result from incomplete fusion or incomplete canalization of this organ system during development.
- The female pelvic organs have a rich blood supply and complex innervation. The ureter's path through the pelvis puts it in close proximity to most of the pelvic organs.
- The hypothalamic/pituitary/ovarian axis is responsible for the hormonal regulation of the menstrual cycle. Pulsatile GnRH release from the hypothalamus causes release of FSH and LH from the pituitary. These hormones, in turn, cause the cyclic changes in levels of estrogen and progesterone released from the ovary.
- Pelvic inflammatory disease is caused by an ascending infection of the lower genital tract, causing polymicrobial infection and inflammation of the pelvic organs. The most common causative organisms are *Neisseria gonorrhoeae* or *Chlamydia trachomatis*, although vaginal and enteric organisms have also been associated. Treatment involves broad-spectrum antibiotics. Evidence of a tuboovarian abscess is an indication for inpatient management.
- Endometriosis is characterized by endometrial implants outside of the endometrial cavity. It can cause widespread inflammation and scarring, infertility, and pelvic pain. Treatment of endometriosis may be medical (involving suppression of cyclic hormonal levels) or surgical (involving removal or ablation of implants and lysis of adhesions).
- Endometrial carcinoma is the most common gynecologic malignancy in the United States. Increased exposure to estrogen is the major predisposing factor for endometrial cancer. The incidence of endometrial cancer is likely to continue to increase secondary to the obesity epidemic. Postmenopausal bleeding should always be evaluated in order to rule out malignancy.
- Ovarian carcinoma is the leading cause of death from gynecologic malignancies in the United States. Epithelial tumors are the most common type of ovarian carcinoma, although sex cord stromal tumors and germ cell tumors also exist. Epithelial ovarian carcinoma is usually diagnosed in advanced stages. Treatment involves surgical debulking as well as adjuvant chemotherapy.
- The Pap test is the primary screening tool for cervical cancer. Precancerous changes of cervical epithelial cells are closely related to exposure to high-risk HPV types. The Bethesda classification system is the most common descriptive terminology used in the evaluation of Pap tests.
- Ectopic pregnancy may lead to fallopian tube rupture, hemodynamic instability, and death. Ectopic pregnancy must be ruled out in all women with a positive serum hCG test complaining of abdominal pain and/or vaginal bleeding. Medical management may be indicated for treatment of ectopic pregnancy in specific situations. Surgical management is indicated in any situation involving hemodynamic instability.
- The best initial diagnostic test for evaluating the female reproductive organs is transvaginal ultrasonography. CT and MRI may have utility in specific circumstances for further diagnosis.

Obstetricians and gynecologists specialize in diseases of the female reproductive tract. The female reproductive tract is in proximity to both the genitourinary and the gastrointestinal tracts. Therefore, the most common complaints relating to these organ systems are often similar—gynecologic pathology may present with gastrointestinal or urinary symptoms and vice versa. As a result, general surgeons must be aware of the anatomy and pathophysiology of the female reproductive tract in order to treat the variety of disease that their patients' symptomatology may represent.

EMBRYOLOGY

The female reproductive tract is derived from the müllerian duct system (paramesonephric duct), and the male reproductive tract is derived from the wolffian duct system (mesonephric duct). If the embryo possesses a Y chromosome, differentiation from the indifferent gonad to male reproductive organs begins during gestational weeks 6 through 9. The testes produce testosterone and anti-müllerian hormone (AMH), which lead to regression of the müllerian system during the 8th week of gestation. In the absence of testicular differentiation, the müllerian duct system persists and the wolffian system regresses leading to female reproductive organs. In the female embryo, the müllerian ducts fuse by the 10th week of gestation to form the three distinct zones of the female reproductive tract: the fallopian tubes, the uterus, and the upper two thirds of the vagina (Fig. 28.1). Incomplete regression of the wolffian system can result in paratubal cysts along the length of the fallopian tubes in the developed female reproductive tract. The lower third of the vagina is derived from the urogenital sinus, which is an inclusion of the ectoderm.

Congenital abnormalities of the müllerian ducts occur in approximately 0.1% to 3.2% of women. The two most common types of defects related to the embryologic development of the

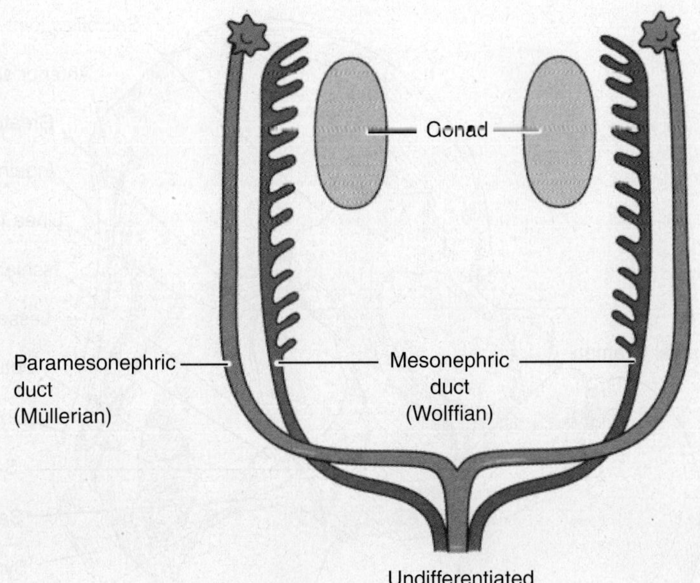

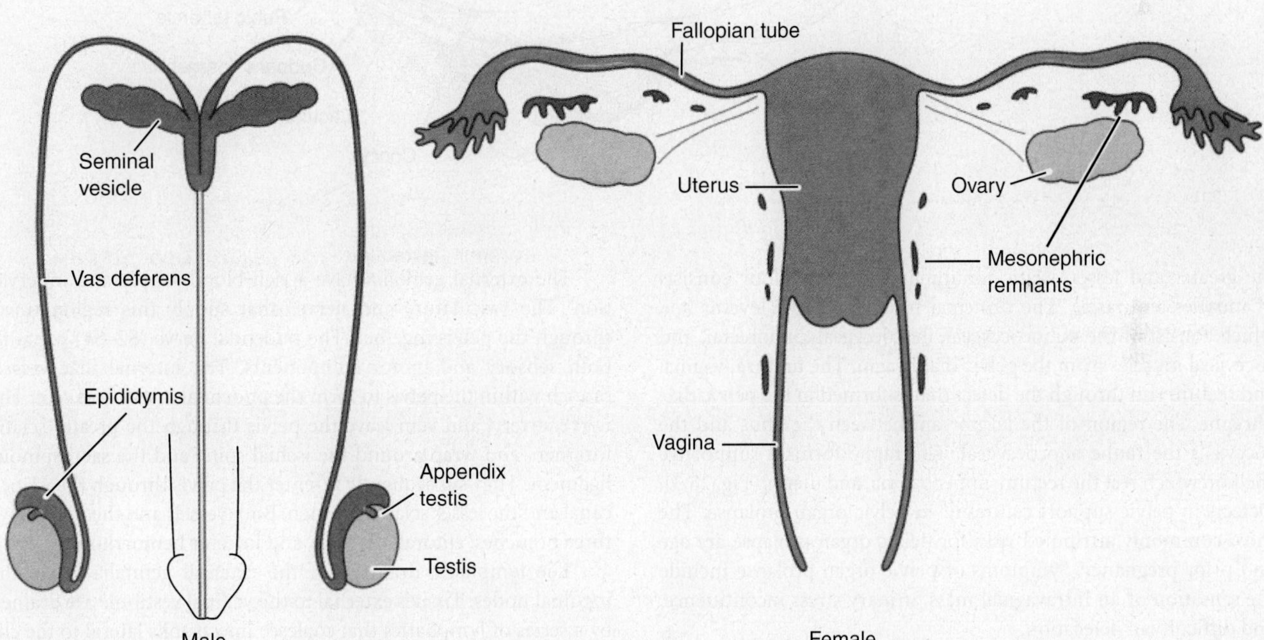

FIGURE 28.1 Development of the normal male and female reproductive tract. (From Speroff L, Glass RH, Kase N, eds. *Clinical Gynecologic Endocrinology and Infertility*. 5th ed. Baltimore: J.B. Lippincott; 1994:323, with permission.)

female genital tract involve fusion and canalization. Fusion defects are responsible for duplications in the organs such as a bicornuate uterus and uterus didelphys. These conditions may be asymptomatic, although they are sometimes associated with pelvic pain and infertility. Failure of canalization may result in the presence of transverse vaginal septa or incomplete formation of the uterine cavity or cervical canal. A buildup of sloughed endometrium and blood in the vagina (hematocolpos) and the uterus (hematometra) may result due to occlusion of the outlet tract. Patients may present complaining of primary amenorrhea, and/or cyclic pain, or may have a mass detected on abdominal or pelvic examination. In this case, ultrasound (US) or magnetic resonance imaging (MRI) of the abdomen and pelvis demonstrates an enlarged vagina and uterus filled with blood.

ANATOMY

Bony Pelvis

The *bony pelvis* is formed by the union of the sacrum and coccyx with the ileum, the ischium, and the pubis (Fig. 28.2). The sacrospinous and sacrotuberous ligaments delineate the margins of

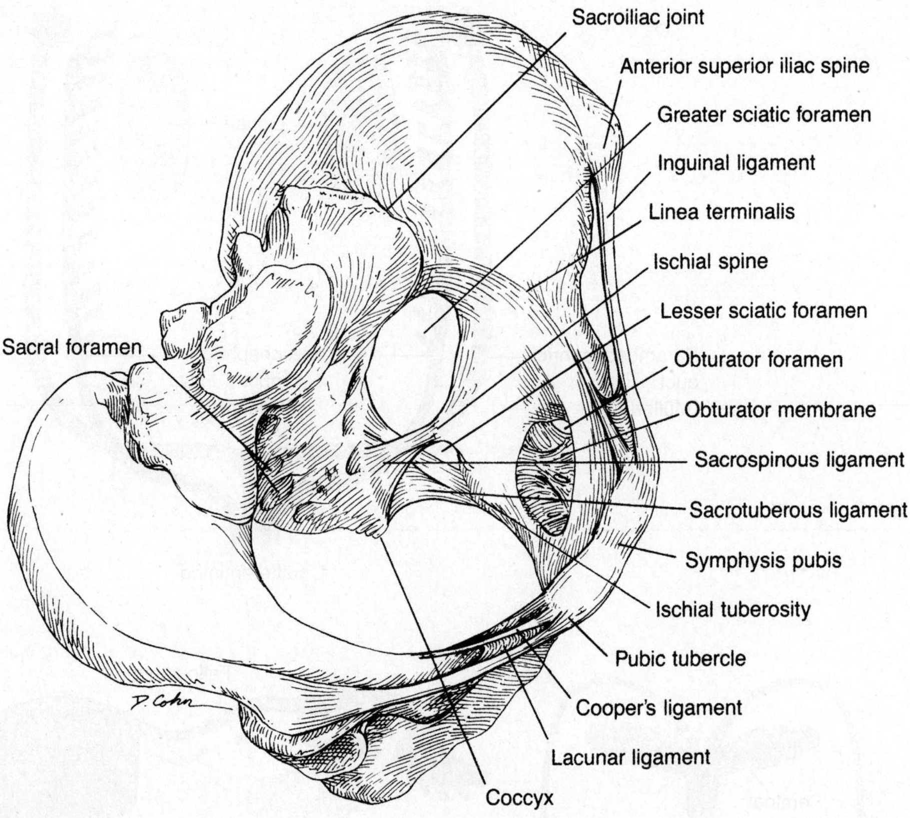

FIGURE 28.2 The female pelvis. (From Berek JS, Adashi EY, Hillard PA, eds. *Novak's Gynecology*. 12th ed. Baltimore: Lippincott-Raven; 1996:72, with permission.)

the greater and lesser sciatic foramina. The pelvic floor consists of muscles and fascia. The principal muscles are the levator ani, which consist of the pubococcygeal, iliococcygeal, puborectal, and coccygeal muscles from the pelvic diaphragm. The urethra, vagina, and rectum run through the defect that is formed in the pelvic diaphragm. The region of the levator ani between the anus and the coccyx is the raphe anococcygeal. The raphe forms a supportive shelf on which rest the rectum, upper vagina, and uterus (Fig. 28.3). Defects in pelvic support can result in pelvic organ prolapse. The most commonly attributed risks for pelvic organ prolapse are age and prior pregnancy. Symptoms of pelvic organ prolapse include the sensation of an intravaginal mass, urinary stress incontinence, and difficulty in defecation.

External Genitalia

The external genitalia are comprised of the *vulva*, which is the hair-bearing skin and adipose tissue underneath the skin. The vulva consists of two portions, the labia majora and the labia minora. Between the labia minora are the vestibule of the vagina, the urethra, and the clitoris. The erectile bodies and their associated muscles lie underneath the subcutaneous tissue and above the fascial layer.

The perineal membrane is the underlying fascial layer. It consists of a dense sheet of fibromuscular tissue that spans the anterior portion of the pelvic outlet. Posteriorly, the perineal body is a condensation of connective tissue that separates the lower vagina and the anus. The perineal membrane connects the vagina and the perineal body. The perineal membrane supports the pelvic floor against increases in intra-abdominal pressure.

The external genitalia have a rich blood supply and innervation. The vasculature and nerves that supply this region travel through the pelvis together. The pudendal nerve (S2–S4) contains both sensory and motor components. The internal iliac vessels branch within the pelvis to form the pudendal artery and vein. The nerve, artery, and vein leave the pelvis through the greater sciatic foramen, and wrap around the ischial spine and the sacrospinous ligament. They subsequently re-enter the pelvis through the Alcock canal and the lesser sciatic foramen. Both vessels and the nerve have three branches: clitoral, perineal, and inferior hemorrhoidal.

The lymphatic drainage of the external genitalia is via the inguinal nodes. Tissues external to the vaginal vestibule are drained by a series of lymphatics that coalesce into trunks lateral to the clitoris. These, in turn, drain into the superficial inguinal nodes. The urethral lymphatics also drain into the superficial inguinal nodes. These superficial lymph nodes drain into and communicate with the deep inguinal lymph nodes, which are found under the fascia cribrosa in the femoral triangle.

Female Genital Organs

The *female genital organs* consist of the vagina, cervix, uterus, fallopian tubes, and ovaries (Fig. 28.4).

The *vagina* is a fibromuscular canal that connects the vestibule distally to the cervix and uterus proximally. Its anatomic position is almost in the horizontal plane when a woman is standing. This orientation occurs due to the obtuse angle formed by the pelvic diaphragm on the retroperitoneal margin on the vagina. This angle is used to delineate the margin of the lower third and upper two

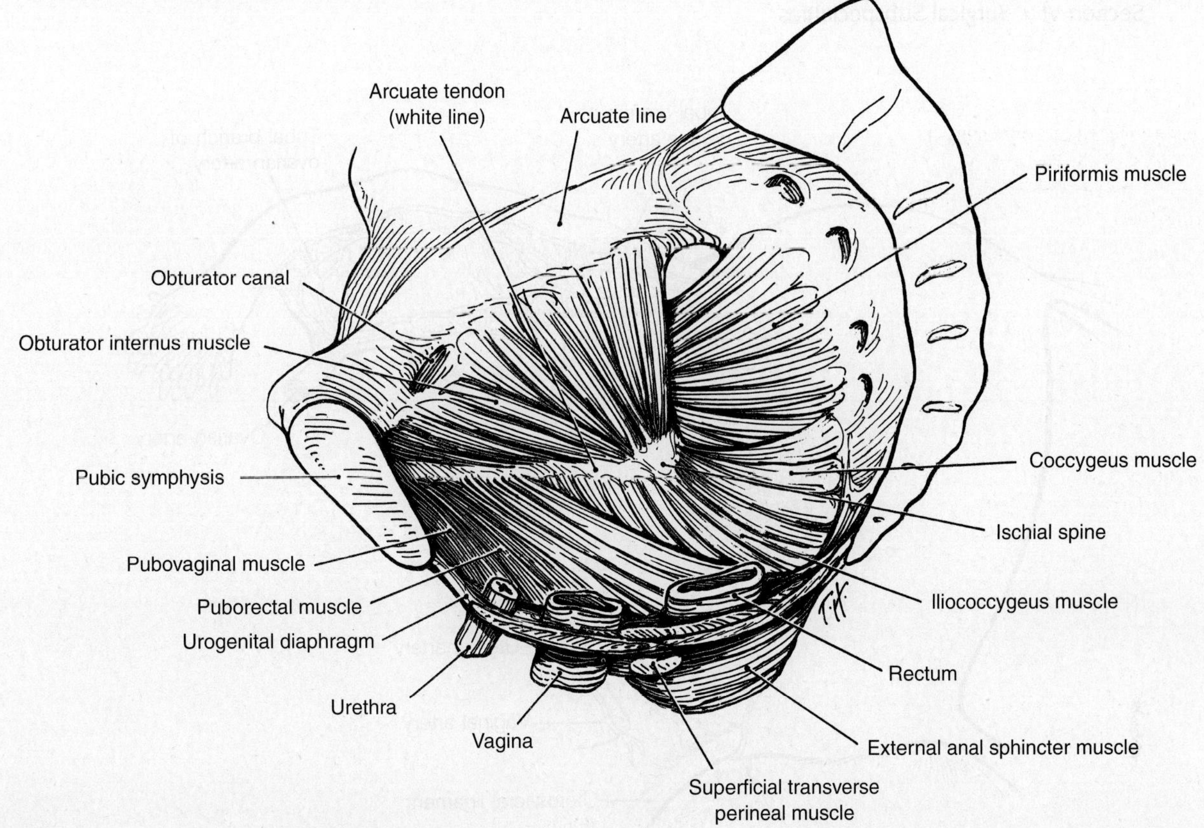

FIGURE 28.3 Muscles of the pelvic floor. (From Berek JS, Adashi EY, Hillard PA, eds. *Novak's Gynecology*. 12th ed. Baltimore: Lippincott-Raven; 1996:77, with permission.)

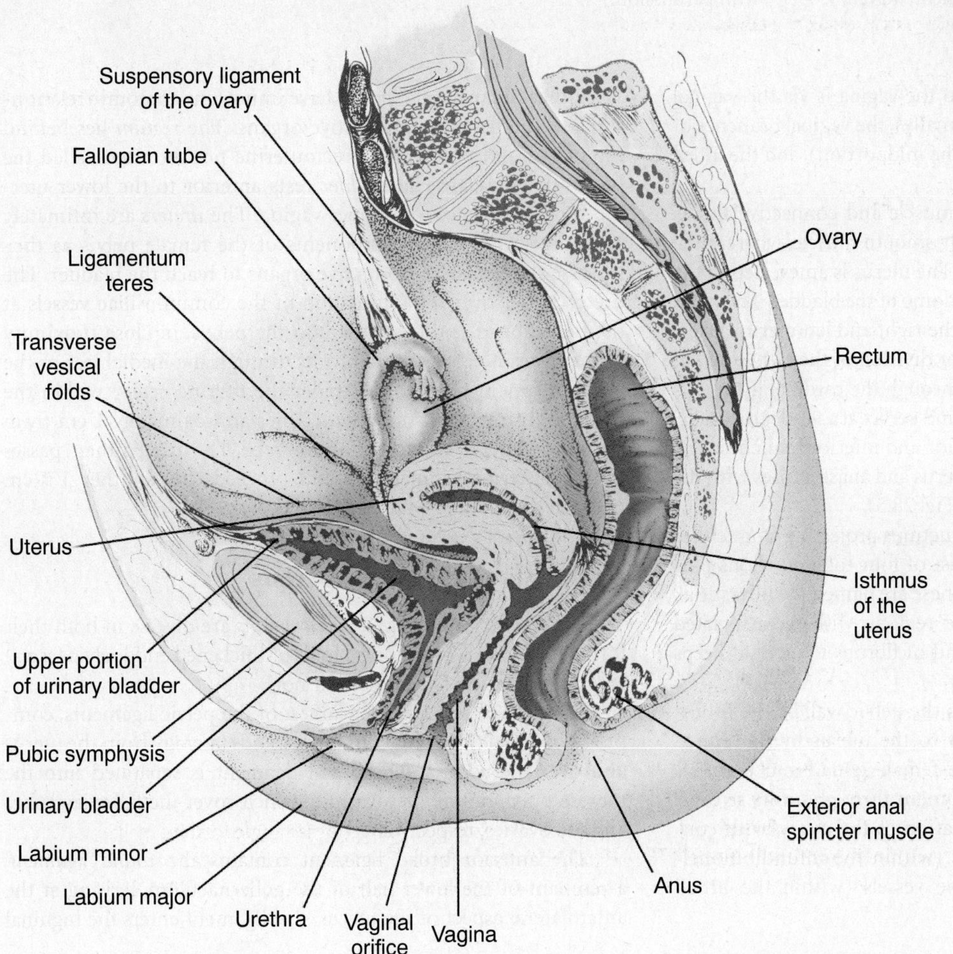

FIGURE 28.4 The pelvic viscera. (From Berek JS. *Berek & Novak's Gynecology*. 14th ed. Philadelphia: Lippincott Willams & Wilkins; 2007: 104, with permission)

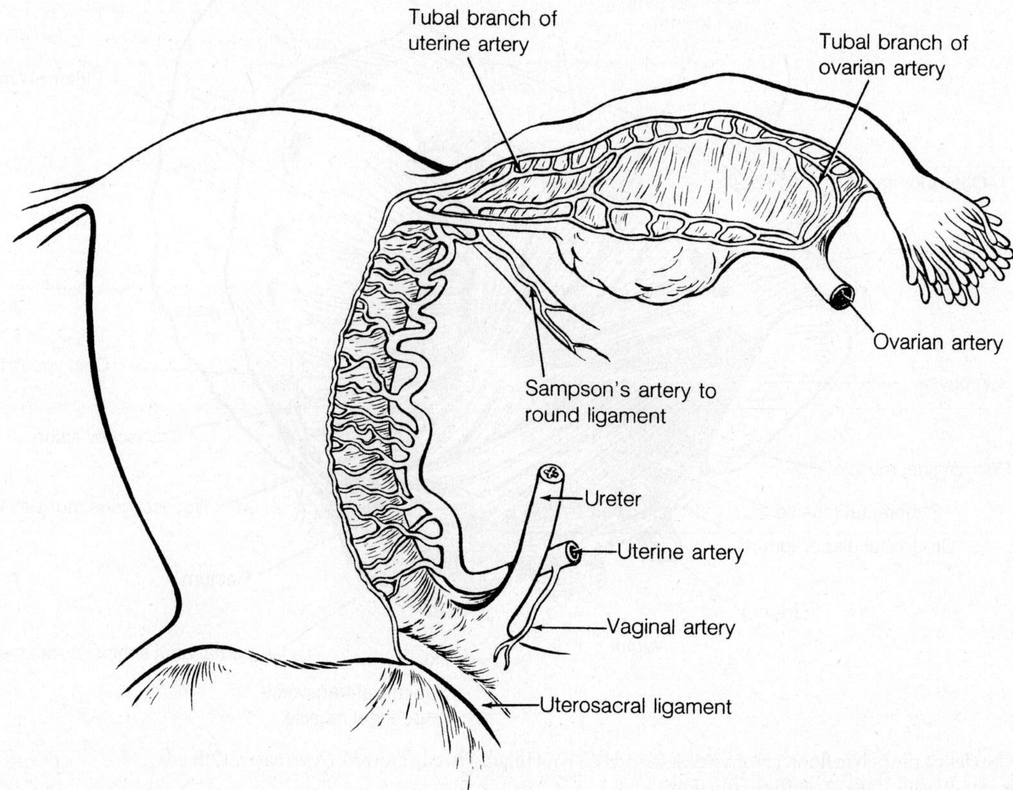

FIGURE 28.5 The vascular supply of the female pelvis. (From Rock J, Thompson JD, eds. *TeLinde's Operative Gynecology*. 8th ed. Philadelphia: Lippincott-Raven; 1997:73, with permission.)

thirds of the vagina. Blood supply to the vagina is via the vaginal branches of the uterine artery (proximally), the vaginal branches of the middle hemorrhoidal artery (in the midportion), and the internal pudendal vessels (distally).

The *uterus* consists of smooth muscle and connective tissue. The uterine corpus consists of mainly smooth muscle, whereas the cervix is composed of fibrous tissue. The uterus is anteverted in the majority of women and lies over the dome of the bladder. The main arterial supply to the uterus is from the right and left uterine arteries, which are branches of the anterior division of the right and left internal iliacs. These vessels course through the cardinal ligaments at the junction of the uterine corpus and cervix at a 90-degree angle. They subsequently divide into superior and inferior branches. The marginal arteries run lateral to the uterus and anastomoses with the ovarian arteries in the mesosalpinx (Fig. 28.5).

The *fallopian tubes* are paired structures projecting from either side of the uterine fundus and consist of four tubal portions plus the fimbriae: from medial to lateral, these are named the interstitial, isthmic, ampullary, and infundibular regions, with the associated fimbria. The fimbria ovarica is a band of fibrous tissue that keeps the fimbria apposed to the ovary.

The *ovary* is attached laterally to the pelvic wall by the infundibulopelvic ligament and medially to the uterus by the utero-ovarian ligament. The ovary is the female gonad and contains follicles in various stages of development throughout its stroma. There is a complex collateral circulation to the ovary, with contributions from the ovarian vessels (within the infundibulopelvic ligament) and from the uterine vessels (within the broad ligament).

Other organs in the pelvis have important anatomic relationships to the female reproductive organs. The *rectum* lies behind the uterus and posterior to rectouterine pouch, often called the pouch of Douglas. The *bladder* rests anterior to the lower uterine segment, cervix, and upper vagina. The *ureters* are intimately associated with many components of the female pelvis as they traverse the female reproductive organs to reach the bladder. The ureter passes over the bifurcation of the common iliac vessels at the pelvic brim and descends into the pelvis, in close proximity to the ovarian vessels. It then runs through the medial leaf of the broad ligament and crosses under the uterine artery within the cardinal ligament. At this point, it lies approximately 1 cm from the anterolateral surface of the cervix. The ureter then passes on the anterior vaginal wall and proceeds for another 1.5 cm through the bladder wall (Fig. 28.6).

Ligaments of the Pelvic Organs

The *ligaments of the internal pelvic organs* are diverse in both their form (comprised of peritoneal folds or thickened endopelvic fascia) and their function (suspensory or not).

The *broad ligament* is the largest of the pelvic ligaments, comprised of a fold of peritoneum that extends laterally from the uterus and over the adnexa. The broad ligament is separated into the mesosalpinx and the mesovarium, which cover the fallopian tubes and the ovaries, respectively.

The anterior broad ligament contains the *round ligament*, a remnant of the lower half of the gubernaculum. Arising at the anterolateral aspect of the uterus, this ligament enters the inguinal

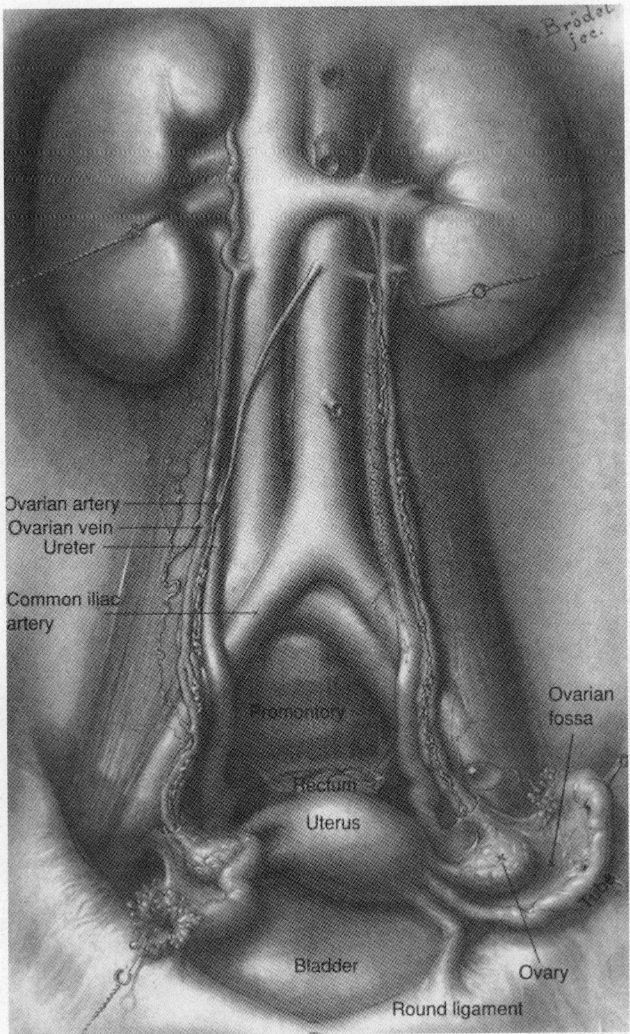

FIGURE 28.6 The relationship of the ureters to the female reproductive organs. (From Rock J, Thompson JD, eds. *TeLinde's Operative Gynecology*. 8th ed. Philadelphia: Lippincott-Raven; 1997:82, with permission.)

canal at the internal inguinal ring and exits the canal to insert into the subcutaneous tissue of the labia majora.

The *infundibulopelvic ligaments* attach the ovary and fallopian tubes to the pelvic sidewall. The ovarian artery and vein run through these ligaments.

The *uterosacral ligaments* are a condensation of ligaments from the second, third, and fourth segments of the sacrum to the cervix. These ligaments hold the cervix posteriorly over the levator plate.

Finally, the *cardinal ligaments* (transverse cervical) run from the lateral wall of the cervix and vagina to the pelvic sidewall and provide the primary support for the uterus in the pelvis. The uterine artery and vein reside within the cardinal ligaments.

The lymphatic vessels of the upper two thirds of the vagina and the uterus drain into the obturator, internal, and external iliac lymph nodes, which then proceed to the common iliac lymph nodes and the para-aortic lymph nodes. Accessory channels also include uterine drainage along the round ligaments to the superficial inguinal lymph nodes and from the posterior surface of the uterus along the uterosacral ligaments to the lateral sacral lymph nodes. Lymphatic channels from the ovaries follow the course of the ovarian vessels and drain into the para-aortic lymph nodes.

The autonomic nerves of the pelvis lie in the presacral space. The uterus receives its innervation from the uterovaginal plexus (Frankenhäuser ganglion), which is one of three divisions emanating from the superior hypogastric plexus. This plexus runs within the connective tissue of the cardinal ligament. The fallopian tubes and ovaries receive their innervation from the plexus of nerves that accompany the ovarian vessels having originated from the renal plexus.

ENDOCRINOLOGY OF THE HYPOTHALAMIC/PITUITARY/OVARIAN AXIS

The menstrual cycle is mediated centrally via gonadotropin-releasing hormone (GnRH). GnRH is produced in the hypothalamus and transported to the pituitary gland via the local portal blood system. The amplitude and frequency of the pulsatile secretion of GnRH vary throughout the menstrual cycle and are the essential components in the control of the cycle. Follicle-stimulating hormone (FSH) and luteinizing hormone (LH) are secreted from the anterior pituitary in response to GnRH signaling. They are responsible for estrogen and progesterone production from the ovary and the corpus luteum (after ovulation), respectively. Depending on the phase of the cycle, FSH and LH may have negative and/or positive feedback relationships with the hypothalamus and the pituitary, which result in regulation of hormone levels.

The *normal menstrual cycle* lasts 21 to 35 days with 2 to 6 days of flow and an average blood loss of 20 to 60 mL. The cycle consists of two phases: the follicular phase and the luteal phase. During the follicular phase, hormonal feedback promotes the recruitment of follicles and ultimately the development of a single dominant follicle. This phase lasts from 10 to 14 days. During the luteal phase, the endometrium is prepared for the possibility of pregnancy. This occurs by production of progesterone from the corpus luteum, which leads to coiling and folding of secretory glands and blood vessels. This phase lasts approximately 14 days and encompasses the events from ovulation to the first day of menstrual flow.

The hormonal, ovarian, and endometrial changes of the menstrual cycle are illustrated in Figure 28.7. The follicular phase begins with day 1 of the menstrual cycle, which corresponds with the first day of menses and the start of the proliferative phase of the endometrium. Low levels of estradiol and progesterone lead to an increase in GnRH pulsatility, which subsequently causes a modest rise in FSH. This stimulates the recruitment of a cohort of ovarian follicles, which secrete estrogen, which serves as the stimulus for endometrial proliferation. The increased estrogen level during this phase has a negative feedback on pituitary FSH secretion and a positive feedback on pituitary LH secretion. After sufficient estrogen stimulation, there is an LH surge, which causes ovulation of a single mature oocyte to occur 24 to 36 hours later, around day 14. At the same time, there is progressive mitotic growth of the superficial two thirds of the endometrium in response to increasing levels of estrogen. During this period, the endometrial glands become elongated and tortuous.

The luteal phase is dominated by the production of progesterone by the corpus luteum. The rise in progesterone leads to organization of the endometrial glands and a decrease in LH pulsatility. The estrogen level declines through the early luteal phase and begins to rise again at the end of the luteal phase as a result of corpus luteum secretion. Both estrogen and progesterone levels remain elevated throughout the life span of the corpus luteum, and their

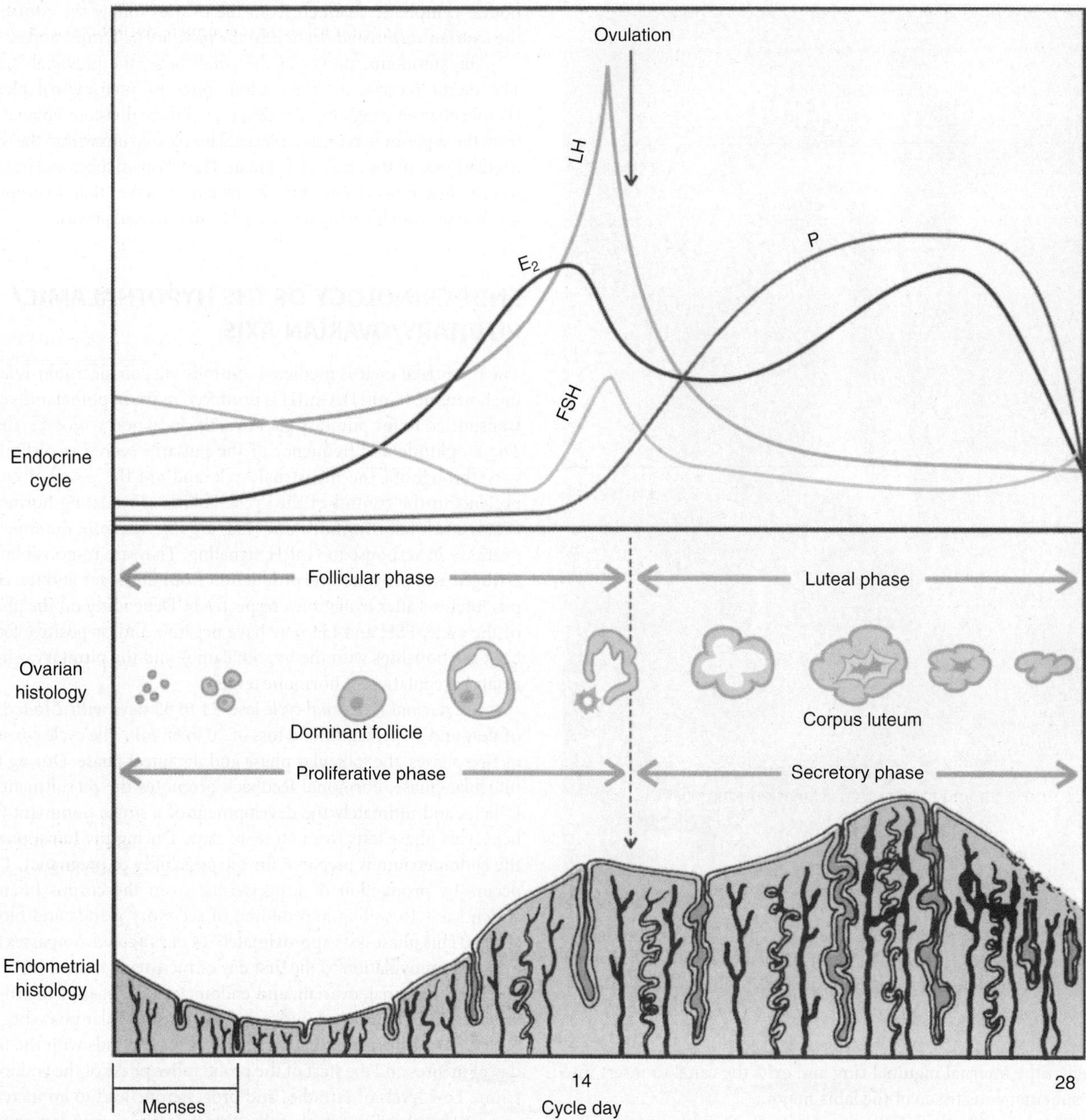

FIGURE 28.7 The menstrual cycle. (From Berek JS, Adashi EY, Hillard PA, eds. *Novak's Gynecology*. 12th ed. Baltimore: Lippincott-Raven; 1996:160, with permission.)

levels wane with its demise if fertilization does not occur. This fall in gonadal steroids causes the breakdown of the superficial endometrium and the beginning of menstrual flow. It also permits the level of FSH to rise, thus beginning the next cycle.

INFECTIOUS DISEASES

The majority of vaginal infections are *lower genital tract infections* such as cervicitis and vaginitis and are readily treatable with minimal long-term sequelae. In contrast, *pelvic inflammatory disease* (PID) usually results from an infection of the endocervix with bacteria that ascend to the endometrium and the fallopian tubes, causing polymicrobial infection and inflammation. Approximately one half of all PID is caused by an infection due to *Neisseria gonorrhoeae* or *Chlamydia trachomatis*. However, normal vaginal flora such as *Escherichia coli* and group B streptococcus may also be involved.

The symptoms of PID include pelvic pain, purulent vaginal discharge, fever, nausea, and vomiting. Gonococcal PID typically manifests as an abrupt onset of fever and pain that worsens with movement. Associated arthralgia has been reported with gonococcal infection. Chlamydial PID can have a more insidious course. The diagnosis of PID is usually based on the triad of signs: abdominal tenderness with or without peritoneal signs, cervical motion tenderness, and adnexal tenderness. Other softer markers for PID include pyrexia, elevated leukocyte count, Gram stain of the cervical discharge, and the presence of a pelvic or adnexal collection on US and/or bimanual examination. A physician should have a low

TABLE 28.1 Current recommendations for treatment of PID

Outpatient—suitable for mild-to-moderate acute PID

A. Ceftriaxone (250 mg i.m. in a single dose) plus doxycycline (100 mg p.o. b.i.d. for 14 d) with or without metronidazole (500 mg p.o. b.i.d. for 14 d)
B. Cefoxitin (2 g i.m. in a single dose) and probenecid, 1 g orally administered in a single dose plus doxycycline (100 mg p.o. b.i.d. for 14 d) with or without metronidazole (500 mg p.o. b.i.d. for 14 d)
C. Other parenteral third-generation cephalosporin, such as ceftizoxime or cefotaxime plus doxycycline (100 mg p.o. b.i.d. for 14 d) with or without metronidazole (500 mg p.o. b.i.d. for 14 d)

Inpatient—recommended for severe PID and for patients who do not respond to outpatient therapy

A. Cefoxitin (2 g IV q6 h) OR cefotetan (2 g IV q12 h), plus doxycycline (100 mg IV q12 h)
B. Clindamycin (900 mg IV q8 h) and gentamicin (2 mg/kg IV or i.m. load then 1.5 mg/kg IV q8 h; Or single daily dosing 3 to 5 mg/kg)

i.m., intramuscular; p.o., per os; b.i.d., twice a day; q.i.d., four times a day; IV, intravenous.
Centers for Disease Control (CDC) Sexually Transmitted Diseases Guidelines, 2010.

threshold to treat PID, as the consequences of untreated PID can be devastating and include infertility and chronic pelvic pain.

Treatment of this disease requires broad-spectrum antibiotics. Both outpatient and inpatient treatment options exist (Table 28.1). Indications for inpatient therapy include pregnancy, severe clinical presentation, pelvic abscess, persistent nausea and vomiting precluding compliance with oral medication, and failure to respond to an outpatient regimen after 48 hours of treatment. Intravenous therapy is continued until there is complete resolution of abdominal pain, and the patient has been afebrile for 48 hours.

PID may occur early in the first trimester of pregnancy. By 12 weeks of gestation, however, the fetal membranes have sealed over the internal cervical os, protecting the upper genital tract from infection. Gonorrhea and chlamydia may cause cervicitis throughout pregnancy.

A *tuboovarian abscess* (TOA) is a variant of acute PID. The agglutination of inflamed fallopian tubes, ovaries, and sometimes bowel with inflammatory exudates forms a palpable complex. Diagnosis requires the finding of a palpable mass on physical exam in a woman with PID. This finding is usually confirmed by US (Fig. 28.8). A TOA is treated initially with a broad-spectrum intravenous antibiotic regimen covering sexually-transmitted organisms and anaerobes; a combination of parenteral ampicillin, gentamicin, and clindamycin is a common first-line treatment. Seventy-five percent of patients treated with triple antibiotics will respond to therapy with resolution of fever and abdominal pain. Percutaneous drainage of the abscess should also be considered, if possible. Treatment failure requires surgical exploration for possible abscess drainage or hysterectomy and bilateral salpingo-oophorectomy. With current antibiotic regimens and early initiation of treatment, and with the improvement of percutaneous drainage techniques, the need for surgical exploration has decreased considerably.

MANAGEMENT OF BENIGN GYNECOLOGIC CONDITIONS

Endometriosis

Endometriosis is the ectopic growth of endometrial tissue outside the uterine cavity. This is thought to be caused both by metaplastic transformation of peritoneal tissue and retrograde

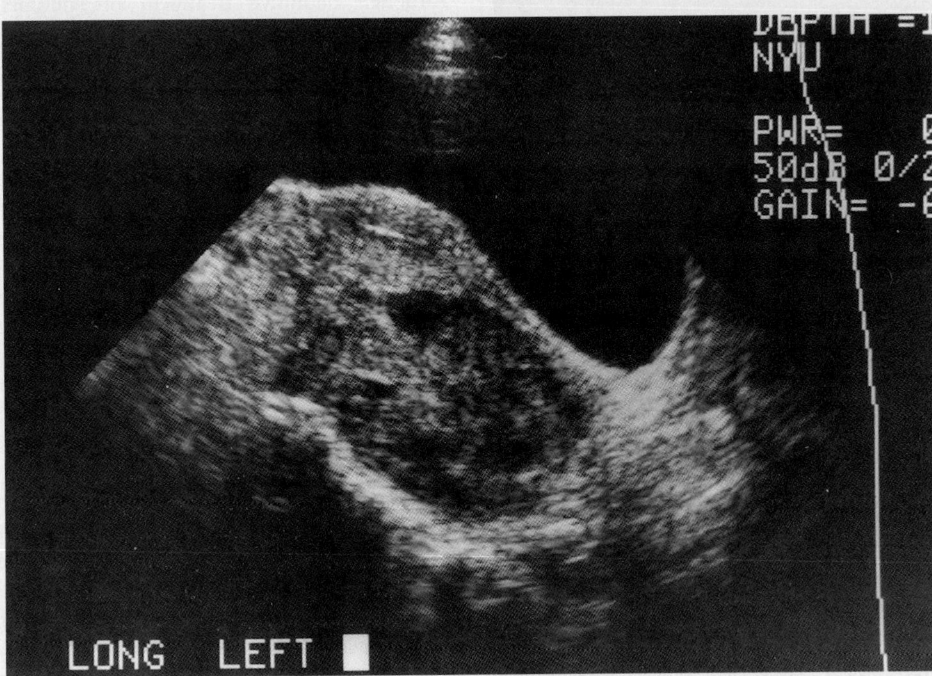

FIGURE 28.8 Transvaginal ultrasonogram of bilateral tuboovarian abscesses. (From Berek JS. *Berek & Novak's Gynecology*. 14th ed. Philadelphia: Lippincott Willams & Wilkins; 2007:477, with permission)

menstruation with subsequent peritoneal implantation. The most prevalent site for endometriosis is the pelvis. Other sites include the ovary, bowel, bladder, omentum, umbilicus, and lungs. Endometriosis is found in 7% of reproductive-age women and may present as pelvic pain, infertility, dysmenorrhea, dyschezia, or dyspareunia. Endometriosis may also be asymptomatic. There does not appear to be a correlation between the degree of endometriosis and the severity of pelvic pain, dyspareunia, and infertility. The typical lesions present as black, brown, or blue nodules surrounded by various degrees of fibrosis. In addition, ovarian cysts, called "chocolate cysts," containing thick, viscous brown fluid may occur as a result of endometriosis (Figs. 28.9 and 28.10).

Extrapelvic endometriosis is uncommon and is suspected when a palpable mass associated with pain that occurs in a cyclic monthly pattern is found outside the pelvis. The most common site for extrapelvic endometriosis is the gastrointestinal tract, particularly the colon and rectum. These patients usually present with abdominal pain, back pain, abdominal distension, and cyclic rectal bleeding. Other less common sites of involvement include the ureters, bladder, umbilicus, and lungs.

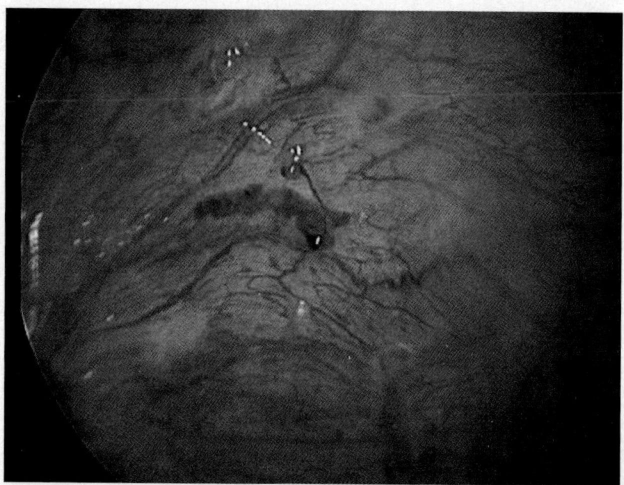

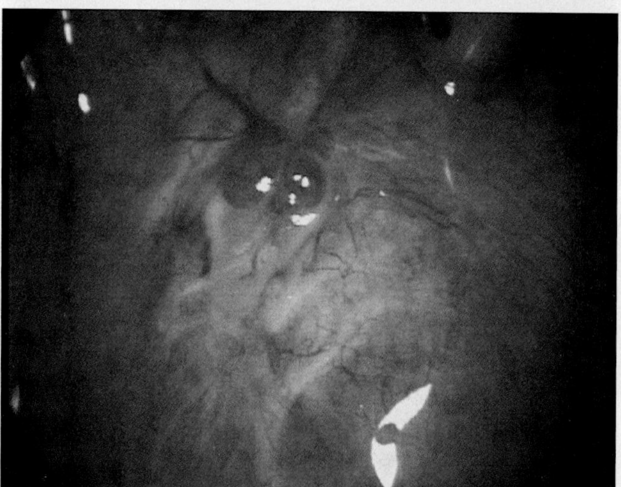

FIGURE 28.9 Typical and subtle endometriotic lesions on peritoneum. (From Berek JS. *Berek & Novak's Gynecology*. 14th ed. Philadelphia: Lippincott Willams & Wilkins; 2007:1149, with permission)

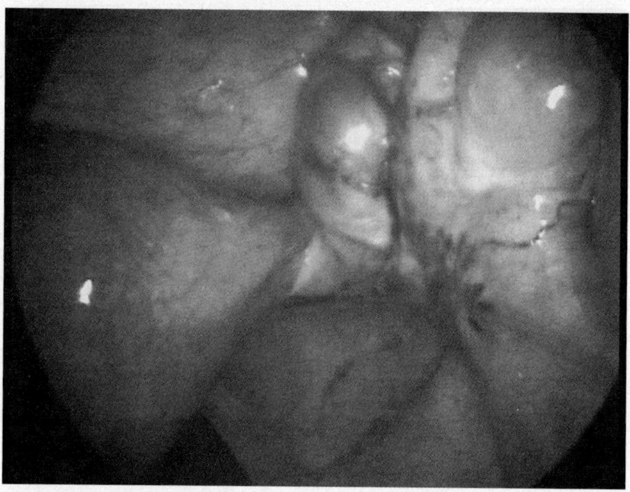

FIGURE 28.10 Laparoscopic image of the uterus and right ovary with dark endometrioma. (From Berek JS. *Berek & Novak's Gynecology*. 14th ed. Philadelphia: Lippincott Willams & Wilkins; 2007:1151, with permission)

Endometriosis can be treated medically and surgically. Medical treatment involves hormonal manipulation that suppresses cyclic estrogen synthesis and promotes atrophy of the endometrial implants. Drugs that have been used with variable success include oral contraceptive pills, oral and injectable progestins, and GnRH agonists. Surgical therapy includes both laparoscopy and laparotomy. Laparoscopy involves the ablation of the endometrial implants using bipolar coagulation, excision, or laser. The goal is to remove all implants and adhesions in an attempt to discontinue the associated chronic inflammatory state and restore the pelvis to its normal anatomy. Laparotomy is reserved for severe cases. In extreme cases, a total abdominal hysterectomy and bilateral salpingo-oophorectomy with lysis of adhesions is performed. Although definitive treatment of endometriosis necessitates removal of both ovaries to halt all cyclic hormonal processes, this is usually reserved for severe and recalcitrant cases as it results in early surgical menopause.

Benign Adnexal Masses

The relative frequency of adnexal masses (both benign and malignant) varies with age (Table 28.2). Following a thorough history and physical examination, evaluation of adnexal masses must proceed with imaging. Transvaginal US is the most useful radiographic tool in the preliminary evaluation of the adnexa, although MRI may be used for further classification. Characteristics that should be evaluated using US include size and location of the mass, presence of cystic or solid components, presence of septations within the mass, Doppler flow within the mass, and the presence or absence of associated ascites and intraperitoneal nodularity. In general, expectant management is indicated in premenopausal women with small (<5 cm), simple, asymptomatic cysts. Surgery is indicated in premenopausal women for the management of cysts that are large (>5 cm), symptomatic, persistent over the course of one to two menstrual cycles or have ultrasonographic findings suspicious for malignancy. In postmenopausal women, small, simple, asymptomatic cysts may be managed expectantly. Any masses not meeting these criteria should be managed surgically.

TABLE 28.2 Common adnexal masses

Age	Most Common	Other Common Adnexal Masses
0–19 y	Benign cystic teratoma	Wilms tumor Malignant germ cell tumor Neuroblastoma
20–44 y	Benign cystic teratoma	Serous cystadenoma Endometrioma
45–74 y	Serous cystadenoma	Mucinous cystadenoma Adenofibroma Endometrioma Brenner tumor Primary and metastatic malignancies

Adnexal masses can cause abdominal distension, pain, pelvic pressure, and urinary or gastrointestinal symptoms. Acute abdominal pain and peritoneal signs in the presence of an adnexal mass can result from adnexal torsion (a surgical emergency), or rupture of a cyst. Laparoscopy can be considered in hemodynamically stable patients with smaller, relatively benign-appearing masses. Laparoscopy may also be considered for small masses concerning for malignancy, as staging may also be performed laparoscopically; however, masses that are too large to be amenable to laparoscopic resection without intra-abdominal rupture should be removed via laparotomy.

The most common adnexal mass is a *functional ovarian cyst.* Functional ovarian cysts include follicular cysts and corpora lutea. Follicular cysts are more common and are usually less than 8 cm. They are often asymptomatic, found incidentally during a pelvic examination, and resolve within one or two menstrual cycles. Occasionally, they can rupture and cause acute abdominal pain and peritoneal signs. A follicular cyst that exceeds 3 cm in size is called a *corpus luteum cyst.* If a luteal cyst does not resolve in subsequent menstrual cycles, it can also rupture, causing hemoperitoneum and sometimes requires surgical intervention.

Mucinous cystadenomas are benign adnexal masses that may become quite large—tumors greater than 300 pounds have been reported. On gross inspection, they are smooth and loculated with a clear viscid fluid. Of major concern is that spillage of the cyst contents into the peritoneum, on removal of the tumor or spontaneously, can result in pseudomyxoma peritonei. Pseudomyxoma peritonei is the transformation of peritoneal epithelium to mucin-secreting epithelium and results in the gradual accumulation of gelatinous material in the abdomen and pelvis.

Benign cystic teratomas (dermoids) result from neoplastic growth of totipotent cells, which cause a mass composed of any or all of the following: skin, bone, teeth, hair, and dermal tissue. They characteristically contain calcium deposits and fat. Dermoids are bilateral in 10% of cases and have a relatively high incidence of torsion. Malignant transformation occurs in less than 2% of these masses. More than 75% of these transformations will occur in women older than 40 years. In all women for whom fertility is an important consideration, the surgical procedure of choice is an ovarian cystectomy with conservation of as much normal ovarian cortex as possible.

Benign Uterine Conditions

Uterine neoplasms are predominately benign in origin and are extremely common in women of all age groups. The most common of these are leiomyomas (fibroids). These tumors increase in incidence with age until menopause. Because leiomyomas are estrogen sensitive, there is a gradual decrease in size after menopause. Their incidence is higher in the African American population, affecting approximately 50% of the population at age 50, and is lowest in the Asian population. Fibroids can present in many ways, including lower abdominal pain, sensations of mass, urinary/bowel symptoms, and abnormal vaginal bleeding.

Treatment of fibroids can vary depending on the presentation, age, position, number, and desire to preserve fertility in the individual patient. The treatment modalities include surgical and medical management. Surgical management can include hysteroscopy, laparoscopy, and laparotomy, either to resect the fibroids (myomectomy) or perform a hysterectomy. Uterine artery embolization, performed by interventional radiologists, is a less-invasive option for the treatment of symptomatic fibroids. Patients who are poor surgical candidates, or who wish to preserve their uterus (although effect on future pregnancy is unclear), and those with relatively smaller, less numerous myomas, are good candidates for this treatment. Medical management is predominately in the form of a GnRH agonist, which inhibits the hypothalamic–pituitary axis and results in the inhibition of estrogen production by the ovaries. Nonsteroidal anti-inflammatory drugs (NSAIDs) have also been used for symptomatic pain in fibroids. Bleeding due to myomas can also be treated with NSAIDS, oral contraceptives (OCPs), GnRH analogs, or surgery.

Adenomyosis is a benign uterine condition in which the endometrial glands and stroma exist within the myometrium of the uterus. This causes hypertrophy of the myometrial tissue, resulting in a diffusely enlarged uterus, often having a globular appearance. The most common presenting symptoms are menorrhagia (heavy menstrual bleeding) and dysmenorrhea (painful menses). While a definitive diagnosis of adenomyosis can be made only with histologic confirmation, a presumptive diagnosis is often made based on symptoms and radiographic features. MRI is the most useful radiographic tool for the diagnosis of adenomyosis—there is generally increased signal intensity in areas of adenomyosis on T2-weighted imaging. Many treatment options have been proposed and used with some efficacy, although none are well tested. These include intrauterine progestin-containing devices, oral contraceptives, uterine artery embolization, and laparoscopic resection of adenomyosis. The only definitive treatment for adenomyosis is hysterectomy (with or without ovarian conservation).

Ectopic Pregnancy

Ectopic pregnancy is responsible for 15% of all maternal deaths in this country. In the United States, there are 16 ectopic pregnancies per 1,000 pregnancies annually. The major risk factors for ectopic pregnancy are tubal damage from tubal inflammation, infection, use of tobacco, or prior abdominal surgery. Therefore, previous PID, prior ectopic pregnancy, and previous tubal surgery (tubal ligation or tubal reanastomosis) are risk factors for ectopic pregnancy.

The presentation of this condition is variable, ranging from an incidental diagnosis in an asymptomatic patient to hemorrhagic shock. However, common symptoms include amenorrhea, abdominal cramping, and abnormal vaginal bleeding. Serial β-hCG measurements and transvaginal US are helpful in establishing the diagnosis. In a normal intrauterine pregnancy, the β-hCG level increases by at least 66% every 48 hours. If the β-hCG level rises appropriately, US should be performed when a level of 1,500 to 2,000 IU/mL is reached, in order to diagnose an intrauterine pregnancy. This range, called the discriminatory zone, is the earliest that an intrauterine pregnancy can be reliably visualized by *transvaginal* US. If the β-hCG level fails to rise appropriately, ectopic pregnancy must be suspected.

The natural progression for an ectopic pregnancy may lead to expulsion from the fimbriated end of the fallopian tube (tubal abortion), involution of the conceptus within the tube, or tubal rupture. If the diagnosis remains uncertain following initial evaluation of a hemodynamically stable patient, serial β-hCG levels may be followed until the location of the pregnancy can be confirmed on US. However, emergent laparotomy or laparoscopy is indicated in patients with hemodynamic instability.

The treatment options for a diagnosed ectopic pregnancy include both medical and surgical management. Medical management is reserved for patients who fulfill the following strict clinical criteria:

- Hemodynamic stability
- β-hCG < 5,000 mIU/mL
- Tubal/mass size less than 3 cm on US
- No evidence of fetal cardiac activity
- Ability and reliability to present for posttreatment monitoring

Options for surgical intervention are linear salpingostomy or salpingectomy via laparoscopy or laparotomy. After diagnosis and treatment of an ectopic pregnancy, it is imperative that β-hCG levels are followed until they are undetectable in the blood, as there are failure rates with both medical and surgical management. If the entire ectopic pregnancy is removed by salpingectomy, it can be presumed that all pregnancy tissue has been excised, and β-hCG levels do not need to be followed. If one fallopian tube is removed, and the other fallopian tube is normal, patients do not suffer any appreciable decrement to future fertility.

Infertility

Infertility is a complex disorder that has economic, psychological, and medical implications. Approximately 33% of infertility is attributed to female factors, 33% is attributed to male factors, and 33% is of unknown etiology. The most common causes of female factor infertility are ovulatory dysfunction, fallopian tube dysfunction (secondary to pelvic adhesions and infection), endometriosis, congenital uterine abnormalities, and cervical factors. While *in vitro* fertilization has decreased the overall impact of obstructive and anatomic factors on infertility, there are still many surgical procedures designed to restore normal anatomy in the pelvis in an attempt to improve a patient's fertility. In the setting of pelvic adhesions from previous surgery, appendicitis, or PID, *diagnostic laparoscopy* with lysis of adhesions is an early step in the treatment of infertility. *Chromopertubation* is a diagnostic and sometimes therapeutic procedure in which dye is injected via the cervix through the fallopian tubes to evaluate their patency under direct laparoscopic visualization. Hydrosalpinges, which are dilated fallopian tubes caused by distal tubal obstruction, are known to decrease the success rate of *in vitro* fertilization, and so are often surgically removed prior to treatment. *Myomectomy* and *resection of uterine septae/horns* are performed either abdominally or hysteroscopically to restore a normally shaped endometrial cavity. Lastly, in patients with previous tubal ligation or known tubal occlusion, *tubotubo reanastomosis* and *tuboplasty* are infrequently performed to restore the patency of the fallopian tubes. In general, obstructions due to pelvic adhesive disease should be prevented—timely treatment of appendicitis and PID in young women may obviate the need for future fertility-restoring procedures.

MANAGEMENT OF MALIGNANT GYNECOLOGIC CONDITIONS

Uterine Malignancies

Endometrial carcinoma is the most common pelvic malignancy in the United States. There are approximately 49,500 new cases and 8,200 deaths due to endometrial carcinoma annually. In general, exposure to unopposed estrogen increases a woman's risk for endometrial carcinoma. More specifically, the most common risk factors for endometrial carcinoma include nulliparity, menopause after age 52, obesity, prolonged estrogen exposure, use of estrogen replacement without concurrent use of progesterone during menopause, tamoxifen use, and diabetes. Inherited susceptibility to endometrial cancer is also seen in *Lynch syndrome*, which is an autosomal dominant condition that increases the risk of endometrial, ovarian, and colon cancer due to defects in mismatch repair genes (see Chapter 12). Lynch syndrome accounts for approximately 5% of endometrial cancer cases and can increase a woman's lifetime risk of endometrial cancer to 70%.

Endometrial carcinoma is typically classified into two types: Type I, the most common and estrogen associated, includes low and moderate-grade endometrioid adenocarcinoma, which accounts for 80% of all endometrial cancers. Type II cancers, which include papillary serous, clear cell, and undifferentiated carcinoma, are more aggressive and have risk factors, molecular etiology, and recurrence patterns distinct from type I cancers. Histologic grading of endometrial cancer is performed based on the International Federation of Gynecology and Obstetrics (FIGO) system. In general, as tumors become less differentiated and higher grade, they exhibit more solid and less glandular components.

Ninety percent of women with endometrial carcinoma present with vaginal bleeding or discharge; however, only 10% of postmenopausal women with these symptoms actually have endometrial carcinoma. In order to obtain a tissue diagnosis, the patient should first undergo an office endometrial biopsy, where a small piece of endometrial tissue is removed from the uterus using a thin curette. If the tissue obtained is insufficient, or if the biopsy is not feasible due to body habitus, anatomic factors, or medical history, a dilation and curettage ± hysteroscopy should be performed. In this procedure, a survey of the endometrial cavity may be made using the hysteroscope in order to evaluate for anatomic abnormalities (e.g., polyp, fibroid, etc.). The endometrium is then thoroughly sampled using a curette, and the tissue is sent for pathologic evaluation. The results may indicate normal endometrium, benign polyps, endometrial atrophy, endometrial hyperplasia, or carcinoma. Transvaginal ultrasonography is also highly accurate in determining the thickness of the endometrial stripe and may be helpful as an adjunctive study. A sonographic endometrial thickness of greater than or equal to 5 mm or a polypoid endometrial mass are considered suspicious findings for endometrial pathology in postmenopausal woman who are not taking exogenous hormones. Endometrial cancer is very rarely diagnosed when the endometrial thickness is 4 mm or less.

Endometrial carcinoma is surgically staged (Table 28.3). The procedure requires total hysterectomy, bilateral salpingo-oophorectomy, and pelvic and para-aortic lymph node sampling in selected patients. Any extrauterine lesions may also be debulked. Traditionally, surgery is accomplished via laparotomy, but appropriate candidates may undergo minimally invasive surgery via laparoscopic-assisted vaginal hysterectomy or total laparoscopic hysterectomy and laparoscopic staging. Robotic surgery is an increasingly utilized option as well. Because of the exfoliative nature of the tumor, patients with uterine papillary serous carcinomas undergo extended surgical staging and cytoreduction, similar to that performed for patients with ovarian cancer. This includes omentectomy, peritoneal biopsies, nodal sampling, and peritoneal washings. If obvious extrauterine tumor is noted, debulking of all gross tumor is the goal. Following surgical staging and treatment, some women may require adjuvant chemotherapy and/or radiation therapy.

Adjuvant radiation treatment of early stage, intermediate risk disease decreases the risk of local recurrence from 15% to nearly 7%. External beam radiation therapy is indicated for cervical involvement, pelvic lymph node metastases, or pelvic disease outside the uterus. Vaginal brachytherapy may also be utilized. Women with para-aortic lymph node metastases receive extended field radiation therapy to include the common iliac and para-aortic lymph nodes. Chemotherapy and hormonal therapy may be utilized for the treatment of advanced or recurrent disease. Whole abdominal radiation therapy was historically performed for women with stage III or IV disease, but recent evidence suggests that chemotherapy is equally or more effective and less morbid.

Posttreatment surveillance is performed by serial examination and symptom review, with imaging if indicated. The most common sites of recurrence are locoregional at the vaginal cuff and pelvis. Distant recurrence may also be seen, specifically in the lung, abdomen, lymph nodes, liver, brain, and bone.

Uterine sarcomas represent a small percentage of uterine malignancies, with an annual incidence of 1.7 per 100,000 women greater than 20 years of age. Sarcomas generally present with abdominal pain and a rapidly enlarging uterus. Leiomyosarcomas are commonly misdiagnosed preoperatively as benign uterine fibroids. Women who have received pelvic irradiation are at increased risk for developing uterine sarcomas. There are three major histologic variants: endometrial stromal sarcoma, leiomyosarcoma, and malignant mixed müllerian tumor. Endometrial stromal sarcoma produces an enlarged uterus with a soft yellow-gray necrotic and hemorrhagic

TABLE 28.3 Staging and grading of endometrial carcinoma

2010 FIGO surgical staging for endometrial carcinoma	
Stage I	Tumor confined to the corpus uteri
IA	No or less than half myometrial invasion
IB	Invasion equal to or more than half the myometrium
Stage II	Tumor invades cervical stroma but does not extend beyond the uterus[a]
Stage III	Local and/or regional spread of the tumor
IIIA	Tumor invades the serosa of the corpus uteri and/or adnexae[b]
IIIB	Vaginal and/or parametrial involvement[b]
IIIC	Metastases to pelvic and/or para-aortic lymph nodes[b]
IIIC1	Positive pelvic nodes
IIIC2	Positive para-aortic lymph nodes with or without positive pelvic lymph nodes
Stage IV	Tumor invades the bladder and/or bowel mucosa, and/or distant metastases
IVA	Tumor invasion of the bladder and/or bowel mucosa
IVB	Distant metastases, including intra-abdominal metastases and/or inguinal lymph nodes

[a]Endocervical glandular involvement only should be considered as stage I and no longer as stage II.

[b]Positive cytology has to be reported separately without changing the stage.

mass. Leiomyosarcoma originates from uterine smooth muscle and is differentiated from a leiomyoma by the number of mitotic figures per high-power field, cytologic atypia, and necrosis. Although leiomyomas may coexist with a leiomyosarcoma, they are distinct entities, and leiomyosarcomas have never been reported to arise from a leiomyoma. Malignant mixed müllerian tumors, now more commonly known as carcinosarcomas, consist of both sarcomatous elements and malignant epithelial elements. Based on their epidemiology and behavior, it is now believed that carcinosarcomas are better classified as an aggressive variant of endometrial carcinoma, rather than a uterine sarcoma, as it has been traditionally classified. Uterine sarcoma is generally treated with total hysterectomy and bilateral salpingo-oophorectomy. The utility of adjuvant treatment is controversial, depends on the cell type, and may consist of hormonal therapy, chemotherapy, and/or radiation.

Ovarian Malignancies

In the United States, ovarian carcinoma is the second most common gynecologic malignancy after endometrial carcinoma, but it is the most frequent cause of death from any pelvic malignancy. The higher death rate is due, in part, to the late stage at which ovarian carcinoma is typically detected.

Although most cases of ovarian cancer are sporadic, approximately 10% to 15% of ovarian cancer cases are due to inherited causes such as mutations in *BRCA1* and *BRCA2* (*BRCA1/2*) as well as Lynch syndrome. These conditions cause a marked increase in a woman's lifetime risk of ovarian cancer, and thus, these patients are followed closely and often undergo early risk-reducing salpingo-oophorectomy. These conditions also cause an increased risk of cancers that a general surgeon may commonly encounter, such as the breast and pancreas (*BRCA1/2*) and colon (Lynch). This underscores the importance of taking a thorough family history, as it may lead to lifesaving preventive measures for patients and their families.

There are three major histologic types of ovarian cancer: epithelial, germ cell, and sex cord stromal. Epithelial tumors arise from the fimbriated ends of the fallopian tube or ovarian surface epithelial cells and account for 70% of all ovarian malignancies. Germ cell tumors originate from embryonic and extraembryonic tissues and are responsible for 15% of ovarian malignancies. Sex cord stromal tumors contain elements that recapitulate the ovary or the testis and account for 10% of ovarian malignancies. They have the capacity to stimulate sex steroid hormone secretion or may themselves be hormonally active. Gonadoblastomas are tumors composed of both sex cord elements and germ cell elements. They are found in dysgenic gonads, particularly when a Y chromosome is present in the patient's karyotype. Women with these genotypic abnormalities require removal of their gonads to prevent this rare tumor. Five percent of cancers in the ovary are metastatic lesions, most commonly from the gastrointestinal tract, breast, or endometrium.

Epithelial ovarian cancer (EOC) is a very heterogeneous disease and is often broadly classified into two categories. Type I tends to be more indolent and encompasses the low-grade carcinomas, such as mucinous, and low-grade serous carcinoma. Type II EOC, which is the most common, aggressive, and lethal, is composed mainly of high-grade serous carcinoma, which clinically behaves identically to fallopian tube and primary peritoneal carcinoma. These entities are often challenging to distinguish from one another and are treated identically. In recent years, there has been increasing evidence that most high-grade serous ovarian carcinomas may in fact originate from distal fallopian tube precursor lesions.

There are many risk factors that increase the chance of developing EOC. In general, an increase in the number of ovulatory cycles in a patient's lifetime increases the risk of developing ovarian carcinoma. For example, frequent ovulation, late menopause, infertility, and nulliparity increase a woman's risk of this malignancy. In contrast, multiparity, breast-feeding, and the use of hormonal contraceptive methods decrease a woman's risk for this disease. Tubal ligation and hysterectomy with ovarian conservation are also associated with a decreased risk of ovarian cancer, but this may be due to the opportunity to directly visualize the ovaries at the time of surgery and to intervene if otherwise asymptomatic abnormalities are identified.

Epithelial ovarian carcinoma spreads by direct extension along peritoneal surfaces throughout the abdomen and pelvis. Because the ovaries are intrapelvic organs and ovarian tumors are usually asymptomatic, the disease has usually spread beyond the ovaries before any signs or symptoms of the malignancy are present. Patients may complain of a distended abdomen and vague gastrointestinal symptoms such as bloating and early satiety. Physical examination may reveal ascites and an abdominal or pelvic mass. The preoperative evaluation includes basic laboratory studies, a CA125 level, and imaging of the abdomen and pelvis (usually a CT).

Staging of ovarian carcinoma is performed surgically (Table 28.4). During this procedure, ascites or peritoneal washings are sent for cytologic examination, the undersurface of the diaphragm is sampled, all suspicious nodules are removed, random peritoneal biopsies, pelvic and para-aortic lymph node sampling, omentectomy, and a total abdominal hysterectomy with bilateral salpingo-oophorectomy are performed. Up to 30% of cases that appear clinically to be confined to the ovary actually have occult spread to lymph nodes or the upper abdomen, making correct staging critical for determining the appropriate postoperative treatment.

Twenty percent of all ovarian epithelial carcinomas are classified as borderline. These tumors consist of malignant cells that are not invasive. Women with this condition require an appropriate staging procedure. In young women desirous of retaining reproductive capacity, unilateral salpingo-oophorectomy can be performed if the tumor is confined to one ovary, and the contralateral ovary appears normal. With resection alone, the 5-year survival rate approaches 90%. Adjuvant chemotherapy and radiation therapy are reserved for patients whose tumor demonstrates invasive implants.

For patients with advanced disease, the goal of surgery is not merely to stage the cancer but to perform maximal cytoreduction of all visible lesions. This may include bowel resection or radical procedures such as diaphragm stripping or splenectomy at the discretion of the surgeon. Patients who achieve optimal cytoreduction have improved overall survival and a better response to adjuvant chemotherapy.

Patients with high-risk stage I disease as well as those with stage II–IV disease benefit from adjuvant postoperative chemotherapy. For advanced disease, first-line chemotherapy often consists of combination taxane and platinum administered every 3 weeks for six to eight cycles. Patients who are able to achieve optimal cytoreduction may be candidates for combination intravenous and intraperitoneal chemotherapy, which is administered through an implanted intraperitoneal Port-a-Cath. Patients are followed with serial physical examinations, CT examinations, and serum CA125 levels. Exponential regression of a patient's CA125 level suggests response to this regimen.

TABLE 28.4 2014 FIGO staging of primary carcinoma of the ovary, fallopian tube, and peritoneum

Stage I	Tumor confined to the ovaries or fallopian tube(s)
IA	Tumor limited to one ovary (capsule intact) or fallopian tube; no tumor on surface, negative washings
IB	Tumor involves both ovaries or fallopian tubes, otherwise like IA
IC	Tumor limited to one or both ovaries or fallopian tubes, with any of the following:
IC1	Surgical spill
IC2	Capsule rupture before surgery or tumor on ovarian or tubal surface
IC3	Malignant cells in the ascites or peritoneal washings
Stage II	Tumor involves one or both ovaries or fallopian tubes with pelvic extension (below the pelvic brim) or primary peritoneal cancer
IIA	Extension and/or implant on the uterus and/or fallopian tubes and/or ovaries
IIB	Extension to other pelvic intraperitoneal tissues
Stage III	Tumor involves one or both ovaries or fallopian tubes, or primary peritoneal cancer, with cytologically or histologically confirmed spread to the peritoneum outside the pelvis and/or metastasis to the retroperitoneal lymph nodes
IIIA	Positive retroperitoneal lymph nodes and/or microscopic metastasis beyond the pelvis
IIIA1	Positive retroperitoneal lymph nodes only
IIIA1(i)	Metastasis ≤10 mm in greatest dimension
IIIA1(ii)	Metastasis >10 mm in greatest dimension
IIIA2	Microscopic, extrapelvic (above the pelvic brim) peritoneal involvement ± positive retroperitoneal lymph nodes
IIIB	Macroscopic, extrapelvic, peritoneal metastasis ≤2 cm ± positive retroperitoneal lymph nodes. Includes extension to capsule of the liver/spleen
IIIC	Macroscopic, extrapelvic, peritoneal metastasis >2 cm ± positive retroperitoneal lymph nodes. Includes extension to capsule of the liver/spleen
Stage IV	Distant metastasis excluding peritoneal metastases
IVA	Pleural effusion with positive cytology
IVB	Hepatic and/or splenic parenchymal metastasis, metastasis to extra-abdominal organs (including inguinal lymph nodes and lymph nodes outside of the abdominal cavity)

Germ cell tumors generally occur in young, reproductive-age women. These tumors originate from the primitive germ cells and differentiate into embryonic (endoderm, mesoderm, and ectoderm) or extraembryonic (yolk sac or trophoblast) tissues. Dysgerminomas account for 45% of all malignant germ cell tumors, and immature teratomas and endodermal sinus tumors are the second most frequently occurring malignant germ cell tumors. Germ cell tumors are typically managed with conservative surgical resection (staging surgery with removal of the affected ovary and preservation of the contralateral ovary and uterus) in reproductive-age women followed by adjuvant chemotherapy in most situations.

Dysgerminomas are composed of primitive germ cells infiltrated by lymphocytes. They represent approximately 1% of all ovarian malignancies. Dysgerminomas are found primarily in women younger than 30 years old. In 10% of the patients, they are found on both ovaries. Conservative surgical resection of the affected ovary along with surgical staging is performed. While these tumors are very sensitive to radiation therapy, multiagent chemotherapy with cisplatin, bleomycin, and etoposide is the adjuvant therapy of choice given that almost all patients are of reproductive age.

Endodermal sinus tumors (yolk sac tumors) account for approximately 10% of malignant germ cell tumors. This tumor resembles the extraembryonic tissue of the yolk sac and secretes α-fetoprotein (AFP), which is used as a marker to follow disease progression and response to treatment. Before the development of multiagent chemotherapy, endodermal sinus tumors were universally fatal. At present, they may be successfully treated with cisplatin, bleomycin, and etoposide.

Choriocarcinoma of the ovary is a highly malignant, rare form of germ cell tumor. This tumor resembles the extraembryonic tissue of the cytotrophoblast and the syncytiotrophoblast. Human chorionic gonadotropin (hCG) is the tumor marker used to follow disease progression and response to treatment. In the past, choriocarcinoma was also a universally fatal disease; however, multiagent chemotherapy now provides improved response rates for this disease.

The histology of *sex cord stromal tumors* resembles the sex cord and specialized stroma of the developing gonad. In the ovary, the granulosa cells represent the sex cord tissue and the theca cells represent the specialized stroma. Granulosa theca cell tumors are low-grade malignancies that often secrete estrogen. This excess estrogen can be responsible for a range of symptoms from precocious puberty to postmenopausal bleeding and necessitates endometrial sampling as resulting endometrial hyperplasia or carcinoma may be found in up to 30% of patients with granulosa cell tumors. These tumors are identified histologically by the presence of *Call–Exner bodies*, which are eosinophilic bodies surrounded by granulosa cells. Sertoli–Leydig tumors are also low-grade malignancies that replicate testicular elements. In 75% to 80% of patients, these tumors produce androgens. As a result, women may present with amenorrhea, breast atrophy, acne, hirsutism, clitoromegaly, increased muscle tone, deepening of the voice, and male pattern baldness. Treatment for both of these tumors requires surgical excision followed by multiagent chemotherapy. Once a patient has completed childbearing, the contralateral ovary should be removed.

Malignancies Metastatic to the Ovary

Most tumors metastatic to the ovary originate from malignancies of other pelvic organs such as the uterus or the fallopian tube. The most common distant sites of origin include the breasts and the gastrointestinal tract. A *Krukenberg tumor* is a specialized type of gastrointestinal tumor metastatic to the ovary. This tumor contains signet ring cells filled with mucin in an acellular stroma. The stomach and the large intestine are the most common sites of origin. Bilateral ovarian masses with surface deposits should warrant suspicion of metastatic disease and a thorough evaluation for an extraovarian primary.

Vaginal Carcinoma

Vaginal carcinomas are rare and make up less than 2% of all gynecologic malignancies. Eighty percent of these carcinomas are squamous cell, and the remaining are adenocarcinomas, melanomas, and sarcomas. For women with a history of cervical or vulvar carcinoma, a vaginal lesion appearing at least 5 years after the initial malignancy is considered a primary vaginal cancer and not a recurrence of their original disease. Most women present with abnormal vaginal bleeding or abnormal vaginal discharge. This malignancy spreads by direct extension to the pelvic soft tissues. Hematogenous dissemination to the lungs, liver, and bone occurs late in the disease. The diagnosis is confirmed by a biopsy of the vaginal lesion. The mainstay of treatment is radiation therapy to the vagina with surgical therapy as an option only for young women whose disease is limited to the upper vagina.

Vulvar Carcinoma

Squamous cell carcinoma accounts for 90% of vulvar malignancies. Five percent of vulvar malignancies are melanomas. Another 5% are adenocarcinomas, verrucous carcinomas, basal cell carcinomas, and sarcomas. Most women complain of perineal bleeding, a lesion that fails to heal, and pruritus. On physical examination, a polypoid mass may be found on the vulva; clinically suspicious lesions should be biopsied as early treatment can be curative and considerably less morbid. This tumor spreads via the lymphatic system to the superficial inguinal femoral lymph nodes and to the deep pelvic, obturator, and iliac lymph nodes. Treatment consists of a radical vulvectomy with a gross 1- to 2-cm margin. Flap reconstruction may be necessary to fill in the defect created by resection, and a unilateral or bilateral gracilis flap is usually employed depending on the size of the defect. If the primary lesion demonstrates more than 1 mm of invasion, superficial and deep inguinofemoral lymphadenectomy is performed as well. Sentinel lymph node sampling may be performed in place of full lymphadenectomy for initial evaluation of lymphatic spread. Bilateral lymphadenectomy or sentinel lymph node sampling is indicated if the primary lesion is within 2 cm of the midline given the decussation of the lymphatics in the area. Adjuvant radiation therapy to the primary tumor bed and the groins may be considered in certain circumstances.

Gestational Trophoblastic Disease

Gestational trophoblastic disease (GTD) is composed of a rare spectrum of tumors that includes complete hydatidiform mole, partial hydatidiform mole, placental site trophoblastic tumor, and choriocarcinoma. In the United States, the incidence of GTD is 0.6 to 1.1 per 1,000 pregnancies. Risk factors for GTD include maternal age less than 15 and greater than 40 years, prior history of GTD, and vitamin A deficiency. A higher incidence is seen in many Asian countries.

Complete hydatidiform moles lack fetal tissue but contain chorionic villi with hydatidiform swelling and trophoblastic hyperplasia. In 90% of cases, the karyotype is 46XX; however, all of the chromosomes are of paternal origin, either by fertilization of an egg by a single sperm cell or two sperm cells in an ovum devoid of maternal DNA. Partial hydatidiform moles have chorionic villi with focal hydatidiform swelling and trophoblastic hyperplasia, but in this scenario, identifiable fetal parts may be present with this form of GTD. Partial moles have a triploid karyotype, and the extra set of chromosomes is of paternal origin. Complete and partial molar pregnancies usually present with abnormal bleeding. Molar pregnancies may also present with excess uterine size, hyperemesis gravidarum, hyperthyroidism, and prominent theca lutein ovarian cysts. An abnormally elevated β-hCG level and transvaginal US usually confirm the diagnosis. A complete mole has a characteristic vesicular sonographic pattern, whereas a partial mole has cystic spaces in the placental tissue and an increase in the transverse diameter of the gestational sac (Fig. 28.11.) Treatment begins with evacuation of the uterine contents by suction curettage. Women are followed after uterine evacuation with serial β-hCG levels. Concurrent contraception is prescribed to prevent a subsequent pregnancy, which will interfere with the monitoring of the disease. If the β-hCG level does not fall to zero or begins to increase, the patient is presumed to have persistent disease and may be at risk for distant metastases. In complete moles, local invasion occurs in 15% of patients and metastases occur in 4% of patients. In contrast, partial molar gestations will have a persistent nonmetastatic tumor in 4% of the patients. Persistent or low-risk metastatic GTD is considered the most treatable gynecologic malignancy and is frequently cured with single-agent methotrexate. High-risk metastatic disease is treated by using combination chemotherapy.

Cervical Malignancies

Most neoplastic changes of the cervix occur in the "transformation zone," the area of squamous metaplasia at the boundary of the endocervical canal and the ectocervix. The premalignant changes of the cervix are considered a continuum from mild-to-severe dysplasia. The predominant descriptive pathologic system used to describe these changes on screening Pap tests is the Bethesda system. The Bethesda system classifies premalignant changes into atypical squamous cells of undetermined significance (ASCUS), low-grade squamous intraepithelial lesion (LGSIL), and high-grade squamous

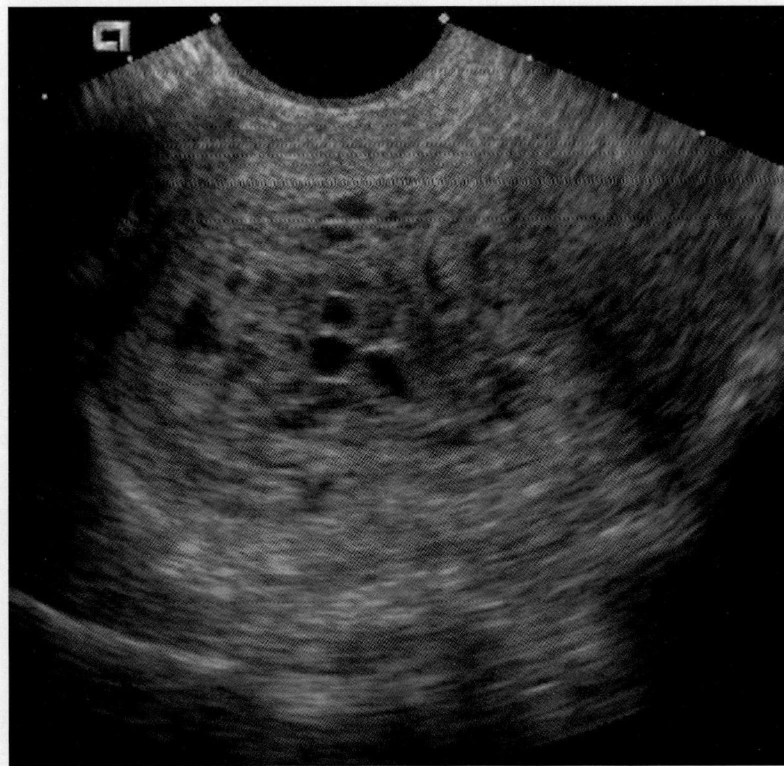

FIGURE 28.11 Ultrasonogram of a uterus showing a typical pattern of a complete hydatidiform mole. (From Berek JS. *Berek & Novak's Gynecology*. 14th ed. Philadelphia: Lippincott Willams & Wilkins; 2007:1589, with permission)

intraepithelial lesion (HGSIL). LGSIL indicates koilocytotic change and mild dysplasia. HGSIL indicates moderate-to-severe dysplasia.

The major risk factor for cervical neoplastic changes is infection with a high-risk type of human papillomavirus (HPV). Because exposure to HPV is via sexual contact, other risk factors include early age at first sexual intercourse, multiple sexual partners, early childbearing (<20 years of age at first birth), prostitution, sexually transmitted diseases, and immunocompromised states. HPV subtypes 16, 18, 31, 33, 35, 39, 45, 51, 52, 56, and 58 are associated with cervical carcinoma. The quadrivalent HPV vaccine is designed to prevent primary infection with the most common high-risk subtypes, 16 and 18, which are responsible for 70% of cervical cancers, as well as two common condyloma causing low-risk subtypes, 6 and 11.

The Pap test is the primary screening test for cervical dysplasia. If a Pap test demonstrates abnormal cytology or the presence of high-risk HPV subtypes, a colposcopy is usually performed accompanied by cervical biopsies. The colposcope is a binocular microscope that can magnify the cervix 10 to 16 times. The Pap test, findings on colposcopy, and histology from the cervical biopsies are used together to form a diagnosis. Mild dysplasia (cervical intraepithelial neoplasia grade 1, or CIN1) has a spontaneous regression rate of up to 70% and can be followed by regular Pap tests with colposcopic examinations if warranted. CIN2 and 3 are generally treated with excisional or ablative therapies. There are multiple techniques that can be used for excisional therapy such as cold knife cone biopsy or loop electrocautery excision. Laser and cryotherapy can also be used to destroy certain lesions, but a biopsy specimen is not produced to confirm the diagnosis. Ablative methods also preclude the ability to rule out microinvasive cancers and thus are not utilized when there is any suspicion of cancer or when lesions are present in the endocervical canal (and not visible). HIV-positive patients and other immunosuppressed patients may have particularly aggressive disease and may experience unpredictable progression. Therefore, curative surgery is initiated sooner in these patients.

Cervical carcinoma is the third most frequently occurring gynecologic malignancy in the United States. There are 12,000 new cases and 4,000 deaths due to cervical carcinoma annually. Most women present with abnormal bleeding, classically postcoital bleeding, or brown vaginal discharge after intercourse or between menstrual cycles. The diagnosis of cervical carcinoma is made by biopsy of the tumor, and the extent of cervical involvement is determined by a cone biopsy of the cervix.

Seventy percent of cervical carcinomas are squamous cell carcinomas, and 25% are adenocarcinomas, with the incidence of the latter increasing in recent decades. This malignancy infiltrates locally, and disease spreads laterally and inferiorly from the cervix to the vagina and paracervical and parametrial tissues. Lymphatic spread is not uncommon, though hematogenous metastases are a late complication of cervical carcinoma and most commonly involve the lung, liver, and bone.

Cervical carcinoma is staged clinically (Table 28.5). Initial evaluation of cervical carcinoma includes a history and physical examination, laboratory studies, an intravenous pyelogram or computerized tomography (CT), and a chest x-ray. An examination under anesthesia, cystoscopy, and proctoscopy with biopsies as needed are then performed. These examinations provide information about the spread of disease to the parametrial tissues, bladder, and rectum. Once the evaluation has been completed, the patient is assigned a clinical stage and a course of therapy is determined.

Women with stage Ia_1 cervical carcinoma have microinvasive disease and may be treated with a cone biopsy (if the ability to retain potential for childbearing is important) or a simple extrafascial hysterectomy. Women with stage Ia_2, Ib, or IIa may be treated

TABLE 28.5 2010 FIGO staging of carcinoma of the cervix uteri

Stage I	The carcinoma is strictly confined to the cervix (extension to the corpus would be disregarded)
IA	Invasive carcinoma that can be diagnosed only by microscopy, with deepest invasion ≤5.0 mm and largest extension ≥7.0 mm
IA1	Measured stromal invasion of ≤3.0 mm in depth and horizontal extension of ≤7.0 mm
IA2	Measured stromal invasion >3.0 mm and not >5.0 mm with an extension of not >7.0 mm
IB	Clinically visible lesions limited to the cervix uteri or preclinical cancers greater than stage IA[a]
IB1	Clinically visible lesion ≤4.0 cm in greatest dimension
IB2	Clinically visible lesion >4.0 cm in greatest dimension
Stage II	Cervical carcinoma invades beyond the uterus but not to the pelvic wall or to the lower third of the vagina
IIA	Without parametrial invasion
IIA1	Clinically visible lesion ≤4.0 cm in greatest dimension
IIA2	Clinically visible lesion >4.0 cm in greatest dimension
IIB	With obvious parametrial invasion
Stage III	The tumor extends to the pelvic wall and/or involves lower third of the vagina and/or causes hydronephrosis or nonfunctioning kidney[b]
IIIA	Tumor involves lower one third of the vagina, with no extension to the pelvic wall
IIIB	Extension to the pelvic wall and/or hydronephrosis or nonfunctioning kidney
Stage IV	The carcinoma has extended beyond the true pelvis or has involved (biopsy proven) the mucosa of the bladder or rectum. A bullous edema, as such, does not permit a case to be allotted to stage IV
IVA	Spread of the growth to adjacent organs
IVB	Spread to distant organs

[a]All macroscopically visible lesions—even with superficial invasion—are allotted to stage IB carcinomas. Invasion is limited to a measured stromal invasion with a maximal depth of 5.00 mm and a horizontal extension of not >7.00 mm. Depth of invasion should not be >5.00 mm taken from the base of the epithelium of the original tissue—superficial or glandular. The depth of invasion should always be reported in millimeters, even in those cases with "early (minimal) stromal invasion" (~1 mm). The involvement of vascular/lymphatic spaces should not change the stage allotment.

[b]On rectal examination, there is no cancer-free space between the tumor and the pelvic wall. All cases with hydronephrosis or nonfunctioning kidney are included, unless they are known to be due to another cause.

with either radical hysterectomy and lymph node dissection or primary radiation therapy combined with radiosensitizing chemotherapy. Primary radiation and chemotherapy is the preferred route of treatment for older women with multiple medical problems, but radical hysterectomy with ovarian preservation is usually the best choice for younger women. Radical trachelectomy may also be considered if fertility preservation is paramount.

Surgery generally commences with exploratory laparotomy, though rates of minimally invasive radical hysterectomy are increasing steadily. Biopsy of any suspicious extrauterine lesions is performed for frozen section analysis. Additionally, para-aortic lymph nodes are also sampled for frozen section analysis. If disease is present outside of the pelvis, the procedure is aborted, and the patient is treated with primary radiation and chemotherapy. If biopsies are negative, the surgeon will proceed with radical hysterectomy. Radical hysterectomy includes removal of the uterus and cervix *en bloc* with the entire parametria out to the pelvic side wall and the upper third of the vagina. The uterine artery is ligated at its origin from the hypogastric artery, and the ureters are tunneled out from the parametria. Pelvic lymphadenectomy is also performed. The ovaries may be retained in younger patients to avoid surgical menopause. Uncommon postoperative complications include urinary fistulas or urinary retention due to severing of the nerves traveling near the uterosacral ligaments innervating the bladder. If examination of the lymph nodes demonstrates metastatic disease, the margins are positive, or deep penetration of the tumor is noted, then postoperative radiation and chemotherapy is warranted. Women with stage IIb or greater disease are treated with primary radiation and chemotherapy as definitive treatment.

One third of patients have recurrence of disease 6 months or more after primary treatment, 50% of which occur in the pelvis. Other common sites for recurrent disease include para-aortic lymph nodes, lung, liver, or bone. Surgical failures are treated with radiation alone or chemotherapy in combination with radiation therapy. Palliative chemotherapy regimens that include cisplatin and 5-fluorouracil may also be used as treatment for recurrent disease.

If preoperative evaluation can identify no metastatic disease, pelvic exenteration may be considered for patients with an isolated central pelvic recurrence that has failed radiation therapy. Patients undergo exploratory laparotomy with extensive biopsies. Frozen section analysis is performed on any suspicious lesions as well as both pelvic and para-aortic lymph node biopsies. Proven metastatic disease in any of these areas is sufficient indication to abort the procedure. Next, the pararectal and paravesical spaces are developed. Biopsies along the pelvic sidewalls in the area of the tumor are also sent for frozen section. If at any point metastatic disease is detected, the procedure is aborted. If no evidence of unresectable disease is found, the bladder with distal ureters, uterus/cervix (if still present), vagina, and rectum are removed *en bloc* with the accompanying parametria. Varying degrees of the vulva and perineum may also be resected depending on the distal extent of the tumor. Generally, two teams of surgeons are necessary to facilitate dissection from both the intra-abdominal and the perineal approaches. The reconstructive portion of the procedure generally involves end colostomy with urinary diversion. Typically, incontinent diversion with an ileal conduit is performed, or a continent urinary diversion may be performed via a modified Miami or Indiana pouch utilizing the distal ileum and ascending colon so that the ileal–cecal junction may be employed as a continence mechanism. Vaginal reconstruction may be performed with a myocutaneous flap, generally utilizing either unilateral or bilateral gracilis flaps depending on the size of the defect.

Occasionally, depending on the location of the lesion, either anterior (resection of the bladder, uterus/cervix, and vagina) or posterior (resection of the rectum, uterus/cervix, and vagina), exenteration is possible. However, if a prior radical hysterectomy has been performed, these more conservative procedures are often very difficult due to distortion of the anatomy and postoperative and/or postradiation adhesions, leaving total pelvic exenteration as the only option.

Suggested Readings

Barakat RR, Berchuck A, et al. eds. *Principles and Practice of Gynecologic Oncology*. 6th ed. Philadelphia: Lippincott Williams & Wilkins; 2013.

Berek JS, Novak E, eds. *Berek & Novak's Gynecology*. 15th ed. Philadelphia: Lippincott Williams & Wilkins; 2012.

Fritz MA, Speroff L, eds. *Clinical Gynecologic Endocrinology and Infertility*. 8th ed. Philadelphia: Lippincott Williams & Wilkins; 2011.

Hurt KJ, Guile MW, et al., eds. *The Johns Hopkins Manual of Gynecology and Obstetrics*. 4th ed. Philadelphia: Lippincott Williams & Wilkins; 2011.

Lentz GM, Lobo RA et al., eds. *Comprehensive Gynecology: Expert Consult—Online and Print*. 6th ed. Philadelphia: Mosby; 2012.

Morrow CP. *Morrow's Gynecologic Cancer Surgery*. 2nd ed. Encinitas: South Coast Medical Publishing; 2013.

Rock JA, Jones HW, eds. *TeLinde's Operative Gynecology*. 10th ed., updated. Philadelphia: Lippincott Williams & Wilkins; 2011.

Smith JR, Del Priore G, et al., eds. *An Atlas of Gynecologic Oncology*. 3rd ed. New York: Informa Healthcare; 2011.

CHAPTER

29 Otorhinolaryngology

ELIZABETH A. NICOLLI, SRI KIRAN CHENNUPATI, AND ARA A. CHALIAN

KEY POINTS

- Hearing loss is characterized as conductive, sensorineural, or mixed. Management varies based on etiology.
- Paranasal sinus infections are common. Surrounding structures, such as the eye, cavernous sinus, and brain, can become involved in untreated or inadequately treated cases.
- Approximately 80% of parotid neoplasms are benign. The most common parotid neoplasm is a pleomorphic adenoma. The most common parotid malignancy is mucoepidermoid carcinoma.
- The majority of cancers of the upper aerodigestive tract are squamous cell carcinomas. Tobacco and alcohol were traditionally implicated in their pathogenesis, but today, HPV plays a prominent role in these cancers.
- Malignancies from different subsites within the head and neck tend to metastasize to specific cervical lymph node chains, and understanding lymphatic drainage is important in management.
- Trauma to the face, mandible, and larynx can be associated with airway obstruction, which may require a surgical airway (tracheostomy).

INTRODUCTION

Otorhinolaryngology–head and neck surgery is a unique specialty that encompasses the management of disorders of hearing and balance, smell and taste, swallowing and voice, the skin and the neck, and more. There is collaboration with several other specialties as well as the opportunity to care for patients of all ages and types of diagnoses. Technically, the procedures can range from short in-office procedures to complex surgeries involving intricate microanatomy and multiple surgical teams. Moreover, otolaryngologists are called on to treat a variety of both common and rare disorders.

OTOLOGY

The Auditory System

The human auditory system is capable of hearing sounds from 20 to 20,000 Hz, with typical speech-exhibiting frequencies in the 500- to 4,000-Hz range. Sound intensities are measured on a logarithmic scale from 0 to 120 decibels (dB). An individual with normal hearing has a threshold for perception of sounds at 0- to 20-dB intensity. Normal conversational speech is in the 20- to 50-dB range. Amplification of sound is accomplished because of the ratio of vibrating tympanic membrane area to stapes footplate area (17:1) and the lever function of the ossicles (Fig. 29.1). These two factors yield an approximate 25-fold amplification of signal intensity delivered to the cochlea.

Conductive hearing loss may occur secondary to cerumen impaction, tympanic membrane perforation, middle ear effusion, or ossicular discontinuity. Otosclerosis, another cause of conductive hearing loss, is due to fixation of the stapes footplate at its articulation with the oval window. Otosclerosis is a disorder that affects predominantly middle-aged, white patients in an autosomal dominant fashion, with females being affected roughly twice as often as males. For surgical candidates, the stapes is mobilized or removed and replaced with a prosthesis.

Evidence of an asymmetric sensorineural hearing loss on audiogram merits workup to exclude tumors or masses of the vestibulocochlear nerve and cerebellopontine angle. In addition, both bacterial and viral infections such as meningitis can affect the cochlea and cochlear nerve. Neurologic and autoimmune conditions can also cause hearing loss, as can neoplasms and bone disorders such as osteogenesis imperfecta and Paget disease.

Several medications are known to be ototoxic and/or vestibulotoxic, including aminoglycosides, vancomycin, loop diuretics (furosemide), salicylates, nonsteroidal anti-inflammatory drugs (NSAIDs), and chemotherapeutic agents (cisplatin). With respect to ototoxicity, the hearing loss is typically bilateral (although it can be unilateral), begins after several days of treatment (although it may occur after one dose or even several months after the completion of therapy), and may be permanent. Patients requiring long-term treatment with ototoxic medications should therefore undergo baseline audiometric testing prior to treatment. In the elderly, when an etiology cannot be identified, the disorder is termed "presbycusis," or age-related hearing loss.

Treatment of hearing loss depends upon the etiology. With bacterial infections, appropriate antibiotic therapy is initiated. Autoimmune hearing loss may improve with steroids. Hearing loss from ototoxic medications or noise exposure is first managed by removing the offending agent. Tumors may require surgical excision, and congenital deafness may be improved with cochlear implantation or hearing aids.

In cases of stable, sensorineural hearing loss, hearing amplification devices can be worn in one or both ears. When patients have profound sensorineural hearing loss and receive minimal benefit from traditional hearing aids, they can be candidates for a cochlear implant. In a simplified description, these devices employ a wire

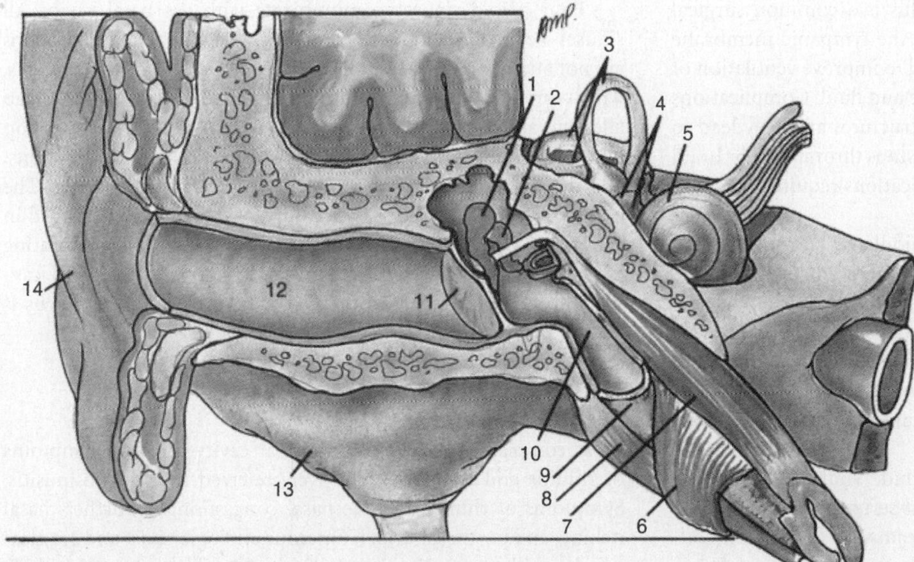

FIGURE 29.1 Structures of the ear: (*1*) malleus, (*2*) incus, (*3*) semicircular canals, (*4*) utricle and saccule, (*5*) cochlea, (*6*) dilator tubae muscle, (*7*) tensor tympani muscle, (*8*) levator veli palatini muscle, (*9*) cartilaginous auditory tube, (*10*) eustachian tube, (*11*) tympanic membrane, (*12*) external auditory canal, (*13*) mastoid, and (*14*) pinna.

electrode that is threaded into the cochlea and attached to a receiver that is anchored to the skull under skin flaps. The receiver converts sound into electrical impulses that are transmitted along the wire electrode into the cochlea, which are then relayed to the brain.

Balance and the Vestibular System

The perception of position, spatial orientation, acceleration, and rotation is accomplished through the synthesis of sensory input from peripheral muscles and ocular cues, as well as from the vestibular structures of the inner ear. Linear acceleration results in displacement of otoconia, small crystals of calcium carbonate in the saccule and utricle, producing neural impulses from the hair cells of the saccule and the utricle. This information is processed with impulses generated in the right and left semicircular canals, which perceive angular acceleration. Asymmetric firing of right and left vestibular systems produces the subjective sensation of rotation, or vertigo.

Common causes of vertigo include viral infection (vestibular neuritis), vascular compromise (stroke), benign paroxysmal positional vertigo (BPPV), and Meniere's disease. BPPV is a syndrome of recurrent short episodes of vertigo elicited by certain changes in head position. It is caused by otoconia, where tiny calcium crystals become dislodged and settle in one of the semicircular canals (most often the posterior semicircular canal). Treatment involves the Epley maneuver, a series of head motions that direct the crystals back into the utricle. Meniere's disease is a syndrome of unclear etiology, which presents with vertigo, tinnitus, aural fullness, and hearing loss. Seventy percent of cases are unilateral, with 30% of these cases developing contralateral symptoms within several years. Many treatments have been described to address the most distressing symptoms associated with intractable vertigo. These include fluid restriction, diuretics, intratympanic gentamicin injections, and labyrinthectomy.

Otologic Infection

Infections of the external and middle ear are common. Otitis externa is an infectious condition that typically affects the external auditory canal. Etiologic factors include water exposure ("swimmer's ear") and local trauma to the ear canal, which typically occurs when patients insert objects in the canal in an attempt to remove wax. The patient presents with symptoms of ear pain (otalgia) and ear drainage (otorrhea). On physical examination, the auricle and external canal may be erythematous and tender upon manipulation. The causative organisms are usually *Pseudomonas aeruginosa* and *Staphylococcus aureus*. Management includes debridement of the ear canal and application of antibiotic drops; severe cases may warrant the addition of oral antibiotics and insertion of a cotton wick to both stent open the ear canal and draw the medication to the medial surfaces of the external ear. Malignant otitis externa is a more serious infection of the external auditory canal seen in poorly controlled diabetics or immunocompromised patients. Infection can spread beyond the external auditory canal to involve the skull base, which may lead to cranial neuropathies, meningitis, venous sinus thrombosis, and death. Management includes strict glucose control, long-term antibiotics, surgical debridement of diseased bone, and drainage of any associated abscesses.

Inflammation of the middle ear is broadly referred to as otitis media. Briefly, the middle ear space houses the ossicles and is connected to the mastoid air cells posteriorly and to the nasopharynx via the eustachian tube anteriorly. This connection to the nasopharynx is what allows ventilation of an otherwise sealed space. When the eustachian tube is blocked or its function impaired, ventilation of the middle ear is disrupted and fluid accumulates. When sterile, this condition is referred to as serous otitis media. Acute otitis media results when the fluid becomes secondarily infected, and pain, fever, and possibly otorrhea from tympanic membrane rupture may be reported. Treatment consists of oral antibiotics directed at the usual pathogens: *Streptococcus pneumoniae, Haemophilus influenzae*, and *Moraxella catarrhalis*.

Acute otitis media in children is a common problem and is secondary to several factors. Adenoid hypertrophy blocks the eustachian tube orifice and also serves as a reservoir for bacteria, which may travel in a retrograde fashion into the middle ear. This is further facilitated by anatomic differences in the pediatric eustachian tube that make this retrograde travel easier. In children who experience recurrent bouts of acute otitis media or who have persistent sterile middle ear fluid causing speech and language delays, pressure equalization tubes may be indicated. This is a common surgical procedure where an incision is made in the tympanic membrane (myringotomy) and a small tube is placed to improve ventilation of the middle ear and relieve excess pressure and fluid. Complications of acute otitis media can involve local structures and may lead to facial nerve paralysis, meningitis, venous sinus thrombosis, or brain abscess. These potentially serious complications require aggressive medical and surgical management.

Chronic negative pressure in the middle ear can lead to the development of a cholesteatoma, which is an epithelial-lined cyst containing desquamated keratin. Growth of this histologically benign lesion can lead to erosion of the ossicles and may proceed to involve the semicircular canals, the facial nerve, and the brain. Surgical resection of the cholesteatoma with reconstruction of ossicles and tympanic membrane is required to restore functional hearing.

Additional infections of the ear include viral infections harbored in cranial nerve ganglia. The most serious is caused by the reactivation of the *varicella-zoster* virus leading to *herpes zoster oticus*, which is associated with *Ramsay Hunt syndrome*. The syndrome includes herpetic lesions seen in the external canal and in the distribution of CN VII. Also, facial nerve edema with associated paresis and loss of taste are often noted. The infections typically respond well to antiviral agents and oral steroids.

Otologic Neoplasms

Neoplastic processes affecting the inner ear and cerebellopontine angle are rare. Tumors arising in the internal auditory canal can compress any of four nerves that travel via this canal to the central nervous system: the facial nerve, the cochlear nerve (a division of CN VIII), or the inferior and superior vestibular nerves (also divisions of CN VIII). Vestibular schwannomas, are the most common. Other masses of the cerebellopontine angle include gliomas, meningiomas, epidermoid cysts, and arachnoid cysts. Compression of CN VII or the divisions of CN VIII can produce various symptoms necessitating diagnostic evaluation. Treatment involves surgical excision or stereotactic radiation.

The overwhelming majority of malignancies of the external ear are squamous cell and basal cell carcinomas developing secondary to sun exposure on the auricle. Tumors of the external auditory canal and temporal bone are also overwhelmingly squamous cell carcinomas, although adnexal tumors are possible. Surgical management is the mainstay of treatment for both locations. This may range from a wide local excision for small, nonbony tumors to more extensive temporal bone resections for larger tumors.

RHINOLOGY

Anatomy of the Nose and Paranasal Sinuses

The external nose consists of a bony skeleton forming the upper one third of the nose and a cartilaginous skeleton forming the lower two thirds. The internal nose is divided by the septum, which is composed of four structures: the perpendicular plate of the ethmoid bone, the vomer bone, the quadrilateral cartilage, and the crest of the maxillary bone. The lateral nasal walls consist of 3 turbinates (inferior, middle, and superior) and corresponding meatuses or spaces that provide drainage for the sinuses and the nasolacrimal duct. All of these structures are covered by mucoperichondrium or mucoperiosteum.

Four paired sinuses communicate with the nasal cavity. All sinuses begin development in utero; however, adult dimensions are not attained until late adolescence. Each sinus produces mucus, which serves to warm and humidify inspired air, as well as to trap allergens and fine particulate matter. The maxillary sinuses develop beneath the orbits, the frontal sinuses anterosuperior to the orbits, and the sphenoid sinuses midline and posterior to the orbits. The ethmoid sinuses consist of two groups of 8 to 12 cells arranged in a honeycomb configuration between the orbits. Ciliary beating directs mucus to the natural sinus openings, into the nasal cavity, and then posteriorly to the nasopharynx, where the mucus is swallowed.

Rhinitis

Most complaints related to the nasal cavity concern symptoms of rhinitis and sinusitis, collectively referred to as rhinosinusitis. Symptoms of rhinitis include nasal congestion, rhinorrhea, nasal itching, and postnasal drip. Numerous etiologies exist and are classified as either nonallergic or allergic. Nonallergic causes include infections, medications, pregnancy, and systemic disease states. Allergic rhinitis may be perennial or seasonal, depending on the allergen involved. Treatment of nonallergic rhinitis is directed at the underlying cause of the disease. Infectious rhinitis, which may be viral, bacterial, or both, may require antibiotics. Likewise, medications, most commonly sympathetic-blocking agents and birth control pills, may need to be changed. Additional pharmacotherapy for nonallergic rhinitis includes nasal and systemic decongestants. Nasal decongestant sprays must not be used for more than 3 days, as prolonged use can cause *rhinitis medicamentosa*, a rebound nasal congestion that becomes a challenge to treat.

In addition to minimizing the offending allergens (often pets, cigarette smoke, or molds), nasal steroids are the first-line therapy for allergic rhinitis. They act to blunt the allergic response by stabilizing mast cells, inhibiting formation of inflammatory mediators, and blocking chemotaxis of inflammatory cells. Topical administration has little systemic absorption, and side effects are usually local, including nasal irritation, crusting, and epistaxis. Other treatment modalities include antihistamines, the newer of which have less central nervous system penetration and are therefore less sedating. Leukotriene antagonists, used in the management of reactive airways disease, are finding a more defined role in the treatment of allergic rhinitis as well. In addition to pharmacotherapy for allergic rhinitis, identification of allergens through allergy testing is essential in refractory cases. Once identified, immunotherapy, which is aimed at desensitization of the immune system against a particular allergen, may also be employed if the allergens cannot be avoided.

Paranasal Sinus Infections

Sinus infections stem from impaired sinonasal mucociliary transport and/or blockage of sinus ostia. The former may occur from a viral infection that damages ciliary action, while the latter may be secondary to blockage from a deviated septum, turbinate hypertrophy, or nasal polyps. In either case, the infection may manifest as facial pain or pressure, nasal obstruction, postnasal drip, rhinorrhea, and fever. Diagnosis is based on history and physical examination. Imaging is not indicated for acute sinusitis unless a complication extending beyond the sinuses is suspected.

Acute sinusitis is defined as sinusitis with symptoms lasting less than 4 weeks, whereas chronic sinusitis is defined as sinus disease with persistent symptoms lasting more than 12 weeks. Chronic sinusitis, wherein symptoms persist, should be differentiated from recurrent sinusitis, in which patients get recurrent attacks of acute sinusitis, each lasting less than 4 weeks, with symptom-free intervals between acute attacks.

Postobstructive sinusitis merits some additional consideration. It is sinusitis that occurs as a result of blockade of the natural drainage sinus tracts. Frequently, nasal polyps are the cause of this obstruction, but sinonasal neoplasm can also be the culprit. Unilateral sinusitis especially should raise suspicion of a mass lesion. Endoscopic exam and/or imaging of the sinuses should be undertaken. MRI in this setting is helpful to differentiate blocked secretions from a solid mass.

First-line therapy for acute bacterial sinusitis involves decongestants and antibiotics. Management of chronic sinusitis includes nasal irrigations, antibiotics, and treatment of an allergy when present. In patients who fail medical management, endoscopic sinus surgery may be indicated to enlarge natural sinus ostia and to resect areas of obstructing bony overgrowth and sinonasal polyps. This allows for better drainage as well as improved access to the sinuses for topical irrigations.

Complications of Sinusitis

The most serious complication of sinus infections involves spread of infection to the orbits and central nervous system. The mode of spread from the sinuses is via the bloodstream or direct extension. Orbital complications of sinus disease most commonly originate from the ethmoid sinuses and progress along a spectrum from preseptal cellulitis to orbital cellulitis, orbital abscess, and cavernous sinus thrombosis (Fig. 29.2). Symptoms may include proptosis, chemosis (conjunctival edema), extraocular muscle entrapment, and vision loss. Diagnosis is based on physical examination and contrast-enhanced imaging. Patients with periorbital cellulitis typically can be managed successfully with broad-spectrum, intravenous antibiotics. Orbital abscesses require surgical drainage and opening of the involved sinuses. An ophthalmology consultation is necessary to document baseline vision and any progression of visual compromise or ocular entrapment that would prompt more urgent surgical intervention.

Intracranial spread of sinusitis most commonly stems from the frontal sinuses, especially in adolescent males; this is thought to be related to the rich vascularity of the diploic veins in this population. Intracranial involvement may present as meningitis, epidural abscess, subdural empyema, intracerebral abscess, venous sinus thrombosis, or osteomyelitis (Pott puffy tumor). Diagnosis is again made by physical examination plus contrast-enhanced imaging, often employing MRI. Treatment is multidisciplinary and utilizes the skills of an otolaryngologist, an infectious disease specialist, and a neurosurgeon and involves drainage of the involved sinuses as well as any intracranial collection when appropriate, while covering with appropriate antibiotics.

Epistaxis

Epistaxis represents a common yet potentially serious medical condition that can affect airway stability and hemodynamic stability. Information regarding prescription and nonprescription medications (warfarin, aspirin, and nonsteroidal anti-inflammatories), history of hypertension, coagulopathy, hepatic disease, prior bleeding episodes, and recent trauma should be elicited. Pharmacologic control of blood pressure should be initiated in the hypertensive patient and laboratory studies, including complete blood count and coagulation panels, should be ordered as well. In the presence of significant bleeding with anemia, blood products should be available, particularly in the elderly patients or those with significant cardiac histories.

Of all nosebleeds, approximately 90% originate from the anterior septum in a region called the Kiesselbach plexus, which comprises a rich anastomotic network of vessels. Local factors predispose to bleeding from this area, including digital or mechanical trauma, dry indoor heat in the wintertime, and chemical irritants. Anterior rhinoscopy (using either nasal speculum and headlight or an otoscope) will often reveal excoriated septal mucosa with exposed vessels. If pressure applied across the nose in conjunction with correction of coagulopathy and control of hypertension does not stop the bleeding, cauterization with silver nitrate sticks may suffice. If this is not possible secondary to copious bleeding or

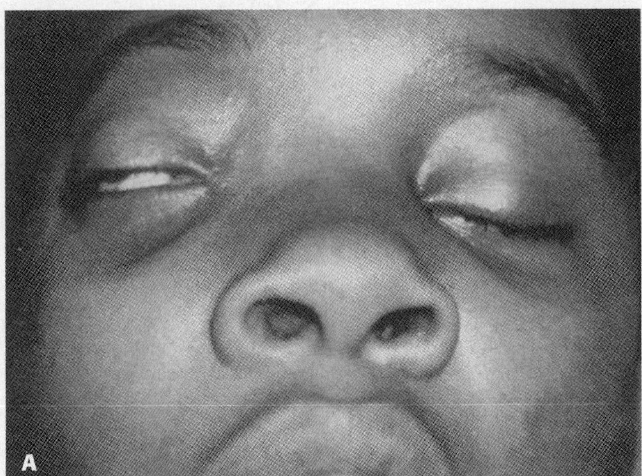

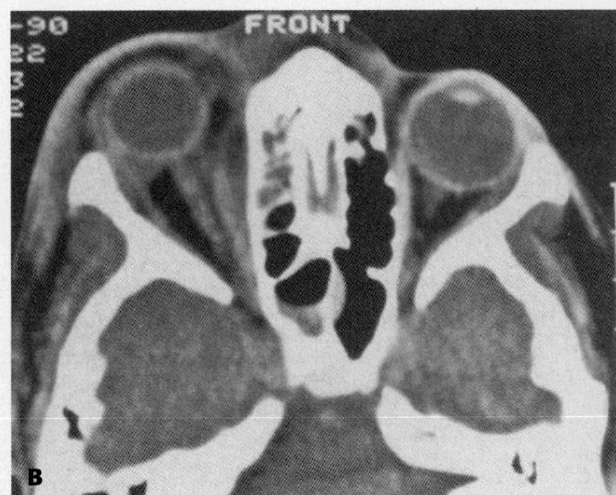

FIGURE 29.2 **A.** Patient with asymmetric proptosis secondary to a subperiosteal abscess. **B.** Axial computed tomography scan of the same patient.

patient discomfort, placement of nasal packing may be required. Packs are left in place for 3 days, antistaphylococcal antibiotics are administered (to prevent toxic shock syndrome), and blood-thinning agents are held if medically possible.

In the extreme case, ligation of the internal maxillary, anterior ethmoid, and/or posterior ethmoid arteries may be required. Angiography and embolization are also useful in identifying responsible vessels and controlling bleeding. However, the anterior and posterior ethmoid arteries are not routinely embolized because of the risk of blindness due to their origin off of the ophthalmic artery.

As discussed above for unilateral sinusitis, sinonasal neoplasm must also be considered in the differential diagnosis of epistaxis. Patients with recurrent or persistent epistaxis should undergo an endoscopic examination and/or CT of the sinuses to rule out a tumor.

LARYNGOLOGY

The Larynx

Anatomically, the larynx is described as having three divisions: the supraglottis, glottis, and subglottis (Fig. 29.3). The supraglottis is bounded superiorly by the tip of the epiglottis and inferiorly by the floor of the laryngeal ventricle (the space between the true and false vocal folds). The glottis contains the true vocal folds. The subglottis begins 5 mm below the free edge of the true vocal folds and extends to the inferior border of the cricoid cartilage. The glottis serves as a sphincter to protect the airway from aspiration and to provide phonation. These structures are enclosed by the cricoid and thyroid cartilages, to which the intrinsic muscles of the glottis are attached. The actions of these intrinsic muscles serve to abduct and adduct the vocal folds, as well as modulate vocal fold tension. The internal branch of the superior laryngeal nerve, a branch of the vagus nerve, provides sensory innervation to the supraglottis; stimulation in this region triggers a strong cough reflex. Inability to detect sensation in this area places an individual at risk for aspiration. The external branch of superior laryngeal nerve provides motor innervation to the cricothyroid muscle, which relaxes and tenses the vocal folds. The recurrent laryngeal nerve innervates the remaining intrinsic muscles of the larynx.

Unilateral vocal fold paralysis usually manifests as hoarseness and may be caused by a variety of pathologic conditions. Laryngeal cancer invading the intrinsic muscles and thoracic or neck masses compressing the recurrent laryngeal nerve can present with vocal fold paralysis. Iatrogenic causes include cardiothoracic surgery, anterior approaches to the cervical spine, and thyroid surgery. Other causes include stroke, carcinomas of the left upper lobe of the lung with adenopathy in the aortopulmonary window, blunt neck trauma, and viral infections. Although hoarseness and voice changes can significantly impact patient quality of life, the main concern with a unilateral paralysis is aspiration due to a weak cough and inability to close a glottic gap. Some patients with a unilateral paralysis can actually compensate, with the functioning vocal fold crossing midline to meet the paralyzed vocal fold. Several surgical options exist to medialize a paralyzed vocal fold if a patient cannot adequately compensate and the glottic gap persists. Injection thyroplasty involves injecting one of several available materials into the true vocal fold to bring it toward the midline. More permanent medialization can be achieved with laryngeal framework thyroplasty. Bilateral vocal fold paralysis is an airway emergency and usually requires a tracheostomy.

Hoarseness does not always imply vocal fold paralysis or paresis. Lesions of the larynx, such as glottic tumors (both benign and malignant) and vocal cord nodules, may cause voice changes without impairing overall vocal cord mobility but by impairing apposition of the true vocal cord surfaces. Chronic changes of the larynx from gastroesophageal reflux or postnasal drip may also cause voice changes secondary to laryngeal irritation and inflammation. In addition to history, office endoscopy is essential in the evaluation of hoarseness. Flexible nasopharyngolaryngoscopy (NPL) is relatively quick and well tolerated. If suspicious lesions are seen,

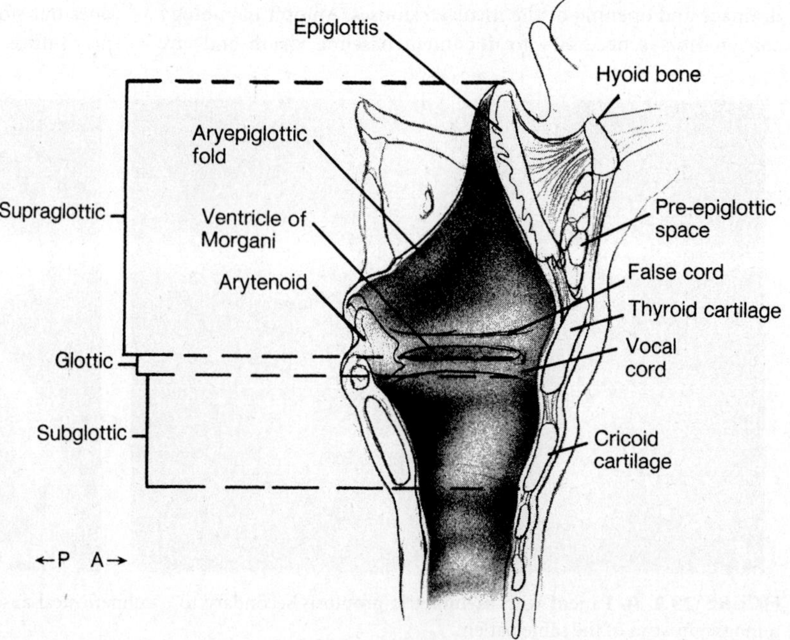

FIGURE 29.3 Midline sagittal section of the larynx, demonstrating the supraglottic, glottic, and subglottic regions, as well as the pre-epiglottic space. *A*, anterior; *P*, posterior.

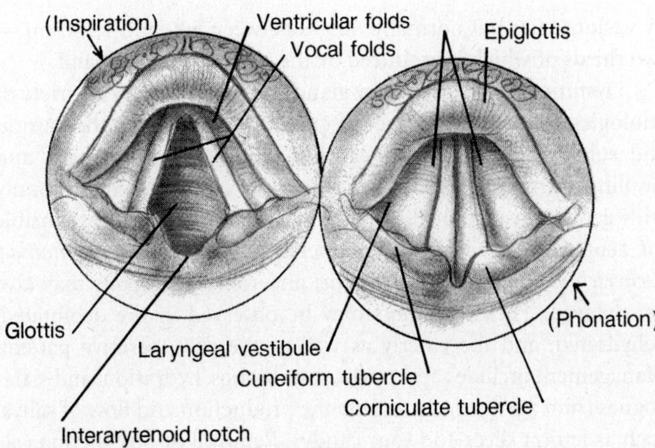

FIGURE 29.4 Endoscopic view of the larynx.

more extensive evaluation may be performed in the operating room utilizing direct laryngoscopy with rigid laryngoscopes and bronchoscopy (Fig. 29.4).

Stridor is a high-pitched sound during inspiration and/or expiration due to turbulent airflow in the upper airway. Principal causes of stridor include infectious etiologies, foreign bodies, and angioedema. The presence of stridor mandates an assessment of the airway. Flexible NPL can be extremely helpful in assessing the patency of the upper airway and the possible need for intubation or tracheostomy. Viral or bacterial infections can be managed with humidification, appropriate antibiotics, and steroids. Angioedema is an unusual entity presenting as a rapid onset of swelling in some or all parts of the upper airway (lips, tongue, or larynx). It occurs most commonly in response to food (peanuts) or medication allergies (angiotensin-converting enzyme inhibitors). Management includes high-dose systemic steroids, histamine blockers, subcutaneous epinephrine, and observation in a monitored setting. Securing the airway in these patients can be a challenge due to airway swelling; fiberoptic nasotracheal intubation and even emergent tracheostomy may be necessary. An additional cause of acute-onset stridor is an aspirated foreign body. More common in the pediatric population, airway foreign bodies may be pieces of food, toy parts, or other objects. Because organic matter is often radiolucent, plain films are of little use, although they may demonstrate air trapping with lung hyperinflation. Bronchoscopy can be both diagnostic and therapeutic in these situations.

A common cause of neonatal stridor and airway distress is laryngotracheomalacia. In these patients, the immature cartilage of the larynx and trachea is unable to maintain its shape and collapses with forceful breathing (Fig. 29.5). Laryngomalacia may exist separately from tracheomalacia, and each presents differently. With laryngomalacia, inspiratory stridor is noted as the epiglottis and arytenoids collapse into the glottic airway with inspiration. During expiration, these structures are propelled back to their normal supraglottic positions. Conversely, expiratory stridor is heard in tracheomalacia as the tracheal cartilage collapses as air is expelled; with inspiration, inspired air fills the trachea and stents it open. In most cases, as the cartilage matures with age, the breathing becomes quieter and more comfortable. In severe cases of laryngomalacia with respiratory distress, supraglottoplasty may be performed to release the epiglottis from the aryepiglottic folds and prevent collapse. For severe tracheomalacia with respiratory distress, tracheostomy may be required.

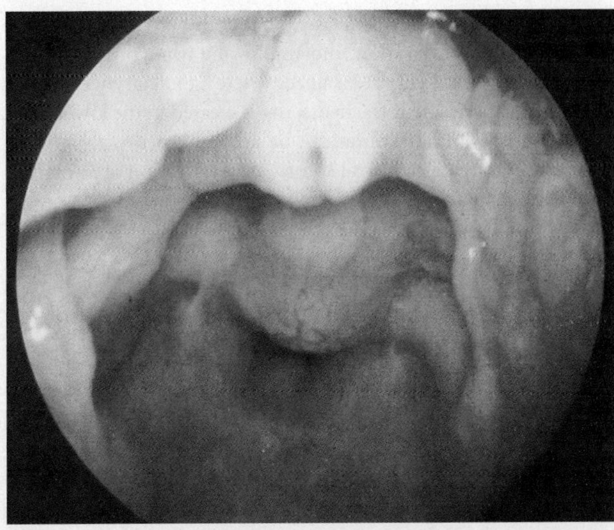

FIGURE 29.5 Endoscopic view of laryngomalacia during inspiration with folding inward of the epiglottis, shortened aryepiglottic folds, and collapse of the cuneiform cartilages completely obstructing the laryngeal introitus. (From Bailey BJ, Johnson JT, eds. *Head and Neck Surgery—Otolaryngology*. 4th ed. Philadelphia: Lippincott Williams & Wilkins; 2006:1104, with permission.)

Other causes of chronic respiratory distress and stridor in pediatric patients include vascular malformations, which compress the trachea, subglottic cysts and hemangiomas, and subglottic stenosis. An open surgical procedure usually is required to repair vascular rings or anomalous vessels if compressive signs or symptoms are present, while cysts are usually resected endoscopically. Hemangiomas, which typically enlarge in the first few years of life before involution, may produce symptoms of airway compromise as well. In cases of severe airway compromise, tracheostomy or laser resection of the hemangioma can be used to improve the airway. Subglottic stenosis, which may be primary or acquired from prolonged intubation, typically causes biphasic stridor. For patients with respiratory distress, tracheostomy may be necessary until a laryngotracheoplasty can be performed to resect the stenosis.

Cancers of the Larynx

Approximately 11,000 laryngeal cancers are diagnosed each year in the United States. Peak incidence occurs in the fifth through seventh decades with men affected more commonly than women. As with other head and neck cancers, principal risk factors include tobacco and alcohol use. Presenting symptoms include hoarseness, dyspnea, hemoptysis, dysphagia, and odynophagia.

Extensive lymphatics from the supraglottic larynx drain anteriorly to the pre-epiglottic space and bilaterally to the cervical lymph nodes resulting in metastases frequently found at the time of diagnosis. On the other hand, glottic cancers, representing the majority of laryngeal cancers, tend to have relatively infrequent lymph node involvement because of typically earlier presentation due to early symptomatology and anatomic barriers to spread. Finally, subglottic cancers represent less than 5% of laryngeal tumors and carry a poor prognosis because patients develop symptoms late in the course of the disease and nodal metastases are common.

Treatment for laryngeal cancer includes resection, radiation, and/or chemotherapy. Organ preservation procedures such as partial laryngectomies (open, laser, or robotic) are utilized to preserve phonation, respiration, and swallowing while providing successful cancer treatment. In instances where a total laryngectomy is performed, a permanent tracheostoma is created in the lower neck. Postoperative communication can be accomplished with an electrolarynx, through esophageal speech, or via creation of a tracheoesophageal fistula with the placement of a voice prosthesis.

HEAD AND NECK SURGERY

Salivary Gland Anatomy, Physiology, and Pathology

There are three paired groups of major salivary glands: parotid, submandibular, and sublingual. The parotid gland is located over the masseter muscle of the cheek and extends from its superior most point at the zygoma to an inferior point that curves around the angle of the mandible (Fig. 29.6). Saliva produced by this gland is mostly serous and is directed through Stensen duct with its opening located opposite the second upper molar. The facial nerve divides the parotid gland into superficial and deep lobes.

The submandibular gland courses around the mylohyoid muscle and the mandible. It produces mostly seromucous saliva that is directed via Wharton duct to an orifice in the floor of the mouth adjacent to the frenulum. The mandibular division of the facial nerve and the facial artery and vein lie superficial to the submandibular gland and must be identified during any procedure involving the gland.

The sublingual gland is the smallest of the major salivary glands and secretes mostly mucous saliva through approximately 10 small ducts that drain directly into the floor of mouth along the sublingual fold. The remainder of saliva is produced by the 600 to 1,000 minor salivary glands distributed in the cheek, lips, and hard and soft palates. The quantity of saliva produced daily is influenced by various cues but normally ranges between 500 and 1,500 mL—two thirds of which is produced by the submandibular gland.

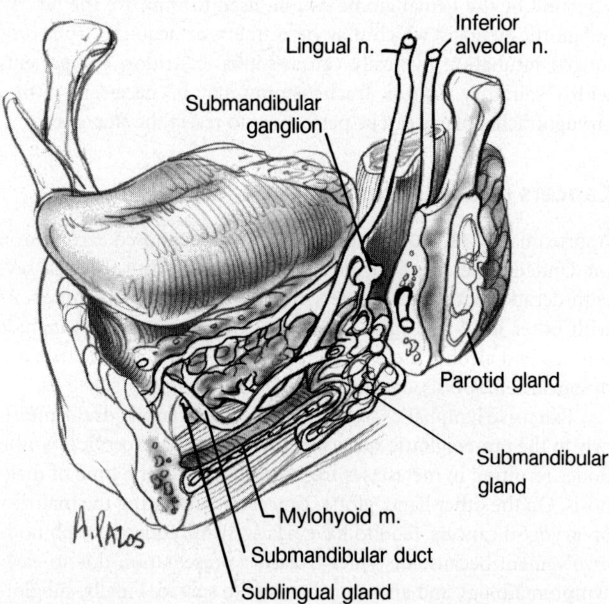

FIGURE 29.6 The superficial and deep lobes of the submandibular gland are separated by the mylohyoid muscle. The sublingual gland has multiple ducts that open along the plica of the floor of the mouth. (From Bailey BJ, Johnson JT, eds. *Head and Neck Surgery—Otolaryngology*. 4th ed. Philadelphia: Lippincott Williams & Wilkins; 2006:521, with permission.)

Dysfunction of the salivary glands can be caused by a variety of etiologies. Acute suppurative infections typically affect the parotid and submandibular glands, causing induration, tenderness, and swelling. Purulent discharge can frequently be expressed intraorally with gentle massage of the gland. Bacterial organisms responsible for acute infections commonly include *S. aureus*, *S. pneumoniae*, *Escherichia coli*, and *H. influenzae*; anaerobic organisms may also be involved. These disorders may be observed in the debilitated, dehydrated, and the elderly as well as the postoperative patient. Management includes appropriate antibiotics, hydration, and sialagogues (oral agents that promote the production and flow of saliva, such as lemon slices and sour candy). Removal of obstructing calculi, when present, is also indicated to restore salivary flow. Incision and drainage of associated abscesses and/or removal of the acutely affected gland may also be necessary. Viral parotitis, or mumps, is most frequently caused by the *Paramyxovirus*, but this entity has become less common with the introduction of mumps vaccinations. Additionally, granulomatous diseases and actinomycosis are prevalent especially in the HIV-positive population.

Benign salivary disease also includes sialolithiasis, or ductal stones. Of parotid calculi, 65% to 90% are radiolucent, while 65% to 90% of submandibular gland stones are radiopaque on conventional plain films. Painful swelling is temporally associated with meals, and frequent bouts may lead to acute suppurative infections as described previously. Traditionally, these were treated by directly opening the duct to remove the stones or removing the entire offending gland. More recently, sialendoscopy has emerged as a minimally invasive technique to remove stones and clear the ducts. Tiny endoscopes are passed through the ducts to visualize and retrieve calculi, wash out the duct, or even dilate a stenotic duct.

Autoimmune processes frequently involve the salivary glands. One example is *Sjögren syndrome*, a disorder seen in the middle aged and the elderly, with women outnumbering men by a ratio of 9:1. Symptoms include xerostomia (dry mouth), keratoconjunctivitis sicca (dry eyes), glandular swelling, and papillary atrophy of the tongue. Histopathologic diagnosis is made on the basis of a minor salivary gland biopsy, usually from the lower lip, which demonstrates plasma cell and histiocytic infiltration with acinar atrophy. Other causes of xerostomia include previous irradiation to the head and neck as well as a variety of pharmacologic agents, such as anticholinergics, diuretics, antihistamines, antispasmodics, and antiparkinsonian agents.

Neoplastic disorders of the salivary glands include benign and malignant lesions and account for approximately 3% to 5% of tumors arising in the head and neck. Approximately 70% of tumors arise from the parotid gland, 15% to 20% from the submandibular gland, and the remaining 8% to 15% from minor salivary glands of the head and neck. As a general rule, the larger the gland, the more likely the neoplasm is to be benign.

Benign neoplasms tend to progress slowly, are painless, and rarely cause facial nerve dysfunction. Pleomorphic adenomas (benign mixed tumor) are the most common salivary tumors (approximately 50% of all salivary neoplasms). Surgical management includes superficial parotidectomy as these lesions carry a risk of malignant degeneration to carcinoma ex-pleomorphic adenoma. Warthin tumors (papillary cystadenoma lymphomatosum) represent the second most common type of benign salivary neoplasm. They occur more commonly in men and are associated with cigarette smoking. They can be bilateral or multicentric.

Malignant tumors of the salivary glands constitute approximately 35% to 45% of all salivary masses. The likelihood of malignancy is inversely proportional to the size of the gland: parotid (20%), submandibular (50%), and minor (80%). Of the minor salivary gland neoplasms, approximately 40% arise in the palate. The most common malignant tumor of the salivary glands is mucoepidermoid carcinoma. Patients note a slowly enlarging painless mass with rare facial nerve involvement; 30% to 40% of patients have lymph node metastases on presentation and thus require a cervical lymph node dissection in addition to parotidectomy. Adenoid cystic carcinoma is the most common malignant tumor of the submandibular and minor salivary glands. Classically, this tumor is associated with perineural invasion and can recur many years after initial diagnosis and treatment. The most common mode of failure in adenoid cystic carcinoma is distant metastasis, specifically in the lung. Other salivary gland malignancies include acinic cell carcinomas, malignant mixed tumors, and adenocarcinoma. The remaining 1% fall within various cell types including squamous cell carcinoma, salivary duct carcinoma (which resembles breast cancer), and lymphomas. The presence of intraparotid lymph nodes allows for metastases to the parotid gland, usually from cutaneous malignancies of the head and neck.

The diagnosis of parotid neoplasms incorporates elements of patient history (pain, paresis, and progress of growth), physical examination (tenderness, compressibility, fixation, erythema, and edema), cytopathology and histopathology, and radiology. Superficial parotidectomy is indicated for all parotid tumors, unless deep lobe extension is noted, in which case total parotidectomy is performed with sparing of the facial nerve. Because of the presence of pseudopod extensions from neoplasms, enucleation alone carries a higher rate of recurrence. Malignant neoplasms may require elective or therapeutic neck dissections according to tumor type and histologic grade. Management of minor salivary gland tumors also requires wide surgical margins, and postoperative radiation is recommended for malignancies with aggressive characteristics.

Temporary facial nerve paresis is not unusual after parotid surgery and most often involves the temporal and mandibular branches. The integrity of the nerve may be assessed at the termination of the procedure with a nerve stimulator. If intact, return to normal function can be predicted with confidence. When tumor involvement requires sacrifice of CN VII, nerve grafting to distal branches is recommended although complete return of function is rare.

Frey syndrome, or gustatory sweating, is a phenomenon that can arise after parotidectomy when severed parasympathetic fibers initially supplying the parotid gland aberrantly reinnervate sweat glands on the skin. Thus, actions that would normally trigger salivation instead produce perspiration. The incidence of gustatory sweating is unknown, although it is estimated to be 35% to 60%. Treatment includes topical anticholinergic creams (scopolamine), antiperspirants, and injection of botulinum toxin.

Oral Cavity and Pharynx

The oral cavity/oropharynx is involved in three principal functions: phonation, ingestion, and respiration. Anatomically, the oral cavity is defined as the area including the lips, upper and lower alveolar ridges, buccal mucosa, floor of the mouth, retromolar trigone, hard palate, and anterior two thirds of the tongue. Motor functions of the oral cavity are provided by the tongue and the masticatory muscles. The muscles of mastication are innervated by CN V_3 and include the masseter, temporalis, lateral pterygoid, and medial pterygoid. The tongue receives motor innervation from the hypoglossal nerve (CN XII). Tactile sensation of the tongue is provided by the lingual nerve (a branch of CN V_3), while taste is provided by the chorda tympani nerve (from CN VII) to the anterior two thirds of the tongue and the glossopharyngeal nerve (CN IX) for posterior two thirds of the tongue.

The pharynx includes three distinct regions. The nasopharynx extends from the base of the skull to the level of the junction of hard and soft palates. The oropharynx begins at the undersurface of the soft palate and includes the palatine tonsils, tonsillar fossae, base of tongue, and the vallecula. Finally, the hypopharynx extends from the level of the floor of the vallecula and pharyngoepiglottic folds to the inferior border of the cricoid cartilage. It includes the pharyngoesophageal junction and pyriform sinuses.

Multiple benign processes may produce inflammation of the oral cavity and pharynx. These include bacterial, viral, and fungal infections, autoimmune disorders, nutritional deficiencies, and toxin or chemical exposure. Oral candidiasis, or thrush, is seen frequently in the HIV population and in postirradiation patients with diminished salivary production. The most concerning infections, however, are those that can lead to airway compromise. Odontogenic infections, for example, can spread rapidly to the floor of the mouth, tongue base, and submandibular space causing airway compromise. This is known as *Ludwig angina*, and sometimes, a tracheostomy is necessary to secure the airway (Fig. 29.7). Bacterial collections adjacent to the palatine tonsils within the tonsillar capsule, known as peritonsillar abscesses, can cause airway compromise if submucosal extension proceeds inferiorly toward the larynx. Common signs and symptoms of peritonsillar abscess include trismus, odynophagia, dysphagia, dehydration, "hot potato" voice, uvular deviation to the contralateral side, and bulging of the anterior tonsillar pillar secondary to infection. Management includes broad-spectrum antibiotics and bedside drainage of the abscess

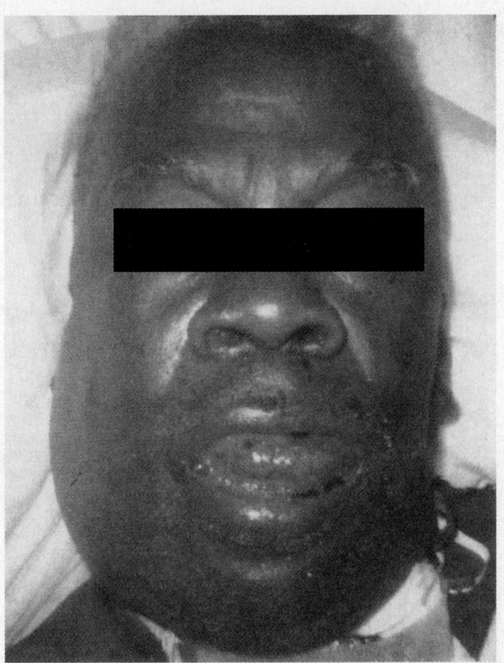

FIGURE 29.7 The Ludwig angina. Note the cuff of bilateral submandibular and submental swelling enveloping the upper neck and elevation of the floor of the mouth causing protrusion of the tongue. (From Bailey BJ, Johnson JT, eds. *Head and Neck Surgery—Otolaryngology*. 4th ed. Philadelphia: Lippincott Williams & Wilkins; 2006:619, with permission.)

after topical anesthesia is applied. Care must be taken to avoid the great vessels located in the parapharyngeal space while draining the infection. Other noninfectious lesions include recurrent aphthous ulcers, erythema multiforme, pemphigus vulgaris, and pemphigoid.

Malignant Lesions of the Oral Cavity and Pharynx

Approximately 31,000 new cancers of the oral cavity and pharynx are diagnosed each year in the United States. Greater than 90% of these neoplasms are squamous cell carcinomas, and overall, these tumors constitute 65% of all malignancies of the head and neck. Despite advances in radiotherapy and chemotherapy protocols, survival rates are little improved from those of the 1960s, with a generalized 5-year survival rate of 50%. Factors implicated in the etiology of these carcinomas include tobacco, alcohol, betel nut, and human papillomavirus infection. In addition, exposure to ultraviolet light has been associated with carcinomas of the lower lip.

At a minimum, diagnostic evaluation should include a chest x-ray and liver function tests because distant metastases may be present in advanced disease. Panendoscopy (direct laryngoscopy, bronchoscopy, and esophagoscopy) is advocated before definitive treatment to rule out synchronous primary lesions of the aerodigestive tract. Moreover, postoperatively, these patients carry an elevated risk of developing a second upper aerodigestive tract primary tumor most commonly in the head and neck (50%) and the lungs (20%). So, continued surveillance is imperative.

Oral cavity cancers are treated surgically with adjuvant radiation and/or chemoradiation for advanced disease. Surgical resection can range from simple excision of a tongue mass to radical resection of a large part of the tongue, floor of mouth, and mandible. Significant advances have been made in reconstructive surgery, allowing the creation of bulky or pliable surfaces and contours in the oral cavity with pedicled and free flaps to permit deglutition after extensive resections. In addition, mandibular reconstruction can be accomplished with titanium plates or osteocutaneous free flaps from the fibula, scapula, and iliac crest. Nevertheless, the inability to recreate delicate motor movements performed by the tongue can carry significant morbidity with respect to swallowing competency and articulate speech.

Optimal treatment of oropharyngeal cancers remains a topic of debate. Historically, to access these tumors, surgeons would have to split the lip or mandible leading to significant patient morbidity. With advances in radiation and chemotherapy, there was a movement away from primary surgical treatment of these tumors. Within the last decade, advances in transoral laser surgery and transoral robotic surgery have brought primary surgical treatment back into the discussion. HPV-positive tumors seem to be especially responsive to radiation and chemotherapy but overall have a better prognosis than HPV-negative tumors regardless of treatment modality.

Nasopharyngeal Carcinoma

Nasopharyngeal carcinoma comprises only 0.2% of newly diagnosed malignancies in the United States. However, in certain regions of China, it represents 25% of all diagnosed cancers. This disparity in incidence is thought to be related to environmental exposure to specific types of Epstein–Barr virus (EBV), to food-preserving nitrosamines, and to the prevalence of specific human leukocyte antigen genotypes. Demographically, peak incidence occurs in the fifth and sixth decade, although 20% of patients are younger than 30 years at diagnosis.

Tumors may cause obstruction of the eustachian tube and result in persistent unilateral serous otitis media (Fig. 29.8). The presence of a neck mass, which represents cervical metastasis, is also a common

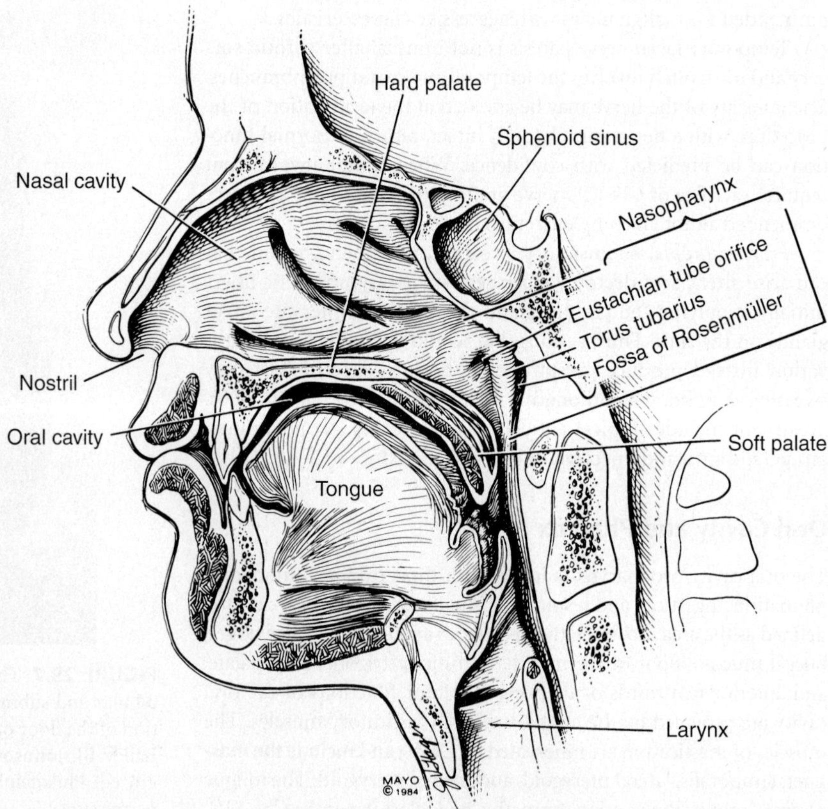

FIGURE 29.8 The nasopharynx and its anatomic relationships.

presenting complaint owing to the silent nature of this malignancy. Other presenting symptoms may include nasal congestion, eye pain, diplopia, hypesthesia in the CN V_1 or V_2 distribution, epistaxis, and headache secondary to intracranial extension. Endoscopic examination may not detect submucosal spread; therefore, MRI examination should be obtained if uncertainty persists. The mainstay of treatment is radiation with chemotherapy. Resection may be employed for patients with radiation failure or tumor recurrence.

Other Head and Neck Masses

Lymphomas also frequently present as head and neck masses. Extranodal sites commonly include the lymphoid tissue of Waldeyer ring (adenoids, palatine tonsils, and lingual tonsils); however, other sites may include the paranasal sinuses, nasal cavity, oral cavity, salivary glands, and larynx. Non-Hodgkin lymphoma of the head and neck commonly presents as cervical adenopathy, although extranodal disease is present in 10% to 25% of patients. In contrast, it is unusual for Hodgkin disease of the head and neck to present in extranodal sites; rather, cervical adenopathy alone is the rule. When fine-needle aspirate (FNA) is inconclusive, diagnosis is made on the basis of excisional lymph node biopsy.

In the pediatric population, developmental anomalies can account for a large proportion of neck masses. Branchial cleft cysts are typically found along the anatomic line that extends inferiorly from the external auditory canal along the anterior border of the sternocleidomastoid muscle. A patent ductal remnant frequently communicates with the aerodigestive tract, resulting in intermittent swelling associated with upper respiratory tract infections. Treatment involves excision of the cyst along with its tract.

In contrast to branchial cleft cysts, thyroglossal duct cysts are found in the midline neck along the course of the thyroid gland descent from the tongue base at the foramen cecum. Management includes removal of the cyst, its tract, and the midportion of the hyoid bone—the *Sistrunk procedure.* A preoperative ultrasound of the neck should be ordered to ensure that normal thyroid tissue is present because in rare instances, the thyroglossal duct cyst represents the only functioning thyroid tissue in an individual; in these patients, counseling regarding the need for thyroid hormone replacement must occur preoperatively. Additionally, carcinomas have been reported within thyroglossal duct cysts, and adjunctive thyroidectomy in these cases is controversial.

Lymphatics of the Head and Neck

Six lymph node groups or levels have been defined in the neck and various regions of the head and neck (Fig. 29.9). Level I nodes are located in the submental and submandibular triangles and drain the oral cavity and submandibular gland. Level II nodes are found from the skull base to carotid bifurcation at the hyoid bone. Drainage from the nasopharynx, oropharynx, the parotid gland, and supraglottic structures first involves these nodes. Level III nodes are located between the carotid bifurcation and the intersection of the omohyoid muscle with the internal jugular vein at the level of the cricothyroid membrane. Level III nodes drain the oropharynx, hypopharynx, and supraglottic larynx. Level IV nodes are present inferior to level III and extend to the level of the clavicles. These nodes drain the subglottic larynx, hypopharynx, esophagus, and thyroid. The level V (posterior triangle) nodal group is bounded anteriorly by the posterior border of the sternocleidomastoid muscle and posteriorly by the anterior border of the trapezius muscle. This

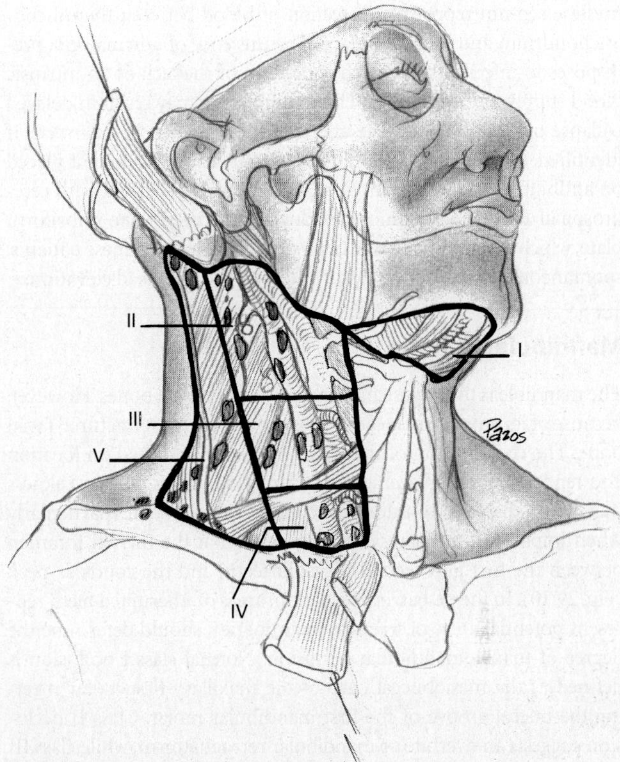

FIGURE 29.9 Lymph node regions of the neck. Level VI (central compartment) is not shown. (From Bailey BJ, Johnson JT, eds. *Head and Neck Surgery—Otolaryngology.* 4th ed. Philadelphia: Lippincott Williams & Wilkins; 2006:1589, with permission.)

nodal group is a frequent site of metastases from tumors of the nasopharynx. Finally, level VI (central compartment) nodes are located between the medial borders of the carotid sheath and drain thyroid and parathyroid malignancies.

The term "neck dissection" refers to procedures for surgical excision of lymph nodes and fibrofatty tissue from any or all of the nodal groups in the neck. The most extensive procedure is the *radical neck dissection*, which involves resection of lymph node levels I to V and sacrifice of the internal jugular vein, sternocleidomastoid muscle, and spinal accessory nerve (CN XI). A *modified radical neck dissection* spares one or more of these vital structures to lessen morbidity, while a *selective neck dissection* removes only the lymph nodes most likely to be involved in draining the primary tumor site.

Therapeutic neck dissection is performed when nodal disease is clinically apparent. Elective neck dissection is performed in patients with cancers where the risk of occult cervical metastases is high, such as oral tongue or supraglottic cancers. In tumors associated with a low risk of cervical spread, patients are often observed clinically for development of cervical metastases.

TRAUMA

Nasal Trauma

The nasal bones are the most commonly fractured bones of the face. Presenting symptoms of nasal fractures may include epistaxis, pain, and nasal obstruction. Clinical exam is the mainstay of diagnosis, and radiographic studies are not necessary in cases of isolated nasal fractures. In all cases of nasal trauma, an inspection of the nasal cavity is required to rule out a septal hematoma. This bluish swelling of the midline septum represents dissection of blood between the mucoperichondrium and septal cartilage. The presence of a hematoma predisposes to infection and necrosis because of the lack of an intrinsic blood supply of the cartilage. This combination may result in delayed collapse of the nasal cartilage and lead to a *saddle nose deformity*. If identified, the hematoma should be evacuated and the patient placed on antibiotics. In rare instances, nasal trauma is associated with cerebrospinal fluid (CSF) rhinorrhea due to fracture of the cribriform plate, which is connected to the bony septum. In most of these patients, spontaneous resolution will occur with bed rest and head elevation.

Mandibular Trauma

The mandible is the largest and strongest of the facial bones. However, because of its prominent location, it is the second most fractured facial bone. The classification of mandibular fractures is based on location and tendency for displacement or distraction. The sites of weakness that are predisposed to fracture include the third molar (particularly when impacted), the parasymphyseal region at the mental foramen between the first and second bicuspid teeth, and the condylar neck (Fig. 29.10). In the pediatric population, areas of unerupted teeth represent potential areas of fracture. Examination should determine the degree of maxillomandibular occlusion. Normal class I occlusion is defined as the mesiobuccal cusp of the maxillary first molar meeting the buccal groove of the first mandibular molar. Class II occlusion suggests an overbite or mandibular retrognathism, while class III occlusion suggests an underbite or mandibular prognathism. Presence of teeth on both sides of the fracture facilitates interdental wire fixation. An intact molar in the fracture line should be left untouched to maximize repositioning surface. A mobile tooth is usually removed as it can be a source of infection. Condylar fractures may be associated with external auditory canal laceration or bloody otorrhea.

A simple fracture does not communicate with the oral cavity, while a complex fracture is associated with violation of mucous membranes or skin and carries increased risk of infection. A maxillofacial CT scan provides a complete view of the mandible and is optimal for diagnosing fractures. Although isolated fractures occur in children, the overwhelming majority of fractures in adults are multiple; in fact, when one fracture is identified on radiography, additional fractures should be ruled out. In general, surgical management for mandible fractures, when indicated, includes maxillo-mandibular fixation with or without open reduction and internal fixation of involved bone fragments.

Additional factors influence healing and morbidity. The elderly edentulous population or patients with poor dentition represent a greater challenge to fixation due to the lack of repositioning surface areas provided by the teeth. In general, any form of compression plating increases the risk of intraoperative damage to the inferior alveolar nerve, which runs in the mandibular canal and exits the mental foramen. Damage to this nerve can result in hypesthesia of the ipsilateral anterior chin and lower lip. Other complications, such as infection and osteomyelitis, are unlikely to occur with good reduction.

Emergencies resulting from mandibular fractures are rare. One such emergency is airway obstruction due to bilateral body fractures or multisegment fractures causing the tongue base to fall posteriorly. A jaw thrust or pulling the tongue anteriorly can relieve the obstruction and open the airway. If intubation of a patient with major facial fractures or suspected cervical spine injury is not possible, emergent tracheostomy or cricothyroidotomy is indicated. As a general rule, cricothyroidotomy offers the advantage of rapid airway access with a decreased risk of thyroid hemorrhage. However, there is a greater likelihood of injury to the recurrent laryngeal nerve, which pierces the cricothyroid membrane and an elevated risk of subglottic stenosis.

Otologic Trauma

The temporal bone is one of the hardest in the human body, and fractures affecting this structure are rare. Those that do occur are typically the result of a high-speed motor vehicle accident, a fall,

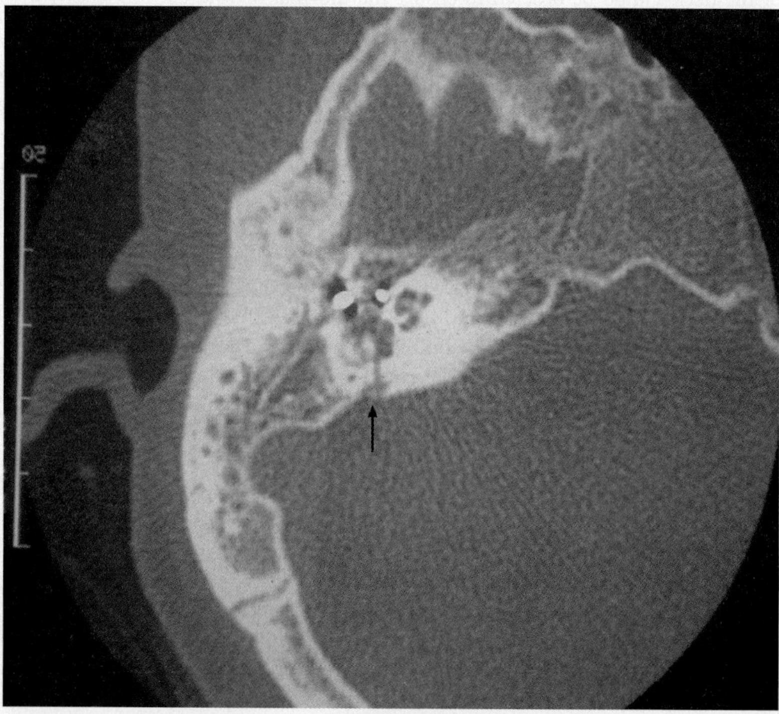

FIGURE 29.10 Axial cut high-resolution computed tomography demonstrating a transversely oriented fracture, secondary to a gunshot injury, disrupting the otic capsule. *Black arrow* point along the fracture line. (From Bailey BJ, Johnson JT, eds. *Head and Neck Surgery—Otolaryngology*. 4th ed. Philadelphia: Lippincott Williams & Wilkins; 2006:2060, with permission.)

or assault. Two principal classifications have been described with the diagnosis made on the basis of noncontrast temporal bone CT scans. Longitudinal fractures are caused by lateral trauma to the head and extend from the posterosuperior portion of the external auditory canal through the eardrum (Fig. 29.11). Delayed paresis of the facial nerve due to edema occurs in approximately 10% to 20% of cases. If the nerve is intact, this weakness should resolve. Physical examination findings may include ecchymosis overlying the mastoid bone (battle sign), blood in the external auditory canal, CSF otorrhea, and tympanic membrane perforation. Conductive hearing loss is common due to disruption of middle ear ossicles, eardrum perforation, and hemotympanum (blood in the middle ear). Vestibular symptoms and sensorineural hearing loss are uncommon and are usually due to the concussive effect on the cochlea and inner ear. An audiogram should be obtained when possible to assess hearing loss.

Transverse fractures represent 10% to 20% of injuries and occur with trauma to either the occiput or frontal area (Fig. 29.12). They typically are associated with higher mortality rates secondary to the level of impact required to cause them. The fracture line extends across the petrous pyramid and through the internal auditory canal. Facial nerve injury occurs in approximately 50% of cases and is due to crush injury or laceration of the nerve. Vestibular complaints including vertigo occur because of concussion of the semicircular canals. A CSF leak may not manifest as otorrhea due to an intact eardrum but rather as clear rhinorrhea as the CSF gains access to the nose through the eustachian tube. When present, CSF leaks are usually managed conservatively with bed rest, head of bed elevation, and possible lumbar drain placement. Exploration and surgical repair are indicated when these conservative measures are

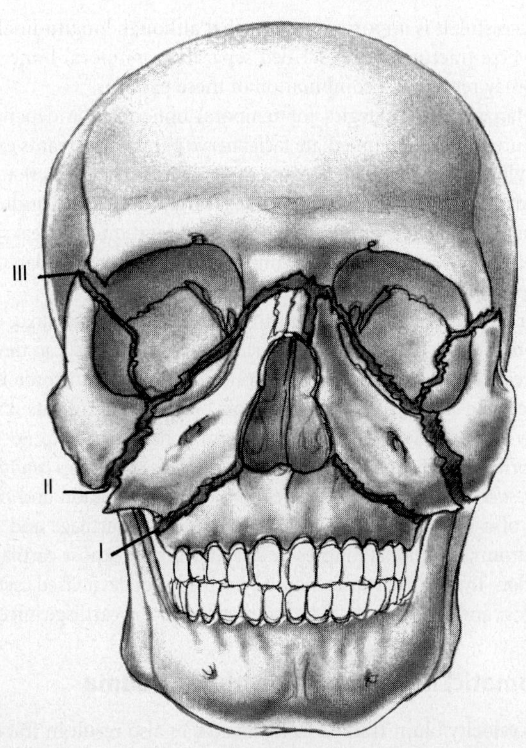

FIGURE 29.11 Le Fort fracture levels. (From Bailey BJ, Johnson JT, eds. *Head and Neck Surgery—Otolaryngology*. 4th ed. Philadelphia: Lippincott Williams & Wilkins; 2006:977, with permission.)

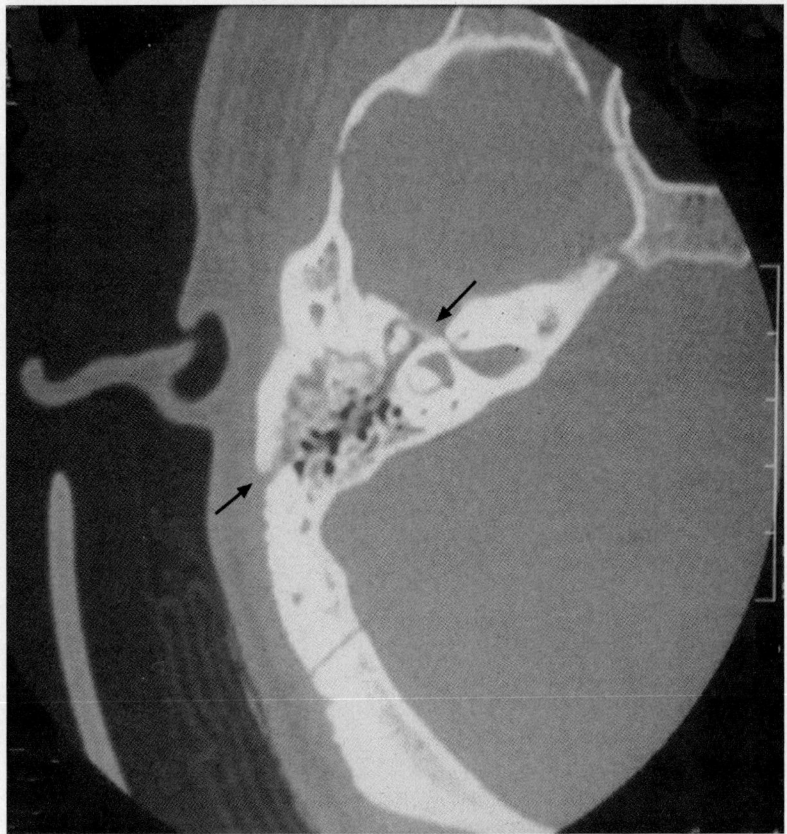

FIGURE 29.12 Axial cut high-resolution computed tomography demonstrating a longitudinally oriented fracture that is sparing the otic capsule. *Black arrows* point along the fracture line. (From Bailey BJ, Johnson JT, eds. *Head and Neck Surgery—Otolaryngology*. 4th ed. Philadelphia: Lippincott Williams & Wilkins; 2006:2060, with permission.)

unsuccessful. It is important to note that although longitudinal and transverse fractures are described separately, temporal bone fractures may represent a combination of these patterns.

Management strategies for temporal bone trauma depend on structures involved. Immediate facial nerve paralysis warrants exploration but is often delayed because of concomitant injuries that take precedence. Sensorineural hearing loss is rarely reversible. Conductive hearing loss due to tympanic membrane perforation may heal spontaneously or require delayed tympanoplasty, while ossicular chain disruption often requires surgical repair at a later date.

Trauma can also be localized to the external ear and canal, especially in athletes. Typically, a subperichondrial hematoma can develop between the cartilage and the perichondrium. If the hematoma is not drained, the cartilage becomes ischemic because it derives its oxygen supply from the adjacent perichondrium. Ischemia leads to necrosis, scar formation, and loss of the helical shape. This results in a *cauliflower* or *wrestler ear*. Treatment involves hematoma evacuation and placement of a bolster to maintain approximation of cartilage and perichondrium. Additional injuries or lacerations may expose cartilage to infection. Traumatized areas should be debrided of devitalized cartilage and skin, and antibiotics may be required to prevent cartilage infection.

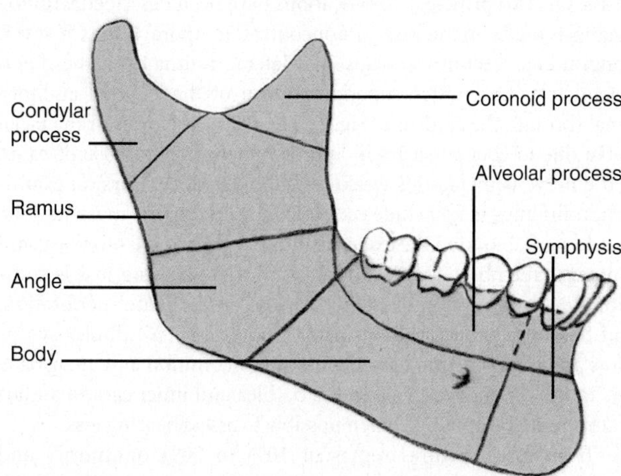

FIGURE 29.13 The anatomic components of the mandible include the symphysis, parasymphysis, body, angle, ramus, coronoid process, condyle, and alveolus. (From Bailey BJ, Johnson JT, eds. *Head and Neck Surgery—Otolaryngology*. 4th ed. Philadelphia: Lippincott Williams & Wilkins; 2006:961, with permission.)

Zygomatic, Maxillary, and Orbital Trauma

High-velocity blunt trauma to the head can also result in fractures of the zygomatic arch, the maxilla, and the orbits. To fully understand the management of facial fractures requires a review of the structural support systems of the face. The middle one third of the facial skeleton consists of an intersecting system of buttresses that distributes forces generated through mastication. The vertical dimensions are maintained by the nasomaxillary, zygomaticomaxillary, and pterygomaxillary buttresses. These vertical supports are interconnected via the horizontal buttresses, which include the orbital rims, maxillary alveolus and palate, zygomatic process, greater wing of the sphenoid, and medial and lateral pterygoid plates. If sufficient force is directed at the anterior face, predictable patterns of structural collapse are observed.

In 1901, Rene Le Fort described these patterns, which bear his name (Fig. 29.13). Each of the three classifications involves a fracture of the pterygoid plates. The Le Fort I fracture line passes horizontally along the palate inward to the pterygoid plates. The Le Fort II fracture line incorporates the nasofrontal suture line, traverses the medial orbital wall, and then proceeds across the orbital floor inferiorly beneath the zygomatic arch toward the palate. The Le Fort III fracture is the most serious and involves each of the three vertical buttresses, resulting in craniofacial disassociation. The fracture line extends from the nasofrontal suture line posteriorly along the cribriform plate/anterior skull base, travels through the root of the zygoma, and disrupts the junction of the pterygoid plates with the skull base.

The classic finding indicative of a Le Fort fracture is a mobile palate. Le Fort II and III fractures are commonly associated with CSF rhinorrhea, profound epistaxis, visual loss, and upper airway obstruction. As with mandibular fractures, a tracheostomy may be necessary to secure the airway. Most Le Fort fractures are repaired in a delayed fashion following stabilization of the patient. Correction is directed at re-establishing vertical and horizontal buttresses through open reduction and internal fixation. Common postoperative complications include malocclusion and, less frequently, facial asymmetry.

The zygomaticomaxillary complex, or tripod, fracture is the most common fracture of the midface. The principal fracture sites include the frontozygomatic suture line, the zygomatic arch, and the maxilla extending from the inferior orbital rim to the palate. Findings include posterior displacement of the complex producing a flattened appearance of the malar eminence. Compression of the infraorbital nerve may produce hypesthesia in the CN V_2 distribution. In addition, impingement upon the coronoid process of the mandible, which courses deep to the zygomatic arch, may cause trismus. The tripod fracture and isolated fractures of the zygomatic arch are easily identified on head CT. Surgical correction of the tripod fracture requires reapproximation and plating of the orbital rim, zygomatic arch, and maxilla.

Orbital floor fractures or "blowout" fractures are caused by inferiorly directed forces producing a fracture of the thin orbital floor along the infraorbital canal (Fig. 29.14). A coronal CT scan can identify intraorbital free air, which suggests violation of the bony orbit. It is also useful to identify herniation of the inferior rectus muscle into the maxillary sinus, which may result in enoph-

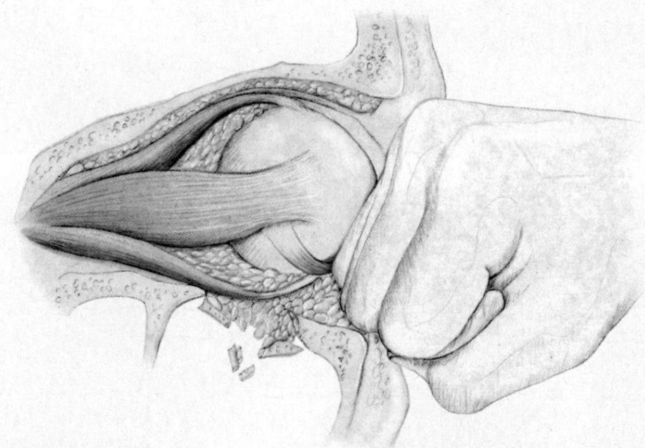

FIGURE 29.14 Fisticuffs resulting in a "classic" orbital blowout fracture. (From Bailey BJ, Johnson JT, eds. *Head and Neck Surgery—Otolaryngology*. 4th ed. Philadelphia: Lippincott Williams & Wilkins; 2006:979, with permission.)

thalmos and diplopia on upward gaze due to entrapment. If orbital injury is suspected, an ophthalmology consultation is mandated to assess ocular entrapment and globe projection and document visual acuity. Autologous bone, titanium mesh, Silastic, or absorbable gelatin film can be used to reconstruct the orbital floor. Most fractures should be repaired within 7 to 10 days, prior to scar formation and bone fusion, to prevent slow downward herniation of orbital contents (enophthalmos). Optic nerve compression and orbital hemorrhage, however, necessitate emergent exploration.

Penetrating Trauma of the Pharynx

Penetrating trauma of the oropharynx is relatively rare in the adult population but not uncommon in the pediatric age group. Children who fall while an object is in their mouth may sustain injury to the soft palate. Impalement is most dangerous when it occurs in the lateral soft palate near the course of the internal carotid artery, which can sustain either puncture or blunt injury. Radiographic imaging of the great vessels is indicated in cases where parapharyngeal space violation has occurred or is suspected. Regardless, most such injuries are associated with a minimal amount of self-limited bleeding, and the lacerations themselves usually heal by secondary intention.

Laryngeal Trauma

Laryngeal injury should be considered in all patients sustaining blunt or sharp trauma to the neck. Signs of acute laryngeal trauma include voice change, stridor, respiratory distress, dysphagia, odynophagia, and hemoptysis. Examination of the neck may demonstrate tenderness over the thyroid cartilage, subcutaneous emphysema, hematoma, or ecchymosis. Initial management consists of securing an adequate airway. When laryngeal or tracheal injury is apparent and airway compromise is imminent, a controlled open tracheostomy should be performed. A cricothyroidotomy (access through the cricothyroid membrane) should not be used because of further potential injury to the larynx and upper trachea (Fig. 29.15). Oral endotracheal intubation is also not recommended because additional injury may result, such as creating a false passage.

In cases where trauma has occurred but the airway is stable, the mainstay of evaluation includes flexible fiberoptic laryngoscopy to assess vocal cord motion, integrity of mucosa, and evidence of laryngeal swelling, ecchymosis, or hematoma. In the absence of obvious injury, management should include elevation of the head of the bed, humidified oxygen, steroids, and airway observation in a monitored setting. If there is evidence of significant mucosal edema, a tracheostomy is performed emergently, as the stable airway can be rapidly lost with progressive swelling. Following stabilization of the airway, a CT scan is obtained to identify any fractures of the thyroid and cricoid cartilages. If a fracture is present, exploration of the neck is performed with open reduction and internal fixation, employing nonabsorbable suture, wires, or miniplates. Finally, depending on the extent of mucosal injury, a temporary laryngeal stent may be placed to prevent endolaryngeal scarring.

Facial Nerve Injury

Injury to the facial nerve can accompany head trauma. After exiting the stylomastoid foramen, the nerve courses posteriorly around the angle of the mandible and enters the parotid gland. At this point, the nerve divides into superior and inferior divisions at the

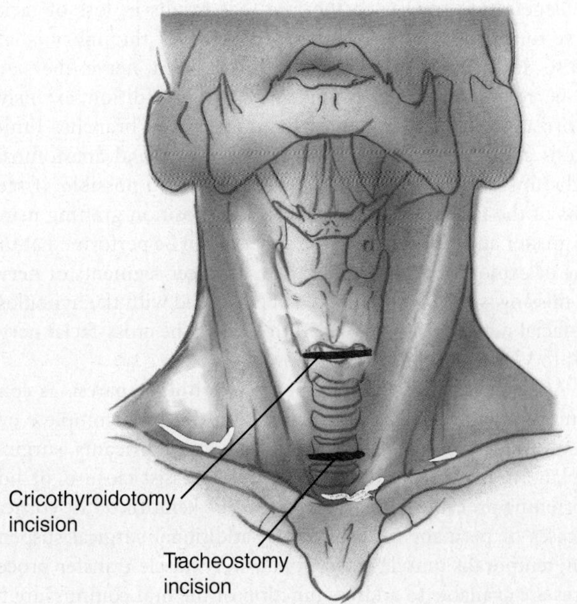

FIGURE 29.15 Cricothyroidotomy versus traditional tracheostomy. (From Bailey BJ, Johnson JT, eds. *Head and Neck Surgery—Otolaryngology*. 4th ed. Philadelphia: Lippincott Williams & Wilkins; 2006:809, with permission.)

pes anserinus. From here, the nerve splits into five main branches: temporal, zygomatic, buccal, marginal mandibular, and cervical (Fig. 29.16). Each subdivision of the facial nerve should be assessed when performing a cranial nerve examination.

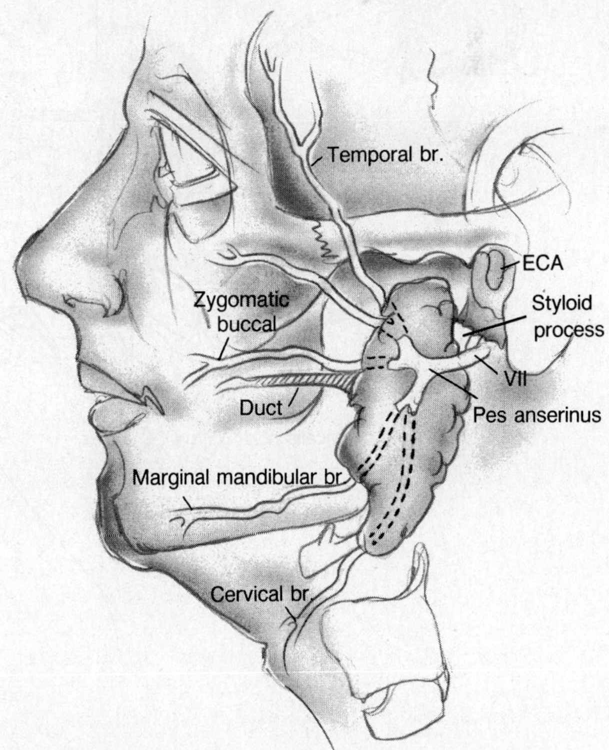

FIGURE 29.16 Anatomy of the parotid gland and facial nerve. (From Bailey BJ, Johnson JT, eds. *Head and Neck Surgery—Otolaryngology*. 4th ed. Philadelphia: Lippincott Williams & Wilkins; 2006:518, with permission.)

Penetrating trauma to the face that results in loss of facial nerve function should be repaired surgically if the injury is lateral to the lateral canthus. Medial to this point, nerve fibers are too narrow to be surgically approximated; in addition, extensive arborization between the buccal and zygomatic branches limits paresis affecting these divisions. Direct end-to-end anastomosis of disrupted nerve branches is performed when possible. If sections of the facial nerve are missing, interposition grafting using the greater auricular nerve or sural nerve can be performed at the time of exploration or at a later date. If larger segments of nerve are missing, some innervation can be restored with the hypoglossal–facial nerve anastomosis (XII to VII) or the cross-facial nerve (VII to VII) technique (Fig. 29.17).

Aside from cosmetic asymmetry, facial nerve paresis is concerning for potential corneal desiccation due to incomplete eye closure. This problem can be addressed with lubricants, surgical implantation of upper lid gold weights to assist closure, or lid-shortening procedures to prevent exposure keratitis of the cornea. In cases of permanent nerve injury, additional surgical suspension, temporalis muscle transfer, and free muscle transfer procedures are available to address function of the oral commissure to prevent drooling.

Salivary Gland Trauma

Injury to salivary glands may be blunt, penetrating, intraoral or extraoral. Of the major salivary glands, the parotid is the most commonly injured because of its superficial location. Lacerations of the face posterior to the anterior margin of the masseter muscle may injure the parotid (Stensen) duct. If a lacerated or transected duct is identified during wound exploration, end-to-end anastomosis over a stent is indicated. Identification of the injured duct can be facilitated by passing a probe intraorally through the duct orifice and identifying it within the wound. Postoperative stenosis of the duct may require dilation with ophthalmic lacrimal probes. Smaller lacerations to salivary gland parenchyma can be repaired with careful closure of the gland capsule. Facial nerve injury is also possible, as discussed earlier.

The principal complications of salivary gland trauma include sialocele (cystic collection of saliva) and salivary–cutaneous fistula. Management includes aspiration of the cyst and application of a pressure dressing; repeat aspirations are often required in the case of sialoceles, and recurrent cases may indicate ductal obstruction. Persistent collections are best addressed by gland excision. Similar management strategies apply to the submandibular and sublingual glands; however, ductal injuries are much less common owing to the protective effects of the mandible.

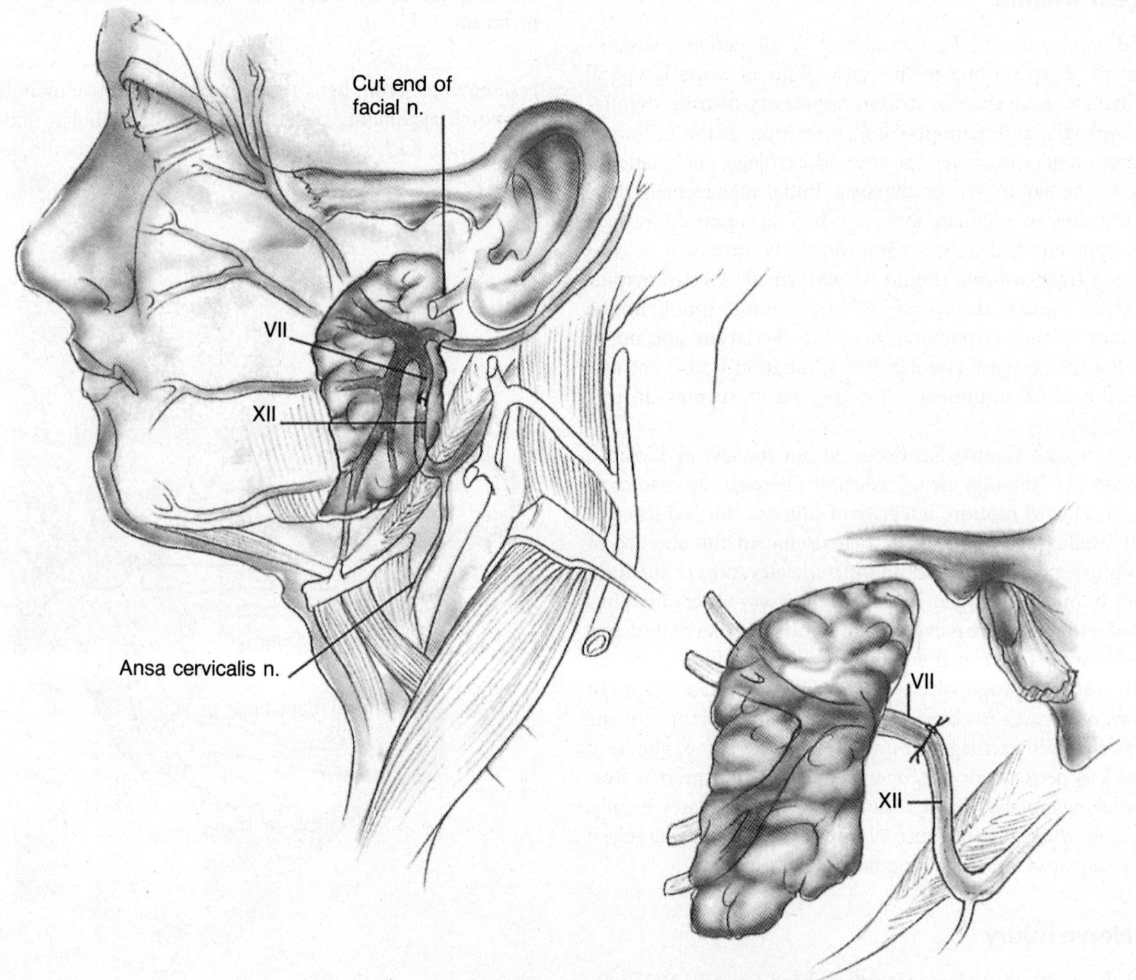

FIGURE 29.17 Nerve crossover using the proximal trunk of the hypoglossal nerve to the distal trunk of the facial nerve. (From Bailey BJ, Johnson JT, eds. *Head and Neck Surgery—Otolaryngology*. 4th ed. Philadelphia: Lippincott Williams & Wilkins; 2006:2472, with permission.)

Suggested Readings

Bailey BJ, Johnson JT, eds. *Head and Neck Surgery—Otolaryngology*. 5th ed. Philadelphia: Lippincott Williams & Wilkins; 2013.

Cummings CW, ed. *Otolaryngology: Head and Neck Surgery*. 6th ed. St. Louis: Mosby; 2014.

Lalwani AK, ed. *Current Diagnosis and Treatment in Otolaryngology*. 3rd ed. New York City: McGraw-Hill; 2011.

Lee KJ, ed. *Essential Otolaryngology*. 10th ed. New York: McGraw-Hill; 2012.

Pasha R, Golub J. *Otolaryngology – Head and Neck Surgery: Clinical Reference Guide*. 4th ed. San Diego: Plural Publishing; 2013

Ruckenstein MJ. *Comprehensive Review of Otolaryngology*. Philadelphia: WB Saunders; 2004.

CHAPTER

30 Orthopaedic Surgery

MATTHEW P. SULLIVAN, RYAN M. TAYLOR, AND SAMIR MEHTA

KEY POINTS

- There are several true orthopaedic emergencies that all surgeons must be familiar with as they will be encountered in both trauma and general surgery patients. These include fractures associated with a dysvascular limb, acute compartment syndrome, hemodynamic instability due to pelvic ring trauma, necrotizing fasciitis, and pyogenic flexor tenosynovitis.
- External fixation is a method of fracture fixation in which pins and bars are applied to the skeleton and maintained outside of the skin. It is indicated when there are concerns about the ability of the soft tissue to handle a surgical incision or when rapid fixation needs to be applied in a critically ill patient.
- Damage control orthopaedics is a concept of temporizing long bone fractures with provisional fixation techniques, such as external fixation, in order to minimize the systemic insult to a critically injured patient.
- Compartment syndrome is a clinical diagnosis made when a patient experiences symptoms such as pain with passive stretch, pain out of proportion to injury, and tense compartments. The most reliable objective measurement parameter used to assist in the diagnosis of acute compartment syndrome is delta P (pressure) equation. The equation suggests that acute compartment syndrome exists if the diastolic pressure minus compartment pressure is *less* than 30. Compartment pressure measurements must always be used in conjunction with clinical exam to make the diagnosis.
- Joint dislocations are common orthopaedic injuries. The joints most frequently dislocated are the glenohumeral joint (shoulder), ulnohumeral joint (elbow), metacarpophalangeal joint (finger), and patellofemoral joint (kneecap). Prompt reduction of a dislocated joint is important in order to limit additional damage to the articular cartilage. Hip dislocations and knee dislocations (tibiofemoral joint) are orthopaedic emergencies; the former because of the risk of damaging the delicate vessels that provide blood to the femoral head and the latter because of the extremely high association of vascular injury.

INTRODUCTION

The practice of orthopaedic surgery is based on the fundamental principles governing musculoskeletal injury and its medical and surgical treatment. As with all surgical specialties, proper diagnosis of the orthopaedic patient requires a thorough history and physical examination. Radiographic analysis using plain radiographs as well as computed tomography (CT) and magnetic resonance imaging (MRI) is essential in providing additional information as they correlate to the clinical examination. The following chapter is dedicated to highlighting principles utilized to evaluate the orthopaedic trauma patient and detailing surgical emergencies that all general surgeons should be familiar with when evaluating a patient with a concomitant orthopaedic complaint. A working knowledge of this list of diagnoses and treatment regimens is critical in avoiding significant morbidity and mortality in the patient with orthopaedic pathology.

EVALUATION OF THE ORTHOPAEDIC TRAUMA PATIENT

Advanced Trauma Life Support (ATLS) is the cornerstone of evaluation and management of trauma patients and should be adhered to closely when treating patients in the trauma bay and emergency department. orthopaedic injuries are extremely common in the traumatically injured patient population. In fact, nearly 60% of all trauma patients have an orthopaedic or musculoskeletal injury. Typically, orthopaedic injuries are diagnosed during the secondary survey; however, patients with severe musculoskeletal injuries that compromise hemodynamic stability may be diagnosed during the primary survey.

A thorough understanding of the injury mechanism in a trauma patient may greatly aid in the physician's understanding of injury patterns and potential complications (Fig. 30.1). The mechanism of injury allows for a high index of suspicion for specific injury patterns as well as associated injuries. For example, a fall from a height should raise suspicion for foot and ankle as well as lumbar spine trauma. Blunt high-energy mechanism trauma (e.g., motor vehicle or motorcycle collisions) with hemodynamic instability raises concern for a pelvic ring injury or spinal cord injury. The two most common orthopaedic causes of hemorrhagic shock overall are pelvic ring injuries and, to a lesser extent, femoral shaft fractures.

Physical Exam of the Orthopaedic Trauma Patient

All patients presenting after sustaining a traumatic injury should undergo a primary survey focused on airway, breathing, and circulation. Once this is complete and the patient stabilized, a secondary survey should take place. In the polytraumatized patient, orthopaedic injuries are often diagnosed during the secondary survey. Gross deformity or instability of the involved extremity or large soft tissue

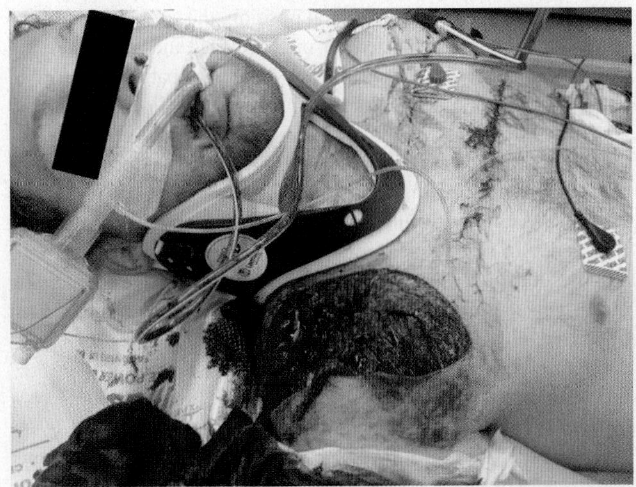

FIGURE 30.1 Clinical picture of a 25 year old male involved in a high speed motorcycle crash in which he was thrown from the motorcycle into a tree shoulder first. Knowledge of this mechanism in combination with the physical exam findings of a massive anterior shoulder laceration and diminished pulse exam points toward the devastating scapulothoracic dissociation injury. This patient went on to require revascularization of the subclavian artery which was complicated by an acute compartment syndrome, ultimately resulting in a transhumeral amputation. Approximately 50% of scapulothoracic dissociation injuries result in a flail extremity and an associated 10% mortality rate.

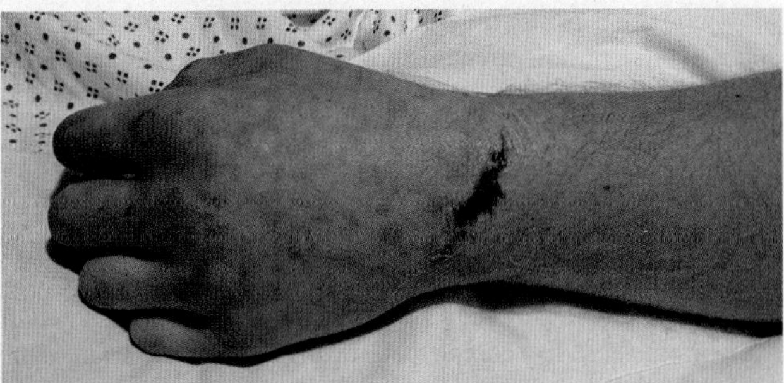

FIGURE 30.2 Clinical picture of a 20 year old male who presented to the trauma bay following a narcotic overdose. This patient had been down for 12 hours unconscious on his forearm. On secondary survey he was noted to have a cool and mottled hand without a palpable radial pulse or capillary refill. These physical exam findings prompted more advanced vascular studies, which demonstrated radial and ulnar artery occlusion.

defects with bone or joint involvement may be obvious on observation; however, other more subtle physical exam findings often go unnoticed. Lacerations, abrasions, ecchymosis, or crepitus should increase the clinician's suspicion for an underlying osseous injury and should lead to further workup with the appropriate radiographs. All patients should also undergo a more detailed tertiary survey once stabilized, awake, and alert to ensure that no injuries are missed. Often times, the pain and disorientation caused by a traumatic injury can distract from more minor injuries, ultimately leading to a delay in diagnosis.

During the secondary survey, an orthopaedic exam should be performed. All joints should be taken through a range of motion to assess for instability and mechanical blocks. In addition, all extremities should be palpated to elicit tenderness and evaluate for crepitus. Furthermore, all peripheral pulses should be palpated and assessed for inadequacy and asymmetry. If the patient is able, motor and sensory testing of the upper and lower extremity to assess the major peripheral nerves should also be performed. Finally, in the adequately resuscitated trauma patient, capillary refill should be less than 2 seconds. An overall assessment of the perfusion of the extremity is critical. Skin temperature and appearance should be evaluated. Mottling and coolness point toward a major vascular insult (Fig. 30.2).

The upper extremity examination should include range of motion of the shoulder, elbow, and wrist as well as palpation of the above-mentioned joints. In addition, the long bones and hand should be assessed for stability and pain. Nerves tested should include the radial, ulnar, median, musculocutaneous, and axillary nerve. The radial nerve is assessed by testing for active elbow, wrist, or thumb extension as well as sensation in the first dorsal webspace. Distal 1/3 humeral shaft fractures are sometimes associated with radial nerve palsies. The ulnar nerve is tested by assessing intrinsic hand musculature by asking the patient to spread his fingers and cross over the long and index finger. The ulnar nerve gives sensation to the small and ulnar half of the ring fingers. The median nerve is tested by asking the patient to flex the wrist or flex the IP and DIP joints of the thumb and index finger, respectively. The median nerve supplies sensation to the palmar aspect of the thumb, index, long, and half of the ring finger. The axillary nerve innervates the deltoid and can be tested by asking the patient to lift their arm. It also supplies a small sensory zone on the anterolateral aspect of the deltoid. Finally, the musculocutaneous nerve innervates the flexors of the elbow and can be tested by asking the patient to flex their elbow against resistance. Its sensory component can be tested at the lateral aspect of the forearm.

The principles of the lower extremity exam are similar to those of the upper extremity exam. Each joint should be taken through range of motion, all joints and osseous structures should be palpated, motor and sensory exams should be performed when feasible, and vascularity of the limbs should be assessed. Range of motion testing should be performed for the hip, knee, and ankle, and the vascular examination should include palpation of the femoral artery at the groin, the popliteal artery in the popliteal fossa, the posterior tibial artery just posterior to the medial malleolus, and the dorsalis pedis artery over the dorsum of the foot. The neurologic examination includes testing the terminal branches of the sciatic nerve as well as the femoral and obturator nerves. The terminal branches of the sciatic nerve are the common peroneal nerve and the tibial nerve, which innervate the majority of the muscles in the lower extremity. The common peroneal nerve is further subdivided into a superficial and deep branch. The superficial peroneal nerve can be tested by observing foot eversion strength and intact sensation over the dorsum of the foot. The deep peroneal nerve motor function can be evaluated by testing ankle dorsiflexion or great toe extension with sensation tested in the first dorsal webspace.

Direct blows, lacerations, or rotational forces to the proximal fibula can result in injury to the common or deep peroneal nerves leading to both sensory and motor dysfunction distally. This manifests as a "foot drop" on the affected side with the foot resting inverted and in a plantar flexed position with the inability to dorsiflex or evert the foot and loss of sensation.

The tibial nerve innervates the superficial and deep posterior compartments of the lower leg as well as the intrinsic muscles in the foot via its terminal branches, the medial and lateral plantar nerves.

Motor function of the tibial nerve is tested by demonstration of ankle plantar flexion strength through the gastrocnemius–soleus muscle complex, while sensation should be intact on the plantar aspect of the foot. Any injury to the sciatic nerve proximally, either at the level of the lumbar spine or hip, may result in motor and sensory functional loss of the lower extremity distal to the knee. The only area of the foot where sensory innervation is not supplied by the branches of the sciatic nerve is the medial aspect of the ankle. This area is supplied by the saphenous nerve, which is a branch of the femoral nerve. In a complete sciatic nerve palsy, sensation to the medial aspect of the ankle should remain intact.

Assessment and documentation of neurologic deficits is essential. If a provider is unable to assess neurologic function, this should be documented on the medical record as well. There can be several causes of neurologic dysfunction or deterioration—some requiring urgent surgical management (e.g., compartment syndrome). Having a well-documented neurologic examination is critical in this continuous assessment process.

Physical Exam of the Spinal Cord Injured Patient

Every trauma patient must receive a detailed cervical, thoracic, and lumbar spine examination. This is performed during the secondary survey and consists of the patient carefully being log rolled to the lateral position. A trained physician at the head of the bed is in charge of the turn and controlling the head/neck. There must be several additional caregivers supporting the trunk and upper/lower extremities during the turn. Once in the lateral position, the entire length of the vertebral column is inspected for open injuries and palpated along the spinous processes for tenderness. Before the patient is returned to the supine position, a rectal examination with a clean-gloved hand is performed. It is essential that a clean glove be used to ensure accurate identification of blood in the rectum. If after the formal inspection and palpation exam of the spine there is no immediate concern for spinal trauma, a detailed neurologic exam may be deferred until completion of the secondary survey. However, if there is concern for a spine injury, a thorough neurologic examination documenting motor and sensory findings of the cervical and lumbar spine must be carried out prior to leaving the resuscitation area. The clinical outcome of a patient with a spinal cord injury is based on the initial functional level (lowest functioning motor and sensory root level of function) and thus necessitates its accurate documentation.

A detailed motor and sensory examination of bilateral upper and lower extremities needs to be conducted to completely evaluate spinal cord function. This examination should be performed in a systematic fashion at the examiner's discretion. Refer to Table 30.1 for a detailed description of the motor, sensory, and reflex exams. The examination commences at the level of the shoulders and progresses distally. Motor strength is graded on a standard 0 to 5 scale as follows: 0/5 is no muscle contraction. 1/5 is muscle flickering. 2/5 is movement when gravity is removed. 3/5 is movement against gravity only. 4/5 is some resistance against the examiner. This is the only category in which a minus and plus may be added for a more detailed description. And 5/5 is normal strength. Sensation may initially

TABLE 30.1 Detailed description of thorough cervical, thoracic, lumbar spine neurological exam

Level	Motor (Motion and Muscle)	Sensory	Reflex
C4	Shoulder shrug/trapezius	Sternal notch	X
C5	Shoulder abduction/deltoid	Anterior shoulder	Biceps
C6	Elbow flexion/biceps Wrist extension/Extensor Carpi Radialis Longus	Lateral shoulder	Brachioradialis
C7	Elbow extension/triceps Wrist flexion/Flexor Carpi Radialis	Index finger Long finger	Triceps
C8	Finger flexion/Flexor digitorum Superficialis	Small finger	X
T1	Finger abduction and adduction Dorsal and palmar interossei	Medial elbow	X
T4	X	Nipple line	X
T8	X	Xyphoid process	X
T10	X	Umbilicus	X
L2/L3	Hip flexion/iliopsoas Hip adduction/adductor magnus	Proximal medial thigh	X
L3/L4	Knee extension/quadriceps	Medial knee (L3)	Quadriceps (L4)
L4/L5	Ankle dorsiflexion/tibialis anterior	Anterior knee (L4) Lateral knee (L5)	X
S1	Ankle plantar flexion	Posterior lateral calf	Achilles
S2	Great toe plantar flexion	Posterior medial calf	X

be evaluated based on light touch, and if there are any identifiable abnormalities, vibration and pinprick sensation should be evaluated to examine the dorsal column and spinothalamic tracts, respectively.

There are a series of reflexes that should also be tested and documented to complete a thorough spinal cord evaluation. The biceps, brachioradialis, and triceps reflexes of the upper extremity demonstrate an intact spinal cord reflex at the level of C5, C6, and C7, respectively. The patellar and Achilles reflexes of the lower extremity demonstrate an intact spinal cord reflex at the level of L4 and S1, respectively. The presence of a Hoffman sign (involuntary flexion of the thumb with flicking of the distal long finger) or a Babinski sign (upward extension of the toes with posterior to anterior, lateral to medial irritation of the plantar foot) signifies an upper motor neuron lesion.

Finally, if there is concern for spinal cord injury, a rectal examination is essential. A sensory and motor exam of the rectum may be performed simultaneously. Perianal sensation should be evaluated as well as the bulbocavernosus reflex. This is performed by pulling of the Foley catheter with a finger in the rectum. The absence of this anal contraction classifies the patient to be in a state of spinal shock and may last up to 48 hours following the injury. Spinal shock is a state in which the spinal cord has been severely traumatized and the neurologic exam is not reliable. A repeat examination at 48 hours with restoration of the bulbocavernosis reflex signifies that the patient is no longer in spinal shock and the neurologic examination is reliable.

Injuries Associated with Vascular Injuries/Fractures with Neurovascular Compromise

Any laceration that results in arterial bleeding should be addressed early on in the resuscitation of a polytraumatized patient. The bleeding should be initially managed with direct pressure and, if necessary, tourniquet applied proximal to the injury. Arterial injuries almost invariably need to be treated in the operating room, and necessary arrangements should be initiated as soon as the injury is identified and the patient stabilized.

Vascular injuries that are not associated with external bleeding and large lacerations are more subtle in their presentation. Physical exams findings such as a pale, cool limb with an attenuated or absent pulse are indicative of an arterial injury. Pulses should be compared bilaterally for symmetry, and an ankle–brachial index (ABI) should also be performed if there is any suspicion for a vascular injury. If there is any difference in pulses or the ABI is less than 0.9, further investigation is warranted, usually in the form of formal angiography or CT angiography.

All patients with orthopaedic injuries should have thorough neurovascular exam to rule out vascular injury, and this should be dutifully documented in the chart. There is a subset of injuries that one should be more aware of the possibility of vascular injuries. Any dislocation or fracture dislocation of a joint should raise awareness for a vascular injury. Fractures associated with penetrating injuries, crush injuries, or high-energy trauma also have a high probability of being associated with a vascular injury (Fig. 30.3).

Should a patient need combined intervention with both the vascular and orthopaedic surgery teams, the usual sequence of events begins with stabilization of the fracture followed by repair or grafting by the vascular team. This gives an added measure of stability to the limb and allows the vascular surgery team to complete their procedure without having to deal with the instability of a fractured limb and further protects their repair in the postoperative period.

Gross deformities of an extremity identified in a trauma patient mandate the documentation of a detailed neurovascular examination, especially distal to the site of the deformity. A patient who presents with a neurovascular deficit distal to an extremity injury should undergo fracture reduction and/or gentle traction to pull the extremity out to length. It is imperative that a repeat neurovascular examination of the extremity be performed after any manipulation of the injured limb. If the neurovascular examination returns to normal following manipulation, the initial deficit noted on physical examination was likely due to traction or tension on the neurovascular structures resulting from the deformity. The extremity should at this point be splinted appropriately to avoid any additional undue stress on the neurovascular structures traversing the injury site. Ideally, patients should have radiographs obtained prior to manipulation of any deformed extremity. However, there should be no delay in waiting for radiographs if there is a neurovascular deficit, and manipulation should be attempted without formal X-rays. Following manipulation, radiographs of the deformity site as well as of the joint proximal and distal to the injury should be obtained and reviewed thoroughly for associated bony injuries.

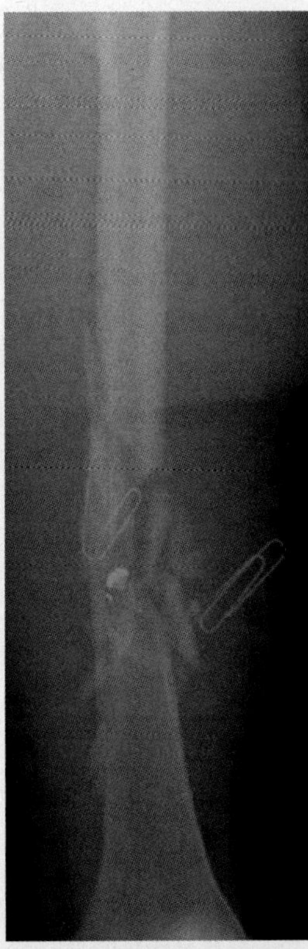

FIGURE 30.3 Radiograph of 23 year old male who sustained a high energy gun shot injury to the left mid shaft femur. There is extensive comminution due to the energy imparted by the bullet. A small fragment of bullet is seen about the fracture site. The closed paperclip indicates an anterior wound and the open paperclip indicates a posterior wound. The oblique trajectory of the bullet centered over the femur and the severe comminution raise concern for injury to the femoral artery. A thorough vascular examination in the trauma bay including an ankle-brachial index is imperative for this patient.

Patients with persistent neurovascular deficit following manipulation of a deformed extremity require additional evaluation. Nerve deficits sustained at the time of injury are often neuropraxic in nature as a result of the nerve stretching. These types of injuries typically are self-limited and may take anywhere from 3 to 6 months to completely resolve. Electromyography is the gold standard to monitor improvement of nerve function and may show activity or improvement as early as 6 weeks following the inciting event. Fractures that result from high-energy injuries may result in nerve laceration and complete disruption of the neuronal axons. In this situation, the decision may be made to explore the nerve at the time of definitive treatment and perform a primary repair.

Vascular deficits that do not return after limb manipulation are considered vessel injuries until proven otherwise and require additional formal studies and imaging to confirm the diagnosis. The initial step is to determine the ankle–brachial index. This noninvasive measure of distal blood flow is done by measuring the blood pressure at the level of the elbow and at the ankle at which blood flow returns to the distal upper and lower extremity, respectively. A Doppler signaling device is typically used to hear the pulsatile nature of arterial flow around each joint. A ratio (index) of the ankle to brachial systolic blood pressure of less than 0.9 is considered positive and points in the direction of a vessel injury. In these patients, a more formal study is required to identify intimal injuries to the arterial wall versus a complete disruption of the vessel. The finding of an abnormal ankle–brachial index mandates further workup (e.g., angiogram), which can be conducted in an interventional radiology suite or in the operating room at the time of surgical treatment of the injury.

DIAGNOSIS AND CONSIDERATIONS OF SPECIFIC TRAUMATIC INJURIES

Open Fractures

An open fracture, historically referred to as a compound fracture, is defined as any fracture that communicates with the external environment through a defect in the soft tissue envelope. Open fractures are commonly the result of high-energy trauma. The soft tissue injury can be as significant, if not more significant, than the bony injury, which may range from a "poke" hole to complete soft tissue devitalization with periosteal stripping and exposed bone. When a patient arrives in the trauma bay with an obvious extremity deformity and a large soft tissue injury, the diagnosis of an open fracture is self-evident (Fig. 30.4). However, in the patient that presents with a deformed extremity and a small abrasion or laceration, an open fracture may be easily missed. It is here that a thorough physical examination in which the entire limb is circumferentially exposed and evaluated is most critical.

Open fractures are considered urgent orthopaedic injuries requiring intervention within 6-24 hours of arrival to limit or prevent complications such as infection and soft tissue necrosis. Initially, tetanus prophylaxis should be administered if a tetanus booster has not been given in the previous 5 years. In addition, intravenous antibiotics should be administered immediately upon recognition of the injury. Following diagnosis of an open fracture and documentation of a detailed neurovascular examination, the fracture site should be thoroughly irrigated with sterile normal saline and covered with a povidone–iodine-soaked gauze. Historically, open fractures were considered surgical emergencies with recommendation of operative debridement within 6 hours of presentation. However, a recent debate in the orthopaedic literature has questioned the merits of emergent surgery if it means mobilizing a call team in the middle of the night that is unfamiliar with orthopaedic procedures or if the debridement and initial treatment will be performed by those with limited experience. The quality of the initial debridement and stabilization has a significant impact on the final outcome. Upon diagnosis, the involved extremity should be splinted appropriately prior to subjecting the patient to further imaging studies (e.g., additional radiographs or CT scans for periarticular fractures) as well as for transport to the operating room. Splinting minimizes further injury to the soft tissue envelope.

Open fractures are classified based on the Gustilo and Anderson classification, which considers the soft tissue trauma a critical component of the injury picture. This classification system is based on the degree of energy imparted to the limb at the time of the injury and the resulting soft tissue trauma. Type I injuries

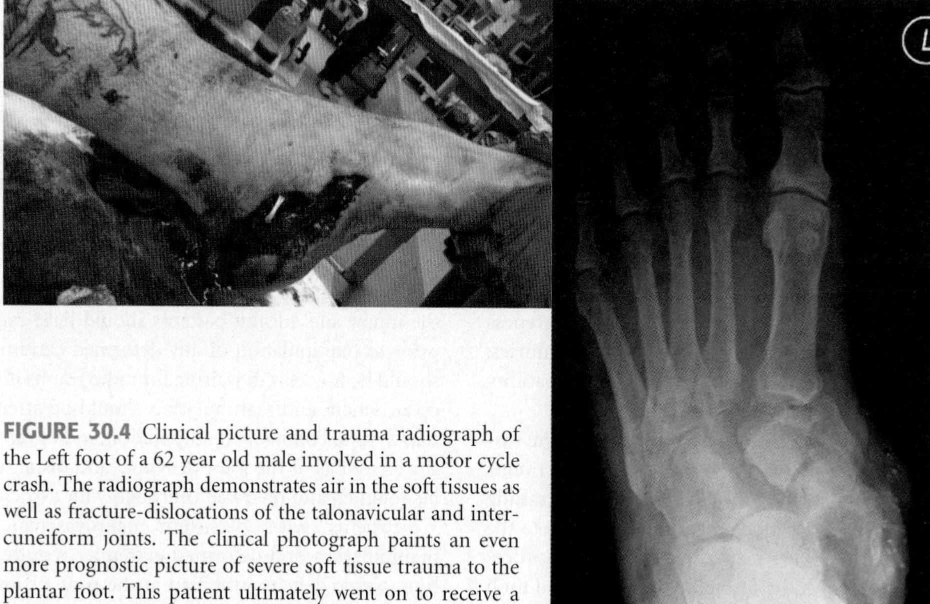

FIGURE 30.4 Clinical picture and trauma radiograph of the Left foot of a 62 year old male involved in a motor cycle crash. The radiograph demonstrates air in the soft tissues as well as fracture-dislocations of the talonavicular and intercuneiform joints. The clinical photograph paints an even more prognostic picture of severe soft tissue trauma to the plantar foot. This patient ultimately went on to receive a trans-tibial amputation due to overwhelming infection that could not be controlled with serial debridements.

are low-energy open fractures associated with a soft tissue defect less than 1 cm. Type II injuries are also low-energy injuries with an associated soft tissue defect between 1 and 10 cm. Type III injuries are high-energy injuries and are subcategorized on the degree of soft tissue injury. Subcategorization of type III open fractures cannot accurately be made until the wound has been explored in the operating room and the maximal degree of soft tissue trauma fully assessed. Type IIIa injuries are high energy as determined by the mechanism of injury and degree of comminution. Type IIIb injuries have more severe damage to the soft tissue and require soft tissue coverage in the way of rotational flaps or free tissue transfer. Skin grafting does not define an injury as being type IIIb. Type IIIc injuries require emergent vascular repair for a dysvascular limb. Types I and II open fractures require prompt administration of a third-generation cephalosporin such as cefazolin. All type III fractures require the administration of cefazolin plus the addition of an aminoglycoside such as gentamicin. Patients who have sustained open fractures with severe contamination (e.g., "barnyard" injuries) require the addition of penicillin to cover gas-forming bacteria such as *Clostridium perfringens*. The major concern with open fractures is the increased incidence of infection associated with these injuries due to the degree of wound contamination as well as the degree of soft tissue loss.

Initial treatment in the operating room involves thorough debridement and irrigation of the wound with delivery of the bony edges of the fracture site for debridement. The laceration is typically extended in a proximal and distal fashion to gain adequate access to the fracture site. Depending on the fracture type, the associated soft tissue defect, and the extent of wound contamination, the treatment may include definitive internal fixation or temporary stabilization with external fixation. As mentioned in the preceding text, open fractures associated with a vessel injury (i.e., type IIIC injuries) may require external fixation of the fracture prior to definitive vascular repair to avoid undue tension on the repair.

Compartment Syndrome

Compartment syndrome occurs when the intracompartmental pressure (ICP) exceeds the perfusion pressure leading to tissue ischemia and ultimately tissue death. Increased ICP can be the result of either increased pressure from within the compartment, secondary to swelling or bleeding, or increased pressure outside of the compartment, such as extrinsic compression from a cast, circumferential burn, or elastic dressing. Increased pressure first leads to increased venous pressure leading to further increase in the ICP that eventually leads to arteriolar collapse, loss of perfusion gradient, and cellular anoxia and death.

Compartment syndrome is diagnosed clinically in the awake and alert patient and a high index of suspicion must be maintained at all times. The five classic signs of compartment syndrome (colloquially known as the 5 Ps) are pain out of proportion to the injury or examination, paresthesias, paralysis/paresis, pulselessness, and pallor. These signs, however, are not reliable in the diagnosis of compartment syndrome. In the absence of vascular injury, pulses may be present and pallor absent in a developing compartment syndrome. In addition, paralysis and paresis are hard to determine in the acute setting especially when there are multiple painful injuries to the extremity. The most reliable indications of an evolving compartment syndrome are both pain out of proportion to the examination and worsening or unalleviated pain with increasing narcotic pain medication requirement. Pain with passive stretch is also a strong indicator for impending compartment syndrome. In younger patients, persistent fussiness and agitation could be indications of developing compartment syndrome. The diagnosis of compartment syndrome may be extremely difficult when the patient is obtunded requiring invasive compartment pressure monitoring.

The treatment of acute compartment syndrome is emergent fasciotomies to decrease the ICP and restoration of perfusion to the ischemic muscle tissue. Each extremity has unique anatomic compartments that must be released to avoid tissue necrosis. The two most common areas for compartment syndrome are the leg and the forearm. Complete fasciotomies of the leg must include releases of the anterior, lateral, superficial posterior, and deep posterior compartments, through either one or two incisions. A fasciotomy of the forearm includes the volar compartment and the carpal tunnel. In the forearm, once the volar compartment is released, the pressure in the dorsal compartment and mobile wad compartment usually decreases significantly; however, a separate dorsal incision with fascial release can be performed if elevated pressures persist. Fasciotomy incisions are rarely closed at the time of initial release as the skin can be constricting as well. When closure is performed, only skin should be closed, leaving the fascia open. Often times, multiple trips to the operating room for serial debridements are necessary, and it is not uncommon to need a skin graft over the fasciotomy site. Negative pressure wound therapy, wet to dry dressings, and dermatotraction techniques with vessel loops are all common means to manage fasciotomy wounds to aid in closure.

There are a few misconceptions about compartment syndrome, which should be clarified. First, a compartment syndrome may occur in the setting of an open fracture. Even though the fracture has penetrated part of the fascial envelope, typically, not enough of the compartment has been decompressed to prevent a compartment syndrome. Second, the sensitivity of compartment "compressibility" is quite poor and therefore clinical suspicion and overall presentation should guide decision making more than whether or not a compartment is compressible. Missed or undertreated compartment syndrome is one of the most common orthopaedic-related causes for litigation, and a high index of suspicion must be kept at all times.

The following patient scenarios should increase the likelihood of the possible diagnosis of compartment syndrome: (a) high-energy closed fractures, (b) prolonged external pressure on the compartment (e.g., patients found down for a prolonged period of time) (Fig. 30.5), (c) intravenous iodinated dye extravasation (e.g., patients receiving contrast dye for a CT scan that extravasates out of the intravascular system into a fascial compartment), (d) crush injuries, (e) reperfusion injuries (e.g., repair of arterial injuries resulting in reconstitution of blood flow and thus increased inflammation), (f) concomitant arterial and venous injuries to an extremity, and (g) limb ischemia greater than 6 hours.

The diagnosis of compartment syndrome is more difficult to make in the unconscious patient or in the pediatric population. Again, the most important concept in making the diagnosis, even in the unconscious patient, is a high index of suspicion. Specifically in the pediatric population, even though the child may be awake, compliance with the physical examination and ability to answer questions may be the limiting factor. In addition, the administration of intravenous narcotic medications for pain control may also obscure the physical examination findings. In those patients in whom the

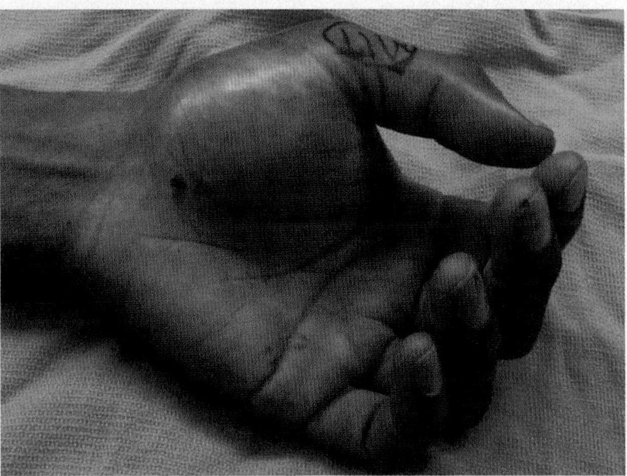

FIGURE 30.5 Clinical photograph of a 46 year old construction worker who had a 15 lb brick fall onto his hand from 5 feet. Radiographs showed an unimpressive nondisplaced fracture of the base of the thumb metacarpal. Clinical exam was much more concerning demonstrating tense thenar and first dorsal compartments and severe pain with passive extension of the thumb. The clinical diagnosis of acute compartment syndrome was made and the patient was emergently taken to the operating room for decompressive fasciotomy.

index of suspicion is high but the physical examination is equivocal, a more invasive diagnostic measure, intra-compartmental pressure assessment, may be performed.

Several commercially available needle devices can be used to measure ICPs. In general, a small amount of saline is introduced into the compartment under interrogation that then equilibrates within the compartment. The pressure measurement reading is then taken as the pressure within the fascial compartment. Typically, the forearm requires pressure measurement in three separate compartments: the flexor compartment, the extensor compartment, and the mobile wad (fascial compartment containing the brachioradialis, extensor carpi radialis longus, and extensor carpi brevis muscles). For the lower leg, the anterior, lateral, superficial posterior, and deep posterior fascial compartments should be measured. Each compartment measurement should be documented as well as the patient's diastolic pressure at the time of the measurement.

There are several measurement thresholds that can be used to determine whether an ICP is high and requires emergent treatment. Some authors recommend an absolute value greater than 30 mm Hg as the threshold value. The intracapillary pressure required for the forward flow of blood into a fascial compartment is 25 mm Hg. Therefore, an ICP greater than or equal to 30 mm Hg most likely impedes the forward flow of arterial blood into the compartment. However, other authors have demonstrated that each compartmental measurement should take into account the hemodynamics of the patient at the time of the measurement. With this in mind, an ICP that is within 30 mm Hg of the diastolic pressure of the patient should be considered a high pressure. Regardless of the technique used to define a high compartmental pressure, the method should be clearly recorded in the patient record, and the decision making should reflect the documented pressure measurements or pressure differentials. Measurement of elevated compartment pressures mandates immediate treatment, which consists of fasciotomy and complete release of the involved fascial compartments.

Pelvic Ring Injuries

Fractures of the pelvic ring can be devastating injuries and are often the cause of hypotension and hemodynamic instability in the polytraumatized patient. The AP pelvis radiograph should be part of the initial trauma series and will reveal the presence and pattern of any pelvic ring injury. Patients with acute symphyseal disruption or an "open-book" pelvic ring injury are at extremely high risk for massive hemorrhage leading to hemorrhagic shock secondary to venous plexus injuries and less commonly arterial bleeding. The pelvis is examined by applying gentle pressure on the anterior superior iliac spines in an anterior to posterior direction with the palm of both hands. This will assess for pubic disruption and overall pelvic ring instability. In a pelvis that is already widened or "booked open," gentle medial pressure is applied from the lateral aspect of each iliac wing with both hands. These maneuvers should only be performed once by an experienced examiner. The more an unstable pelvis is manipulated, the more likely the initial hematoma will be disrupted, leading to increased bleeding. Patients with pelvic ring injuries should also be examined for possible open injuries. This includes a thorough genitourinary exam to rule out urethral disruption, bladder rupture, or vaginal wall perforation. A rectal exam should also be performed to rule out rectal wall lacerations.

The reduction of the intrapelvic volume is a critical step in stabilization of these patients and must be accomplished expeditiously. A circumferential wrap (e.g., bedsheet or commercially available binder) can be wrapped around the patient's pelvis, centered over the greater trochanters, and secured anteriorly. The feet can also be internally rotated and taped together to aid in reduction. During application of the circumferential wrap, there should be no folds in order to prevent excessive pressure on one area of skin and distribute the load in an even distribution to aid in reduction. Commercially available devices (e.g., T-pods) also serve this purpose (Fig. 30.6). They must be closely inspected after placement for any related soft tissue damage due to over aggressive compression.

The circumferential wrap should be applied early during resuscitation, and aggressive fluid and blood resuscitation should be undertaken. Most often, intrapelvic bleeding is the result of venous bleeding secondary to fracture or venous plexus sheering. There can also be arterial contributions to the hemorrhage, most often from the superior gluteal artery. In the event of arterial bleeding, formal angiography and embolization may play some role in the overall resuscitation. However, angiography and embolization should be used only after adequate stabilization of the pelvic ring and appropriate fluid resuscitation.

Spinal Cord Injury

A complete physical examination must be conducted on all patients with a suspected spinal cord injury as was discussed previously in the evaluation of the trauma patient. There are several incomplete spinal cord injury patterns, which are associated with predictable neurologic deficits. Brown–Séquard syndrome is a hemicord transection, often by a penetrating injury (e.g., knife wound). An injury pattern of this nature results in ipsilateral motor, proprioception, and light touch loss with a contralateral loss of pain and temperature sensation distal to the injury level. Central cord syndrome is typically seen in elderly patients with a history of degenerative disease of the cervical spine. A hyperextension moment caused by a

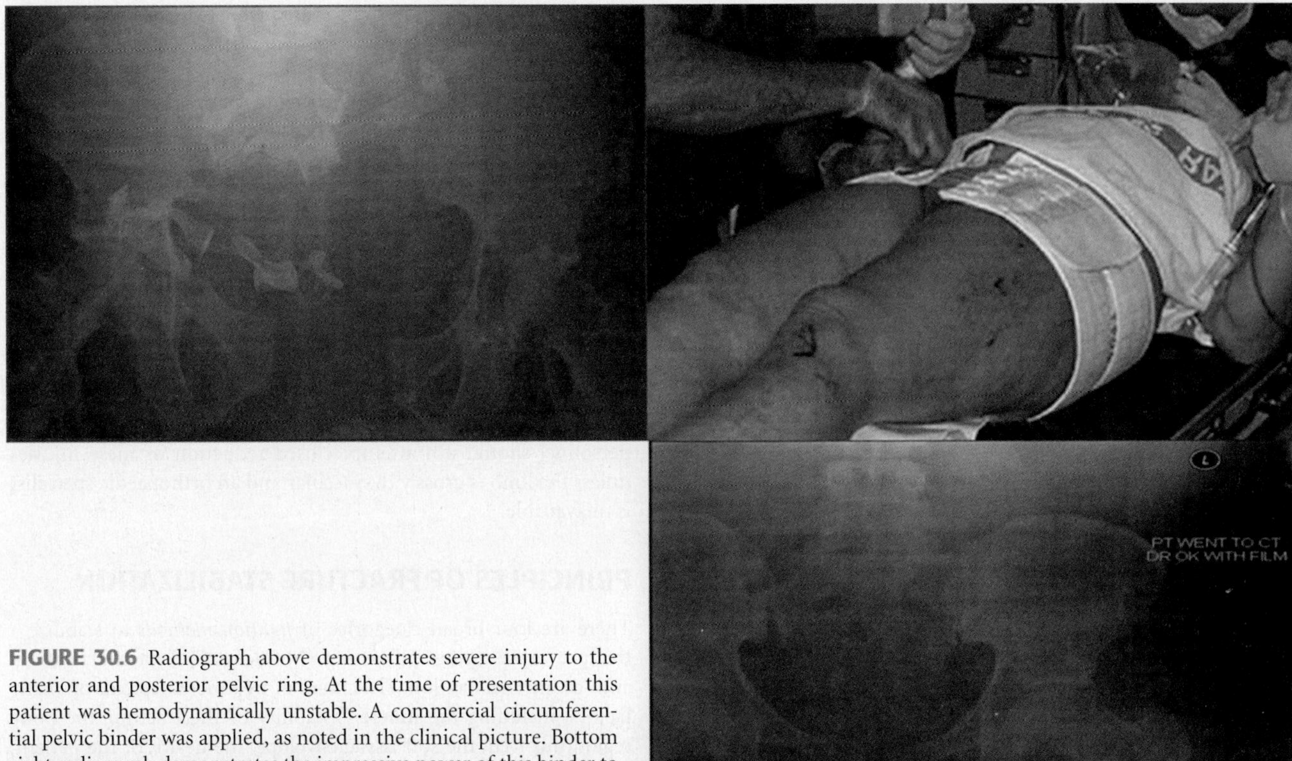

FIGURE 30.6 Radiograph above demonstrates severe injury to the anterior and posterior pelvic ring. At the time of presentation this patient was hemodynamically unstable. A commercial circumferential pelvic binder was applied, as noted in the clinical picture. Bottom right radiograph demonstrates the impressive power of this binder to close down the pelvic ring allowing for restoration of hemodynamic stability.

fall in which the forehead hits a counter or railing is a common mechanism. This injury pattern results in bilateral upper extremity motor weakness with relative sparing of the lower extremities. Anterior cord syndrome is usually the result of a vascular insult to the anterior spinal cord (anterior spinal artery distribution). The deficit pattern is a loss of bilateral motor function, and loss of pain and temperature sensation caudal to the level of injury. Of the three described incomplete spinal cord injuries, Brown–Séquard syndrome has the best prognosis with nearly all patients recovering some degree of ambulation, whereas anterior cord syndrome has the worst prognosis with less than 25% of patients recovering motor function.

Traumaic Amputation

Traumatic amputation of an extremity is not an uncommon injury in the orthopaedic trauma population and can be the result of various mechanisms ranging from a young child getting their finger caught in the door to industrial accidents to high-speed motor vehicle collisions. Resulting traumatic amputations can range in size and severity from distal fingertip soft tissue avulsions to transfemoral or transhumeral amputations (Fig. 30.7).

Technical advances in microvascular surgery have made replantation a reasonable option in the treatment of upper extremity traumatic amputations; however, there are several factors that must be considered when deciding whether someone is a good replant candidate. Lower extremity replantations are rarely undertaken given the excellent clinical results achieved with prostheses.

Ischemia time is an important factor in tissue viability, therefore making it a major factor in the success of a replantation. Warm ischemia times should be under 6 hours for the replantation of a limb, while cold ischemia times up to 12 hours are acceptable. When an amputated limb is placed on ice, it should first be wrapped in damp, sterile gauze, placed in a plastic bag, and then packed in ice. Direct contact between the amputated limb and ice can cause increased tissue damage and could further compromise viability. Wounds that have a wide zone of injury or are the result of a crush or avulsion are usually poor replantation candidates. Other

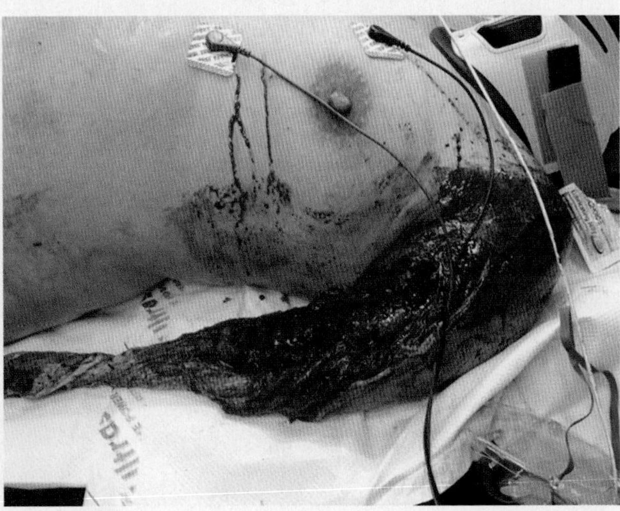

FIGURE 30.7 Clinical photograph of a 35 year old female restrained driver involved in a role-over motor vehicle crash with her left arm out of the window. Due to the severe shear and crush trauma to the upper extremity, completion amputation was urgently performed.

factors to consider include whether the patient is an active smoker, has a history of peripheral vascular disease, or has a psychiatric history making them not amenable to following strict postoperative protocols.

The replantation procedure must achieve bony stability, arterial inflow and outflow, nervous innervation, and soft tissue repair. Immediate postoperative monitoring should include both Doppler pulse checks and visual inspection to assess for blanching or venous congestion, which would indicate arterial occlusion and venous outflow obstruction, respectively. Anticoagulants, such as heparin, are often used in the postoperative period to maintain arterial patency and prevent thrombosis at the repair or graft site, and leech therapy can also be employed to help alleviate venous congestion. Pharmacologic agents with vasoconstrictive properties should also be avoided in the postoperative period, as should chocolate, caffeine, and nicotine.

Fracture–Dislocations

Fracture–dislocations are fractures that occur around a joint resulting in a fracture of the bone with an associated dislocation of the joint. This type of injury has several variations based on the fracture pattern, the bone that is involved, and the joint that is involved. Dislocations, in general, require prompt reduction due to the stress imparted on the traversing neurovascular structures and soft tissue. In addition, articular regions that are left dislocated for a prolonged period of time, typically greater than 6 hours, may result in irreversible chondral (cartilage) damage and increase the risk for posttraumatic arthritis of the involved joint. Following reduction of a fracture dislocation, the limb is splinted to prevent any further damage during patient transport and often requires definitive operative fixation of the fracture as well as repair/reconstruction of any associated soft tissue disruption (e.g., ligaments).

Fractures surrounding a joint (periarticular fractures), whether associated with a dislocation or not, often require advanced imaging to fully delineate the injury pattern. CT scans are helpful in identifying the bony pattern of injury, while MRI is used to determine soft tissue (i.e., ligament or tendon) injuries. MRI is more useful when delayed treatment of the injury is undertaken since obtaining an MRI in the acute setting usually demonstrates a great deal of edema and little soft tissue detail. Periarticular fractures should be imaged with a CT scan after an adequate closed reduction in the acute setting to aid in preoperative planning.

There are a few "bad actors" when it comes to dislocations and fracture–dislocations that have extremely high rates of neurovascular compromise and gross instability requiring prompt temporary stabilization. Such injuries include pure tibiofemoral dislocation (Fig. 30.8), isolated medial tibial plateau fractures (Fig. 30.9), posterior acetabular wall fractures with hip dislocation, proximal humerus fracture–dislocations, and elbow dislocations with associated radial head and coronoid fractures. In general, emergency personnel should not attempt closed reduction of these injuries unless the limb is grossly dysvascular and an orthopaedic specialist is unavailable.

PRINCIPLES OF FRACTURE STABILIZATION

There are four broad categories of *fixation methods* to stabilize a fracture: (a) splinting and casting, (b) traction, (c) external fixation, and (d) internal fixation. The choice of treatment depends on many factors, including the inherent stability of the fracture, the body region involved, the soft tissue envelope, the health of the patient, and the resources available such as an orthopaedic surgeon, traction supplies, and orthopaedic implants. For the most part, the initial injury, particularly the amount of displacement and comminution, will determine the maximal degree of fracture instability. There are many fractures in which splinting or casting is the treatment of choice (e.g., clavicle, humerus, distal radius, and ankle). In addition, many pediatric fractures can be treated successfully in a cast because of the rapid healing and remodeling potential in pediatric patients.

A general principle of splinting or casting a fracture is to immobilize the joint above and below the fracture site. For example, a tibial shaft fracture may be temporarily or definitively treated with a splint

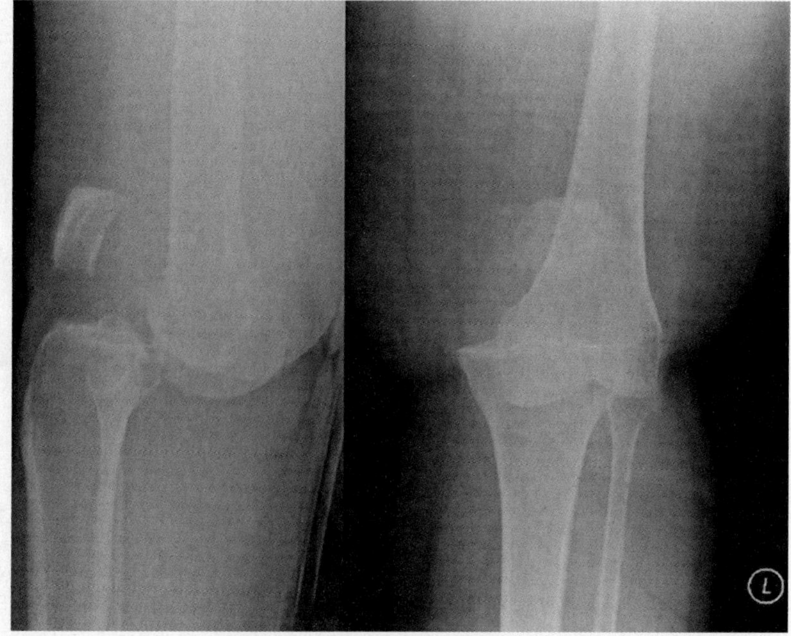

FIGURE 30.8 Radiographs of a 53 year old male who presented to the emergency department with severe knee pain after twisting his knee sliding into second base playing softball. Plain radiographs clearly demonstrate a tibio-femoral dislocation however clinical examination of this patient was subtle due to body habitus. Close evaluation of the plain films reveals a massive soft tissue envelope about the knee. Fortunately, after emergent reduction under sedation in the emergency department ankle-brachial index was 0.98, suggesting normal vascular flow at the time of the exam.

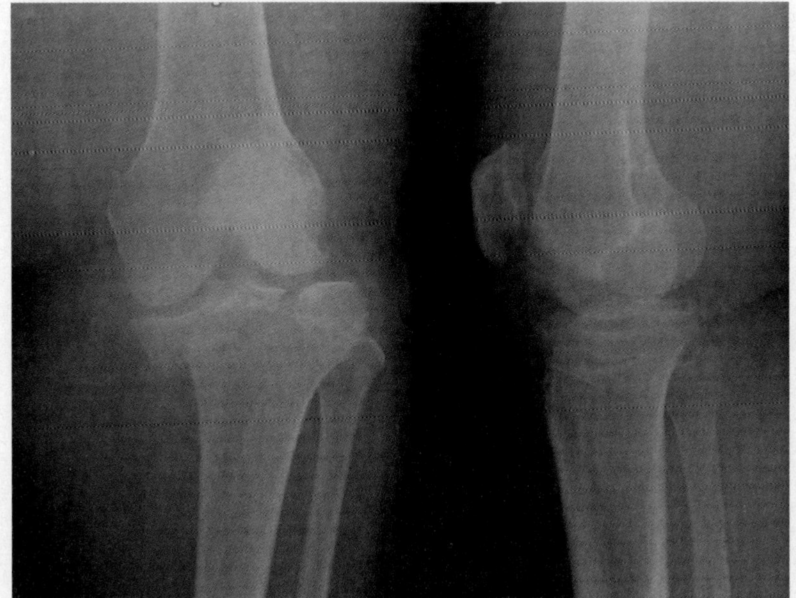

FIGURE 30.9 Radiographs of a 20 year old male involved in a motor cross accident in which he crashed from a height of 20 feet. Though innocuous appearing at first glance, these radiographs demonstrate a tibiofemoral fracture-dislocation which was likely massively displaced at the moment of impact. Note that the medial tibial plateau is congruent with the distal femur while the lateral tibial plateau and remaining shaft is grossly displaced. This injury warrants a full vascular injury work up in the trauma bay.

or cast extending from the mid thigh to the foot. The main disadvantages of this form of stabilization are the inability to rigidly hold a reduction, joint stiffness from prolonged immobilization, and danger of skin ulcerations at bony prominences. Traction is used mostly in the lower extremity, in which longitudinal traction is applied through a pin inserted through the distal femur or the proximal tibia. It is generally used as a temporizing measure in patients with femoral, acetabular, or pelvic ring injuries prior to surgery. In the rare instance in which skeletal traction is used as definitive management, the need for prolonged immobilization (3 to 6 weeks) can lead to development of pressure ulcers, joint stiffness, pulmonary disease, and blood clots.

External fixation is indicated in fractures with segmental bone loss, associated vascular injuries, and soft tissue trauma in which early surgical intervention increases the risk of infection or wound complication (Fig. 30.10). In addition, because of the efficiency with which an external fixator can be applied and the relatively minimal systemic physiologic insult, external fixation is also indicated in the multiply injured patient with extremity injuries and in the hemodynamically unstable patient. The main complications of external fixators are the risk of pin tract infection and prolonged healing time as a result of being less rigid compared to internal fixation.

The final and most versatile method of fracture fixation is internal fixation. There are four main types of internal fixation devices: pins and wires, screws, plates, and intramedullary implants. Pins can be inserted percutaneously and are often used to stabilize fractures in the hand and foot and to supplement fixation elsewhere. There are many types of screws and screw techniques. Lag screws, for example, are designed to compress across a fracture and are used to treat fractures with simple patterns such as femoral neck fractures and medial malleolus fractures. Plates and plating techniques are a cornerstone of orthopaedic traumatology and have a role in the operative management of countless fracture patterns. Intramedullary nailing is likewise an extremely versatile method of fracture management. The IM nail is inserted from one end of a long

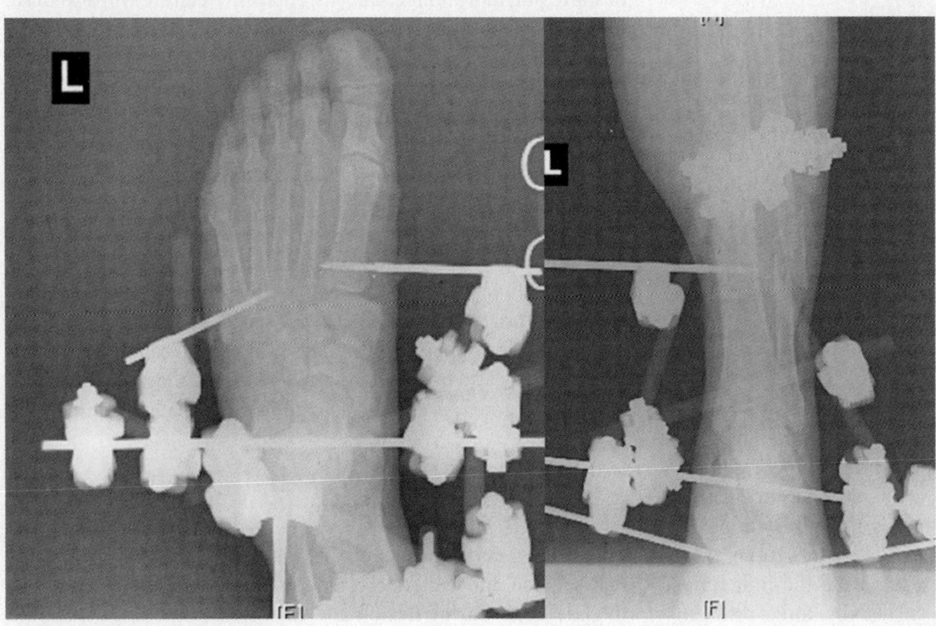

FIGURE 30.10 Radiographs demonstrating an ankle spanning external fixator with extension to the midfoot. This construct was placed in order to temporize a distal tibia fracture with combined severe midfoot fracture-dislocation in the setting of an internal degloving soft tissue injury to the anterior ankle and plantar foot.

bone down the IM canal transfixing the fracture site and providing translational, axial, and rotational stability. The smaller incision used to insert the IM nail avoids extensive soft tissue dissection and allows rapid healing and early return to function. Most commonly, the IM canal is reamed to allow for insertion of a larger (and hence, stiffer) rod, and it is important to note that there have been reports of embolization of fat and marrow elements during IM reaming and rodding; however, a multicenter prospective, randomized controlled trial comparing reamed tibial nails to unreamed tibial nails showed no difference in pulmonary disease between the groups.

ATRAUMATIC ORTHOPAEDIC EMERGENCIES

There are a number of orthopaedic emergencies that may be encountered in the nontraumatized patient. These emergencies often times affect systemically ill general surgery and general medicine inpatients. An important concept that has been mentioned throughout this chapter pertains to this set of diseases as well—it is imperative to have a high index of suspicion. In the general surgery patient, the most common scenario may involve an intensive care unit (ICU) patient with systemic disease (sepsis) with eventual spread to a region of the musculoskeletal system.

Necrotizing Fasciitis

Necrotizing fasciitis is an infection originating in the subcutaneous tissue overlying the fascia of an extremity. It can be extremely aggressive and does not respect tissues planes and fascial compartments. The most common organism involved in this type of infection is group A *Streptococcus* sp.; however, wound cultures are generally polymicrobial. Patients may present with a superficial skin infection that appears benign. However, the index physical examination finding is pain out of proportion to the clinical examination. Furthermore, these patients tend to rapidly progress to an extremely ill state.

Cellulitis is a superficial infection of the epidermis and may present in similar fashion to necrotizing fasciitis. However, necrotizing fasciitis is often associated with an elevated body temperature and hemodynamic instability (hypotension). In the early stages, hemodynamic instability may be absent, and by the time hypotension is present, the infection may have become more extensive. A missed diagnosis of necrotizing fasciitis is fatal.

Any patient with the diagnosis of necrotizing fasciitis requires emergent surgical debridement of the affected region. An extensile exposure is utilized to expose from the level of the skin to the underlying deep fascia. The infectious exudate is commonly described as "dishwater" pus and requires thorough irrigation and debridement. Patients typically require vasopressor support and close ICU care in the immediate postoperative period to optimize their hemodynamic status. Repeat irrigation and debridement is the standard of care and allows for exploration of the wound for evaluation of infection spread. Intravenous antibiotics, serial debridements, and supportive care are the mainstays of treatment.

Septic Arthritis

Septic arthritis is another orthopaedic emergency that requires expeditious diagnosis and subsequent irrigation and debridement in the operating room. Septic arthritis is the bacterial inoculation of a native or prosthetic joint, which leads to an immunologic response resulting in increased joint destruction due to enzymes released from the hosts' white blood cells during the inflammatory response. The joint may be inoculated by three different mechanisms: (a) direct seeding, (b) contiguous spread, and (c) hematogenous seeding. The most commonly affected joints are the knee, hip, and elbow, but any articulation can be infected.

Septic arthritis is diagnosed by physical exam and confirmed by laboratory testing. On physical exam, a septic joint may appear red, warm, and swollen secondary to a large effusion. There may be overlying cellulitis or skin lesions over the affected joint. Short arc range of motion testing will illicit micromotion pain, as the inflamed synovium responds to any intra-articular disturbance. A patient with a septic hip will feel most comfortable with their hip flexed and internally rotated, while those with a septic knee will feel most comfortable in slight flexion and often place a pillow or blankets behind their knee to keep it from going into full extension.

Radiographs are helpful in ruling out other causes for a painful, swollen joint, but cannot diagnose septic arthritis. An ultrasound evaluation can help identify an effusion especially in joints that cannot be directly evaluated, such as the hip. Finally, in a patient with high clinical suspicion for septic arthritis but no significant effusion, an MRI will be helpful in showing small effusions, synovitis, abscesses, and osteomyelitis.

If there is any suspicion for a septic joint, the joint must be aspirated under sterile conditions and the synovial fluid sent for analysis. Care should be taken not to violate an area of compromised skin or existing cellulitis during the aspiration as there is a risk for inoculation of a sterile joint or obtaining a false-positive result. All synovial fluid specimens should be sent for cell count with differential, culture, and crystal analysis. Though inflammatory arthritis can present like septic arthritis, the presence of inflammatory arthritis does not rule out septic arthritis, as superinfection of an inflammatory arthritis is not uncommon. The patient should also have an erythrocyte sedimentation rate, a C-reactive protein, and a complete blood count drawn. Though these labs can be negative in the setting of a septic joint, this does not completely rule one out. In immunocompromised patients, the resulting inflammatory response may not be as vigorous leading to an equivocal physical exam and deceiving lab data. In addition, patients with peripheral neuropathy, altered mental status, or previously infected joints may present much more subtly.

The diagnosis of native joint septic arthritis is made when the synovial fluid white blood cell count is greater than 50,000, with 85% or more polymorphonuclear cells. A positive culture will also make the diagnosis of septic arthritis. Extremely high synovial white blood cell counts can be associated with inflammatory arthritis and crystal disease; however, most surgeons would still proceed to irrigation and debridement emergently to minimize damage to a native joint.

The surgical treatment of septic arthritis includes thorough irrigation and debridement of the affected joint in conjunction with bacteria-specific antibiotics obtained from cultures. Irrigation and debridement can be performed both arthroscopically and open, depending on the preference of the practitioner, and often times, drains are left in place to allow for continued egress of synovial fluid.

The most common bacteria associated with native joint septic arthritis is *Staphylococcus aureus*; however, gonococcal septic arthritis must also be high in the differential in those that are sexually active. Lyme arthritis is also common especially in areas where Lyme disease is endemic.

Pyogenic Flexor Tenosynovitis

The flexor tendon sheaths of the hand are synovial-lined sheaths that provide nutrients to the tendon as well as allow the tendons to glide freely during flexion and extension of the fingers. Should this space be inoculated with bacteria, a devastating infection could result. Acute infection within the flexor tendon sheath is known as pyogenic flexor tenosynovitis and given the communication of the flexor tendon sheaths with the deep spaces of the palm and wrist, the infection can quickly spread more proximally. The threat of proximal spread as well as the devastating complications of delayed or missed pyogenic flexor tenosynovitis makes this diagnosis an orthopaedic surgical emergency.

The events leading up to inoculation of the tendon sheath are often obscure but could be a recent superficial abrasion or puncture wound to the hand. The four classic physical exam findings leading to the diagnosis are known as Kanavel's signs and include (a) a finger held in a flexed position, (b) tenderness to palpation over the flexor tendon sheath, (c) fusiform swelling, and (iv) pain with passive extension. In addition, general signs of infection may be present, including warmth, redness, fever, and possibly even drainage from a wound that could be the source of inoculation. The presence of all four Kanavel's signs almost invariably coincides with a diagnosis of pyogenic flexor tenosynovitis.

Complications from delayed or missed pyogenic flexor tenosynovitis include flexor tendon adhesions leading to decreased range of motion, deep abscesses of the hand or forearm, and systemic infection. The most common organism responsible for pyogenic flexor tenosynovitis is *S. aureus* with an ever-increasing percentage being methicillin resistant. Initial antibiotic treatment should cover for Methicillin Resistant Staphylococcus aureus.

The treatment for flexor tenosynovitis is emergent irrigation and debridement of the tendon sheath in the operating room combined with appropriate parenteral antibiotic coverage. Preoperative workup should also include C-reactive protein and erythrocyte sedimentation rate, which can help postoperatively for monitoring the effectiveness of treatment and possible need for repeat irrigation and debridement.

PATHOLOGIC FRACTURES

Fractures that occur through abnormal bone under normal loading conditions are described as pathologic fractures (Fig. 30.11). Pathologic fractures have many etiologies including metastatic lesions, primary bone tumors, osteoporosis, bone cysts, and abnormal architecture related to metabolic disorders. In these cases, one needs to first and foremost rule in or out an underlying neoplasm. The diagnosis of a musculoskeletal neoplasm requires a multidisciplinary approach including involvement of the radiologist, oncologist, radiation oncologist, pathologist, and general and orthopaedic surgeons. In addition to a thorough history and physical examination, radiographic imaging is a powerful adjunct.

All patients suspected to have a bone lesion should undergo radiographic imaging, starting with an anteroposterior (AP) and a lateral X-ray. Additional detail of the bony architecture can be evaluated via CT scan. MRI is imperative in evaluation of musculoskeletal tumors. Bone scans can be helpful in determining the presence of multiple lesions throughout the skeleton. The radiographic evaluation chosen for each patient must be individualized to the specific bony lesion.

Initially, bone tumors are classified as being benign or malignant. In general, benign bone tumors are less aggressive, while malignant tumors will typically result in destruction of the cortical bone and often extend into the adjacent soft tissues. Malignant bone tumors most commonly metastasize to the lungs. Patients suspected of having a malignant bone tumor require an appropriate staging evaluation that includes a CT scan of the chest, abdomen, and pelvis.

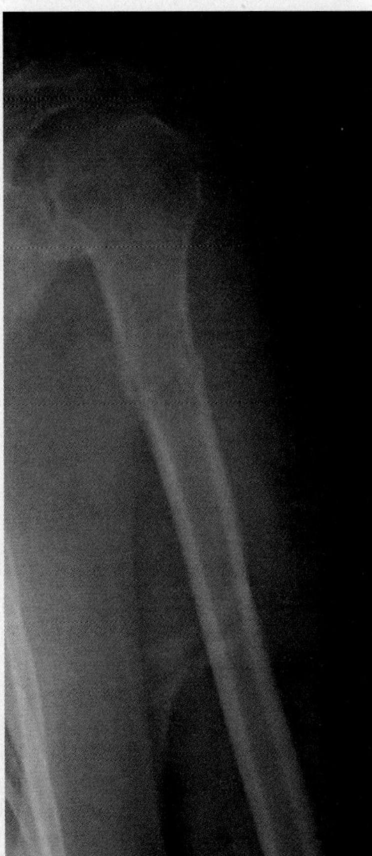

FIGURE 30.11 Radiograph of an 86 year old male with a history of Large B-Cell lymphoma and 3 weeks of worsening L shoulder pain without any known trauma. There is a meta-diaphyseal proximal humerus fracture with pathologic characteristics. A tissue biopsy from the time of surgical stabilization confirmed this was a pathologic fracture due to his known lymphoma.

In patients older than 55 years with a new bone lesion present on imaging studies, a diagnosis of a metastatic lesion from a distant source must be considered until proven otherwise. The most common primary tumors with metastatic potential to bone include breast, lung, prostate, thyroid, and kidney.

Additional pathologic fracture scenarios, which warrant extensive workup, include a low-energy long bone fracture in a healthy young adult, recurrent fractures in an otherwise healthy patient, and low-energy fractures in geriatric patients such as femoral neck, proximal humerus, and distal radius fractures. These specific scenarios warrant extensive endocrine and metabolic bone workup including vitamin D analysis, thyroid and parathyroid evaluation, bone mineral density testing, and additional tests dictated by a multispecialty approach.

COMPLICATIONS

Posttraumatic arthritis is a common complication that occurs after an intra-articular fracture. Articular displacement of greater than 2 mm is associated with an increased risk of subsequent arthritis. Anatomic reduction and fixation can help to minimize this risk.

Loss of fixation after either closed or open treatment can lead to malunions and nonunions. *Malunion* results from fracture malalignment or failure of fixation. There are many possible causes of *delayed union* and *nonunion*: (a) poor fixation leading to motion at the fracture site, (b) large gap at the fracture site,

(c) infection, (d) poor vascular supply, (e) soft tissue interposition, (f) significant bone loss, and (g) host factors such as nutritional status and smoking habits. There are a few important fractures that are notorious for becoming nonunions including open tibia fractures, scaphoid fractures, and young femoral neck fractures. Patient risk factors include smoking, diabetes, obesity, and noncompliance with the weight-bearing limitations. In addition, infection and inherent fracture instability due to fracture comminution can lead to a loss of fixation. Lastly, poor technique or inappropriate choice of internal fixation might also result in a loss of fixation.

Postoperative *wound infections* and *osteomyelitis* are frequently related to high-energy mechanisms causing trauma to the soft tissue envelope. Other risk factors include prolonged open wound time, inadequate fixation, and extensive surgical dissection and periosteal stripping, which compromise blood flow to the wound. *S. aureus* is the most common offending organism. Treatment for osteomyelitis consists of debridement of infected and dead tissue followed by intravenous antibiotics. Temporary implantation of antibiotic-impregnated cement beads and hyperbaric oxygen can help with more resistant cases of infection.

Heterotopic ossification is the formation of ectopic bone adjacent to the fracture site and within the soft tissues. This is a debilitating posttraumatic complication because of pain and loss of motion that may occur if the ectopic bone crosses a joint or encases neurovascular structures. It is mainly associated with fractures of the elbow, acetabulum, hip, and shoulder (Fig. 30.12). Although the exact causes of heterotopic ossification are not known, risk factors include spinal cord injury and traumatic brain injury, burns, and extensive soft tissue dissections particularly about the hip.

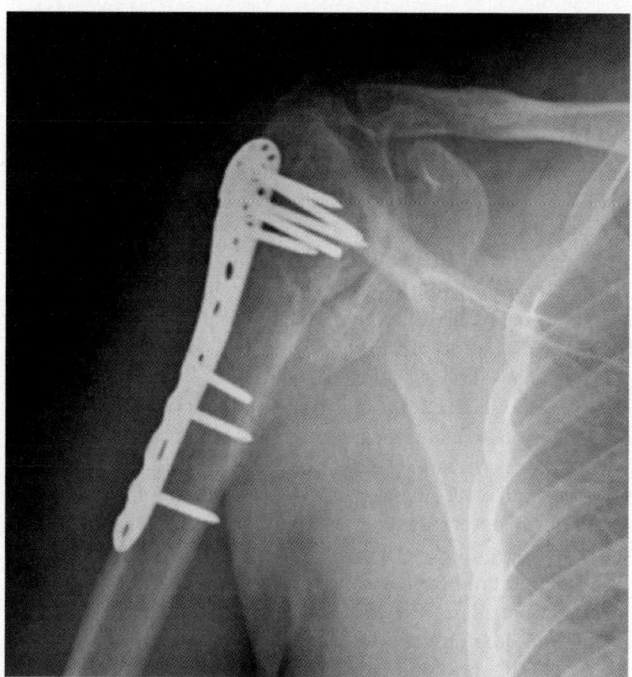

FIGURE 30.12 Radiograph of a 32 year old male with shoulder stiffness following open reduction and internal fixation of a proximal humerus fracture. This patient also sustained a traumatic brain injury. This radiograph demonstrates bridging heterotopic ossification between the scapula and the humerus. Heterotopic ossification is unfortunately extremely common in patients sustaining orthopaedic injuries in the setting of traumatic brain injuries and spinal cord injuries.

AVN (avascular necrosis), which is also known as "osteonecrosis" or "aseptic" necrosis, describes the death of bone cells due to impairment in circulation. Posttraumatic AVN occurs when the amount of displacement from the fracture or dislocation is severe enough to disrupt the blood supply to the bone. Sites that are more susceptible to AVN are the scaphoid, humeral head and femoral head, talus, and odontoid. Nontraumatic causes of AVN include sickle cell disease, corticosteroid use, radiation therapy, and alcohol abuse. The end result of AVN is collapse of the articular surface, leading to end-stage osteoarthritis.

Deep venous thrombosis (DVT) can occur in up to 50% to 60% of trauma patients and is most frequently seen in patients with spinal cord injury and fractures of the pelvis and femur. Prophylaxis against DVT and the potential sequelae of pulmonary embolism are important in all trauma patients. If there are no contraindications, subcutaneous heparin, low molecular weight heparin, or low-dose warfarin can be used, along with compression or pneumatic stockings.

In the multiply injured patient, *fat embolism* is an important cause of adult respiratory distress syndrome (ARDS) and a major source of morbidity and mortality. Fat embolism syndrome is clinically apparent in 10% of polytrauma patients, although the actual incidence rate is probably much higher. It may not appear until 2 to 3 days after the injury and may present as respiratory distress (shortness of breath and tachypnea), arterial hypoxemia, tachycardia, fevers, and a deterioration of neurologic status (restlessness, confusion, or coma). In addition, petechiae (which may be short lived) can appear across the chest and axilla. Treatment consists of supportive care. Arguably, the most important aspect of managing polytraumatized patients with fat embolism syndrome is determining appropriate time and type of surgical stabilization. The strategy of damage control orthopaedic (DCO) has gained significant popularity over the past decade. DCO is the concept of provisionally stabilizing long bones in the multiply injured patient quickly and affectively without causing additional insult to the cardiopulmonary system. External fixation of lower extremity injuries and splinting of upper extremity injuries at the time of presentation is the cornerstone of DCO. The system is allowed to "cool down" over 7 to 10 days at which time definitive management of the injuries with open reduction internal fixation is performed. The second hit phenomenon is the result of orthopaedic surgical intervention too soon after the index trauma (usually around day 3) overwhelming the system from an inflammatory perspective resulting in multiorgan failure and death.

Suggested Readings

McQueen MM, Court-Brown CM. Compartment monitoring in tibial fractures. The pressure threshold for decompression. *J Bone Joint Surg.* 1996;78(1):99–104.

Mills WJ, Barei DP, McNair P. The value of the ankle-brachial index for diagnosing arterial injury after knee dislocation: a prospective study. *J Trauma.* 2004;56(6):1261–1265.

Schenker ML, Yannascoli S, Baldwin KD, et al. Does timing to operative debridement affect infectious complications in open long-bone fractures? A systematic review. *J Bone Joint Surg.* 2012;94(12):1057–1064. doi:10.2106/JBJS.K.00582

Sirkin M, Sanders R, DiPasquale T, et al. A staged protocol for soft tissue management in the treatment of complex pilon fractures. *J Orthop Trauma.* 1999;13(2):78–84.

INDEX

Note: Page numbers followed by *t* indicate tables; those followed by *f* indicate figures.

C